NELSON
Essentials of
PEDIATRICS

WITHDRAWN

W9-BFI-107

NELSON
Essentials of
PEDIATRICS

RICHARD E. BEHRMAN, M.D.
Senior Vice President for Medical Affairs
Lucile Packard Foundation for Children's Health
and
Clinical Professor of Pediatrics
Stanford University
Stanford, California
and the University of California, San Francisco
San Francisco, California

ROBERT M. KLIEGMAN, M.D.
Professor and Chair
Department of Pediatrics
Medical College of Wisconsin
Pediatrician-in-Chief
Pamela and Leslie Muma Chair in Pediatrics
Children's Hospital of Wisconsin
Milwaukee, Wisconsin

FOURTH EDITION

W.B. SAUNDERS COMPANY
A Division of Harcourt Health Sciences
Philadelphia London New York St. Louis Sydney Toronto

W.B. SAUNDERS COMPANY
A Harcourt Health Sciences Company

The Curtis Center
Independence Square West
Philadelphia, Pennsylvania 19106

Library of Congress Cataloging-in-Publication Data

Nelson essentials of pediatrics / [edited by] Richard E. Behrman, Robert M. Kliegman. – 4th ed.
     p. ; cm.
  Includes bibliographical references and index.
  ISBN 0-7216-9406-3
     1. Pediatrics. I. Title: Essentials of Pediatrics. II. Behrman, Richard E., 1931 – III. Kliegman, Robert. IV. Nelson, Waldo E. (Waldo Emerson), 1898 – Textbook of pediatrics
     [DNLM: 1. Pediatrics. WS 100 N425 2002]
  RJ45 .N418 2002
  618.92—dc21
                            2001042607

Acquisitions Editor: William Schmitt
Developmental Editor: Ellen Baker Geisel
Project Manager: Patricia Tannian
Production Editor: Larry State
Book Design Manager: Gail Morey Hudson
Cover Designer: Teresa Breckwoldt

NELSON ESSENTIALS OF PEDIATRICS   ISBN 0-7216-9406-3

Last digit is the print number: 9   8   7   6   5   4   3   2   1

Dedicated to

Children and their families

*The tomorrow we all look forward to
depends on their health and well-being today*
REB
RMK

Contributors

HERBERT T. ABELSON, M.D.
George M. Eisenberg Professor and Chairman
Department of Pediatrics, University of Chicago
Pritzker School of Medicine
Physician-in-Chief, Children's Hospital
Chicago, Illinois
Oncology

DAVID M. ALLEN, M.D.
Resident
Department of Dermatology (Pediatric)
Children's Hospital of Wisconsin
Milwaukee, Wisconsin
Pediatric Dermatology

R. STEPHEN S. AMATO, M.D., Ph.D.
Chief of Pediatrics
Director of Medical Genetics
Eastern Maine Medical Center
Bangor, Maine
Clinical Professor of Pediatrics
Tufts University College of Medicine
Boston, Massachusetts
Human Genetics and Dysmorphology

IRA BERGMAN, M.D.
Professor of Pediatrics and Neurology
Department of Pediatrics
University of Pittsburgh School of Medicine
Attending Physician, Division of Child Neurology
Children's Hospital of Pittsburgh
Pittsburgh, Pennsylvania
Neurology

DENNIS D. BLACK, M.D.
Scientific Director
Crippled Children's Foundation Research Center
Memphis, Tennessee
The Gastrointestinal Tract

MICHAEL M. BROOK, M.D.
Assistant Professor
Department of Pediatrics (Cardiology)
Associate Director, Pediatric Echocardiography
University of California, San Francisco
School of Medicine
Attending Pediatric Cardiologist
The Medical Center at the University of California
Moffett-Long Hospitals
San Francisco, California
Cardiovascular System

NIENKE P. DOSA, M.D.
Departmental Fellow
University of Rochester Medical Center
Rochester, New York
Developmental and Behavioral Pediatrics

BETH A. DROLET, M.D.
Associate Professor
Department of Dermatology (Pediatric)
Children's Hospital of Wisconsin
Milwaukee, Wisconsin
Pediatric Dermatology

AARON L. FRIEDMAN, M.D.
Professor, Department of Pediatrics
University of Wisconsin Medical School
Chairman Department of Pediatrics
University of Wisconsin Hospital and Clinics
Madison, Wisconsin
Nephrology: Fluids and Electrolytes

NICOLE S. GLASER, M.D.
University of California Davis Medical Center
Division of Endocrinology
Department of Pediatrics, School of Medicine
Davis, California
Endocrinology

CAROLYN M. KERCSMAR, M.D.
Associate Professor, Department of Pediatrics
Case Western Reserve University School of Medicine
Director, Children's Asthma Center
Rainbow Babies and Children's Hospital
Cleveland, Ohio
The Respiratory System

BARBARA S. KIRSCHNER, M.D.
Professor, Department of Pediatrics
University of Chicago, Pritzker School of Medicine
Attending Physician, Children's Hospital
Chicago, Illinois
The Gastrointestinal Tract

ROBERT M. KLIEGMAN, M.D.
Professor and Chair, Department of Pediatrics
Medical College of Wisconsin
Pediatrician-in-Chief
Pamela and Leslie Muma Chair in Pediatrics
Children's Hospital of Wisconsin
Milwaukee, Wisconsin
Fetal and Neonatal Medicine

CHERYL M. KODJO, M.D., M.P.H.
Senior Instructor in Adolescent Medicine
University of Rochester
Rochester, New York
Adolescent Medicine

RICHARD E. KREIPE, M.D.
Professor of Pediatrics
Chief, Division of Adolescent Medicine
University of Rochester
School of Medicine and Dentistry
Rochester, New York
Adolescent Medicine

STEVEN E. KRUG, M.D.
Associate Professor, Department of Pediatrics
Northwestern University Medical School
Head, Division of Emergency Medicine
Children's Memorial Hospital
Chicago, Illinois
The Acutely Ill or Injured Child

JAMES B. NACHMAN, M.D.
Assistant Professor of Clinical Pediatrics
University of Chicago Children's Hospital
Chicago, Illinois
Oncology

JOHN F. NICHOLSON, M.D.
Associate Professor of Pediatrics and Pathology
Columbia University
College of Physicians and Surgeons
Attending Physician, Babies' and Children's Hospital
New York, New York
Inborn Errors of Metabolism

JUDYANN C. OLSON, M.D.
Associate Professor, Department of Pediatrics
Medical College of Wisconsin
Pediatric Rheumatologist
Children's Hospital of Wisconsin
Milwaukee, Wisconsin
Rheumatic Diseases of Childhood

MICHAEL J. PAINTER, M.D.
Professor of Neurology and Pediatrics
University of Pittsburgh School of Medicine
Chief, Division of Child Neurology
Children's Hospital of Pittsburgh
Pittsburgh, Pennsylvania
Neurology

ALICE PRINCE, M.D.
Professor, Department of Pediatrics
Columbia University
College of Physicians and Surgeons
Attending Pediatrician, Babies and Children's Hospital
Columbia-Presbyterian Medical Center
Department of Pediatrics
New York, New York
Infectious Diseases

J. PAUL SCOTT, M.D.
Professor, Department of Pediatrics
Medical College of Wisconsin
Head, Department of Pediatric Hematology
Children's Hospital of Wisconsin
Milwaukee, Wisconsin
Hematology

VIRGINIA A. STALLINGS, M.D.
Associate Professor, Department of Pediatrics
University of Pennsylvania School of Medicine
Senior Physician
The Children's Hospital of Philadelphia
Philadelphia, Pennsylvania
Pediatric Nutrition and Nutritional Disorders

DENNIS M. STYNE, M.D.
Professor, Department of Pediatrics
University of California Davis School of Medicine
Davis, California
Endocrinology

STEPHEN B. SULKES, M.D.
Associate Professor of Pediatrics
University of Rochester
School of Medicine and Dentistry
Pediatric Discipline Coordinator
The Strong Memorial Hospital
Center for Developmental Disabilities
Children's Hospital at Strong, Rochester, New York
Developmental and Behavioral Pediatrics

ELIZABETH C. TePAS, M.D.
Graduate Student
Stanford University
Stanford, California
Immunology and Allergy

ANDREW M. TERSHAKOVEC, M.D.
Assistant Professor, Department of Pediatrics
University of Pennsylvania School of Medicine
Associate Physician, Children's Hospital of Philadelphia
Philadelphia, Pennsylvania
Pediatric Nutrition and Nutritional Disorders

GEORGE H. THOMPSON, M.D.
Professor, Department of Orthopaedic Surgery
Case Western Reserve University
Director, Department of Pediatric Orthopaedics
Rainbow Babies' and Children's Hospital
Cleveland, Ohio
Common Orthopaedic Problems of Children

DALE T. UMETSU, M.D.
Professor of Pediatrics
Chief, Division of Allergy and Clinical Immunology
Department of Pediatrics
Stanford University School of Medicine
Director, Center for Allergy, Asthma, and Immunology
Lucile Packard Hospital at Stanford
Stanford, California
Immunology and Allergy

Preface

Nelson Textbook of Pediatrics, edition 16, incorporates the full range and depth of content of pediatrics at the start of the 21st century. It thus serves as the major reference textbook for those caring for children, encompassing progress in clinical care and biomedical science and technology. The exponential expansion of information and understanding about normal growth and development and about the diagnosis, management, and prevention of the diseases and disorders of childhood has, however, made it difficult for many students to read the entire text during pediatric clerkships and courses. In publishing *Nelson Essentials of Pediatrics,* we have addressed this issue by focusing on core aspects of pediatric health and illness within the context of the special educational needs of medical students and starting house officers.

Nelson Essentials is primarily intended to introduce important pediatric problems and diseases, representing both the common illnesses in childhood and the less common disorders of special educational importance that exemplify pathophysiologic mechanisms and disease processes. This book is not a "primer," and is not a synopsis of or a comparison to the *Nelson Textbook of Pediatrics.* The term "essential" does not mean "superficial" or "outlined." Rather, in a readable text with a simplified format and array of tables and figures, *Nelson Essentials* provides students with sufficient information to improve their understanding of representative pediatric problems and clinical decisions, enabling them to gain a basic knowledge of the particular disease process and to develop a clinical approach to a child's problem. In addition, the relatively short text can be digested during the usual length of a core pediatric clerkship.

The contents of this fourth edition have been significantly updated, and it incorporates many helpful suggestions made by students and faculty who used the third edition. We have organized each chapter in a way that reflects the clinical approach to patients. The student or house officer first should learn to generate a broad differential diagnosis based on the data obtained by taking a history and performing a physical examination; second, to perform an initial analysis of this information, which is facilitated by thinking in terms of the course of illness (acute or chronic), the organ system involved, and the evidence suggesting that a particular pathophysiologic process may be present (e.g., infection or neoplasm); and third, to use the clinical information and its analysis to determine the kind of laboratory data that will further modify and narrow the list of diagnostic possibilities and lead to more specific diagnostic testing.

Besides organizing the chapters to reflect this logical process, we have emphasized the physiologic and pathophysiologic aspects of pediatric disease and, when applicable, the genetic bases, since the understanding of this biology is critical for clinical decision making. Each new contact the student has with a sick child and the child's family should reinforce an understanding of the pathophysiologic basis of a disease and the psychosocial dynamics of illness.

Presenting the essentials of pediatric medicine does not always permit detailed discussion of the range of variations of each pediatric illness or disease or coverage of all the less common disorders. To facilitate a student's interest in obtaining additional knowledge, cross-references to the relevant chapters in the 16th edition of *Nelson Textbook of Pediatrics,* as well as selected references to other literature, are provided.

The editors especially wish to express their gratitude and appreciation to the hard-working and dedicated authors of the individual chapters. In addition, we thank the many medical students, house staff, and faculty who provided constructive criticism that has improved the final text.

Richard E. Behrman
Robert M. Kliegman

Contents

NELSON
Essentials of
PEDIATRICS

CHAPTER 1

Developmental and Behavioral Pediatrics

Stephen B. Sulkes ▼ Nienke P. Dosa

GROWTH AND DEVELOPMENT

Knowledge of the normal growth and development of children is essential for preventing and detecting disease by recognizing overt deviations from normal patterns. Although the processes of growth and development are not completely separable, it is convenient to refer to "growth" as the increase in the size of the body as a whole or the increase in its separate parts, and to reserve "development" for changes in function, including those influenced by the emotional and social environments. The development of the human organism is a large, complex topic. To identify and treat underlying disorders, all who care for children must be familiar with normal patterns of growth and development so that they can recognize abnormal variations.

Within the broad limits that characterize normal development, every individual's path of growth and development through the life cycle is unique, with a range of complex, interrelated changes occurring from the molecular to the behavioral level. One goal of pediatrics is to help each child achieve his or her individual potential for growth and development and thus become a mature adult. Periodically monitoring each child for the normal progression of growth and development and screening for abnormalities are important means of accomplishing this goal (Fig. 1–1).

Normal Growth Patterns

Deviations in growth patterns are nonspecific but important indicators of serious medical disorders. Deviations often provide the first clue that something is wrong, occasionally even when the parents do not suspect a problem. An accurate measurement of height, weight, and head circumference should be obtained at every health supervision visit. Serial measurements are much more useful than single measurements because they can help detect deviations from a particular child's growth pattern even if the value remains within statistically defined normal limits (e.g., between the 3rd and 97th percentiles).

Normal growth patterns have spurts and plateaus, so some shifting on percentile graphs can be expected; however, large shifts warrant attention. Large discrepancies among height, weight, and head circumference percentiles also deserve attention. For example, when caloric intake is inadequate, the weight percentile falls first, then the height, and last the head circumference. Similarly, an increasing weight percentile in the face of a falling height percentile suggests hypothyroidism. Head circumference may be disproportionately large when there is familial megalencephaly (knowing the sizes of the parents' heads is essential), hydrocephalus, or merely "catch-up" growth in a neurologically normal premature infant. A child is considered microcephalic if head circumference is at less than the 5th percentile, even if length and weight measurements are also proportionally low. Serial measurement of head circumference is critical during early brain development and should be plotted regularly until the child is 3 years old.

Whenever possible, growth should be assessed by plotting accurate measurements on growth charts (Figs. 1–2 to 1–10) and comparing each set of measurements with previous measurements. The CDC Growth Charts 2000 are based on nationally representative data collected from 1971 to 1994. They consist of 16 charts, including "Body mass index (BMI)-for-age percentiles" for boys and girls aged 2–20 years. The BMI is defined as body weight in kilograms divided by height in meters squared. The BMI is an index for classifying adiposity in adults and is recommended as a screening tool for children and

Recommendations for Preventive Pediatric Health Care
Committee on Practice and Ambulatory Medicine

Each child and family is unique; therefore, these **Recommendations for Preventive Pediatric Health Care** are designed for the care of children who are receiving competent parenting, have no manifestations of any important health problems, and are growing and developing in satisfactory fashion. **Additional visits may become necessary** if circumstances suggests variations from normal.

These guidelines a represent a consensus by the Committee on Practice and Ambulatory Medicine in consultation with national committees and sections of the American Academy of Pediatrics. The Committee emphasizes the great importance of **continuity of care** on comprehensive health supervision and the need to avoid **fragmentation of care.**

INFANCY / EARLY CHILDHOOD

AGE[5]	PRENATAL[1]	NEWBORN[2]	2-4d[3]	By 1mo	2mo	4mo	6mo	9mo	12mo	15mo	18mo	24mo	3y	4y
HISTORY														
Initial/Interval	•	•	•	•	•	•	•	•	•	•	•	•	•	•
MEASUREMENTS														
Height and Weight		•	•	•	•	•	•	•	•	•	•	•	•	•
Head Circumference		•	•	•	•	•	•	•	•	•	•	•		
Blood Pressure													•	•
SENSORY SCREENING														
Vision		S	S	S	S	S	S	S	S	S	S	S	O[8]	O
Hearing		O[7]	S	S	S	S	S	S	S	S	S	S	S	O
DEVELOPMENTAL/ BEHAVIORAL ASSESSMENT[8]		•	•	•	•	•	•	•	•	•	•	•	•	•
PHYSICAL EXAMINATION[9]		•	•	•	•	•	•	•	•	•	•	•	•	•
PROCEDURES-GENERAL[10]														
Hereditary/Metabolic Screening[11]		←——→	←——→											
Immunization[12]		•	•	•	•	•	•	•	↑	•	•	•	•	•
Hematocrit or Hemoglobin[13]							•	↕	•					
Urinalysis														
PROCEDURES-PATIENTS AT RISK														
Lead Screening[16]								★↑				★	★	★
Tuberculin Test[17]									★	★	★	★	★	★
Cholesterol Screening[18]														
STD Screening[19]														
Pelvic Exam[20]														
ANTICIPATORY GUIDANCE[21]														
Injury Prevention[22]		•	•	•	•	•	•	•	•	•	•	•	•	•
Violence Prevention[23]		•	•	•	•	•	•	•	•	•	•	•	•	•
Sleep Positioning Counseling[24]		•	•	•	•	•	•							
Nutrition Counseling[25]		•	•	•	•	•	•	•	•	•	•	•	•	•
DENTAL REFERRAL[26]												↓	•	

MIDDLE CHILDHOOD

AGE[5]	5y	6y	8y	10y
HISTORY				
Initial/Interval	•	•	•	•
MEASUREMENTS				
Height and Weight	•	•	•	•
Head Circumference				
Blood Pressure	•	•	•	•
SENSORY SCREENING				
Vision	O	O	O	O
Hearing	O	O	O	O
DEVELOPMENTAL/ BEHAVIORAL ASSESSMENT[8]	•	•	•	•
PHYSICAL EXAMINATION[9]	•	•	•	•
PROCEDURES-GENERAL[10]				
Hereditary/Metabolic Screening[11]				•
Immunization[12]				
Hematocrit or Hemoglobin[13]	★			
Urinalysis	•	•		

ADOLESCENCE

AGE[5]	11y	12y	13y	14y	15y	16y	17y	18y	19y	20y	21y
HISTORY											
Initial/Interval	•	•	•	•	•	•	•	•	•	•	•
MEASUREMENTS											
Height and Weight	•	•	•	•	•	•	•	•	•	•	•
Head Circumference											
Blood Pressure	•	•	•	•	•	•	•	•	•	•	•
SENSORY SCREENING											
Vision	S	O	S	S	O	S	S	O	S	S	S
Hearing	S	O	S	S	O	S	S	O	S	S	S
DEVELOPMENTAL/ BEHAVIORAL ASSESSMENT[8]	•	•	•	•	•	•	•	•	•	•	•
PHYSICAL EXAMINATION[9]	•	•	•	•	•	•	•	•	•	•	•
PROCEDURES-GENERAL[10]											
Hereditary/Metabolic Screening[11]											
Immunization[12]	←——→		[14]			[15]					
Hematocrit or Hemoglobin[13]	←——————→					[15]					
Urinalysis											

PROCEDURES-PATIENT AT RISK	Age columns →
Lead Screening[16]	★ ★ ★ ★ ★ ★ ★ ★ ★ ★ ★ ★
Tuberculin Test[17]	★ ★ ★ ★ ★ ★ ★ ★ ★ ★ ★ ★
Cholesterol Screening[18]	★ ★ ★ ★ ★
STD Screening[19]	★ ★ ★ ★ ★
Pelvic Exam[20]	★ ←—20—→
ANTICIPATORY GUIDANCE[21]	
Injury Prevention[22]	• • • • • • • • •
Violence Prevention[23]	• • • • • • •
Sleep Positioning Counseling[24]	• •
Nutrition Counseling[25]	• • • • • • •
DENTAL REFERRAL[26]	←—→

1. A prenatal visit is recommended for parents who are at high risk, for first-time parents, and for those who request a conference. The prenatal visit should include anticipatory guidance, pertinent medical history, and a discussion of benefits of breastfeeding and planned method of feeding per AAP statement "The Prenatal Visit" (1996).

2. Every infant should have a newborn evaluation after birth. Breastfeeding should be encouraged and instruction and support offered. Every breastfeeding infant should have an evaluation 48-72 hours after discharge from the hospital to include weight, formal breastfeeding evaluation, encouragement, and instruction as recommended in the AAP statement "Breastfeeding and the Use of Human Milk" (1997).

3. For newborns discharged in less than 48 hours after delivery per AAP statement "Hospital Stay for Healthy Newborns" (1995).

4. Developmental, psychosocial, and chronic disease issues for children and adolescents may require frequent counseling and treatment visits separate from preventive care visits.

5. If a child comes under care for the first time at any point on the schedule, or if any items are not accomplished at the suggested age, the schedule should be brought up to date at the earliest possible time.

6. If the patient is uncooperative, rescreen within 6 months.

7. All newborns should be screened per the AAP Task Force on Newborn and Infant Hearing statement, "Newborn and Infant Hearing Loss: Detection and Intervention" (1999).

8. By history and appropriate physical examination; if suspicious, by specific objective developmental testing. Parenting skills should be fostered at every visit.

9. At each visit, a complete physical examination is essential, with infant totally unclothed, older child undressed and suitably draped.

10. These may be modified, depending upon entry point into schedule and individual need.

11. Metabolic screening (e.g., thyroid, hemoglobinopathies, PKU, galactosemia) should be done according to state law.

12. Schedule(s) per the Committee on Infectious Diseases, published annually in the January edition of Pediatrics. Every visit should be an opportunity to update and complete a child's immunizations.

13. See AAP Pediatric Nutrition Handbook (1998) for a discussion of universal and selective screening options. Consider earlier screening for high-risk infants (e.g., premature infants and low birth weight infants). See also "Recommendations to Prevent and Control Iron Deficiency in the United States". MMWR. 1998;47 (RR-3):1-29.

14. All menstruating adolescents should be screened annually.

15. Conduct dipstick urinalysis for leukocytes annually for sexually active male and female adolescents.

16. For children at risk for lead exposure consult the AAP statement "Screening for Elevated Blood Levels" (1998). Additionally, screening should be done in accordance with state law where applicable.

17. TB testing per recommendations of the Committee on Infectious Diseases, published in the current edition of Red Book: Report of the Committee on Infectious Diseases. Testing should be done upon recognition of high-risk factors.

18. Cholesterol screening for high-risk patients per AAP statement "Cholesterol in Childhood" (1998). If family history cannot be ascertained and other risk factors are present, screening should be at the discretion of the physician.

19. All sexually active patients should be screened for sexually transmitted diseases (STDs).

20. All sexually active females should have a pelvic examination. A pelvic examination and routine pap smear should be offered as part of preventive health maintenance between the ages of 18 and 21 years.

21. Age-appropriate discussion and counseling should be an integral part of each visit for care per the AAP Guidelines for Health Supervision III (1998).

22. From birth to age 12, refer to the AAP injury prevention program (TIPP*) as described in A Guide to Safety Counseling in Office Practice (1994).

23. Violence prevention and management for all patients per AAP statement "The Role of the Pediatrician in Youth Violence Prevention in Clinical Practice and at the Community Level" (1999).

24. Parents and caregivers should be advised to place healthy infants on their backs when putting them to sleep. Side positioning is a reasonable alternative but carries a slightly higher risk of SIDS. Consult the AAP statement "Changing Concepts of Sudden Infant Death Syndrome: Implications for Infant Sleeping Environment and Sleep Position" (2000).

25. Age-appropriate nutrition counseling should be an integral part of each visit per the AAP Handbook of Nutrition (1998).

26. Earlier initial dental examinations may be appropriate for some children. Subsequent examinations as prescribed by dentist.

Key: • = to be performed   ★ = to be performed for patients at risk
S = subjective, by history   O = objective, by a standard testing method
←——→ = the range during which a service may be provided, with the dot indicating the preferred age.

NB: Special chemical, immunologic, and endocrine testing is usually carried out upon specific indications. Testing other than newborn (e.g., inborn errors of metabolism, sickle disease, etc) is discretionary with the physician.

FIG. 1–1

Recommendations for preventive pediatric health care. (From Committee on Practice and Ambulatory Medicine, American Academy of Pediatrics: *Pediatrics*, 96[2]: 2000, Copyright American Academy of Pediatrics, 2000.)

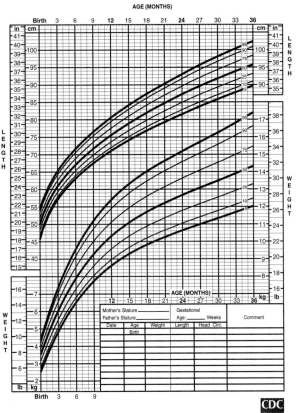
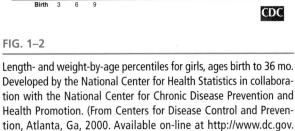

FIG. 1–2

Length- and weight-by-age percentiles for girls, ages birth to 36 mo. Developed by the National Center for Health Statistics in collaboration with the National Center for Chronic Disease Prevention and Health Promotion. (From Centers for Disease Control and Prevention, Atlanta, Ga, 2000. Available on-line at http://www.dc.gov.growthcharts.)

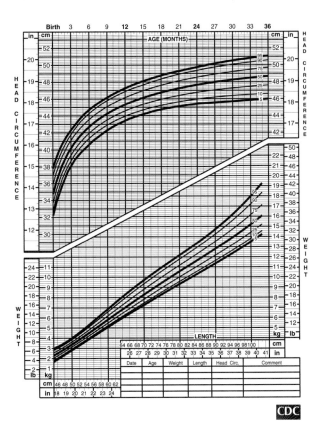

FIG. 1–3

Head circumference and weight-by-length percentiles for girls, ages birth to 36 mo. Developed by the National Center for Health Statistics in collaboration with the National Center for Chronic Disease Prevention and Health Promotion. (From Centers for Disease Control and Prevention, Atlanta, Ga, 2000. Available on-line at http://www.cdc.gov.growthcharts.)

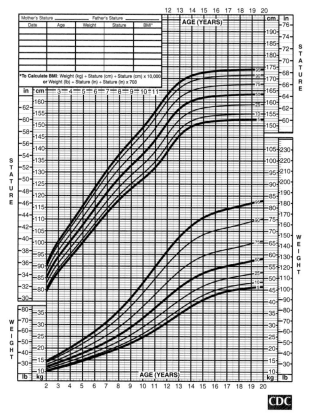

FIG. 1–4

Stature-for-age and weight-for-age percentiles for girls, ages 2–20 years. Developed by the National Center for Health Statistics in collaboration with the National Center for Chronic Disease Prevention and Health Promotion. (From Centers for Disease Control and Prevention, Atlanta, Ga, 2000. Available on-line at http://www.cdc.gov.growthcharts.)

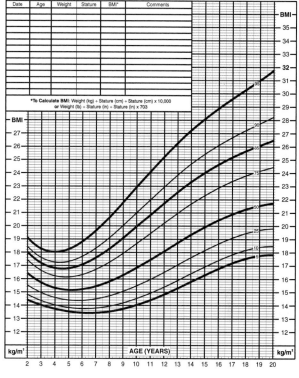

FIG. 1–5

Body mass index–for–age percentiles for girls, ages 2–20 years. Developed by the National Center for Health Statistics in collaboration with the National Center for Chronic Disease Prevention and Health Promotion. (From Centers for Disease Control and Prevention, Atlanta, Ga, 2000. Available on-line at http://www.cdc.gov.growthcharts.)

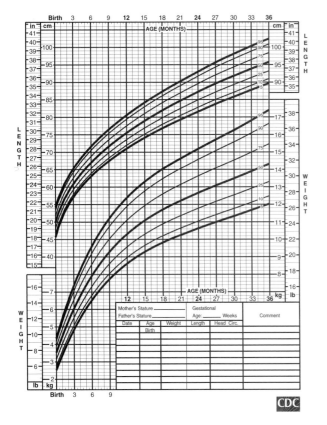

FIG. 1–6

Length- and weight-by-age percentiles for boys, ages birth to 36 mo. Developed by the National Center for Health Statistics in collaboration with the National Center for Chronic Disease Prevention and Health Promotion. (From Centers for Disease Control and Prevention, Atlanta, Ga, 2000. Available on-line at http://www.cdc.gov.growthcharts.)

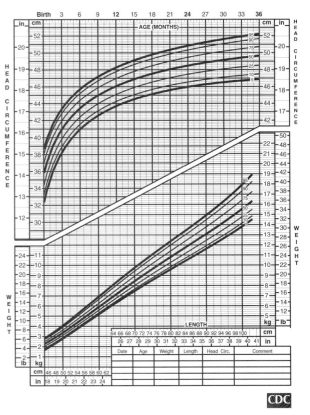

FIG. 1–7

Head circumference and weight-by-length percentiles for boys, ages birth to 36 mo. Developed by the National Center for Health Statistics in collaboration with the National Center for Chronic Disease Prevention and Health Promotion. (From Centers for Disease Control and Prevention, Atlanta, Ga, 2000. Available on-line at http://www.cdc.gov.growthcharts.)

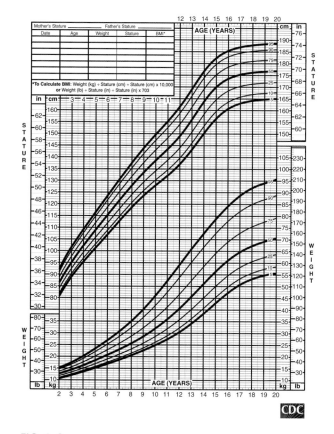

FIG. 1–8

Stature-for-age and weight-for-age percentiles for boys, ages 2–20 years. Developed by the National Center for Health Statistics in collaboration with the National Center for Chronic Disease Prevention and Health Promotion. (From Centers for Disease Control and Prevention, Atlanta, Ga, 2000. Available on-line at http://www.cdc.gov.growthcharts.)

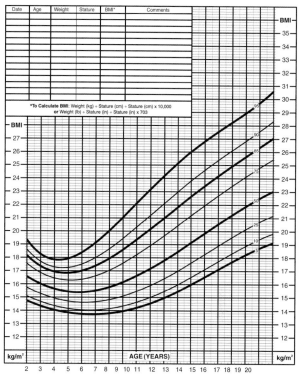

FIG. 1–9

Body mass index–for–age percentiles for boys, ages 2–20 years. Developed by the National Center for Health Statistics in collaboration with the National Center for Chronic Disease Prevention and Health Promotion. (From Centers for Disease Control and Prevention, Atlanta, Ga, 2000. Available on-line at http://www.cdc.gov/growthcharts.)

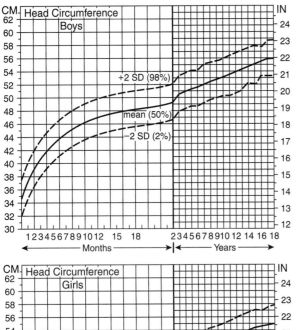

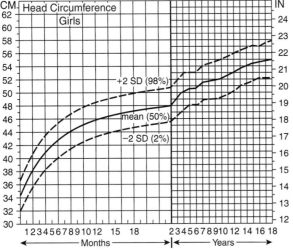

FIG. 1–10

Changes in head circumference with age for boys and girls. (From Nellhaus G: *Pediatrics* 41[1]:106–114, 1968.)

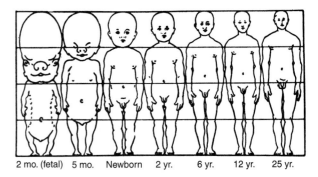

FIG. 1–11

Changes in body proportions from second fetal month to adulthood. (From Robbins WJ et al: *Growth*, New Haven, Conn, 1968, Yale University Press.)

TABLE 1–1
Rules of Thumb for Growth

Weight
1. Weight loss in first few days: 5–10% of birth weight
2. Return to birth weight: 7–10 days of age
   Double birth weight: 4–5 mo
   Triple birth weight: 1 yr
   Quadruple birth weight: 2 yr
3. Average weights: 3.5 kg at birth
   10 kg at 1 yr
   20 kg at 5 yr
   30 kg at 10 yr
4. Daily weight gain: 20–30 g for first 3–4 mo
   15–20 g for rest of the first yr
5. Average annual weight gain: 5 lb between 2 yr and puberty (spurts and plateaus may occur)

Height
1. Average length: 20 inches at birth, 30 inches at 1 yr
2. At age 3 yr, the average child is 3 ft tall
3. At age 4 yr, the average child is 40 in tall (double birth length)
4. Average annual height increase: 2–3 inches between age 4 yr and puberty

Head Circumference (HC)
1. Average HC: 35 cm at birth (13.5 inches)
2. HC increases: 1 cm/mo for first yr (2 cm/mo for first 3 mo, then slower); 10 cm for rest of life

adolescents to determine whether an individual is overweight (BMI above the 95th percentile for age) or at risk for being overweight (BMI between the 85th and 95th percentile for age). The most common reasons for deviant measurements are technical (faulty equipment and human errors in measurement or plotting), so the first step in investigating a deviant measurement should be to repeat it. It also helps to know some rough rules of thumb, as presented in Table 1–1. Separate growth charts are available for very low birth weight (VLBW) infants (weight <1500 g) and for children with Turner syndrome, Down syndrome, achondroplasia, and other dysmorphology syndromes.

Variability in body proportions occurs from fetal to adult life (Fig. 1–11). There is also considerable vari-ation in body form among normal children, often following familial patterns. Differences in body proportions depend on variations in the growth rates of parts of the body or organ systems. Certain growth disturbances result in characteristic changes in the proportional sizes of the trunk, extremities, and head.

The distinctive patterns of proportionate growth rates for several body systems correlate closely with function. Growth of the nervous system is most rapid in the first 2 years, whereas the growth rate for lymphoid tissue peaks at about 12 years. Osseous maturation (bone age) is determined from roentgenograms on the basis of the number and size of epiphyseal centers; the size, shape, density, and sharpness of outline of the ends of bones; and the distance separating the epiphyseal center from the zone of provisional calcification. Functional correlations also exist between growing systems. Thus bone age corresponds more closely to sexual maturity, which is dependent on the growth and development of the endocrine system, than to chronologic age. The heart is relatively large at birth, and a pubertal growth spurt in the size of the heart parallels the general growth spurt. Pulse rate and blood pressure vary with age and growth, as do a great many metabolic and nutritional changes.

REFERENCES

Behrman RE, Kliegman RM, Jenson HB, editors: *Nelson textbook of pediatrics*, ed 16, Philadelphia, 2000, WB Saunders, Chapters 7–16.

International Obesity Task Force: Assessment of childhood and adolescent obesity, *Am J Clin Nutr* 70(1):117S–175S, 1999 (supplement).

National Center for Health Statistics: Growth Chart Information. Available on-line at http://www.cdc.gov/nchs/about/major/nhanes/growchart.htm.

Developmental Milestones and Theories

The use of developmental milestones to assess development focuses on discrete behaviors that the clinician can observe or accept as present by parental report. This approach is based on comparing the patient's behavior with that of many normal children whose behaviors evolve in a uniform sequence and within specific age ranges. A behavior is the response of the neuromotor system to a specific situation. The development of the neuromotor system, like that of other organ systems, is first determined by genetic endowment and then molded by environmental influences.

Norms for discrete behaviors provide a convenient way to monitor development (Fig. 1–12 and later in the chapter), but they provide an incomplete picture. Although a sequence of specific, easily measured behaviors can adequately represent some areas of development (e.g., gross motor, fine motor, and language), other areas, particularly social and emotional development, are not adequately assessed by this means. In addition, easily measured developmental milestones are well established only

through the 6th year of age. Many other types of assessment (e.g., intelligence tests, achievement tests, personality profiles, and neurodevelopmental assessments) that expand the developmental milestone approach beyond the age of 6 years are available for all ages; however, these tests generally require time and expertise in administration and interpretation that are not available in the primary care medical setting. Pediatricians therefore need to supplement their screening of developmental milestones with less precise but possibly more important surveillance of psychosocial issues that are pertinent at each age. The following brief presentation of some developmental theories is intended as an introduction to these important areas.

Piaget

Piaget's theory is the major theory of cognitive development. Cognition is defined as the process of knowing in the broadest sense, including perception, memory, judgment, and reasoning. Piaget contended that cognitive ability develops in a fixed sequence of qualitatively different stages—that is, a child's mind works in different ways in each stage. Table 1–2 presents an outline of the major characteristics of each stage (see p. 12). Unrealistic parental expectations often result from a lack of understanding about how a child's logic differs from that of an adult. Helping the parent see an episode of problem behavior from the child's perspective can often improve a behavioral problem.

Piagetian theory includes the concept of **equilibration,** the mechanism for the formation of knowledge. Equilibration involves two processes that are set in motion when a person is confronted with a new situation that he or she does not fully understand: **assimilation** involves attempts to reshape the new experience to make it fit with accustomed ways of thinking, and **accommodation** involves revisions in the accustomed ways of thinking to fit with the new experience. When the disequilibrium produced by the new experience is resolved by the use of both processes, a new equilibration is achieved at a higher level of cognitive organization. Disequilibrium is thus a necessary stimulus for development. Avoiding new or unfamiliar experiences limits the chances for cognitive growth. An important related concept is **cognitive dissonance,** the degree to which a new stimulus differs from familiar stimuli. Novelty attracts children, but if the cognitive dissonance is too great, they will be frightened or frustrated and will not achieve a new equilibrium (cognitive growth).

Freud

Freudian theory contains a number of concepts that are helpful in understanding child development. The principle of *psychic determinism* holds that no

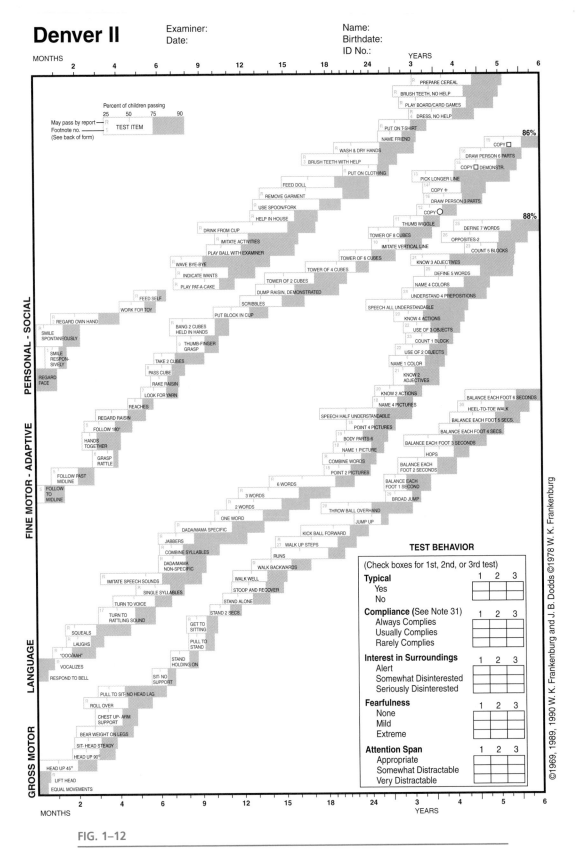

FIG. 1–12

Scoring form for Denver II. (From Frankenburg WK: *Denver II Developmental Screening Test,* ed 2, Denver, 1990, Denver Developmental Materials.)

1. Try to get child to smile by smiling, talking or waving. Do not touch him/her.
2. Child must stare at hand several seconds.
3. Parent may help guide toothbrush and put toothpaste on brush.
4. Child does not have to be able to tie shoes or button/zip in the back.
5. Move yarn slowly in an arc from one side to the other, about 8" above child's face.
6. Pass if child grasps rattle when it is touched to the backs or tips of fingers.
7. Pass if child tries to see where yarn went. Yarn should be dropped quickly from sight from tester's hand without arm movement.
8. Child must transfer cube from hand to hand without help of body, mouth, or table.
9. Pass if child picks up raisin with any part of thumb and finger.
10. Line can vary only 30 degrees or less from tester's line.
11. Make a fist with thumb pointing upward and wiggle only the thumb. Pass if child imitates and does not move any fingers other than the thumb.

   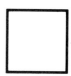

12. Pass any enclosed form. Fail continuous round motions.
13. Which line is longer? (Not bigger.) Turn paper upside down and repeat. (pass 3 of 3 or 5 of 6)
14. Pass any lines crossing near midpoint.
15. Have child copy first. If failed, demonstrate.

When giving items 12, 14, and 15, do not name the forms. Do not demonstrate 12 and 14.

16. When scoring, each pair (2 arms, 2 legs, etc.) counts as one part.
17. Place one cube in cup and shake gently near child's ear, but out of sight. Repeat for other ear.
18. Point to picture and have child name it. (No credit is given for sounds only.)
    If less than 4 pictures are named correctly, have child point to picture as each is named by tester.

 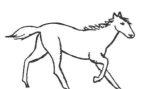 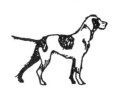 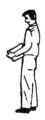

19. Using doll, tell child: Show me the nose, eyes, ears, mouth, hands, feet, tummy, hair. Pass 6 of 8.
20. Using pictures, ask child: Which one flies?… says meow?… talks?… barks?… gallops? Pass 2 of 5, 4 of 5.
21. Ask child: What do you do when you are cold?… tired?… hungry? Pass 2 of 3, 3 of 3.
22. Ask child: What do you do with a cup? What is a chair used for? What is a pencil used for?
    Action words must be included in answers.
23. Pass if child correctly places <u>and</u> says how many blocks are on paper. (1, 5).
24. Tell child: Put block **on** table; **under** table; **in front of** me, **behind** me. Pass 4 of 4.
    (Do not help child by pointing, moving head or eyes.)
25. Ask child: What is a ball?… lake?… desk?… house?… banana?… curtain?… fence?… ceiling? Pass if defined in terms of use, shape, what it is made of, or general category (such as banana is fruit, not just yellow). Pass 5 of 8, 7 of 8.
26. Ask child: If a horse is big, a mouse is __? If fire is hot, ice is __? If the sun shines during the day, the moon shines during the __? Pass 2 of 3.
27. Child may use wall or rail only, not person. May not crawl.
28. Child must throw ball overhand 3 feet to within arm's reach of tester.
29. Child must perform standing broad jump over width of test sheet (8 1/2 inches).
30. Tell child to walk forward, ∞∞∞→ heel within 1 inch of toe. Tester may demonstrate.
    Child must walk 4 consecutive steps.
31. In the second year, half of normal children are non-compliant.

OBSERVATIONS:

FIG. 1–13

Instructions for the Denver II. Numbers are coded to scoring form (Fig. 1–12). "Abnormal" is defined as two or more delays (failure of an item passed by 90% at that age) in two or more categories, or two or more delays in one category with one other category having one delay and an age line that does not intersect one item that is passed. A "suspect" or "questionable" score is given if one category has two or more delays or if one or more categories have one delay and in the same category the age line does not pass through one item that is passed. (From Frankenburg WK: *Denver II Developmental Screening Test,* ed 2, Denver, 1990, Denver Developmental Materials.)

TABLE 1–2
Jean Piaget's Stages of Cognitive Development

Stage	Description	Major Developments
Sensorimotor Birth to 2 yr	Learning occurs through activity, exploration, and manipulation of the environment. Motor and sensory impressions form the foundation of later learning.	Learns to differentiate self from world—beginning sense of self-identity. Formation and integration of schemes—as in learning that sucking on a nipple produces milk or that shaking a rattle produces a noise. Achieves object permanence—that things exist even when not visible. Simple tool use.
Preoperational 2 to 6 or 7 yr	Child is capable of symbolic representations of world, as in use of language, play, and deferred imitation; still not capable of sustained, systematic thought.	Engages in symbolic play—can represent something with something else. Some decline in egocentricity—can take greater account of others' points of view. Develops language and drawing as modes of representing experience.
Concrete Operations 6 or 7 to 11 yr	Child becomes capable of limited logical thought processes, as in seeing relationships and classifying, as long as manipulable, concrete materials are available.	Becomes aware that some aspects of things remain the same despite changes in appearance (conservation). Can mentally reverse a process or action (reversibility). Can focus on more than one aspect of a situation at a time (decentration). Can deduce new relationships from sets of earlier ones (transitivity). Can order things in sequence (seriation). Can group objects on the basis of common features (classification).
Formal Operations 12 yr through adulthood	Child can reason logically and abstractly. Can formulate and test hypotheses. Thought no longer depends on concrete reality. Can play with possibilities.	Can deal with abstract ideas. Can manipulate variables in a scientific situation. Can deal with analogies and metaphors. Can reflect on own thinking. Can work out combinations and permutations.

Adapted from Stone LJ, Church J: *Childhood and adolescence*, New York, 1979, Random House.

psychic event happens in a chance or random way but instead is determined by preceding psychic events. "Freudian slips" (e.g., forgetting a meeting that is expected to be stressful) illustrate this principle. At a conscious level, these slips seem to be simple mistakes with no apparent explanation. According to the theory, however, unconscious mental processes are responsible for their occurrence. A patient's explanation for a behavior or recounting of an event taps only the conscious level; probing questions may bring more information to the conscious level. The concept of innate sexual and aggressive drives that provide "psychic energy" also is central to Freudian theory. Freud proposed five stages of psychosexual development, with different parts of the body serving as the focus of gratification of the sexual drive at different ages (Table 1–3).

One of Freud's most enduring contributions is his hypothesis about the organization of mental processes into id, ego, and superego. The **id** is the source of a person's impulses and drives and is dominant at birth. The **ego** is the pragmatic, rational part of the mind, consisting of those functions that have to do with an individual's relationship to the environment (sensory perception, motor control, memory, affect, and thinking). Initially the ego serves the id, finding ways to achieve gratification of the id impulses. Gradually the ego exerts increasing control over the id in the service of greater long-term gratification and avoidance of discomfort. The

TABLE 1–3
Stage Theories of Socioemotional Development

	Birth–18 mo	18 mo–3 yr	3–6 yr	6–12 yr	Adult
Piaget (see Table 1–2)	*Sensorimotor*	*Preoperational*		*Concrete*	*Formal*
Freud (psychosexual development)	*Oral Stage* Infants obtain gratification through stimulation of the mouth, as they suck and bite.	*Anal Stage* Children obtain gratification through exercise of the anal musculature during elimination or retention.	*Phallic Stage (Oedipal)* Children develop sexual curiosity and obtain gratification through masturbation. They have sexual fantasies about the parent of the opposite sex and guilt about their fantasies.	*Latency Stage* Children's sexual urges are submerged; they put their energies into acquiring cultural skills.	*Genital Stage* Adolescents have adult heterosexual desires and seek to satisfy them.
Erikson (psychosocial development)	*Trust versus Mistrust* Infants learn to trust, or mistrust, that their needs will be met by the world, especially by the mother.	*Autonomy versus Shame, Doubt* Children learn to exercise will, to make choices, to control themselves, or they become uncertain and doubt that they can do things by themselves.	*Initiative versus Guilt* Children learn to initiate activities and enjoy their accomplishments, acquiring direction and purpose. If they are not allowed initiative, they feel guilty for their attempts at independence.	*Industry versus Inferiority* Children develop a sense of industry and curiosity and are eager to learn, or they feel inferior and lose interest in the tasks before them.	*Identity versus Role Confusion* Adolescents come to see themselves as unique and integrated persons with an ideology, or they become confused about what they want out of life.

Adapted from Clarke-Stewart A, Koch JB: *Children: development through adolescence,* New York, 1983, John Wiley & Sons; Stone LJ, Church J: *Childhood and adolescence,* New York, 1979, Random House.

superego, or conscience, comprises the moral precepts of an individual's mind and his or her ideal aspirations.

Identification is one of the hypothesized processes by which the ego gains mastery over the id; it is manifested as a child's identification of himself or herself with people or things that are highly charged with psychic energy. Identification is apparent in the observation that children behave according to what they see and experience rather than what they are told. Fantasized gratification is another process by which the ego gains mastery over the id. A *fantasy* (dream or daydream) in which the wishes of the id are represented as fulfilled results in partial gratification of id impulses. The id impulse may be so nearly satisfied that it is easy for the ego to control the impulse afterward. This is the idea behind play therapy.

The most important factor in the control of id impulses is *anxiety.* "Automatic anxiety" develops whenever a child's psyche is overwhelmed by a flood of stimuli too great to be mastered or discharged. These stimuli may be external, but most often they are internal, arising from the id. This type of anxiety is characteristic of infancy because of the immaturity of the ego, but it also is found in adult life in cases of anxiety neurosis. In the course of development the ego acquires the capacity to produce "signal anxiety" when a potential danger situation arises (i.e., the threat of a traumatic situation), which enables the ego to inhibit id impulses. Freud proposed the following sequence of danger situations in early and later childhood that persist unconsciously to some degree throughout life:
1. Loss of the object—separation from a person or thing that is an important source of gratification
2. Loss of the object's love
3. Loss of sexual gratification
4. Guilt, or disapproval of the superego

Defense mechanisms are unconscious ego processes that focus narrowly on the reduction of anxiety through the control of id impulses. *Repression* occurs when the ego bars from consciousness the unwanted id impulse. *Suppression* is the conscious equivalent of repression. In *reaction formation* one of a pair of ambivalent attitudes is made unconscious and kept unconscious by an overemphasis on the other (e.g., love/hate, cruelty/gentleness, and stubbornness/compliance). Reactions to a new sibling may include the use of defense mechanisms such as *repression* (of hostile wishes toward the sibling) and *reaction formation* (love instead of hate), as well as other ego processes such as *identification* with the mother (imitating caregiving). Other common defense mechanisms are *denial* (the disavowal of an unpleasant or unwanted piece of external reality) and

projection (the attribution of one's own wish or impulse to another person, such as the imaginary friend in early childhood).

Defense mechanisms are both evidence of healthy coping and a sign of anxiety. Therefore in the treatment of anxiety, the aim is not to attack the defense mechanism directly, but rather to understand the source of the anxiety that creates the need for the defense mechanism and work toward the removal of the source.

According to Freud, resolving the *Oedipus complex* between the ages of 3 and 6 years results in development of the superego. The Oedipus complex involves contrasting attitudes toward the parents, regardless of the gender of the child (e.g., a wish to eliminate the jealously hated father and take his place in a sensual relationship with the mother). Such wishes arouse fears of retaliation and the loss of love, resulting in the formation of the superego to control the impulses. Subsequently, the superego becomes the principal source of anxiety, guilt, and unconscious feelings of inferiority but may also produce feelings of joy and self-satisfaction.

Erikson

Erikson revised and expanded Freud's psychosexual stages into psychosocial stages that span the life cycle. His theory emphasized the development of the ego within a social context rather than the instinctual drives of the id. Erikson's stages start with a focus on a particular part of the body and expand to a consideration of the social context of the child's behavior (see Table 1–3). For example, in Freud's oral stage the major mode of gratification involves sucking and feeding. In Erikson's parallel stage the major psychosocial issue involves the development of "basic trust versus basic mistrust" that the mother will meet the infant's needs. Similarly, in the next stage Erikson goes beyond Freud's narrow focus on bowel control (anal stage) and proposes "autonomy versus shame and doubt" as the central psychosocial issue. Toilet training is a specific behavior that may serve as the focus of the child's struggle with this psychosocial issue, but this struggle may be generalized to other behaviors that involve control of the body and the environment, especially when the child has physical disabilities.

Normal resolution of each psychosocial issue involves the development of a balance between the positive and negative attitudes that characterize the issue, with a ratio favoring the positive. Each issue is never completely resolved but instead becomes part of the developmental history of the individual, which influences the resolution of each subsequent stage. The sequence of issues proposed by Erikson coincides with the widening circle of societal exposures and demands that are common to all human cultures. Individuals may **regress** to an earlier stage when a previously attained balance is disrupted by new events and stresses (e.g., the birth of a sibling, beginning of school, illness, separation from loved ones, moves, and family turmoil). Puberty and adolescence frequently upset balances achieved in preceding stages and necessitate a reworking of the issues to achieve new balances.

REFERENCES

Behrman RE, Kliegman RM, Jenson HB, editors: *Nelson textbook of pediatrics,* ed 16, Philadelphia, 2000, WB Saunders, Chapters 7–13.
Brenner C: *An elementary textbook of psychoanalysis,* Garden City, NY, 1973, Doubleday.
Erikson EH: *Childhood and society,* ed 2, New York, 1963, WW Norton.
Ginsburg H, Opper S: *Piaget's theory of intellectual development,* ed 2, Englewood Cliffs, NJ, 1979, Prentice-Hall.

Bonding and Attachment

Bonding and attachment are terms that describe the affectional relationships between parents and infants. **Bonding** occurs rapidly and shortly after birth and reflects the feelings of the parents toward the newborn (unidirectional); **attachment** involves reciprocal feelings between parent and infant and develops gradually over the first year. Effective bonding in the postpartum period may enhance the development of attachment. An increased awareness of the importance of bonding has led to significant improvements in routine birthing procedures and postpartum parent-infant contact.

Attachment to a specific, stable parent figure is crucial for a child's normal mental and physical development. Beyond mere feeding and protection, attachment to a primary caregiver also serves to promote exploration of the environment and learning.

Between the ages of 9 and 18 months, children normally become insecure about separation from the primary caregiver. This insecurity coincides with the child's increasing cognitive and motor abilities. The child is beginning to understand simple, immediate, cause-and-effect relationships and thus can anticipate separations (e.g., after Mommy gets her coat) but still has an inadequate appreciation of time and delayed gratification. In addition, the child's new motor skills and attraction to novelty may lead to headlong plunges into new adventures that result in fright or pain followed by frantic efforts to find and cling to the primary caregiver. This often results in dramatic swings from stubborn independence to clinging dependence that can be frustrating and confusing to parents. With a secure

attachment, the period of ambivalence may be shorter and less tumultuous.

REFERENCES

Behrman RE, Kliegman RM, Jenson HB, editors: *Nelson textbook of pediatrics,* ed 16, Philadelphia, 2000, WB Saunders, Chapters 10, 11, 90.
Crittenden PM: Attachment and risk for psychopathology: the early years, *J Dev Behav Pediatr* 16(3 Suppl):S12, 1995.
Kennell JH, Klaus MH: Bonding: recent observations that alter perinatal care, *Pediatr Rev* 19(1):4–12, 1998.

Behavior Theory

Behavior theory postulates that behavior is primarily a product of external environmental determinants and that manipulation of the environmental antecedents and consequences of behavior can be used to modify maladaptive behavior and to increase desirable behavior. **Conditioning** is the process through which behavior is modified by environmental manipulations.

Respondent (classic) conditioning is illustrated by Pavlov's famous experiment, in which a dog's salivary response was conditioned to occur at the sound of a bell. The experiment starts with an automatic stimulus-response relationship—food (unconditioned stimulus) stimulating salivation (unconditioned response). Conditioning occurs when another stimulus (a bell ringing in Pavlov's experiment) is presented just before or with the unconditioned stimulus (food). After many presentations of the two stimuli together, the bell (conditioned stimulus) alone will elicit the response: salivation (conditioned response). Respondent conditioning has been used to explain **phobic behavior,** in which a previously unfeared object or stimulus now arouses fear because it is associated with the occurrence of an unconditioned fearful stimulus (e.g., an episode of falling off a diving board leads to a fear of all swimming). Phobias can be treated by *desensitization,* a process involving training in relaxation techniques, later coupled with gradual exposure to stimuli associated more and more closely with the feared stimulus. The most effective treatment currently available for nocturnal enuresis involves respondent conditioning (see Enuresis).

Operant conditioning modifies behavior by manipulating the antecedents or the consequences of the behavior. The four major methods of operant conditioning are positive reinforcement, negative reinforcement, extinction, and punishment. Many common behavioral problems of children can be improved by these methods.

Positive reinforcement increases the frequency of a behavior by following the behavior with a favorable event (e.g., a child eats vegetables more often after being rewarded with dessert). **Negative reinforcement** increases the frequency of a behavior by following the behavior with the removal or avoidance of an unpleasant event (e.g., a child avoids a parent's wrath by staying away from the stove). Conversely, reinforcement also may occur unintentionally, increasing the frequency of an undesirable behavior. Differential reinforcement of incompatible behavior encourages activities that make an undesirable behavior impossible (e.g., rewarding keeping hands in pockets to avoid nail biting). **Extinction** occurs when there is a decrease in the frequency of a previously reinforced behavior because the reinforcement is withheld. This is the principle behind the common advice to ignore such behavior as crying at bedtime or temper tantrums that parents may unwittingly reinforce through attention and comforting. **Punishment** decreases the frequency of a behavior through unpleasant consequences.

REFERENCES

Behrman RE, Kliegman RM, Jenson HB, editors: *Nelson textbook of pediatrics*, ed 16, Philadelphia, 2000, WB Saunders, Chapters 5, 7, 28.
Parrish JM: Child behavior management. In Levine MD, Carey WB, Crocker AC, editors: *Developmental-behavioral pediatrics*, ed 3, Philadelphia, 1999, WB Saunders.

Individual Differences

Normal children differ widely in behavior. If this fact is not appreciated and an expected pattern of behavior is too narrowly defined, normal behavior may be labeled as abnormal or pathologic. Although there are always gray areas between clearly normal and clearly abnormal behavior, in clinical situations the differentiation between abnormal and normal (although perhaps unusual) behavior frequently rests on a judgment of whether the behavior is adaptive. This judgment must be made in the context of the environment in which the individual functions, as well as in the context of the unique physical and mental characteristics of the individual. However, the physician must avoid explaining away serious problems by attributing them to individual variations in behavior. Significant individual differences exist within the normal development of **temperament** (behavioral style). There are three common constellations of temperamental characteristics:

1. The "easy child" (applying to 40% of children) is characterized by regularity of biologic functions (i.e., consistent, predictable times for eating, sleeping, and elimination), a positive approach to new stimuli, high adaptability to change, mild or moderate intensity in responses, and a positive mood.
2. The "difficult child" (10%) is characterized by irregularity of biologic functions, negative withdrawal from new stimuli, poor adaptability, intense responses, and a negative mood.
3. The "slow-to-warm-up child" (15%) is characterized by a low activity level, withdrawal from new stimuli, slow adaptability, mild intensity in responses, and a somewhat negative mood.

The remaining percentage of children have more mixed temperaments. The individual temperament of a child has important implications for parenting and for the advice a pediatrician may give in anticipatory guidance or behavior problem counseling (see Management of Developmental and Behavioral Problems).

Although temperament may be to some degree "hard wired" (nature) in each child, the environment (nurture) in which the child grows has a strong effect on the child's adjustment ("goodness of fit"). Social and cultural factors can have marked effects on the child through differences in parenting style, educational approaches, and behavioral expectations. Although we are only beginning to understand the multitude of ways in which the environment can influence development, aspects of the environment clearly play an important role in the etiology and management of many behavioral problems of children.

Gardner noted variable patterns in cognitive processes, described as "multiple intelligences." Based on observations of geniuses and individuals with unique skills, this theory suggests that most people have unique mixes of innate strengths and weaknesses. Recognizing the strengths and weaknesses of an individual can be useful in planning for school, career, and recreational aspects of life.

REFERENCES

Behrman RE, Kliegman RM, Jenson HB, editors: *Nelson textbook of pediatrics*, ed 16, Philadelphia, 2000, WB Saunders, Chapter 7.
Chess S, Thomas A: The development of behavioral individuality. In Levine MD, Carey WB, Crocker AC, editors: *Developmental-behavioral pediatrics*, ed 3, Philadelphia, 1999, WB Saunders.
Gardner H: *Multiple intelligences: the theory in practice*, New York, 1993, BasicBooks.

Adolescence

Early, middle, and late adolescence are characterized by different behavioral and developmental issues (see Table 7–3). The age at which each issue becomes manifest and the importance of these issues vary widely among individuals, as do the rates of cognitive, psychosexual, psychosocial, and physical development.

During *early adolescence*, a young person undergoes maximal somatic and sexual growth. Thinking is focused on the present and on the peer group. Identity is focused primarily on the physical changes, and concern is about normality. Exploratory, undifferentiated sexual behavior resulting in physical contact with same-sex peers is normal during early adolescence, although heterosexual interests can also develop. Strivings for independence are ambivalent.

Middle adolescence can be a most difficult time for both adolescents and the adults who have contact with them. Cognitive processes are more sophisticated. Through formal operational thinking, middle adolescents can experiment with ideas, consider things as they might be, develop insight, and reflect on their own feelings and those of others. As they mature cognitively and psychosocially, these adolescents focus on issues of identity not limited solely to the physical aspects of the body. As middle adolescents socialize with peers, experiment sexually, engage in risk-taking behaviors, and develop employment and interests outside the home, they augment their unique, developing identities. As a result of experimental, risk-taking behaviors, they may experience unwanted pregnancies, drug addiction, or motor vehicle accidents. The strivings of middle adolescents for independence, testing of limits, and need for autonomy are maximal and often distressing to their families, teachers, or other authority figures.

Late adolescence is usually marked by full formal operational thinking, including thoughts about the future (educationally, vocationally, and sexually). Late adolescents are usually more committed to their sexual partners than are middle adolescents. Unresolved separation anxiety from previous developmental stages may emerge at this time as the young person begins to move physically away from the family of origin to college or vocational school, a job, or military service.

REFERENCES

Behrman RE, Kliegman RM, Jenson HB, editors: *Nelson textbook of pediatrics,* ed 16, Philadelphia, 2000, WB Saunders, Chapter 14.

Ford CA, Coleman WL: Adolescent development and behavior: implications for the primary care physician. In Levine MD, Carey WB, Crocker AC, editors: *Developmental-behavioral pediatrics,* ed 3, Philadelphia, 1999, WB Saunders.

Litt IF: Pubertal and psychosocial development implications for pediatricians, *Pediatr Rev* 16(7):243–247, 1995.

McAnarney E, Kreipe R, Orr DP, et al, editors: *Textbook of adolescent medicine,* Philadelphia, 1992, WB Saunders.

ASSESSMENT
Primary Care Setting
Initial History and Observations

Developmental and behavioral problems are more common than any category of problems in pediatrics except acute infections and trauma. Parents often neglect to mention these problems because they think the physician is uninterested or cannot help. Therefore there is a need to screen for the presence of such problems in every health supervision visit, particularly in the preschool years when the pediatrician may be the only professional to evaluate the child. The limited time allotted to each health supervision visit will not allow a detailed assessment, but at least a few questions must be asked to supplement observations of the child's behavior during the visit. This will also encourage parents to express behavioral and developmental concerns about the child that can then be the focus of anticipatory guidance or early problem solving. The outline in Table 1–4 suggests topics for screening in health supervision visits.

The environment in which the child grows and develops is a crucial component of the causes and manifestations of problems, especially behavioral and developmental problems. Furthermore, appropriate approaches to managing these problems depend on the environmental context. Ignorance of the context will result in ineffective and perhaps inappropriate management suggestions from the physician. Table 1–5 lists some of the contextual factors that should be considered in the etiology of a child's behavioral problem.

Building rapport with the parents and the child is a prerequisite for obtaining the often sensitive infor-

---

TABLE 1–4
Topics for Health Supervision Visits

Focus on the Child
Concerns (parent's or child's)
Past problem follow-up
Immunization and screening test update
Routine care (e.g., eating, sleeping, elimination, and
  health habits)
Developmental progress
Behavioral style and problems

Focus on the Child's Environment
Family
Caregiving schedule for caregiver who lives at home
Parent-child and sibling-child interactions
Extended family role
Family stresses (e.g., work, move, finances, illness,
  death, marital and other interpersonal relationships)
Family supports (relatives, friends, groups)
Community
Caregivers outside the family
Peer interaction
School and work
Recreational activities
Physical Environment
Appropriate stimulation
Safety

TABLE 1–5
Context of Behavioral Problems

Child Factors
Health (past and current)
Developmental status
Temperament (e.g., difficult, slow to warm up)
Coping mechanisms

Parental Factors
Misinterpretations of stage-related behaviors
Mismatch of parental expectations and characteristics
of child
Parental characteristics (e.g., depression, lack of interest, rejection, overprotectiveness)
Coping mechanisms

Environmental Factors
Stress (e.g., marital discord, unemployment, personal loss)
Support (e.g., emotional, material, informational, child care)

Parent-Child Interactions
The common pathway through which the listed factors interact to influence the development of a behavior problem
The key to resolving the behavior problem

mation that is essential for understanding a behavioral or developmental problem. Rapport usually can be quickly established if the parents sense that the clinician respects them and is genuinely interested in listening to their concerns. Rapport with the child can be developed by engaging the child in developmentally appropriate conversation or play, providing toys while interviewing the parents, and being sensitive to the fears the child may have. Too often the child is ignored until it is time for the physical examination. Like their parents, children will feel more comfortable if they are greeted by name and involved in pleasant interactions before they are asked sensitive questions or threatened with examinations. Young children can be engaged in conversation on the parent's lap, which provides security and places the child at the eye level of the examiner.

With adolescents, emphasis should be placed on building a doctor-patient relationship that is distinct from the relationship with the parents. This does not mean the parents should be excluded; however, the adolescent should have the opportunity to express concerns to and ask questions of the clinician in confidence. This confidence can be achieved by meeting with the adolescent alone for at least part of each visit. However, confidentiality has limits, and parents must be informed when the clinician has concerns about the health and safety of the child. Often the clinician can convince the child to inform the parents directly of a problem or can reach an agreement with the child about how the parents will be informed.

Expanded History and Observations

Because the initial health supervision visit is brief, it is best to explore developmental and behavioral problems during subsequent visits when more comprehensive information and observations can be obtained, unless the problem is simple and the clinician knows the family well.

Specific interviewing practices enhance the collection of behavioral information. Responses to open-ended questions often provide clues to underlying, unstated problems and identify the appropriate direction for further, more directed questions. Sensitivity to the way something is said, not just to what is said, provides important clues for content areas to pursue. The interviewer may restrict the scope of the discussion unintentionally by prematurely using directed questions. Histories about developmental and behavioral problems are often vague and confusing; to reconcile apparent contradictions, the interviewer frequently must request clarification (to ascertain the meaning of a word to the patient), more detail, or mere repetition. By summarizing an understanding of the information at frequent intervals and by recapitulating at the close of the visit, the interviewer and patient can ensure that they understand each other. To build trust and to encourage the patient to talk about difficult issues, the physician must convey respect and empathy for the patient. Empathy is apparent when the physician recognizes the emotions that underlie the patient's responses and communicates this understanding both verbally and nonverbally.

Other techniques for improving the quality of information include the detailed description of a typical day (including parental responses to problem behaviors) and discussion of the physician's observations of the child's behavior and of parent-child and physician-child interactions during the visit. Although the child's behavior during the visit may be unrepresentative of his or her typical behavior, the physician's observations will serve as a springboard for discussion.

One very useful technique is to ask the parents to keep a diary of the occurrence and duration of problem behaviors and the antecedents and parental responses, if possible. This practice often reveals a pattern to the behavior that was not previously apparent to the parents. Projective techniques may provide additional useful information (e.g, "What are your happiest, saddest, and maddest moments?" or "If you could have any three wishes, what would they be?"). Third-person techniques (e.g., "Most boys your age are concerned about . . ." or asking about the drinking behavior of friends) may permit a child to talk about an issue that would be too difficult to handle if confronted directly.

If the clinician's impression of the child differs markedly from the parent's description, there may be a crucial parental concern that has not yet been expressed. The parent may fail to express a concern for several reasons: because it may be difficult to talk about (e.g., marital problems), because it is unconscious, or because the parent overlooks its relevance to the child's behavior. Alternatively, the physician's observations may be atypical, even with multiple visits. The observations of teachers, relatives, and other regular caregivers may be crucial in sorting out this possibility. The parent may also have a distorted image of the child, rooted in parental psychopathology. A sensitive, supportive, and noncritical approach to the parent may facilitate referral for appropriate therapy.

REFERENCES

Behrman RE, Kliegman RM, Jenson HB, editors: *Nelson textbook of pediatrics*, ed 16, Philadelphia, 2000, WB Saunders, Chapters 5, 6, 17.

Coleman WL: The interview. In Levine MD, Carey WB, Crocker AC, editors: *Developmental-behavioral pediatrics*, ed 3, Philadelphia, 1999, WB Saunders.

Developmental Screening and Surveillance

Developmental screening is a brief evaluation of developmental skills that is applied to a total population of children to identify children with suspected delays who require further diagnostic assessment. Developmental screening involves the use of standardized screening tests. In contrast, developmental surveillance is an informal, continuous process that may or may not involve the use of formal measures. Developmental screening or a combination of surveillance and screening is generally preferred over surveillance alone, since it has been demonstrated that office-based informal assessments by physicians are highly inaccurate. The ideal screening test must be highly sensitive (i.e., detect nearly all children with problems) and reasonably specific (i.e., not mislabel). It must also be relatively quick to administer and inexpensive. As with any screening test, a failed developmental screen implies the need for more conclusive "gold standard" evaluation. Finally, a prerequisite of any screening program is that an effective intervention be available. Early intervention

(EI) services for children with documented developmental delays are available free to families through a combination of state and federal funds. The benefits of EI services for children with a variety of disabilities has been well documented.

Screening tests can be categorized as general screening tests that cover all behavioral domains or as targeted screens that focus on one area of development. They can be administered in the office setting by professionals or completed at home by parents.

The **Denver Developmental Screening Test II** (Figs. 1–12 and 1–13) assesses the development of children from birth to 6 years in four domains: (1) personal-social, (2) fine motor–adaptive, (3) language, and (4) gross motor. Its items were carefully selected for their reliability and consistency of norms across subgroups. The Denver II is useful as a screening instrument, but it cannot adequately assess the complexities of socioemotional development. In addition, the criteria for passing are set low to minimize labeling normal children as abnormal; this may result in a failure to identify children with mild but significant developmental problems. Children with "suspect" or "questionable" scores therefore must be followed carefully.

An abbreviated Denver screen has been validated using only 12 items per subject (the three items in each category falling immediately to the left of, but not touching, the age line). This abbreviated test is helpful in busy clinical settings. A two-stage screening procedure can be used in which the abbreviated screen is used with every child, and a full Denver screen is used only with those who have suspect or abnormal scores. Another adaptation of this screen is a parental questionnaire using 97 of the original DDST items (this is the Prescreening Developmental Questionnaire, or PDQ). There was a high agreement rate between parent responses and the full Denver Screening Test scores in a largely middle-class sample. The **Clinical Linguistic and Auditory Milestone Scale and Clinical Adaptive Tests (CALMS/CAT)** can be administered quickly. They correlate well with "gold standard" tests for language delay and mental retardation.

Other parent-completed measures include the **Ages and Stages Questionnaires** and **Child Development Inventories**. Parent report screens have good validity when compared with office-based measures. They may have the added benefit of promoting parental involvement with the child's development.

Speech and Language Screening. Language screening is important because it correlates best with cognitive development in the early years. Table 1–6 provides some rules of thumb for language development that focus on speech production (expressive language). Receptive language is not assessed by these rules and only incompletely assessed by the

TABLE 1–6
Rules of Thumb for Speech Screening

Age (Yr)	Speech Production	Articulation (Amount of Speech Understood by a Stranger)	Following Commands
1	1–3 words		One-step commands
2	2- to 3-word phrases	½	Two-step commands
3	Routine use of sentences	¾	
4	Routine use of sentence sequences; conversational give-and-take	Almost all	
5	Complex sentences; extensive use of modifiers, pronouns, and prepositions	Almost all	

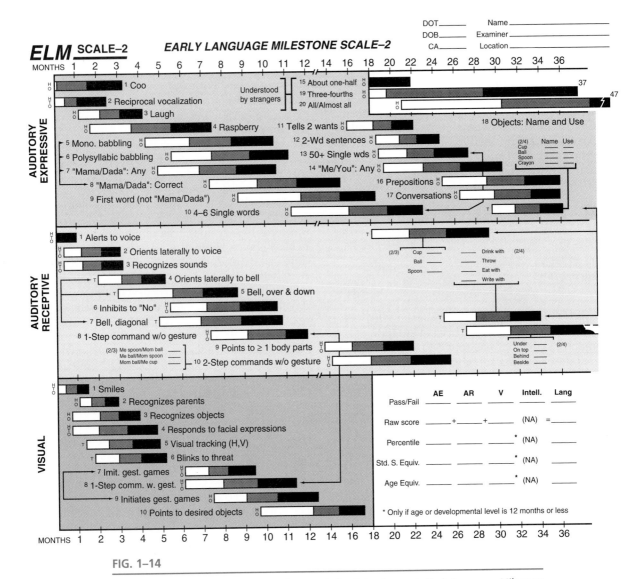

FIG. 1–14

Early language milestone scales for auditory and visual development. (Early Language Milestone Scale—2 [ELM Scale—2]: A language screening instrument that covers auditory expressive, auditory receptive, and visual language development from birth to 36 mo, and intelligibility of speech up to 4 yr of age, Austin, Tex, PRO-ED, 1987. Copyright 1983, 1993 by James Coplan, M.D.)

TABLE 1–7
Conditions Considered High Risk for Associated Hearing Deficit

Congenital hearing loss in first cousin or closer relative

Bilirubin level of 20 mg/dL or above

Congenital rubella or other nonbacterial intrauterine infection

Defects in the ear, nose, or throat

Birth weight of 1500 g or less

Multiple apneic episodes

Exchange transfusion

Meningitis

5-min Apgar score of 5 or less

Persistent fetal circulation (primary pulmonary hypertension)

Treatment with ototoxic drugs (e.g., aminoglycosides and loop diuretics)

Denver II. Although expressive language (speech) is the most obvious language element, the most dramatic changes in language development in the first years involve recognition and understanding (receptive language). Also, much language up to the age of 2 years is visually mediated (e.g., pointing). Thus language screening deserves focused attention. One useful tool is the Early Language Milestone (ELM) Scale (Fig. 1–14), which screens visual and auditory receptive and expressive skills.

Whenever there is a language delay, a hearing deficit must be considered (see Hearing Impairment). Conditions that present a high risk for an associated hearing deficit are listed in Table 1–7. Early clues that indicate a need for audiologic and speech evaluation are listed in Table 1–8.

Dysfluency ("stuttering") is quite common in 3- and 4-year-olds. Unless the dysfluency is severe, is accompanied by tics or unusual posturing, or occurs after the age of 4 years, parents should be counseled that it is normal and to accept it calmly

TABLE 1–8
Clues to When a Child with a Communication Disorder Needs Help

0-11 Months

Before 6 months, the child does not startle, blink, or change immediate activity in response to sudden, loud sounds.

Before 6 months, the child does not attend to the human voice and is not soothed by his or her mother's voice.

By 6 months, the child does not babble strings of consonant + vowel syllables or imitate gurgling or cooing sounds.

By 10 months, the child does not respond to his or her name.

At 10 months, the child's sound-making is limited to shrieks, grunts, or sustained vowel production.

12–23 Months

At 12 months, the child's babbling or speech is limited to vowel sounds.

By 15 months, the child does not respond to "no," "bye-bye," or "bottle."

By 15 months, the child will not imitate sounds or words.

By 18 months, the child is not consistently using at least six words with appropriate meaning.

By 21 months, the child does not respond correctly to "Give me . . .," "Sit down," or "Come here" when spoken without gestural cues.

12–23 Months—cont'd

By 23 months, two-word phrases have not emerged that are spoken as single units ("Whatszit," "Thank you," "Allgone").

24–36 Months

By 24 months, at least 50% of the child's speech is not understood by familiar listeners.

By 24 months, the child does not point to body parts without gestural cues.

By 24 months, the child is not combining words into phrases ("Go bye-bye," "Go car," "Want cookie").

By 30 months, the child does not demonstrate understanding of on, in, under, front, and back.

By 30 months, the child is not using short sentences ("Daddy went bye-bye.").

By 30 months, the child has not begun to ask questions, using where, what, why.

By 36 months, the child's speech is not understood by unfamiliar listeners.

All Ages

At any age, the child is consistently dysfluent with repetitions, hesitations; blocks or struggles to say words. Struggle may be accompanied by grimaces, eye blinks, or hand gestures.

Adapted from Weiss CE, Lillywhite HE: *Communication disorders: a handbook for prevention and early detection,* St Louis, 1976, Mosby.

and patiently. Comments such as "relax," "slow down," or "think before you speak" may be counterproductive for a child who already may be too anxious about a behavior over which he or she has little control.

Temperament Questionnaires. The **Carey Infant Temperament Questionnaire** is widely used to assess temperament in 4- to 8-month-olds. Questionnaires for assessing behavioral style at older ages are also available and can be very helpful in tailoring anticipatory guidance about behavioral issues or management plans for behavioral problems to the individual characteristics of the child. Examples include the **Pediatric Symptom Checklist** and the "trigger questions" that function as informal screens for developmental and behavioral adjustment in **Bright Futures: Guidelines for Health Supervision of Infants, Children, and Adolescents.**

More Extensive Assessment Instruments. Some pediatricians develop expertise in more extensive assessment instruments, including the Brazelton Neonatal Behavioral Assessment Scale, the Pediatric Examination of Educational Readiness, and the Pediatric Early Elementary Examination. These assessments require training for expertise in administration and interpretation.

REFERENCES

Behrman RE, Kliegman RM, Jenson HB, editors: *Nelson textbook of pediatrics*, ed 16, Philadelphia, 2000, WB Saunders, Chapter 607.
Levine MD, Carey WB, Crocker AC, editors: *Developmental-behavioral pediatrics*, ed 3, Philadelphia, 1999, WB Saunders.

Team Assessment of Complex Problems

When the results of screening efforts suggest the presence of significant developmental lags, the pediatrician should take responsibility for coordinating the further assessment of the child that is indicated and providing the continuity in the relationship that has developed with the child and family. The physician should become aware of the facilities and programs for assessment and treatment in his or her area. If the child was considered to be at high risk because of prematurity or another identified illness that might have long-term developmental impact, a structured follow-up program to monitor the child's progress may already exist. Federal laws mandate that special education programs be provided for all children with developmental disabilities from birth through 21 years of age.

Medical Assessment

The physician's main goals in team assessment are to identify the cause of the developmental dysfunction and identify and interpret other medical conditions that have a developmental impact. The comprehensive history (Table 1–9) and physical examination (Table 1–10) should include a careful graphing of growth parameters and an accurate description of dysmorphic features (see Chapter 4).

Motor Assessment

Although the traditional neurologic examination provides an excellent basis for evaluating motor function, it should be supplemented by an adaptive

---

TABLE 1–9
Information to Be Sought During the History Taking of a Child with Suspected Developmental Disabilities

Item	Possible Significance
Parental Concerns	Parents are quite accurate in identifying developmental problems in their children.
Current Levels of Developmental Functioning	Should be used to monitor child's progress
Temperament	May interact with disability or may be confused with developmental delay
Prenatal History	
Alcohol ingestion	Fetal alcohol syndrome; an index of care-taking risk
Exposure to medication, illegal drug, or toxin	Developmental toxin (e.g., phenytoin); may be an index of care-taking risk
Radiation exposure	Damage to central nervous system (CNS)
Nutrition	Inadequate fetal nutrition

TABLE 1–9

Information to Be Sought During the History Taking of a Child with Suspected Developmental Disabilities—cont'd

Item	Possible Significance
Prenatal History—cont'd	
Prenatal care	Index of social situation
Injuries, hyperthermia	Damage to CNS
Smoking	Possible CNS damage
Human immunodeficiency virus (HIV) exposure	Congenital HIV infection
Maternal phenylketonuria (PKU)	Maternal PKU effect
Maternal illness	Toxoplasmosis, rubella, cytomegalovirus, herpesvirus infections
Perinatal History	
Gestational age, birth weight	Biologic risk from prematurity and small for gestational age
Labor and delivery	Hypoxia or index of abnormal prenatal development
Apgar scores	Hypoxia, cardiovascular impairment
Specific perinatal adverse events	Increased risk for CNS damage
Neonatal History	
Illness—seizures, respiratory distress, hyperbilirubinemia, metabolic disorder	Increased risk for CNS damage
Malformations	May represent syndrome associated with developmental delay
Family History	
Consanguinity	Autosomal recessive condition more likely
Mental functioning	Increased hereditary and environmental risks
Illnesses (e.g., metabolic disease)	Hereditary illness associated with developmental delay
Family member died young or unexpectedly	May suggest inborn error of metabolism or storage disease
Family member requires special education	Hereditary causes of developmental delay
Social History	
Resources available (e.g., financial, social support)	Necessary to maximize child's potential
Educational level of parents	Family may need help to provide stimulation
Mental health problems	May exacerbate child's conditions
High-risk behaviors (e.g., illicit drugs, sex)	Increased risk for HIV infection; index of care-taking risk
Other stressors (e.g., marital discord)	May exacerbate child's conditions or compromise care
Other History	
Gender of child	Important for X-linked conditions
Developmental milestones	Index of developmental delay; regression may indicate progressive condition
Head injury	Even moderate trauma may be associated with developmental delay or learning disabilities
Serious infections (e.g., meningitis)	May be associated with developmental delay
Toxic exposure (e.g., lead)	May be associated with developmental delay
Physical growth	May indicate malnutrition; obesity, short stature associated with some conditions
Recurrent otitis media	Associated with hearing loss and abnormal speech development
Visual and auditory functioning	Sensitive index of impairments in vision and hearing
Nutrition	Malnutrition during infancy may lead to delayed development
Chronic conditions such as renal disease	May be associated with delayed or anemia development

From Liptak G: Mental retardation and developmental disability. In Kliegman RM, editor: *Practical strategies in pediatric diagnosis and therapy,* Philadelphia, 1996, WB Saunders.

TABLE 1–10
Information to Be Sought During the Physical Examination of a Child with Suspected Developmental Disabilities

Item	Possible Significance
General Appearance	May indicate significant delay in development or obvious syndrome
Stature	
Short stature	Williams syndrome, malnutrition, Turner syndrome; many children with severe retardation have short stature
Obesity	Prader-Willi syndrome
Large stature	Sotos syndrome
Head	
Macrocephaly	Alexander syndrome, Sotos syndrome, gangliosidosis, hydrocephalus, mucopolysaccharidosis, subdural effusion
Microcephaly	Virtually any condition that can retard brain growth (e.g., malnutrition, Angelman syndrome, de Lange syndrome, fetal alcohol effects)
Face	
Coarse, triangular, round, or flat face; hypo- or hypertelorism, slanted or short palpebral fissure; unusual nose, maxilla, and mandible	Specific measurements may provide clues to inherited, metabolic, or other diseases such as fetal alcohol syndrome, cri du chat (5p-syndrome), or Williams syndrome
Eyes	
Prominent	Crouzon syndrome, Seckel syndrome, fragile X
Cataract	Galactosemia, Lowe syndrome, prenatal rubella, hypothyroidism
Cherry-red spot in macula	Gangliosidosis (GM1), metachromatic leukodystrophy, mucolipidosis, Tay-Sachs disease, Niemann-Pick disease, Farber lipogranulomatosis, sialidosis III
Chorioretinitis	Congenital infection with cytomegalovirus, toxoplasmosis, or rubella
Corneal cloudiness	Mucopolysaccharidosis I and II, Lowe syndrome, congenital syphilis
Ears	
Pinnae, low set or malformed	Trisomies such as 18, Rubinstein-Taybi syndrome, Down syndrome, CHARGE association, cerebro-oculo-facial-skeletal syndrome, fetal phenytoin effects
Hearing	Loss of acuity in mucopolysaccharidosis; hyperacusis in many encephalopathies
Heart	
Structural anomaly or hypertrophy	CHARGE association, CATCH-22, velo-cardio-facial syndrome, glycogenosis II, fetal alcohol effects, mucopolysaccharidosis I; chromosomal anomalies like Down syndrome; maternal PKU; chronic cyanosis may impair cognitive development

TABLE 1–10
Information to Be Sought During the Physical Examination of a Child with Suspected Developmental Disabilities—cont'd

Item	Possible Significance
Liver	
Hepatomegaly	Fructose intolerance, galactosemia glycogenosis types I–IV, mucopolysaccharidosis I and II, Niemann-Pick disease, Tay-Sachs disease, Zellweger syndrome, Gaucher disease, ceroid lipofuscinosis, gangliosidosis
Genitalia	
Macroorchidism	Fragile X syndrome
Hypogenitalism	Prader-Willi syndrome, Klinefelter syndrome, CHARGE association
Extremities	
Hands, feet, dermatoglyphics, and creases	May indicate specific entity like Rubinstein-Taybi syndrome or be associated with chromosomal anomaly
Joint contractures	Sign of muscle imbalance around joints—e.g., with meningomyelocele, cerebral palsy, arthrogryposis, muscular dystrophy; also occurs with cartilaginous problems such as mucopolysaccharidosis
Skin	
Café au lait spots	Neurofibromatosis, tuberous sclerosis, Bloom syndrome
Eczema	Phenylketonuria, histiocytosis
Hemangiomas and telangiectasia	Sturge-Weber syndrome, Bloom syndrome, ataxia-telangiectasia
Hypopigmented macules, streaks, adenoma sebaceum	Tuberous sclerosis, hypomelanosis of Ito
Hair	
Hirsutism	De Lange syndrome, mucopolysaccharidosis, fetal phenytoin effects, cerebro-oculo-facial-skeletal syndrome, trisomy 18
Neurologic	
Asymmetry of strength and tone	Focal lesion, cerebral palsy
Hypotonia	Prader-Willi syndrome, Down syndrome, Angelman syndrome, gangliosidosis, early cerebral palsy
Hypertonia	Neurodegenerative conditions involving white matter, cerebral palsy, trisomy 18
Ataxia	Ataxia-telangiectasia, metachromatic leukodystrophy, Angelman syndrome

From Liptak G: Mental retardation and developmental disability. In Kliegman RM, editor: *Practical strategies in pediatric diagnosis and therapy*, Philadelphia, 1996, WB Saunders.
CHARGE, Coloboma, *h*eart defects, *a*tresia choanae, *r*etarded growth, *g*enital anomalies, *e*ar anomalies (deafness); *CATCH-22*, cardiac defects, *a*bnormal face, *t*hymic hypoplasia, *c*left palate, *h*ypocalcemia-defects on chromosome No. 22; *PKU*, phenylketonuria.

functional evaluation. Watching the child at play can aid in such assessment. In addition, standardized tools for evaluating gross and fine motor abilities are used by physical and occupational therapists to estimate age-appropriate functional levels.

Psychologic Assessment

Psychologic assessment includes the testing of cognitive ability (Table 1–11) and the evaluation of personality and emotional well-being by a skilled evaluator. The intelligence quotient (IQ) and mental age scores, taken in isolation, are only partially descriptive of a person's functional abilities, which are a combination of cognitive, adaptive, and social skills. Tests of achievement are subject to variability based on experience and must be standardized for social factors. Projective and nonprojective tests are useful in understanding the child's emotional status. Although a child should not be labeled as having a problem solely on the basis of a standardized test, such tests do provide important and reasonably objective data for evaluating a child's growth within a particular educational program.

TABLE 1–11
Tests of Cognition

Test	Age Range	Special Features
Infant Scales		
Bayley Scales of Infant Development (ed 2)	2–42 mo	Mental, psychomotor scales, behavior record; weak intelligence predictor
Cattell Infant Intelligence Scale	Birth–30 mo	Used to extend Stanford-Binet downward
Gesell Developmental Schedules	Birth–3 yr	Used by many pediatricians
Ordinal Scales of Infant Psychological Development	Birth–24 mo	Six subscales; based on Piaget's stages; weak in predicting later intelligence
Preschool Scales		
Stanford-Binet Intelligence Scale (ed 4)	2 yr–adult	Four area scores, with subtests and composite IQ score
McCarthy Scales of Children's Abilities	2½–8 yr	6–18 subtests; good at defining learning disabilities; strengths/weaknesses approach
Wechsler Primary and Preschool Test of Intelligence—Revised (WPPSI-R)	3–6½ yr	11 subtests; verbal, performance IQs; long administration time; good at defining learning disabilities
Merrill-Palmer Scale of Mental Tests	2–4½ yr	General test for young children
Differential Abilities Scale	2½ yr–adult	Special nonverbal composite; short administration time
School-Age Scales		
Stanford-Binet Intelligence Scale (ed 4)	2 yr–adult	See above
Wechsler Intelligence Scale for Children (ed 3) (WISC III)	6–16 yr	See comments on WPPSI-R
Leiter International Performance Scale	2 yr–adult	No verbal abilities needed
Wechsler Adult Intelligence Scale—Revised (WAIS-R)	16 yr–adult	See comments on WPPSI-R
Differential Abilities Scale	2½ yr–adult	See above
Adaptive Behavior Scales		
Vineland Adaptive Behavior Scale	Birth–adult	Interview/questionnaire; typical persons and blind, deaf, and retarded
American Association on Mental Retardation (AAMR) Adaptive Behavioral Scale	3 yr–adult	Useful in retardation, other disabilities

IQ, Intelligence quotient.

Educational Assessment

The educational assessment involves the evaluation of areas of specific strengths and weaknesses in reading, spelling, written expression, and mathematical skills. Schools routinely screen children with group tests to aid in problem identification and program evaluation. For the child with special needs, this should ultimately lead to individualized testing and the development of an individualized educational plan (IEP) that will enable the child to progress comfortably in school. Diagnostic teaching, in which the child's response to various teaching techniques is assessed, may also be helpful.

Social Environment Assessment

Assessment of the environment in which the child is living, working, playing, and growing is also important in understanding the child's development. A home visit by a social worker, community health nurse, or home-based intervention specialist can provide valuable information about the child's social milieu.

REFERENCES

Behrman RE, Kliegman RM, Jenson HB, editors: *Nelson textbook of pediatrics,* ed 16, Philadelphia, 2000, WB Saunders, Chapters 16, 29.

Coplan J: Normal speech and language development: an overview, *Pediatr Rev* 16(3):91–100, 1995.

McInerny TK: Children who have difficulty in school: a primary pediatrician's approach, *Pediatr Rev* 16(9):325–332, 1995.

Newton R, Wraith J: Investigation of developmental delay, *Arch Dis Child* 72(5):460–465, 1995.

MANAGEMENT OF DEVELOPMENTAL AND BEHAVIORAL PROBLEMS
Intervention in the Primary Care Setting

After assessment, the clinician must decide whether a problem requires referral for further diagnostic workup and management or whether management in the primary care setting is appropriate. Some of the counseling roles required in caring for these children are listed in Table 1–12 and discussed in the following paragraphs. In this context the word "patient" refers to the child, the parent, or both. When a child is young, much of the counseling interaction takes place between the parents and the clinician; as the child matures, direct counseling shifts increasingly toward the child.

The assessment process (particularly that of expanded history and observations) may be therapeutic in itself. By assuming the role of a nonjudgmental, supportive listener, the clinician creates a climate of trust in which the patient feels free to express difficult or even painful thoughts and feelings. Ventilation of these feelings alone may be helpful; in addition, it may free the patient from a preoccupation with previously unexpressed emotions, allowing the patient to move on to the work of understanding and resolving the problem.

Interview techniques also may facilitate clarification of the problem for the patient, as well as for the clinician. The patient's ideas about the causes of the problem and descriptions of attempts to deal with it can provide a basis for developing strategies for problem management that are much more likely to be implemented because they emanate in part from the patient. Furthermore, the clinician shows respect by endorsing the patient's ideas when appropriate; this can increase the patient's self-esteem and sense of competency. Providing reassurance appropriate to the patient's concern is potentially of great additional benefit, but giving reassurance too hastily and nonspecifically may suggest a lack of regard for the patient.

Educating parents about normal and aberrant development and behavior may prevent problems through early detection and anticipatory guidance. Such education also communicates the physician's interest in hearing parental concerns. Early detection is important because intervention can be started before the problem becomes entrenched and associated problems develop.

Many parents expect and need specific, detailed parenting advice from the clinician. Other parents will work out the details if the clinician first provides some general principles and guidelines. When the parents and child play a relatively passive role in the development of the plan, it is particularly important to give them a written copy of the plan to review, to be certain that the details are fully understood. Specific suggestions for changes in the family environment often are very useful.

TABLE 1–12
Primary Care Counseling Roles
Allow ventilation
Facilitate clarification
Support patient problem solving
Provide specific reassurance
Provide education
Provide specific parenting advice
Suggest environmental interventions
Provide follow-up
Facilitate appropriate referrals
Coordinate care and interpret reports after referrals

One helpful suggestion is to arrange for respite and increased emotional support for the primary caregiver, who usually is discouraged and exhausted by the time the clinician hears about the problem. The clinician also may suggest other community services to relieve pressure and to improve the coping ability of the family (e.g., nursery school, tutors, recreational programs, and parent support and education groups).

The severity of developmental and behavioral problems ranges from variations of normal, to understandable but problematic responses to stressful situations, to frank disorders (e.g., late onset of toilet training, to resumption of wetting in response to birth of a sibling, to diabetes-induced enuresis). The clinician must try to establish the severity and scope of the patient's symptoms so that appropriate intervention can be planned. The DSM-PC, pediatric version, provides useful information on spectra of conditions that can present in similar ways.

Most developmental and behavioral problems appear simple when initially presented, and often a small amount of education and reassurance and a few simple suggestions are sufficient. Follow-up is crucial, because complex problems often present as simple problems. Clinicians must be ready to accept failure of their suggestions without attributing the failure to inadequacy in the parents' application of the recommendations. Indications for referral to developmental disability or mental health specialists will vary according to the expertise of the primary care clinician, but children should not be followed for long periods in the hope that they will "outgrow" the problem. After referral, the clinician is needed to help coordinate and interpret the evaluations and recommendations.

Counseling Principles

Behavioral change must be learned, not imposed. It is easiest to learn when the lesson is simple, clear, and consistent and presented in an atmosphere free of fear or intimidation. Parents often try to impose behavioral change in an emotionally charged atmosphere. Clinicians often try to "teach" parents with hastily presented advice when the parents are distracted by other concerns. The teacher (parent or clinician) must also remember that patient repetition is the basis of learning.

Apart from management strategies directed specifically at the problem behavior, regular times for *positive parent-child interaction* should be instituted. Frequent, brief, affectionate physical contact over the day provides opportunities for positive reinforcement of desirable child behaviors and for building a sense of competence in the child and the parent. The parent should be reminded to "catch the child being good" and to criticize the child's *behavior* rather than the child.

Guilt is felt by almost all parents when their children have a developmental-behavioral problem. This may be caused by the assumption or fear that the problem was caused by inadequate parenting, or guilt about previous angry responses to the child's behavior (e.g., excessive physical punishment or derogatory comments). The clinician should not unwittingly contribute to parental guilt with insensitive comments that may be construed as criticism by the parents. The clinician should, if possible and appropriate, find ways to alleviate guilt. Guilt may be a serious impediment to problem solving. The clinician can diffuse this guilt by honestly pointing out how often other parents have similar problems and by empathizing with the difficulties of coping with the problem.

It is usually beneficial to find ways to increase support for the primary caregiver. A mother is better able to nurture a child well when she is well nurtured herself.

The clinician must be careful of using developmental or behavioral labels, even though they may be helpful in diagnosis and management. These labels can become self-fulfilling prophecies as the people in the child's environment treat the child as "difficult," which becomes part of the child's self-concept.

Interdisciplinary Team Intervention

In many cases a team of professionals is required to provide the breadth and quality of services needed to serve the child who has developmental problems appropriately. This is commonly the case, for example, in follow-up programs for infants leaving intensive care nurseries. Although early intervention programs are now mandated across the United States, the physician may play a key role in guiding the child and family to these services. Once the child reaches school age, the public school system takes increasing responsibility for developmental and educational services, and the physician's role becomes primarily one of consultation on medically related issues.

Educational intervention for the young child begins as home-based infant stimulation, often with an early childhood educator, nurse, or occupational, speech, or physical therapist providing direct stimulation for the child and training the family to provide the stimulation. As the child matures, a center-based nursery program may be indicated. For the school-aged child, special services may range from extra attention given by the classroom teacher to a self-contained special education classroom. Home-based tutoring or residential programs typically are reserved for only the most behaviorally or cognitively impaired children in this age range.

Psychologic intervention may take several forms. Therapy may be parent or family directed or may become, with the older child, purely child directed. Examples of therapeutic approaches are guidance therapies such as directive advice-giving, counseling the family and child in their own solutions to problems, psychotherapy, behavior management techniques, psychopharmacologic methods, and cognitive therapy.

Motor intervention may be performed by a physical or occupational therapist or by another professional under the therapist's direction. Neurodevelopmental therapy (NDT), the most commonly used method, is based on the concept that nervous system development is hierarchical and subject to some plasticity. The focus of NDT is on gait training and motor development, including daily living skills and perceptual abilities such as eye-hand coordination, spatial relationships, and motor sequencing that help guide motor activity. Sensory integration therapy is sometimes used by occupational therapists to structure sensory experience from the tactile, proprioceptive, and vestibular systems to allow for adaptive motor responses.

Speech and language intervention by the speech therapist is usually part of the overall educational program and is based on the tested language strengths and weaknesses of the child. Children needing this type of intervention may demonstrate difficulties in reading and other academic areas and develop social and behavioral problems because of their difficulties in being understood and in understanding others.

Hearing intervention, performed by the audiologist and otolaryngologist, includes monitoring hearing acuity, providing amplification when necessary via hearing aids, and treating ear infections.

Social and environmental intervention generally takes the form of nursing or social work involvement with the family. Frequently the task of coordinating the services of other disciplines falls to these specialists.

Medical intervention for the child with a developmental disability involves providing primary care and specific treatment of conditions associated with disability. Although curative treatment often is not possible because of the irreversible nature of many disabling conditions, functional impairment can be minimized through thoughtful medical management. Certain general medical problems are found more frequently in the mentally retarded and developmentally disabled population (Table 1–13).

TABLE 1–13
Recurring Medical Issues in Children with Developmental Disabilities

Problem	Ask About or Check
Motor	Range of motion examination; scoliosis check; assessment of mobility; interaction with orthopedist, physiatrist, and PT/OT as needed
Diet	Dietary history, feeding observation, growth parameter measurement and charting, supplementation as indicated by observations
Sensory impairments	Functional vision and hearing screening; interaction as needed with audiologist, ophthalmologist
Dermatology	Examination of *all* skin areas for decubitus ulcers or infection
Dentistry	Examination of teeth and gums; confirmation of access to dental care
Behavioral problems	Aggression, self-injury, pica; sleep problems; psychotropic drug levels and side effects
Advocacy	Educational program, family supports, financial supports
Seizures	Major motor, absence, other suspicious symptoms; monitoring of anticonvulsant levels and side effects
Infectious diseases	Ear infections, diarrhea, respiratory symptoms, aspiration pneumonia, immunizations (especially hepatitis B and influenza)
Constipation (GI problems)	Constipation, gastroesophageal reflux, GI bleeding (stool for occult blood)
Sexuality	Sexuality education, hygiene, contraception (when appropriate), genetic counseling
Other syndrome-specific problems	Ongoing evaluation of other "physical" problems as indicated by known MR/DD etiology

GI, Gastrointestinal; *MR/DD,* mental retardation/developmental disability; *PT/OT,* physical therapist/occupational therapist.

REFERENCES

Behrman RE, Kliegman RM, Jenson HB, editors: *Nelson textbook of pediatrics*, ed 16, Philadelphia, 2000, WB Saunders, Chapters 16, 29.

Levine MD, Carey WB, Crocker AC, editors: *Developmental-behavioral pediatrics*, ed 3, Philadelphia, 1999, WB Saunders.

Liptak GS: The pediatrician's role in caring for the developmentally disabled child, *Pediatr Rev* 17(6):203–210, 1996.

Sulkes SB: MD's DD basics: identifying common problems and preventing secondary disabilities, *Pediatr Ann* 24(5):245–248, 1995.

Wolraich MI, Felice ME, Drotar D, editors: *The classification of child and adolescent mental diagnoses in primary care. Diagnostic and statistical manual for primary care (DSM-PC), child and adolescent version*, Elk Grove Village, Ill, 1996, American Academy of Pediatrics.

Crying

The compelling sound of an infant's cry makes it an effective distress signal and appropriate to the human infant's prolonged dependence on a caregiver. However, cries are discomforting and may be alarming to parents, many of whom find it very difficult to listen to their infant's crying for even short periods of time.

Many reasons for crying are obvious, such as hunger and discomfort caused by heat, cold, illness, and a lying position. However, these reasons account for a relatively small percentage of infant crying episodes and usually are recognized quickly and alleviated. In the absence of a discernible reason for the behavior, crying often stops when the infant is held. In most infants, there are frequent episodes of crying with no apparent cause, and holding or other soothing techniques seem ineffective. Infants cry and fuss for a mean of 1¾ hours per day at the age 2 weeks, 2¾ hours per day at the age of 6 weeks, and 1 hour per day at the age of 12 weeks. Counseling about normal crying may relieve guilt and diminish concerns, but for some parents the distress caused by the crying cannot be suppressed by logical reasoning. For these parents, respite from exposure to the crying may be necessary to allow them to cope appropriately with their own distress. Without relief, fatigue and tension may result in an inappropriate parental response such as leaving the infant in the house alone or abusing the infant.

Acute crying that persists for more than 2 hours and is not relieved by holding may be the result of serious medical conditions (e.g., surgical abdomen, infections, trauma-abuse, and testicular torsion), hair tourniquets, corneal abrasion, intussusception, or reactions to drugs or vaccines. Infants with these symptoms require prompt medical attention.

Colic

Colic is characterized by periods of unexplained paroxysmal bouts of crying lasting more than 3 hours per day, for more than 3 days per week, for more than 3 weeks in a healthy, well-fed infants. The crying may be intense, and it may be brief or last for hours. The episodes typically recur in the late afternoon or evening but may occur at any time. The onset is usually in the first 2–3 weeks with resolution by 3 months, although it sometimes lasts much longer. Colic occurs in 16–26% of infants. Its etiology, although unknown, is probably multifactorial, with the infant, the parent, and environmental factors playing potentially important roles.

Management begins with sympathetic listening to the parents' frustration and concern, which should not be quickly dismissed with vague reassurance that lots of crying is to be expected. Education about normal crying patterns, specific reassurance about health concerns, suggestions about techniques for consoling the infant, and recommendations for increased support and respite for the primary caregiver often are helpful. The clinician should also underscore to parents that colic is a self-limited condition and that symptoms usually resolve by 3 months of age.

The most effective and appropriate intervention for a crying episode is to pick up and soothe the infant. Greater maternal responsiveness to cries in the first 3 months is associated with decreased crying and increased use of other forms of communication by the infant later in the first year. However, this is impractical for some parents, particularly if the infant must be carried virtually all the time to control crying. Also, when a crying infant does not respond to holding, prolonged attempts to soothe the infant may be counterproductive, serving only to increase parental fatigue and guilt. The interactions may become tense, abrupt, and even hostile, with resulting escalation of the infant's irritability. To optimize parents' ability to be sensitive and responsive to their infants, parents need to be well rested and have some time for themselves.

The clinician should discuss with parents the amount and quality of stimulation a colicky infant is exposed to during the day. Some infants exposed to chaotic environments do better in quieter settings. Other techniques that may work are burping, gentle motion (e.g., automatic rockers or stroller or car rides), continuous monotonous noise or music (e.g., a mechanical alarm clock or radio), a pacifier, or a warm water bottle next to the abdomen. Naturopathic interventions have not been well studied. Although only a small percentage of colic cases may be caused by food intolerance, the practice of changing formulas remains popular because it allows time for the colic to resolve on its own. Hypoallergenic formula is superior to soy formula for truly allergic infants. Sedatives may be indicated for a limited time to break the cycle of crying and loss of sleep when the family can no longer cope with the problem; choices include diphenhydramine (1 mg/kg) 1 hour before the worst period of crying each day (or before the parents' bedtime) for 1–2 weeks. An often effective alternative is to encourage the parents to arrange for a weekend away from the infant.

REFERENCES

Behrman RE, Kliegman RM, Jenson HB, editors: *Nelson textbook of pediatrics*, ed 16, Philadelphia, 2000, WB Saunders, Chapter 41.
Garrison MM, Christakis DA: A systematic review of treatments for infant colic, *Pediatrics* 106(1 pt 2):184–190, 2000.
Fleisher DR: Coping with colic, *Contemp Pediatr* 15(6):144–156, 1998.

Discipline

Discipline involves teaching, not merely punishment. The ultimate goal is the child's self-control. Overbearing punishment to control a child's behavior will interfere with the learning process and focus on external control at the expense of the development of self-control.

Commonly used and effective techniques to control undesirable behavior in children include scolding, physical punishment, and threats. However, these techniques have potential adverse effects on children's sense of security and self-esteem. The effectiveness of scolding diminishes the more it is used, and it should not be allowed to expand from an expression of displeasure about a specific event to derogatory statements about children that may be interpreted as loss of love for them. Scolding also may escalate to the level of psychologic abuse. Frequent mild physical punishment also may become less effective and tempt the parent to escalate the physical punishment, increasing the risk of child abuse. Threats by parents to leave or give up the child are perhaps the most powerful and psychologically damaging ways to control a child's behavior. Children of any age may remain fearful and anxious about loss of the parent long after the threat is made. A common alternative technique is positive reinforcement for desirable behavior. This reinforcement is a powerful tool for molding a child's behavior, particularly when it is given immediately after the behavior occurs. It fosters self-control and self-esteem.

Parenting involves a dynamic balance between *setting limits* on the one hand and allowing and encouraging freedom of expression and exploration on the other. Children whose behavior is out of control improve when clear limits on their behavior are set and enforced. In general, children find comfort and security in clear limits. However, parents must agree on where the limit will be set and how it will be enforced. The limit and the consequence of breaking the limit must be clearly presented to the child. Enforcement of the limit should be consistent and firm. Too many limits will be hard to learn and may thwart the normal development of autonomy. The limit must be reasonable in terms of the child's age, temperament, and developmental level.

Extinction is a systematic way to eliminate a frequent, annoying, and relatively harmless behavior by ignoring it. First, parents record the frequency of the behavior in the baseline phase in order to appreciate realistically the magnitude of the problem and to evaluate progress in eliminating the problem. To determine what reinforces the behavior (and therefore what needs to be consistently eliminated), it is essential to record the consequences of the behavior before any changes are made in the parental response or in other environmental factors. An appropriate behavior is identified to give the child a positive alternative that the parents can reinforce. Parents should be warned that the annoying behavior usually increases in frequency and intensity (and may last for weeks) before it decreases when the parent ignores it (removes the reinforcement).

The *time-out procedure* is another quite useful technique to modify inappropriate behavior that cannot be ignored. The procedure consists of a short period of isolation that interrupts the behavior and requires considerable effort by the parents initially. A simple isolation technique, such as making a child stand in the corner or sending a child to his or her room, may be effective. If such a technique is not helpful, a more systematic procedure may be needed. For example, one very effective protocol for the time-out procedure involves interrupting the child's play when the behavior occurs and having the child sit in a dull, isolated place for a brief period, measured by a portable kitchen timer. This inescapable and unpleasant consequence of the undesired behavior motivates the child to learn to avoid the behavior. If used matter-of-factly and with a minimum of expressed anger by the parent, such a time-out procedure is a potent teaching tool with less chance for adverse side effects than other commonly used discipline techniques. Parents often report that they have tried limit-setting, extinction, and time-out, but that the child responds angrily when parents impose their wills. The child's foreseeable frustration can be minimized if the parents are prepared to *redirect* the child to more acceptable activities and then follow up with attention and other rewards.

REFERENCES

Berhman RE, Kliegman RM, Jenson HB, editors: *Nelson textbook of pediatrics*, ed 16, Philadelphia, 2000, WB Saunders, Chapter 5.
Parrish JM: Child behavior management. In Levine MD, Carey WB, Crocker AC, editors: *Developmental-behavioral pediatrics*, ed 3, Philadelphia, 1999, WB Saunders.

Toilet Training

Toilet training involves the child's mastery of bowel and urinary control while the child is awake and asleep. The ages at which these tasks are mastered vary widely in different cultures, as well as within cultures (see Enuresis and Encopresis). The decision about when to start toilet training should be based on the following readiness signals: dry periods lasting several hours; interest in the potty chair; desire to be changed when wet or dirty; and ability to carry out a series of simple commands. Some general principles about approaching toilet training are as follows:

1. Anger or punishment for lack of performance on the potty chair or for accidents off the potty chair is usually counterproductive and inappropriate.
2. When the child resists sitting on the potty chair, allow her or him to get up and try again after a meal.
3. If resistance is persistent, postpone training for at least several weeks.
4. Power struggles should be avoided. The result may be stool retention, chronic constipation, encopresis, or strained parent-child relations. It is almost impossible to win a battle of wills with a toddler, and imposing the will of the adult may interfere with the child's developing autonomy and increase feelings of shame and doubt.
5. A key to successful toilet training is to approach it so that the child sees it as his or her own accomplishment.
6. The age at which daytime training is likely to be successful varies according to individual characteristics of the child: predictability of the child's elimination schedule; ability of the child to anticipate elimination and to understand the steps involved in toileting (getting to the bathroom on time, undressing, sitting on the potty chair, eliminating, wiping, flushing, and redressing); and motivation of the child to toilet train.
7. Many children find it difficult to relax enough while on the potty chair to allow urine or stool to flow. Distracting the child by reading to him or her may be helpful.

One of the many possible approaches to toilet training is the method presented in Table 1–14. This method works well for children with predictable elimination schedules. Children with irregular elimination schedules may need to be able to anticipate the need to go themselves before they can be trained. Complete daytime toilet training should be expected to take a long time. Success is sporadic initially, and occasional accidents are common long after toilet training is accomplished.

TABLE 1–14
Timing Method for Toilet Training

After demonstrating readiness signals, child is introduced to potty chair.

Child initially sits on potty chair briefly, fully clothed.

Child then sits on potty chair with pants down for gradually increasing lengths of time (1 min, up to a maximum of 10 min).

Simple explanations of toileting procedure are given repeatedly and emphasized by placing wet or soiled diapers in the potty.

Parent attempts to anticipate child's need to go (hence "timing method"), puts child on potty chair, and provides positive reinforcement for successful elimination on potty chair (praise, hug, star chart, stickers, or some other sufficiently motivating reward that can be given repeatedly).

REFERENCES

Behrman RE, Kliegman RM, Jenson HB, editors: *Nelson textbook of pediatrics*, ed 16, Philadelphia, 2000, WB Saunders, Chapters 5, 12.

Howe AC, Walker CE: Behavioral management of toilet training, enuresis, and encopresis, *Pediatr Clin North Am* 39(3):413–432, 1992.

Enuresis

Enuresis is urinary incontinence at any age at which urinary continence is considered normal. Enuresis is primary when the child has never been continent of urine for a prolonged period and secondary when incontinence recurs after a prolonged period of continence (3–6 months). *Primary nocturnal enuresis* is the most common type. It is defined as the occurrence of involuntary voiding at night in a child aged 5 years or older. At least one episode of bedwetting per month occurs in 15–30% of 6-year-olds (higher in boys and black children) and 4–16% of 12-year-olds. About 20% of bedwetters have *secondary nocturnal enuresis*, which warrants a more careful evaluation. *Daytime enuresis* has a prevalence rate of 3–4% in 5–12-year-olds and is more common in girls than it is in boys. Most children are continent of urine during waking hours by the age of 3–4 years.

An organic *etiology* is present in fewer than 5% of children with primary enuresis and in only 1% of children with primary nocturnal enuresis. The reason for almost all primary enuresis is a delay in the maturation of urethral sphincter control. This immaturity may be prolonged by a psychologic overlay related to the parents' and child's concerns about the problem. Holding urine until the last minute is the most common cause of primary day-time enuresis. Secondary enuresis usually is the result of a psychologically stressful event or condition but also is more likely than primary enuresis to have an organic cause. A urinary tract infection is the most common organic cause. Uncommon causes include chemical distal urethritis (e.g., from a bubble bath), congenital anomalies (e.g., spina bifida), severe lower urinary tract obstruction (e.g., from posterior urethral valves, urethral cyst, or urethral duplication), ectopic ureter, diabetes mellitus or insipidus, and pelvic masses (e.g., presacral teratoma, fecal impaction, hydrocolpos).

In addition to incontinence, other related *clinical manifestations* of organic causes include dysuria, frequency, hematuria, straining on urination, dribbling, small-caliber stream, stress incontinence (with coughing, lifting, or running), gait disturbance, poor bowel control, and continuous dampness. A careful history and physical examination can rule out unusual causes. Urinalysis and a urine culture should be performed at the initial visit.

Treatment is usually not recommended before 6 years of age because spontaneous cure rates are high. Even after 6 years of age, the spontaneous cure rate for primary enuresis is 15%/year; for secondary enuresis without an organic cause, spontaneous cure rates are also high.

Four commonly used treatments are counseling (Table 1–15), enuresis alarms, desmopressin acetate (DDAVP), and imipramine. The simplest initial approach is the use of fluid restriction and motivational measures such as a star chart. Enuresis alarms are effective for older children. Cure rates are about 70%, with relapse rates of 10–15% in 5- to 15-year-olds. Complete success often takes several months. Pharmacologic treatments provide symptomatic relief but are not curative. Desmopressin acetate, a synthetic analog of antidiuretic hormone, reduces urine output. It is available as a tablet or nasal spray that is administered before bedtime. The lowest effective dose should be prescribed, and the drug should not be used if the child has a systemic illness with vomiting or diarrhea. A 3–4-month course is effective in 40–60% of children. This medication may also be prescribed for occasional use—for example, when a child is away at camp or for a sleepover. The tricyclic antidepressant imipramine is an effective treatment for enuresis in 30–60% of children. Untoward effects include anticholinergic symptoms, bone marrow suppression, and life-threatening accidental ingestions. This medication necessitates periodic monitoring of electrocardiogram, blood pressure, and cell blood counts.

TABLE 1–15
Enuresis Counseling

Child assumes active, responsible role
  Keeps calendar of wet and dry nights
  Talks to physician
  Urinates just before bedtime
  Changes wet clothes and bedding
Fluids not given after dinner
Punishments and angry parental responses avoided
Positive reinforcement given for each dry night (star chart or other reward, depending on age)
Reassurance given about etiology and prognosis (aim is to remove blame and guilt)

REFERENCES

Behrman RE, Kliegman RM, Jensen HB, editors: *Nelson textbook of pediatrics*, ed 16, Philadelphia, 2000, WB Saunders, Chapters 20, 551.
Moffatt ME: Enuresis. In Levine MD, Carey WB, Crocker AC, editors: *Developmental-behavioral pediatrics*, ed 3, Philadelphia, 1999, WB Saunders.
Robson LM: Diurnal enuresis, *Pediatr Rev* 18(12):407–412, 1997.

Encopresis

Encopresis is incontinence of fecal material at any age at which fecal continence is considered normal. In the United States, bowel control is usually achieved between 2 and 3 years of age, and encopresis usually refers to regular fecal incontinence after 4 years of age. It involves a continuum from mild fecal soiling of underwear to the passage of larger amounts of fecal material. Encopresis has a prevalence of about 1% in first- and second-graders; about 80% of those with encopresis are boys.

The *pathogenesis* of encopresis is based on retention of stool. The retention may be intermittent or partial, with the child having regular but incomplete defecation. With increasing retention, sensory feedback from the bowel is reduced, the rectal wall is stretched and loses contractile strength, and water absorption from fecal material increases, resulting in larger and harder feces. The result is a vicious cycle in which the child has less control of his or her bowel movements.

Etiologic factors that contribute to the development of encopresis include constitutional predisposition for inefficient intestinal motility, overly aggressive and prolonged medical management (laxatives, enemas, and suppositories), dietary manipulation for perceived constipation, anal fissures and rashes that cause pain on defecation, decreased physical mobility, and surgical procedures for imperforate anus and other anorectal conditions. Parental overreaction to irregular frequency or form of bowel movements may result in inappropriate use of medications or diet changes or counterproductive demands on the child. Not only may demands be impossible for the child to meet (i.e., he or she may not yet be ready for toilet training), but parental coercion also may stimulate the negativism and resistance that characterize the toddler's budding autonomy. The child may perceive toileting as a negative experience and withhold stool out of a need to exercise control or out of fear for the consequences of soiling. The resulting increased retention exacerbates the problem. During the preschool years, irrational fears of the toilet also often result in withholding. Reading to the child and providing a potty seat or a step that allows the feet to be on a firm surface may help the child relax enough to allow stool to pass. During the school years, rigid or hurried schedules or reluctance to use the school bathroom may cause alterations in bowel habits. At any age, psychosocial stresses or illness may cause a regression in toilet training or a change in bowel habits that may potentiate encopresis.

Although encopresis may be more prevalent in children with severe behavioral and developmental disorders, it usually occurs in children and families without significant psychopathology. However, encopresis may result in ridicule and shame for the child and family and carries a significant risk of secondary isolation, depression, and low self-esteem. Because parents and children may not spontaneously mention this problem during the interview, the clinician should specifically inquire about it.

Diagnosis is based on a comprehensive assessment, with particular emphasis on a description of bowel patterns since birth, the age of onset of bowel-related symptoms, the effects of attempts to manage the symptoms, associations of the onset or exacerbations of symptoms with psychosocial stresses in the family, and the effects of the problem on the child and other family members. The clinician or parents should talk to the child directly about the child's perception of the problem and feelings about management plans. Hirschsprung disease must also be considered in the differential diagnosis of encopresis (see Chapter 11).

A comprehensive approach to *treatment* is presented in Table 1–16. This approach involves reassurance about the commonness of the problem and emphasis on the need for patience. Relapses are common, most often related to new or recurrent psychosocial stresses or illnesses. Refractory cases may involve complex underlying psychologic issues that warrant further investigation, organic disease that warrants reevaluation, or inadequate evacuation of a chronic impaction.

REFERENCES

Abi-Hanna A, Lake AM: Constipation and encopresis in childhood, *Pediatr Rev* 19(1):23-30, 1998.

Behrman RE, Kliegman RM, Jensen HB, editors: *Nelson textbook of pediatrics*, ed 16, Philadelphia, 2000, WB Saunders, Chapters 20, 306.

Rockney R: Encopresis. In Levine MD, Carey WB, Crocker AC, editors: *Developmental-behavioral pediatrics*, ed 3, Philadelphia, 1999, WB Saunders.

Recurrent Pain Disorders

Chronic, recurrent pain syndromes in childhood most commonly involve abdominal pain, headache, limb pain, or chest pain. It is unusual for children to exhibit more than one such pain syndrome at the same time, although they often may have had chronic, recurrent pain in a different location of the body in the past. An organic etiology is found in only about 10% of children. The diagnosis of psychogenic pain, however, should be based not only on the absence of adequate physical findings to explain the pain but also on evidence specific for the etiologic role of psychologic factors. Most chronic, recurrent pain syndromes have no clear organic or emotional origin.

Diagnosis is based on a careful physical examination and history, including a comprehensive psychosocial assessment. In addition to the location, quality, and chronology of the pain, attention must be focused on the circumstances in which the pain is felt. Signs and symptoms indicating increased likelihood of an organic etiology include constant pain; pain that awakens the child from sleep; well-localized pain; and physical findings such as fever, weight loss, jaundice, changes in the color, consistency, or frequency of stools, and urinary tract symptoms.

Psychologic conditions that preceded the onset of the recurrent pain syndrome must be distinguished from those that followed onset, because evidence of psychologic stress usually is found by the time the child exhibits a chronic problem. The nurturing responses of the family may provide secondary gain that prolongs the pain complaints. Alternatively, frustration with failure to find a specific cause may lead to accusations of malingering and to increased stress on the child, which may serve as additional reasons for chronic pain. Diagnostic studies should be undertaken in response to specific findings that suggest an organic etiology.

Counseling with reassurance of the benign nature of the pain is the primary treatment for the nonorganic diagnosis. Symptom diaries (including the events that immediately precede and follow the pain episode) are helpful in the ongoing management of the problem, as well as in the initial assessment. Minimizing secondary psychologic consequences of recurrent pain syndromes is important.

TABLE 1–16
Management of Encopresis*

Treatment Phase	Treatment Program	Comments
Initial counseling	Education and "demystification" of the problem Removal of blame Establishment and explanation of treatment plan	Include a diagram, review of colonic function, shared observation and x-ray views. Emphasize the need for intestinal "muscle building."

Initial catharsis
  Inpatient
	High normal saline enemas (750 ml bid), 3–7 days
	Bisacodyl (Dulcolax) suppositories bid, 3–7 days
	Use of bathroom for 15 min after each meal
		Patient admitted when:
		  Retention is very severe.
		  Home compliance is likely to be poor.
		  Parents prefer admission.
		  Parental administration of enemas is inadvisable psychologically.

At home	For moderate to severe retention, three–four cycles as follows: Day 1: hypophosphate enemas (Fleet's Adult) twice Day 2: bisacodyl suppositories twice Day 3: bisacodyl tablet once For mild retention: senna or danthron, one tablet daily for 1–2 weeks Follow-up abdominal x-ray examination to confirm adequate catharsis	Dosages or frequency may need alteration if child experiences excessive discomfort. Admission should be considered if there is inadequate yield. No lubricant is used during this phase.
Maintenance regimen	Child sits on toilet twice a day at same times each day for 10 min each time Light mineral oil (at least 2 tablespoons) twice a day, usually for at least 4–6 mo Multiple vitamins, 2/day, between doses of mineral oil High-roughage diet: bran, cereal, vegetables, fruits Use of an oral laxative (senna or danthron) for 2–3 wk, then alternate days of mineral oil for 1 mo (given between doses); then laxative is discontinued; lubricant is continued	A kitchen timer can be helpful. A chart with stars for sitting may be good for children younger than 7 yr. Bathroom reading encouraged. Mineral oil can be put in juice, soft drinks, or any other medium. Vitamins can be used to compensate for alleged problems with absorption secondary to mineral oil. Diet should be applied but not to the point of coercion.

Follow-up pattern	Visits every 4-10 wk, depending on severity, need for support, compliance, and associated symptoms
	Telephone availability to adjust doses when needed
	In case of relapse:
	  Check compliance
	  Use of oral laxative (e.g., Senokot) for 1–2 wk
	  Adjust dosage of mineral oil
	Counseling or referral for associated psychosocial and developmental issues
	Continuing use of demystification diagram to continue to document progress
		Duration of treatment can be as long as 2–3 yr or as short as 6 mo.
		Signs of relapse:
		  Excessive oil leaks
		  Large-caliber stools
		  Abdominal pain
		  Decreased frequency of defecation
		  Soiling
		The physician should spend time alone with the child.
		In patients who are slow to respond, the physician should sustain optimism; persistence cures almost all cases (eventually).

Modified from Levine MD: Encopresis. In Levine MD, Carey WB, Crocker AC, editors: *Developmental-behavioral pediatrics*, ed 2, Philadelphia, 1992, WB Saunders.
*All dosages and frequencies are for an average-sized 7-year-old child. Appropriate adjustments should be made for smaller and larger patients.

REFERENCES

Behrman RE, Kliegman RM, Jensen HB, editors: *Nelson textbook of pediatrics,* ed 16, Philadelphia, 2000, WB Saunders, Chapters 19, 154, 306.

Frazer CH, Rappaport LA: Recurrent pains. In Levine MD, Carey WB, Crocker AC, editors: *Developmental-behavioral pediatrics,* ed 3, Philadelphia, 1999, WB Saunders.

Failure to Thrive

Failure to thrive (FTT) is a term used to describe an inadequate growth rate in a young child. This may refer to weight below the 3rd percentile on a standard growth chart; however, many children below the 3rd percentile are normal, and some above it may have fallen from a much higher percentile and be failing to thrive. Growth percentile changes demonstrated over time, although meaningful, can be misleading in the first year or two, when wide fluctuations in percentile position are not uncommon in normal children. For example, it is quite common for a child who is above the 75th percentile in weight in the first 6–9 months to fall to the 50th percentile or lower from 9–18 months and then to maintain that percentile position. When the percentile drop is great, it is helpful to compare the child's weight percentile to height and head circumference percentiles. It is not a concern when the weight falls from a disproportionately high percentile position to a position consistent with height and head circumference. A fall to a disproportionately low weight percentile is a cause for concern.

In the short term a child who is failing to thrive as a result of inadequate caloric intake will drop in weight percentile before dropping in height and head circumference percentiles. Over time the height percentile also will fall, but the head circumference is usually spared, unless the FTT is severe. In comparison, the child with poor growth as the result of hypothyroidism will exhibit slowed height growth with relative sparing of weight growth. FTT also may be defined as a weight of less than 80% of the median weight for height. Weight-by-height charts (Figs. 1–3 and 1–6) are particularly helpful when adequate serial measurements are unavailable.

An etiologic approach to the *differential diagnosis* of FTT is presented in Table 1–17 along with some of the common causes. Almost every chronic or serious condition in childhood may cause FTT. It is the diagnosis for 3–5% of children admitted to teaching hospitals. *In most children with inadequate growth, both organic and nonorganic risk factors are present.* Children with primarily environmental causes of FTT may exhibit physical signs and symptoms because of nutritional deficiency, unusual diets, recurrent infection, and perhaps neuroendocrine responses to stress (e.g., diarrhea, vomiting, depressed growth hormone levels, delayed bone age, iron or zinc deficiency, lead poisoning, elevated serum transaminase levels, and

TABLE 1–17
Etiology of Failure to Thrive

Mechanism	Disorders
Psychosocial	Poor maternal-child interaction, poor feeding technique, psychologically disturbed mother, unusual maternal nutritional beliefs, errors in formula preparation, emotional deprivation (dwarfism), child neglect
Inability to suck, swallow, or masticate	CNS pathology (psychomotor retardation), neuromuscular disease (Werdnig-Hoffmann, myotonia congenita, dysautonomia)
Maldigestion, malabsorption	Cystic fibrosis, celiac disease, Schwachman-Diamond syndrome, chronic diarrhea
Poor nutrient use	Renal failure, renal tubular acidosis, inborn errors of metabolism
Vomiting	CNS abnormality (e.g., tumor, infection, or increased pressure), metabolic toxin (e.g., inborn errors of amino or organic acid metabolism), intestinal obstruction (e.g., pyloric stenosis, malrotation), renal tubular disease
Regurgitation	Gastroesophageal reflux, hiatal hernia, rumination syndrome
Elevated metabolic rate	Thyrotoxicosis, chronic disease (bronchopulmonary dysplasia, heart failure), cancer, inflammatory lesions (SLE, inflammatory bowel disease, chronic infection), immunodeficiency diseases, burns
Reduced growth potential	Chromosomal disorders, primordial dwarfism, skeletal dysplasia, specific syndromes (e.g., fetal alcohol)
Combinations	Human immunodeficiency virus infection

CNS, Central nervous system; *SLE,* systemic lupus erythematosus.

glucose intolerance). Conversely, the environmental stresses faced by the family of a child with a chronic illness may adversely affect the adequacy of nutritional and psychologic nurturing of the child, as in the parents of the child with recurrent vomiting who exhibit stress around feeding that further impedes intake. Infection with the human immunodeficiency virus (HIV) often is associated with complex combinations of both biologic and environmental factors that result in poor growth.

In early infancy, feeding difficulties are the predominant cause of FTT, including lactation failure, inadequate feeding frequency or volume, and formula-mixing errors. A calorically inadequate diet at any age may be the result of ignorance or neglect by the caregivers. It also may result from irregular caregiving arrangements that involve many caregivers, who are sometimes themselves children. Retrospective diet histories often do not coincide with actual intake, particularly when there are multiple caregivers. Even a competent parent simply may not know the actual intake of the child unless a detailed contemporaneous diary is kept by all caregivers.

Among children with milder growth abnormalities, systemic disease is less likely as a primary cause. It is important to observe caregiver-child interactions (in a natural environment, if possible) and to obtain complete historical data. Causes include postpartum depression; maternal depression related to a significant loss (e.g., a spouse or parent); a social environment characterized by many stresses and poor social support; and caregiver-child interaction patterns that are hostile, rejecting, or aloof.

History and observation are the most important aspects of the *diagnostic evaluation* of FTT. If possible, the attitudes and interactions of important caregivers with each other and with the child should be observed or obtained by history. Any behavioral problems the child or siblings have (e.g., excessive crying, discipline problems, sleep disturbances, and feeding problems) are often associated with family dysfunction. *Clinical manifestations* in children experiencing environmental deprivation include "frozen watchfulness," minimal smiling, decreased vocalization, resistance to being held, and self-stimulating rhythmic behaviors. Observing the child during a meal is also useful to watch for food-specific problems such as gagging, choking, refusal to accept a particular food, or unusual parent-child interactions.

If a careful history and physical examination fail to identify a cause or clue that suggests specific diagnostic procedures, it is unlikely that any tests will reveal a cause. In one study of children admitted to a teaching hospital with FTT of unknown etiology, fewer than 2% of tests performed during the hospitalization contributed to a diagnosis, and all of the positive tests were associated with a positive finding in the initial history and physical examination. Still, it is standard procedure to obtain a few screening tests: a complete blood count, urinalysis, serum electrolyte level, and perhaps an erythrocyte sedimentation rate. If even mild gastrointestinal symptoms are present, a stool culture, pH, reducing substances test, and guaiac test are indicated.

Treatment of FTT by hospitalization of the child may be particularly stressful when the parent-child attachment is insecure. If the cause appears to be inadequate caloric intake, a reasonable initial ambulatory plan may be to provide dietary advice and have caregivers keep a detailed diary of feedings and the frequency, volume, and consistency of stools and vomitus. If the picture remains unclear and the child fails to exhibit catch-up growth within several weeks, hospitalization is necessary because adequate nutrition is crucial for brain development during the first 2 years of life.

One common approach to FTT of unknown etiology, after outpatient attempts to manage the problem have failed, is to admit the child to the hospital and to observe for weight gain after the child demonstrates adequate caloric intake. Most children will grow if given 120 kcal × the median weight in kilograms for the child's measured length over each 24-hour period. If the child gains weight, FTT resulting from inadequate intake is assumed and steps are taken to monitor and support the environment and the child's nutrition after discharge. If the child fails to gain, an organic cause is more aggressively sought. However, as noted above, environmental and organic factors usually occur together. Table 1–18 presents data from one study demonstrating the time required in the hospital before catch-up weight gain was observed in children with calorie-deprivation FTT.

TABLE 1–18

Time Required in Hospital for Accelerated Weight Gain in Children with Calorie-Deprivation Failure to Thrive

Age younger than 6 months
   Most gaining by 2–3 days
   All gaining by 9 days
Age 6–24 months
   Gaining by 2–17 days
   2 of 25 required more than 2 weeks
Age 2 years or more
   All gaining in 2–7 days

Adapted from Ellerstein NS, Ostrov BE: *Am J Dis Child* 139(2):164-166, 1985.

TABLE 1–19
Hospital Protocol for Failure to Thrive of Unknown Etiology

Defer all investigations for at least 1 week (assuming no clues for organic etiology on comprehensive history and physical examination).

Aim to provide 120 kcal/24 hr × median weight (kg) for *measured* length.

Record the following data daily:
  Weight before breakfast (unclothed)
  Total calories consumed in the previous 24 hours
  Calories/kg of *ideal weight* in the previous 24 hours
  Output (stool, urine, vomitus)

Record observations of the child's behavior and interactions of the child with the parents and the staff.

Provide an organized program of stimulation, including regular affectionate interaction with adults.

Involve the parents from the start in the feeding and stimulation interventions.

Begin interdisciplinary evaluations on admission (e.g., social worker, nurse, nutritional support team or dietitian, and behavioral/developmental specialist).

Table 1–19 presents a protocol for management in or out of the hospital. Deferring investigations decreases the stress of hospitalization, which may shorten the time required to achieve adequate caloric intake and thereby to test the hypothesis that the FTT is caused by inadequate caloric intake. Because catch-up growth must be demonstrated, more calories should be provided than normally required for the child's current depressed weight. A positive change in the mood of a child usually is followed by accelerated weight gain in 1–2 days. The parents should be involved in the development and implementation of the management plan.

The *prognosis* for children hospitalized for nonorganic FTT in the first 2 years of life shows a high percentage of retardation (15–67%), school learning problems (37–67%), and behavioral disturbances (28–48%) at 3–11 years of age. Continued FTT is a much less frequent problem.

REFERENCES

Behrman RE, Kliegman RM, Jensen HB, editors: *Nelson textbook of pediatrics*, ed 16, Philadelphia, 2000, WB Saunders, Chapters 35, 36.

Casey PH: Failure to thrive. In Levine MD, Carey WB, Crocker AC, editors: *Developmental-behavioral pediatrics*, ed 3, Philadelphia, 1999, WB Saunders.

Frank D, Silva M, Needleman R: Failure to thrive: mystery, myth, and method, *Contemp Pediatr* 10:114, 1993.

Zenel JA: Failure to thrive: a general pediatrician's perspective, *Pediatr Rev* 18(11):371–378, 1997.

Child Abuse and Neglect

Child maltreatment is a frequent, serious problem that the federal government and every state government have addressed through creation of laws. The Child Abuse Prevention and Treatment Act (Public Law 93–247) defines child abuse and neglect as "the physical or mental injury, sexual abuse, negligent treatment, or maltreatment of a child under the age of eighteen by a person who is responsible for the child's welfare under circumstances which indicate that the child's health and welfare is harmed or threatened thereby." In most cases, child abuse must be understood as a symptom of family dysfunction that spans generations. Studies indicate that child abuse occurs in 33–77% of families in which there is abuse of adults. Identifying and intervening on behalf of battered women may be one of the most effective means by which pediatricians can prevent child abuse. Only by understanding the factors that contribute to its occurrence can a logical management plan be developed (Fig. 1–15).

Estimates of the *incidence* of child abuse and neglect vary widely, depending on the definition and the source. Approximately 1% of children are reported to be abused or neglected each year. Child neglect is the most common form of child maltreatment, accounting for more than 50% of all cases reported to child protective services (CPS) agencies. Child neglect is legally defined as parental omissions in care that result in actual or potential harm to the child. This includes failure to provide for a child's basic needs (i.e., adequate food, health care, clothing, nurturance, protection, supervision, and a home). Physical abuse, sexual abuse, and emotional abuse constitute approximately 25%, 13%, and 5% of confirmed maltreatment cases, respectively. Failure to thrive because of underfeeding and **Munchausen by proxy** are less common situations. Estimates of the incidence of child abuse based on household surveys range from 5–14%. Abuse is less likely to be reported if it involves children from white, nonpoor families; if the mother is alleged to be responsible for the abuse; and if the abuse is emotional rather than physical.

Physicians may be reluctant to report cases because they are uncomfortable in the role of accuser, the antithesis of their usual role of compassionate helper, or because of time constraints, concern over possible court appearances, and lack of knowledge about the problem or how to proceed once child abuse is suspected. Laws that govern reporting attempt to overcome this reluctance by mandating the report of "suspected" abuse, by making physicians immune from suits related to a report made in good faith, and by making it the responsibility of protection agencies (not physicians) to determine whether abuse has actually occurred. Physicians thus can at-

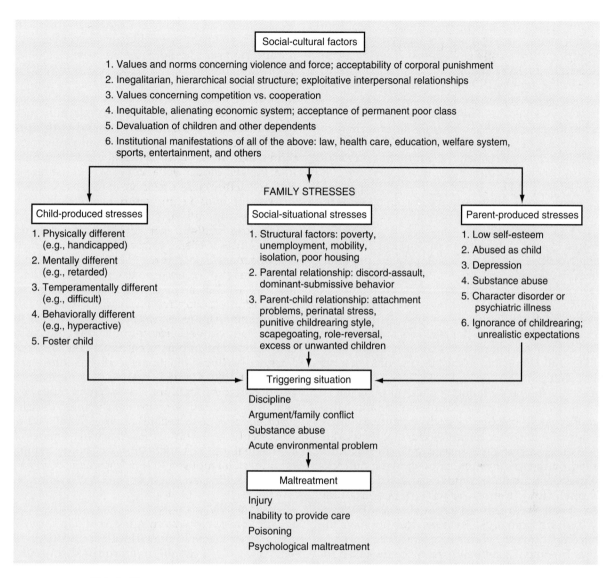

FIG. 1–15

Model for understanding child abuse. (From Bittner S, Newberger EH: *Pediatr Rev* 2:198, 1981.)

tempt to maintain a helping relationship with the family by telling the family that as physicians they are obligated by law to make a report but that their aim is to help find ways to prevent a recurrence of the injury or condition. Only a few states currently require that medical professionals report domestic violence, which is known to place a child at risk for abuse. Physicians can identify unsafe settings by asking about family violence as part of anticipatory guidance and by referring battered women to appropriate community resources. Some families react with anger or hurt, but others welcome the opportunity to find help for their difficult situation.

To detect less obvious cases of child abuse, the physician must be sensitive to the more subtle signs and must take the time to obtain an expanded history and behavioral observations. Because a determination of whether a report is warranted may take more time or expertise than the physician has, the use of a social worker who specializes in child abuse or preferably a child abuse team may be invaluable.

Physical Abuse

Conservative estimates indicate that 1–2% of children in the United States are physically abused at some time during childhood and that 10% of injuries seen in a hospital emergency room in children younger than 5 years of age are caused by abuse. About one third of physical abuse cases occur in children under 1 year of age and another one third between the ages of 1 and 6 years. Approximately 2000 deaths per year in the United States are the result of physical abuse. The most common perpetrators are the father (21%), mother (21%), boyfriend of the mother (9%), baby sitter (8%), and stepfather (5%). Physical abuse usually occurs in the context of increased socioenvironmental stresses and often is triggered by child behaviors such as persistent crying, wetting or soiling, spilling, or disobedience. Fewer than 10% of abusive parents have psychotic or criminal personalities.

Some *clinical manifestations* of physical abuse are unequivocal. Distinctive bruising patterns are often caused by blunt instruments, belts, cords, hand slaps, pinches, choke holds, and bites. Burn patterns from cigarettes, irons, hot plates, and forced submersion into scalding water are also distinctive. A circular burn limited to the buttocks and genitalia with no involvement of the hands or feet is incompatible with falling into or mistakenly entering a tub of hot water.

Usually, the presentation of child abuse is not so clear. Bruises, burns, and fractures may be accidental and often are dismissed as such without adequate consideration of other causes. Accidental bruises are most common over the forehead, anterior tibia, and bony prominences; bruises confined to the buttocks or lower back are most commonly caused by abuse. Anaphylactoid (Henoch-Schönlein) purpura may present with ecchymoses over the buttocks, but usually purpura from organic causes does not have the limited distribution of bruising characteristic of child abuse. Healing cigarette burns may be mistaken for impetigo or atopic or contact dermatitis.

Some presentations of serious child abuse may not suggest the diagnosis at all. In the absence of injury to the skull or scalp, subdural hematomas may be caused by violent shaking that has led to the tearing of bridging cerebral vessels. Serious abdominal injuries (e.g., rupture of the liver, spleen, intestines, or blood vessels; traumatic pancreatitis; or intramural hematomas) may be caused by striking or squeezing the abdomen; children with these injuries may exhibit signs and symptoms of an acute abdomen but may not have evidence of external trauma to raise the suspicion of child abuse.

Table 1–20 outlines the *diagnostic evaluation* for suspected child abuse. The history is crucial when the injury is not pathognomonic for abuse. The interviewer should strive to be a supportive listener and avoid making judgmental statements that may arouse increased defensiveness. After beginning the interview with nonthreatening general conversation, the interviewer should focus on concrete details about how the injury occurred. Key questions are whether the family's explanation for the injury is compatible with the physical findings and whether the explanation is consistent among family members, including the injured child, and with subsequent interviews with the same family member. If old enough to be interviewed, the child should be interviewed alone. The interviewer must be very sensitive to the child's feelings of fear or guilt.

Description of the injury and identification of the probable cause are the relatively easy aspects of a child abuse workup. The skeletal survey is mandatory in all cases of suspected physical abuse in children younger than 2 years of age. Radionucleotide bone scans provide increased sensitivity for detecting rib fractures, subtle shaft fractures, and areas of early periosteal elevation but may not identify bilateral or subtle spine injuries. All children with suspected intracranial injury should undergo cranial computed tomography (CT) or magnetic resonance imaging (MRI) examination. Bleeding studies should be obtained if bruising is present. A comprehensive evaluation of the family and social environment is essential to guide subsequent management decisions when the diagnosis is child abuse. Hospital admission may be necessary to treat the child's injuries and to ensure the child's safety until it can be determined that it is safe for the child to return home or to an alternative setting.

Sexual Abuse

Sexual abuse involves engaging a child in sexual activities that the child often does not understand, to which the child cannot give informed consent, or that violate the sexual social taboos. This definition includes a broad range of sexual activities (e.g., exhibitionism; fondling; child pornography; and oral, anal, and genital contact), both inside and outside the family. Some reserve the term "sexual abuse" to refer to forced sexual contact between a victim and perpetrator, while using the term "sexual misuse" for instances in which a child is exposed to sexual stimulation inappropriate for the child's role in the family. **Incest** is sexual abuse by a close relative that involves intercourse. **Molestation** is sexual abuse by a stranger, with or without penetration. **Rape** involves forced genital contact. **Sexual assault** involves violent or nonviolent manual, oral, or genital contact with the genitalia of the victim or the perpetrator. Activities that are considered to be normal sexual exploratory behavior among children of similar age may be considered sexual abuse or misuse if the ages

---

TABLE 1–20
Initial Diagnostic Evaluation for Suspected Child Abuse

History

Obtain separate histories from parents, other adults, and child (if possible).

Record history precisely.

  Record direct quotations.

  Clarify ambiguous statements.

  Use qualifiers like "the mother alleges that . . ." rather than "the child was . . ."

Record the following:

  Data and time of evaluation

  Date, time, and place of alleged abuse

  Informant

  How alleged abuse occurred and who allegedly caused it

  History of abuse

Physical Examination

Perform a careful, complete examination.

List bruises by site, size, shape, and color.

Check the retina, eardrums, oral cavity, and genitalia for signs of occult trauma.

Check bones and joints for tenderness and range of motion.

Record height and weight percentiles.

Physical Examination—cont'd

Obtain color photographs of injuries (include paper with patient's name, date, and time in the photograph).

Laboratory Tests

Obtain a radiologic bone survey (skull, thorax, spine, long bones) for children under the age of 5 years who are suspected victims of child abuse.

Obtain bleeding studies (platelet count, bleeding time, prothrombin time [PT], and partial thromboplastin time [PTT]) when bruising is present.

Disposition

Consult immediately with a social worker or child abuse team to arrange comprehensive multidisciplinary evaluation.

Report the situation to the mandated agency if indicated.

Inform parents of the need to report and desire to be helpful.

Hospitalize the child if further investigation is necessary to determine the safety of the home or to treat injuries.

Establish a multidisciplinary follow-up plan (e.g., with health and social services).

---

are discrepant. Approximately 1% of children experience some form of sexual abuse each year, resulting in the sexual victimization of 12–25% of girls and 8–10% of boys by age 18. Most recognized sexual offenders are male, and about 20% are adolescents.

The *clinical manifestations* of sexual abuse may be more difficult to recognize than those of physical abuse. Early warnings may take the form of simulation of sexual acts with dolls, inclusion of genitalia in drawings, precocious flirtation, and verbalization of concern about sexual molestation in general. Direct statements from children about abusive behaviors should be taken seriously. Most sexually abused children are reluctant to break the secrecy of the abuse because of fear and guilt; many who do make a statement recant it later. Many nonspecific behavioral problems may be associated with sexual abuse, including sleeping and eating disorders, school dysfunction, phobias, depression, acting out behaviors, conversion reactions, and suicide attempts.

The presence in prepubertal children of genital and anal trauma or diseases that are usually sexually transmitted (e.g., gonorrhea, syphilis, lym-phogranuloma venereum, trichomoniasis, genital herpes, and chlamydial infections) should raise a strong suspicion of sexual abuse. Recurrent urinary tract infections, recurrent nonspecific vaginitis, genital warts, or early pregnancy may also be the result of sexual abuse.

The diagnostic evaluation in Table 1–20 may need to be modified for sexual abuse. Because the diagnosis of sexual abuse has legal ramifications, investigative interviews should be conducted by the designated agency or individual in the community. Efforts should also be made to minimize repetitive questioning of the child. Occasionally, children spontaneously describe their abuse to the physician, and such information should be documented in the chart as evidence. Generally, only professionals trained in interviewing children should use drawings, dolls, or other aids. Most expert interviewers do not interview children younger than 3 years old.

The physician should obtain a focused history to guide the examination. Particularly important points include the type and time of the alleged abusive act and subsequent events that may alter the presence of evidence (e.g., bathing, urinating, defecation, brushing teeth, or changing clothes). It is best to obtain this information from someone other than the child. The examination should proceed just like a normal general examination, with special attention given to any evidence of physical abuse, trauma, or the presence of blood or semen on body parts or clothing. The knee-chest position may provide better visualization of the vagina and anus in prepubertal girls, although the lithotomy position is usually better as girls approach puberty. Findings that are concerning but that in isolation are not diagnostic of sexual abuse include abrasions and bruising of the inner thighs and genitalia, scarring or tears of the labia minora, and enlargement of the hymenal opening. Findings that are more concerning are scarring, tears, or distortion of the hymen; a decreased amount of or absent hymenal tissue; scarring of the fossa navicularis; injury or scarring of the posterior fourchette; and anal lacerations or an anterior-posterior diameter with immediate anal dilatation greater than 20 mm. Wood lamp inspection of the body and clothing is indicated to look for the fluorescence of sperm. Laboratory evaluation for suspected sexual abuse includes gonorrhea and *Chlamydia* cultures from the mouth, anus, and genitals. Serologic tests for syphilis, HIV, and hepatitis B should also be used. Certain laboratory findings are considered diagnostic of sexual abuse. Table 1–21 lists the implications of commonly encountered sexually transmitted diseases for the diagnosis and reporting of sexual abuse. Many hospital emergency departments have standardized protocols and kits for specimen collection that have been developed in collaboration with law enforcement agencies.

Treatment of sexually transmitted diseases is discussed in Chapter 7. Pregnancy can be prevented within 72 hours of intercourse by giving the patient two norgestrel and ethinyl estradiol (Ovral) tablets at the time of examination and two more tablets 12 hours later. The physician will need the help of social workers and perhaps mental health professionals to immediately assess child and family functioning, the family's social environment, and their needs for services. A child victim will need extensive counseling. Hospital admission may be warranted for treatment of injuries, for mental health evaluation, or to ensure safety. Subsequently, the effectiveness of health and social services to which the child and family have been referred should be monitored and close communication maintained among the professionals involved in the evaluation and continuing care of the family. Medical follow-up must ensure adequate treatment of injuries and infections; serology tests for syphilis should be rechecked in 6 weeks.

TABLE 1–21
Implications of Commonly Encountered Sexually Transmitted Diseases for the Diagnosis and Reporting of Sexual Abuse of Infants and Prepubertal Children

STD Confirmed	Sexual Abuse	Suggested Action
Gonorrhea*	Diagnostic†	Report‡
Syphilis*	Diagnostic	Report
HIV§	Diagnostic	Report
Chlamydia*	Diagnostic†	Report
Trichomonas vaginalis	Highly suspicious	Report
Condylomata acuminata (anogenital warts)*	Suspicious	Report
Herpes (genital location)	Suspicious	Report‖
Bacterial vaginosis	Inconclusive	Medical follow-up

*If not perinatally acquired.
†Use definitive diagnostic methods such as culture or DNA probes.
‡To agency mandated in community to receive reports of suspected sexual abuse.
§If not perinatally or transfusion acquired.
‖Unless there is a clear history of autoinoculation. Herpes 1 and 2 are difficult to differentiate by current techniques.

REFERENCES

Behrman RE, Kliegman RM, Jenson HB, editors: *Nelson textbook of pediatrics*, ed 16, Philadelphia, 2000, WB Saunders, Chapters 34, 35.
Committee on Child Abuse and Neglect, American Academy of Pediatrics: Guidelines for the evaluation of sexual abuse of children: subject review (AAP policy statement RE9819), *Pediatrics* 103(1):186–191, 1999.
Committee on Child Abuse and Neglect, American Academy of Pediatrics: The role of the pediatrician in recognizing and intervening on behalf of abused women (AAP policy statement RE9748), *Pediatrics* 101(6):1091–1092, 2000.

Separation from One or Both Parents
Hospitalization

About 30% of children are hospitalized at least once during childhood, and about 5% have multiple hospital admissions. Along with separation from parents, hospitalization stresses include the illness itself (with discomfort, pain, fear, uncertainty, and parental anxiety), separation from almost everything that is familiar (e.g., siblings, home, friends, school, and customary routines), and exposure to many strange and threatening experiences (e.g., painful and uncomfortable procedures, many new people, and sick or disabled people experiencing pain and emotional upset).

Hospitalization of a child can result in distress during the hospitalization, disturbance on the return home, and long-term sequelae. Distress during hospitalization is most marked between 6 months and 4 years of age. Distress is related to the degree of separation from all people to whom the child is attached, the lack of opportunity to form new attachments (large numbers of frequently changing caregivers), and the strangeness of the environment. For children younger than age 5–6 years, parents should room with the child if feasible. A preadmission visit may also allay fears. Finally, families should be encouraged to participate in the hospital's child-life support programs, if available. Child-life personnel offer therapeutic play and socialization opportunities and explain procedures and hospital routines to children and families.

On returning home, many children exhibit regressive, withdrawn, ambivalent, or labile behavior. Parents may also experience psychologic disturbances. A posttraumatic stress response is not unusual, particularly among parents whose children were critically ill. This may be minimized during the hospital stay by providing frequent updates on diagnosis, prognosis, and treatment options and if possible by offering parents the opportunity to actively participate in the child's care, such as by bathing or reading to their child.

Prolonged and serious illnesses in children place great stress on the parents (e.g., in marital relationships, parenting of siblings, and work performance) and siblings, who are often neglected to some degree while the parents are consumed by the care of and anxiety over the sick child. Even with conditions that are judged as relatively mild by health care providers, the behavior of the parents toward the sick child may be altered for a long time after the illness resolves. The so-called vulnerable child syndrome includes difficulties with separations, infantilization, preoccupation with bodily functions, and decreased school achievement.

Divorce

The problems associated with divorce are usually chronic and often devastating for both the children and the parents. Divorce is usually not a single event but a sequence of difficult changes and adjustments that span years. For years before a divorce, children may be exposed to family turmoil that may include violent arguments and physical violence, involving their parents, other family members, and perhaps themselves. Alternatively, some children, particularly young ones, may be completely unaware that a problem exists until one of the parents leaves. For the parents, the period between the separation and the formal divorce can be particularly acrimonious, making it very difficult for them to help the children cope with their losses, fears, and disruptions in the usual pattern of family life.

Complicating the family's emotional adjustment to the divorce are the untoward economic results that affect many of these families. Often ex-husbands fail to provide child support payments. Women, who are usually the custodial parents, may lack the education, job skills, or experience to obtain adequately compensated and secure jobs. When a mother who has remained in the home to care for a preschool child must start work, that child suffers a second loss. The custodial parent also must assume household responsibilities that previously were shared. In addition, relocation to cheaper housing often is necessary, frequently involving a loss of friends and familiar school and neighborhood. Worsening parent-child relations are often a result of these additional stresses. It is usually not until after the first year of divorce that reduced tension and an increased sense of well-being begin to emerge in the children of divorced parents. Because many divorced women and men remarry, there are further periods of adjustment as stepparents and often stepchildren join the family. Divorced and blended families are becoming increasingly common and approach the norm in some communities. Little is known about the long-term effects of these changes in social demographics.

The most important determinant of how a child initially responds to divorce is the child's age (Table 1–22). More than one third of children are psychologically troubled and distressed 5 years after the divorce. The most frequent clinical finding is depression. Poor psychologic adjustment in children is more likely when parental fighting continues and when the children remain in the custody of a lonely, depressed, or emotionally disturbed parent. Many children of divorced parents are reluctant to form intimate relationships as they enter adulthood.

Children who are told about the divorce before the actual separation and who are reassured that they will continue to see both parents are calmer at the time of separation. Children should be told the details about what their living arrangements and daily routines will be after the separation. The children also need to be told repeatedly that they did not cause the divorce and that their efforts cannot mend it. Young children may be told that the divorce is

TABLE 1–22
Related Responses of the Child of Divorced Parents

Age	Common Reactions of Child	Role of Physician
2–5 yr	Regression, irritability, sleep disturbance	Encourage restabilization of household and bedtime routines. Reassure the child. Urge restoration of contact with the departed parent.
6–8 yr	Open grieving, feelings of rejection	Support maintenance of the child's relationship to both parents. Reassure the child.
9–12 yr	Fear, anger at one or both parents	Express interest and availability to the child.
Adolescence	Worried about own future; depressed and/or acting-out behavior	Offer opportunity for private discussion.

From Wallerstein JS: Separation, divorce, and remarriage. In Levine MD, Carey WB, Crocker AC, editors: *Developmental-behavioral pediatrics*, ed 2, Philadelphia, 1992, WB Saunders.

necessary to bring an end to fighting or unhappiness between the parents. Older children may have more specific questions that should be answered simply without the parents going beyond a concrete, superficial response unless they are questioned further. Children need to be assured that neither parent expects them to take sides, and they need to be allowed to love both parents. They also need to be allowed to express feelings of anger, sadness, and disappointment. Children have a continuing need for reassurances after the separation. Children who receive additional attention from grandparents, family, and friends do better than those who do not.

REFERENCES

Behrman RE, Kliegman RM, Jenson HB, editors: *Nelson textbook of pediatrics*, ed 16, Philadelphia, 2000, WB Saunders, Chapter 33.
Emery RE, Coiro MJ: Divorce: consequences for children, *Pediatr Rev* 16(8):306–310, 1995.
Leslie LK, Boyce T: The vulnerable child, *Pediatr Rev* 17(9):323–326, 1996.

Sleep Disorders

Sleep patterns in children follow a typical developmental sequence, with the gradual increase of deep sleep and the development of regular sleep cycles. Sleep stages are defined by electroencephalographic, electromyographic, and electrooculographic characteristics, such as waking, rapid eye movement (REM), and non-REM sleep. Most infants (up to 70%) will sleep through the night (at least 5 hours at a stretch) by 3 months postterm, at which time they have assumed schedules of about four sleep periods within 24 hours. Premature infants take longer to assume the patterns typical of full-term infants. Most children reach a point later in the first year of life, often associated with an intercurrent illness, when they begin to wake at night again, sometimes falling into patterns of night waking that persist for years and that require behavioral interventions for correction.

Common sleep disruption disorders may be organic in nature or related to environmental factors that usually are easily remedied once their features are recognized. Table 1–23 lists several common sleep disruption patterns and their treatments. When schedules need to be regularized, imposing a routine bedtime and naptime for the child, along with a usual presleep routine, and firmly but supportively maintaining it despite protests can be very successful. When parental work and lifestyles result in children being awakened early and going to bed late, the schedule must be arranged so that the child gets enough sleep. In children with delayed sleep phase onset, the circadian clock is probably set so that the child is not ready for sleep at the prescribed bedtime; treatment involves either gradually moving the bedtime backward 15–30 min/day or forward by 2–3 hr/night over a week. A short course of over-the-counter melatonin may also be helpful.

Obstructive sleep apnea occurs in children and in adults and frequently is associated with a predisposing physical condition, such as tonsillar hypertrophy. It is characterized by snoring, may be associated with enuresis or obesity, and may be associated with hyperactivity and school dysfunction in some children. Weight reduction and otolaryngologic surgery may be indicated.

TABLE 1–23
Childhood Sleep Disruption Disorders

Type	Cause	Symptoms	Treatment
Organic			
Colic	Unknown	Crying, irritability	Rocking, pacifier, nursing Support until resolution
Medications	Stimulants Bronchodilators Anticonvulsants	Failure to fall asleep; restless sleep	Adjust dosage/timing; change medication
Illness	Any chronically irritating disorder (e.g., otitis, dermatitis, asthma, or esophageal reflux)	Painful crying out	Treat disease symptomatically
Central nervous system disorders	Variable; rule out seizures	Decreased sleep	Evaluate environment Sedatives as last resort
Parasomnias			
Sleepwalking, sleep terrors Confusional arousals	Stage IV (deep) sleep instability	Awakening 1–3 hr after falling asleep Intense crying, walking, disorientation, talking	Reassurance; protective environment
Enuresis	? Stage IV instability Metabolic disease (e.g., diabetes) Urinary tract infection Urinary anatomic anomaly	Bedwetting	Rule out medical conditions Fluid limitation Prebed voiding Behavioral approaches (bell and pad) Emotional support Medication (e.g., imipramine, DDAVP) Reassurance
Sleep-Wake Schedule Disorders			
Irregular sleep-wake pattern	No defined schedule	Variable waking and sleeping	Regularize schedule
Regular but inappropriate sleep-wake schedule	Napping at wrong times Prematurely eliminated nap	Morning sleepiness Night wakenings	Rework schedule
Delayed sleep phase	Late sleep onset with resetting of circadian rhythm	Late sleep onset Morning sleepiness Not sleepy at bedtime	Enforce wake-up time Gradually move bedtime earlier or keep awake overnight to create drowsy state
Environmental and Psychosocial Factors			
Inappropriate sleep-onset associations	No defined bedtime routine Child falls asleep in conditions different from those of the rest of the night	Night wakings requiring intervention	Regularize routine Minimize nocturnal parental response
Excessive nocturnal fluid	Child gets food/drink with each awakening	Night waking or wanting drink	Gradually decrease nocturnal fluid
Inconsistent limit setting	Parental anxiety	Delayed bedtime Excessive expression of "needs" by child	Modify parental behavior to improve limit setting Gradually increase limits
Anxieties; fears	Separation anxieties	Night waking Refusal to sleep	Reassurance when appropriate Counseling in severe cases
Social disruptions	Family stressors	Night waking Refusal to sleep	Family counseling Regularize routines

Night terrors (pavor nocturnus), bedwetting (enuresis), and sleepwalking are common deep-sleep phenomena that are developmentally normal and usually do not represent pathologic processes. Similarly, head rolling, head banging, and rocking are seen in many normal children between 9 months and 3 years of age and usually are benign, self-limited phenomena. If these behaviors persist or are associated with other developmental lags, they should be further evaluated.

REFERENCES

Behrman RE, Kliegman RM, Jenson HB, editors: *Nelson textbook of pediatrics*, ed 16, Philadelphia, 2000, WB Saunders, Chapters 5, 20.

Blum NJ, Carey WB: Sleep problems among infants and young children, *Pediatr Rev* 17(3):87–92, 1996.

Shapiro HL: Sleep disorders. In Levine MD, Carey WB, Crocker AC, editors: *Developmental-behavioral pediatrics*, ed 3, Philadelphia, 1999, WB Saunders.

Mental Retardation

Mental retardation (MR) is significantly subaverage general intellectual functioning for a child's developmental stage, existing concurrently with deficits in adaptive behavior. MR is defined statistically as tested cognitive performance that is two standard deviations below the mean (roughly below the 3rd percentile) of the general population. This implies that as many as 8.5 million persons in the United States can be characterized as having mental retardation; clinical estimates range from 2.2 to 10 million (the higher number includes persons with so-called borderline intelligence and poor social adaptation). About 60,000 individuals with cognitive impairment live in public residential facilities.

Levels of MR from intelligence quotient (IQ) scores derived from two typical tests are shown in Table 1–24. These categories do not necessarily reflect the actual functional level of the tested individual. In school, a child with mild MR may, because of poor social (adaptive) abilities, be better served in a class for children defined as "trainable," whereas another child who tests in the moderate range of retardation but who has especially good language abilities may be more stimulated in a class for children defined as "educable." Persons who perform in the severe or profound ranges of MR are also capable of responding to some educational interventions.

The etiology of the central nervous system (CNS) insult resulting in MR may involve genetic disorders, teratogenic influences, perinatal insults, acquired childhood disease, and environmental and social factors (Table 1–25). Although a single organic cause may be found, each individual's performance should be considered a function of the interaction of environmental influences with the individual's organic substrate. Thus it is common for a child with MR to have behavioral difficulties resulting from both the retarding condition itself and the family's reaction to the child and his or her condition. In general, more severe forms of retardation can be traced to biologic factors, and the earlier the cognitive slowing is recognized, the more severe the deviation from normal is likely to be. The pattern of an individual's development can aid in making a diagnosis, but at any given point in time it may be quite difficult to predict future performance accurately.

In approaching to the diagnosis of MR, the first step is to provide interdisciplinary evaluations to identify functional strengths and weaknesses. Expertise from several disciplines is needed to characterize the child functionally for purposes of medical and habilitative therapies (see earlier topics of Interdisciplinary Team Assessment and Intervention). Once the developmental lags have been identified, the history and physical examination may suggest the point in development at which a CNS insult may have taken place and minimize the need for laboratory tests. Almost one third of individuals with mental retardation do not have readily identifiable reasons for their disability. However, in many cases enough factors can be ruled out to allay the guilt and anxiety of families about their responsibility in causing the disability. With advances in genetic diagnosis and the completion of the Human Genome Project, more genetic etiologies will be possible in coming years.

TABLE 1–24
Levels of Mental Retardation

Level of Retardation	Stanford-Binet IQ Score	WISC-III IQ Score	Educational Label
Mild	67–52	70–55	"Educable (EMR)"
Moderate	51–36	54–40	"Trainable (TMR)"
Severe	35–20	39–25	
Profound	Below 20	Below 24	Severe-profound

IQ, Intelligence quotient; *WISC-III,* Wechsler Intelligence Scale for children (ed 3).

TABLE 1–25
Mechanisms of Developmental Disabilities*

Disorder	Total in Group with Mental Retardation (%)
Hereditary disorders: preconceptual origin, variable expression, multiple somatic effects, frequently a progressive course	5
Inborn errors of metabolism (e.g., Tay-Sachs disease, Hurler disease, and phenylketonuria)	
Other single gene abnormalities (e.g., muscular dystrophy, neurofibromatosis, and tuberous sclerosis)	
Chromosomal aberrations, including translocation and fragile X syndrome	
Polygenic familial syndromes	
Early alterations of embryonic development: sporadic events affecting embryogenesis, phenotypic changes, usually a stable developmental handicap	32
Chromosomal changes, including trisomy (e.g., Down syndrome)	
Prenatal influence syndromes (e.g., intrauterine infections, drugs, alcohol, or unknown	
Other pregnancy problems and perinatal morbidity: impingement on progress of fetus during last two trimesters or on newborn, neurologic abnormalities frequent, handicap stable or occasionally worsening	11
Fetal malnutrition and placental insufficiency	
Perinatal difficulties (e.g., prematurity, hypoxia, and trauma)	
Acquired childhood diseases: acute modification of developmental status, variable potential for functional recovery	4
Infection (e.g., encephalitis, and meningitis)	
Cranial trauma	
Other (e.g., cardiac arrest, drowning, and intoxications)	
Environmental and social problems: dynamic influences, operational throughout development, commonly combined with other handicaps	18
Deprivation	
Parental neurosis, psychosis	
Childhood neurosis	
Childhood psychosis	
Unknown causes: no definite hereditary, gestational, perinatal, acquired, or environmental issues; or else multiple elements present	

Adapted from Crocker AC, Nelson RP: Mental retardation. In Levine MD, Carey WB, Crocker AC, editors: *Developmental-behavioral pediatrics,* ed 2, Philadelphia, 1992, WB Saunders.
*Mental retardation, cerebral palsy, seizure disorders, and sensory handicaps.

REFERENCES

Behrman RE, Kliegman RM, Jenson HB, editors: *Nelson textbook of pediatrics,* ed 16, Philadelphia, 2000, WB Saunders, Chapter 37.

Crocker AC, Nelson RP: Mental retardation. In Levine MD, Carey WB, Crocker AC, editors: *Developmental-behavioral pediatrics,* ed 3, Philadelphia, 1999, WB Saunders.

Liptak GS: The pediatrician's role in caring for the developmentally disabled child, *Pediatr Rev* 17(6):203–210, 1996.

Palmer FB, Capute AJ: Mental retardation, *Pediatr Rev* 15(12):473–479, 1994.

Vision Impairment

Significant visual impairment is a problem in many children. *Partial vision* (defined as visual acuity between 20/70 and 20/200) occurs in 1 in 500 school-children in the United States, with about 35,000 children having visual acuity between 20/200 and total blindness. Legal blindness is defined as distant visual acuity of 20/200 in the better eye or a visual field that subtends an angle not greater than 20°. Although this definition allows for considerable residual vision, such impairment can be a major barrier to optimal educational development.

The most common cause of severe visual impairment in children is retinopathy of prematurity (see Chapter 6). Congenital cataracts caused by a variety of causes occur in 1 of 250 newborn infants and can lead to significant amblyopia. Cataracts are also associated with other ocular abnormalities and developmental disabilities. Optic atrophy, retinal degeneration (Leber congenital amaurosis and retinitis pigmentosa), retinoblastoma, and congenital glaucoma are other common causes of significant visual impairment in childhood.

The *diagnosis* of visual impairment is commonly made when the child is between 4 and 8 months of age. Diagnosis is based on parental suspicions aroused by unusual behavior, such as lack of smiling in response to appropriate stimuli or motor delays in beginning to reach for objects. Fixation and visual tracking behavior can be seen in most children by 6 weeks postterm and by many infants at birth. This behavior can be assessed by moving a brightly colored object or the examiner's face across the visual field of a quiet but alert infant at a distance of 1 foot. The eyes should be examined for red reflexes and pupillary reactions to light, although optical alignment should not be expected until the child is beyond the newborn period. Persistent nystagmus is abnormal at any age. If abnormalities are seen, referral to an ophthalmologist should be made.

The developmental implications of visual impairment are many. Perceptual development is abnormal in terms of body image, and imitative behavior such as smiling is delayed. Delays in mobility may occur in children who are visually impaired from birth, although their postural milestones usually are achieved appropriately. Social bonding with the parents also is limited. Stereotypic behaviors ("blindisms") occur in these children and may at times be self-injurious, requiring intensive behavioral interventions to reduce trauma to eyes, periorbital structures, or other body parts.

Treatment of children with vision impairments is aimed at maximizing available visual skills and developing compensatory methods for individualized education. Classroom settings may be augmented with resource-room assistance to present material in a nonvisual format; some schools consult with an experienced teacher of the blind. Noninclusive programs sometimes are necessary in training for mobility and for individuals with multiple disabilities. Fine motor activity development, listening skills, and Braille reading and writing are intrinsic to successful educational intervention with the child who has severe visual impairment.

REFERENCES

Behrman RE, Kliegman RM, Jenson HB, editors: *Nelson textbook of pediatrics*, ed 16, Philadelphia, 2000, WB Saunders, Chapters 626–640.

Davidson PW, Burns CM: Vision impairment and blindness. In Levine MD, Carey WB, Crocker AC, editors: *Developmental-behavioral pediatrics*, ed 3, Philadelphia, 1999, WB Saunders.

Moller MA: Working with visually impaired children and their families, *Pediatr Clin North Am* 40(4):881–890, 1993.

Repka MX: Common pediatric neuro-ophthalmologic conditions, *Pediatr Clin North Am* 40(4):777–788, 1993.

Hearing Impairment

The clinical significance of hearing loss varies with its type (conductive versus sensorineural), its frequency distribution, and its severity as measured in number of decibels (Table 1–26). The most common *cause* of mild to moderate hearing loss in children is a conduction abnormality caused by acquired middle-ear disease. This abnormality may have significant effect on the development of speech and other aspects of language, particularly if there is chronic fluctuating middle-ear fluid. Sensorineural hearing loss is more common as an etiologic factor as hearing loss becomes more severe. The age of onset of the hearing loss may suggest the etiology as well. Other causes of deafness are congenital infection with rubella or cytomegalovirus, meningitis, birth asphyxia, perinatal complications such as kernicterus, ototoxic drugs such as aminoglycoside antibiotics, and tumors and their treatments. Genetic deafness may be either dominant or recessive in inheritance pattern; this is the main cause of hearing impairment in schools for the deaf. In Down syndrome there is a predisposition to both conductive loss caused by middle-ear infection and sensorineural loss caused by cochlear disease.

Screening of children who are at risk may allow early appropriate intervention. Hearing can be screened by means of an office audiogram, but other techniques are needed (e.g., auditory evoked brainstem potential or otoacoustic emission testing) for the young, neurologically immature or impaired, behaviorally difficult, or severely cognitively impaired child. The typical audiologic *assessment* includes pure-tone audiometry over a variety of sound frequencies (pitches), especially over the range of frequencies in which most speech takes place. The response to actual speech at various volumes (decibel levels) is also tested. Tympanometry is used in the assessment of middle ear function and the evaluation of tympanic membrane compliance for pathology in the middle ear, such as fluid, ossicular dysfunction, and eustachian tube dysfunction. For the young infant or less cooperative child who nevertheless can consistently turn his or her eyes to sound stimuli, pure-tone and speech audiometry can be done in a sound field, with and without masking of one ear at a time. A list of indications for referral is shown in Table 1–8.

Treatment of hearing impairment may be medical or surgical. The audiologist may believe that amplification is indicated, in which case hearing aids can be tuned to preferentially amplify the frequency

TABLE 1–26
Neurodevelopmental-Behavioral Complications of Hearing Loss

Severity of Hearing Loss	Possible Etiologic Origins	Complications			Types of Therapy
		Speech-Language	Educational	Behavioral	
Slight 15–25 db (ASA)	Serous otitis media Perforation of tympanic membrane Sensorineural loss Tympanosclerosis	Difficulty with distant or faint speech	Possible auditory learning dysfunction May reveal a slight verbal deficit	Usually none	May require favorable class setting, speech therapy, or auditory training Possible value in hearing aid
Mild 25–40 dB (ASA)	Serous otitis media Perforation of tympanic membrane Sensorineural loss Tympanosclerosis	Difficulty with conversational speech over 3–5 feet May have limited vocabulary and speech disorders	May miss 50% of class discussions Auditory learning dysfunction	Psychologic problems May act inappropriately if directions are not heard well Acting out behavior Poor self-concept	Special education resource help Hearing aid Favorable class setting Lip reading instruction Speech therapy
Moderate 40–65 dB (ASA)	Chronic otitis media Middle ear anomaly Sensorineural loss	Conversation must be loud to be understood Defective speech Deficient language use and comprehension	Learning disability Difficulty with group learning or discussion Auditory processing dysfunction Limited vocabulary	Emotional and social problems Behavioral reactions of childhood Acting out Poor self-concept	Special education resource or special class Special help in speech-language development Hearing aid and lip reading Speech therapy
Severe 65–95 dB (ASA)	Sensorineural loss Middle ear disease	Loud voices may be heard 2 ft from ear Identification of environmental sounds Defective speech and language No spontaneous speech development if loss present before 1 yr	Marked educational retardation Marked learning disability Limited vocabulary	Emotional and social problems that are associated with handicap Poor self-concept	Full-time special education for deaf children Hearing aid, lip reading, speech therapy Auditory training Counseling Cochlear implant
Profound 95 dB or more (ASA)	Sensorineural or mixed loss	Relies on vision rather than hearing Defective speech and language Speech and language will not develop spontaneously if loss present before 1 yr	Marked learning disability because of lack of understanding of speech	Congenital and prelingually deaf may show severe emotional problems	As above Oral and manual communication Counseling

From Gottleib MI: Otitis media. In Levine MD, Carey WB, Crocker AC, et al, editors: *Developmental-behavioral pediatrics*, Philadelphia, 1983, WB Saunders. *ASA,* Acoustical Society of America; *dB,* decibel.

ranges in which the patient has decreased acuity. Educational intervention typically includes speech-language therapy and manual communication. For some children with significant language impairment, manual communication may be used as an adjunct to aid in language concept formation (Total Communication), even in the absence of severe hearing impairment. Even with amplification, many hearing-impaired children demonstrate deficits in processing information presented through the auditory pathway, requiring special educational services for help in reading and other academic skills. Cochlear implants may benefit some children, but they remain controversial within the deaf culture community.

Speech and Language Impairment

Among the most common and difficult developmental problems is the child with speech delay. The most common causes are MR, hearing impairment, social deprivation, autism, and oral-motor abnormalities. If a problem is suspected based on screening with tests such as the Denver Developmental Screening Test (Denver II) or the Early Language Milestone Scale, a referral to a specialized hearing and speech center should be arranged.

Language development may be characterized by progress in both receptive and expressive areas of auditory and visual functioning. Simply assessing speech quality, although important, does not suffice for identification of significant language impairments. A child with severe motor impairments may, for example, have speech delays but have normal auditory reception and understanding, whereas a deaf child may lack the capability of speech and be unresponsive to auditory stimuli but have excellent communication abilities via the visual pathway (Table 1–27).

REFERENCES

Behrman RE, Kliegman RM, Jenson HB, editors: *Nelson textbook of pediatrics*, ed 16, Philadelphia, 2000, WB Saunders, Chapters 10, 11, 16, 29, 643, 644.
Coplan J: Normal speech and language development: an overview, *Pediatr Rev* 16(3):91–100, 1995.
Kelly DP: Hearing impairment. In Levine MD, Carey WB, Crocker AC, editors: *Developmental-behavioral pediatrics*, ed 3, Philadelphia, 1999, WB Saunders.
Kelly DP, Sally JI: Disorders of speech and language. In Levine MD, Carey WB, Crocker AC, editors: *Developmental-behavioral pediatrics*, ed 3, Philadelphia, 1999, WB Saunders.

Cerebral Palsy

The term cerebral palsy (CP) includes a variety of nondegenerating neurologic disabilities caused by abnormal CNS development, as well as injuries in the prenatal, perinatal, and early postpartum period that result in abnormalities of motor function. The live-birth prevalence rate is approximately 2.5:1000. Since the advent of neonatal intensive care units, prematurely born children with very low birth weight (those weighing less than 1500 g) have come to represent nearly half of the childhood cases of CP. Approximately one third of children with CP have epilepsy, and 30–70% have significant cognitive impairments.

Risk factors associated with CP are presented in Table 1–28. These are based on epidemiologic studies and often do not establish the cause of CP for the individual child. Nearly 50% of children with CP have no identifiable risk factors.

Two classification systems are used to describe the clinical manifestations of CP. *Classification by physiologic type* identifies forms of motor impairments, including abnormalities of movement and abnormalities of muscle tone. *Classification by distribution* identifies the location of musculoskeletal involvement.

Classification by Physiologic Type

Spastic cerebral palsy is the most common form of CP, occurring in 70–80% of individuals with CP. It results from injury to the upper motor neurons of the pyramidal tract. Children with this form of CP often exhibit truncal hypotonia in the first year of life. Spasticity, which is a velocity-dependent resistance to stretch, becomes apparent in the second year of life and is typically associated with increased deep tendon reflexes and clonus.

Dyskinetic cerebral palsy occurs in 10–15% of individuals with CP. It is characterized by variable tonal abnormalities that involve the whole body. Involuntary movements are also present. Athetosis is an involuntary writhing movement, often also associated with involuntary jerky movements called chorea. This form of CP is the result of injury to the basal ganglia and is classically associated with kernicterus. It has become less common with aggressive management of neonatal hyperbilirubinemia. There are fewer seizures and more normal cognitive function than in other forms of CP, although hearing impairment is more common and motor-speech disorders may mimic retardation.

Ataxic cerebral palsy accounts for less than 5% of CP cases. This rare form of CP results from cerebellar injury. It is characterized by abnormalities of voluntary movement and balance. Children with ataxic CP have a wide-based, unsteady gait and often also have abnormalities of muscle tone.

Mixed cerebral palsy (10–15% of all cases) is a term that is used when more than one type of motor

TABLE 1–27
Language Disorders, Evaluative Techniques, and Interventions

Disorder	Etiology	Evaluation	Treatment
Disorders of Resonance			
Hypernasality	Increased air through nose because of incompetent velopharyngeal seal	Examine for clefts (open or submucous)	ENT, dental evaluation Functional therapy
Hyponasality	Decreased air through nose because of mucosal or lymphoid obstruction of nasal passage	Look in nose for edema Look for tonsillar or adenoidal hypertrophy	ENT evaluation Speech therapy not indicated
Disorders of Voice			
Abnormality of voice quality, pitch, or loudness	Vocal nodules Voice misuse Prolonged endotracheal intubation Neuropathy Nonmalignant tumors Laryngeal trauma Anxiety	History and physical Listen to and describe voice quality Laryngoscopy, direct and indirect	Voice therapy Surgical intervention, when needed Antihistaminic medications for allergy
Disorders of Fluency			
Stuttering	Normal development Response to anxiety Neurogenic (aphasic disorders)	History from family Speech observation Speech pathology evaluation in presence of severe stutter, attempts to hide behavior, avoidance of speaking, or muscle tension	Observation in mild cases Speech therapy referral in moderate-severe cases Psychologic evaluation if emotional stressors present Decrease stress of speaking, slow pace of conversation
Disorders of Receptive/Expressive Language			
Auditory attention Auditory discrimination Narrative organization Syntax abnormalities Vocabulary problems Word-finding problems	Hearing loss Neurogenic causes Unknown (functional problem in isolation) Social/cultural factors	General: History and physical Oral examination Speech pathology evaluation	Speech therapy

ENT, Ear, nose, and throat.

TABLE 1–28
Risk Factors for Cerebral Palsy in Populations

Before Pregnancy
History of fetal wastage
Long menstrual cycles
Maternal thyroid disorder
Family history of mental retardation

During Pregnancy
Low socioeconomic status
Treatment of mother with thyroid hormone, estrogen, or progesterone
Maternal seizure disorder
Polyhydramnios
Eclampsia
Bleeding in third trimester
Twin gestation
Congenital malformation
Fetal growth retardation
Abnormal fetal presentation

During Labor and Delivery
Premature separation of the placenta

During the Early Postnatal Period
Newborn encephalopathy

Adapted from Kuban KCK, Leviton A: *N Engl J Med* 330(3): 188–195, 1994.

pattern is present and when one pattern does not clearly dominate another. It is typically associated with more complications, including sensory deficits, seizures, and cognitive-perceptual impairments.

Classification by Distribution

Dyskinetic and ataxic CP typically present with total body involvement, whereas spastic cerebral palsy often presents with limited regional involvement.

Spastic diplegia (25–35% of individuals with CP) involves the lower extremities and typically occurs in low-birth-weight infants. It is related to cerebral asphyxia, with or without intraventricular hemorrhage from the immature germinal matrix. Seizures may be present along with other impairments such as learning disabilities and language problems. Severe MR is less common than in other forms of CP. Hip, knee, and ankle contractures can interfere with ambulation.

Spastic quadriplegia (40–45%) involves all four extremities. It is associated with low birth weight and severe asphyxia and can result in MR, seizures,

feeding difficulties, scoliosis, and other orthopaedic problems.

Spastic hemiplegia (25–40%) is associated with the situations just described but also may be caused by cerebrovascular insults, such as embolic phenomena or vascular malformations. Seizures are common, but cognitive function may be spared because only one side of the brain is involved. Motor impairments and language processing difficulties can be significant.

Prognosis in CP depends on the individual's spectrum of disability and on the type and intensity of habilitative intervention.

Treatment depends on the pattern of dysfunction that is present. Physical and occupational therapy can facilitate optimal positioning and movement patterns, increasing function of the affected parts. Spasticity management may also include oral medications, botulinum toxin injections, and implantation of intrathecal baclofen pumps. Management of seizures, spasticity, orthopedic impairments, and sensory impairments all help provide optimal educational stimulation. Family support is essential to allow emotional growth.

REFERENCES

Behrman RE, Kliegman RM, Jenson HB, editors: *Nelson textbook of pediatrics*, ed 16, Philadelphia, 2000, WB Saunders, Chapter 607.
Dormans JP, Pellegrino L: *Caring for children with cerebral palsy: a team approach*, Baltimore, Md, 1998, Brookes Publishing.
Kuban KCK, Leviton A: Medical progress: cerebral palsy, *N Engl J Med* 330(3):188–195, 1994.

School Dysfunction

The inability to function normally in school may be caused by a variety of problems (Table 1–29). This dysfunction may itself result in somatic complaints such as headache, abdominal pains, sleep disorders, and other problems. Learning disabilities and the attention deficit disorders are particularly important causes of school dysfunction that are discussed here.

Learning Disabilities

Learning disabilities occur in 5–15% of school-aged children. Parents may become aware of behavioral difficulties that may interfere with learning in the preschool years when a child demonstrates hyperactivity and inattention, but usually learning disabilities do not become evident until the child enters the primary grades. Teachers in the primary grades may identify weaknesses in specific areas of school performance or behavior that interfere with learning. The physician may be asked to evaluate the child for evidence of neurologic impairment or other medical illness.

TABLE 1–29
Causes of School Dysfunction

Systemic medical illness
Learning disability
Medication effects (e.g., chronic administration of
    bronchodilators, anticonvulsants, decongestants,
    and drug abuse)
Anxiety caused by social and emotional factors (e.g.,
    child abuse or neglect, sexual abuse, and parental
    divorce)
Sensory impairments
Classroom-student mismatch (e.g., language barriers,
    classwork too simple, or classwork too hard)
Conduct disorder
Attention-deficit/hyperactivity disorder
Occult seizure activity
Environmental toxins (e.g., lead poisoning)
Sleep disorders

Vision and hearing should be screened, but they are usually normal. In an extended neurologic examination, markers of neurologic immaturity ("soft signs") and gross and fine motor incoordination may be observed. These findings are physical concomitants that suggest that many learning disabilities are neurologically based at some level; the findings should be used only in conjunction with other tests to describe the child's strengths and weaknesses. They are not predictive of learning disorders because they may occur in the absence of educational disability. An expanded neurodevelopmental examination can better describe skills, whereas specialized psychoeducational testing must be done to characterize particular learning disabilities.

Attention-Deficit/Hyperactivity Disorder

The diagnosis of attention-deficit/hyperactivity disorder (AD/HD) is based on the presence of a complex of behaviors that characterize the child as inattentive, easily distracted, overactive, and impulsive to such an extent that his or her behavior interferes with the ability to function socially and academically. Restlessness and fidgeting (hyperactivity) are common but not essential concomitants of this syndrome. Current classifications include the predominantly impulsive-overactive type (more common in boys), the predominantly inattentive type, and mixed combination forms. Specific learning disabilities also are commonly associated, and some children may display aggressive or oppositional behavior.

The *clinical manifestations* of AD/HD usually are obvious to teachers. Inattentiveness is demonstrated by failure to complete tasks once begun, failure to grasp directions, and making errors through inattention rather than lack of understanding of the material presented. Impulsivity refers to the child's difficulty in controlling reactions and responses when he or she faces uncertainty or the need to attend carefully. Impulsive children commonly act without thinking, shifting quickly from one activity to another, and often exhibit the right behavior at the wrong time, such as calling out in class with an inappropriate answer. They often get into trouble with their peers because they seem socially inept. Distractibility presents as a reaction to environmental noises or visual stimuli that others can ignore. Distractible children also may be distracted by their own bodies, clothing, or other objects (e.g., touching clothes or hair or running their hands over furniture or walls).

Overactivity, although the most noticeable feature of AD/HD, is not uniformly present. Children with AD/HD commonly can be observed swinging their legs, rocking their bodies, tapping fingers, or making odd noises. In more obvious cases they may be in near-constant motion, darting around the room and often ignoring their own or others' safety. The male-to-female ratio in overactivity is 4:1. Girls more typically demonstrate inattention but without hyperactivity.

The physical examination findings typically are normal, although there may be a suggestion of neurologic immaturity. Cranial imaging and electroencephalographic examination are not beneficial in diagnosing or treating AD/HD or other forms of school dysfunction. They should be performed only when seizures or focal neurologic findings are suggested by history and physical examination.

Some infants and preschool children who are later characterized as having AD/HD are colicky, irritable, and occasionally more active than their peers, spending a shorter time than normal playing with a given toy and requiring more supervision than other children.

As the child with AD/HD ages, neurologic maturation may result in symptomatic improvement. However, adolescents who have had AD/HD in their early school years often continue to demonstrate school dysfunction, low self-esteem, and social inappropriateness, and many benefit from ongoing medical treatment.

Primary *treatment* of the child with AD/HD combines pharmacologic and environmental interventions. However, such management is often complicated by the presence of associated learning disabilities that require specific educational interventions. Moreover, many such children have developed emotional reactions to what may be years of social inappropriateness and school dysfunction, and both family behavior patterns and the child's psychologic reactions must be assessed to avoid continuation of undesirable stereotyping. The beneficial effects of medication decrease significantly in the presence of unaddressed emotional or educational needs.

The drugs most commonly used in treating AD/HD are presented in Table 1–30. They are presumed to have their neuropharmacologic effects on dopaminergic neurons in the brainstem reticular activating system. Such psychostimulants are most effective when used in conjunction with behavior modification techniques. Major side effects of these drugs are sleep and appetite impairment, elevation of pulse rate and blood pressure, rebound overactivity, irritability on withdrawal of the medication, and attentional overfocusing. Motor tics may be exacerbated by these drugs. The child should play an active role in decisions about medications in terms of administration and monitoring the effect of the drug, both to give the child a measure of control in managing his or her problem and to prevent noncompliance.

There are no significant beneficial effects of specific dietary interventions in children with AD/HD or other forms of school dysfunction.

REFERENCES

Behrman RE, Kliegman RM, Jenson HB, editors: *Nelson textbook of pediatrics,* ed 16, Philadelphia, 2000, WB Saunders, Chapter 29.

Committee on Quality Improvement, Subcommittee on Attention-Deficit/Hyperactivity Disorder, American Academy of Pediatrics: Clinical practice guideline: diagnosis and evaluation of the child with attention-deficit/hyperactivity disorder, *Pediatrics* 105(5):1158–1170, 2000.

Diagnostic and statistical manual of mental disorders: DSM-IV, ed 4, Washington, DC, 1994, American Psychiatric Association.

Levine MD, Carey WB, Crocker AC, editors: *Developmental-behavioral pediatrics,* ed 3, Philadelphia, 1999, WB Saunders.

Children With Special Health Care Needs

"Children with special health care needs" is an umbrella term that includes children with disabilities (e.g., CP or spina bifida), children with chronic illnesses (e.g., diabetes, AIDS, or asthma), children with congenital defects (e.g., cleft lip and palate or congenital heart defect), and children with health-related educational and behavior problems (e.g., AD/HD or a learning disability). With the exception of asthma, most of these conditions are rare. Yet many of these children share a broad group of experiences and encounter similar problems, such as school difficulties and family stress. The phrase "children with special health care needs" defines these children noncategorically, without regard to specific diagnoses, in terms of increased service needs. It is estimated that 18% of U.S. children younger than 18 have special health care needs, defined as a physical, developmental, behavioral, or emotional condition requiring health and related services of a type or amount beyond that required by children generally. If the definition of chronic illness is restricted to a condition that lasts or is expected to last more than 3 months and limits age-appropriate social functioning such as school performance or recreational activities, about 6% of U.S. children are affected. Approximately 0.1% of U.S. children are limited in activities of daily living such as feeding and bathing.

The goal in managing children with special health care needs is to maximize the children's potential for productive adult functioning by treating the primary diagnosis and by helping the patient and family deal with the stresses incurred because of the disease or disability. Factors that influence responses to chronic conditions include disease-related factors (e.g., pain, treatment, and visibility of condition), age of onset, age and developmental level of the child, and family attitudes and stress.

Whenever a chronic disease is diagnosed, family members typically go through grieving processes similar to those seen at the time of death, including anger, denial, negotiation in an attempt to forestall the inevitable, and depression. However, because the child with special health care needs is a constant reminder of the object of this grief, it may take family members a long time to accept the condition. An understanding and supportive physician can facilitate this process by sharing both the known and the unknown and by allaying guilty feelings and fear. To minimize denial, it is helpful to confirm the family's observations about the child. Once the diagnosis has been presented, the family may not be able to absorb any additional information, so written material and the option for further discussion at a later date should be offered.

The primary pediatrician must provide a "medical home" to maintain close oversight of treatments and subspecialty services, provide preventive care, and facilitate interactions with school and community agencies. The pediatrician must also recognize that the family is the one constant in a child's life, whereas service systems and support personnel within those systems fluctuate. A major goal of "family-centered care" is that the family and child feel in control of the situation. Although the medical management team typically directs treatment in the acute health care setting, the locus of control should shift to the family as the child moves into a more routine, home-based life. Treatment plans should be organized to allow the greatest degree of normalization of the child's

TABLE 1–30
Stimulant Medications for Attention-Deficit–Hyperactivity Disorders

Medication	Dose Schedule	Range	Onset and Duration	Potential Side Effects and Cautions
Methylphenidate (MPH)				
Ritalin or generic 5-, 10-, or 20-mg tablets	Initial: 5 mg or 0.3 mg/kg/dose Increase: 2.5–5 mg weekly Frequency: 2–3 doses/d	5–80 mg/d 0.3–0.8 mg/kg per dose	Onset: 20–30 min Duration: 3–5 hr	Anorexia, insomnia, stomach aches, headaches, irritability, "rebound," flattened affect, social withdrawal, weepiness, tics, weight loss, reduced growth velocity
Ritalin SR or generic 10- or 20-mg sustained-release tablets only	Initial: 20 mg Increase: 20 mg Frequency: 1 or 2 doses/day; sometimes combined with regular in morning	20–80 mg/d 0.6–2 mg/kg per dose	Onset: 60–90 min Duration 5–8 hr	Same as regular MPH; may release unevenly Do not chew or cut in half 20 mg SR may be equivalent to 12–15 mg regular released over 5–8 hr
Concerta 18-, 36-, or 54-mg sustained-release tablets	Initial: 18 mg in AM Increase: 18 mg Frequency: 1 dose in AM	18–56 mg/day 0.6–2.5 mg/kg/dose	Onset: 20–30 min Duration: 8–12 hr	Same as regular MPH Do not chew or cut Depleted tablets may pass in stool
Dextroamphetamine (DEX)				
Dexedrine 5-mg tablets Dextrostat 5, 10-mg tablets Elixir no longer available	Initial: 2.5–5 mg (0.15 mg/kg per dose) Increase: 2.5–5 mg weekly Frequency: 1–2 doses/d	5–40 mg/d 0.3–0.8 mg/kg per dose	Onset: 60–90 min Duration: 6–10 hr	Anorexia, insomnia, stomach aches, headaches, irritability, "rebound," tics, sterotypies, weight loss, reduced growth velocity Avoid decongestants Monitor height, weight, blood pressure, and pulse
Dexedrine Spansules 5-, 10-, 15-mg capsules No generic available	Initial: 5 mg in AM (0.3 mg/kg/dose) Increase: 5 mg weekly Frequency: 1–2 doses/d	5–40 mg/d 0.3–0.8 mg/kg per dose	Onset: 60–90 min Duration: 6–10 hr	Anorexia, insomnia, stomach aches, headaches, irritability, social withdrawal, weepiness, stereotypies, tics, weight loss, reduced growth velocity Avoid decongestants Monitor height, weight, blood pressure, and pulse
Mixed Amphetamine Salts				
Adderall 5-, 7.5-, 10-, 12.5-, 15-, 20-, 30-mg tablets (limited data available)	Initial: 2.5–5 mg in AM Increase: 2.5–5 mg weekly Frequency: 1–2	2.5–40 mg/d	Onset: 30 min Duration: 5–7 hr	Presumed to be similar to dextroamphetamine Appears to be better tolerated by some

Used with permission of Karen J. Miller, MD (2001).
Medications approved by the Food and Drug Administration for use in children with AD/HD.

TABLE 1–31
Predictable Crises and Stress in the Medical Course of Chronic Disease

Onset and diagnosis
Disease-specific, emotionally distressing medical symptoms
Hospitalization(s)
Response to appearance of initial major complication
Confrontation with significant therapeutic choices
Failure(s) of an expected therapeutic response
Threat of imminent death
Unpredictable complications

From Hamburg BA: Chronic illness. In Levine MD, Carey WB, Crocker AC, et al, editors: *Developmental-behavioral pediatrics*, Philadelphia, 1983, WB Saunders.

---

life. As the child matures, self-management programs that provide health education, self-efficacy skills, and practical techniques such as symptom monitoring help promote good long-term health habits. These programs should be introduced at age 6 or 7, or when a child is at a developmental level to take on chores and benefit from being given responsibility. Self-management minimizes "learned helplessness" and "vulnerable child syndrome," both of which occur commonly in families with chronically ill or disabled children. The pediatrician should also be aware of predictable times in the course of a chronic illness when family stress is greatest (Table 1–31). A proactive approach is essential to providing chronic health care services.

REFERENCES

Behrman RE, Kliegman RM, Jenson HB, editors: *Nelson textbook of pediatrics*, ed 16, Philadelphia, 2000, WB Saunders, Chapter 37.
Liptak GS, Weitzman M: Children with chronic conditions need your help at school, *Contemp Pediatr* 12(9):64–80, 1995.
Nichols RE, Desch LW: *The physician's guide to caring for children with disabilities and chronic conditions*, Baltimore, Md, 2000, Brookes Publishing.

Autism and Psychoses in Childhood

Autism and childhood psychosis may have a distinctive early onset in infancy and preschool years or an adult-like presentation in older children.

Autism spectrum conditions are clinical disorders of a variety of causes and variable prognoses that usually are characterized by significant impairment of the child's ability to relate to people, including parents. They affect 0.7–4.5:10,000 children. *Clinical manifestations* typically include that, as an infant, the autistic child was noticeably "uncuddly," with delayed or absent smiling. Later the young child may spend hours in solitary play and be withdrawn in the presence of other children or adults and indifferent to attempts to communicate. Intense, absorbing interests, ritualistic behavior, and compulsive routines are characteristic, and disruption of these may invoke tantrum or rage reactions. Eye contact is abnormal or absent. Head banging, teeth grinding, rocking, diminished responsiveness to pain and external stimuli, and even self-mutilation may be noted. Speech often is delayed; when present, it is frequently dominated by echolalia, pronoun reversal, nonsense rhyming, and other unusual language forms. The child's IQ is difficult to evaluate because of language and socialization deficits and often falls in the functional retarded range by conventional testing. Some children with autism spectrum disorders show remarkable isolated abilities (savant skills). Suspicion of this diagnosis requires referral to a specialist for further evaluation and treatment. Higher measured intelligence and the presence of meaningful language by the age of 5 years are favorable prognostic indicators. Early intensive intervention may dramatically improve outcomes. A relationship between autism and schizophrenia has been suspected, but these children rarely go on to develop classic schizophrenic symptoms.

The onset of *affective psychosis* and *schizophrenia* in older children resembles that in adults. The same diagnostic criteria are applied but must be interpreted in terms of the developmental stage of the child. Long-term psychiatric care often is required for these chronic disorders.

REFERENCES

Bauer S: Autism and the pervasive developmental disorders: part 1, *Pediatr Rev* 16(4):130–136, 1995.
Bauer S: Autism and the pervasive developmental disorders: part 2, *Pediatr Rev* 16(5):168–176, 1995.
Behrman RE, Kliegman RM, Jenson HB, editors: *Nelson textbook of pediatrics*, ed 16, Philadelphia, 2000, WB Saunders, Chapters 18–28.
Brent D, Rabinovich H, Birmaher B, et al: Major psychiatric disorders in childhood and adolescence. In Levine MD, Carey WB, Crocker AC, editors: *Developmental-behavioral pediatrics*, ed 3, Philadelphia, 1999, WB Saunders.
Teplin SW: Autism and related disorders. In Levine MD, Carey WB, Crocker AC, editors: *Developmental-behavioral pediatrics*, ed 3, Philadelphia, 1999, WB Saunders.

CHAPTER 2

Pediatric Nutrition and Nutritional Disorders

Andrew M. Tershakovec ▼ Virginia A. Stallings

Proper nutrition is central in promoting the normal growth and development of children. Rapidly growing infants, children, and maturing adolescents have specific but not necessarily fixed requirements for macronutrients (protein, fat, carbohydrates, and fluids) and micronutrients (vitamins, trace elements, and minerals). Pathophysiologic mechanisms that are present during various disease states may adversely affect nutritional status, retarding growth and development even in the presence of normal recommended intakes of both macronutrients and micronutrients. Diseases associated with inflammation (e.g., infectious diseases, systemic lupus erythematosus, and inflammatory bowel disease), with trauma such as fractures and burns, with malignancy, with malabsorption (e.g., cystic fibrosis, celiac disease, and sprue), with inborn errors of metabolism (e.g., galactosemia and maple syrup urine disease), and with chronic cardiopulmonary insufficiency (heart failure, bronchopulmonary dysplasia) place additional stress on nutritional balance, may alter energy and nutrient needs, and thus may require nutrient supplementation or special diets (Fig. 2–1). These diseases may limit the genetic potential and may even modify the eventual expression of growth.

Nutritional disorders are not confined to children living in areas of famine and starvation. Deficiencies and excesses of nutrient intake are common problems among infants and children in the United States at all income levels, as evidenced by the continued existence of iron deficiency anemia and the increasing rate of childhood obesity, respectively. Furthermore, specific nutritional deficiency syndromes are relatively common among low-weight infants, children with malabsorption (syndromes such as cystic fibrosis, short bowel syndrome, and cholestatic jaundice), breast-fed infants of strict vegetarian parents, and acutely or chronically ill hospitalized children with multiorgan system dysfunction necessitating intensive care.

BODY COMPOSITION AND GROWTH

Nutrition plays a central role in growth and the changing body composition. Growth and maturation begin at the moment of conception and cease with the end of puberty. Prenatal growth is part of a continuous developmental and genetic process modified by maternal variables. During postnatal growth this process is also dependent on familial, socioeconomic, and environmental factors. The normal growth patterns after birth are shown in Chapter 1, Figs. 1–2 to 1–19. The velocity (rate of change) of body mass and length accretion is greater at 32 weeks' gestation (15 kg/yr and 65 cm/yr, respectively) than in any subsequent period, including puberty. Growth in length reflects the differential growth of the head, trunk, and long bones of the legs (see Fig. 1–11). Head size increases most rapidly after 28 weeks of gestation, and growth slows before 2–3 years of age. The trunk increases during the same period but continues to lengthen at a slower rate from 2 years through puberty. The legs grow fastest during the period covering the last 14 weeks of gestation through the first 6 months of life (18 cm/yr). This rate far exceeds that of leg growth in male puberty (4 cm/yr). Linear growth and mass growth are differentially reduced by malnutrition, but both types of growth are increased by obesity. (See Chapters 1 and 17 for measurement of growth.)

Height and weight measurements provide only a crude estimation of body composition. Organ weights increase with maturation; some organs assume a smaller proportion of body mass (such as the

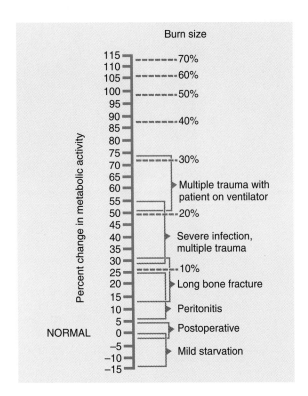

FIG. 2–1

Increased energy needs with stress. (Adapted from Witmore D: *The metabolic management of the critically ill*, New York, 1977, Plenum Publishing. Revised in Walker W, Watkins J, editors: *Nutrition in pediatrics: basic science and clinical application*, Boston, 1985, Little, Brown.)

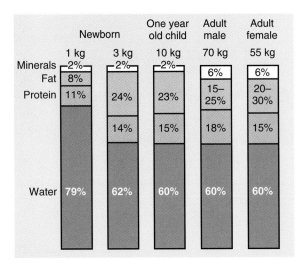

FIG. 2–2

The changes in the proportions of body composition with growth. (Adapted from Pencharz P: Body composition and growth. In Walker W, Watkins J, editors: *Nutrition in pediatrics: basic science and clinical application*, Boston, 1985, Little, Brown.)

brain), whereas muscle and adipose tissue make up an increasing percentage of body mass as the child grows. Little adipose tissue is deposited during early fetal development, but a rapid deposition occurs during the last 3 months of gestation. The body of the term infant contains approximately 20–25% adipose tissue, of which 80% is subcutaneous and 20% visceral. After early infancy, the percentage of fat decreases moderately and is fairly constant until the acceleration during pubertal growth. During puberty, the proportion of fat increases to 20–30% in the average girl (Fig. 2–2). The largest amount tissue of the body is skeletal muscle, which makes up 25% of body mass during fetal life and increases to 45% in the adult. The rate of increase is greatest between birth and 5 years of age, with an additional, small increase in boys at puberty.

Different organ systems develop at different times and rates. Seventy-five percent of brain growth is completed by 3 years of age, and 90% is completed by the age of 7 years; the reproductive system grows little until puberty. The effect of malnutrition on development depends on the stage of development. Because the brain develops early, it is relatively protected from malnutrition in later childhood; delayed puberty is seen in malnourished adolescents.

The embryo contains 95% water, which decreases to 80% at 28 weeks' gestation. During the third trimester, as significant fat (which is anhydrous) is deposited, the proportion of body water decreases further to 72%. By 8 years of age, body water has reached the adult proportion of 60%. The extracellular fluid compartment is substantially greater than the intracellular fluid compartment during fetal life. Before 6 months of age, intracellular fluid increases and extracellular fluid decreases so that the components become equal. This trend continues so that by adulthood the intracellular fluid compartment has twice the volume of the extracellular compartment (Fig. 2–3). The relatively high extracellular fluid volume in the young infant results in a vulnerability to abnormal fluid losses during illness.

The chemical composition of lean body mass (LBM) changes with growth. The concentrations of nitrogen and potassium increase and the concentration of chloride decreases as the relationship between extracellular and intracellular water compartments changes. After the seventh month of gestation, the fall in the level of total extracellular sodium is counterbalanced by an increase in the

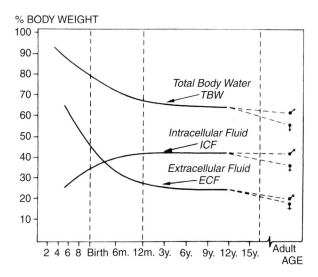

% BODY WEIGHT

FIG. 2–3

Change with age in total body water (TBW) and its major subdivisions. (Data from Friis-Hansen: *Pediatrics* 28:169, 1961; revised in Winter RW, editor: *The body fluids in pediatrics*, Boston, 1973, Little, Brown.)

level of total sodium in bone. Calcium is confined primarily to bone, but phosphorus is an equally important constituent of soft tissues. During the first 2 months of gestation, the phosphorus concentration is greater than that of calcium. Skeletal calcification begins thereafter, and body calcium concentration increases more rapidly than that of phosphorus. At term, 98% of body calcium, 80% of phosphorus, and 60% of magnesium are in bones. During the adolescent growth period, a male accumulates 12 kg of protein, 1.2 kg of calcium, 0.7 kg of phosphorus, 26 g of magnesium, 4 g of iron, and 1.5 g of zinc. These nutrients are accumulated in specific tissues, which cease to grow when they reach a size proportional to the total body length and mass. The genetic coordination of tissue accretion is remarkable, but various dietary deficiencies may limit the rate of growth for any of these growth processes.

Energy and nutrient requirements generally are proportional to LBM; these requirements increase as children grow and attain more LBM. Because women have proportionally more fat mass and less LBM, their requirements usually are less than those of men. For some nutrients, women have equal (vitamin C) or greater (iron) needs than men. To meet the daily recommended intake (DRI), a woman needs to ingest a more nutrient-dense diet than does a man. Thus women are at greater risk for deficiencies of some of those specific nutrients.

DIET OF THE NORMAL INFANT

In the first 6 months of life, human milk or various infant formulas can provide complete nutrition to the growing infant. However, breast milk is the recommended source of nutrition for almost all children. Nonetheless, few infants are exclusively breast-fed beyond 6 months of age. Every effort should be made to encourage and promote breast feeding.

Although infant formulas simulate the composition of human milk, human milk has several subtle nutritional and nonnutritional advantages over infant formula. From a practical point of view, breast milk does not need to be warmed, is ready to serve, does not need a clean water supply, is generally free of microorganisms, and does not need a clean serving container. These issues are significant concerns in less developed areas of the world. Breast feeding also encourages maternal-infant bonding. By limiting the exposure to potential antigens, human milk may reduce the incidence of cow's-milk protein allergy and eczema. Breast milk also contains protective bacterial and viral antibodies (e.g., immunoglobulin A) and macrophages, which helps limit infections. Although the iron content of human milk is relatively low, the iron is more biologically available than that in cow's milk. Human milk also contains lactoferrin, an iron-binding whey protein that inhibits the growth of *Escherichia coli.* In addition, there are other nutrients contained in breast milk that are not present in significant amounts in most formulas (e.g., cholesterol and omega-3 fatty acids), whose function or importance is not well understood. Breast feeding is recommended for children from 6–12 months of age.

The alternative to human milk is iron-fortified formula, which permits adequate growth of most infants. No vitamin or mineral supplements, other than fluoride, are needed with such formulas. Cow's milk should not be introduced until after the first year of life.

After 6 months, solid foods (beikost) and juices are introduced (using these nutrient sources initiates weaning), progressively replacing some of the calories and nutrients provided by human milk or formula. Although the growth rate of the child is decreasing, energy needs for greater activity increase (Fig. 2–4). A relatively high-fat and calorically dense diet (e.g., milk) still is needed to deliver adequate calories. Nutritional supplements, including fortified foods such as iron-fortified cereal, become an important source of some nutrients (e.g., iron) in the second 6 months of life.

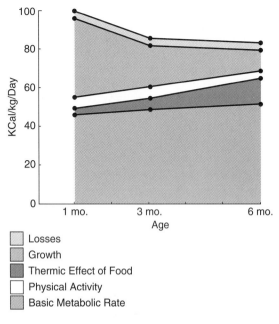

FIG. 2–4

Energy requirements of infants. (From Waterlow JC: Basic concepts in the determination of nutritional requirements of normal infants. In Tsang RC, Nichols BL, editors: *Nutrition during infancy*, Philadelphia, 1988, Hanley & Belfus.)

REFERENCES

American Academy of Pediatrics Committee on Nutrition (1996–1997): *Pediatric nutrition handbook,* ed 4, Elk Grove Village, Ill, 1998, The Academy.

Behrman RE, Kliegman RM, Jenson HB, editors: *Nelson textbook of pediatrics,* ed 16, Philadelphia, 2000, WB Saunders, Chapter 40.

Walker WA, Watkins JB, editors: *Nutrition in pediatrics,* ed 2, Philadelphia, 1997, WB Saunders.

Nutrient Needs

Dietary Reference Intakes (DRI) are estimates for recommended nutrient intakes developed by the Food and Nutrition Board of the Institute of Medicine, National Academy of Sciences. The DRI includes four components: *Recommended Daily Allowance (RDA), Adequate Intake, (AI), Tolerable Upper Intake Level (UL),* and *Estimated Average Requirement* (EAR).

The *RDA* is the average daily dietary intake level that is sufficient to meet the nutrient requirement of nearly all (97–98%) healthy individuals in a particular life stage and gender group. The *AI* is the recommended daily intake value based on observed or experimentally determined approximations of nutrient intake by a group (or groups) of healthy people that are assumed to be adequate. The AI is used when RDA cannot be determined. The *UL* is the highest level of daily nutrient intake that is yet likely to pose no risk of adverse health effects to almost all individuals in the general population. As intake increases above the UL, the risk of adverse effects increases. The *EAR* is a daily nutrient intake value that is estimated to meet the requirement of half of the healthy individuals in a group.

The DRI for children and adults are listed in Table 2–1. Note that the recommendations are age specific and that some are gender specific. The minimum daily requirement (MDR) of a nutrient is set at a level of consumption below which signs of deficiency develop. The RDA (now DRI) is generally 2–6 times the MDR and takes into consideration modifications needed for weight, sex, age, pregnancy, and lactation. The DRI for nutrients usually is two standard deviations above the mean requirement for each food group, whereas it is at the mean for energy requirements. Caloric needs are determined by counting resting energy expenditure plus energy needed for exercise, growth, and the thermic effect of food. More often, caloric needs are estimated by the following rule of thumb: 100 kcal/kg for the first 10 kg, 50 kcal/kg for the next 10–20 kg, and 20 kcal/kg for weight above 20 kg (see Chapter 6); or by the use of World Health Organization (WHO) or other prediction equations and a factor adjusting for such factors as physical activity and stress.

Breast-Feeding

Mothers usually decide before delivery whether to breast-feed or bottle-feed their infants. When they choose breast-feeding, mothers should be assisted to develop appropriate infant feeding skills and practices. The optimal goal is to produce sufficient milk to breast-feed an infant for 6–12 months (see Chapter 6, Table 6–28 for composition of human milk). However, even short-term breast-feeding is probably beneficial.

Beginning Breast-Feeding

The mother should be comfortable and the infant positioned so that nothing interferes with mouth-to-breast contact. The breast from which the infant nurses should be supported with the opposite hand, with the thumb and index finger above the nipple to allow the infant easy access to the nipple. The *rooting reflex* should be explained to the parents to make initiation of breast-feeding easier. The nipple should be stroked against the infant's cheek nearest the nipple. The infant will turn toward the nipple (rooting reflex) and open the mouth, allowing the introduction of the nipple and areola. The entire nipple and most of the areola should be placed in the infant's mouth. The infant "latches on" by compressing the

TABLE 2–1
Food and Nutrition Board, Institute of Medicine—National Academy of Sciences
Dietary Reference Intakes: Recommended Intakes for Individuals

Life Stage Group	Calcium (mg/day)	Phosphorus (mg/day)	Magnesium (mg/day)	Vitamin D (µg/day)*†	Fluoride (mg/day)	Thiamin (mg/day)	Riboflavin (mg/day)	Niacin (mg/day)‡	Vitamin B$_6$ (mg/day)	Folate (µg/day)§	Vitamin B$_{12}$ (µg/day)	Pantothenic Acid (mg/day)	Biotin (pg/day)	Choline (mg/day)‖
Infants														
0–6 mo	210	100	30	5	0.01	0.2	0.3	2	0.1	65	0.4	1.7	5	125
7–12 mo	270	275	75	5	0.5	0.3	0.4	4	0.3	80	0.5	1.8	6	150
Children														
1–3 yr	**500**	**460**	**80**	5	0.7	**0.5**	**0.5**	**6**	**0.5**	**150**	**0.9**	2	8	200
4–8 yr	**800**	**500**	**130**	5	1	**0.6**	**0.6**	**8**	**0.6**	**200**	**1.2**	3	12	250
Males														
9–13 yr	**1300**	**1250**	**240**	5	2	**0.9**	**0.9**	**12**	**1.0**	**300**	**1.8**	4	20	375
14–18 yr	**1300**	**1250**	**410**	5	3	**1.2**	**1.3**	**16**	**1.3**	**400**	**2.4**	5	25	550
19–30 yr	**1000**	**700**	**400**	5	4	**1.2**	**1.3**	**16**	**1.3**	**400**	**2.4**	5	30	550
31–50 yr	**1000**	**700**	**420**	5	4	**1.2**	**1.3**	**16**	**1.3**	**400**	**2.4**	5	30	550
51–70 yr	**1200**	**700**	**420**	10	4	**1.2**	**1.3**	**16**	**1.7**	**400**	**2.4¶**	5	30	550
>70 yr	**1200**	**700**	**420**	15	4	**1.2**	**1.5**	**16**	**1.7**	**400**	**2.4¶**	5	30	550

Note: This table presents recommended dietary allowances (RDAs) in **bold type** and adequate intakes (AIs) in ordinary type. RDAs and AIs may both be used as goals for individual intake. RDAs are set to meet the needs of almost all (97–98%) individuals in a group. For healthy breast-fed infants, the AI is the mean intake. The AI for other life-stage and gender groups is believed to cover needs of all individuals in the group, but lack of data or uncertainty in the data prevents being able to specify with confidence the percentage of individuals covered by this intake.

*As cholecalciferol. 1 pg cholecalciferol = 40 IU vitamin D.

†In the absence of adequate exposure to sunlight.

‡As niacin equivalents (NE). 1 mg of niacin = 60 mg of tryptophan; 0–6 months = preformed niacin (not NE).

§As dietary folate equivalents (DFE). 1 DFE = 1 µg food folate = 0.6 µg of folic acid from fortified food or as a supplement consumed with food = 0.5 µg of a supplement taken on an empty stomach.

‖Although AIs have been set for choline, there are few data to assess whether a dietary supply of choline is needed at all stages of the life cycle, and it may be that the choline requirement can be met by endogenous synthesis at some of these stages.

¶Because 10–30% of older people may malabsorb food-bound B$_{12}$, it is advisable for those older than 50 years to meet their RDA mainly by consuming foods fortified with B$_{12}$ or a supplement containing B$_{12}$.

Continued

TABLE 2–1
Dietary Reference Intakes: Recommended Intakes for Individuals—cont'd

Life Stage Group	Calcium (mg/day)	Phosphorus (mg/day)	Magnesium (mg/day)	Vitamin D (µg/day)*†	Fluoride (mg/day)	Thiamin (mg/day)	Riboflavin (mg/day)	Niacin (mg/day)‡	Vitamin B$_6$ (mg/day)	Folate (µg/day)§	Vitamin B$_{12}$ (µg/day)	Pantothenic Acid (mg/day)	Biotin (pg/day)	Choline (mg/day)‖
Females														
9–13 yr	1300	240	240	5	2	0.9	0.9	12	1.0	300	1.8	4	20	375
14–18 yr	1300	360	360	5	3	1.0	1.0	14	1.2	400#	2.4	5	25	400
19–30 yr	1000	310	310	5	3	1.1	1.1	14	1.3	400#	2.4	5	30	425
31–50 yr	1000	320	320	5	3	1.1	1.1	14	1.3	400#	2.4	5	30	425
51–70 yr	1200	320	320	10	3	1.1	1.1	14	1.5	400	2.4¶	5	30	425
>70 yr	1200	320	320	15	3	1.1	1.1	14	1.5	400	2.4¶	5	30	425
Pregnancy														
≤18 yr	1300	1250	400	5	3	1.4	1.4	18	1.9	600**	2.6	6	30	450
19–30 yr	1000	700	350	5	3	1.4	1.4	18	1.9	600**	2.6	6	30	450
31–50 yr	1000	700	360	5	3	1.4	1.4	18	1.9	600**	2.6	6	30	450
Lactation														
≤18 yr	1300	1250	360	5	3	1.4	1.6	17	2.0	500	2.8	7	35	550
19–30 yr	1000	700	310	5	3	1.4	1.6	17	2.0	500	2.8	7	35	550
31–50 yr	1000	700	320	5	3	1.4	1.6	17	2.0	500	2.8	7	35	550

Note: This table presents recommended dietary allowances (RDAs) in **bold type** and adequate intakes (AIs) in ordinary type. RDAs and AIs may both be used as goals for individual intake. RDAs are set to meet the needs of almost all (97–98%) individuals in a group. For healthy breast-fed infants, the AI is the mean intake. The AI for other life-stage and gender groups is believed to cover needs of all individuals in the group, but lack of data or uncertainty in the data prevents being able to specify with confidence the percentage of individuals covered by this intake.

#In view of evidence linking folate intake with neural-tube defects in the fetus, it is recommended that all women capable of becoming pregnant consume 400 µg from supplements or fortified foods in addition to intake of food folate from a varied diet.

**It is assumed that women will continue consuming 400 µg from supplements or fortified foods until their pregnancy is confirmed and they enter prenatal care, which ordinarily occurs after the end of the periconceptional period—the critical time formation of the neural tube.

lips. The mechanics of normal suckling include: (1) suction of 4–6 cm of the areola, (2) compression of the nipple against the palate, (3) stimulation of milk ejection by initial rapid nonnutritive sucking, and (4) extraction of milk from the lactiferous sinuses by a slower suck-swallow rhythm of approximately one per second. The infant may be removed from the breast by placing a clean finger between the baby's gums and the areola to release suction. The mean feeding frequency during the first 2 weeks is 8–12 times per day.

Exclusive Breast-Feeding

Breast-feeding is the recommended method for feeding normal infants during the first 6 months of life. Alerting the new breast-feeding mothers and their families about possible nursing problems that may arise shortly after hospital discharge may avert many cases of lactation failure. *Colostrum,* a high-protein and low-fat lactose product, is produced in small amounts during the first few postpartum days. It has some nutritional value but primarily has important immunologic and maturational properties. Primiparous women usually experience breast engorgement on the third postpartum day; the breasts become hard and are painful, the nipples become nonprotractile, and the mother's temperature may increase slightly. Enhancement of milk flow is the best management. If severe engorgement occurs, areolar rigidity may prevent the infant from grasping the nipple and areola. Attention to proper latch-on and hand expression of milk assist drainage. The first appetite spurt of the infant is noted at 8–10 days of life in an increase in the demand for nursing, which serves to stimulate the production of a greater volume of milk. The hydration status of the infant is an index of the adequacy of intake. A well-hydrated infant voids 6–8 times a day. Each voiding should soak, not merely moisten, a diaper. Parents should be advised to contact the pediatrician if the infant voids less than 6 times a day. Telephone follow-up is valuable during the interim between discharge and the first pediatric visit in order to monitor the progress of lactation. Initial weight loss in the neonatal period is greater in the breast-fed than in the bottle-fed infant, but birth weight should be regained by 2 weeks of age.

The duration of attempted nursing varies widely. Longer nursing may be an adaptation to inadequate milk production or ineffective latch-on. Most of the milk is consumed in the first few minutes of nursing at each breast. Milk volume increases rapidly during the first 2 weeks after parturition. Women who exclusively breast-feed their infants commonly produce up to 750 mL/day. This level of production declines in response to decreased nursing or other factors.

The characteristics of the stools of breast-fed infants often alarm parents. Stools are unformed; yellow, brown, or green; and seedy in appearance. Parents commonly think their breast-fed baby has diarrhea. Stool frequencies are variable, although breast-fed babies tend to produce stool more frequently than do formula-fed infants.

In the newborn period, elevated concentrations of serum bilirubin are present more often in breast-fed infants than in formula-fed infants. Feeding frequency during the first 3 days of life of breast-fed infants is related inversely to the level of bilirubin; frequent feedings stimulate meconium passage and excretion of bilirubin in the stool. The use of water supplements in breast-fed infants has no effect on serum bilirubin levels. If the concentration of serum bilirubin rises sufficiently to be of clinical concern, formula feedings should be temporarily substituted, which may prevent further increases in bilirubin levels. A temporary discontinuation of breast-feeding for 24–72 hours is of diagnostic value in identifying *breast milk jaundice* (see Chapter 6). Slight elevations in serum bilirubin commonly are observed when breast-feeding is resumed, and a less severe level of jaundice may persist for several weeks. Few detrimental effects of breast milk jaundice have been reported. If temporary formula feeding is introduced, the mother's milk production can be maintained by manual milk expression.

Supplementation

Breast-fed term infants require supplementation with vitamin K (by intramuscular injection) at birth. Oral vitamin D supplements should also be considered, especially for mothers and infants with darker skin pigmentation or limited skin sun exposure. After 6 months of age, fluoride supplements should be started. Iron or iron-fortified formula should be added at 4–6 months of life. Vitamin B_{12} should be provided if the mother is a strict vegan (one who consumes no animal products). Formula and water supplements in addition to breast milk are usually not necessary for term breast-fed infants.

When nursing from an artificial nipple, the infant positions the tongue differently than when breast-feeding. If the infant has difficulty breast-feeding after nursing from a bottle, the mother should make certain that the infant's mouth is positioned well over the areola. Bottle feedings that are introduced before breast-feeding is well established may interfere with the continuation of breast-feeding.

When the mother is physically unable to be present to breast-feed the infant, the mother may express her milk and store it frozen for use by other caregivers. Alternatively, iron-fortified infant formula can be used for infants younger than 12 months of age. However, the mother must continue expressing her breast milk to maintain milk production.

Solid foods may be added to the diet when the child is 6 months old. After 6 months of age, the nutrients often found somewhat lacking in the diet of the exclusively breast-fed infant are likely to be protein, iron, and zinc; total calories may also be lacking. Thus the most appropriate first food to add to the diet of exclusively breast-fed infants may be iron-fortified (rice) cereals.

Common Breast-Feeding Problems

Problems such as breast tenderness, engorgement, and cracked nipples are the most common problems encountered by mothers who are breast-feeding. Meeting with a breast-feeding consultant may help minimize these problems and allow the successful continuation of breast-feeding.

If a lactating woman reports fever, chills, and malaise, *mastitis* should be considered. Treatment includes frequent and complete emptying of the breast. Breast-feeding usually should not be stopped because the mother's mastitis commonly has no adverse effects on the breast-fed infant. Antibiotic therapy (using antibiotics that are safe for the infant) is indicated. Untreated mastitis may progress to a *breast abscess*. If an abscess is diagnosed, breast-feeding should be discontinued from the affected breast until the condition is successfully treated. Milk expression from the affected breast should continue, but the milk should be discarded.

Certain maternal infections, such as active tuberculosis, syphilis, human immunodeficiency virus (HIV), typhoid, rubella, mumps, cytomegalovirus, or localized cutaneous herpesvirus, are contraindications for breast-feeding. When the mother has active tuberculosis or syphilis, restarting breast-feeding may be considered after therapy is initiated.

The mother should be advised against the use of unprescribed drugs, including alcohol, nicotine, caffeine, or "street drugs." No medications (including over-the-counter drugs) should be taken without consulting a physician.

Lactation failure resulting in malnutrition, failure to thrive (FTT), and hypernatremic dehydration is a serious problem that may be caused in part by poor parent education and inadequate follow-up with an infant after discharge from the nursery.

REFERENCES

Behrman RE, Kliegman RM, Jansen HB, editors: *Nelson textbook of pediatrics*, ed 16, Philadelphia, 2000, WB Saunders, Chapter 41.
Joint Food and Agriculture Organization/World Health Organization/United Nations University Expert Consultation: *Energy and protein requirements*, Geneva, 1985, World Health Organization.
Satter E: *Child of mine: feeding with love and good sense*, Palo Alto, Calif, 2000, Bull Publishing.
Schofield WN: Predicting basal metabolic rate: new standards and review of previous work, *Hum Nutr Clin Nutr* 39(Suppl):1–41, 1985.
Standing Committee on the Scientific Evaluation of Dietary Reference Intakes and its Panel on Folate, Other B Vitamins, and Choline and Subcommittee on Upper Reference Levels of Nutrients (Food & Nutrition Board, Institute of Medicine): *Dietary reference intakes for thiamin, riboflavin, niacin, vitamin B_6, folate, vitamin B_{12}, pantothenic acid, biotin, and choline*, Washington, DC, 1998, National Academy Press.
Work Group on Breast Feeding, American Academy of Pediatrics: Breastfeeding and the use of human milk, *Pediatrics* 100(6): 1035–1039, 1997.

Weaning Foods

Substitutes for and supplements to human milk are regarded as weaning foods in this section.

Cow's Milk–Based Formulas

Cow's milk formulas (see Table 6–28) are composed of reconstituted, skimmed cow's milk or a mixture of skimmed cow's milk and electrolyte-depleted cow's milk whey or casein proteins. The fat used in infant formulas is a mixture of vegetable oils, commonly including soy, palm, coconut, corn, oleo, or safflower oils; all contain lactose. Modern cow's milk–based formulas are generally equivalent to human milk in promoting growth during the first 6 months of life, although information suggests formula-fed infants may gain weight slightly more rapidly than breast-fed infants. Complete cow's milk–based infant formulas are used as substitutes for breast milk for infants whose mothers choose not to or cannot breast-feed, as *supplements* for breast-feeding, as supplements for breast-fed infants whose mothers choose to omit occasional feedings, or as *complementary* feedings if breast-feeding alone does not result in normal growth or if other signs of malnutrition are present. Breast milk fortifiers which, when mixed with breast milk, boost the caloric and nutrient content, also are available for use in special situations (as in the premature infant when breast milk's nutrient composition is inadequate for growth).

Soy Formula

Soy protein–based formulas are used if cow's milk–based formula intolerance occurs either from protein hypersensitivity or from lactose intolerance. However, a significant proportion of infants allergic to cow's milk protein are also allergic to soy protein. These formulas are nutritionally sound and safe alternatives to cow's milk–based formulas (see Table 6–28). The soy protein is supplemented with l-methionine to improve its nutritional qualities. The carbohydrate in soy formulas is glucose oligomers (smaller molecular weight corn starches) and sometimes sucrose. The fat mixture is similar to that used in cow's milk formulas.

Soy protein formulas do not prevent the development of allergic disorders in later life, and clinical intolerances to soy milk proteins or cow's milk occur with equal frequency (see Chapter 11). Soy protein formulas can be recommended for use by vegetarian families choosing not to serve animal protein formulas and in the management of galactosemia and primary and secondary lactose intolerance. Although safe for the normal child, soy-based formula has been associated with protein malnutrition in patients with cystic fibrosis and with neonatal rickets in premature infants. Too often, soy and other "special" formulas are used indiscriminately to "treat" poorly evaluated patients with colic, formula intolerance, or more serious diseases.

Premature Infant Formulas

See Chapter 6.

Therapeutic Formulas

The composition of infant formulas has been further modified to meet specific therapeutic requirements (see Table 6–28). Therapeutic formulas designed to prevent digestive insufficiency or protein hypersensitivity contain hydrolyzed casein, whole casein, soy protein, or synthetic-free amino acids as a source of amino acids. These formulas are also lactose free; some contain glucose oligomers and soluble starches, and some contain medium-chain triglycerides. Modular formulas allow stepwise introduction of specific carbohydrates and fats into the diet in a logical sequence for the purpose of therapeutic feeding trials. Modular formulas are nutritionally incomplete, are often hyperosmolar, and should be used only under close, professional supervision. Therapeutic and modular formulas also tend to be very expensive, and thus should be used only when indicated.

Whole Cow's Milk

Whole cow's milk should not be introduced into the diet before the age of 1 year. The high solute load of cow's milk and its low iron content make it inappropriate to use earlier. Cow's milk ingested before the child is 12 months old may cause gross or microscopic intestinal bleeding, leading to iron-deficiency anemia.

Baby Foods

Commercially prepared or homemade foods help fulfill the nutritional needs of the infant older than 6 months. Because infant foods are usually calorically less dense than milk, they do not "fatten up" an infant. Furthermore, oropharyngeal coordination is immature before 3 months, making feeding with solid foods difficult. Vitamin- and mineral-enriched dry cereals are used as a source of calories (approximately 375 calories/100 g), vitamins, and minerals (particularly iron) to supplement the diet of infants whose needs for these nutrients are not met by human milk or formula after 6 months of age. The manufacture of infant dry cereals involves the enzymatic hydrolysis of cereal flour and heat to precook and gelatinize the starches. Cereals are commonly mixed with milk or water, and later with fruits such as bananas and apple sauce. To help identify possible allergies or food intolerances that may arise when new foods are added to the diet, single-grain cereals (e.g., rice, oatmeal, and barley) are recommended as starting cereals. Mixed cereal (oat, corn, wheat, and soy) provides greater variety to older infants. High-protein cereal (soy, oat, wheat) offers the advantages of low cost and high protein in addition to variety.

Pureéd fruits, vegetables, and meats are available in containers that provide an appropriate serving size. Fruit and vegetable juices usually provide a small amount of the total caloric intake of infants; however, some children do develop a habit or are given an inappropriately high level of juice. The juices are strained, homogenized, and supplemented with vitamin C to achieve a uniform nutrient level that is equivalent to that of fresh orange juice. Excessive milk (more than 24 oz/day) or juice intake should be avoided in infants over 1 year of age, because these products may reduce the intake of nutritionally important solid foods or support excessive caloric intake. Foods with high allergic potential that should be avoided during early infancy include fish, peanuts, and egg whites. Hot dogs, grapes, and nuts also present a risk of aspiration and airway obstruction. All foods with the potential to obstruct the young child's airway should be cut into sizes smaller than a young child's main airway.

REFERENCES

Curran JS, Barness LA: The feeding of infants and children. In Behrman RE, Kliegman RM, Jenson HB, editors: *Nelson textbook of pediatrics*, ed 16, Philadelphia, 2000, WB Saunders, Chapter 41.

DIET OF THE NORMAL CHILD AND ADOLESCENT

Nutrient needs for children and adolescents are shown in Table 2–1.

OBESITY

Epidemiology. The prevalence of obesity in children has increased dramatically in the last 2–3 decades. From 1988–1991, 22% of American children were considered overweight (above the 85th percentile). In addition, the prevalence of obesity has

TABLE 2–2
Complications of Obesity

Complication	Effects
Psychosocial	Peer discrimination, teasing, reduced college acceptance, isolation, reduced job promotion*
Growth	Advance bone age, increased height, early menarche
Central nervous system	Pseudotumor cerebri
Respiratory	Sleep apnea, pickwickian syndrome
Cardiovascular	Hypertension, cardiac hypertrophy, ischemic heart disease,* sudden death*
Orthopedic	Slipped capital femoral epiphysis, Blount disease
Metabolic	Insulin resistance, type II diabetes mellitus, hypertriglyceridemia, hypercholesterolemia, gout,* hepatic steatosis, polycystic ovary disease, cholelithiasis

*Complications unusual until adulthood.

increased in children as young as 4–5 years. The largest increases in the prevalence of obesity were seen in the most overweight classifications, and in certain ethnic groups, such as African-American and Mexican-American children.

Many obese children become obese adults. The risk of remaining obese increases with age and the degree of obesity. For example, 11-year-old children who are overweight are more than twice as likely to remain overweight at the age of 15 than are 7-year-old overweight children. The risk of becoming obese as a child and remaining obese as an adult is also influenced by family history. Forty percent of children with one overweight parent become overweight, and 80% of children with two overweight parents become overweight. Only 10% of children with no overweight parents become overweight.

Obesity runs in families; this could be related to genetic influences or the influence of a common, shared environment. Cases of truly "inherited" obesity caused by a simple genetic defect, as demonstrated by individuals who are leptin deficient, are very rare in humans. Other influences of genetics have been addressed in studies of twins. In comparisons of adopted twin pairs, up to 80% of the variance in weight for height or skin fold thickness may be explained on the basis of genetics. A strong relationship exists between the body mass index (BMI) of adoptees and that of their biologic parents; a weaker relationship exists between the BMI of adoptees and that of their adoptive parents. This supports the influence of genetics. However, the association between obesity and television watching and dietary intake, the different rates of obesity observed in urban versus rural areas, and changes in obesity with seasons also support the influence of environment. Furthermore, although genetic influences are associated with obesity, it is difficult to explain the recent epidemic of obesity in the United States purely on genetic grounds.

Clinical Manifestations. Severe complications of obesity in children and adolescents are rare but are more frequently recognized (Table 2–2). For example, the prevalence of pediatric type-2 diabetes has increased 10-fold in a 12-year period. The clinician should direct the history and physical examination toward screening for many potential complications noted among obese patients (Table 2–2) in addition to specific diseases associated with obesity (Table 2–3). During childhood, children develop increasing awareness of body types and generate negative stereotypic attitudes toward obesity; even preschool children will begin to tease and otherwise single out obese children. Medical complications are usually somewhat related to the degree of obesity and usually decrease in severity or resolve with weight reduction.

The diagnosis of obesity is specifically related to the measurement of excess body fat. However, actual measurement of body composition is not practical in most clinical situations. Most clinicians are also not prepared to complete proxy measures of adiposity, such as skinfold thickness. In addition, skinfold thickness measurement may not be accurate with very obese individuals. BMI (weight [kg]/ height [m]^2) has been widely used in adults as a measure of relative weight. In adults, a BMI above 25 is overweight, and a BMI over 30 defines obesity. In children, BMI changes with age; therefore, it is not possible to define a specific BMI cutpoint to define overweight or obesity. Newly released BMI age- and

TABLE 2–3
Diseases Associated With Childhood Obesity*

Syndrome	Manifestations
Alström syndrome	Hypogonadism, retinal degeneration, deafness, diabetes mellitus
Carpenter syndrome	Polydactyly, syndactyly, cranial synostosis, mental retardation
Cushing syndrome	Adrenal hyperplasia or pituitary tumor
Fröhlich syndrome	Hypothalamic tumor
Hyperinsulinism	Nesidioblastosis, pancreatic adenoma, hypoglycemia, Mauriac syndrome (poor diabetic control)
Laurence-Moon-Bardet-Biedl syndrome	Retinal degeneration, syndactyly, hypogonadism, mental retardation; autosomal recessive
Muscular dystrophy	Late onset of obesity
Myelodysplasia	Spina bifida
Prader-Willi syndrome	Neonatal hypotonia, normal growth immediately after birth, small hands and feet, mental retardation, hypogonadism; some have partial deletion of chromosome 15
Pseudohypoparathyroidism	Variable hypocalcemia, cutaneous calcifications
Turner syndrome	Ovarian dysgenesis, lymphedema, web neck; XO chromosome

*These diseases represent fewer than 5% of cases of childhood obesity.

gender-specific percentile curves allow an assessment of BMI percentile. A BMI above the 85th percentile is labeled "at-risk for overweight," and a BMI above the 95th percentile is labeled overweight.

Treatment. Obesity is difficult to treat, and management often includes a combination of education, behavior modification, exercise, and diet. A balanced diet with an approximate 30% decrease in caloric intake (total calories adjusted to body size, but generally 1000–1500 kcal/day) is an appropriate starting point for most obese patients. Because fat is more calorically dense than carbohydrate and protein, dietary fat and thus total calories are reduced; portion size and meal patterns also are modified. More severe dietary restriction, such as the very-low-calorie diet or "protein modified fast," may be needed when a life-threatening complication (e.g., alveolar hypoventilation, sleep apnea, or significant hypertension) is present. Such restrictive diets require close supervision; supplementation with potassium, magnesium, calcium, and multiple vitamins; and the use of high-quality protein sources. Pharmacotherapy is currently not approved for use in children, although clinical trials are ongoing. The cardiac complications associated with the use of phentermine/fenfluramine for weight loss emphasize the need to scrutinize any potential weight loss drug therapy very carefully. Surgical therapy for morbid obesity includes gastric stapling or ileal bypass; this is rarely indicated in children or adolescents.

Prevention. There is no recognized method of prevention, although increasing exercise and decreasing fat intake may be helpful. Despite constant energy intake per unit weight, there are large differences among normal children for rate of fat accumulation. Thus an appropriate level of calories for a given child may be difficult to specify, especially considering the fact that all people, and particularly obese persons, commonly underreport their caloric intake significantly. Dietary and exercise recommendations, therefore, should be based on decreasing the rate of weight gain. Decreasing the rate of weight gain while maintaining an appropriate rate of growth in height is an acceptable goal for children and adolescents in many situations. However, any such interventions must be implemented with care. Some studies suggest that attempts by parents to restrict the child's caloric intake may be counterproductive.

REFERENCES

Barlow SE, Dietz WH: Obesity evaluation and treatment: expert committee recommendations, *Pediatrics* 102(3):e29, 1998.

Curran JS, Barness LA: Obesity. In Behrman RE, Kliegman RM, Jenson HB, editors: *Nelson textbook of pediatrics*, ed 16, Philadelphia, 2000, WB Saunders, Chapter 43.

Hill JO, Trowbridge FL: The causes and health consequences of obesity in children and adolescents, *Pediatrics* 101(3)(March Supplement), 1998.

Whitaker RC, Wright JA, Pepe MS, et al: Predicting obesity in young adulthood from childhood and parental obesity, *N Engl J Med* 337(13)869–873, 1997.

EATING DISORDERS
Anorexia Nervosa

The prevalence of anorexia nervosa has been estimated to be 1–5% in teenage girls. The female-to-male ratio is approximately 20:1, and the condition shows a familial pattern. The cause of anorexia nervosa is unknown.

Clinical Manifestations. The clinical manifestations of weight loss usually begin with moderate efforts to lose weight, which progress to a fear of obesity and a preoccupation with being inappropriately thin (Table 2–4). Predisposing factors include perfectionist behavior, low self-esteem, and in many cases a history of being mildly overweight. A classic feature of anorexia is the person's altered body image. The person may be very thin and undernourished yet describe herself or himself as being fat and needing to lose weight. Any weight gain may generate anxiety, and weight loss reduces this anxiety. Vitamin and nutrient deficiency disorders are relatively rare. Nonetheless, scalp hair loss is common; fine, lanugo-like hair commonly grows on the face and the trunk. The skin may become rough and scaly, which may be a sign of essential fatty acid deficiency.

Two types of dieting prevail: (1) the fasting, abstaining, or restricting type, and (2) the so-called bulimic type. In the bulimic type of dieting, binge-eating initially occurs in spurts but gradually becomes a habit. Binge-eating ends with self-induced vomiting, either alone or in combination with laxative and/or diuretic abuse, as a means to get rid of excess weight. Intense, compulsive exercise is another weight-control method.

TABLE 2–4
Diagnostic Criteria for Anorexia Nervosa

A. Refusal to maintain body weight at or above a minimally normal weight for age and height (e.g., weight loss leading to maintenance of body weight less than 85% of that expected or failure to make expected weight gain).

B. Intense fear of gaining weight or becoming fat, even though underweight.

C. Disturbance in the way in which one's body weight or shape is experienced, undue influence of body weight or shape on self-evaluation, or denial of the seriousness of the current low body weight.

D. In postmenarchal females, amenorrhea (i.e., the absence of at least three consecutive menstrual cycles). A woman is considered to have amenorrhea if her periods occur only following hormone (e.g., estrogen) administration.

Additional features of anorexia include bradycardia, osteopenia, delayed gastric emptying, lymphopenia, low voltage on electrocardiogram, decreased 1-second forced expiratory volume (FEV_1), hypothermia, myopathy, neuropathy, and, if anorexia is severe, organic brain syndrome.

Endocrine changes are malnutrition induced (Table 2–8). For most female patients, amenorrhea, which occurs when body weight drops below the normal range, occurs because of low plasma luteinizing hormone levels, low estradiol levels, and low progesterone levels. The hypothalamic-pituitary-thyroid axis changes are similar to those in marasmic patients. Weight gain to the normal, premorbid level generally reverses the endocrine changes in patients with anorexia nervosa.

Diagnosis. The *differential diagnosis* includes Addison disease, hyperthyroidism, diabetes mellitus, inflammatory bowel disease, malignancy (including brain tumors), drug abuse, primary depression, hypothalamic lesions, schizophrenia, and obsessive/compulsive disorders.

Treatment and Prognosis. *Treatment* requires a multidisciplinary approach consisting of a feeding program and individual and family therapy. Therapy is difficult because the patients and families involved often deny the severity of the illness and may conceal symptoms. Goals of therapy are to restore normal function and body weight and to reestablish normal eating patterns. Adequate caloric and nutrient intake is of lifesaving importance in the acutely ill, severely underweight patient; weight restoration and refeeding require the patient's cooperation if this therapy is to succeed. Bradycardia and hypothermia are usually warning signs of severe, potentially life-threatening malnutrition. Though instituting some nutrient delivery is an urgent matter in such cases, refeeding too rapidly may be dangerous.

When vital signs are stable, discussion and negotiation of a detailed treatment contract with the patient and the parents are essential before further treatment begins. The first step is to restore body weight; the patient's weight should be increased to more than 80% of normal levels for height and age. This is accomplished through voluntary intake of regular foods or of a nutritional formula ingested orally or by nasogastric tube. Occasionally, parenteral nutrition is indicated to improve the nutritional status to a safe level. During the second step, the patient is given freedom to gain weight at a personal pace. Hospitalization should be considered in the following conditions:

1. Weight loss exceeds 25% of ideal body weight.
2. Personal and family dynamics place the patient at excessive risk for suicide, abuse, bradycardia, or hypothermia.

3. Metabolic disturbances (e.g., dehydration; hypokalemia; severe dysrhythmias; severe, recurrent induced vomiting; or laxative abuse) are noted.
4. Outpatient therapy fails.

Antidepressant drug therapy may be indicated for depressed patients.

The *prognosis* includes a 3–5% mortality (suicide, malnutrition) rate, the development of bulimic symptoms (in 30% of individuals), and persistent anorexia nervosa syndrome (in 20% of individuals).

Bulimia Nervosa

The diagnostic indicators in the behavior of a patient with bulimia nervosa are binge-eating episodes and the loss of control during overeating (Table 2–5). Although this condition is often considered a symptom of anorexia nervosa, the term "bulimia" also is applied to a distinct eating disorder. Previous dieting is usually a precondition for the development of bulimia. The disorder occurs predominantly in young women of normal weight or in slightly overweight women. The prevalence may be as high as 5% of female college students; the female-to-male ratio is 10:1.

During binge-eating episodes, patients tend to consume large volumes of "forbidden" foods that are high in carbohydrate and fat content; others may eat leftovers of unpalatable foods. The individual consumes the food rapidly and secretly without dwelling on the taste. Vomiting eventually becomes coupled to binge-eating. Most patients overeat with the forethought of vomiting afterward. Most metabolic abnormalities are the result of excessive vomiting. The excessive use of laxatives or diuretics also increases the risks of metabolic disturbance such as hypokalemia.

In contrast to patients with anorexia nervosa, patients with bulimia are more likely to exhibit personality disturbances, impulse-control difficulties (e.g., stealing, drug abuse, and sexual promiscuity), personal and family histories of affective disorders, and a positive response to antidepressant therapy. These patients often feel embarrassed, guilty, and ashamed. Repetitive binge-eating and vomiting can result in salivary gland enlargement, esophagitis, fluid and electrolyte imbalance, callus formation on knuckles caused by abrasion from the teeth while vomiting was induced with the hand, and erosion of dental enamel by acidic gastric contents. Ipecac abuse (to induce emesis) may cause cardiomyopathy.

A combination of nutritional, educational, and self-monitoring techniques is used to increase awareness of the maladaptive behavior, after which efforts are made to change the eating behavior. Antidepressants have a place in the treatment of bulimia. Up to 5% of patients complete a suicide, and many more patients attempt suicide.

TABLE 2–5
Diagnostic Criteria for Bulimia Nervosa

A. Recurrent episodes of binge eating are characterized by the following:
　　1. Eating in a discrete period of time (e.g., within any hour period) an amount of food that is definitely larger than most people would eat during a similar period of time under similar circumstances
　　2. A sense of lack of control over eating during the episode (e.g., a feeling that one cannot stop eating or control what or how much one is eating).
B. The individual engages in recurrent inappropriate compensatory behavior in order to prevent weight gain, such as self-induced vomiting; misuse of laxatives, diuretics, enemas, or other medications; fasting; or excessive exercise.
C. The binge eating and inappropriate compensatory behaviors both occur, on average, at least twice a week for 3 months.
D. Self-evaluation is unduly influenced by body shape and weight.
E. The disturbance does not occur exclusively during episodes of anorexia nervosa.

REFERENCES

American Psychiatric Association Task Force on DSM-IV: *Diagnostic and statistical manual of mental disorders,* ed 4, Washington, DC, 2000, The Association.
Litt IF: Anorexia nervosa and bulimia. In Behrman RE, Kliegman RM, Jenson HB, editors: *Nelson textbook of pediatrics,* ed 16, Philadelphia, 2000, WB Saunders, Chapter 112.

ARTERIOSCLEROSIS

Evidence suggests that prevention of adult cardiovascular disease should begin in childhood. Elevated low-density lipoprotein (LDL) cholesterol levels are associated with heart disease in adults; dietary modification reduces LDL cholesterol levels in adults and children. The childhood origin of atherosclerosis is suggested by the finding of vascular atherosclerotic lesions in young soldiers killed in wars and in autopsies of younger children. High cholesterol levels in childhood are associated with subsequent high cholesterol levels and heart disease in adulthood. Given the known influences (diet, exercise, and smoking) on blood

TABLE 2–6
Characteristics of Step-One and Step-Two Diets for Lowering Blood Cholesterol

Nutrient	Recommended Intake	
	Step-One Diet	Step-Two Diet
Total fat	Average of no more than 30% of total calories*	Same
Saturated fatty acids	Less than 10% of total calories	Less than 7% of total calories
Polyunsaturated fatty acids	Up to 10% of total calories	Same
Monounsaturated fatty acids	Remaining total fat calories	Same
Cholesterol	Less than 300 mg/day	Less than 200 mg/day
Carbohydrates	About 55% of total calories	Same
Protein	About 15–20% of total calories	Same
Calories	To promote normal growth and development and to reach or maintain desirable body weight	Same

From National Cholesterol Education Program: Report of the expert panel on blood cholesterol levels in children and adolescents, *Pediatrics* 89(3 pt 2):525–584, 1992.
*The American Academy of Pediatrics suggests that the fat intake of children should not be below 20% of total calories.

lipid levels and the development of heart disease and the resistance of many adults to behavioral intervention, children should be encouraged to adopt healthier lifestyles to reduce the risk of atherosclerotic heart disease. The Prudent or Step-One Diet (Table 2–6) is proposed for all children over 2 years of age, especially for those with elevated cholesterol levels, whereas the Step-Two Diet is reserved for those with elevated LDL cholesterol levels that have not responded to the original dietary intervention. Drug therapy is reserved for older children (older than 10 years) who have severe elevations in LDL cholesterol after 6–12 months of dietary management has failed to lower the level. Drug therapy in children should be considered only after consultation with a pediatric lipid specialist.

Several questions have been raised about the safety and efficacy of dietary interventions in children. Some children fail to thrive when put on very low-fat, low-calorie diets by well-meaning but misguided parents. Dietary intervention should be undertaken with appropriate guidance (a registered dietitian with pediatric experience) to ensure that the diet has sufficient calories and nutrients for growth while fulfilling the guidelines of the Prudent Diet.

There is concern about the psychosocial consequences of labeling children as hypercholesterolemic (i.e., the development of the "sick child" role). To prevent this, intervention programs should focus on the positive changes the child and family can make to limit their risk. Another concern is the mislabeling of children based on a single or inaccurate screening test as a result of inherent biologic and laboratory variability in cholesterol testing. Any measure of cholesterol should be completed with adequate quality assurance; repeated measurements are required to define a child's lipid status (Table 2–7).

The current National Cholesterol Education Program guidelines recommend screening children with a positive family history of early (before 55 years of age) cardiovascular disease or of hypercholesterolemia (>240 mg/dL). Children with unknown histories or other cardiovascular risk factors may be screened at the physician's discretion. To prevent heart disease it is also important to focus on lifestyle interventions to minimize other risk factors, such as smoking, hypertension, obesity, diabetes mellitus, and physical inactivity.

REFERENCES

Committee on Nutrition, American Academy of Pediatrics: Cholesterol in childhood, *Pediatrics* 101(1):141, 1998.
National Cholesterol Education Program: Report of the expert panel on blood cholesterol levels in children and adolescents, *Pediatrics* 89(3 pt 2):525–584, 1992.
Tershakovec AM, Rader DJ: Disorders of lipoprotein metabolism and transport. In Behrman RE, Kliegman RM, Jenson HB, editors: *Nelson textbook of pediatrics*, ed 16, Philadelphia, 2000, WB Saunders, Chapter 83.

TABLE 2–7
Cutpoints of Total and Low-Density Lipoprotein (LDL) Cholesterol for Dietary Intervention in Children and Adolescents with a Family History of Hypercholesterolemia or Premature Cardiovascular Disease

Category	Total Cholesterol (mg/dL)	LDL Cholesterol (mg/dL)	Dietary Intervention
Acceptable	<170	<110	Recommended population eating pattern
Borderline	170-199	110-129	Step-One Diet prescribed, other risk factor intervention
High	≥200	≥130	Step-One Diet prescribed, then Step-Two if necessary

From National Cholesterol Education Program: *Pediatrics* 89(3 pt 2):525–584, 1992.

PITFALLS IN CHILD AND ADOLESCENT NUTRITION

When dietary intakes are compared with recommendations (Table 2–1), the intake of preschool children in the United States is deficient in zinc. The deficiency is profound in the diets of children living in families of low socioeconomic status (70% in 1–3-year-olds and 79% in 4–5-year-olds). Calcium intake also is inadequate for many children. Latent calcium and zinc deficiencies are likely to be buffered by adaptive mechanisms; however, illness may precipitate clinical signs and symptoms of deficiency.

Iron intake tends to be inadequate in children between 1 and 3 years of age in the United States. The incidence of iron-deficiency anemia has decreased in young children in the United States, in part as a result of participation in the Women, Infants and Children (WIC) program, but is still significant. Dietary iron deficiency is the major nutritional risk for the children in the first year of life.

Osteoporosis (osteopenia) caused by poor dietary calcium or vitamin intake or absorption of ingested calcium in children and adolescents is becoming more clinically recognized and treated. Poor calcium intake during adolescence may predispose adults to osteoporotic hip fractures in later life.

In the United States, 20% of all children and 50% of all black and Hispanic children live in families of low socioeconomic status. Among those families who participate in federal assistance programs, 2–3 times the expected number of children have weight/height measurements below the 5th percentile. This problem is evident in infants from 3 months through the second year of life. Surveillance of growth velocity is essential in this population, and evidence for macronutrient and micronutrient deficiencies should be sought in all children placed below the 5th percentile for weight or height.

REFERENCES

Popkin B, Siega-Riz A, Haines P: A comparison of dietary trends among racial and socioeconomic groups in the United States, *N Engl J Med* 335(10):716–720, 1996.
Subar AF, Krebs-Smith SM, Cook A, et al: Dietary sources of nutrients among US children, 1989-1991, *Pediatrics* 102(4):913–923, 1998.

MACRONUTRIENT DEFICIENCIES

Worldwide, protein-energy malnutrition (PEM) is a leading cause of death among children younger than 5 years of age. PEM is a spectrum of conditions caused by varying levels of protein and calorie deficiencies. Primary PEM is caused by social or economic factors that result in a lack of food. Secondary PEM occurs in children with various conditions associated with increased caloric requirements (e.g., infection, trauma, and cancer), increased caloric loss (e.g., malabsorption and cystic fibrosis), reduced caloric intake (e.g., anorexia, cancer, oral intake restriction, and social factors), or a combination of these three variables.

Marasmus

Marasmus is the most common form of primary PEM and is caused by severe caloric depletion. Many secondary forms of marasmic PEM are associated with such diseases as cystic fibrosis, tuberculosis, cancer, acquired immunodeficiency syndrome (AIDS), or celiac disease.

The principal *clinical manifestation* in a child with severe malnutrition is emaciation with a body weight below 60% of that expected for age or below 70% of the ideal weight for height and depleted body-fat stores. Although growth stunting may be observed with longer-term malnutrition, the ratio of observed to expected weight to height reveals a reduction in body mass exceeding that caused by any coexisting growth stunting. Loss of muscle mass and subcutaneous fat stores is confirmed by inspection or palpation and quantified by anthropometric measurements. The head may appear large but generally is proportional to the body length. Edema usually is absent. The skin is dry and thin, and the hair may be thin, sparse, and easily pulled out. Marasmic children are generally apathetic and weak. Bradycardia and hypothermia signify severe and life-threatening malnutrition. Atrophy of the filiform papillae of the tongue is common, and monilial stomatitis is frequent. Recent weaning of the child or inappropriate weaning practices and chronic diarrhea are common findings in developing countries.

Role of Chronic Diarrhea

Malnutrition often is associated with chronic diarrhea as a result of the effects of malnutrition on the gastrointestinal tract (mucosal atrophy and secondary malabsorption) and the increased susceptibility to viral, bacterial, protozoal, and parasitic infections related to a secondary T- and B-cell immunodeficiency state. Recurrent episodes of diarrhea treated with prolonged periods of fasting or oral electrolyte solutions reduce caloric intake and contribute to malnutrition. Diarrhea may worsen during rehabilitation as a result of excessive refeeding or formula intolerance (transient lactose or monosaccharide malabsorption or milk protein intolerance). Nonetheless, cow's-milk formulas are used routinely to rehabilitate malnourished children, with good results. In severe cases of diarrhea, malabsorption, and malnutrition, intravenous refeeding may be necessary.

Kwashiorkor

Kwashiorkor, presenting with pitting edema that starts in the lower extremities and ascends with increasing severity, is caused by inadequate protein intake in the presence of fair to good caloric intake. It is common in developing countries if children are weaned to low-protein foods, but it also may be a complication of critical illness (e.g., burns, cancer, acute and chronic infections, multiorgan system failure, inflammatory bowel disease, anorexia nervosa, and postoperative surgery) when inadequate amounts of protein are provided for a prolonged time.

The major *clinical manifestation* of kwashiorkor is that the body weight of the child ranges from 60–80% of the expected weight for age; weight may not represent the nutritional status because of the presence of edema. Physical examination reveals a relative maintenance of subcutaneous adipose tissue and a marked atrophy of muscle mass. Edema varies from a minor pitting of the dorsum of the foot to generalized edema with involvement of the eyelids and scrotum. The hair is sparse, easily pluckable, and appears dull brown, red, or yellow-white. Adequate protein intake restores hair color (flag sign), leaving a band of hair with altered pigmentation followed by a band with normal pigmentation. Skin changes are common and range from hyperpigmented hyperkeratosis to an erythematous macular rash on the trunk and extremities. In the most severe form of kwashiorkor, a superficial desquamation occurs over pressure surfaces. Angular cheilosis and the atrophy of the filiform papillae of the tongue are common. Monilial stomatitis is frequent. Examination of the abdomen may reveal a large, soft liver with an indefinite edge. Lymphatic tissue commonly is atrophic. Chest examination may reveal basilar rales. The abdomen is distended, and bowel sounds tend to be hypoactive.

Treatment of Malnutrition

The basal metabolic rate and immediate nutrient needs decrease in cases of malnutrition. When nutrients are provided, the metabolic rate increases, stimulating anabolism and thus increasing nutrient requirements. The body of the malnourished child may have compensated for vitamin and mineral deficiencies with lower metabolic and growth rates; refeeding may unmask these deficiencies. Furthermore, the gastrointestinal tract may not tolerate a rapid increase in intake. Nutritional rehabilitation, therefore, should be initiated and advanced slowly to minimize these complications. Fluid and solute load must be monitored to avoid stressing the compromised myocardial function. If edema develops in the child during refeeding, caloric intake should be kept stable until the edema begins to resolve.

When nutritional rehabilitation is initiated, calories can be safely started at 20% above the child's recent intake. If no estimate of the caloric intake is available, 50–75% of the normal energy requirement is safe. Caloric intake can be increased 10–20% per day, with monitoring for electrolyte imbalances, poor cardiac function, edema, or feeding intolerance. If any of these occurs, further caloric increases are not made until the child's status stabilizes. Caloric intake is increased until appropriate regrowth is initiated. This may require 150% or more of the recommended calories for an age-matched, well-nourished child. Protein needs also are increased as anabolism begins and are provided in proportion to the caloric intake.

In most cases, cow's-milk–based formulas are tolerated and provide an appropriate mix of nutrients. Other easily digested foods, appropriate for the age, also may be introduced slowly. If feeding intolerance occurs, lactose-free elemental formulas or other regimens (e.g., parenteral nutrition) should be considered (see Marasmus earlier in this chapter). During 2–3 weeks of dietary rehabilitation and rapid growth, a *hypermetabolic nutritional recovery syndrome* may develop that is characterized by postprandial diaphoresis, hepatic glycogenesis, and eosinophilia.

Vitamin and mineral intake in excess of the daily recommended intake is provided to account for the increased requirements. Potassium, phosphorus, calcium, and magnesium status are carefully monitored. Potassium is a major component of lean body tissue and is thus needed during growth and healing; serum potassium levels may decrease dangerously in response to a glucose load, with subsequent insulin-induced transcellular shift of potassium. Phosphorus is needed for phosphorylated intermediates because it becomes "trapped" intracellularly by such phosphorylation in response to a glucose load, increased anabolism, and increased metabolic rate. Magnesium, a cofactor for adenosine triphosphatase, is needed when the metabolic and anabolic rates increase. Hypomagnesemia blunts the parathyroid response to hypocalcemia, which may be exacerbated by the vitamin D and calcium deficiencies associated with malnutrition (see Chapter 17). Electrolyte imbalances can further alter cardiac function, exacerbating heart failure. Overzealous refeeding has been documented to cause life-threatening abnormalities of these and other nutrients.

REFERENCES

Curran JS, Barness LA: Nutrition. In Behrman RE, Kliegman RM, Jenson HB, editors: *Nelson textbook of pediatrics*, ed 16, Philadelphia, 2000, WB Saunders, Chapter 42.

Torun B, Chew F: Protein-energy malnutrition. In Shils ME, Olson JA, Shike M, et al, editors: *Modern nutrition in health and disease*, ed 9, Philadelphia, 1999, William & Wilkins.

Complications of Malnutrition

Malnourished children are more susceptible to infection, especially sepsis, pneumonia, and gastroenteritis. Hypoglycemia is common after periods of severe fasting but also may be a sign of sepsis. Hypothermia may signify infection or, with bradycardia, may signify a decreased metabolic rate to conserve energy. Bradycardia and poor cardiac output predispose the malnourished child to heart failure, which is exacerbated by acute fluid or solute loads. Vitamin deficiencies also can complicate malnutrition. Vitamin A deficiency is common in the developing world and is an important cause of altered immune response and increased morbidity (e.g., infections and blindness) and mortality (especially from measles). Depending on the age at onset and the duration of the malnutrition, malnourished children may suffer permanent growth stunting (from malnutrition in utero, infancy, or adolescence) and delayed development (from malnutrition in infancy or adolescence). Environmental (social) deprivation may interact with the effects of the malnutrition to further impair development and cognitive function.

Pathophysiology of Macronutrient Deficiencies

PEM represents a complex relationship between reduced protein and calorie intake, inciting events such as weaning or gastrointestinal infection, some chronic illnesses, and the complications associated with PEM and infection. The child's adaptation to reduced protein and calorie intake is typical for that of starvation, and secondary immune dysfunction and continued exposure to infectious diseases increase the morbidity and mortality of PEM.

Endocrine Adaptation

The hormonal responses to malnutrition are noted in Table 2–8. The net effects of nutrient deficiency and these hormonal events are to reduce (spare) tissue glucose utilization and to increase alternate fuel mobilization and use (proteolysis, lipolysis, ketogenesis). Initially, free fatty acids and ketones may spare proteolysis, but with profound deficiencies muscle breakdown continues and net protein synthesis is reduced.

Metabolic Substrates

There are several stages of metabolic adaptation in PEM. The first stage is a reduction in voluntary energy expenditure used for spontaneous physical activity, the second is a reduction in the rate of gain of body mass and length, and the last is a reduction in resting energy expenditure. The marasmic form of malnutrition results in a more striking reduction in resting energy expenditure than the reduction produced by kwashiorkor.

Inadequate macronutrient intake, especially when amplified by concurrent infection, results in growth arrest. Normal nitrogen balance may be sustained if protein intake has not been exceeded by excessive nitrogen losses; in both healthy children and those with PEM, the efficiency of nitrogen balance is greater than 95%. Protein turnover is a measure of

TABLE 2–8
Summary of Selected Hormonal Changes and Their Main Metabolic Effects Usually Seen in Severe Protein-Energy Malnutrition (PEM)

Hormone	Influenced in PEM by	Hormonal Activity in		Metabolic Effects of Changes in PEM
		Energy Deficit	Protein Deficit	
Insulin	Low food intake ($\downarrow$ glucose) ($\downarrow$ amino acids)	Decreased	Decreased	$\downarrow$ muscle protein synthesis $\downarrow$ lipogenesis $\downarrow$ growth
Growth hormone	Low protein intake ($\downarrow$ amino acids) Reduced somatomedin synthesis	Normal or moderately increased	Increased	$\uparrow$ visceral synthesis $\downarrow$ urea synthesis $\uparrow$ lipolysis
Somatomedins (IGF-I)	Low protein intake?	Variable	Decreased	$\downarrow$ muscle and cartilage protein synthesis $\downarrow$ collagen synthesis $\downarrow$ lipolysis $\downarrow$ growth $\uparrow$ production of growth hormone
Epinephrine	Stress of food deficiency, infections ($\downarrow$ glucose)	Normal but can increase	Normal but can increase	$\uparrow$ lipolysis $\uparrow$ glycogenolysis inhibits insulin secretion
Glucocorticoids	Stress of hunger Fever ($\downarrow$ glucose)	Increased	Normal or moderately increased	$\uparrow$ muscle protein catabolism $\uparrow$ visceral protein turnover $\uparrow$ lipolysis $\uparrow$ gluconeogenesis
Aldosterone	$\downarrow$ blood volume $\uparrow$ extracellular K? $\downarrow$ serum Na?	Normal	Increased	$\uparrow$ sodium retention and $\uparrow$ water retention contributes to appearance of edema
Thyroid hormones	?	T_4 normal or decreased; T_3 decreased	T_4 usually decreased; T_3 decreased	$\downarrow$ glucose oxidation $\downarrow$ basal energy expenditure $\uparrow$ reverse T_3
Gonadotropins	Low protein intake? Low energy intake?	Decreased	Decreased	Delayed menarche

From Shils M, Young V: *Modern nutrition in health and disease,* ed 7, Philadelphia, 1988, Lea & Febiger.
$\downarrow$, Low or reduced; $\uparrow$, high or increased; *IGF-I,* insulin-like growth factor-I.

total endogenous protein synthesis and degradation. In normal adults the rate of turnover is influenced only modestly by starvation; in children with kwashiorkor, however, the rate of turnover is strikingly reduced. In contrast, turnover rates in normal children are increased in response to the stress of an infection.

The turnover of individual proteins is reduced under modest dietary restrictions. In both well-nourished and malnourished children, a reduced protein intake results in a few days in reduced rates of albumin synthesis. Later, if the reduction continues, the intake reduction results in decreased concentrations of serum albumin transferrin, retinol-binding protein, and pre-albumin. However, because of differences in half-life, serum albumin concentrations do not decrease for 1–2 weeks, whereas pre-albumin levels decrease within a few days. Thus, to assess short-term nutritional status, it is preferable to use serum markers with a shorter half-life, such as pre-albumin. Although the synthesis of hepatic acute albumin levels decreases within a few days, the synthesis of hepatic acute-phase proteins (e.g., C-phase proteins such as C-reactive protein) nonetheless is preserved under these conditions. In addition to the hepatic synthetic adaptations, the degradation of muscle proteins is increased. In the marasmic child, these mechanisms maintain the plasma levels of free amino acids and hepatic secretory proteins. In the child with kwashiorkor, the adaptation fails to maintain serum amino acid levels and hepatic protein synthesis, and the plasma levels of branched-chain amino acids decrease.

Macronutrient deficiency and specific infections (e.g., measles and rotavirus) also decrease the rate of synthesis of pancreatic enzymes and intestinal mucosa brush-border hydrolases, which can retard later dietary rehabilitation.

Body water content is increased in kwashiorkor as a result of reduced adipose tissue mass and fluid retention. Blood osmolality and serum sodium concentrations may be low, and serum concentrations of potassium and magnesium may be reduced. Total body magnesium and potassium levels are reduced in all malnourished children as the result of loss of muscle mass. In kwashiorkor there also are defects in the maintenance of the normal sodium-potassium membrane gradients in soft tissues. Calcium and phosphorus are uniformly low, but tetany is rare. Concentrations of serum zinc and copper are strikingly reduced in kwashiorkor but are normal in marasmus. If adequate micronutrient dietary supplements are not provided, serum zinc and copper concentrations fall rapidly during nutritional rehabilitation.

REFERENCES

Hoffer LJ: Metabolic consequences of starvation. In Shils ME, Olson JA, Shike M, et al, editors: *Modern nutrition in health and disease*, ed 9, Philadelphia, 1999, Williams & Wilkins.

Immune Function

Cell-mediated immunity is depressed in patients with PEM. Severely malnourished children fail to respond to tuberculin or *Candida albicans* skin tests, which reveals an inability of their system to demonstrate prior sensitization. They also do not react to dinitrofluorobenzene sensitization, indicating that noncommitted lymphocytes are unresponsive. Thymic, lymph node, tonsil, and splenic tissues are atrophic in malnourished children. This immuno-compromised status improves with dietary rehabilitation; functional recovery occurs within 2 weeks, and the total lymphocyte count recovers within 4 weeks. The response of polymorphonuclear (PMN) leukocytes to chemotactic stimulation is normal, but that of the macrophages is reduced in PEM. Malnourished children have reduced secretory immunoglobulin A (sIgA) levels in nasal washings, duodenal fluids, and tears, despite the elevated serum IgA level.

Infection

A triangle of interactions exists among host defenses, infection, and macronutrient malnutrition. PEM may be initiated by primary dietary deficiencies or by illnesses that induce a secondary dietary deficiency. Infections induce anorexia and increase caloric requirements as a result of hypermetabolism during the febrile response. Contributing infections may be bacterial (e.g., *E. coli* enteritis or pneumococcal pneumonia), viral (e.g., rotavirus or measles), protozoal (e.g., malaria or *Giardia*), or a result of intestinal helminths (e.g., roundworms, flukes or tapeworms). The results of infection are catabolism and a loss of body nutrient stores, leading to clinical malnutrition. The impaired host defenses associated with PEM are important factors in determining the frequency and severity of infection. Gastrointestinal infections also exacerbate intestinal malabsorption, mucosal atrophy, and micronutrient losses.

REFERENCES

Walker WA, Watkins JB, editors: *Nutrition in pediatrics,* ed 2, Philadelphia, 1997, WB Saunders, Chapter 19.
Yoshida SH, Keen CL, Ansari AA: Nutrition and the immune system. In Shils ME, Olson JA, Shike M, et al, editors: *Modern nutrition in health and disease,* ed 9, Philadelphia, 1999, Williams & Wilkins.

MICRONUTRIENT DEFICIENCIES

The causes of micronutrient deficiencies are diverse and relate to unusual diets; various malabsorption or maldigestion syndromes; drugs that alter nutrient absorption, metabolism, and excretion or that compete with vitamin action; and various genetic disorders associated with specific nutrient metabolic defects (Tables 2–9 and 2–10).

Water-Soluble Vitamins

Ascorbic Acid

The first recognized micronutrient deficiency disease was that caused by a deficiency in ascorbic acid (vitamin C). The principal forms of vitamin C are L-ascorbic acid and the oxidized form, dehydroascorbic acid. Ascorbic acid accelerates hydroxylation reactions in many biosynthetic reactions. The needs of full-term infants for ascorbic acid and dehydroascorbic acid are calculated by estimating the availability of this vitamin in human milk. Commercially available cow's–milk-based formulas are fortified to a comparable level of 5.5 mg/dL (8 mg/100 kcal).

A deficiency of ascorbic acid results in the clinical manifestations of **scurvy.** Infantile scurvy is manifested by irritability, bone tenderness with swelling, and pseudoparalysis of the legs. The disease may

TABLE 2–9
Etiology of Vitamin and Nutrient Deficiency States

Etiology	Deficiency
Diet	
Vegans (strict)	Protein, vitamins B_{12}, D, riboflavin
Breast-fed infant	Vitamins K, D
Cow's milk–fed infant	Iron
Bulimia, anorexia nervosa	Electrolytes, other deficiencies
Parenteral alimentation	Essential fatty acid, trace elements
Alcoholism	Calories, vitamin B_1, B_6, folate
Medical Problems	
Malabsorption syndromes	Vitamins A, D, E, K, zinc, essential fatty acids
Cholestasis	Vitamins E, D, K, A, zinc, essential fatty acids
Medications	
Sulfonamides	Folate
Phenytoin, phenobarbital	Vitamins D, K, folate
Mineral oil	Vitamins A, D, E, K
Antibiotics	Vitamin K
Isoniazid	Vitamin B_6
Antacids	Iron, phosphate, calcium
Digitalis	Magnesium, calcium
Penicillamine	Vitamin B_6
Specific Mechanisms	
Transcobalamin II or intrinsic factor deficiency	Vitamin B_{12}
Other digestive enzyme deficiencies	Carbohydrate, fat, protein
Menkes kinky hair syndrome	Copper
Acrodermatitis enteropathica	Zinc
Reduced exposure direct sunlight	Vitamin D

TABLE 2–10
Characteristics of Vitamin Deficiencies

Vitamin	Purpose	Deficiency	Comments	Source
Water Soluble				
Thiamine (B_1)	Coenzyme in ketoacid decarboxylation (e.g., pyruvate →acetyl-CoA trans-ketolase reaction)	*Beri-beri:* polyneuropathy, calf tenderness, heart failure, edema, ophthalmoplegia	Inborn errors of lactate metabolism; boiling milk destroys B_1	Liver, meat, milk, cereals, nuts, legumes
Riboflavin (B_2)	FAD coenzyme in oxidation-reduction reactions	Anorexia, mucositis, anemia, cheilosis, nasolabial seborrhea	Photosensitizer	Milk, cheese, liver, meat, eggs, whole grains, green leafy vegetables
Niacin (B_3)	NAD coenzyme in oxidation-reduction reactions	*Pellagra:* photosensitivity, dermatitis, dementia, diarrhea, death	Tryptophan is a precursor	Meat, fish, live, whole grains, green leafy vegetables

DNA, Deoxyribonucleic acid; *FAD,* flavin adenine dinucleotide; *G6PD,* glucose-6-phosphate dehydrogenase; *NAD,* nicotinamide adenine dinucleotide.

TABLE 2–10
Characteristics of Vitamin Deficiencies—cont'd

Vitamin	Purpose	Deficiency	Comments	Source
Water Soluble—cont'd				
Pyridoxine (B$_6$)	Cofactor in amino acid metabolism	Seizures, hyperacusis, microcytic anemia, nasolabial seborrhea, neuropathy	Dependency state: deficiency secondary to drugs	Meat, liver, whole grains, peanuts, soybeans, meat
Pantothenic acid	Coenzyme A in Krebs cycle	None reported		Meat, vegetables
Biotin	Cofactor in carboxylase reactions of amino acids	Alopecia, dermatitis, hypotonia, death	Bowel resection, inborn error of metabolism,* and ingestion of raw eggs	Yeast, meats; made by intestinal flora
B$_{12}$	Coenzyme for 5-methyl-tetrahydrofolate formation; DNA synthesis	Megaloblastic anemia, peripheral neuropathy, posterior lateral column disease, vitiligo	Vegans; fish tapeworm; transcobalamin or intrinsic factor deficiencies	Meat, fish, cheese, eggs
Folate	DNA synthesis	Megaloblastic anemia	Goat milk deficient; drug antagonists; heat inactivates	Liver, greens, vegetables, cereals, cheese
Ascorbic acid (C)	Reducing agent; collagen metabolism	*Scurvy:* irritability, purpura, bleeding gums, periosteal hemorrhage, aching bones	May improve tyrosine metabolism in preterm infants	Citrus fruits, green vegetables; cooking destroys it
Fat Soluble				
A	Epithelial cell integrity; vision	Night blindness, xerophthalmia, Bitot spots, follicular hyperkeratosis	Common with protein-calorie malnutrition; malabsorption	Liver, milk, eggs, green and yellow vegetables, fruits
D	Maintain serum calcium, phosphorus levels	*Rickets:* reduced bone mineralization	Prohormone of 25- and 1,25-vitamin D	Fortified milk, cheese, liver
E	Antioxidant	Hemolysis in preterm infants; areflexia, ataxia, ophthalmoplegia	May benefit patients with G6PD deficiency	Seeds, vegetables, germ oils, green leafy vegetables
K	Posttranslation carboxylation of clotting factors II, VII, IX, X and proteins C, S	Prolonged prothrombin time; hemorrhage; elevated PIVKA (protein induced in vitamin K absence)	Malabsorption; breast-fed infants	Liver, green vegetables; made by intestinal flora

*Biotinidase deficiency.
DNA, Deoxyribonucleic acid; *FAD,* flavin adenine dinucleotide; *G6PD,* glucose-6-phosphate dehydrogenase; *NAD,* nicotinamide adenine dinucleotide.

TABLE 2–11
Recommended Daily Dose Ranges for Treatment of Vitamin-Related Diseases

Vitamin	Treatment of Vitamin Deficiency	Treatment of Deficiency in Patients with Malabsorption	Treatment of Dependency Syndrome
A (IU)	5000–10,000	10,000–25,000	—
D (IU)	400–5000	4000–20,000	50,000–200,000
Calcifediol (μg)	—	20–100	50–100
Calcitriol (1,25-[OH]$_2$-D) (μg)	—	1–3	1–3
E (IU)	—	100–1000	—
K (mg)	1*	5–10*	—
Ascorbic acid (C) (mg)	250–500	500	—
Thiamine (mg)	5–25	5–25	25–500
Riboflavin (mg)	5–25	5–25	—
Niacin (mg)	25–50	25–50	50–250
B$_6$ (mg)	5–25	2–25	10–250
Biotin (mg)	0.15–0.3	0.3–1.0	10
Folic acid (mg)	1	1	—†
B$_{12}$ (μg)	—*	—*	1–40

From AMA Council on Scientific Affairs: *JAMA* 257(14):1929-1936, 1987.
*To be used parenterally as needed.
†To be used only in conjunction with multivitamin mixtures.

occur if infants are fed unsupplemented cow's milk in the first year of life. Subperiosteal hemorrhage, hyperkeratosis of hair follicles, and a succession of mental changes characterize the progression of the illness. Anemia secondary to decreased iron absorption or to abnormal folate metabolism also is seen in chronic scurvy.

Treatment is presented in Table 2–11.

Thiamine

Vitamin B$_1$ functions as a coenzyme in biochemical reactions related to carbohydrate metabolism, to decarboxylation of alpha-keto acids and pyruvate, and to transketolase reactions of the pentose pathway. Thiamine also is involved in the decarboxylation of branched-chain amino acids. Thiamine is lost during milk pasteurization and sterilization. The thiamine content of commercial formulas for full-term and preterm infants is 59–156 μg/100 kcal and 100–250 μg/100 kcal, respectively.

Infantile beriberi occurs between 1 and 4 months of life in breast-fed infants whose mothers have a thiamine deficiency, in infants with protein-calorie malnutrition, in infants receiving unsupplemented hyperalimentation fluid, or in infants receiving boiled milk. Acute cardiac symptoms and signs predominate. Anorexia, apathy, vomiting, restlessness, and pallor progress to dyspnea, cyanosis, and death from congestive heart failure. Infants with beriberi

have a characteristic aphonic cry; they appear to be crying, but no sound is uttered.

Treatment is noted in Table 2–11.

Riboflavin

Vitamin B$_2$ is a constituent of two coenzymes, riboflavin 5'-phosphate and flavin-adenine dinucleotide. These coenzymes are essential components of glutathione reductase and xanthine oxidase, which are involved in electron transport. A deficiency of riboflavin affects glucose, fatty acid, and amino acid metabolism. Riboflavin and its phosphate are decomposed by exposure to light and by strong alkaline solutions. The intake of riboflavin from standard infant formulations is significantly greater than from human milk; the processes of pasteurization, evaporation, and condensation of milk do not destroy riboflavin.

Ariboflavinosis is characterized by an angular stomatitis; glossitis; cheilosis; seborrheic dermatitis around the nose and mouth; and eye changes that include reduced tearing, photophobia, corneal vascularization, and the formation of cataracts. Subclinical riboflavin deficiencies have been found in diabetic subjects, children in families with low socioeconomic status, children with chronic cardiac disease, and infants undergoing prolonged phototherapy for hyperbilirubinemia.

Treatment is presented in Table 2–11.

Niacin

Niacin consists of the compounds nicotinic acid and nicotinamide (niacinamide). Nicotinamide, the predominant form of the vitamin, functions as a component of the coenzymes nicotinamide adenine dinucleotide (NAD) and nicotinamide adenine dinucleotide phosphate (NADP). Niacin is involved in multiple metabolic processes, including fat synthesis, intracellular respiratory metabolism, and glycolysis.

In determining the needs for niacin, the content of tryptophan in the diet must be considered because tryptophan is converted to niacin. Niacin is stable in foods and can withstand heating and prolonged storage. The concentration of niacin in human milk remains stable throughout lactation. Approximately 70% of the total niacin equivalents in human milk are derived from tryptophan. The deficiency disease **(pellagra)** related to a niacin deficiency is characterized by weakness, lassitude, dermatitis, inflammation of mucous membranes, diarrhea, vomiting, dysphagia, and, in severe cases, dementia.

Treatment is noted in Table 2–11.

Vitamin B₆

Vitamin B_6 refers to three naturally occurring pyridines: pyridoxine (pyridoxol), pyridoxal, and pyridoxamine. The phosphates of the latter two pyridines are metabolically and functionally related and are converted in the liver to the coenzyme form, pyridoxal phosphate.

The metabolic functions of vitamin B_6 include interconversion reactions of amino acids, conversion of tryptophan to niacin and serotonin, metabolic reactions in the brain, carbohydrate metabolism, immune development, and the biosynthesis of heme and prostaglandins. The pyridoxal and pyridoxamine forms of the vitamin are destroyed by heat; heat treatment has been responsible for vitamin B_6 deficiency and seizures in infants fed improperly processed formulas. For this reason, heat-stable pyridoxine is presently used for the fortification of milk. The vitamin B_6 content in human milk reflects the mother's nutritional status. Full-term infants become deficient in vitamin B_6 when fed human milk containing 9–12 μg/100 kcal. Goat's milk is deficient in vitamin B_6.

Dietary deprivation or *malabsorption* of vitamin B_6 in children results in hypochromic microcytic anemia, vomiting, diarrhea, failure to thrive, listlessness, hyperirritability, and seizures. Children receiving isoniazid may require additional vitamin B_6 because the drug binds to the vitamin.

Treatment is noted in Table 2–11.

Biotin

Biotin has coenzyme functions in the metabolism of fat and carbohydrates (e.g., it is a component of several carboxylase enzymes). Biotin is synthesized by intestinal bacteria, and thus a deficiency state is uncommon. Biotin deficiencies have been reported when biotin was omitted from parenteral nutrition solutions. A deficiency of biotinidase, the enzyme needed for conservation of metabolically active biotin, produces a biotin deficiency.

Clinical manifestations of biotin deficiency include anorexia, nausea, glossitis, pallor, mental changes, alopecia, and a fine maculosquamous dermatitis that becomes exfoliative. Antibiotics may increase biotin requirements by decreasing enteric synthesis of the vitamin. The protein avidin, found in raw eggs, binds biotin.

Treatment is noted in Table 2–11.

Vitamin B₁₂

For a discussion of vitamin B_{12} deficiency, see the discussion of Nutritional Anemia in the section on Minerals later in this chapter.

REFERENCES

Behrman RE, Kliegman RM, Jenson HB, editors: *Nelson textbook of pediatrics,* ed 16, Philadelphia, 2000, WB Saunders, Chapter 44.
Shils ME, Olson JA, Shike M, et al, editors: *Modern nutrition in health and disease,* ed 9, Philadelphia, 1999, Williams & Wilkins, Chapter 30.

Fat-Soluble Vitamins

Vitamin A

The basic constituent of the vitamin A group is retinol. Ingested plant carotene or animal-tissue retinol esters release retinol after hydrolysis by pancreatic and intestinal enzymes. Chylomicron-transported retinol esters are stored in the liver as retinol palmitate. Retinol is transported from the liver to target tissues by retinol-binding protein (RBP). After free retinol is delivered to the target tissues, the RBP is excreted by the kidney. Diseases of the kidney diminish excretion of RBP, whereas liver parenchymal disease or malnutrition lowers the synthesis of RBP. The uptake of retinol by target tissues is facilitated by specific cellular binding proteins. In the eye, retinol is metabolized to form rhodopsin; the action of light on rhodopsin is the first step of the visual process. Retinol also influences the growth and differentiation of epithelia and serves as a cofactor in glycoprotein synthesis. Retinoic acid can substitute for retinol in all functions except those for maintaining tissue growth and vision.

The *clinical manifestations* of vitamin A deficiency in humans appear as a group of ocular signs termed **xerophthalmia.** The earliest symptom is night blindness, which is followed by xerosis of the conjunctiva and cornea. Untreated, xerophthalmia can result in ulceration, necrosis, keratomalacia, and a permanent corneal scar. Clinical and subclinical vitamin A deficiencies are associated with immunodeficiency; increased risk of infection, especially measles; and increased risk of mortality, especially in developing nations. Xerophthalmia and vitamin A deficiency should be urgently treated.

Treatment is noted in Table 2–11. Hypervitaminosis A also has serious sequelae, including dry skin, alopecia, headaches, and hepatotoxicity. Death may occur (Table 2–12). Excessive vitamin A is also teratogenic.

Vitamin E

There are eight naturally occurring compounds with vitamin E activity. The most active of these, α-tocopherol, accounts for 90% of the vitamin E present in human tissues and is commercially available as an acetate or succinate. The other compounds of importance are β- and γ-tocopherol, which possess 33% and 10%, respectively, of the activity of α-tocopherol.

In humans, vitamin E acts as a biologic antioxi-

TABLE 2–12
Toxic Effects of Vitamins and Other Nutrients

Nutrient	Effects	Comments
Fat-Soluble Vitamins		
		Toxicity noted at lower multiples of RDA than water-soluble vitamins
A		
Acute	Lethargy, headache, papilledema, bulging fontanel	Megadoses used to prevent cancer,* treat acne
Chronic	Scaly, dry skin; alopecia; sore tongue; hyperostoses; anorexia; increased intracranial pressure (pseudotumor cerebri); teratogenic	Consumption of polar bear liver; toxicity with chronic 20,000–50,000 IU/24 hr
D		
Acute	Hypercalcemia, muscle weakness, anorexia, emesis, headache, polyuria	Hypercalcemia produces arrhythmias, hypertension, renal water wasting
Chronic	Nephrocalcinosis, bone pain, vascular calcification, renal insufficiency; idiopathic infantile hypercalcemia	Toxicity with chronic 3000–4000 IU/24 hr
E	Muscle weakness, diarrhea, antagonism of vitamin K, enhanced anticoagulant drug action	Megadoses used to improve libido and prevent heart disease and cancer*; toxicity with 300–800 IU/24 hr
K	Water-soluble analogs produce neonatal jaundice	Menadione induces neonatal hemolysis
Water-Soluble Vitamins		
C	Uricosuria, oxalate stones, G6PD-deficient hemolysis, rebound scurvy in infants; false-positive test for glycosuria; false-negative test for hematochezia	Prevention of upper respiratory tract infections*
Niacin	Histamine release, ulcers, asthma, flushing, pruritus, gout, hepatotoxic	Used to treat hypercholesterolemia; orthomolecular treatment of schizophrenia; toxicity with 200–1000 mg/24 hr
Pyridoxine (B₆)	Peripheral sensory neuropathy; fetal-neonatal dependency and seizures	Treat depression and premenstrual syndrome; toxicity with 2–6 g/24 hr
Tryptophan	Eosinophilia, myositis, fasciitis, scleroderma	Treat depression* and premenstrual syndrome*; possible toxic metabolite; toxicity with 0.5–4.0 g/24 hr

*No established benefit.
G6PD, Glucose-6-phosphate dehydrogenase; *RDA,* recommended daily allowance.

dant by inhibiting the peroxidation of polyunsaturated fatty acids (PUFAs) present in cell membranes. It scavenges free radicals generated by the reduction of molecular oxygen and by the action of oxidative enzymes. In the process, the α-tocopherol is oxidized to a quinone, which is excreted in the urine.

Human milk has a lower content of α-tocopherol and a lower ratio of vitamin E to PUFAs compared with currently used formulas. Nevertheless, term and preterm infants have higher serum α-tocopherol levels when fed human milk. The vitamin E requirement is increased in diets that have high concentrations of PUFAs or iron, both of which facilitate membrane peroxidation and generation of free radicals.

Tocopherol deficiency occurs in children with prolonged and profound fat malabsorption secondary to biliary atresia, cystic fibrosis, and abetalipoproteinemia; in these children a syndrome of progressive sensory and motor neuropathy may develop late in the first decade of life. Deficient preterm infants at 1–2 months of age have hemolytic anemia characterized by an elevated reticulocyte count, an increased sensitivity of the erythrocytes to hemolysis in hydrogen peroxide, peripheral edema, and thrombocytosis. All the abnormalities are corrected after oral vitamin E therapy (see Table 2–11). Toxic conditions caused by excess vitamin E are noted in Table 2–12.

Vitamin D

Cholecalciferol (vitamin D_3) is the mammalian form of vitamin D and is produced by ultraviolet irradiation of inactive precursors in the skin. Ergocalciferol (vitamin D_2) is derived from plants. Both vitamin D_2 and vitamin D_3 require further metabolism to become active. They are of equivalent potency. Clothing, lack of sunlight exposure, and skin pigmentation decrease the generation of vitamin D in the epidermis and dermis.

Vitamin D (D_2 and D_3) is metabolized in the liver to calcidiol, or 25-(OH)-D; this metabolite, which has little intrinsic activity, is transported by a plasma-binding globulin to the kidney, where it is converted to the most active metabolite calcitriol, or 1,25-$(OH)_2$-D. The molecular action of 1,25-$(OH)_2$-D results in a decrease in the concentration of messenger ribonucleic acid (mRNA) for collagen in bone and an increase in the concentration of mRNA for vitamin D–dependent calcium-binding protein in the intestine (directly mediating increased intestinal calcium transport). The antirachitic action of vitamin D is probably mediated by provision of appropriate concentrations of calcium and phosphate in the extracellular space of bone and by enhanced intestinal absorption of these minerals. The effect of vitamin D on bone is probably similar to that of parathyroid hormone and results in bone resorption. Vitamin D also may have a direct anabolic effect on bone. 1,25-$(OH)_2$-D also has direct feedback to the parathyroid gland and inhibits secretion of parathyroid hormone.

Vitamin D deficiency appears as **rickets** in children and as **osteomalacia** in postpubertal adolescents. Inadequate direct sun exposure and vitamin D intake are sufficient causes, but other factors (e.g., high cereal intake, a vegetarian diet, or various drugs [phenobarbital, phenytoin]) also may increase the risk of development of vitamin-deficiency rickets. Breast-fed infants, especially infants with dark-pigmented skin, are also at risk for vitamin D deficiency.

The *pathophysiology* of rickets results from defective bone growth, especially marked at the epiphyseal cartilage matrix, which fails to mineralize. The uncalcified osteoid results in a wide, irregular zone of poorly supported tissue, the rachitic metaphysis. This soft rather than hardened zone produces many of the skeletal deformities through compression and lateral bulging or flaring of the ends of bones.

The *clinical manifestations* of rickets are most common during the first 2 years of life and may become evident only after several months of a vitamin D–deficient diet. Craniotabes is caused by thinning of the outer table of the skull, which when compressed feels to the touch like a Ping-Pong ball. Enlargement of the costochondral junction (the rachitic rosary) and thickening of the wrists and ankles may be palpated. The anterior fontanel is enlarged, and its closure may be delayed. In advanced rickets, scoliosis and exaggerated lordosis may be present. Bowlegs or knock-knees may be evident in older infants, and greenstick fractures may be observed in long bones.

The *diagnosis* of rickets is based on a dietary history of poor vitamin D intake and a history of little exposure to direct ultraviolet sunlight. The serum calcium usually is normal but may be low, the serum phosphorus level always is reduced, and the serum alkaline phosphatase activity is elevated. When serum calcium levels decline below 7.5 mg/dL, tetany may occur. Levels of 24,25-$(OH)_2$-D are undetectable, and serum 1,25-$(OH)_2$-D levels are commonly below 7 ng/mL, although 1,25-$(OH)_2$-D levels may also be normal. The best measure of vitamin D status is the level of 25-(OH)-D. Characteristic roentgenologic changes of the distal ulna and radius include widening, concave cupping, and frayed, poorly demarcated ends. The increased space between the distal ends of the radius and ulna and the metacarpal bones is the enlarged, nonossified metaphysis.

The *treatment* of vitamin D–deficiency rickets and osteomalacia is indicated in Table 2–11. Breast-fed infants born of mothers with adequate vitamin D stores usually maintain adequate serum vitamin D levels for the first 6 months, but rickets may subsequently develop if these infants are not exposed to the sun or do not receive supplementary vitamin D. Toxic effects of vitamin D are noted in Table 2–12.

Vitamin K

The plant form of vitamin K is phylloquinone, or vitamin K_1. Another form is menaquinone, or vitamin K_2; this is one of a series of compounds with unsaturated side chains synthesized by the intestinal bacteria. Plasma factors II (prothrombin), VII, IX, and X in the cascade of blood coagulation factors depend on vitamin K for synthesis and for posttranslational conversion of their precursor proteins. The post-translational conversion of glutamyl residues to carboxyglutamic acid residues of a prothrombin molecule creates effective calcium-binding sites, making the protein active.

Other vitamin K–dependent proteins include proteins C, S, and Z in plasma and γ-carboxyglutamic acid (Gla)–containing proteins in the kidney, spleen, lung, uterus, placenta, pancreas, thyroid, thymus, testes, and bone. Bone contains a major vitamin K–dependent protein, osteocalcin, as well as lesser amounts of other glutamic acid–containing proteins.

Phylloquinone is absorbed from the intestine and transported by chylomicrons. The rarity of dietary vitamin K deficiency in humans with normal intestinal function suggests that the absorption of menaquinones is possible. Vitamin K deficiency has been observed in subjects with impaired fat absorption caused by obstructive jaundice, pancreatic insufficiency, and celiac disease; often these problems are combined with the use of antibiotics that change intestinal flora. Absorption of vitamin K also may be inhibited by mineral oil and high dietary intakes of vitamins A and E.

Hemorrhagic disease of the newborn, a disease more common among breast-fed infants, occurs in the first few weeks of life. It is rare in infants who receive prophylactic vitamin K on the first day of life. Hemorrhagic disease of the newborn usually is marked by generalized ecchymoses, gastrointestinal hemorrhage, or bleeding from a circumcision or umbilical stump; intracranial hemorrhage can occur, but is uncommon (see Chapter 6).

REFERENCES

Behrman RE, Kliegman RM, Jenson HB, editors: *Nelson textbook of pediatrics,* ed 16, Philadelphia, 2000, WB Saunders, Chapter 44.
Shils ME, Olson JA, Shike M, et al, editors: *Modern nutrition in health and disease,* ed 9, Philadelphia, 1999, Williams & Wilkins, Chapter 30.

Minerals

Calcium

Ninety-nine percent of calcium is in the skeleton; the remaining 1% is in extracellular fluids, intracellular compartments, and cell membranes. The 1% nonskeletal calcium serves a role in nerve conduction, muscle contraction, blood clotting, and membrane permeability. There are two distinct bone calcium phosphate pools, a large, crystalline form and a smaller, amorphous phase. Bone calcium constantly turns over, with concurrent bone resorption and formation. Bone mass peaks in the late teens and is influenced by prior and concurrent dietary calcium intake, exercise, and hormone status (testosterone, estrogen).

Dietary calcium intake depends on the consumption of dairy products. The calcium equivalent of 1 cup of milk is ¾ cup plain yogurt, 1½ oz cheddar cheese, 2 cups ice cream, ⅔ cup almonds, and 2½ oz sardines. Other sources of calcium include some leafy green vegetables (e.g., broccoli, kale, and collards), lime-processed tortillas, and calcium-precipitated tofu ("bean curd" from soybeans).

There is no classical calcium deficiency syndrome, because blood and cell levels are closely regulated. The body can mobilize skeletal calcium and increase the absorptive efficiency of dietary calcium. Osteoporosis occurs in childhood and is related to protein-calorie malnutrition, vitamin C deficiency, steroid therapy, endocrine disorders, immobilization and disuse, osteogenesis imperfecta, or calcium deficiency (in premature infants) (see Chapter 6). It is believed that the primary method of prevention of postmenopausal osteoporosis is to ensure maximum peak bone mass by providing optimal calcium intake during childhood and adolescence. Bone mineral status can be monitored by dual-energy x-ray absorptiometry.

No adverse effects are observed in adults with dietary calcium intakes of up to 2.5 g/day. There is concern that higher intakes may increase the risk for urinary stone formation, constipation, and decreased renal function and inhibit intestinal absorption of other minerals (e.g., iron and zinc).

REFERENCES

Behrman RE, Kliegman RM, Jenson HB, editors: *Nelson textbook of pediatrics,* ed 16, Philadelphia, 2000, WB Saunders, Chapter 49.
Shils ME, Olson JA, Shike M, et al, editors: *Modern nutrition in health and disease,* ed 9, Philadelphia, 1999, Williams & Wilkins, Chapter 7.

Nutritional Anemia

(See Chapter 14)

The recognition of anemia in infancy requires knowledge of normal age-related and birth weight–related changes in hemoglobin concentration. Reference values are given in Table 14–2.

Iron-Deficiency Anemia

In infancy, the major causes of iron-deficiency anemia are a decrease of body iron stores by rapid growth and an iron-poor diet. Blood loss results in more severe iron-deficiency anemia than is seen with the other two causes. Blood loss may be caused by conditions such as fetal/maternal transfusion, placenta previa, rupture of umbilical vessels, and twin/twin transfusion. Intestinal bleeding may be caused by the ingestion of cow's milk in early infancy, or rarely, by pulmonary hemosiderosis, a bleeding Meckel diverticulum or polyp, esophagitis, or peptic ulcer. The removal of blood for laboratory studies in infants requiring intensive care also may result in iron-deficiency anemia.

Iron is used in the synthesis of hemoglobin, myoglobin, and enzyme iron. Iron-deficiency anemia occurs when a lack of iron is sufficient to restrict the production of hemoglobin, and the hemoglobin concentration falls below the normal range. Body iron content is regulated primarily through modulation of iron absorption, which depends on the state of body iron stores, the form and amount of iron in foods, and the mixture of foods in the diet. Iron excretion occurs through the feces.

There are two categories of iron in food. The first is heme iron, present in hemoglobin and myoglobin; it is supplied by meat and rarely accounts for more than a quarter of the iron ingested by infants. The absorption of heme iron is relatively efficient and is not influenced by other constituents of the diet. The second category is nonheme iron, which represents the preponderance of iron intake consumed by infants and exists in the form of iron salts. The absorption of nonheme iron is influenced by the composition of consumed foods. The fractional intestinal absorption of the small amount of iron in human milk is 50%, in contrast to 10% of iron absorbed from unfortified cow's-milk formula and 4% absorbed from iron-fortified cow's-milk formula. About 4% of the iron from iron-fortified infant dry cereals is absorbed. Enhancers of nonheme iron absorption are ascorbic acid, meat, fish, and poultry. Inhibitors are bran, polyphenols (including the tannates in tea), and phosphate. During pregnancy, iron is efficiently transported from the maternal circulation to the fetus, and transport is not impaired by maternal iron-deficiency anemia. In the *term infant,* there is little change in total body iron and little need for exogenous iron before 4 months of age. Iron deficiency is rare among term infants during the first 4 months unless there has been substantial blood loss.

After 4 months of age, iron reserves become marginal for the remainder of infancy. In term infants who receive unfortified cow's-milk formula, depletion of storage iron can occur as early as 4 months of age. Breast-fed infants rarely deplete their iron stores until after 6 months of age. *Premature infants* have a lower amount of stored iron because significant amounts of iron are transferred from the mother in the third trimester. In addition, their postnatal iron needs are greater because of rapid rates of growth.

Term breast-fed infants need an alternative source of iron after 4–6 months of age. Some pediatricians recommend ferrous sulfate supplementation, whereas others introduce iron-containing solid foods. Under normal circumstances, iron-fortified formula is the only alternative to breast milk in the child younger than 1 year old.

Premature infants fed human milk may develop iron-deficiency anemia unless they receive iron supplements. Formula-fed preterm infants should receive iron-fortified formula.

In older children, iron deficiency is often the result of blood loss from such sources as menses or gastric ulceration. It is important to note that iron deficiency affects many tissues (e.g., muscle and central nervous system) in addition to producing anemia. Iron deficiency and anemia have been associated with lethargy, altered development, and decreased work capacity.

The *diagnosis* of iron-deficiency anemia is established by the presence of a microcytic hypochromic anemia, low serum ferritin levels, low serum iron levels, reduced transferrin saturation, normal to elevated red-cell width distribution (RDW), and enhanced iron-binding capacity. The mean corpuscular volume (MCV) and red cell indices are reduced, and the reticulocyte count is low. Iron deficiency may be present without anemia (see Chapter 14). *Clinical manifestations* are noted in Table 2–13.

Treatment of iron-deficiency anemia requires changes in the diet to provide adequate iron, as well as the administration of 2–6 mg iron/kg/24 hr (as ferrous sulfate). Reticulocytosis is noted within 3–7 days of starting treatment. Oral treatment should be continued for 5 months. Rarely, intramuscular or intravenous iron therapy is needed if oral iron cannot be given. Such parenteral therapy carries the risk of anaphylaxis.

Megaloblastic Anemia

In infancy, the rare anemias discussed in this chapter are caused by folate deficiency, vitamin B_{12} deficiency (discussed in the next section), and inborn errors of metabolism. *Folate deficiency,* which may result from a low dietary intake, malabsorption, or vitamin-drug interactions, can develop within a few weeks of birth, because infants require 10 times as

TABLE 2–13
Characteristics of Mineral Deficiencies

Mineral	Function	Manifestations of Deficiency	Comments	Sources
Iron	Heme-containing macromolecules (e.g., hemoglobin, cytochrome, and myoglobin)	Anemia, spoon nails, reduce muscle and mental performance	History of pica, cow's milk, gastrointestinal bleeding	Liver, eggs, grains
Copper	Redox reactions (e.g., cytochrome oxidase)	Hypochromic anemia, neutropenia, osteoporosis, hypotonia, hypoproteinemia	Inborn error, Menkes kinky hair syndrome	Liver, oysters, meat, nuts, grains, legumes, chocolate
Zinc	Metalloenzymes (e.g., alkaline phosphatase, carbonic anhydrase, DNA polymerase); wound healing	*Acrodermatitis enteropathica:* poor growth, acroorificial rash, alopecia, delayed sexual development, hypogeusia, infection	Protein-calorie malnutrition; weaning; malabsorption syndromes	Meat, grains, cheese, nuts
Selenium	Antioxidant; glutathione peroxidase	Keshan cardiomyopathy in China	Endemic areas; long-term TPN	Meat, vegetables
Chromium	Insulin cofactor	Poor weight gain, glucose intolerance, neuropathy	Protein-calorie malnutrition, long-term TPN	Yeast, breads
Fluoride	Strengthening of dental enamel	Caries	Supplementation during tooth growth, narrow therapeutic range, fluorosis may cause staining of the teeth	Seafood, water
Iodine	Thyroxine, triiodothyronine production	Simple endemic goiter *Myxedematous cretinism:* congenital hypothyroidism *Neurologic cretinism:* mental retardation, deafness, spasticity, normal thyroxine level at birth	Endemic in New Guinea, the Congo; endemic in Great Lakes area prior to use of iodized salt	Seafood, iodized salt, most food in nonendemic areas

TPN, Total parenteral nutrition; *DNA,* deoxyribonucleic acid.

much folate as adults per kilogram of body weight but have scant stores of folate in the newborn period. **Heat-sterilizing** the home-prepared formula can decrease the folate content by half. **Evaporated milk** and **goat's milk** are low in folate. Folate deficiency has been reported in healthy low-weight infants who are fed formulas based on heated or boiled evaporated or pasteurized milk. In proprietary infant formulas the presence of ascorbic acid decreases the loss of folic acid. Infants who are fed human milk

or proprietary cow's-milk formulas are not at risk for nutritional folate deficiency.

Patients with chronic hemolysis (sickle cell anemia or thalassemia) may require extra folate to avoid deficiency caused by increased production of red blood cells.

Folate deficiency should be suspected when hypersegmented neutrophils or elevation of the MCV is observed. The *diagnosis* is confirmed by the determination of both serum and red cell folate and serum vitamin B_{12}. A therapeutic dose is given when the diagnosis of folate deficiency is established (Table 2–11).

Treatment is monitored through the reticulocyte response and the rise in hemoglobin and hematocrit, responses similar to those noted during the iron treatment of iron-deficiency anemia. Folate therapy may mask the hematologic manifestations of vitamin B_{12} deficiency. Folate supplementation in very early pregnancy decreases the risk of fetal neural-tube defects. The window of opportunity for folate supplementation is so early in pregnancy that it has passed by the time most women learn they are pregnant. Folate supplementation of the food supply in the United States has been instituted in an attempt to prevent neural-tube defects. In addition, low folate intake has been associated with elevated homocysteine levels, which are associated with an increased risk of cardiovascular disease in adults.

Vitamin B_{12} Deficiency

Vitamin B_{12} deficiency is a rare disorder. Early diagnosis and treatment of this disorder in childhood are important because of the danger of irreversible neurologic damage. Most cases in childhood result from a specific defect in absorption (Tables 2–9 and 2–10). Such defects include congenital pernicious anemia (absent intrinsic factor), juvenile pernicious anemia (autoimmune), and deficiency of transcobalamin II transport. Intestinal resection, small bowel bacterial overgrowth, and the fish tapeworm *Diphyllobothrium latum* also cause vitamin B_{12} deficiency. An exclusively breast-fed infant ingests adequate vitamin B_{12} unless the mother is a strict vegetarian. The absorption of vitamin B_{12} depends on the formation of a complex between the vitamin and a mucoprotein, intrinsic factor. The complex is absorbed in the distal ileum. In the plasma, vitamin B_{12} is bound to a specific serum transport protein, transcobalamin II. The vitamin is stored in the liver. These stores are large in the newborn and are rarely depleted before 1 year of age or longer, even with inadequate vitamin B_{12} intake.

Depression of serum vitamin B_{12} below 100 pg/mL and the appearance of hypersegmented neutrophils are the earliest *clinical manifestations* of deficiency. Late findings of vitamin B_{12} deficiency are similar to the findings of folate deficiency; these finding include megaloblastic anemia, leukopenia, and thrombocytopenia. Neurologic manifestations include peripheral neuropathy, posterior spinal column signs, dementia, and eventual coma; these signs do not occur in folate deficiency, but administration of folate in excess of 0.1 mg/24 hr to vitamin B_{12}–deficient individuals may aggravate the neurologic manifestations.

The *diagnosis* of vitamin B_{12} deficiency is made by history and the presence of a macrocytosis accompanied by a megaloblastic bone marrow. Serum folate is normal, but red-cell folate may be reduced with vitamin B_{12} deficiency. Serum vitamin B_{12} levels are reduced. Patients with vitamin B_{12} deficiency also have increased urine levels of methylmalonic acid.

In nondietary deficiencies, resection of the terminal ileum without parenteral vitamin B_{12} should be considered as a cause of vitamin B_{12} deficiency. In unusual cases a Schilling test should also be considered to identify those patients with pernicious anemia and bacterial overgrowth. Vitamin B_{12} (radiolabeled) is ingested, and 2 hours later a flushing intravenous dose of vitamin B_{12} is given. If inadequate radiolabeled vitamin B_{12} is excreted in urine, the test is repeated with the addition of oral intrinsic factor. Normal excretion after the addition of intrinsic factor confirms the diagnosis of pernicious anemia (absent endogenous intrinsic factor). If urinary excretion of labeled vitamin B_{12} remains low, an intestinal lesion such as bacterial overgrowth may be present; pretreatment with antibiotics and repetition of the test with subsequent normal results confirms the diagnosis of bacterial overgrowth. Elevated breath hydrogen levels or culture of small bowel aspirates may also confirm the diagnosis of small bowel overgrowth.

Most cases of vitamin B_{12} deficiency in infants and children are not of dietary origin and require *treatment* throughout life. Maintenance therapy consists of repeated monthly intramuscular injections, although a new form of vitamin B_{12} that is administered intranasally has been released.

REFERENCES

Behrman RE, Kliegman RM, Jenson HB, editors: *Nelson textbook of pediatrics*, ed 16, Philadelphia, 2000, WB Saunders, Chapters 460, 461.

Shils ME, Olson JA, Shike M, et al, editors: *Modern nutrition in health and disease*, ed 9, Philadelphia, 1999, Williams & Wilkins, Chapter 88.

Stallings VA, Fung EB: Nutrition assessment of infants and children. In Shils ME, Olson JA, Shike M, et al, editors: *Modern nutrition in health and disease*, ed 9, Philadelphia, 1999, Williams & Wilkins.

Trace Elements

Trace element deficiencies are important clinical syndromes in persons who have malabsorption or are receiving parenteral nutrition. Many of these elements have a narrow therapeutic range and may cause toxicity.

Copper. Copper, as a constituent of many enzymes, is involved in energy production via oxidative phosphorylation, in the protection of cell membranes against oxidative damage, in the oxidation of iron released from storage, in erythropoietin synthesis, and in cerebral protein and myelin deposition. Some of the better known cuproenzymes are cytochrome oxidase, superoxide dismutase, ceruloplasmin, ferroxidase II, lysyl oxidase, tyrosinase, and dopamine β-hydroxylase.

Because copper is present in many foods (Table 2–13), adequate intake levels are easily achieved. Large amounts of copper are deposited in the fetal liver during the third trimester and gradually are depleted when ceruloplasmin synthesis and secretion begin. Transcuprein is the predominant vehicle of copper transport to the liver in the portal circulation. The liver of term infants contains a copper concentration 10- to 20-fold greater than that in the liver of adults. After its uptake from the portal circulation, copper is bound to hepatic metallothionein, from which it is released for enzyme synthesis in mitochondria and cytosol, transferred to the nuclei, and then incorporated into ceruloplasmin, which is released into the plasma compartment. Copper in plasma is found in four fractions: transcuprein and albumin, each 15%; ceruloplasmin, 60%; and various low-molecular-weight components, 10%. Synthesis and secretion in the liver occur with ceruloplasmin-bound copper, the preferred transport form to other tissues (e.g., brain, muscle, and bones). Copper breakdown products normally are sequestered in lysosomes and excreted in bile; copper overload may occur in patients with cholestasis. Children with cholestasis who are receiving parenteral nutrition should have the copper removed or reduced in their parenteral nutrition solution and serum copper and ceruloplasmin levels followed. Urinary excretion of copper normally is minimal.

Serum levels of copper and ceruloplasmin are low at birth and remain low for several weeks in preterm infants. Levels rise, however, as ceruloplasmin synthesis begins between the 6th and 12th postnatal weeks, varying with the gestational age of the infant. Concentrations are not affected by the levels of oral copper intake.

Copper deficiency was first reported in infants recuperating from PEM whose diet was based on cow's milk. It also has been noted in infants and patients receiving total parenteral nutrition containing inadequate amounts of copper, with chronic antacid use, and after ingesting large amounts of zinc.

The *clinical manifestations* of copper deficiency may be traced to the specific cuproenzyme affected—depigmentation (such as of hair or skin) and tyrosinase; hypothermia and hypotonia and cytochrome C; altered elastin and collagen and lysyl oxidase deficiency; central nervous system degeneration (e.g., hypotonia or psychomotor retardation) and dopamine

β-hydroxylase. Other signs include apnea, scurvy-like hemorrhage, blood vessel rupture, failure to thrive, flaring of anterior ribs, fractures, osteoporosis, periosteal reaction, metaphyseal spurs, hypercholesterolemia, edema, diarrhea, altered glucose tolerance, anemia, and neutropenia.

Wilson disease, an autosomal-recessive disease (1:200,000 births) caused by defective mobilization of copper from lysosomes, is characterized by increased copper deposition in the brain, liver, kidney, and cornea and low serum copper and ceruloplasmin levels. Hepatic failure with cirrhosis, hepatitis, Fanconi renal syndrome, hemolytic anemia, and Kayser-Fleischer corneal pigmented rings and neurologic signs such as behavioral problems, tremor, spasticity, and poor fine-motor control are noted after the age of 5 years. Treatment is a low-copper diet and lifelong chelation therapy with D-penicillamine.

Menkes kinky hair syndrome, a lethal X-linked neurodegenerative condition caused by a defect in copper absorption and transport across the intestines, is characterized by low serum copper and ceruloplasmin levels and increased copper levels in fibroblasts and urine. Manifestations include hypotonia; myoclonic seizures; spasticity; failure to thrive; steely, depigmented hair; osteoporosis; and arterial tortuosity. There is no specific therapy.

Excessive copper intake is associated with **Indian childhood cirrhosis.** Copper *toxicity* may produce nausea, hemolysis, and hepatic necrosis. Unfortunately, no perfect measure of copper status exists. Thus serum copper and ceruloplasmin levels and trends in these levels must be considered in the patient evaluation.

Zinc. Zinc is important in protein metabolism and synthesis, in nucleic acid metabolism, and in the stabilization of cell membranes. Zinc metalloenzymes include erythrocyte carbonic anhydrase, alcohol dehydrogenase, carboxypeptidases A and B, alkaline phosphatase, DNA and RNA polymerase, various dehydrogenases, and retinene reductase (Table 2–13); many other enzymes use zinc as a cofactor.

Dietary zinc is absorbed (20–80%) in the duodenum and proximal small intestine. In zinc sufficiency, an increasing zinc pool triggers synthesis of intestinal mucosal metallothionein, which binds intracellular zinc. Protein-bound zinc and human milk zinc are the most readily absorbed forms of the mineral. Histidine and cysteine facilitate absorption, whereas phytase and fiber inhibit it. Excess dietary copper, iron, or cadmium decreases zinc absorption by competing for cellular uptake and metallothionein binding. After cellular uptake, the metal is secreted into the portal circulation, where it binds primarily to albumin. Zinc transported from the intestine is taken up rapidly by the liver, pancreas, kidneys, and spleen. Excretion occurs through fecal losses. In the presence of ongoing losses, such as chronic diarrhea, requirements can drastically increase.

The original account of **zinc deficiency dwarfism** syndrome was described in a group of children with low levels of zinc in their hair, poor appetite, diminished taste acuity, hypogonadism, and short stature.

Acute acquired zinc deficiency may occur in patients receiving total parenteral nutrition without zinc supplementation and in premature infants fed human milk. Transient zinc deficiency rarely has been reported in full-term, breast-fed infants. Mild *clinical manifestations* of zinc deficiency in infants include failure to thrive; in children and adolescents, manifestations include decreased growth velocity, anorexia, and hypogeusia. Moderately severe manifestations include delayed sexual maturation, rough skin, pica, and hepatosplenomegaly. The severe signs include acral and periorificial skin lesions, failure to thrive, diarrhea, mood changes, alopecia, night blindness, and photophobia.

Acrodermatitis enteropathica is an autosomal recessive disorder that begins within 2–4 weeks after infants have been weaned from breast milk. It is characterized by an acute perioral and perianal dermatitis, alopecia, and failure to thrive. The disease is caused by severe zinc deficiency from an undefined but specific defect of intestinal zinc absorption. Plasma zinc levels are reduced, and serum alkaline phosphatase activity is low. Treatment is provided with oral zinc supplementation.

Zinc excess produces nausea, emesis, abdominal pain, headache, vertigo, and seizures.

Selenium. The only well-defined function of selenium is as part of the enzyme glutathione peroxidase (GSHPx), one of the enzyme systems that, with catalase, superoxide dismutase, and vitamin E, protect cells from oxidative damage by destroying cytosolic hydrogen peroxide (Table 2–13). Selenium is well absorbed. The primary route of excretion is in the urine. The intake of selenium by exclusively breast-fed infants is approximately 10 mg/24 hr, compared with 7 mg/24 hr by formula-fed infants. Concentrations in human milk reflect selenium levels in the mother. Infants and children who receive total parenteral nutrition may have a rapid drop of blood selenium levels unless adequate amounts are provided in the solution.

A **selenium deficiency syndrome** (Keshan disease) has been reported in rural China and is characterized by necrosis and fibrosis of the myocardium, which results in potentially fatal acute or chronic heart failure. Those most at-risk individuals include infants, young children, and women of childbearing age. Fatal cardiomyopathy has been reported in adults receiving long-term total parenteral nutrition

and in a 2-year-old child whose diet was very low in both selenium and animal protein. Low blood selenium levels in orally fed preterm infants also are associated with increased erythrocyte fragility. Muscle pain, myopathy, and nail bed changes may occur.

Iodine. Iodine is an integral part of the thyroid hormones (Table 2–13). Circulating iodine is taken up avidly by the thyroid gland, where it is bound to thyroglobulin, an iodinated glycoprotein from which the hormones thyroxine (T_4) and triiodothyronine (T_3) are formed. In iodine deficiency, the synthesis and release of thyroid hormones are decreased, low blood levels of T_4 and T_3 result, and the feedback mechanism involving the thyroid-hypothalamus-pituitary axis is stimulated. This sequence of events produces an increased output of thyroid-stimulating hormone (TSH) by the pituitary, which ultimately results in enlargement of the thyroid gland, or **goiter.**

Ingested iodine is readily absorbed; the main route of excretion is in the urine. Fifty percent of an adequate iodine intake is retained by healthy infants. For infants of iodine-sufficient mothers, additional iodine is not necessary during short-term intravenous feeding. Because of its potential for toxicity, all sources of iodine to the infant should be considered before supplementation is initiated.

Moderate *iodine deficiency* may produce a euthyroid state accompanied by hyperplasia and hypertrophy of the thyroid gland or goiter. Severe dietary iodine deficiency results in hypothyroidism. **Endemic cretinism** is seen in the same geographic areas as endemic goiter and may be characterized by ataxia, spasticity, deaf-mutism, mental retardation with or without short stature, and little or no impairment of thyroid function. This variant affecting the nervous system is probably caused by early fetal iodine deficiency. The **myxedematous type** of cretinism is characterized by retarded growth, delayed mental and sexual function, and the presence of myxedema in the absence of abnormal neurologic signs. This variant may be caused by late fetal and postnatal iodine deficiency, which results in low thyroid hormone levels, elevated TSH concentration, and markedly delayed bone age. Both syndromes are prevented by iodine supplementation. Excessive iodine treatment may produce thyrotoxicosis or goiter.

Fluoride. Dental enamel is strengthened when fluoride is substituted for hydroxyl ions in the hydroxyapatite crystalline mineral matrix of the enamel. The resulting fluorapatite is more resistant to both chemical and physical damage. Fluoride is incorporated into the enamel during the mineralization stages of tooth formation and also by surface interaction after the tooth has erupted. Fluoride is similarly incorporated into bone mineral and may protect against osteoporosis later in life. Approximately 80% of fluoride in foods and fluids is absorbed; as much as 97% is absorbed from soluble supplements such as sodium fluoride. Fluoride is excreted mainly in the urine, with less than 10% of the intake appearing in the feces.

Because of concern about the risk of **fluorosis**, infants should not receive fluoride supplements before 6 months of age. In the formula-fed infant, the need for supplementation depends on the type of formula used. Commercial formulas now are made with defluoridated water and contain small amounts of fluoride. An infant older than 6 months who receives only ready-feed formula should be given supplemental fluoride. The fluoride content of human milk is low, 5–15 ng/mL, and intakes by exclusively breast-fed infants are about 4–5 μg/day in optimally fluoridated areas. Breast-fed infants older than 6 months should receive fluoride supplements. Fluoride levels of the water supply to which the child is exposed should be determined before fluoride supplements are prescribed. Fluorosis commonly stains the teeth.

REFERENCES

Behrman RE, Kliegman RM, Jenson HB, editors: *Nelson textbook of pediatrics*, ed 16, Philadelphia, 2000, WB Saunders, Chapter 40.
Walker WA, Watkins JB, editors: *Nutrition in pediatrics*, ed 2, Philadelphia, 1997, WB Saunders, Chapter 7.

NUTRITIONAL MANAGEMENT DURING ILLNESS

Nutritional Assessment

Pediatric nutritional assessment includes consideration of medical and nutrition history, dietary intake, factors that alter nutrient use and absorption, physical examination (including growth patterns and current anthropometry), and laboratory assessment. The assessment is used to define nutritional status and nutrient needs in children.

Macronutrient depletion can be assessed by comparing height, weight, and head circumference measurements of the patient with normal standards. Recent weight loss or failure of normal growth is an important consideration. A low percentage of expected weight for height suggests recent macronutrient deficiency (usually calories), whereas low height for age suggests chronic deficiency. Loss of body fat is measured by determining triceps skinfold thicknesses, and loss of muscle mass is reflected in reduced arm circumference measurements corrected for skinfold thicknesses. Measurements of the triceps skinfold and the circumference of the upper arm are made at the midpoint of the distance between the palpated head of the humerus and the bony promi-

nence of the elbow on the extensor (dorsal) surface when the elbow is flexed 90°. Additional physical signs are noted in Table 2–14. Useful laboratory tests include measurement of hepatic secretory proteins in serum (Table 2–15). Albumin, retinol-binding protein, prealbumin, and transferrin are depleted during inadequate protein or calorie intake. Albumin is affected by nonnutritional influences; these other proteins have a shorter half-life and reflect recent (days to weeks) macronutrient intake. Reduced total lymphocyte count and a failure of T-cell function are reflected in anergy in skin tests.

The nutritional management of the ill patient is accomplished by enteral or parenteral feeding. Priority should be given to oral feedings, followed by intragastric, duodenal, or jejunal tube delivery; peripheral intravenous infusions; and, finally, central intravenous infusions. The complexity and expense of nursing and dietary care increase exponentially with the progression through this management sequence. The immunologic and metabolic effects of malnutrition make the delayed introduction of adequate feeding a clinical risk that must be aggressively addressed.

REFERENCES

Hubbard VS, Hubbard LR: Clinical assessment of nutritional status. In Walker WA, Watkins JB, editors: *Nutrition in pediatrics*, ed 2, Hamilton, Ontario, 1996, BC Decker.
Lo CW: Laboratory assessment of nutritional status. In Walker WA, Watkins JB, editors: *Nutrition in pediatrics*, ed 2, Hamilton, Ontario, 1996, BC Decker.

Enteral Nutrition

Contraindications to oral feeding include an obstructive ileus, gastric retention, intestinal perforation, anatomic obstruction, severe acute gastrointestinal hemorrhage, and severe diet-induced diarrhea. When conditions may limit tolerance of enteral feedings, feeding should begin with a diet appropriate for age, given first in diluted form or in a limited amount. When tolerance is established, there should be as rapid a progression as reasonable toward full concentration and nutritional adequacy. The rate of this progression is governed by gastrointestinal tolerance as determined by emesis, abdominal distention, and diarrhea.

When intestinal digestion is abnormal or when protein hypersensitivity is suspected, an oligomeric or elemental enteral product can be used. In older children this commonly is administered by a continuous intragastric drip because of the objectionable taste. Some of these products have an increased osmolarity and may produce intestinal luminal water sequestration if delivered into the jejunum at rates adequate to meet nutrient requirements. The level of

TABLE 2–14
Physical Signs of Nutritional Deficiency Disorders

System	Sign	Deficiency
General appearance	Reduced weight for height	Calories
Skin and hair	Pallor	Anemias (iron, B_{12}, vitamin E, folate, and copper)
	Edema	Protein, thiamine
	Nasolabial seborrhea	Calories, protein, vitamin B_6, niacin, riboflavin
	Dermatitis	Riboflavin, essential fatty acids, biotin
	Photosensitivity dermatitis	Niacin
	Acrodermatitis	Zinc
	Follicular hyperkeratosis (sandpaperlike)	Vitamin A
	Depigmented skin	Calories, protein
	Purpura	Vitamins C, K
	Scrotal, vulval dermatitis	Riboflavin
	Alopecia	Zinc, biotin, protein
	Depigmented, dull hair, easily pluckable	Protein, calories, copper
Subcutaneous tissue	Decreased	Calories
Eye (vision)	Adaptation to dark	Vitamins A, E, zinc
	Color discrimination	Vitamin A
	Bitot spots, xerophthalmia, keratomalacia	Vitamin A
	Conjunctival pallor	Nutritional anemias
	Fundal capillary microaneurysms	Vitamin C
Face, mouth, and neck	Angular stomatitis	Riboflavin, iron
	Cheilosis	Vitamins B_6, niacin, riboflavin
	Bleeding gums	Vitamins C, K
	Atrophic papillae	Riboflavin, iron, niacin, folate, vitamin B_{12}
	Smooth tongue	Iron
	Red tongue (glossitis)	Vitamins B_6, B_{12}, niacin, riboflavin, folate
	Parotid swelling	Protein
	Caries	Fluoride
	Anosmia	Vitamins A, B_{12}, zinc
	Hypogeusia	Vitamin A, zinc
	Goiter	Iodine
Cardiovascular	Heart failure	Thiamine, selenium, nutritional anemias
Genital	Hypogonadism	Zinc
Skeletal	Costochondral beading	Vitamins D, C
	Subperiosteal hemorrhage	Vitamin C, copper
	Cranial bossing	Vitamin D
	Wide fontanel	Vitamin D
	Epiphyseal enlargement	Vitamin D
	Craniotabes	Vitamin D, calcium
	Tender bones	Vitamin C
	Tender calves	Thiamine, selenium, vitamin C
	Spoon-shaped nails (koilonychia)	Iron
	Transverse nail line	Protein
Neurologic	Sensory, motor neuropathy	Thiamine, vitamins E, B_6, B_{12}
	Ataxia, areflexia	Vitamin E
	Ophthalmoplegia	Vitamin E, thiamine
	Tetany	Vitamin D, Ca^{2+}, Mg^{2+}
	Retardation	Iodine, niacin
	Dementia, delirium	Vitamin E, niacin, thiamine
	Poor position sense, ataxia	Thiamine, vitamin B_{12}

TABLE 2–15
Screening Tests for Nutritional Deficiency Disorders*

Test	Deficiency
Hemoglobin + RBC indices	Iron, folate, vitamins B_{12}, B_6, copper
Lymphocyte count	Protein, calories
Delayed hypersensitivity skin tests	Protein, calories
Retinol-binding protein, prealbumin, transferrin	Protein, calories
Albumin	Protein; affected by fluids, renal and hepatic dysfunction
Calcium, phosphate	Vitamin D
Prothrombin time	Vitamin K
Thyroxine	Iodine
Bone radiographs	Iodine, vitamins D and C, copper
Alkaline phosphate	Zinc
Ceruloplasmin	Copper

RBC, Red blood cell count.
*Specific assays are available for most vitamins. Macronutrients and trace elements are determined when indicated by the history, physical examination, and screening tests.

tolerance for oligomeric diets varies with each patient and the etiology of the gastrointestinal disease. Glucose polymers, medium-chain and long-chain triglycerides, and oligopeptides and free amino acid formulas are available when needed for specific patients. Care must be taken to ensure the overall quality of the therapeutic diet. In moderately to severely affected patients, enteral feeding should be supplemented with peripheral intravenous nutrition until acceptable nutrient absorption and weight gain are established.

A number of complications can occur as a consequence of enteral feeding. Enteral catheter complications include erosion of the nasal septum; displacement of the catheter tip into the esophagus, lung, or duodenum; and perforation of the gastric wall. Silastic catheters reduce irritation and the likelihood of perforation. A percutaneously placed gastrostomy feeding tube should be considered for long-term enteral feeding.

Parenteral Nutrition

Total parenteral nutrition (TPN) is indicated when enteral nutrients cannot meet the nutritional needs for nutritional rehabilitation or normal growth. Enteral nutrition is preferred because it is more physiologic, less expensive, and associated with fewer complications. Often the parenteral nutrition is used to supplement the enteral intake until the latter route provides sufficient nutrients for growth. Indications for TPN include congenital gastrointestinal anomalies, necrotizing enterocolitis, short bowel syndrome, and

intractable diarrhea unresponsive to enteral alimentation. TPN also is useful in patients with trauma, burns, malignant disease, multiple organ system failure, and severe inflammatory bowel disease.

Generally, TPN by peripheral venous access is instituted first, with central access established when peripheral access becomes unavailable or when it is required to allow greater calorie delivery. In patients who need long-term TPN, a central venous line is placed early in the course of care. With few exceptions (e.g., marked fluid limitations), adequate nutritional support can be provided by either central or peripheral line TPN. Intravenous nutrient solutions provide all of the protein, calorie, electrolyte, vitamin, mineral (except iron), trace element, and essential fatty acid requirements. Iron can be added or given separately in most situations. The nonprotein calories are provided by both carbohydrates (dextrose) and a 20% lipid emulsion.

Peripheral Intravenous Nutrition

Peripheral TPN is based on a 10–12% dextrose solution with 2–3% amino acids solution to provide about 0.8–2.0 g protein/kg/24 hr for older children, 1.5–3.0 g/kg/24 hr for full-term and older infants, and 2.5–3.5 g/kg/24 hr for preterm infants. The caloric density of glucose- and amino acid–based solutions is limited by the solution's osmolality (10% glucose = 550 mOsm). Higher-osmolality solutions are associated with phlebitis of peripheral veins. The high caloric density but low osmolar lipid emulsion usually provides additional calories in excess of the 3–5% of total calories needed to prevent essential

TABLE 2–16
Potential Complications of Total Parenteral Alimentation

Catheter-Related	Electrolyte (Minerals)—cont'd
Superior vena cava syndrome (thrombosis)	Metabolic acidosis
Pulmonary thromboembolism	Trace mineral deficiency (zinc, copper)
Pulmonary hypertension	Aluminum toxicity
Pneumothorax	
Pleural effusions (extravasated solution)	Metabolic
Cardiac arrhythmias	Hypoglycemia (infusion stopped)
Pericardial effusion	Hyperglycemia (hyperosmolar state)
Mural thrombosis (cardiac)	Hyperaminoacidemia (↑ protein intake)
Intramyocardial infusion	Hyperammonemia (↑ protein intake)
Tricuspid valve injury	Azotemia (↑ protein intake)
Hemorrhage	Hypoalbuminemia (↓ protein intake)
Flocculation precipitation of nutrients	Essential fatty acid deficiency
	Hypertriglyceridemia
Infections	Carnitine deficiency
Bacterial (staphylococcal; gram negative)	Vitamin deficiencies (biotin)
Candida sepsis	Acanthocytosis (lipids)
Malassezia furfur (intralipid)	
Aspergillosis sepsis	Systemic
Entry, exit site, tract infections	Cholestasis (hepatic dysfunction)
Contaminated solutions (rare organisms)	Cirrhosis
	Fatty infiltration (liver, monocytes, lung; intralipid)
Electrolyte (Minerals)	Intestinal mucosal atrophy
Hypocalcemia	Osmotic diuresis (hyperglycemia)
Hypercalcemia	Metabolic bone disease (osteopenia)
Hyponatremia	Increased extracellular fluid space
Hypernatremia	White blood cell dysfunction (phosphate depletion, lipids)
Hypokalemia	Poor sucking, swallowing (NPO)
Hypophosphatemia	Fat overload syndrome (high dose, rapid lipid infusion)
Hypomagnesemia	

NPO, Nothing by mouth.

fatty acid deficiency. The rate of lipid infusion is initiated at 0.5–1.0 g/kg/24 hr but is advanced to 2–3 g/kg/24 hr as appropriate. The intravenous caloric requirement is approximately 10% less than the enteral requirement because of the omission of the caloric expenditure for the thermic effect of feeding (Fig. 2–4).

Central Venous Nutrition

Central TPN primarily differs from peripheral TPN in the dextrose concentration; usually 20% with central TPN versus 10% with peripheral TPN. In situations involving severe fluid limitations or lipid intolerance, up to 25–30% dextrose may be used centrally. For longer-term central access, a silicon-rubber cuffed catheter is surgically placed in a large vein tunneled subcutaneously to an exit site on the anterior chest wall and threaded to the superior vena cava into the right atrium.

Careful monitoring of the venous line site and placement, fluid and electrolyte balance, growth, and metabolic response is essential to the safety and efficacy of TPN. Laboratory evaluation includes measurement of the levels of blood glucose, urea nitrogen, creatinine, calcium, phosphorus, magnesium, bilirubin, albumin, liver enzymes, and triglycerides. These are obtained before initiation of TPN and weekly during infusion. Serum triglycerides are monitored as the amount of lipids infused is increased from 1–2 g/kg/24 hr to the level required for caloric needs (3 g/kg/24 hr).

Complications of TPN are categorized as metabolic, technical (catheter-related), or infectious (Table 2–16). *Hepatobiliary dysfunction* is seen in some patients who require long-term TPN. Cholestasis is associated with conjugated hyperbilirubinemia, modest elevation in the hepatocellular enzymes, and, rarely, irreversible hepatic failure. Although several factors (e.g., fasting, amino acids) have been implicated in the pathogeneses of hepatobiliary dysfunction, no single causal factor has been identified. The diagnosis of TPN-induced cholestasis is one of exclusion; other causes of hyperbilirubinemia must be considered, such as sepsis, structural abnormalities, antitrypsin deficiency, cystic fibrosis, viral hepatitis, and inborn errors of metabolism (galactosemia, tyrosinemia). The development of cholestasis increases the urgency of establishing enteral support and discontinuing TPN as soon as enteral intake is adequate. To prevent infection, trained personnel clean the catheter site with aseptic solutions; entry into the system is avoided, and if entry is necessary, it is performed with sterile technique.

Delays in behavioral development may result from the long-term administration of enteral nasogastric or parenteral feedings to young infants, in part because the development of oral feeding patterns is bypassed. The opportunity for nonnutritive sucking (i.e., the provision of a pacifier) may prevent this complication. When the infant has not learned to suck or swallow, a team approach is required to teach the infant these functions.

REFERENCES

Mascarenhas MR, Stallings VA: Enteral and parenteral nutrition. In Walker WA, Durie PR, Hamilton JR, et al, editors: *Pediatric gastrointestinal disease: pathophysiology, diagnosis and management,* ed 3, Hamilton, Ontario, 2000, BC Decker.

Wyllie R, Hyams JS, editors: *Pediatric gastrointestinal disease,* ed 2, Philadelphia, 2000, WB Saunders, Chapter 59.

CHAPTER 3

The Acutely Ill or Injured Child

Steven E. Krug

RECOGNITION OF SHOCK AND RESPIRATORY FAILURE

The care of the acutely ill or injured child requires an evaluation and management approach that is quite different than that used to assess the well child or the child with a chronic or minor illness. The assessment of the acutely ill child centers on the rapid identification of physiologic derangement in organ-system function rather than the immediate development of a differential diagnosis. The goal of this efficient assessment is *triage,* or identifying children at risk for critical illness or injury. Because suspicion of critical illness warrants immediate management such as resuscitation, such action may need to be based on very limited information.

Cardiopulmonary failure is rarely a spontaneous event in children. It is typically the end result of progressively deteriorating respiratory or circulatory function. Unfortunately, once cardiopulmonary arrest has occurred, the outcome is generally poor, with 75–80% dying and 75% of the survivors sustaining permanent disability. The strategy for successful pediatric resuscitation relies on the recognition of a prearrest state, such as impending respiratory failure or shock. This recognition depends on an individual's ability to identify the symptoms or signs of those conditions or to determine which children are at special risk for these life-threatening events.

The initial evaluation of the acutely ill child requires rapid cardiopulmonary assessment. This evaluation should take less than 60 seconds to complete, follow the "ABC" (*a*irway, *b*reathing, and *c*irculation) approach used in cardiopulmonary resuscitation (Table 3–1), and integrate pertinent physical findings and physiologic data into one of the following clinical impressions:
1. Stable
2. Impending respiratory failure or shock

3. Definite respiratory failure or shock
4. Cardiopulmonary failure
5. Cardiopulmonary arrest

This assessment will then determine the priorities and urgency of patient management and their urgency. Initial treatment is directed toward the physiologic derangement (e.g., shock) rather than what might be the underlying cause (e.g., sepsis).

After the initial evaluation, objective data are used both to assess the response to stabilization procedures and to make the ultimate diagnosis. Collecting such data requires ongoing *monitoring of vital organ functions,* including the brain, heart, kidney, bone marrow, lung, and liver. By using a combination of monitoring and therapeutic interventions, the physician is able to anticipate the further progression of the illness and can manage ongoing physiologic derangements (Table 3–2).

Respiratory failure is the most common cause of cardiopulmonary arrest in children and is characterized by inadequate oxygenation or ventilation. It may be caused by intrinsic lung or airway disease, airway obstruction, or poor respiratory effort resulting from central nervous system dysfunction. It is generally preceded by respiratory distress, a compensated state characterized by signs of increased work of breathing (e.g., tachypnea, nasal flaring, intercostal muscle retraction, grunting, and accessory respiratory muscle use) (see Chapter 12).

Shock is defined as a physiologic state with insufficient delivery of oxygen and metabolic substrates to meet the metabolic needs of tissues. Shock is characterized by signs of inadequate tissue perfusion (e.g., pallor, cool skin, poor pulses, delayed capillary refill, oliguria, and abnormal mentation) and may be further classified on the basis of the presence of a normal (compensated) or low (uncompensated) blood pressure.

The clinical signs of respiratory failure and shock

TABLE 3–1
Rapid Cardiopulmonary Assessment

Airway Patency
  Patent, able to be maintained independently
  Maintainable with positioning, suctioning
  Unmaintainable, requires assistance
Breathing
  Rate
  Mechanics
    Retractions
    Grunting
    Use of accessory muscles
    Nasal flaring
  Air entry
    Chest expansion
    Breath sounds
    Stridor
    Wheezing
    Paradoxical chest motion
  Color
Circulation
  Heart rate
  Peripheral pulses
    Present/absent
    Volume/strength
  Skin perfusion
    Capillary refill time
    Skin temperature
    Color
    Mottling
  Blood pressure
    Central pulse strength
CNS perfusion
  Responsiveness (AVPU)
  Recognition of parents or caregivers
  Muscle tone
  Pupil size
  Posturing

AVPU, Alert, responds to voice, responds to pain, unresponsive.

TABLE 3–2
Elements of Acute Care

Examine
Perform an initial assessment followed by complete and systematic evaluation.
Focus examination on areas of chief complaints; determine life-threatening and organ-threatening conditions.
Synthesize findings to plan further evaluation.

Monitor
Monitor vital signs.
Monitor the physiologic parameters required to:
1. Make a diagnosis
2. Ascertain response to therapy or progression of disease
Prospectively determine allowable limits for changes in monitored parameters; generate and record objective data to guide therapy.

Intervene
Before initiating therapy, determine therapeutic goals and endpoints.
Prioritize life-threatening and organ-threatening conditions.
Initiate therapy based on recognized pathophysiologic derangements.
Adjust therapeutic strategies to individual patient needs.
Use objective data to guide changes in therapy.

Anticipate
Anticipation requires understanding of the underlying pathophysiology.
Always plan for the "worst-case" scenario.
Use data obtained through examination and monitoring to update prognostic impressions continually.

---

are caused by tissue hypoxia and the resulting metabolic or mixed (metabolic and respiratory) acidosis. Early in the course of critical illness, respiratory failure and shock may be clinically distinct entities. As both states progress, they deteriorate to a state of cardiopulmonary failure. Irregular respiration, bradycardia, and hypotension are ominous findings in acutely ill children, suggestive of impending cardiopulmonary arrest.

The goals of management of acutely ill patients are to recognize the early signs of impending respiratory failure or shock and to intervene before further deterioration occurs. This requires careful observation and may be aided by the use of various clinical severity scoring systems (e.g., trauma, coma, or acute injury scores). One system, PRISM (*p*ediatric *r*isk of *m*ortality), combines physiologic (heart and respiratory rates, blood pressure, Glasgow Coma Scale, and pupillary signs) and biochemical (PaO_2/FiO_2 and $PaCO_2$, coagulation tests, bilirubin, potassium, ionized calcium, glucose, and bicarbonate) data to help predict the risk of critical illness progression.

Common causes of death among children over one month of age include sudden infant death syndrome (SIDS), trauma (e.g., motor vehicle crashes, falls, child abuse, or violence), burns, drowning, toxic ingestion, respiratory diseases (e.g., asthma), severe infections (e.g., meningitis, sepsis, human immunodeficiency virus [HIV] pneumonia, or gastroenteritis), metabolic disorders (e.g., diabetes), and the consequences of treating congenital anomalies or malignancy.

REFERENCES

Behrman RE, Kliegman RM, Jenson HB, editors: *Nelson textbook of pediatrics*, ed 16, Philadelphia, 2000, WB Saunders, Chapter 56.

Chameides L, Hazinski MF, editors: *Textbook of pediatric advanced life support*, Dallas, 1997, American Heart Association, Chapter 2.

Strange GR, editor: *The pediatric emergency medicine course*, ed 3, Elk Grove Village, Ill, 1998, American Academy of Pediatrics, Chapters 1, 3.

EMERGENCY MEDICAL SERVICES FOR CHILDREN

The outcome of the critically ill or injured child's condition depends on the provision of timely and appropriate emergency care. This care begins with the early recognition of a life-threatening problem and continues through prehospital, in-hospital, and rehabilitative care. Because the occurrence of critical illness is much lower in children than in adults and because the presenting signs of critical illness in children may be difficult to recognize, existing components of emergency medical services (EMS) may not be prepared to meet the unique needs of children. With the development of modern-day EMS and trauma systems, dramatic reductions have been realized in adult cardiac and trauma mortality and disability rates; these reduction have not been as dramatic with children. Efforts to integrate EMS for children (EMS-C) and the special needs of children (via education and training, equipment, and protocols) into existing EMS systems will improve the outcome of pediatric acute illness and injury.

REFERENCES

Behrman RE, Kliegman RM, Jenson HB, editors: *Nelson textbook of pediatrics*, ed 16, Philadelphia, 2000, WB Saunders, Chapter 58.

Durch JS, Lohr KN: *Emergency medical services for children*, Washington, DC, 1993, Institute of Medicine, National Academy Press.

Seidel J: Emergency medical services for children, *Emerg Med Clin North Am* 13(2):255-266, 1995.

Seidel JS, Knapp JF, editors: *Childhood emergencies in the office, hospital, and community: organizing systems of care*, Elk Grove Village, Ill, 2000, American Academy of Pediatrics.

MAJOR TRAUMA
Epidemiology

Injury is the leading cause of death in children 1–14 years of age. Almost 50% of these are caused by motor vehicle crashes. A majority of the rest are the result of falls (25–30%) and burns (10–15%). Gunshot wounds, assaults, and ingestions account for 5–10% of pediatric trauma. More than 50% of trauma fatalities occur at the scene of the injury rather than at a secondary site to which the victim may be transported, such as a hospital or the home. These scene deaths occur with patients who receive injuries to the brainstem, head, aorta, heart, and upper cervical spine. The next substantial group of deaths occurs within several hours of arrival in the emergency department; survival depends on the severity of shock at the time of arrival and the length of time the shock state has been present. If the patient is taken to a center at which definitive care can be provided and is stabilized within an hour of the time of the injury, the outcome is likely to be optimal. A final peak in mortality occurs days to weeks after the initial injury and results from multi–system-organ failure or other severe, life-threatening complications that have not responded to medical and surgical management.

Education for Preventing Injuries

The recognition that much of morbidity and mortality are determined at the scene of an injury has stimulated the development of prevention measures throughout the United States, including a decrease in the speed limit, the imposition of more stringent automobile safety standards, mandatory use of automobile child-restraining devices and bicycle helmets, promotion of cardiopulmonary resuscitation (CPR) training, and more frequent use of the Heimlich maneuver for choking victims. Regional poison-control centers throughout the United States provide the lay public and medical professionals with information regarding toxic ingestions and exposures. Other primary prevention efforts have included fire safety programs, water safety and swimming programs, and legislative efforts ranging from requirements for the reporting of suspected child abuse to the control of the temperature of hot water in order to prevent children from being scalded.

Providing Prehospital Care

Trauma care begins at the scene of the injury. The prehospital phase of care is focused on a rapid assessment of the ABCs and initiation of basic or advanced life

TABLE 3–3
Children Requiring Pediatric Trauma Center Care

Patients with serious injury to more than one organ or system

Patients with one-system injury who require critical care or monitoring in an intensive care unit

Patients with signs of shock who require more than one transfusion

Patients with fracture complicated by suspected neurovascular or compartment injury

Patients with fracture of axial skeleton

Patients with two or more long-bone fractures

Patients with potential replantation of an extremity

Patients with suspected or actual spinal cord or column injuries

Patients with head injury with any one of the following:
    Orbital or facial bone fracture
    Cerebrospinal fluid leaks
    Altered state of consciousness
    Changing neural signs
    Open head injuries
    Depressed skull fracture
    Requiring intracranial pressure monitoring

Patients suspected of requiring ventilator support

TABLE 3–4
Pediatric Trauma Score*

Category Component	+2	+1	−1
Size	>20 kg	10–20 kg	<10 kg
Airway	Normal	Maintainable	Unmaintainable
Systolic BP†	>90 mm Hg	50–90 mm Hg	<50 mm Hg
CNS	Awake	Obtunded/ LOC	Coma/ decerebrate
Skeletal	None	Closed fracture	Open/ multiple fractures
Cutaneous/ wounds	None	Minor	Major/ penetrating

Modified from Tepas J, Mollitt D, Talbert J, et al: *J Pediatr Surg* 22:14, 1987.

+2, Palpable pulse at wrist; +1, palpable pulse at groin; −1, no palpable pulse; *BP*, blood pressure; *CNS*, central nervous system; *LOC*, loss of consciousness.

*If score <8, refer to Pediatric Trauma Center.

†If proper size BP cuff is not available

support interventions at the scene or en route to the hospital. The scope of care provided in the field is determined by the nature of the injured child's physiologic state and associated injuries, the anticipated transit time to the hospital, and the skill level or scope of practice of the prehospital care providers. The general goal of prehospital trauma care is rapid assessment, support of the ABCs, immobilization, and transportation.

Prehospital care providers, with the assistance of protocols and on-line medical direction, must also determine which injured children require transport to a trauma center (Table 3–3). A number of trauma triage scoring tools have been developed to assist the evaluation of injury severity, trauma center triage decision making, and patient prognosis. The most appropriate objective scoring system for children is the Pediatric Trauma Score (Table 3–4).

Evaluating and Managing the Trauma Patient in the Emergency Department

When the patient arrives at the emergency department, the responding trauma team must initiate an organized and synchronized response. The initial assessment of the seriously injured child should involve a systematic approach that includes the following: a primary survey, resuscitation, secondary survey, postresuscitation monitoring, and definitive care.

The *primary survey* focuses on the "ABCDEs" of emergency care, as modified for trauma from the ABCs of cardiopulmonary resuscitation: "A" stands for *airway*, accompanied by *cervical spine control*. Effective care of the traumatized child should ensure spinal immobilization. If cervical spine stability is a concern, orotracheal intubation, when indicated, should be performed with the neck immobilized in the neutral position. Nasotracheal intubation is extremely difficult in children and may be contraindicated in facial trauma or basilar skull fracture, because the tube may enter the cranial vault. Needle cricothyrotomy and transtracheal ventilation also may be used in instances of facial trauma or cervical spine fracture.

"B" stands for assessment of *breathing*, which is critical in the traumatized patient, even if an artificial airway is already in place. Ventilation can be assessed by observation, palpation, and auscultation. As a component of the primary survey, major thoracic injuries (Table 3–5) must be assessed and treated immediately to ensure a successful resuscitation.

TABLE 3–5
Life-Threatening Chest Injuries

Tension Pneumothorax
One-way valve leak from lung parenchyma
Complete collapse with mediastinal and tracheal shift
  to side opposite the leak
Compromises venous return and decreases ventilation
  of other lung
Clinically, manifests as respiratory distress, unilateral
  absent breath sounds, tracheal deviation, distended
  neck veins, tympany to percussion of involved side,
  and cyanosis
Relieve first with needle aspiration, then with chest
  tube drainage

Open Pneumothorax (Sucking Chest Wound)
Effect on ventilation depends on size

Major Flail Chest
Usually caused by blunt injury resulting in multiple rib
  fractures

Major Flail Chest—cont'd
Loss of bone stability of thoracic cage
Major disruption of synchronous chest wall motion
Mechanical ventilation and positive end-expiratory
  pressure required

Massive Hemothorax
Must be drained with large-bore tube
Initiate drainage only with concurrent vascular volume
  replacement

Cardiac Tamponade
Beck triad:
1. Decreased or muffled heart sounds
2. Distended neck veins from increased venous
   pressure
3. Hypotension with pulsus paradoxus (decreased
   pulse pressure during inspiration)
Must be drained

"C" stands for *circulation and hemorrhage control.* Circulation can be assessed via observation (of heart rate, skin color, and mental status) and palpation (of pulse quality, capillary refill, and skin temperature). Control of bleeding is one of the primary responsibilities in the acute care of the traumatized child. Once identified, hemorrhage should be stopped by the use of direct pressure or careful use of extremity tourniquets.

In trauma care, "D" stands for *disability,* which serves as a reminder to assess and monitor neurologic status, a condition that may be changing constantly. The rapid neurologic assessment in the primary survey has two components: (1) examination of pupil size and reactivity, and (2) a brief mental status assessment (AVPU: *a*lert; responds to *v*oice; responds to *p*ain; *u*nresponsive). These changes may provide important diagnostic and prognostic information, as well as therapeutic direction. Another common tool for assessing neurologic injury is the Glasgow Coma Scale (GCS). This scale has been modified for use in preverbal children (Table 3–6). The GCS can direct decisions regarding the initiation of cerebral resuscitation (e.g., hyperventilation or osmolar therapy) in patients with suspected closed head injuries. Head injury is present in 80% of all patients with multiple traumas, and in 60% of pediatric cases the head is the most severely affected part of the body. The mortality rate in multiple traumas accompanied by head injuries is 16%, but it is only 6% in the absence of significant head injury.

"E," for *exposure,* has been added to the mnemonic as a reminder that for a full assessment of the patient, the child must be completely disrobed so that the entire body can be examined in detail. In doing this, the examiner should ensure a neutral thermal environment is maintained to prevent hypothermia.

On completion of the primary survey, a more detailed head-to-toe examination (the *secondary survey*) should ensue. The purpose of this careful reexamination is to identify life- and limb-threatening and less serious injuries. Coincident with the secondary survey and dependent in part on the assessed physiologic status of the patient, certain procedures and resuscitative measures (e.g., large-bore vascular access and fluid therapy) are initiated. The prioritization of definitive care needs is determined by the injury findings collected from the primary and secondary surveys, the child's physiologic response to resuscitative care, and data from continuous monitoring.

Specific Organ Injuries

The initial physical examination in the emergency department, which is augmented by screening laboratory data (Table 3–7), should provide information

TABLE 3–6
Glasgow Coma Scales

Glasgow Coma Scale			Modified Coma Scale for Infants		
Activity	Best Response	Score	Activity	Best Response	Score
Eye opening	Spontaneous	4	Eye opening	Spontaneous	4
	To verbal stimuli	3		To speech	3
	To pain	2		To pain	2
	None	1		None	1
Verbal	Oriented	5	Verbal	Coos, babbles	5
	Confused	4		Irritable, cries	4
	Inappropriate words	3		Cries to pain	3
	Nonspecific sounds	2		Moans to pain	2
	None	1		None	1
Motor	Follows commands	6	Motor	Spontaneous movements	6
	Localizes pain	5		Withdraws to touch	5
	Withdraws to pain	4		Withdraws to pain	4
	Flexion to pain	3		Abnormal flexion	3
	Extension to pain	2		Abnormal extension	2
	None	1		None	1

TABLE 3–7
Initial Laboratory Evaluation of the Major Trauma Patient

Hematology
Complete blood count
Platelet count
Type and cross-match

Urinalysis
Gross
Microscopic

Clinical Chemistry
Amylase
SGOT/SGPT

Radiology
Cervical spine films
AP chest roentgenogram
Roentgenograms of all apparent fractures
CT scans where indicated for head, chest, and abdominal trauma

AP, Anteroposterior; *CT,* computed tomography; *SGOT/SGPT,* serum glutamic oxaloacetic transaminase/serum glutamic pyruvic transaminase.

and direction for further diagnostic evaluation. When the physician is subsequently focusing on various organ systems, evaluating and treating severe *head injury* are given a high priority. Major trauma to the *chest* and *mediastinal structures* frequently requires immediate surgical intervention; with the exception of pulmonary contusion, these injuries have a significant mortality. The *musculoskeletal system* also may require immediate attention. Fractures contribute most to the long-term morbidity associated with multiple trauma and, if inappropriately assessed, may lead to loss of limb or life. The failure rate in the diagnosis of significant fractures is approximately 12% in and around the time of injury. Most fractures may be managed by closed reduction and splinting techniques.

Head Trauma

See Chapter 18.

Abdominal Trauma

Penetrating trauma must be distinguished from blunt trauma. The former accounts for less than 10% of pediatric abdominal trauma. Pediatric patients with penetrating trauma may be asymptomatic or in hypovolemic shock. Performing serial physical examinations is the primary method of obtaining information on which to base decisions regarding operative intervention. Abdominal computed tomography (CT) scanning is invaluable for assessing hemody-

TABLE 3–8
Criteria for a Positive Paracentesis

Free aspiration ≥10 mL gross blood
Turbid or bloody fluid that prevents reading
  newsprint
Free egress through indwelling urinary catheter or
  chest tube
Presence of >500 WBCs/mL or >100,000 RBCs/mL
Amylase >175 U/mL
Presence of gross stool or food debris

RBCs, Red blood cells; *WBCs,* white blood cells.

namically stable children with intraabdominal trauma. Gunshot wounds to the abdomen, an important category of abdominal trauma, involve multiple organs in 80% of cases and have a mortality rate greater than 12%. Operative exploration is based on CT and physical findings and may be indicated when peritoneal irritation, hypovolemia, free air on plain film, or positive results of paracentesis (Table 3–8) are present.

Blunt abdominal trauma occurs far more often in children than does penetrating abdominal trauma. The most frequently injured organs, in descending order, are the spleen, liver, genitourinary tract, stomach, intestine, colon, pancreas, pelvis, and major vessels. Optimal management in stable children with injuries in these organs requires serial physical examinations with CT to confirm the presence and severity of organ injury. Operative intervention may be required in patients whose vital signs are persistently unstable in the face of aggressive fluid resuscitation, even in the absence of extravascular volume loss or an enlarging abdomen. The presence of peritoneal irritation or abdominal wall discoloration, together with signs of intravascular volume loss, indicates the need for laparotomy. Abdominal CT is an especially important adjunct in the patient who is unconscious as a result of a head injury. The use of high-fluid volumes to resuscitate this type of patient may exacerbate brain swelling; therefore, CT confirmation of organ injury or occult blood loss can be most important.

Injury to the Spleen

Splenic injuries often are signaled by pain at the tip of the left shoulder or in the left chest, accompanied by respiratory distress, nausea, and vomiting. A positive *Kehr sign* (pressure on the left upper quadrant eliciting left shoulder pain) also strongly suggests this diagnosis. No other consistent clinical or laboratory findings suggest a splenic injury.

Nonoperative management is the treatment of choice for most serious splenic injuries. This treatment includes intensive care and serial observation by CT, radionuclide scan, or follow-up ultrasound examination. Surgery may be indicated for patients who have an estimated blood loss greater than 40 mL/kg of transfused blood in 24–36 hours. The operative approach often involves repair of the lesion rather than removal of the spleen, but splenectomy is required if the organ is totally separated from its blood supply; if a severe head injury exists for which rapid, high-volume circulatory support might be hazardous; or if an increase in blood loss of unknown cause has occurred in the presence of fecal contamination of the peritoneal contents. If a splenectomy is performed, patients should continue receiving penicillin prophylaxis and should also receive pneumococcal and *Haemophilus influenzae* vaccines, because morbidity and mortality increase as a result of overwhelming sepsis in asplenic patients.

Renal Injury

The kidney commonly is injured by blunt abdominal trauma, and more than 40% of children with injured kidneys have other internal injuries. A young child's kidney is more vulnerable to trauma than an adult's because it is positioned more anteriorly in the peritoneal cavity, the child's rib cage is more compliant, and the child's abdominal muscle development is immature. When minor trauma has led to major renal injury in a child, congenital renal anomalies also should be suspected. The diagnosis of renal injury is based on history and physical examination, coupled with a urinalysis showing blood and increased protein levels. An intravenous pyelogram (IVP) may be diagnostic; however, CT scans with renal contrast also are very useful. In more than 80% of the children with positive IVP results, simple monitoring is all that is required; in the remaining patients, surgery usually is indicated for falling hemoglobin levels, refractory shock, or urinary obstruction caused by clots.

Liver Trauma

Major trauma to the liver is a serious cause of morbidity and accounts for 40% of all deaths associated with blunt abdominal trauma in children. Almost 90% of these injuries involve the right lobe of the liver, and the diagnosis is usually based on the presence of pain in the right shoulder or right upper quadrant. Patients may have hypotension secondary to blood loss; hematobilia is rare. The site of the traumatic lesion may determine its severity. Subcapsular hematomas are less serious than capsular tears, which in turn are less serious than minor or deep lacerations. Burst injuries, with or without major vascular injury, are the most severe of all traumatic injuries to the liver and almost invariably are fatal.

For most children who have liver trauma, conservative management is recommended. This management involves admission to an intensive care unit (ICU) and the monitoring of ongoing blood loss, hepatic function, and liver structure with serial CT scans or ultrasound examinations. Operative management should be reserved for life-threatening situations.

Injuries of the Pancreas and Biliary Tree

Injuries of the pancreas and biliary tree are less common in children than in adults. Pancreatic injuries usually are present in association with injury to overlying structures, including the stomach, duodenum, extrahepatic biliary tree, and spleen. Pancreatic injury generally is identified by the presence of diffuse abdominal tenderness, pain, and vomiting. A pseudocyst, or midepigastric mass, may also be present. Hemodynamic instability, secondary to retroperitoneal hemorrhage, may be the presenting sign. Hyperamylasemia may not occur until 3–5 days after the injury. In the management of these patients, nasogastric suction and parenteral nutrition are indicated. Surgical removal of part or all of the necrotic pancreas may be required in one third of the patients who have a pseudocyst or a persistent fistula. CT or ultrasound examination may reveal pancreatic injury, abscess formation, or pseudocyst.

Injury to the biliary tree is evident in children through the appearance of hematobilia after right-upper-quadrant trauma. The diagnosis usually is confirmed by the presence of bile in the peritoneal cavity or retroperitoneal space. When children with this condition do not have an acute injury, their chronic course is characterized by anorexia, weight loss, the development of bilious ascites, jaundice, and acholic stools. Biliary tree injury generally requires prompt surgical repair once it is identified.

Intestinal Injury

In children, injury to the intestine usually is associated with other injuries requiring surgical treatment. The risk of intestinal injury varies with the amount of intestinal contents. A full bowel is likely to shear more easily than an empty bowel, and the shearing occurs at points of fixation (i.e., the ligament of Treitz, the ileocecal valve, and the ascending and descending peritoneal reflections). Perforation is more common in the jejunum and ileum than in the colon or stomach. Pneumoperitoneum that exists in association with intestinal perforation occurs in only 20% of patients. This diagnosis can be missed by CT and

often is established by paracentesis that is positive for bowel contents. Prompt surgical intervention is required.

REFERENCES

Behrman RE, Kliegman RM, Jenson HB, editors: *Nelson textbook of pediatrics,* ed 16, Philadelphia, 2000, WB Saunders, Chapter 57.
Chameides L, Hazinski MF, editors: *Pediatric advanced life support,* Dallas, 1997, American Heart Association, Chapter 8.
Fleisher GR, Ludwig S, editors: *Textbook of pediatric emergency medicine,* ed 4, Philadelphia, 2000, Lippincott, Williams & Wilkins, Chapters 103–107.
Polhgeers A, Ruddy RM: An update on pediatric trauma, *Emerg Med Clin North Am* 13(2):267–289, 1995.
Quayle KS: Minor head injury in the pediatric patient, *Pediatr Clin North Am* 46(6):1189–1199, 1999.
Strange GR, editor: *APLS: the pediatric emergency medicine course,* ed 3, Dallas, 1998, American College of Emergency Physicians, Chapters 5–7.
Yurt RW: Triage, initial assessment, and early treatment of the pediatric trauma patient, *Pediatr Clin North Am* 39(5):1083–1091, 1992.

BURNS

Burn injury results in over 25,000 hospital admissions and nearly 3000 deaths each year for children, making it the third leading mechanism of injury death. Overall, nearly 1% of all children sustain a burn injury each year. Burn risk is related to age, with a 2.5-fold increase in risk for children younger than 5 years of age. Mortality is primarily associated with burn severity (extent of body surface area and depth), although the presence of inhalation injury and young age are also predictors for mortality.

The upper extremities are the areas most frequently involved in burns (71% of cases), followed by the head and neck (52%). Scalding injuries are most common and inhalation injuries least common in pediatric patients.

The pathophysiology of burn injury is caused by disruption of the three key functions of the skin: regulation of heat loss, preservation of body fluids, and barrier to infection. Burn injury releases inflammatory and vasoactive mediators and promotes a number of hemodynamic changes, including increased capillary permeability, decreased plasma volume, and decreased cardiac output. Shock is common in children with burns that involve more than 10–12% of the total body surface area. For treatment of severe burns, admission to a qualified burn center is necessary.

Classification

Burns usually are classified on the basis of four criteria:
1. Depth of injury
2. Percent of body surface area involved

3. Location of the burn
4. Association with other injuries

Most burn surgeons recommend that the depth of injury be assessed solely on the clinical criteria of appearance.

First-degree burns are red, painful, and dry. These burns are superficial, with damage limited to the epidermis. They are commonly seen with sun exposure or with mild, hot solid, or scald injuries. They heal in 3–6 days without scarring. They are not included in burn surface area calculations. *Second-degree,* or partial-thickness, burns may be superficial (red, painful, mottled, blistered) and heal in 10–21 days with little or no scarring, or deep dermal (pale, painful, and yellow, taking ≥3 weeks to heal, and possibly resulting in scarring). They may result from immersion or flames. *Third-degree burns* are full thickness and require grafts if they are more than 1 cm in diameter. They are avascular and are characterized by coagulation necrosis. *Fourth-degree* burns involve underlying fascia, muscle, or bone.

A *severe burn* is one that covers greater than 15% of the body surface area or involves the face or perineum. Second-degree and third-degree burns of the hands or feet, as well as circumferential burns of the extremities, also are classified as severe. Inhalation injuries resulting in bronchospasm and impaired pulmonary function also must be considered severe burns. A method for estimating the percentage of skin surface area involved in burns in children of various ages is presented in Fig. 3–1. The extent of skin involvement of older adolescent and adult patients is estimated as follows: each upper extremity, 9%; each lower extremity, 18%; anterior trunk, 18%; posterior trunk, 18%; the head, 9%; and the perineum, 1%.

The location of the burn is important in assessing the risk for disability. The risk is greatest when the face, eyes, ears, feet, perineum, or hands are involved. With partial-thickness burns, generally no disability results; however, full-thickness burns almost always result in permanent impairment. Inhalational injuries not only cause respiratory compromise but also may result in difficulty in eating and drinking. Inhalational injuries also may be associated with burns of the face and neck.

Initial Evaluation

The triage decision for the physician caring for a burn patient is based on (1) the extent of the burn, (2) the body surface area involved, (3) the type of burn, (4) associated injuries, (5) any complicating medical or social problems, and (6) the availability of ambulatory management (Fig. 3–2). The goal of

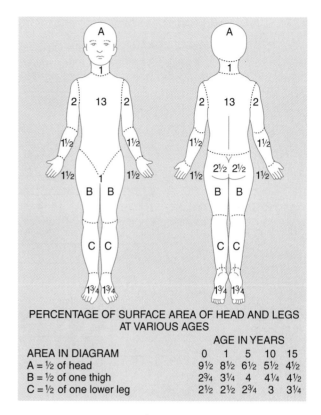

PERCENTAGE OF SURFACE AREA OF HEAD AND LEGS
AT VARIOUS AGES

AREA IN DIAGRAM	AGE IN YEARS				
	0	1	5	10	15
A = ½ of head	9½	8½	6½	5½	4½
B = ½ of one thigh	2¾	3¼	4	4¼	4½
C = ½ of one lower leg	2½	2½	2¾	3	3¼

FIG. 3–1

This chart of body areas, together with the table inserted in the figure showing the percentage of surface area of head and legs at various ages, can be used to estimate the surface area burned in a child. (From Solomon JR: *Crit Care Clin* 1[1]:159–174, 1985.)

initial treatment is to stop the burning process. This includes removing the patient from the site of injury, cleansing away any chemical or injurious contactants, and removing the clothing. The next priority is airway management; the upper airway is susceptible to burn injury, whereas the subglottic space appears protected. Few signs of injury may be present initially, although facial burns, singed nasal hairs or eyebrows, and acute inflammation of the oropharynx suggest inhalation injury. Smoke inhalation may be associated with carbon monoxide toxicity; 100% humidified oxygen should be given if hypoxia or inhalation is suspected. A carboxyhemoglobin assessment should be performed for any suspected inhalation exposure (a house or closed-space fire or a burn victim who requires CPR). Hoarseness on vocalization also is consistent with a supraglottic injury. Some children with inhalation burns require endoscopy, an artificial airway, and mechanical ventilation.

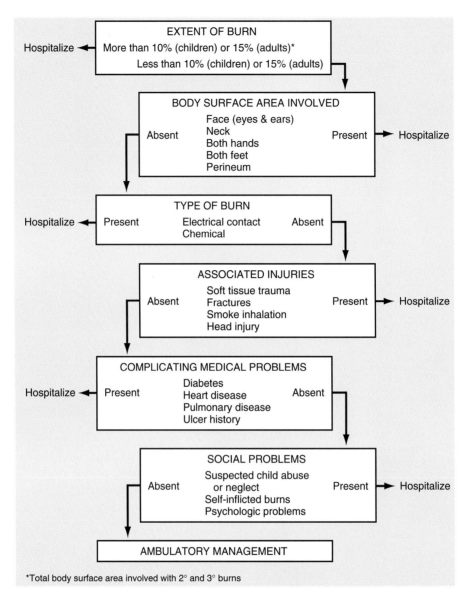

FIG. 3–2

Triage of the burned patient. Additional considerations for hospitalization include involvement of major joints, third-degree burns of greater than 5%, and poor guardianship at home regarding wound care. (From Wachtel TL: *Crit Care Clin* 1[1]:3–26, 1985.)

Fluid, Electrolyte, and Nutrition Management

The initial fluid and electrolyte support of the burned child is critical. The first priority is to support the circulating blood volume, which requires the administration of intravenous fluids to provide both maintenance fluid and electrolyte requirements and to replace ongoing burn-related losses. Children with a significant burn should receive a rapid bolus of 20 mL/kg of lactated Ringer's solution. The resuscitation formula for fluid therapy in the first 24 hours is: 5000 mL/m²/% burned surface + 2000 mL/m² total body surface area (maintenance). This fluid is designed to cover "third space" losses associated with capillary leaking. Half the estimated burn requirement is administered during the first

8 hours after admission, and the remaining burn fluid requirement is divided over the subsequent 16 hours. This estimated fluid replacement should be titrated so that it results in ≥1 mL/kg/hr of urine output. During the second 24 hours, dextrose water in 0.25 normal saline is substituted for this regimen. Controversy exists over whether and when to administer colloid during fluid resuscitation. Colloid therapy may be needed only for burns covering more than 30% of body surface area; this therapy is given 8–24 hours after injury as 12.5 g of albumin in each liter of Ringer's lactated solution.

Because burn injury produces a hypermetabolic response, children with significant burns require immediate nutritional support. Although enteral feeding may be resumed on the second or third day of therapy, children with critical burn injury may require parenteral nutritional support. The hypermetabolic state can be modulated to a degree through the effective management of anxiety and pain (with sedation and analgesia) and the prevention of hypothermia by maintenance of a neutral thermal environment.

Initial Wound Care

Wound care requires careful surgical management. The treatment is simple and noninvasive, and the involved areas should be covered with a sterile sheet. Wrapping the involved area with plastic, particularly for circumferential burns, may increase the child's comfort. Initial surgical attempts focus on relieving any pressure on the peripheral circulation by the developing eschar; then débridement is required for reclassifying the injury, a procedure that must occur before any topical therapy is administered. After débridement, burns are generally covered with silver sulfadiazine (1%) applied to fine-mesh gauze or, if the burn is shallow, with polymyxin B/bacitracin–neomycin (Neosporin) ointment. Silver nitrate (0.5%) and 11.1% mafenide acetate (which is painful, produces metabolic acidosis, and penetrates eschar) are alternative antimicrobial agents. Such agents inhibit but do not prevent bacterial growth. Various grafts, such as cadaver allografts; porcine xenografts; artificial bilaminate (cross-linked chondroitin-6-sulfate and silicone) skin substitute; and cultured patient's keratinocytes, also have been used initially to cover wounds. For full-thickness burns, skin autografting and artificial skin substitutes are required for eventual closure. Burn management and rehabilitation are highly specialized skills, involving the recognition of many complications of burns (Table 3–9) and evaluation of the wound and its cause for suspected child abuse or neglect. Tetanus toxoid and, if needed, immune globulin are indicated in the nonimmunized patient.

TABLE 3–9 **Complications of Burns**	
Problem	**Treatment**
Sepsis	Monitor for infection, avoid prophylactic antibiotics
Hypovolemia	Fluid replacement
Hypothermia	Adjust ambient temperature: dry blankets in field
Laryngeal edema	Endotracheal intubation, tracheostomy
Carbon monoxide poisoning	100% O_2
Cyanide poisoning	100% O_2 plus amyl nitrate, sodium nitrate, and sodium thiosulfate
Cardiac dysfunction	Inotropic agents, diuretics
Gastric ulcers	H_2-receptor antagonist, antacids
Compartment syndrome	Escharotomy incision
Contractures	Physical therapy
Hypermetabolic state	Enteral and parenteral nutritional support
Renal failure	Supportive care, dialysis
Transient antidiuresis	Expectant management
Anemia	Transfusions as indicated
Psychologic trauma	Psychologic rehabilitation
Pulmonary infiltrates	
Burn injury	PEEP, ventilation, O_2
Pulmonary edema	Avoid overhydration, give diuretics
Pneumonia	Antibiotics
Bronchospasm	Beta agonist aerosols

PEEP, Positive end-expiratory pressure.

Prevention

More than 600,000 children suffer burns each year; 94% occur in the home. Prevention is possible by using smoke and fire alarms, having identifiable escape routes and a fire extinguisher, and reducing hot water temperature to 120° F (49° C). Immersion full-thickness burns develop after 1 second at 158° F (70° C), after 5 seconds at 140° F (60° C), after 30 seconds at 130° F (54.5° C), after 60 seconds at 127° F (53° C), after 5 minutes at 122° F (50° C), and after 10 minutes at 120° F (49° C).

REFERENCES

Behrman RE, Kliegman RM, Jenson HB, editors: *Nelson textbook of pediatrics,* ed 16, Philadelphia, 2000, WB Saunders, Chapter 70.

Herndon DN, Rutan RL, Rutan TC: Management of the pediatric patient with burns, *J Burn Care Rehab* 14(1):3–8, 1993.

Monafo WW: Initial management of burns, *N Engl J Med* 335(21):1581–1586, 1996.

Nguyen TT, Gilpin DA, Meyer NA, et al: Current treatment of severely burned patients, *Ann Surg* 223(1):12–25, 1996.

Strange GR, editor: *APLS: the pediatric emergency medicine course,* ed 3, Dallas, 1998, American College of Emergency Physicians, Chapter 8.

POISONING

Ingestions

Unintentional ingestions are most common in the 1–5-year-old age group, an incidence that reveals the inquisitiveness of young children and the carelessness of adults in leaving drugs and household chemicals within reach. In older children, drug overdoses (poisonings) most often are associated with suicide attempts. Most ingestions are unintentional (88%), occur in the home (92%), and produce no (82%) or minor (17%) toxicity; 0.01% are fatal. Common agents in young children include family members' medications, cleaning or polishing solutions, plants, and cosmetics. Fatal childhood poisonings are commonly caused by carbon monoxide, medications (cardiovascular drugs, cyclic antidepressants), drugs of abuse, hydrocarbons, and pesticides.

Clinical Assessment

Poisoning is usually a diagnosis of exclusion, but the history and physical examination often provide sufficient clues to distinguish between toxic ingestion and organic disease (Table 3–10). The comatose child should be considered to have ingested a poison until the facts prove otherwise. Because the comatose patient's history and physical examination may be unrevealing, using the toxicology laboratory to obtain information sometimes is helpful. Nonetheless, no toxicology screen can substitute for careful physical examination by someone who understands the signs and symptoms of various ingestions.

For a number of agents, the diagnosis can be established by evaluating the level of consciousness; determining the pupillary size; and validating the presence of muscle fasciculations, cardiac arrhythmias, seizures, or hypothermia. Certain complexes of symptoms and signs are relatively specific to a given class of drugs (Table 3–11). Even in the absence of an obvious toxidrome, a careful and thorough examination is helpful in suggesting a diagnosis of poisoning. It also is important to determine whether the patient's vital signs are unstable, which warrants immediate supportive cardiopulmonary care.

The recognition of additional clinical manifestations is helpful in determining poisoning involving a particular agent (Table 3–11). For example, an elevated body temperature may be related to sepsis or

---

TABLE 3–10
Historical and Physical Findings in Poisoning

Odor	
Bitter almonds	Cyanide
Acetone	Isopropyl alcohol, methanol, paraldehyde, salicylate
Alcohol	Ethanol
Wintergreen	Methyl salicylate
Garlic	Arsenic, thallium, organophosphates
Violets	Turpentine
Ocular Signs	
Miosis	Narcotics (except meperidine), organophosphates, muscarinic mushrooms, clonidine, phenothiazines, chloral hydrate, barbiturates (late), PCP
Mydriasis	Atropine, alcohol, cocaine, amphetamines, antihistamines, cyclic antidepressants, cyanide, carbon monoxide
Nystagmus	Phenytoin, barbiturates, ethanol, carbon monoxide
Lacrimation	Organophosphates, irritant gas or vapors
Retinal hyperemia	Methanol
Poor vision	Methanol, botulism, carbon monoxide

TABLE 3–10
Historical and Physical Findings in Poisoning—cont'd

Cutaneous Signs

Needle tracks	Heroin, PCP, amphetamine
Bullae	Carbon monoxide, barbiturates
Dry, hot skin	Anticholinergic agents, botulism
Diaphoresis	Organophosphates, nitrates, muscarinic mushrooms, aspirin, cocaine
Alopecia	Thallium, arsenic, lead, mercury
Erythema	Boric acid, mercury, cyanide, anticholinergics

Oral Signs

Salivation	Organophosphates, salicylate, corrosives, strychnine
Dry mouth	Amphetamine, anticholinergics, antihistamine
Burns	Corrosives, oxalate-containing plants
Gum lines	Lead, mercury, arsenic
Dysphagia	Corrosives, botulism

Intestinal Signs

Cramps	Arsenic, lead, thallium, organophosphates
Diarrhea	Antimicrobials, arsenic, iron, boric acid
Constipation	Lead, narcotics, botulism
Hematemesis	Aminophylline, corrosives, iron, salicylates

Cardiac Signs

Tachycardia	Atropine, aspirin, amphetamine, cocaine, cyclic antidepressants, theophylline
Bradycardia	Digitalis, narcotics, mushrooms, clonidine, organophosphates, beta-blockers, calcium channel blockers
Hypertension	Amphetamine, LSD, cocaine, PCP
Hypotension	Phenothiazines, barbiturates, cyclic antidepressants, iron, beta-blockers, calcium channel blockers

Respiratory Signs

Depressed respiration	Alcohol, narcotics, barbiturates
Increased respiration	Amphetamines, aspirin, ethylene glycol, carbon monoxide, cyanide
Pulmonary edema	Hydrocarbons, heroin, organophosphates, aspirin

CNS Signs

Ataxia	Alcohol, antidepressants, barbiturates, anticholinergics, phenytoin, narcotics
Coma	Sedatives, narcotics, barbiturates, PCP, organophosphates, salicylate, cyanide, carbon monoxide, cyclic antidepressants, lead
Hyperpyrexia	Anticholinergics, quinine, salicylates, LSD, phenothiazines, amphetamine, cocaine
Muscle fasciculation	Organophosphates, theophylline
Muscle rigidity	Cyclic antidepressants, PCP, phenothiazines, haloperidol
Paresthesia	Cocaine, camphor, PCP, MSG
Peripheral neuropathy	Lead, arsenic, mercury, organophosphates
Altered behavior	LSD, PCP, amphetamines, cocaine, alcohol, anticholinergics, camphor

CNS, Central nervous system; *LSD,* lysergic acid diethylamide; *MSG,* monosodium glutamate; *PCP,* phencyclidine.

TABLE 3–11
Toxic Syndromes

Agent	Manifestations
Acetaminophen	Nausea, vomiting, pallor, delayed jaundice–hepatic failure (72–96 hr)
Amphetamine, cocaine, and sympathomimetics	Tachycardia, hypertension, hyperthermia, psychosis and paranoia, seizures, mydriasis, diaphoresis, piloerection, aggressive behavior
Anticholinergics	Mania, delirium, fever, red dry skin, dry mouth, tachycardia, mydriasis, urinary retention
Carbon monoxide	Headache, dizziness, coma, skin bullae, other systems affected
Cyanide	Coma, convulsions, hyperpnea, bitter almond odor
Ethylene glycol (antifreeze)	Metabolic acidosis, hyperosmolarity, hypocalcemia, oxalate crystalluria
Iron	Vomiting (bloody), diarrhea, hypotension, hepatic failure, leukocytosis, hyperglycemia, radiopaque pills on KUB, late intestinal stricture, *Yersinia* sepsis
Narcotics	Coma, respiratory depression, hypotension, pinpoint pupils, hyporeflexia
Cholinergics (organophosphates, nicotine)	Miosis, salivation, urination, diaphoresis, lacrimation, bronchospasm (bronchorrhea), muscle weakness and fasciculations, emesis, defecation, coma, confusion, pulmonary edema, bradycardia, reduced erythrocyte and serum cholinesterase, late peripheral neuropathy
Phenothiazines	Tachycardia, hypotension, muscle rigidity, coma, ataxia, oculogyric crisis, miosis, radiopaque pills on KUB
Salicylates	Tachypnea, fever, lethargy, coma, vomiting, diaphoresis, alkalosis (early), acidosis (late)
Cyclic antidepressants	Coma, convulsions, mydriasis, hyperreflexia, arrhythmia (prolonged QT interval), cardiac arrest, shock

KUB, Kidney-ureter-bladder roentgenogram.

meningitis but also is typical of salicylate and anticholinergic overdose.

The patient's breath odors also may provide valuable clues to potential ingestions (Table 3–10). A fruity smell may signify diabetic ketoacidosis, a silver polish smell is typical of cyanide, and a cleaning fluid–type odor is consistent with carbon tetrachloride ingestion. An evaluation of the lungs may reveal pulmonary edema, which can be caused by cyclic antidepressants, organophosphates, or methaqualone.

Major Patterns of Presentation

The poisoned child can exhibit any one of six basic clinical patterns: coma, toxicity, metabolic acidosis, heart rhythm aberrations, gastrointestinal symptoms, and seizures.

Coma. Coma is perhaps the most striking symptom of a poison ingestion but leads to the greatest confusion because the comatose child is unarousable and unresponsive. Coma may be a result of trauma, a cerebrovascular accident, a global asphyxial event, meningitis, or poisoning. A careful history and clinical examination are needed to distinguish among these alternatives. The rapid loss of brainstem function usually suggests a supratentorial lesion, whereas the persistence of the pupillary light reflex in the presence of diminished respiratory effort and diminished level of consciousness often indicates a metabolic insult to the brain. The level of consciousness in the latter condition often is depressed out of proportion to other neurologic signs. Decorticate posturing strongly suggests structural or metabolic disorders rather than toxic ingestions. Pinpoint pupils suggest either a pontine lesion or the toxic ingestion of opiates, organophosphates, phenothiazines, or chloral hydrate. Dilated pupils often are associated with cyclic antidepressant overdoses (Table 3–10). Structural lesions often may be accompanied by midpoint-fixed pupils or by unilaterally dilated pupils and disturbances of ocular movement.

Systemic and Pulmonary Toxicity. *Hydrocarbon ingestion* may result in systemic and pulmonary (locally by aspiration) toxicity (Table 3–12). Halogenated hydrocarbons or those with toxic additives have the greatest systemic toxicities and should be removed

> **TABLE 3–12**
> **Acute Hydrocarbon Risk Assessments**
>
> Systemic Toxicity Common*
> Trichloroethane (spot remover), trichloroethylene, carbon tetrachloride, methylene chloride, benzene, hydrocarbon additives (camphor, heavy metals, insecticides, aniline), toluene
>
> Local Toxicity by Aspiration Common,† Systemic Toxicity Uncommon
> Mineral seal oil, signal oil, furniture polish, turpentine, gasoline, kerosene, charcoal lighter fluid, toluene
>
> Nontoxic in 95% of Cases
> Asphalt, tar, motor oil, mineral or liquid petroleum, lubricants, baby oil
>
> ---
>
> *Chronic abuse of volatile hydrocarbons (e.g., sniffing) may cause ataxia, tremor, seizures, coma, myopathy, peripheral neuropathy, and renal tubular defects. Lead poisoning also is noted with abuse of lead-containing gasoline.
> †Hydrocarbons of low viscosity (30–60 standard Saybolt Universal Seconds [SUS]), low surface tension, and high volatility have the greatest risk for inducing aspiration pneumonia.

by lavage. Hydrocarbons with low viscosity, low surface tension, and high volatility pose the greatest risk for producing aspiration pneumonia; once swallowed, however, they pose no risk unless emesis is induced. Emesis or lavage should *not* be initiated in the child who has ingested volatile hydrocarbons.

Caustic ingestions may cause dysphagia, epigastric pain, oral mucosal burns, and low-grade fever. Patients with esophageal lesions may have no oral burns or may have significant signs and symptoms. Treatment depends on the agent ingested and the presence or absence of esophageal injury. *Alkali agents* may be solid, granular, or liquid (e.g., Liquid Drano, 9.5% sodium hydroxide [NaOH] or Liquid Plumr, 8% potassium hydroxide [KOH]). Both of these liquid agents are tasteless and produce full-thickness liquefaction necrosis of the esophagus or oropharynx. When the esophageal lesions heal, strictures form. Ingestion of these agents also creates a long-term risk of esophageal carcinoma. Many do not recommend the routine use of diluents as a first aid measure because of the lack of proven efficacy and the potential risk of induced vomiting. Subsequent treatment includes antibiotics if there are signs of infection and dilation of late-forming (2–3 weeks later) strictures.

Ingested button batteries also may produce a caustic mucosal injury from NaOH, KOH, or mercuric oxide. If they pass to the stomach, no further therapy is needed because they are likely to be passed in the stool within a week. Those that remain in the esophagus may cause esophageal burns and erosion and should be removed with the endoscope.

Acid agents, such as Lysol Toilet Bowl Cleaner (8.5% hydrochloric acid [HCl]) or Vanish Toilet Bowl Cleaner (65% sodium acid sulfate), can injure the lungs (with HCl fumes), oral mucosa, esophagus, and stomach. Because acids taste sour, children will usually stop drinking the solution, thus limiting the injury. Acids produce a coagulation necrosis, which limits the chemical from penetrating into deeper layers of the mucosa, and therefore damages tissue less severely than alkali. The signs and symptoms and initial therapeutic measures (e.g., dilution and no emesis or neutralization) are similar to those for alkali ingestion.

Metabolic Acidosis. The poisoned child also may have metabolic acidosis (mnemonic = MUDPIES) (Table 3–13), which is assessed easily by measuring arterial blood gases, serum electrolyte levels, and urine pH. Determining serum sodium, potassium, chloride, glucose, urea nitrogen, and carbon dioxide (CO_2) levels permits the calculation of the serum anion gap (see Chapter 16) and osmolality,

$$Osm = 2 \times Na + (Glucose/18) + (Blood\ urea\ nitrogen\ [BUN]/2.8)$$

which may be compared with measured osmolality. A difference of more than 10 between the measured and calculated osmolality, an **osmolal gap,** strongly suggests the presence of an unmeasured component, such as methanol or ethylene glycol. These ingestions require thorough assessment and prompt intervention; the approach described here allows a tentative diagnosis to be made pending access to the toxicology laboratory.

Rhythm Abnormalities. Rhythm abnormalities may be prominent signs of a variety of toxic ingestions, although ventricular arrhythmias are rare. Prolonged QT intervals may suggest phenothiazine or antihistamine ingestion, and widened QRS complexes are seen with ingestions of cyclic antidepressants and quinidine. Because many drug and chemical overdoses may lead to sinus tachycardia, it is not a useful or discriminating sign; sinus bradycardia, however, suggests digoxin, cyanide, a cholinergic agent, or beta-blocker ingestion. A full 12-lead electrocardiogram should be part of the initial evaluation in all patients suspected of having ingested toxic substances (Table 3–14).

Gastrointestinal Symptoms. Gastrointestinal symptoms of poisoning include emesis, nausea, abdominal

---

TABLE 3–13
Screening Laboratory Clues in Toxicologic Diagnosis

Metabolic Acidosis (Mnemonic = MUDPIES)
Methanol,* carbon monoxide
Uremia*
Diabetes mellitus*
Paraldehyde,* phenformin
Isoniazid, iron
Ethanol,* ethylene glycol*
Salicylates, starvation, seizures

Hypoglycemia
Ethanol
Isoniazid
Insulin
Propranolol
Oral hypoglycemic agents

Hyperglycemia
Salicylates
Isoniazid
Iron
Phenothiazines
Sympathomimetics

Hypocalcemia
Oxalate
Ethylene glycol
Fluoride

Radiopaque Substance on KUB (Mnemonic = CHIPPED)
Chloral hydrate, calcium carbonate
Heavy metals (lead, zinc, barium, arsenic, lithium, bismuth as in Pepto-Bismol)
Iron
Phenothiazines
Play-Doh, potassium chloride
Enteric-coated pills
Dental amalgam

KUB, Kidney-ureter-bladder roentgenogram.
*Indicates hyperosmolar condition.

---

cramps, and diarrhea. These symptoms may be the result of direct toxic effects on the intestinal mucosa or of systemic toxicity following absorption.

Seizures. Seizures are the sixth major mode of presentation for children with toxic ingestions, but poisoning is an uncommon cause of afebrile seizures. When seizures do occur with intoxication,

they may be life threatening and require aggressive therapeutic intervention (Table 3–14).

Initial Therapy

Supportive Care. Prompt attention must be given to protecting and maintaining the airway, establishing effective breathing, and supporting the circulation. This management sequence takes precedence over other diagnostic or therapeutic procedures. If the level of consciousness is depressed and a toxic substance is suspected, glucose (1 g/kg IV), 100% oxygen, and naloxone should be administered. Laboratory studies helpful in the initial management include specific toxin-drug assays; measurement of arterial blood gases and blood electrolytes, osmoles, and glucose; electrocardiogram; and the calculation of the anion or osmolar gap. Urine screens for drugs of abuse or to confirm suspected ingestion of medications in the home may be revealing.

Gastric Decontamination. The intent of gastrointestinal decontamination is to prevent the absorption of a potentially toxic ingested substance and in theory to prevent the poisoning. There has been great controversy about which methods are the safest and most efficacious. Although gut decontamination has historically played a significant role in the management of the poisoned patient, recent data indicate there is no conclusive evidence that any method of gastrointestinal decontamination provides meaningful clinical benefit.

SYRUP OF IPECAC. Syrup of ipecac has previously been advocated as a drug of choice for rapid gastric emptying in patients with an acute ingestion. It was recommended that syrup of ipecac be present in the home of every family, so that it might be administered immediately after the discovery of a suspected ingestion and induce emesis.

The American Academy of Clinical Toxicology (AACT) has recommended that ipecac should not be administered routinely to poisoned patients. In experimental studies the amount of a marker substance removed by ipecac-induced emesis was highly unpredictable. In a position statement, the AACT summarized that there is no evidence from clinical studies that ipecac improves the outcome of poisoned patients and recommends that its routine use in the emergency department be abandoned.

GASTRIC LAVAGE. Gastric lavage is another method of gastrointestinal decontamination historically advocated for the routine management of acute poisonings. This was accomplished through the placement of a large-bore nasogastric or orogastric tube through which large volumes of saline (10 to 15 mL/kg) were instilled and then drained. Many decontamination protocols called for repeated cycles of saline, which

TABLE 3–14
Drugs Associated with Major Modes of Presentation

Common Toxic Causes of Cardiac Arrhythmia	Causes of Coma—cont'd
Amphetamine	Lithium
Antiarrhythmics	Methemoglobinemia*
Anticholinergics	Methyldopa
Antihistamines	Narcotics
Arsenic	Phencyclidine
Carbon monoxide	Phenothiazines
Chloral hydrate	Salicylates
Cocaine	
Cyanide	**Common Agents Causing Seizures (Mnemonic =**
Cyclic antidepressants	**CAPS)**
Digitalis	**C**amphor
Freon	Carbamazepine
Phenothiazines	Carbon monoxide
Physostigmine	Cocaine
Propranolol	Cyanide
Quinine, quinidine	**A**minophylline
Theophylline	Amphetamine
	Anticholinergics
Causes of Coma	Antidepressants (cyclic)
Alcohol	**P**b (lead) (also lithium)
Anticholinergics	Pesticide (organophosphate)
Antihistamines	Phencyclidine
Barbiturates	Phenol
Carbon monoxide	Phenothiazines
Clonidine	Propoxyphene
Cyanide	**S**alicylates
Cyclic antidepressants	Strychnine
Hypoglycemic agents	
Lead	

*Causes of methemoglobinemia: amyl nitrite, aniline dyes, benzocaine, bismuth subnitrate, dapsone, primaquine, quinones, spinach, sulfonamides.

was believed to remove significant amounts of ingested toxin.

The AACT has recommended that gastric lavage not be routinely used in the management of poisoned patients. Similar to ipecac, the amount of marker substances removed in experimental trials of gastric lavage was very unpredictable. The AACT noted that lavage was associated with potential complications (e.g., aspiration, laryngospasm, and esophageal perforation) and summarized that there was no evidence that the use of gastric lavage improved clinical outcomes in poisoned patients.

Gastric lavage should be considered only for patients who have ingested a potentially lethal amount of poison, providing the lavage can be performed within 60 minutes of ingestion. Gastric lavage is contraindicated in children who ingest caustic materials or hydrocarbons or in the presence of neurologic abnormalities likely to impair airway protective mechanisms.

ACTIVATED CHARCOAL. Activated charcoal has been a mainstay of decontamination therapy. Activated charcoal is prepared by pyrolyzing organic materials and then activating them by exposure to oxidizing gas flows at high temperatures. This creates a substance with a large relative surface area and an affinity to bind with certain compounds. By binding with toxins, charcoal may prevent the toxin from being absorbed by the intestinal tract.

Historically, charcoal has been used both as a

single-dose (15–30 g for small children; 50–100 g for children older than 12 years, or 1–2 g/kg) and multiple-dose intervention for poisonings. Multiple-dose therapy was advocated as a means to enhance enterohepatic circulation. Charcoal is known to be ineffective against caustic or corrosive agents, hydrocarbons, heavy metals (e.g., arsenic, lead, mercury, iron, or lithium), glycols, and water-insoluble compounds.

As with lavage, the greatest benefit with activated charcoal is likely achieved within 1 hour of the ingestion. The AACT has recommended that single-dose activated charcoal not be routinely administered in the management of poisoned patients. It is recommended that charcoal be administered only in those situations in which it can be given within 1 hour of the ingestion of a potentially lethal agent that is known to be adsorbed by charcoal.

CARTHARTICS. The administration of a cathartic (e.g., sorbitol or magnesium citrate) alone has no role in the management of the poisoned patient. The AACT has stated that based on available data, the use of a cathartic in combination with activated charcoal is not recommended.

WHOLE-BOWEL IRRIGATION. Whole-bowel irrigation is another method advocated for gastrointestinal decontamination. It involves the use of polyethylene glycol (GoLYTELY) as a nonabsorbable cathartic, and it has been proposed as an effective intervention for toxic ingestion of sustained-release or enteric-coated drugs. To date, there have been no controlled experimental studies demonstrating improved outcome for poisoned patients. The AACT does not recommend the routine use of whole-bowel irrigation, although the method is acknowledged as a theoretical option for potentially toxic ingestions of iron, lead, zinc, or packets of illicit drugs.

Additional Therapy

After the initial resuscitation and gastric decontamination have been achieved, determining whether further therapy is needed is often difficult. There are three basic choices in the subsequent care of the child with a significant ingestion: providing continued supportive care, using specific antidotes where available, and actively removing the toxin from the bloodstream. To make a rational decision regarding these options, a judgment should be made as to whether the drug causes tissue damage (as is the case with methyl alcohol, aspirin, acetaminophen, theophylline, iron, and ethylene glycol). *Tissue damage* is defined as an irreversible or slowly reversible structural or functional change in an organ system as a direct result of ingestion of a poison; this definition precludes indirect effects such as respiratory depression or hypotension.

The decision about possible further therapy should take into consideration the amount of poison ingested; the diagnostic assessment, including the condition of the patient at the time of presentation; and the natural history of the suspected type of ingestion. All of these variables may be influenced by the child's prior clinical status or underlying medical problems. For example, in a patient with underlying severe hepatic or renal impairment, a more aggressive approach involving active removal might be selected, even though the ingestion ordinarily would require only the use of simple supportive care. Moreover, in the presence of a chronic ingestion an acute overdose may cause significant clinical toxicity with a lower dose of the drug.

For most common ingestions, continued supportive care and treatment directed toward specific complications are appropriate for otherwise healthy individuals. Specific antidotes should be used according to prescribed guidelines (Table 3–15). Active removal (e.g., hemoperfusion or dialysis) should be undertaken only for toxins that may cause tissue damage, for toxins that have been ingested by a patient already exhibiting confounding medical problems, or to avoid prolonged supportive care.

Toxicology assays are important for some agents, not only for identifying the specific drug but also for providing guidance for therapy and help in anticipating complications and estimating the prognosis. Serum iron levels below 300 µg/dL following iron ingestion usually are safe, but levels of free iron above 600 µg/dL usually are associated with significant toxicity. The timing of the physician's testing of the plasma level relative to the time of the patient's ingestion of the drug also is useful in predicting the severity of illness for acetaminophen (Fig. 3–3) and salicylate (Fig. 3–4). Patients with drug levels (related to the time after ingestion) in the serious zone require immediate treatment.

Preventing Ingestions

Most ingestions occur in the home, and the toxins involved are common household medications, household cleaning and work solutions, or vitamins. Unintentional poisonings are more frequent in children less than 5 years old, in boys, in families of low socioeconomic status, and during times of family disorganization. These poisonings occur most frequently in the kitchen, bathroom, or garage. Properly educating parents to use childproof medication containers, to store toxic substances in locked cabinets, and to label toxic chemicals properly is necessary for preventing ingestions. Kerosene and other toxic liquids should not be stored in soda pop bottles, and children should not come in contact with clothing exposed to pesticides. Old or unused medications should be

TABLE 3–15
Emergency Antidotes

Poison	Antidote	Dosage	Comments
Acetaminophen	N-Acetylcysteine	140 mg/kg PO initial dose, then 70 mg/kg PO q4h × 17 doses	Most effective within 16 hr of ingestion
Atropine	Physostigmine	Initial dose 0.01–0.03 mg/kg IV	Can produce convulsions, bradycardia; reserve for life-threatening situations only
Benzodiazepine	Flumazenil	0.1–0.2 mg/kg IV	Possible seizures, arrhythmias
Beta-blocking agents	Atropine	0.01–0.10 mg/kg IV	
	Isoproterenol	0.05–5 μg/kg/min IV infusion	
	Glucagon	0.05–0.1 mg/kg IV	
Calcium channel blockers	Glucagon	0.05–0.1 mg/kg IV	Increases cyclic adenosine monophosphate, resulting in positive inotropy and chronotropy
Carbon monoxide	Oxygen	100%; hyperbaric O_2	Half-life of carboxyhemoglobin is 5 hr in room air but 1.5 hr in 100% O_2
Coumarin	Vitamin K	2.5–10 mg IV/IM	Monitor PT; fresh frozen plasma or plasma for acute bleeding; repeated vitamin K for super-warfarin
Cyanide	Amyl nitrite, *then*	1–2 pearls every 2 min	Methemoglobin-cyanide complex
	Sodium nitrite, *then*	4.5–10 mg/kg (0.15–0.33 mL/kg 3% solution)	Causes hypotension; dosage assumes normal hemoglobin
	Sodium thiosulfate	50 mg/kg IV	Forms harmless sodium thiocyanate
Cyclic antidepressants	Sodium bicarbonate	0.5–1.0 mEq/kg IV, titrated to produce pH 7.5–7.55	—
Digoxin, digitoxin	Digoxin-specific Fab antibody fragments	Dose based on serum digoxin concentration and body weight; 1 vial (40 mg) neutralizes 0.6 mg digoxin	With acute life-threatening ingestion, dose and serum concentration are unknown; give contents of 20 vials
Iron	Deferoxamine	Initial dose 10–15 mg/kg/hr IV	Deferoxamine mesylate—forms excretable ferrioxamine complex; hypotension
Isoniazid	Pyridoxine	Give dose equal to the amount of isoniazid ingested, up to 250 mg/kg	For treatment of seizures or coma
Lead	Edetate calcium (calcium disodium versenate [EDTA])	1500 mg/m^2/day × 5 days; divided q6h or by continuous infusion	May lower to 1000 mg/m^2/day if given with BAL; nephrotoxic

Data from Kulig K: *N Engl J Med* 326(25):1677–1681, 1992; Liebelt EL: *Clin Pediatr Emerg Med* 1(3):234–243, 2000; Leikin JB, Paloucek FP, editors: *Poisoning and toxicology compendium,* Cleveland, 1998, Lexi-Comp.
ET, Endotracheal; *IM,* intramuscular; *IV,* intravenous; *PO,* by mouth; *SC,* subcutaneous.
*See Table 3–14 for causes of methemoglobinemia.

Continued

TABLE 3–15
Emergency Antidotes—cont'd

Poison	Antidote	Dosage	Comments
Lead—cont'd	BAL (British anti-Lewisite [dimercaprol])	3–5 mg/kg/dose q4h × 3–7 days	May cause hypertension and sterile abscesses
	Penicillamine	25–40 mg/kg/day PO divided q8h	Requires weekly monitoring for hepatic and bone marrow toxicity; should not be used in the presence of ongoing ingestion
	Succimer (2,3-dimercapto-succinic acid ([DMSA])	10 mg/kg/day PO tid × 5 days then 20 mg/kg/day PO bid × 14 days	Few toxic effects, requires lead-free home plus compliant family
Mercury, arsenic, gold	BAL (British anti-Lewisite)	5 mg/kg IM as soon as possible	Each mL BAL in oil has dimercaprol, 100 mg in 210 mL (21%) benzyl benzoate, and 680 mL peanut oil—forms stable nontoxic excretable cyclic compound
Methyl alcohol (ethylene glycol)	Ethyl alcohol in conjunction with dialysis	1 mL/kg of 100% ethanol initially in glucose solution; maintain blood level of 100 mg/dL	Competes for alcohol dehydrogenase; prevents formation of formic acid and oxalates
	Fomepizole	15 mg/kg loading dose followed by 10 mg/kg q12h × 4 doses	May be a better alternative to ethanol therapy
Nitrites/ methemoglobinemia*	Methylene blue	1–2 mg/kg, repeat in 1–4 hr if needed; treat for levels >30%	Exchange transfusion may be needed for severe methemoglobinemia; methylene blue overdose also causes methemoglobinemia
Opiates, Darvon, Lomotil	Naloxone	0.10 mg/kg IV, ET, SC, IM for children, up to 2 mg	Naloxone causes no respiratory depression (0.4 mg/1 mL ampule)
Organophosphates	Atropine	Initial dose 0.02–0.05 mg/kg IV	Physiologic: blocks acetylcholine; up to 5 mg IV every 15 min may be necessary in the critically ill adult patient
	Pralidoxime (2 PAM; Protopam)	Initial dose 25–50 mg/kg IV	Specific: disrupts phosphate-cholinesterase bond; up to 500 mg/hr may be necessary in the critically ill adult patient
Sympathomimetic agents	Blocking agents: phentolamine; beta-blocking agents; other antihypertensives		Must be used in a setting in which vital signs can be monitored effectively

Data from Kulig K: *N Engl J Med* 326(25):1677–1681, 1992; Liebelt EL: *Clin Pediatr Emerg Med* 1(3):234–243, 2000; Leikin JB, Paloucek FP, editors: *Poisoning and toxicology compendium*, Cleveland, 1998, Lexi-Comp.
ET, Endotracheal; *IM*, intramuscular; *IV*, intravenous; *PO*, by mouth; *SC*, subcutaneous.
*See Table 3–14 for causes of methemoglobinemia.

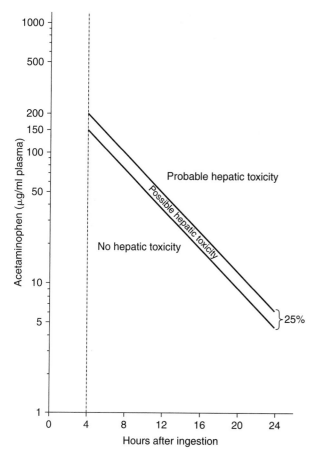

FIG. 3–3

Semilogarithmic plot of plasma acetaminophen levels versus time. Rumack-Mathews nomogram for acetaminophen poisoning. Cautions for use of this chart: (1) the time coordinates refer to time of ingestion; (2) serum levels drawn before 4 hours may not represent peak levels; (3) the graph should be used only in relation to a single, acute ingestion; and (4) the lower solid line, 25% below the standard nomogram, is included to allow for possible errors in acetaminophen plasma assays and estimated time from ingestion of an overdose. (Adapted from Rumack BH, Matthew H: *Pediatrics* 55[6]:871–876, 1975.)

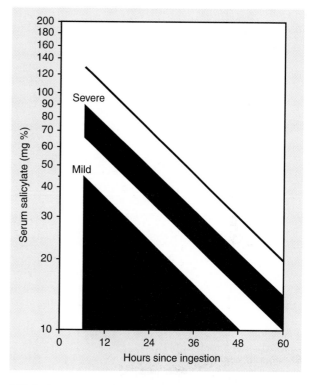

FIG. 3–4

Nomogram relating serum salicylate concentration and expected severity of intoxication at various intervals following the ingestion of a single dose of salicylate. (From Done AK: *Pediatrics* 26:800, 1960.)

Tenenbein M: Recent advances in pediatric toxicology, *Pediatr Clin North Am* 46(6):1179–1188, 1999.
Tenenbein M: Gastrointestinal decontamination of the overdose patient in the year 2000, *Clin Pediatr Emerg Med* 1(3):195–199, 2000.

discarded, and currently used medications should not be left on tabletops or in the mother's purse. If a child has ingested poison, the poison control center should be called.

REFERENCES

Behrman RE, Kliegman RM, Jenson HB, editors: *Nelson textbook of pediatrics,* ed 16, Philadelphia, 2000, WB Saunders, Chapter 722.
Strange GR, editor: *APLS: The pediatric emergency medicine course,* ed 3, Dallas, 1998, American College of Emergency Physicians, Chapter 9.

Bites, Stings, and Envenomations

Toxic reactions to the saliva or venom of living creatures or injuries caused by them are common and depend on exposure, provocation, and the species of insects or animals involved. Most reactions produce local inflammation, with little progression or systemic manifestations. Some reactions may represent allergic responses to insect antigens (papular urticaria), whereas others may result in tissue necrosis, infection, paralysis, and death (Table 3–16).

TABLE 3–16
Bites, Stings, and Envenomations

Species	Characteristics	Agents or Venoms	Treatment
Snakes			
Pit vipers: rattle-snake, copperhead, cottonmouth	Triangular head, elliptical pupils, heat-sensing pits Strike on provocation; site: hand, leg, foot; only 75% of bites have venom release; pain, swelling, ecchymosis ± coagulopathy, rhabdomyolysis, shock, weakness, hemolysis; bites of head and neck are most severe	Phospholipases, proteases, hyaluronidase, thrombin, Mojave (paralytic) toxin	Keep extremity dependent, immobilized; avoid ice, aspirin; mechanically extract venom; gentle tourniquet; treat shock; antivenin (polyvalent) if severe*; tetanus check†; antibiotics‡
Coral snake (cobra, mamba family)	Local pain and edema, hyperesthesia, paresthesia, fasciculations, weakness, bulbar palsy, descending paralysis, respiratory paralysis	Paralytic toxin	Antivenin if severe*
Sea snake	Pinprick lesion, paralysis, myoglobinuria	Neurotoxin, phospholipase	Antivenin,* antibiotics‡
Scorpions			
	Usually benign; local pain, tingling, hyperesthesia; paralysis, agitation, seizures rare; tachycardia, hypertension	Sympathetic and parasympathetic nervous system toxin	No treatment unless severe, then antitoxin; propranolol for tachyarrhythmia
Hymenoptera See Chapter 8 for allergy and anaphylaxis			
Ticks			
	Paralysis (spring, summer); tick located in scalp, groin	Paralytic toxin in saliva	Remove tick with forceps or gauze by constant, gentle, upward motion; prevention: DEET, permethrins
Spiders			
Black widow	Punctate lesions, local erythema, and immediate pain, muscle rigidity, spasms, abdominal pain, periorbital edema, hypertension, diaphoresis; spider has red hourglass marking on abdomen; lives in moist dark outdoor sites	Polypeptides producing spontaneous motor neuron depolarization	Analgesics, diazepam, intravenous calcium; antivenin if severe*

Data from Auerbach PS, editor: Wilderness medicine, ed 3, St Louis, 1995, Mosby, Chapters 28-35, 40, 52; Auerbach PS: *N Engl J Med* 325(7):486–493, 1991; Gentile DA, Kennedy BC: *Pediatrics* 88(5):967–981, 1991.
DEET, Diethyltoluamide; *DIC,* disseminated intravascular coagulation; ?, effect unproved.
*Types of antivenin that are prepared in animals (horse, goat) as hyperimmune serum and as foreign proteins may cause anaphylaxis.
†Tetanus check for all animal bites includes evaluation for need of tetanus immune globulin and booster vaccine.
‡Antibiotics to treat human cutaneous and animal mouth flora.

TABLE 3–16
Bites, Stings, and Envenomations—cont'd

Species	Characteristics	Agents or Venoms	Treatment
Spiders—cont'd			
Brown recluse	Fiddle shape over cephalothorax; lives in dark, indoor dry areas; necrotic painful, pruritic skin lesion; vesiculation, hemorrhage, and eschar formation; hemolysis, DIC, headache, seizures	Sphingomyelinase, protease, esterase, hyaluronidase, hemolysin	Wound débridement; ice; Dapsone; steroids(?)
Tarantula	Local pain, swelling, urticaria from hairs; usually benign	Polyamines, hyaluronidase	Analgesics, ice; remove hair with tape
Marine Envenomation			
Stingray	Defensive attack; laceration, puncture plus venom; pain, edema, bleeding, limb paralysis	Serotonin, phosphodiesterase	Antivenin, hot water immersion, surgical wound exploration
Jellyfish, Portuguese man-of-war	Burning, painful urticaria, pain, lymphadenopathy, anaphylaxis, fever, chills, muscle spasm, paralysis, hypotension	Bradykinin, histamine, hyaluronidase, phosphodiesterase	Remove tentacles, avoid fresh water; topical vinegar, corticosteroids, papain, isopropyl alcohol; calcium IV
Reptiles			
Gila monster	Local pain, edema, cyanosis, hypotension; animal jaws may clamp around the wound	Serotonin, phospholipase, protease, hyaluronidase	Analgesics, ice, immobilization; remove reptile
Toads	Salivation, cyanosis; seizures from placing toads in mouth	Bufotoxin	Supportive care
Mammals			
Humans	Directly from a bite or indirectly from a fist fight; laceration, swelling, erythema, cellulitis	*Eikenella corrodens, Staphylococcus aureus*, streptococcal species	Débridement; tetanus check†; amoxicillin/clavulanate potassium (Augmentin), nafcillin
Dogs	Swelling, erythema, cellulitis, lymphangitis; laceration, crush injury, tenosynovitis	*S. aureus*, streptococci; rabies	Débridement; tetanus check†; antibiotics per culture; rabies check
Cats	Laceration, swelling, cellulitis, osteomyelitis, tenosynovitis	*Pasteurella multocida, S. aureus*, streptococci; rabies	As for dogs; penicillin/ampicillin for *P. multocida*
Rats	Local pain, inflammation (common); rat bite fever (rare) with chills, fever, leukocytosis, rash, arthritis, abscesses, endocarditis, may relapse (*Streptobacillus moniliformis*); *Spirillum minus* produces suppurative bite lesion	Skin, mouth flora; no rabies; *S. moniliformis*; *S. minus*; plague, leptospirosis	Penicillin for rat bite fever
Raccoons, skunks, foxes	Laceration, pain, swelling	Rabies, plus mouth and skin flora	Rabies vaccine and rabies immunoglobulin; tetanus check†

REFERENCES

Behrman RE, Kliegman RM, Jenson HB, editors: *Nelson textbook of pediatrics*, ed 15, Philadelphia, 2000, WB Saunders, Chapter 724.

SHOCK

Shock may result from a number of relatively common childhood disorders or situations, including gastroenteritis, diabetes mellitus, trauma, infection, and unintentional drug ingestion. Early recognition and prompt, appropriate treatment present the best opportunity to improve the clinical outcome of shock.

Oxygen delivery is directly related to the arterial oxygen content (i.e., oxygen saturation and hemoglobin concentration) and to cardiac output. Changes in metabolic needs are met primarily by adjustments in cardiac output, which are determined by the amount of blood ejected from the left ventricle (stroke volume) and by the heart rate (Fig. 3–5). Stroke volume is related to myocardial end-diastolic fiber length (preload), myocardial contractility (inotropy), and resistance of blood ejection from the ventricle (afterload) (see Chapter 13). In the young infant whose myocardium possesses relatively less contractile tissue, increased demand for cardiac output is met primarily

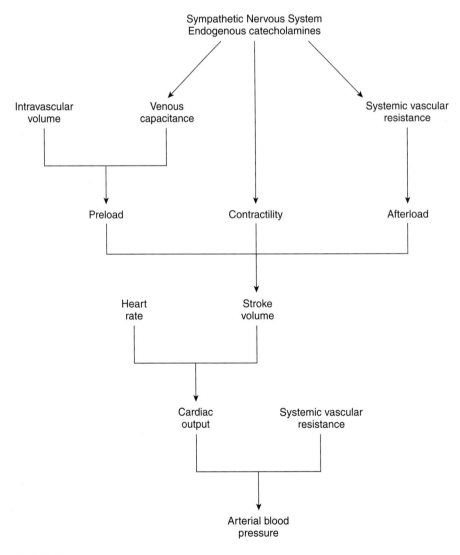

FIG. 3–5

Determinants of cardiac output and arterial blood pressure. (From Witte MK, Hill JH, Blumer JL: *Adv Pediatr* 34:139–174, 1987.)

by a neurally mediated increase in heart rate. In the older child and adult, cardiac output is most efficiently augmented by increasing stroke volume through neurohumorally mediated changes in vascular tone, resulting in increased venous return to the heart (increased preload), decreased arterial resistance (decreased afterload), and increased myocardial contractility.

Shock Syndromes

(Table 3–17 and Fig. 3–6)

Hypovolemic Shock

Acute hypovolemia is the most common cause of shock in pediatric patients. It results from blood loss, fluid and electrolyte depletion secondary to vomiting and diarrhea, third-space fluid losses caused by capillary leak syndromes, and pathologic renal fluid losses (Table 3–17). Hypovolemic shock is distinguished from other causes of shock by history and the absence of signs of heart failure (e.g., hepatomegaly, rales, edema, jugular venous distention, or a gallop) or sepsis (e.g., fever, leukocytosis, or focal infection). Reduced blood volume causes a decreased preload, stroke volume, and cardiac output. Recovery depends on the degree of hypovolemia, the patient's preexisting status, and rapid diagnosis and treatment. The prognosis is good, with a low mortality (<10%) in uncomplicated cases.

One compensatory mechanism for hypovolemic shock is increased sympathoadrenal activity, which produces an increased heart rate and myocardial contractility. Neurohumorally mediated constriction of the arterioles and capacitance vessels also maintains blood pressure, augments venous return to the heart to improve preload, and redistributes blood flow from nonvital to vital organs. An increased heart

---

TABLE 3-17
Classification of Shock and Common Underlying Causes

Type	Primary Circulatory Derangement	Common Causes
Hypovolemic	Decreased circulating blood volume	Hemorrhage Diarrhea Diabetes insipidus Diabetes mellitus Burns Adrenogenital syndrome Capillary leak syndrome
Distributive	Vasodilation → venous pooling → decreased preload Maldistribution of regional blood flow	Sepsis Anaphylaxis CNS/spinal injury Drug intoxication
Cardiogenic	Decreased myocardial contractility	Congenital heart disease Severe heart failure Arrhythmia Hypoxic/ischemic injuries Cardiomyopathy Metabolic derangements Myocarditis Drug intoxication Kawasaki disease
Obstructive	Mechanical obstruction to ventricular outflow	Cardiac tamponade Massive pulmonary embolus Tension pneumothorax Cardiac tumor
Dissociative	Oxygen not released from hemoglobin	Carbon monoxide poisoning Methemoglobinemia

CNS, Central nervous system.

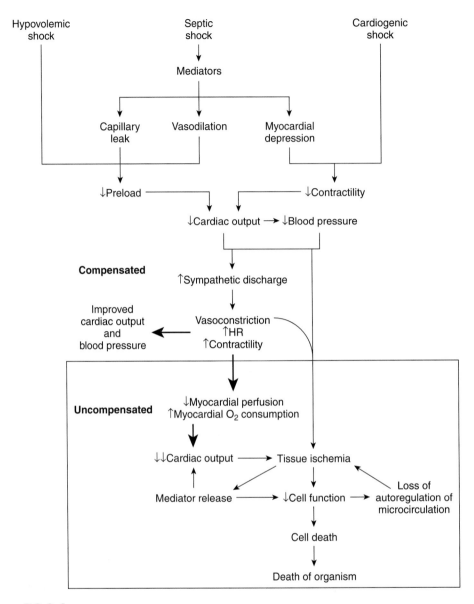

FIG. 3–6

Sequence of pathophysiologic events in the clinical shock state. *HR,* Heart rate. (From Witte MK, Hill JH, Blumer JL: *Adv Pediatr* 34:139–174, 1987.)

rate may impair coronary blood flow and ventricular filling; elevated systemic vascular resistance increases myocardial oxygen consumption, resulting in poorer myocardial function. Intense systemic vasoconstriction and hypovolemia produce tissue ischemia, which impairs cell metabolism and releases potent vasoactive mediators from injured cells. Vasoactive mediators include arachidonic acid metabolites, cytokines, and other vasoactive peptides, all of which can change myocardial contractility, vascular tone, and membrane permeability.

Distributive Shock

Abnormalities in the distribution of blood flow may result in profound inadequacies in tissue perfusion, even in the presence of a normal or high cardiac output. These maldistributions of flow usually result from abnormalities in vascular tone.

Septic shock is the most common type of distributive shock in children. It is commonly a complication of sepsis caused by gram-positive and gram-negative bacteria, as well as by infection resulting from rickettsiae and viruses (Table 3–18 and Fig. 3–7). Patients

---

TABLE 3–18
Definitions of Related Infectious and Shock States

Infection: Microbial phenomenon characterized by an inflammatory response to the presence of microorganisms or the invasion of normally sterile host tissue by those organisms.

Bacteremia: The presence of viable bacteria in the blood.

Systemic inflammatory response syndrome: The systemic inflammatory response to a variety of severe clinical insults. The response is manifested by two or more of the following conditions:

    Temperature >38° C or <36° C
    Heart rate >90 beats/min*
    Respiratory rate >20 breaths/min* or $PaCO_2$ <32 torr
    WBC >12,000 cells/mm^3, <4000 cells/mm^3, or >10% immature (band) forms

Sepsis: The systemic response to infection. This systemic response is manifested by two or more of the following conditions as a result of infection:

    Temperature >38° C or <36° C
    Heart rate >90 beats/min*
    Respiratory rate >20 breaths/min* or $PaCO_2$ <32 torr

    WBC >12,000 cells/mm^3, <4000 cells/mm^3, or >10% immature (band) forms

Severe sepsis: Sepsis associated with organ dysfunction, hypoperfusion, or hypotension. Hypoperfusion and perfusion abnormalities may include, but are not limited to, lactic acidosis, oliguria, or an acute alteration in mental status.

Septic shock: Sepsis with hypotension, despite adequate fluid resuscitation, along with the presence of perfusion abnormalities that may include, but are not limited to, lactic acidosis, oliguria, or an acute alteration in mental status. Patients who are on inotropic or vasopressor agents may not be hypotensive at the time that perfusion abnormalities are measured.

Hypotension: A systolic BP of <90 mm Hg* or a reduction of >40 mm Hg from baseline in the absence of other causes for hypotension.

Multiple organ dysfunction syndrome: Presence of altered organ function in an acutely ill patient such that homeostasis cannot be maintained without intervention.

From American College of Chest Physicians/Society of Critical Care Medicine Consensus Conference: *Crit Care Med* 20(6):864–874, 1992.
BP, Blood pressure; *WBC,* white blood cell count.
*Adults; must use age-appropriate norms.

---

with septic shock usually have fever, lethargy, petechiae or purpura and may have an identified infectious focus. They often have tachycardia and poor peripheral perfusion, with cool, mottled extremities and poor capillary refill time. Hypotension, intense vasoconstriction, and a decreased cardiac index are frequently present. Widespread cellular dysfunction, resulting from inadequate tissue perfusion in the early phases of shock, subsequently leads to diminishing organ function. In the early stages of shock, patients may be febrile and tachycardic, with warm, flushed skin and poor urine output ("warm shock"). Systemic arterial blood pressure is normal, and cardiac output is normal or increased. The diagnosis of warm shock requires a high index of suspicion on the part of the physician and usually involves the presence of a predisposing condition, such as a known infection or immunosuppression (see Chapter 10).

In the systemic inflammatory response syndrome (Table 3–18 and Fig. 3–7), bacterial products stimulate the elaboration of a wide variety of vasoactive and inflammatory mediators. Endotoxins are bacterial cell wall lipopolysaccharides that activate macrophage production of tumor necrosis factor

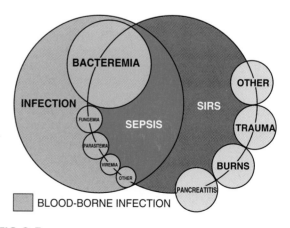

FIG. 3–7

Interrelationship between various host responses to infections and other potential inflammatory injuries (e.g., burns or trauma). The systemic inflammatory response syndrome (SIRS) may be initiated by multiple inciting events; the inflammatory mediators released by these events initiate and perpetuate the SIRS. (From American College of Chest Physicians/Society of Critical Care Medicine Consensus Conference: *Crit Care Med* 20[6]:864-874, 1992.)

(TNF) and interleukin-1 (IL-1) in addition to the complement, kinin, fibrinolytic, and coagulation pathways; injury also causes release of cellular histamine and prostaglandins. Additional inflammatory mediators include cytokines (IL-6), bioactive lipids (e.g., platelet-activating factor and leukotrienes), interferons, and the products of primary and secondary leukocyte granules. Direct injection of TNF produces cardiovascular, inflammatory, metabolic, hematologic, pulmonary, and renal abnormalities identical to those that occur in septic shock. The effect of TNF is blocked by neutralizing antibodies to TNF and only partially blocked by the inhibition of prostaglandin synthesis. Most secondary mediators decrease vascular tone and increase vascular permeability, resulting in the maldistribution of blood flow. Arteriolar vasodilation (vasculopathy) results in reduced systemic vascular resistance, which serves to lower tissue perfusion pressure and impair coronary blood flow. The increased venous capacitance produced by venodilation results in venous stasis and decreased venous return to the heart. Mediator-induced changes in vascular permeability cause capillary leaks and loss of intravascular volume, which impair ventricular filling and thus cardiac output. Activated complement components and arachidonic acid metabolites promote leukocyte and platelet aggregation in capillary beds, producing an obstruction to flow in the microcirculation. Vasculotoxins also directly depress cardiac output by decreasing intrinsic cardiac contractility or by inducing coronary vasospasm.

Cardiogenic Shock

Cardiogenic shock is caused by an abnormality in myocardial function and is expressed as depressed myocardial contractility and cardiac output with poor tissue perfusion. Primary cardiogenic shock occurs in children who have congenital heart disease. Heart failure precedes cardiogenic shock in most patients who have congenital heart disease (except hypoplastic left heart syndrome) and in patients who have circulatory obstruction (e.g., coarctation of the aorta or critical pulmonary stenosis; see Chapter 13).

In cardiogenic shock, compensatory mechanisms may contribute to the progression of shock by further depressing cardiac function. Neurohumoral vasoconstrictor responses increase afterload and add to the work of the failing ventricle. Tachycardia impairs coronary blood flow and decreases myocardial oxygen delivery. Increased central blood volume caused by sodium and water retention and by incomplete emptying of the ventricles during systole results in elevated left ventricular volume and pressure, which impair subendocardial blood flow. Because of this self-perpetuating cycle, congestive heart failure progressing to death may be rapid. As compensatory mechanisms are overcome, the failing left ventricle produces increased ventricular end–diastolic volume and pressure, which leads to increased left atrial pressure, resulting in pulmonary edema. This sequence also contributes to right ventricular failure because of increased pulmonary artery pressure and increased right ventricular afterload. The liver usually enlarges, a gallop is present, and jugular venous distention may be noted. The spleen also may be enlarged. Because renal blood flow is poor, sodium and water are retained, contributing to the formation of peripheral edema.

Generally, *treatment* of cardiogenic shock requires cardiotonic supportive drugs and diuretics to control pulmonary and tissue edema. In cardiogenic shock that develops in infants and children with underlying cardiovascular disease, the *prognosis* is poor.

Cardiogenic shock also may occur in previously healthy children secondary to viral myocarditis, dysrhythmias, toxic or metabolic derangement, or following a hypoxic-ischemic injury. In this circumstance, shock may be reversed by administering cardiotonic drugs.

Obstructive Shock

Obstructive shock results from the patient's inability to produce adequate cardiac output, despite normal intravascular volume and normal myocardial contractility, because the ventricular outflow is mechanically obstructed. The major cause of the obstruction is pericardial tamponade. Clinically, when trauma or previous heart surgery is involved, tamponade should be suspected when a patient has a narrow pulse pressure, a muffled heart tone, an enlarged heart as determined by percussion or roentgenogram, or pulseless electrical activity. Echocardiography may be diagnostic, but in symptomatic patients attempts at needle pericardiocentesis should not await confirmation by diagnostic studies.

Dissociative Shock

Dissociative shock refers to conditions in which tissue perfusion is normal but oxygen cannot be used by the cells because the hemoglobin has an abnormal affinity for oxygen, preventing its release to the tissues (Table 3–17).

Therapy for Shock
General Principles

The key to therapy is the *recognition of shock* in its early state, when many of the hemodynamic and metabolic alterations may be reversible. Therapy for shock is directed largely at treating the signs and symptoms as they appear rather than directly addressing the primary cause or mechanisms involved.

Therapy should minimize cardiopulmonary work while ensuring cardiac output, blood pressure, and gas exchange. Intubation combined with mechanical ventilation with 100% oxygen improves oxygenation and decreases or eliminates the work of breathing but may impede venous return if distending airway pressures (positive end-expiratory pressure [PEEP] or peak inspiratory pressure) (see Chapter 6) are excessive. Blood pressure support is critical because the vasodilation in sepsis may reduce perfusion despite supranormal cardiac output.

Monitoring a critically ill child in shock requires maintaining access to the central venous circulation to record pressure measurements, to perform blood sampling, and to measure systemic blood pressure continuously through an indwelling arterial catheter. These measurements facilitate the estimation of preload and afterload. When knowing the patient's left atrial pressure is critical, the pressure can be measured through a left atrial catheter connected to a pressure monitor or more often estimated by measuring pulmonary capillary wedge pressure with a flow-directed balloon-tip catheter. Directly measuring the cardiac index by thermodilution, injection of indocyanine green, or a Fick procedure also may be helpful. In addition, the management of shock requires monitoring arterial blood gases for oxygenation, ventilation (CO_2), and acidosis and frequently assessing the levels of serum electrolytes, calcium, magnesium, phosphorus, and BUN.

Organ-Directed Therapeutics

Cardiovascular Support. In general, shock states are characterized by some form of primary or secondary impairment of myocardial function. Therefore, efforts to improve cardiac output are a basic component of shock therapy. Cardiovascular therapy should be targeted at fluid resuscitation and at improvement of cardiac output, heart rate and rhythm, preload, afterload, and contractility.

Fluid Resuscitation. Alterations in preload dramatically affect cardiac output. In hypovolemic and distributive shock, decreased preload significantly impairs cardiac output. However, in cardiogenic shock an elevated preload contributes to pulmonary edema. Table 3–19 lists fluids available for volume resuscitation. Plasma volume may be restored successfully with the use of crystalloid solutions, provided that sufficient volumes are used, but edema fluid may accumulate (as a result of capillary leakage) if excessive amounts are infused. This accumulation may be unavoidable but nonetheless may be associated with a good outcome. Colloids contain larger molecules that theoretically may stay in the intravascular space longer than crystalloid solutions and thus exert oncotic pres-

---

TABLE 3–19
Intravenous Fluids Available for Pediatric Volume Resuscitation

Crystalloids
0.9% sodium chloride
Ringer's lactate
Hypertonic saline (3%)

Colloids
5% human serum albumin in 0.9% sodium chloride*
25% human serum albumin in 0.9% sodium chloride*
6% hydroxyethyl starch in 0.9% sodium chloride
10% dextran 40 in 5% dextrose in water
Fresh frozen plasma
Whole blood

---

*Albumin-containing solutions are being used less frequently because of concerns of infection and poor outcomes.

---

sure and draw fluid out of the tissues into the vascular compartment.

Selection of fluids for resuscitation and ongoing use is dictated by clinical circumstances. Crystalloid volume expanders are generally recommended as initial choices because they are effective and inexpensive. Most acutely ill children with signs of shock may safely receive, and usually benefit greatly from, a 20 mL/kg bolus of an isotonic crystalloid over 15 to 30 minutes. However, care must be exercised in treating cardiogenic shock with volume expansion because the ventricular filling pressures may rise without improvement of the cardiac performance. Carefully monitoring cardiac output or central venous pressure helps guide safe volume replacement. In patients with significant cerebral edema the need to improve cardiac output by fluid replacement and the need to maintain an acceptable cerebral perfusion pressure (mean blood pressure − intracranial pressure) should be balanced by the requirement to reduce intracranial pressure; intensive fluid resuscitation may increase intracranial pressure, exacerbating cerebral edema. However, the restoration of blood pressure and cardiac output has the highest priority in this situation.

Cardiotonic and Vasodilator Therapy. In an effort to improve cardiac output after volume resuscitation or when further volume replacement may be dangerous, a variety of cardiotonic and vasodilator drugs may be useful. Therapy is directed first at increasing myocardial contractility and then at decreasing left ventricular afterload. Currently, five sympathomimetic agents are available (Table

3–20). The hemodynamic status of the patient dictates the choice of the agent.

Therapy usually is initiated with dopamine or dobutamine. Combinations of these agents are highly effective. In children who fail to respond to several increases in either the dopamine or dobutamine infusion rate, a more potent cardiotonic agent, such as epinephrine or norepinephrine, may be indicated.

In addition to improving contractility, certain catecholamines may also cause an increase in systemic vascular resistance. The addition of a vasodilator drug may improve cardiac performance by decreasing the resistance against which the heart must pump (i.e., the drug may decrease afterload). Afterload reduction may be achieved with dobutamine, isoproterenol, amrinone, nitroprusside, nitroglycerin, and angiotensin-converting enzyme (ACE) inhibitors. The use of these drugs may be particularly important in late shock, when vasoconstriction is prominent.

Respiratory Support

The lung is a target organ for inflammatory mediators in shock and the systemic inflammatory response syndrome. Respiratory failure may develop rapidly and become progressive. Intervention requires endotracheal intubation and mechanical ventilation accompanied by the use of supplemental oxygen and PEEP. The *acute respiratory distress syndrome* (ARDS) may occur in children who are in shock (see Chapter 12). The mechanism underlying this syndrome is increased vascular permeability (noncardiogenic pulmonary edema) caused by the release of vasoactive mediators. Vascular permeability results from direct damage to the alveolar-capillary endothelium, with leakage of proteinaceous fluid into the interstitium and alveoli, and may interfere with surfactant action. This

is treated with diuretics, cardiotonics, and PEEP to prevent atelectasis and pulmonary edema. Severe cardiopulmonary failure may be managed with inhaled nitric oxide and, if needed, with extracorporeal membrane oxygenation (ECMO) (see Chapter 6).

Renal Salvage

Poor urine output during shock may be the result of acute tubular necrosis (ATN) or of prerenal factors. Hypotension associated with shock may lead to acute renal failure. Prerenal azotemia may be caused by poor cardiac output accompanied by decreased renal blood flow; however, severe hypotension may produce ATN. The azotemia is corrected when blood volume deficits are replaced or myocardial contractility is improved, but ATN does not improve immediately once shock is corrected. Prerenal azotemia is associated with a serum BUN-creatinine ratio of greater than 10:1 and a urine sodium level below 20 mEq/L; ATN has a ratio of 10:1 and a urine sodium level between 40 and 60 mEq/L (see Chapter 16). Aggressive fluid replacement often is necessary to improve the oliguria associated with prerenal azotemia. Because the management of shock requires administering large volumes of fluid (often >50 mL/kg during resuscitation), maintaining urine output greatly facilitates patient management.

Preventing ATN and the subsequent complications associated with acute renal failure (e.g., hyperkalemia, acidosis, hypocalcemia, and edema) is an important goal of shock therapy. Using pharmacologic agents to augment urine output is indicated once the intravascular volume has been replaced. The use of loop diuretics such as furosemide and bumetanide or mannitol or of combinations of a loop diuretic and a thiazide may enhance urine output. Infusion of dopamine, which produces renal artery vasodilation,

---

TABLE 3–20
Catecholamines Used for Cardiopulmonary Resuscitation

	Positive Inotrope	Positive Chronotrope	Direct Pressor	Indirect Pressor	Vasodilator
Dopamine	++	+	±	++	++*
Dobutamine	++	±	−	−	+
Epinephrine	+++	+++	+++	−	−
Isoproterenol	+++	+++	−	−	+++
Norepinephrine	+++	+++	+++	−	−

*Primarily splanchnic and renal in low doses (3–5 μg/kg/min).

also may improve urine output. Nevertheless, if hyperkalemia, refractory acidosis, hypervolemia, or the altered mental status associated with uremia occurs, dialysis or hemofiltration should be initiated. ATN is a self-limited condition that necessitates good supportive care for prevention of potential complications until renal function improves, usually 3–7 days after the renal tubular injury.

REFERENCES

Behrman RE, Kliegman RM, Jenson HB, editors: *Nelson textbook of pediatrics,* ed 16, Philadelphia, 2000, WB Saunders, Chapter 64.

Bone R: Toward an epidemiology and natural history of SIRS (systemic inflammatory response syndrome), *JAMA* 268(24): 3452–3455, 1992.

Carcillo J, Davis A, Zaritsky A: Role of early fluid resuscitation in pediatric shock, *JAMA* 266(9):1242–1245, 1991.

Chameides L, Hazinski MF, editors: *Pediatric advanced life support,* Dallas, 1997, American Heart Association, Chapters 5, 6.

Fleisher GR, Ludwig S, editors: *Textbook of pediatric emergency medicine,* ed 4, Philadelphia, 2000, Williams & Wilkins, Chapter 3.

Gattinoni L, Brazzi L, Pelosi P, et al: A trial of goal-oriented hemodynamic therapy in critically ill patients, *N Engl J Med* 333(16):1025–1032, 1995.

Huskisson L: Intravenous volume replacement: which and why? *Arch Dis Child* 67(5):649–653, 1992.

Strange GR, editor: *APLS: The pediatric emergency medicine course,* ed 3, Dallas, 1998, American College of Emergency Physicians, Chapters 3, 4.

CARDIOPULMONARY RESUSCITATION

Cardiopulmonary resuscitation is rarely needed in pediatric practice. Most infants and children who do need CPR have had an isolated respiratory arrest. The outcome of cardiopulmonary arrest in children is poor; only 10–15% survive, and the majority of the survivors sustain permanent disability. Therefore, the ability to anticipate or recognize prearrest conditions and initiate prompt and appropriate therapy not only may save the child's life but also may preserve the quality of that sustained life.

Hypoxia plays a central role in most of the events leading to cardiopulmonary arrest in children. Furthermore, the presence of hypoxia leads to subsequent organ dysfunction or to ischemic damage, no matter what underlying illness affects the child. Hypoxia may be acute or chronic and may result from either an acquired or a congenital illness. In some children, abnormal pulmonary vasculature or congenital heart disease, leading to right-to-left shunting, contributes to tenuous oxygenation. Physicians should be acutely aware of the potential damage that hypoxia and the resulting ischemia may produce in susceptible organs (Table 3–21) so that their approach to an infant or a child experiencing cardiopulmonary arrest extends beyond CPR to include efforts to preserve vital organ function.

The goal in resuscitating the pediatric patient who has sustained a cardiopulmonary arrest should be to optimize cardiac output and tissue oxygen delivery, which may be accomplished by using artificial ventilation and chest compression and by the judicious administration of pharmacologic agents.

The natural histories and mechanisms of pediatric and adult cardiopulmonary arrest are different. Adult arrests tend to be sudden in onset and cardiac in origin, with ventricular dysrhythmias or asystole preceding respiratory arrest. Children go through a series of physiologic changes before the onset of ventricular fibrillation or asystole, and most often respiration ceases before or concurrently with the cardiopulmonary arrest. Therefore, a child may be recognized as being at risk before cardiopulmonary arrest occurs (Table 3–22).

TABLE 3–21
Target Organs for Hypoxic-Ischemic Damage

Organ	Effect
Brain	Seizures, cerebral edema, infarction, herniation, anoxic damage, SIADH, diabetes insipidus
Cardiovascular	Heart failure, myocardial infarct, tricuspid insufficiency, peripheral gangrene
Lung and pulmonary vasculature	Acute respiratory distress syndrome, pulmonary hypertension
Liver	Infarction, necrosis, cholestasis
Kidney	Acute tubular necrosis, acute cortical necrosis
GI tract	Gastric ulceration, mucosal damage
Hematologic	Disseminated intravascular coagulation

GI, Gastrointestinal; *SIADH,* syndrome of inappropriate secretion of antidiuretic hormone.

TABLE 3–22
Warning Signs and Symptoms Suggesting the Potential Need for Resuscitative Intervention*

CNS	Lethargy, irritability, obtundation, confusion
Respiratory	Apnea, grunting, nasal flaring, dyspnea retracting, tachypnea, poor air movement, stridor, wheezing
Cardiovascular	Arrhythmia, bradycardia, tachycardia, weak pulses, poor capillary refill, hypotension
Skin and mucous membranes	Mottling, pallor, cyanosis, diaphoresis, poor membrane turgor, dry mucous membranes

CNS, Central nervous system.
*Action would seldom be taken if only one or two of these signs and symptoms were present, but the occurrence of several in concert foreshadows grave consequences. Intervention should be directed at the primary disorder.

Airway

On recognizing that a clinical situation requiring resuscitation exists, the physician should first ensure that there is a patent airway. In children, airway patency often is compromised by a loss of muscle tone, allowing the mandibular block of tissue, including the tongue, the bony mandible, and the soft surrounding tissues, to rest against the posterior pharyngeal wall. In adult patients such problems can be corrected by using manual head tilt maneuvers; in infants and young children, however, this correction may result in the excessive overextension of the neck and further narrowing of the tracheal airway. The jaw thrust maneuver is the most effective intervention in children.

Pediatric patients requiring resuscitation should be endotracheally intubated. Oral intubation is the preferred method in a resuscitation and is technically easier than nasal intubation in children. Before intubation, the patient should be ventilated with 100% oxygen using a bag and mask. Cricoid pressure should be used to minimize inflation of the stomach. Many patients may benefit from the use of induction medications (e.g., paralytics and sedatives) to assist intubation. The correct size of the tube may be estimated according to the size of the child's mid-5th phalanx or the following formula:

$$\frac{\text{Patient age in years} + 16}{4}$$

As a result of the presence of a narrow airway segment at the level of the cricoid ring, cuffed endotracheal tubes should not be used in children younger than 8 years of age.

Once the endotracheal tube is in place, the adequacy of ventilation and the position of the tube must be assessed. This is accomplished through assessment of chest wall movement and auscultation of the chest to detect bilateral and symmetric breath sounds. If air exchange is not heard or cyanosis continues, the position or patency of the tube must be reevaluated. This can be accomplished through direct visualization of tube location via laryngoscopy or indirectly through the use of end-tidal CO_2 measurement.

Breathing

The major role of endotracheal intubation is to protect or maintain the airway and ensure the delivery of adequate oxygen to the patient. Because hypoxemia is the final common pathway in pediatric arrests, providing oxygen is more important than correcting the respiratory acidosis that also develops. Thus 100% oxygen at a rate of 20 breaths/min should be delivered through the tube using a tidal volume necessary to produce adequate chest rise and relieve cyanosis. This usually requires a tidal volume equal to 10–15 mL/kg of body weight.

Once a patent airway is established and oxygenation and ventilation are maintained, cardiac output will be reestablished in many children. Thus carefully reassessing the patient before proceeding with other mechanical and pharmacologic maneuvers is essential. This reassessment should include observation of the color of the skin and mucous membranes and palpation of both central and peripheral pulses. If cyanosis persists or the brachial or femoral pulses remain weak or absent, adequate circulation has not been reestablished.

Circulation

Because some children may still have effective circulation early in the history of an acute respiratory arrest, circulation should be independently assessed. Chest compressions should be initiated if a pulse cannot be palpated or if the heart rate is less than 60 beats/min with signs of poor systemic perfusion.

TABLE 3–23
Drug Doses for Cardiopulmonary Resuscitation

Drug	Indication	Dose
Adenosine	Supraventricular tachycardia	0.1–0.2 mg/kg (may repeat at 0.4 mg/kg); maximum 12 mg
Amiodaronc	Pulseless VF/VT	5 mg/kg over 20–60 min
	Perfusing tachyarrhythmias	Maximum dose is 15 mg/kg/day
Atropine	Supraventricular or junctional bradycardia	0.02 mg/kg/dose (minimum dose 0.1 mg); up to 0.5 mg (child), 1.0 mg (adolescent); higher doses needed in anti-cholinesterase poisoning
	Asystole?	
Bicarbonate	Metabolic acidosis?	0.5–1 mEq/kg bolus, if metabolic acidosis present; ensure adequate ventilation; use 4.2% solution in neonates; monitor ABGs, can repeat q 10 min
	Hyperkalemia	
Bretylium	Ventricular tachycardia	5 mg/kg IV bolus (may repeat at 10 mg/kg); may cause hypotension
Calcium	Hypocalcemia	25 mg/kg calcium chloride; stop if bradycardia occurs
	Hyperkalemia	
	Wide QRS pattern?	
Dobutamine	Inotropy	2–30 µg/kg/min
Dopamine	Inotropy	0.5–2 µg/kg/min splanchnic, renal dilation; 2–7 µg/kg/min inotrope; 7–20 µg/kg/min inotrope + pressor
	Renal preservation	
Epinephrine	Chronotropy	0.01 mg/kg bolus q 5 min; 0.1 mg/kg as subsequent doses if 0.01 mg/kg is ineffective; 0.05–2 µg/kg/min drip, inotrope + pressor; may cause subendocardial ischemia and arrhythmias
	Inotropy	
	Hypotension	
Fluid	Hypovolemia	Use crystalloid tailored to patient's physiologic needs
	Sepsis	
Glucose	Hypoglycemia	2 mL/kg 10% dextrose; follow Dextrostix
Isoproterenol	Chronotropy	0.05–1 µg/kg/min inotrope + vasodilator effects; chronotropic response may limit dose; may cause subendocardial ischemia and arrhythmias
	Inotropy	
Lidocaine	Ventricular tachycardia	1 mg/kg/bolus followed by 20–50 µg/kg/min continuous infusion; monitor serum concentration and widening of QRS for toxicity
Nitroprusside	Reduce systemic vascular resistance	0.05–10.0 µg/kg/min by continuous infusion
	Hypertensive crisis	
Oxygen	Hypoxia	100%, humidified
Phenytoin	Ventricular tachycardia, digitalis-induced arrhythmias	15–20 mg/kg slow loading dose; titrate maintenance therapy to serum concentrations of 15–30 µg/mL

Data from Pediatric Working Group of the International Liaison Committee on Resuscitation: *Circulation* 102:I291–I342, 2000.
?, Controversial, uncertain, or unproved efficacy; *ABG*, arterial blood gas; *VF*, ventricular fibrillation; *VT*, ventricular tachycardia.

For compressions to be optimal, the child should be supine on a hard, flat surface. In infants and children the area for compression is the lower half of the sternum. Effective CPR in infants requires a compression depth between 0.5 and 1 inch. The child (ages 1 to 8 years) requires a compression depth of 1 to 1.5 inches. In both cases, the compression rate should be at least 100 per minute, coordinated with assisted ventilation at a ratio of 5:1 compressions to breaths. The effectiveness of compressions should be as-sessed via palpation of the carotid, brachial, or femoral artery.

Drugs

(Table 3–23)
When mechanical means fail to reestablish adequate circulation, pharmacologic intervention is essential. Drug therapy during CPR is directed toward improving cardiac output and the delivery of oxygen to

tissues. The special requirements of drugs used during CPR limit the number of potential routes for their administration. Administration through a central venous line is preferred, although typically this is difficult to achieve in unanticipated arrests. The effectiveness of peripheral intravenous administration is limited by poor circulation. Alternative routes for administration of some drugs are through the endotracheal tube or by intraosseous (bone marrow) infusion.

Perhaps the most important agent used during CPR in children is *oxygen*. Whenever possible, 100% oxygen should be administered through an endotracheal tube. Short periods of exposure to high oxygen tensions cause little pulmonary toxicity, and high oxygen tensions may be required to reverse some of the reactive pulmonary vascular responses to poor cardiac output.

The use of buffers is the subject of considerable controversy. *Sodium bicarbonate* is the most commonly used buffer, but its risk may outweigh its potential benefits. One of the hallmarks of poor cardiac output is acidemia. In pediatric patients, however, this acidemia is often respiratory rather than metabolic. Judicious use of sodium bicarbonate to correct the metabolic component of the acidosis may be beneficial. However, the use of sodium bicarbonate in an attempt to correct what is primarily a respiratory problem can exacerbate respiratory acidosis by inducing the production of more CO_2. Sodium bicarbonate may produce hypernatremia, hyperosmolality, hypokalemia, metabolic alkalosis (shifting the oxyhemoglobin curve to the left and impairing tissue oxygen delivery), reduced ionized calcium level, and impaired cardiac function.

Catecholamines constitute the mainstay of drug therapy for CPR. They are administered both as boluses during the acute phases of resuscitation and by continuous infusions during the maintenance therapy involved in postresuscitative stabilization. Epinephrine is the primary agent used. It is a catecholamine with mixed alpha- and beta-agonist properties. The alpha-adrenergic effects are most important during the acute phases because of the alpha-induced increase in systemic vascular resistance that results in a greater pressure gradient across the coronary bed and an improved coronary blood flow. Vasopressin may have similar effects.

Prompt electrical defibrillation is indicated when ventricular fibrillation is noted (Table 3–24). Bolus administration of lidocaine is recommended before defibrillation, but defibrillation should not be delayed if lidocaine cannot be administered immediately. Defibrillation should be distinguished from *cardioversion* of supraventricular tachycardias that also may compromise cardiac output. Cardioversion requires a lower starting dose and a synchronization

---

TABLE 3–24
Recommendations for Defibrillation and Cardioversion in Children

Defibrillation
Pretreat with 0.01 mg/kg epinephrine (1:10,000) IV.
Place saline gauze or conduction jellied pad at apex and upper right sternal border.
Use 4.5-cm diameter paddles for infants and 8–10-cm diameter paddles for children.
Notify all participating personnel before discharging paddles so that no one is in contact with patient or bed.
Begin with 2 watts/sec/kg (2 joules/kg).
If unsuccessful, double current (4 joules/kg) and repeat rapidly × 3.

Cardioversion
Determine mechanism of the predominant rhythm.
Consider pretreatment with lidocaine, 1 mg/kg IV, for risk of inducing ventricular tachycardia and Valium for sedation.
For symptomatic supraventricular tachycardia* or ventricular tachycardia with a pulse, synchronize signal with electrocardiogram.
Choose paddles, position pads, and notify personnel as above.
Begin with 0.5–1 watts/sec/kg (joules/kg).
If unsuccessful, double the current.

---

*Consider adenosine first (Table 3–23).

---

of the discharge to the electrocardiogram to prevent discharging during a susceptible period, which may convert supraventricular tachycardia to ventricular tachycardia or fibrillation.

Pediatric CPR requires a careful integration of mechanical skills and pharmacotherapy (Table 3–23). Intervention should commence in an anticipatory fashion, and the drug doses provided should serve as a guide rather than a limit to therapy. Resuscitative efforts should be directed toward preserving vital organ function and reversing ongoing tissue damage rather than simply starting the heart. This clinical strategy should continue into the postresuscitative period.

REFERENCES

American Heart Association: Guidelines 2000 for cardiopulmonary resuscitation and emergency cardiovascular care, *Circulation* 102(suppl):I-235, I-291, I-343, 2000.
Behrman RE, Kliegman RM, Jenson HB: *Nelson textbook of pediatrics*, ed 16, Philadelphia, 2000, WB Saunders, Chapter 64.

Chameides L, Hazinski MF, editors: *Pediatric advanced life support*, Dallas, 1997, American Heart Association, Chapters 3–7, 9.

Fleisher GR, Ludwig S, editors: *Textbook of pediatric emergency medicine*, ed 4, Philadelphia, 2000, Williams & Wilkins, Chapter 1.

Patterson M: Resuscitation update for the pediatrician, *Pediatr Clin North Am* 46(6):1285–1303, 1999.

Strange GR, editor: *APLS: the pediatric emergency medicine course*, ed 3, Dallas, 1998, American College of Emergency Physicians, Chapters 1–4.

DRUG THERAPY IN THE ACUTELY ILL CHILD

Drugs cannot create physiologic responses that are not intrinsic to the patient. For this reason, the specific effect that is the goal of pharmacotherapy for the critically ill child is limited to the augmentation, ablation, or modulation of normal physiologic processes.

Two important groups of factors determine the efficacy of drug therapy. *Pharmacokinetic* determinants (Table 3–25) relate to the absorption, distribution, metabolism, and excretion of the drug. *Pharmacodynamic* determinants reflect the drug's mechanism of action and its safety profiles. Effective therapy can be achieved if the selected drug has favorable pharmacokinetic and pharmacodynamic properties.

Various developmental changes affect each phase of pharmacokinetics, as well as drug-receptor interactions and drug safety profiles. Changes in gastric acidity and gastrointestinal motility affect the rate and extent of oral drug *absorption*. Once absorbed, the *distribution* of drug into tissues is influenced by several factors. In the newborn period, it is influenced by the presence of fetal albumin, which has binding characteristics that differ from those of adult albumin. Also in neonates, endogenous substances such as bilirubin and elevated free fatty acids may displace drugs from their albumin-binding sites. Finally, drug distribution in neonates is affected profoundly by the changes in extracellular fluid volume that occur during normal maturation. At birth, water may account for up to 80% of the infant's total body weight, whereas in adults the extracellular fluid volume comprises only 60% of the total body weight. This may account in part for the higher doses that infants and young children require for effects to be obtained, compared with doses required by adults, when assessed on a milligram-per-kilogram basis.

Drug *metabolism* accounts for the major differences between individuals in responses to drugs. In addition, marked changes in the drug-metabolizing enzymes in the liver occur during early infancy and then again at the time of adolescence, when sex differences in drug metabolism may be a result of changes in steroid hormone levels. These changes in drug metabolism coincide with the changes in drug

TABLE 3–25
Pharmacokinetic Considerations in Critically Ill Children

Absorption Phase
Altered gastric emptying
Decreased gastrointestinal blood flow, ileus
Altered gastric pH; exogenous buffers—antacids, H_2-receptor antagonists, maturity
Time delay
Altered biliary function

Distribution Phase
Hemodynamic instability
Inflammation
Decreased protein synthesis/increased protein loss
Synthesis of acute-phase reactants
Extravascular fluid collections—ascites, pleural effusions
Drug interactions
Maturational changes of extracellular fluid space (see Chapter 2)

Metabolism Phase
Hemodynamic instability
Hypoxemia
Substrate deficiencies
Polypharmacy—drug interactions
Use of hormones and autacoids as pharmacologic rather than physiologic agents
Enzyme maturational changes in biotransformation

Excretion Phase
Altered vascular volume
Altered renal blood flow (illness, maturation)
Hypoxemia
Nephrotoxic agents
Altered hepatic function (illness, maturation)

excretion by the kidney, which relate to the maturation of both glomerular filtration and tubular secretion (see Chapter 16).

Changes in the pharmacodynamics of drugs may result from developmental changes in receptor number and affinity or in receptor-effector coupling, so that the dosage producing particular therapeutic and adverse effects will change as the newborn progresses from infancy to childhood, adolescence, and adulthood. This relationship of changing pharmacokinetics and pharmacodynamics to growth and development is complicated further by the effect of the various physiologic derangements during an acute illness (Table 3–25).

Pharmacodynamic changes in critically ill children may result from vascular volume and electrolyte derangements and from the effects of acute alterations in acid-base status. Moreover, acutely ill patients generate endogenous substances that alter drug responsiveness, and the long-term use of certain hormones and autacoids may result in the down-regulation of their various receptors. Finally, patients who already are seriously ill are less likely to tolerate the potential side effects of various drugs, so that the safety profile of the drugs used in a critical care setting may be altered drastically.

The superposition of acute illness on a developmental program controlling drug biodisposition and response presents a challenge to the development of effective therapeutic strategies. One strategy, the *target-concentration strategy,* consists of an attempt to achieve specific plasma levels of a drug. Therapeutic principles emphasize the importance of an awareness of drug pharmacokinetics and active metabolites, having predetermined expectations of the manifestations of drug efficacy and toxicity, awareness of appropriate sampling times for drug levels, treating the patient and *not* the drug level, and, if inconsistencies develop, reevaluating and reexamining the patient. This strategy often is applied to drugs that are used chronically to treat illnesses having intermittent clinical manifestations. Examples of such illnesses include reversible reactive airway disease, seizure disorders, and cardiac arrhythmias. Implementing this strategy requires effective use of the drug analysis laboratory (Table 3–26). The targeted concentrations may relate either to drug efficacy or to toxicity and generally are based on data obtained from large populations rather than from individual patients.

The types of drugs that lend themselves to the target-concentration strategy are those manifesting a wide variation among individuals in drug absorption, distribution, or elimination (Table 3–27). Therapeutic monitoring for drug efficacy is possible for theophylline, anticonvulsants (e.g., phenytoin, phenobarbital, valproate, carbamazepine, and ethosuximide), and antiarrhythmic agents (e.g., procainamide and its metabolite NAPA, quinidine, lidocaine, and amiodarone). This strategy also is useful for administering drugs that have a narrow therapeutic index and for those designed to attain relatively sustained and constant effects over a long period. Such a strategy can be considered only when the concentrations of drug in the plasma relate directly to clinical effects of the drug that can be monitored. Knowing the therapeutic range and toxic level for each drug and the average values for absorption, distribution, and elimination of the drug permits intelligent use of serum drug levels. The pathophysiologic conditions that alter these parameters and the extent of this alteration also must be appreciated.

The *target-effect strategy* is the second approach to the drug treatment of acutely ill children. Two principles are essential to its application: the first relates to the dose-response relationship (i.e., the concept that most drugs show increasing clinical or adverse effects with increasing doses); the second is that, before therapy is initiated, there must be a well-defined clinical endpoint (i.e., the physician prescribing the drug must have a reasonable understanding of the

---

TABLE 3–26
Prerequisites for Therapeutic Drug Monitoring

The analytic method must be specific, sensitive, accurate, and available in an appropriate time frame.
The active drug and important metabolites are measured.
Tolerance does not develop at receptor sites.
The concentration of the drug in serum is proportional to the concentration of the drug at receptor sites.
There must be reasonably good correlation between drug concentration and therapeutic effects.
The therapeutic range must be well defined.
Proper care is taken in interpretation of values.

TABLE 3–27
Drugs Amenable to Therapeutic Monitoring for Drug Toxicity

Antibiotics
Aminoglycosides—gentamicin, tobramycin, and amikacin
Chloramphenicol
Vancomycin

Immunosuppression
Methotrexate
Cyclosporine

Antipyretics
Acetaminophen
Salicylate

Other
Digoxin
Lithium
Theophylline
Anticonvulsant drugs

drug's pharmacodynamic action, including its side effects). There must also be a reasonable understanding of the effect of both ontogeny and disease on these pharmacodynamic actions. Finally, before therapy begins, a system must be in place to monitor both the efficacy and toxicity of the drug.

The target-effect strategy is particularly appropriate in the intensive care setting (Table 3–28). For example, if oxygen is being used as a drug to increase a patient's oxygen saturation in the presence of respiratory failure, the strategy is to choose a clinically acceptable oxygen saturation level (e.g.,

>90%) and to increase the inspired oxygen concentration serially until the patient is receiving the desired oxygen saturation or until the patient is inspiring 100% oxygen. The essence of the target-effect strategy is an increase in dosage until the desired therapeutic effect is achieved. However, if sequential increases produce no increased effect and if the therapeutic effect has not been achieved or if drug toxicity supervenes, changing the drug rather than adding different drugs to the regimen is the appropriate response.

REFERENCES

Behrman RE, Kliegman RM, Jenson HB, editors: *Nelson textbook of pediatrics*, ed 16, Philadelphia, 2000, WB Saunders.

Blumer J: Principles of drug disposition in the critically ill child. In Fuhrman B, Zimmerman J, editors: *Pediatric critical care*, St Louis, 1992, Mosby.

Reed MD, Blumer JL: Therapeutic drug monitoring in the pediatric intensive care unit, *Pediatr Clin North Am* 41(6):1227–1243, 1994.

SEDATION AND ANALGESIA

The critically ill neonate, child, or adolescent may have pain, discomfort, and anxiety resulting from injury, surgery, and invasive procedures (e.g., intubation, bone marrow aspiration, central venous line placement) or during life-sustaining mechanical ventilation. Pain may be expressed by verbal or visible discomfort, crying, agitation, tachycardia, hypertension, and tachypnea. The physician has a commitment to relieve discomfort and treat pain. Common pharmacologic agents used to manage acute and chronic pain are noted in Table 3–29.

TABLE 3–28
Drugs for Using a Target-Effect Strategy in Critically Ill Children

Catecholamines—dopamine, dobutamine, epinephrine, isoproterenol, norepinephrine, and terbutaline

Vasodilators—nitroglycerin, nitroprusside, hydralazine, and angiotensin-converting enzyme inhibitors

Anticoagulants—heparin and warfarin

Beta-lactam antibiotics—penicillins, cephalosporins, carbapenems, and monobactams

Anxiolytics, sedatives—diazepam, lorazepam, midazolam, morphine, fentanyl, chloral hydrate, and secobarbital

Oxygen

Diuretics—furosemide, bumetanide, chlorothiazide, and metolazone

---

TABLE 3–29
Pharmacologic Management of Pain

Agent	Comments
Nonopioid Analgesia	
Nonsteroidal anti-inflammatory drugs (NSAIDs) Ibuprofen Naprosyn Tolectin Ketorolac	Greater efficacy than acetaminophen, equal to or greater than oral opioids; opioid and NSAID combination reduces opioid tolerance and enhances analgesia; *chronic complications:* decreased glomerular filtration rate, fluid retention, gastrointestinal ulceration, bleeding, and perforation; no abuse potential but has ceiling effect
Acetaminophen	Potency equivalent to aspirin; less than NSAIDs; *acute ingestion:* hepatic toxicity

Data from Brill JE: *Crit Care Clin* 8(1):203–218, 1992; Committee on Drugs, American Academy of Pediatrics: *Pediatrics* 89(6 pt 1):1110–1115, 1992; *Med Lett Drugs Ther* 35(887):1–6, 1993; Zeltzer LK, Anderson CT, Schechter NL: *Curr Probl Pediatr* 20(8):409–486, 1990.

Continued

TABLE 3–29
Pharmacologic Management of Pain

Agent	Comments
Opioid Analgesia	
Pure agonists	Have no ceiling effect (e.g., higher dose, greater analgesia) and greater *side effects* (e.g., res-
Morphine	piratory depression, sedation, miosis, nausea, histamine release–pruritus, decreased gut
Codeine	motility, constipation, increased sphincter of Oddi tone, urinary retention, and biliary
Fentanyl, alfentanil, sufentanil	spasm); opioid abstinence syndrome if withdrawn quickly; high abuse potential
Partial agonists/ agonist-antagonists	May produce dysphoria, acute withdrawal symptoms if given with pure agonist opioids; possible reduced biliary spasm
Pentazocine	
Nalbuphine	
Butorphanol	
Buprenorphine	
Propoxyphene	
Methadone	
Meperidine	No histamine release, possibly decreased biliary spasm; toxic, active metabolite— normeperidine—produces seizures
Sedative-Hypnotics	
Benzodiazepines	Produce anxiolysis, sedation, muscle relaxation, amnesia; useful in combination with opi-
Diazepam	oids for painful procedures or postoperative pain; tolerance possible; *acute complications:*
Midazolam (short-acting)	apnea, decreased blood pressure, decreased myocardial function
Lorazepam (long-acting)	
Other agents	
Ketamine	Produces dissociative anesthesia, analgesia, amnesia, increased heart rate, increased blood pressure, increased bronchial secretions (decreased with atropine), bronchodilation and emergent delirium, hallucinations, and vivid dreams (reduced with benzodiazepines); contraindicated with increased intracranial pressure
Propofol	Rapid onset, lipophilic; may decrease cardiovascular function
Chloral hydrate	Predominantly sedative, weak analgesia; *toxicity* includes emesis, gastrointestinal bleed- ing, esophageal stricture, hepatic dysfunction, arrhythmias, decreased blood pressure, possible carcinogenesis
Cyclic antidepressants	Useful as adjuvant analgesia for chronic pain (e.g., cancer pain)
Carbamazepine	Useful as adjuvant for various chronic neuralgias

Data from Brill JE: *Crit Care Clin* 8(1):203–218, 1992; Committee on Drugs, American Academy of Pediatrics: *Pediatrics* 89(6 pt 1):1110–1115, 1992; *Med Lett Drugs Ther* 35(887):1–6, 1993; Zeltzer LK, Anderson CT, Schechter NL: *Curr Probl Pediatr* 20(8):409–486, 1990.

REFERENCES

Behrman RE, Kliegman RM, Jenson HB, editors: *Nelson textbook of pediatrics,* ed 16, Philadelphia, 2000, WB Saunders, Chapter 74.

Committee on Drugs, American Academy of Pediatrics: Guidelines for the monitoring and management of pediatric patients during and after sedation for diagnostic and therapeutic procedures, *Pediatrics* 89(6 pt 1):1110–1115, 1992.

Selbst SM: Sedation and analgesia. In Fleisher GR, Ludwig S, editors: *Textbook of pediatric emergency medicine,* ed 4, Philadelphia, 2000, Lippincott Williams & Wilkins.

Strange GR, editor: *APLS: The pediatric emergency medicine course,* ed 3, Dallas, 1998, American College of Emergency Physicians, Chapter 18.

Zempsky W: Developing the painless emergency department: a systematic approach to change, *Clin Pediatr Emerg Med* 1(4): 253–259, 2000.

CHAPTER 4

Human Genetics and Dysmorphology

R. Stephen S. Amato

Wound healing, susceptibility to infection, risk of environmentally induced cancers, various anemias, and metabolic disorders, as well as adverse reactions to medications, are all functions with major genetic components. Each body cell is governed by its genetic capabilities and its environmental influences and opportunities. Over 6500 specific gene loci of the 30,000 to 60,000 possible genes in the human genome have been identified. A malfunction in any of these genes can theoretically result in the development of a disease. Genetic conditions are common causes of acute and chronic diseases; the onset of disease may occur in the fetus, infant, child, or adult. Molecular diagnostic methods for sequencing genes are available, but the correlation between an individual's genetic makeup (genotype) and the expression of a variation, condition, or disease (phenotype) is only partially understood. Genetic abnormalities may produce congenital malformations (e.g., chromosomal trisomies 13, 18, and 21 [Down syndrome]), metabolic disturbances (e.g., phenylketonuria [PKU] or galactosemia), specific organ dysfunction (e.g., mental retardation or renal failure), or abnormalities of sexual differentiation (e.g., Turner syndrome or virilizing adrenal hyperplasia). Approximately 1% of newborn infants exhibit monogenetic diseases (e.g., cystic fibrosis or sickle cell disease), and 0.5% have chromosomal disorders (e.g., trisomy 21); 1–3% of children have diseases that are multifactorial in pathogenesis (e.g., congenital heart disease, spina bifida, or cleft palate). In a developed country, the majority of infant deaths are the result of genetic disorders and birth defects.

GENE STRUCTURE AND FUNCTION

Each gene is a unique sequence of a deoxyribonucleic acid (DNA) macromolecule, which is arranged as a double-stranded chain of deoxyribose residues linked by complementary base pairs. The purine bases adenine and guanine are paired by hydrogen bonds to the pyrimidine bases thymine and cyto-

sine, respectively. There are about 3 billion of these base pairs in the haploid human genome contained in the 23 chromosomes. A typical gene contains a promoter sequence, an untranslated region, a start codon, the actual gene, and a stop codon, all on the same strand (in *cis* position), running from the 5' end of the DNA to the 3' end. The actual gene consists of *exons*, which are regions containing the code that ultimately corresponds to a sequence of amino acids, and *introns*, which will not become part of the amino acid sequence.

Double-stranded DNA *replicates* to produce new copies of genetic material for daughter cells. *Transcription* is the process of initiating protein synthesis by reading the DNA and copying the future amino acid sequence encoded in the DNA onto a single strand of messenger ribonucleic acid (mRNA). The newly synthesized mRNA must be processed to remove the intron-coded sequences. The intron-derived mRNA pieces are formed into loops and excised. The exon sequences are spliced to yield a shorter, mature mRNA that moves from the nucleus to cytoplasmic ribosomes. The genetic message is *translated* into a polypeptide chain as amino acids are carried to the ribosomal-mRNA complex by transfer RNA (tRNA), small RNA molecules that are specific for each amino acid. *Alternate splicing* of exon sequences is frequent in the human genome; each gene codes for an average of three different proteins. This adds a layer of complexity not found in microbes or lower eukaryotes.

Genes or fragments of DNA from specific genes can be cloned in the laboratory. Specific DNA probes can be labeled to identify the gene's DNA. A probe is a radioactively labeled, single-stranded DNA fragment that selectively binds or hybridizes to complementary DNA of a specific gene, to part of the DNA sequence of a gene, or to parts of the DNA flanking the gene. Specific probes or endonuclease-derived characteristic *restriction fragment length polymorphisms* (RFLPs) can be used to identify mutant or absent genes in patients with genetic disorders. The patient's DNA fragments are separated by gel electrophoresis. A single-stranded ^{32}P-labeled DNA probe then is hybridized to the patient's DNA. An x-ray plate then is exposed to the gel, which produces an autoradiograph and thus demonstrates the sites of ^{32}P-DNA binding.

Because each human chromosome has hundreds of thousands of base pairs, smaller, workable units must be produced to identify genes. *Restriction endonucleases* are enzymes that recognize specific 4–8 base pair sequences and cleave DNA into smaller fragments at these specific sites. Each of the more than 150 endonucleases produces a reproducible and characteristic fragment pattern, and these patterns can be separated by size on an agarose gel. Mutations at the site of cleavage will change the fragmentation pattern, producing an RFLP. DNA from the agarose gel can be transferred to cellulose nitrate, where single-stranded DNA fragments can hybridize with probe DNA to identify the fragment containing the complementary DNA (cDNA). Hybridization of single-stranded DNA to DNA is called *Southern blotting;* hybridization of RNA to DNA is *Northern blotting.* The demonstration of antibody to protein bands is called *Western blotting.*

The combination of cDNA probes, RFLP, and Southern blotting has made it possible to diagnose genetic diseases, to clone genes, to add to our basic understanding of genetic diseases, to offer prenatal diagnoses, and in the future to treat certain genetic disorders by replacing the missing normal gene. Small quantities of genomic DNA can be amplified with the *polymerase chain reaction* (PCR). The PCR is a powerful tool for making many copies of a DNA or RNA segment, which simplifies subsequent analysis.

Automated DNA sequencing can identify the order of bases in a limited-size strand of isolated nucleic acid and can identify base substitutions, deletions, inversions, etc. in specific genes. Automated sequencing combined with computer analysis of overlapping and contiguous segments of DNA has been used to identify over 95% of the human genome. This is helpful in the molecular analysis of candidate genes that are or may be associated with a disease.

INHERITED CONDITIONS

Three basic mechanisms of inheritance exist for single-gene conditions. The three methods of human inheritance are dominant; recessive; and sex-linked, or X-linked. Except for genes on the X and Y chromosomes in males, all genes are duplicated in a normal diploid individual. If a single copy of the gene (a single allele) has a detectable effect when present, the condition is said to be *dominant.* If the effect of the allele is not apparent when only one allele is present and is expressed if two functionally identical alleles

are present, the condition is *recessive.* If an individual has two identical alleles, that individual is said to be homozygous for the gene. If a person has two different alleles, the person is heterozygous for the gene in question. The effects of recessive conditions are seen only in homozygous persons, whereas the effects of dominant conditions are seen in the heterozygous individual. A person who is heterozygous for a hidden recessive allele is described as a *carrier.*

X-linked inheritance is a variation of dominant and recessive inheritance modified by the fact that males have only one X chromosome. Normal XY males will express any genes present on their X chromosome; they are *hemizygous* for genes on the X chromosome. Males also possess a Y chromosome that is passed from father to son (holandric distribution). The Y chromosome is important in determining maleness but appears to do little else.

MENDELIAN INHERITANCE AND CYTOGENICS
Autosomal Dominant Inheritance

The ability to explain gene inheritance during genetic counseling requires an understanding of how a pattern of inheritance occurs. In autosomal dominant conditions (Table 4–1), if one parent displays a dominant condition and is heterozygous for the gene, each child has a 50% chance of receiving the gene's single allele and also of manifesting the condition. Not all patients with the affected gene may be symptomatic. *Penetrance* is the percentage of patients with the gene who manifest symptoms or signs; *expressivity* reflects the spectrum of severity among patients having clinical manifestations.

The *major histocompatibility complex* (MHC) genes illustrate another important type of autosomal dominant inheritance (Fig. 4–1). These genes determine cell surface antigens (proteins) and are located in a cluster close to the middle of the short (p) arm of the number-6 chromosome. Three *human leukocyte antigen* (HLA) genes in the MHC are designated HLA-A, HLA-B, and HLA-C and code for class MHC proteins located on all nucleated cells and platelets. Each HLA gene has a large number of possible alleles; the alleles are designated by number. An unusual feature of the HLA system is that most of the individual alleles have an effect that can be detected on the leukocyte surface. When the effects of each different allele can be detected, the alleles are called "codominants." In this special case, the appearance of the condition produced by the genes (phenotype) corresponds to the allelic composition (genotype). HLA alleles (haplotypes) of gene A are A1, A2, A3, and so forth, continuing past A32; alleles of gene C are C1 to C8; and al-

TABLE 4–1
Autosomal Dominant Diseases

Disease	Frequency	Comments
Achondroplasia Thanatophoric dysplasia Cruzon syndrome with acanthosis Nonsyndromic craniosynostosis	~1:5000	Mutations are in the gene for *fibroblast growth factor receptor-3* on chromosome 4-p16.3. 40% of cases are new mutations. (Different mutations in the same gene cause achondroplasia, thanatophoric dysplasia, Cruzon syndrome with acanthosis, and nonsyndromic craniosynostosis.)
Neurofibromatosis I	1:3000	About 50% of cases result from new mutations in the gene for neurofibromin, a tumor suppressor gene located at 17q11.2. Expression is quite variable.
Neurofibromatosis II (NF II, bilateral acoustic neuromas, Merlin)	Genotype at birth 1:33,000 Phenotype prevalence 1:200,000	The NF II gene is a tumor suppressor gene located at 22q12.2. The protein is called "Merlin."
Huntington disease (HD)	Variable in populations, 1:5000–1:20,000	The disease is caused by a (CAG) repeat expansion in the "Huntington" protein gene on chromosome 4p16.3.
Myotonic dystrophy (DM, Steinert disease)	1:500 in Quebec 1:25,000 Europeans	The disease is caused by a (CTG) repeat expansion in the DM kinase gene at chromosome 19q13.2. The condition shows genetic anticipation with successive generations.
Marfan syndrome (FBN-1)	1:16,000–25,000	The syndrome is caused by mutations in the fibrillin 1 gene on chromosome 15q21.1; there is variable expression.
Hereditary angioneurotic edema (HANE) (C-1 esterase inhibitor that regulates the C-1 component of complement)	1:10,000	The gene is located on chromosome 11q11–q13.2. The phenotype of episodic and variable subcutaneous and submucosal swelling and pain is caused by diminished or altered esterase inhibitor protein, which can result from any one of many mutations in the gene.
Spinocerebellar ataxias (SCAs) (SCA-1, 2, 3, 6, 7), including Machado-Joseph disease (SCA-3)	Uncommon	The following is a list of specific ataxias and their chromosomes: SCA-1: 6p23 SCA-2: 12q241 SCA-3: 14q24.3-q32 SCA-6: 19q13 SCA-7: 3p14.1-p21.1 Progressive conditions are all the result of CAG triplet repeat expansions. All show variability and anticipation.

leles of gene B are B1 to B49. The HLA genes A, B, and C are all codominant, so that an individual will have two alleles for each HLA gene site (A, C, and B) and thus six detectable HLA alleles. (The actual sequence of the genes is A, C, B rather than alphabetical order.)

Myotonic dystrophy, an autosomal dominant disorder, is unusual because a severe congenital form occurs through transmission from the mother and not from the father. In addition, the disease demonstrates *anticipation*—the severity of the disease increases with each subsequent generation. Mutatable expansion of a GCT trinucleotide repeat in a 3' untranslated region of the myotonic protein kinase gene develops with each meiosis (especially maternal), thus explaining the

genetic anticipation (increasing severity) in the next generation. Other conditions result from unstable trinucleotide repeats, including Huntington disease, spinocerebellar ataxias, and fragile X syndrome. This is discussed under A Sex-Linked Condition with a Cytogenetic Marker later in this chapter.

Autosomal Recessive Inheritance

In autosomal recessive conditions, the phenotype is expressed when identical alleles are present. Consanguinity increases the risk of expressing an autosomal recessive disorder. For example, located on the distal segment of the q (long) arm of chromosome 12

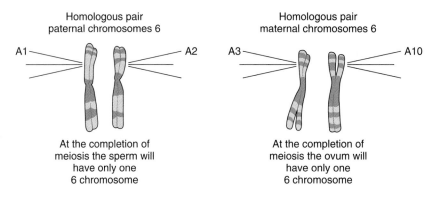

The possibilities for HLA-A alleles in offspring can be diagrammed using the Punnett square method

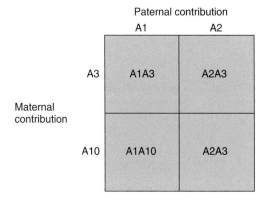

FIG. 4–1

Chromosome 6 showing segregation of HLA-A alleles. *HLA,* Human leukocyte antigen.

is a gene for the enzyme phenylalanine hydroxylase. If an individual is homozygous for a gene that codes for an abnormal enzyme (or for a nonfunctional gene product) in this location, that person is not able to convert the essential amino acid phenylalanine to tyrosine. Under these circumstances, excess phenylalanine cannot be metabolized and accumulates along with phenylalanine metabolic by-products to produce PKU. Elevated levels of phenylalanine can be neurotoxic and can lead to mental retardation (see Chapter 5). The risk of two carriers having a child with PKU is 1 in 4 (25%).

The Hardy-Weinberg equation can be used to determine the frequency of carriers in the population. This is a binomial expansion used in population genetics to assess the relative stability of gene frequencies. The basic equation is expressed as

$$p^2 + 2pq + q^2 = 1$$

This equation is derived from the notion that the homozygous normal genes, "NN," plus the heterozygous genes, "2 NA," plus the abnormal homozygous genes, "AA," equal 100% of the genes in the population. The clinical geneticist takes liberties with the equation to arrive at an estimate of the carrier frequency. The first liberty is the assumption that all the abnormal, homozygous recessive persons are identified, which may or may not be true; for cystic fibrosis this represents about 1 in 2500 persons (among white North Americans of Western European ancestry). This number is the "q^2" in the equation; therefore $q = 50$. The frequency of heterozygote carriers is "2pq." By convention we consider p to be almost "1" (for rare recessives); thus $(2 \times 1) \times (1/50) = 2/50$, which reduces to 1 in 25 as the estimated frequency of carriers for cystic fibrosis in the general population. Although we have taken license with the Hardy-Weinberg equilibrium, the estimates are close to the empiric data for rare recessives in most populations when actual carrier testing is carried out. The short-cut calculation is ½ of the square root of the frequency of affected individuals.

The Hardy-Weinberg equation itself makes some suppositions that are not necessarily true. It assumes

TABLE 4–2
Autosomal Recessive Diseases

Disease	Frequency	Comments
Adrenal hyperplasia, congenital (CAH, 21-hydroxylase deficiency, CA21H, CYP21, cytochrome P450, subfamily XXI)	1:5000	Phenotype variation corresponds roughly to allelic variation. A deficiency causes virilization in females. The gene is located at 6p21.3 within the HLA complex and within 0.005 centimorgans (cM) of HLA B.
Phenylketonuria (PKU, phenylalanine hydroxylase deficiency PAH)	1:12,000–1:17,000	There are hundreds of adverse mutations in the PAH gene located on chromosome 12q22-q24.1. The first population-based newborn screening was a test for PKU because the disease is treatable by diet. Women with elevated phenylalanine will have infants with damage to the central nervous system because high phenylalanine is neurotoxic and teratogenic.
Cystic fibrosis (CF)	1:2500 whites	The gene *CF transmembrane conductance regulator* is on chromosome 7q31.2.
Friedreich ataxia (FA, frataxin)	1:25,000	Frataxin is a mitochondrial protein involved with iron metabolism and respiration. The gene is on chromosome 9q13-q21, and the common mutation is a GAA expanded triplet repeat located in the first *intron* of the gene. FA does not show anticipation.
Gaucher disease, all types (glucocerebrosidase deficiency, acid beta glucosidase deficiency) (a lysosomal storage disease)	1:2500 Ashkenazi Jews	The gene is located on chromosome 1q21. There are many mutations; some mutations lead to neuropathic disease, but most are milder in expression. The phenotypes correspond to the genotypes, but the latter are difficult to analyze.
Sickle cell disease (hemoglobin beta locus, beta 6 glu→val mutation)	1:625 African-Americans	This is the first condition with a defined molecular defect (1959). A single base change results in an amino acid substitution of valine for glutamic acid at position 6 of the beta chain of hemoglobin with resulting hemolytic anemia. The gene is on chromosome 11p15.5. Penicillin prophylaxis reduces death from pneumococcal infections in affected persons, especially in infants.

random mating in a general population, and exceptions to this assumption exist. For example, there are communities that limit the choice of mates within a defined group. In these communities, because carrier testing is available for a severe autosomal recessive condition that is common in the group, social introductions between carriers are intentionally excluded. This exclusion, coupled with the use of pregnancy termination for affected fetuses (as determined by prenatal diagnosis), causes the frequency of homozygous affected children to become virtually zero. However, the corresponding carrier frequency is increasing, and the homozygous "normal" individuals are decreasing

in number. This population is not in equilibrium, and the use of the Hardy-Weinberg equation would be misleading. Nonetheless, in most instances it gives a reasonable approximation. A sample of autosomal recessive conditions is listed in Table 4–2.

Sex-Linked Inheritance

A sex-linked condition occurs when the gene locus is on the X chromosome. There are many more sex-linked recessive conditions than sex-linked dominant conditions, and for this reason males are subject to a much larger number of inherited disorders than are

TABLE 4–3
X-Linked Recessive Diseases

Disease	Frequency	Comments
Fragile X syndrome (FRA, XA, and numerous other names)	1:4000 males	The gene is located at Xq27.3. The condition is attributable to a CGG triplet expansion that is associated with localized methylation (inactivation) of distal genes. Females may have some expression. Instability of the site may lead to tissue mosaicism; therefore, lymphocyte genotype and phenotype may not correlate.
Duchenne muscular dystrophy (DMD, pseudohypertrophic progressive MD, dystrophin, Becker variants)	1:4000 males	The gene is located at Xp21. The gene is relatively large, with 79 exons, and mutations, deletions, etc. may occur anywhere. The gene product is called dystrophin. Dystrophin is absent in DMD but abnormal in Becker MD.
Hemophilia A (factor VIII deficiency, classic hemophilia)	1:5000–1:10,000 males	The gene is located at Xq28. Factor VIII is essential for normal blood clotting. Phenotype depends upon genotype and the presence of any residual factor VIII activity.
Rett syndrome (RTT, RTS autism, dementia, ataxia, and loss of purposeful hand use); gene MECP2 (methyl-CpG-binding protein 2)	1:10,000–1:15,000 girls	The gene is located at locus Xq28. These diseases are a subset of autism. There is a loss of regulation (repression) for other genes, including those in *trans* positions. The disease is lethal in males. Cases represent new mutations or parental gonadal mosaicism.
Color blindness (partial deutan series, green color blindness [75%]; partial protan series, red color blindness [25%])	1:12 males	The gene is located at Xq28 (proximal) for deutan color blindness and at Xq28 (distal) for protan color blindness.
Adrenoleukodystrophy (ALD, XL-ALD, Addison disease, and cerebral sclerosis)	Uncommon	The gene is located at Xq28. The disease involves a defect in peroxisome function relating to *very long chain fatty acid CoA synthetase* with accumulation of C-26 fatty acids. Phenotype is very variable, from rapid childhood progression to later onset and slow progression.
Glucose 6-phosphate dehydrogenase deficiency (G-6-PD)	1:10 African-Americans 1:5 Kurdish Jews A heteromorphism in these and other populations	The gene is located at Xq28. There are numerous variants in which oxidants cause hemolysis. Variants can confer partial resistance to severe malaria.

females (Table 4–3). Hemophilia A, a sex-linked recessive condition, exemplifies this mode of inheritance. The gene for clotting factor VIII is located on the distal q arm of the X chromosome. An absence of normal factor VIII leads to "classic" hemophilia. When the maternal parent is a carrier for hemophilia (factor VIII deficiency), 50% of the male offspring will have hemophilia, and 50% of the female offspring will be carriers, just as their mothers are.

An inspection of the segregation of the sex chromosomes also leads to other important conclusions. The daughters of a man with a sex-linked recessive condition such as hemophilia will all be *obligate carriers* for the condition. Because a man cannot usually pass a sex-linked condition to his sons, male-to-male transmission establishes an autosomal pattern of inheritance.

Males with hemophilia can be identified by an absence of factor VIII, but female carriers are extremely difficult to identify on the basis of factor VIII levels. Direct molecular analysis of the gene is possible using molecular techniques, but this is difficult. The hemophilia gene is relatively quite large; it includes 25 intervening sequences (introns) and 27,000 bases that code for mRNA. The potential exists for a great number of deletions and mutations in many areas of the single gene, all leading to the same disease. Knowledge of the specific deletion in the affected male family member facilitates detection of carriers.

Normally in females, one X chromosome is inactivated, a phenomenon called the *Lyon rule* (*Lyon hypothesis*). According to the Lyon rule, early in embryogenesis one of the two X chromosomes in each cell of a female embryo is randomly inactivated, leaving just one in the active state. All of the subsequent cells developing from this active ancestor have the same active X chromosome. For most of the genes on the X chromosome, females display a phenomenon called *mosaicism*, in which some cells have one X active and other cells have the alternative X active. Therefore, unless a test is available for the presence of the particular gene itself, tests for sex-linked gene products are difficult to interpret. In many cells the inactive X chromosome often can be seen as the Barr body (a clump of heterochromatin) adjacent to the nuclear membrane. There is ordinarily one Barr body for every X chromosome exceeding the active X (e.g., normal females who are 46,XX have one Barr body; a female who is 47,XXX would have two Barr bodies).

A Sex-Linked Condition with a Cytogenic Marker

A number of sex-linked conditions lead to mental retardation, and for many years it was observed that many more males had mental retardation than did females. A chromosome marker called the *fragile X*, so named for a breakage gap that can be induced on the distal q arm of the X chromosome, is present in many of these males. The condition is characterized by the following:
1. The fragile X marker (enhanced by special treatment of the cells in tissue culture)
2. Macroorchidism in the postpubertal male
3. Disproportionately severe delays in expressive language development
4. Mild to moderate mental retardation
5. In general, a normal appearance, except occasionally for some superficial findings such as prominent ears

Fragile X is another example of *anticipation*, with mutable expansion of a CGG trinucleotide repeat. This amplification occurs only during maternal meiosis, which explains why transmission is through carrier mothers and not through unaffected "carrier" fathers. Amplification of CGG trinucleotide repeats creates the heritable, unstable element of the X chromosome. Testing should be accomplished by molecular analysis rather than by cytogenetic methods.

GENES AND LINKAGE

Adjacent genes on the same chromosome are likely to be inherited together unless another genetic event separates the genes from each other. In *recombination*, a genetic event that takes place in meiosis, segments of DNA are exchanged (crossing over) in a reciprocal fashion between homologous chromosomes. The chance of this happening generally is proportional to the distance between the loci. The unit used to describe the distance between loci is the centimorgan (cM). A cM does not represent a specific physical distance; rather, it reflects the chance that recombination will occur between two linked genes. If two loci are separated by 10 cM, recombination between the loci will occur about 10% of the time.

In a clinical situation it is possible to use the concept of linkage to determine genetic composition in a particular individual. If two genes are known to be linked in a particular family and one of the genes is detectable by its normal effect but the other, mutated gene is undetectable, it might be assumed that the individual exhibiting the effect of the linked normal gene has the deleterious one also. The degree of certainty of this assumption depends on the chance that recombination has not occurred between the gene loci.

By applying appropriate methodology using restrictive endonucleases to digest DNA, we may presume a mutated gene to be present based on determination of the presence of a known closely linked DNA RFLP. The degree of certainty still is based on the chance of recombination occurring between the polymorphism and the mutated gene. The use of several closely linked polymorphic DNA fragments, especially those that flank the gene in question, can increase the certainty that recombination has not occurred and that the mutated gene is present. When the actual abnormal DNA sequence responsible for the mutated allele is known and can be tested for directly, there is no uncertainty.

Contiguous gene syndromes occur when multiple neighboring or contiguous genes on a chromosome are deleted, often producing a cytogenetic alteration of chromosomal banding. DiGeorge (velocardiofacial) syndrome is an example of this, manifesting as abnormalities of the heart, thymus, parathyroid glands, and face.

Pedigree Analysis

Constructing a family pedigree is a quick way of surveying family history. The pedigree also helps to

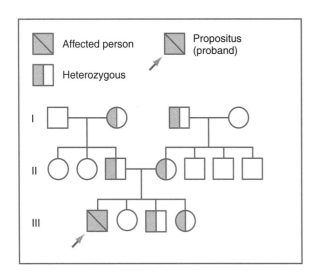

FIG. 4–2

A pedigree showing an autosomal recessive pattern of inheritance.

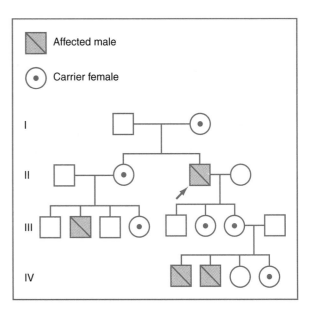

FIG. 4–3

A pedigree showing a sex-linked (X-linked) recessive condition.

analyze the family visually for a specific pattern of inheritance. The conventional symbols used in pedigree construction are shown in Fig. 4–2. *Autosomal dominant conditions* would occur in each generation and would not be passed on by individuals who do not manifest the condition (Table 4–1). (An obvious exception would be an individual in whom there is no detectable expression of the gene, even though the gene is present.) Affected males should approximately equal affected females. An example of this is a pedigree of three generations affected with neurofibromatosis. Each child has a 50% chance of receiving the gene (i.e., one in two will be affected), and male-to-male transmission is present, which excludes a sex-linked condition.

If a child is affected with a condition that is known to follow a dominant mode of inheritance but no family history can be constructed, several possibilities must be considered: the child represents a new mutation; a parent is affected, but the expression cannot be detected or the parental mutation is limited to the germ cells; the condition is genetically heterogeneic and in this family follows another pattern of inheritance, such as an autosomal recessive pattern; this condition is a *phenocopy* with another cause entirely; or an identified parent is not the biologic parent.

Autosomal recessive conditions typically appear without an antecedent family history. Occasionally, the parents will be consanguineous (i.e., they have relatively close ancestors in common). Related persons have a greater chance of sharing the same hidden recessive genes than do unrelated persons. If a

child is found to have a known autosomal recessive condition, the parents are carriers and the risk of recurrence for each subsequent child is 25%. Fig. 4–2 shows a pedigree for autosomal recessive conditions (Table 4–2).

An occasional exception to the biparental carrier state in instances of autosomal recessive conditions has been discovered. This exception, called *uniparental disomy*, must be considered as a possible mechanism in explaining the occurrence of recessive conditions. In uniparental disomy two chromosomes of a pair are derived from one parent. If the two chromosomes in the pair are not just homologs but replicates of each other (a condition called *uniparental isodisomy*, which would happen if the chromosomes failed to separate at metaphase II of meiosis), virtually all genes on the chromosomes are identical (homozygous). If a mutation is present, a recessive disease will occur. If the nondisjunction (failure of the chromosomes to separate) occurs in metaphase I of meiosis, the two chromosomes are uniparental but not identical. Uniparental disomy can also result from a trisomy cell that loses one chromosome from the trisomy set in early embryogenesis. This event is called *trisomy rescue*, which is discussed under Chromosomal Imprinting later in this chapter.

Sex-linked recessive conditions (Table 4–3) are far more common than sex-linked dominant conditions. Males most often are affected, and transmission is through the mother, who often has affected male relatives (brothers or maternal uncles). Fig. 4–3 shows a typical pedigree.

Gonadal mosaicism can result in the unexpected recurrence of autosomal dominant conditions and sex-linked conditions when there is no phenotypic evidence or somatic cell molecular evidence for the condition. Any condition that stems from a new mutation may represent gonadal mosaicism.

MULTIFACTORIAL INHERITANCE: CONDITIONS WITH AN EMPIRIC RISK

For genetic disease inherited by autosomal recessive and by dominant or sex-linkage patterns, the recurrence or inheritance risks are based on classic mendelian genetic laws. However, no definitive genetic explanation exists for the inheritance of multifactorial genetic conditions. Many conditions that occur in children or adults seem also to confer an increased risk of occurrence in siblings, close relatives, and subsequent generations in the family. It is postulated that in this type of genetic disorder a gene or a spectrum of genes confers a vulnerability for the condition in the individual and that some precipitating environmental factors interact to bring the condition about. By evaluating the reproductive outcomes of many families with similar conditions, one can calculate a pooled empiric recurrence risk. For most multifactorial disorders, the recurrence rate is 4–10%. Some disorders involve a predisposition by sex (e.g., pyloric stenosis in males and congenital dislocated hips in females), whereas others involve a predisposition by racial background (e.g., neural tube defects in whites or facial clefts in people of Asian ancestry).

The *inheritance of birth defects* often is multifactorial. The causation of complex birth defects likely is heterogeneous, and the defect may represent a final common pathway with many different causes. Congenital heart anomalies, neural tube defects, and cleft lip and cleft palate have empiric recurrence risks that exceed the general population risk, but the empiric recurrence risk is never as high as the recurrence risk for a classic, specific gene disorder. Congenital heart anomalies affect about 5–10 infants per 1000 live births (0.5–1.0%); the empiric recurrence is probably 5–10%. Neural tube defects, such as anencephaly and meningomyelocele, may affect as few as 1 infant per 1000 live births. There are significant differences in the prevalence of neural tube defects from area to area in the United States and from country to country; the incidence is higher in the United Kingdom and the Republic of Ireland than in the United States. The recurrence risk for neural tube defects is 1–5%; however, the recurrence risk can be lowered by maternal folic acid supplementation in the preconception and early gestation periods.

In evaluations of multifactorial genetic conditions, studies of twins may differentiate genetic from environmental factors. If twins have a disorder in common, they are said to be in *concordance* for their disorder; if they differ, they are described as *discordant* for the finding. With multifactorial genetic disorders, there is never 100% concordance, even in monozygotic twins (twins resulting from cleavage of a single egg). For example, concordance for all types of facial clefts is only about 33% in monozygotic twins and about 7% in dizygotic twins. Thus other factors contribute to producing facial clefts.

Some multifactorial genetic diseases are associated with HLA types. Diabetes mellitus is associated with histocompatibility markers DR3 and DR4, whereas ankylosing spondylitis and postvenereal or enteric spondyloarthropathy are associated with HLA B27. Enteric spondyloarthropathy illustrates an interaction of environmental variables with a genetic predisposition to produce specific diseases.

MITOCHONDRIAL INHERITANCE

Mitochondrial inheritance is another exception to mendelian or nuclear chromosomal inheritance. The mitochondrial genome is not totally autonomous, but must function in concert with nuclear genes to ensure normal mitochondrial function. The majority of mitochondrial proteins are determined by nuclear genes, but there are 37 genes on the circular mitochondrial chromosome (mtDNA). The mtDNA genes encode for 13 polypeptides that form parts of the mitochondrial respiratory complexes, 22 mitochondria-specific transfer RNAs, and two mitochondrial ribosomal RNAs. Mutations, deletions, and other changes in the mtDNA can result in disease. Mitochondria are maternal in origin, with no identified paternal influence. The mature ovum contains about 100,000 mitochondria, which are not necessarily all identical (this condition is called *heteroplasmy*). The replication of mitochondria is controlled by nuclear genes and does not start until later embryogenesis, at about the 1000-cell stage. The mitochondria are distributed randomly among the embryonic cells, and abnormal mitochondria may by chance have low or high prevalence in different cells. The phenotypic consequences depend on the location, function, and proportion of abnormal mitochondria in a tissue or organ. For example, heteromorphisms in the mtDNA gene for mt ribosomal RNA are associated with most cases of aminoglycoside-induced deafness. Specific mtDNA point mutations, deletions, and other changes may be associated with consistent patterns of adverse consequences, but all changes have the capacity to adversely affect separate organ systems (e.g., organs of special senses, the central and peripheral nervous system, muscle function, the heart, endocrine organs, hematologic function, and general metabolism). Point mutations in the mtDNA-tRNA-leucine gene lead to the *MELAS* syndrome, which includes *m*itochrondrial myopathy, *e*ncephalopathy, *l*actic *a*cidosis, and *s*troke-like episodes. The age of onset is variable, and the condition is often associated with episodic vomiting and headache. A muscle biopsy may reveal ragged red fibers. Mutations in the mtDNA-tRNA lysine gene result in the *MERRF* syndrome, which has the phenotype of *m*yoclonic *e*pilepsy and *r*agged *r*ed *f*ibers observable with muscle biopsy. The age of onset is variable, and the condition may be associated with ataxia and a segmental or progressive myopathy. Mutations in subunit 6 of ATP synthetase coded in mtDNA lead to the *NARP* syndrome (*n*europathy, *a*taxia, and *r*etinitis *p*igmentosa). Deletions and duplications of the mtDNA are associated with different, but unpredictable, phenotypes, including Kearns-Sayre syndrome (KSS) (ophthalmoplegia, pigmentary degeneration of the retina, and cardiomyopathy) and the Pearson syndrome (sideroblastic anemia, exocrine pancreatic malfunction, and various components of KSS).

CYTOGENETICS

Cytogenetics, the study of chromosome number and morphology, is an important part of the study of human inheritance. It is possible to analyze the chromosomes of any cell capable of division.

In a clinical setting, most cytogenetic analyses are performed using a mitosis-stimulating agent to cause division of peripheral blood lymphocytes placed in a tissue-culture medium. Fibroblasts, bone marrow cells, amniocytes, and chorionic villi also can be used. Mitotic cells undergoing division are arrested in metaphase and ruptured, and the chromosomes spread out. Each pair of chromosomes has its own pattern of substructure that is expressed as a sequence of light and dark bands when the chromosomes are stained appropriately. The banding relates to the distribution of repetitive spacer DNA, nonrepetitive genomic DNA, and a complex of DNA in association with acidic proteins and histones. These methods of analysis permit the identification of each pair of chromosomes and allow the chromosomes to be studied in detail; more than 1000 bands in a haploid set of chromosomes can be detected for the diagnosis of deletions and duplications of parts of chromosomes. Banding techniques vary; Q banding is detected with quinacrine, G banding with a Giemsa stain, and C banding with staining of the centromere region.

A powerful cytogenetic tool involves in situ chromosome hybridization with a fluorescent-tagged probe specific for a distinct locus on a chromosome. Deletions, translocations, and other small chromo-

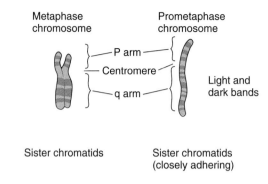

FIG. 4–4

Chromosome morphology.

somal changes can be detected with this method even when conventional banding cannot detect any change. Probes for entire chromosomes are available, which makes it possible to karyotype an entire metaphase based on color analysis, without banding. These techniques are called fluorescent in situ hybridization (FISH), chromosome painting, and spectral analysis.

An understanding of cytogenetics and chromosomal abnormalities requires a special vocabulary and technology (Fig. 4–4).

CHROMOSOMAL ABNORMALITIES

Chromosomal abnormalities may arise de novo during gametogenesis, so that an individual can be conceived with a chromosomal abnormality even though there is no family history of the condition. Chromosomal abnormalities and chromosomal rearrangements also can be present in a parent and passed to an offspring. Sometimes this is associated with a family history of multiple spontaneous abortions or a higher-than-chance frequency of giving birth to children with chromosomal abnormalities. Chromosomal abnormalities or rearrangements also can occur in somatic cells at any time. If they arise early in embryogenesis, they can give rise to a clone, which may have adverse consequences for the mosaic individual. Chromosomal alterations that occur later in life also may have adverse consequences on health; a high percentage of malignant neoplasms are associated with chromosomal abnormalities when the constitutional karyotype of the individual is normal.

Chromosomal abnormalities present at conception often lead to spontaneous abortion; about 50% of first-trimester spontaneous abortions involve chromosomally abnormal fetuses. Even the chromosomal abnormalities that are observed at term, such as trisomy 21 and Turner syndrome (45,X), represent only a fraction of the individuals conceived with these chromosomal problems. In general, abnormalities involving somatic chromosomes have a greater negative effect on the individual than do abnormalities of sex chromosomes.

Indications for obtaining chromosome studies include confirmation of a suspected chromosomal syndrome, multiple organ system malformations, significant developmental delays or mental retardation not otherwise explained, short stature or very delayed menarche in girls, infertility or a history of several spontaneous abortions, ambiguous genitalia, and advanced maternal age (the fetus should be tested). The only way to establish that an individual has a normal karyotype is to perform a chromosome analysis. Higher-resolution banding studies have revealed subtle chromosomal alterations in a number of conditions.

FISH techniques have shown that there are a number of conditions, previously thought to be multifactorial and sporadic, that are caused by chromosomal deletions. Williams syndrome (deletion 7q11.23) and DiGeorge (velocardiofacial) syndrome (deletion 22q11.1–13) are examples of this.

Trisomy 21 (Down Syndrome)

Trisomy 21 is the most common autosomal chromosomal abnormality in humans. A detailed review of this condition serves as a helpful model for understanding other chromosomal abnormalities.

Epidemiology. Trisomy 21 occurs in all areas of the world and among all racial groups. The prevalence is 1 in 700 live births. The incidence of this and other chromosomal aneuploidy increases with increasing maternal age; the incidence is 1:2000 at 20 years and 2–5% after 40 years of age. In many conceptuses, trisomy 21 results in spontaneous abortion. At 20 weeks of gestation, a fetus with trisomy 21 has few phenotypic findings to suggest the diagnosis; at term, however, most affected infants have clinical manifestations suggesting the diagnosis.

Cytogenetics. About 92% of children with Down syndrome have trisomy with an extra 21 chromosome present in all body cells, for a total chromosome count of 47. Chromosomal nondisjunction during *maternal meiosis* is responsible for 80–90% of cases of trisomy 21. About 5% of children have a translocation involving the 21 chromosome; the extra chromosome is attached to another chromosome, most often another acrocentric chromosome (chromosome numbers 13, 14, 15, 21, or 22), and the total chromosome count is 46. The majority of cases of trisomy resulting from translocation represent a new event. However, when a child is found to have trisomy because of a translocation, parental karyotype analysis should be undertaken; it reveals a parent with a balanced translocation 20–40% of the time. If a parent has a balanced translocation, the other immediate family members should be studied to determine who may be at risk for having affected children. About 3% of the time, mosaicism occurs; some cells display trisomy 21, but others have a normal karyotype.

Clinical Manifestations. Infants born with trisomy 21 are the survivors of embryogenesis and fetal development. There is no clinical difference between children with translocation trisomy and those with simple trisomy. In children with mosaicism, the clinical consequences of trisomy depend on the location and percentage of chromosomally normal cells. In many instances of mosaicism, the normal cells represent a minor clone that does not significantly alter the clinical manifestations. Cytogenetic analysis cannot predict the extent of organ malformation.

Children with trisomy 21 have an almost 40% chance of congenital heart disease. Virtually all children with Down syndrome are smaller than their siblings and smaller than peer-age children. The intelligence is adversely affected, but the range of abilities is wide and approximates a bell-shaped curve shifted below the normal mean. Craniofacial manifestations include a small midface with upturned nose, epicanthal folds, brachycephaly, a flat occiput, a speckled iris (Brushfield spots), and palpebral fissures that slant down to the midline. Because of the small mandible and maxillae, the tongue may be prominent and the palate high and narrow. Eighty percent of infants with trisomy 21 are hypotonic at birth, but this feature often disappears with time. Additional neonatal features include a poor Moro reflex (in 85% of affected children), joint hyperflexibility (80%), excess skin at the back of the neck (80%), and flat facies. Table 4–4 lists some of the clinical findings that may be present in trisomy 21.

Other Autosomal Trisomies

Down syndrome accounts for the majority of chromosomal aneuploidy at birth. Trisomy 13 (affecting 1:5000 children) and trisomy 18 (1:8000) are other trisomies that can be differentiated by their spectra of clinical findings (Table 4–5). These trisomies carry a higher risk of spontaneous death in utero than does Down syndrome. Most children with these trisomies die in infancy; very few survive more than 1 year. Definitive diagnosis is obtained through chromosome analysis.

TABLE 4–4
Clinical Findings That May Be Present with Trisomy 21*

Stature smaller than peer age group

Developmental delays

Congenital heart disease (e.g., endocardial cushion defect and ventricular septal defect)

Structural abnormalities of the bowel (e.g., tracheoesophageal atresia, duodenal atresia, annular pancreas, duodenal web, and Hirschsprung disease)

Central hypotonia

Brachycephaly

Delayed closure of fontanels

Small midface, hypoplastic frontal sinuses, myopia, and small (short) ears

Lax joints, including laxity of the atlantoaxial articulation (the latter predisposing the patient to C1- C2 dislocation)

Short, broad hands, feet, and digits; single palmar crease, clinodactyly

Exaggerated space between 1st and 2nd toe

Velvety, loosely adhering mottled skin (cutis marmorata) in infancy; coarse, dry skin in adolescence

Statistically increased risk for leukemia, Alzheimer disease, hypothyroidism

*An individual may exhibit any combination of these findings. There is no correlation between the number of physical findings and eventual level of mental performance. The increased risk for leukemia is significant but probably no greater than 1% for any individual. Alzheimer disease is relatively common in persons with trisomy 21 who die in middle adult life, but the frequency in all adults with Down syndrome is not known.

TABLE 4–5
Findings That May Be Present in Trisomy 13 and Trisomy 18

	Trisomy 13	Trisomy 18
Head and face	Scalp defects (e.g., cutis aplasia)	Small and premature appearance
	Microphthalmia, corneal abnormalities	Tight palpebral fissures
	Cleft lip and palate in 60–80% of cases	Narrow nose and hypoplastic nasal alae
	Microcephaly	Narrow bifrontal diameter
	Sloping forehead	Prominent occiput
	Holoprosencephaly (arhinencephaly)	Micrognathia
	Capillary hemangiomas	Cleft lip or palate
	Deafness	
Chest	Congenital heart disease (e.g., VSD, PDA, and ASD) in 80% of cases	Congenital heart disease (e.g., VSD, PDA, and ASD)
	Thin posterior ribs (missing ribs)	Short sternum, small nipples
Extremities	Overlapping of fingers and toes (clinodactyly)	Limited hip abduction
	Polydactyly	Clinodactyly and overlapping fingers; index over 3rd, 5th over 4th
	Hypoplastic nails, hyperconvex nails	Rocker-bottom feet
		Hypoplastic nails
General	Severe developmental delays and prenatal and postnatal growth retardation	Severe developmental delays and prenatal and postnatal growth retardation
	Renal abnormalities	Premature birth, polyhydramnios
	Nuclear projections in neutrophils	Inguinal or abdominal hernias
	Only 5% live longer than 6 mo	Only 5% live longer than 1 year

ASD, Atrial septal defect; *PDA*, patent ductus arteriosus; *VSD*, ventricular septal defect.

RECURRENCE RISK FOR AUTOSOMAL CHROMOSOMAL ABNORMALITIES

If a mother is younger than 35 years of age, the recurrence risk for de novo chromosome abnormalities is about 1%. For couples in which the mother is older than 35 years, the recurrence risk seems to approximate the empiric age risk.

CHROMOSOMAL IMPRINTING

The sex of the parent contributing a specific chromosome may affect the expression of some of the genes on the chromosome. *Imprinting* is a strong parental (chromosomal) influence on the expression of a particular gene. A small deletion of the q arm adjacent to the centromere of a number 15 chromosome (15 q11–q13) appears to give rise to *Prader-Willi syndrome* (PWS) if the deletion is in the paternal 15 chromosome. A normal gene on the paternal chromosome 15 prevents the syndrome, but two maternal chromosomes 15 (maternal uniparental disomy) produce PWS. Seventy percent of affected children demonstrate a cytogenetically visible deletion. PWS is characterized by transient neonatal hypotonia, hyperphagic obesity (with an onset at 6 months–6 years), almond-shaped palpebral fissures, small hands and feet, and mild to moderate mental retardation. The incidence is 1:15,000. An entirely different condition, *Angelman syndrome*, seems to result if the deletion is in the maternal 15 chromosome.

SEX CHROMOSOME ABNORMALITIES

The clinical consequences of sex chromosome abnormalities in term infants are much less severe than those associated with autosomal chromosomal abnormalities. However, Turner syndrome has a dramatic association with fetal death. Its frequency is about 1 affected individual per 10,000 female live term births; the condition may be present in almost 1% of female fetuses.

Turner Syndrome

Turner syndrome is associated with functional monosomy of the p arm of the X chromosome. The most common karyotype in Turner syndrome is 45,X with the second sex chromosome missing, but many affected females are mosaics. The most common mosaic is 45,X/46,XX, but 45,X/47,XXX and 45,X/46,XY are also observed. Some females with Turner syndrome do have two X chromosomes, but in these instances one X has a missing p arm. The risk of Turner syndrome does not increase with advancing maternal age. These findings suggest an abnormality of embryonic cell division, rather than fertilization by an abnormal gamete, as the cause of Turner syndrome.

In utero mortality in Turner syndrome often is associated with severe edema and cystic hygroma. If swallowing is obstructed, polyhydramnios results. In many instances of severe fetal edema, pulmonary effusions impair lung development. However, liveborn infants have an excellent prognosis. The gonads are present at birth and are appropriately infantile; they often regress during childhood, and they may be absent at puberty.

The main *clinical manifestations* of Turner syndrome are short stature (adult height less than 150 cm in the untreated woman), sexual infantilism, and the consequences of congenital anomalies. Women and girls with Turner syndrome have an increased incidence of bicuspid aortic valve and of coarctation of the aorta. Furthermore, even in the absence of coarctation the frequency of hypertension is higher later in life. In neonates there also may be carpal or pedal edema; this spontaneously resolves but may recur in adolescence when estrogen treatment is initiated. Additional features include a low hairline, a webbed neck, widely spaced hypoplastic nipples, a horseshoe kidney, and cubitus valgus of the elbow. Some children have problems with spatial relationships and geometric visual problem solving. As a consequence of having only one functional X chromosome, females with Turner syndrome exhibit the same frequency of sex-linked conditions as do males with such conditions as hemophilia A or B.

Treatment of short stature has been successful using parenterally administered human growth hormone and orally given anabolic steroids. Secondary sexual characteristics can be developed with estrogen or a combination of estrogen and progesterone (or their synthetic substitutes). A few girls will produce estrogen on their own; most produce no estrogen and have elevated gonadotropins, which reflects ovarian failure. Girls who are mosaic for cells containing a Y chromosome should have their gonads removed in adolescence to eliminate the risk of later gonadal neoplasm. A few women have become pregnant and have carried to term (presumably they had functioning ovaries). Several women with Turner syndrome have had in vitro fertilization with donor eggs and have carried to term.

Klinefelter Syndrome

Klinefelter syndrome occurs at a frequency of about 1:1000 live infant boys, and the frequency at birth appears to increase with advancing maternal age. The typical karyotype is 47,XXY, but Klinefelter syndrome has occurred with multiple X chromosomes and one (or more) Y chromosomes. The condition is not identified in infants and prepubertal boys because recognizable clinical features are absent. In the postpubertal male, infertility results from hypogonadism, with hypospermia or aspermia. Gonadotropin levels usually are elevated unless normal levels of testosterone are produced. Additional clinical manifestations may include mild mental retardation, long limbs, small penis, small and soft testes, and gynecomastia. Testosterone treatment may be indicated at adolescence.

Other Sex Chromosomal Abnormalities

Nature is extremely tolerant of variation in the sex chromosome composition. At least one normal X chromosome is essential for viability, but monosomy of the X chromosome, as in Turner syndrome, is compatible with normal but infertile life. Klinefelter syndrome and all its cytogenetic variants (47,XXY; 48,XXXY; 49,XXXXY; 48,XXYY; and others) are compatible with life, are not associated with elevated fetal loss, and are associated with sterility. Klinefelter syndrome has been associated with personality disorders. Two other relatively frequent sex chromosomal abnormalities occur in humans: the karyotype 47,XXX (the triple-X female) and the karyotype 47,XYY (the double-Y male). Each abnormality occurs with a frequency of about 0.1% and does not lead to sterility or unique phenotypes. Because these karyotypes increase in frequency with maternal age, they are apt to be detected during prenatal diagnosis. The XYY male occasionally has been associated with antisocial behavior.

GENETIC COUNSELING

Inherited conditions and chromosomal abnormalities can create long-term and expensive health problems (e.g., mental retardation, major correctable or noncorrectable congenital anomalies, and multispecialized comprehensive care hospitalization) for the family. Success in the prevention of environmentally caused illness, especially infectious diseases, has led to an increased focus on genetic diseases and birth defects as causes of infant mortality and childhood morbidity. Only some birth defects are inherited, but the scope of clinical genetics includes all conditions with a familial recurrence risk that is higher than normal. Genetic evaluation should be followed by genetic counseling to estimate the recurrence risk for the family and relatives. Treatment for a genetic condition can often be started before a definitive diagnosis is made, but appropriate genetic counseling requires a correct diagnosis.

Genetic counseling is a process of family education about inherited conditions or conditions that may affect future children. Counseling is initiated as soon as a person begins to be evaluated, and it continues for as long as the physician is in contact with the family. The responsibility to communicate also may extend into the indefinite future if a new treatment is found or if new methods for screening or prenatal diagnosis become available. Birth defects, whether genetic or not, and genetic conditions have the potential for significant emotional impact on the family, often because of the potential for parental feelings of guilt. Because these disorders frequently occur without a family history, the family may not understand the nature of the condition and may develop maladaptive coping mechanisms, which will adversely affect the long-term outcome for the child. Genetic counseling can help the family understand the condition, cope with hidden fears and superstitions, and proceed with the process of dealing constructively with the problem. Genetic counseling should include a discussion in understandable terms of the nature of the condition and the mode of inheritance; if the condition is not inherited, this should be explicitly stated. The estimated recurrence risk, the possibilities for prenatal diagnosis, the prognosis, and the treatment alternatives also should be discussed in the counseling.

Recurrence Risk

Conditions inherited in mendelian fashion have a precise recurrence risk that can be described and explained. An empiric risk for recurrence, if present, also should be explained to families. Couples should understand that having no elevated recurrence risk is not the same as having no risk.

Prenatal Diagnosis

A significant number of inherited disorders and virtually all chromosomal abnormalities can be diagnosed prenatally. With the use of fetal ultrasonography, many dysmorphologic conditions with an empiric recurrence risk also can be diagnosed before birth.

Prognosis

Predictions for the outcome of a disease or for the long-term development of a child are approximations at best. Specific predictions often are inappropriate, but the range and variation of a disease or condition can be described.

Treatment Alternatives

Some treatments are dramatic and potentially lifesaving, such as the surgical correction of duodenal atresia. However, other treatments are less dramatic, such as the recommendation for the avoidance of cigarette smoking in an individual with alpha$_1$-antitrypsin deficiency or the dietary and medical management of a person with elevated cholesterol levels and an abnormal pattern of triglycerides and lipoproteins.

EVALUATION OF THE PATIENT: PROBLEMS OF HUMAN SIMILARITIES AND VARIATIONS

Evaluating an individual whose condition potentially is genetic is a challenging diagnostic problem. The pediatrician needs to consider a number of questions, such as the following:

- Is this a "known" inherited condition?
- Is it a chromosomal disorder?
- Is it a "known" syndrome (a combination of nonrandom findings that seem to be associated in affected individuals)?
- Is the condition caused by a disruption of normal development?
- Is the condition one that can arise because of exposure to an environmental agent (e.g., viral, bacterial, chemical, or physical)?
- Is it a condition that may be inherited or that has an elevated recurrence risk, or is it one that is known to occur as a random event without elevated recurrence risk?

If the family history is positive for the condition, the evaluation may be easier than if there is no history; however, many genetic conditions arise without a positive family history. Recessive conditions typically occur in a family without a positive history because most carriers are unaware of their status. New mutation dominant conditions also arise de novo, and even sex-linked conditions can occur as new mutations. In addition, minimal expressivity or nonpenetrance in other family members can result in a genetic condition without an apparent history. Genetic conditions or chromosomal disorders occur regardless of the general health of the mother or father.

In the evaluation of an individual child, several general points about heredity should be kept in mind. Children resemble their parents and other family members, although each individual will have a unique personal appearance. It is therefore a good idea to observe the appearance of parents and siblings. There are also *group or racial similarities among individuals* that may need to be taken into account. Similarity of appearance in population groups may be explained at least partially by geographic and racial clustering of family members and ancestors. Groups originating from limited geographic areas must have had many ancestors in common. It is not surprising, therefore, that limited gene mixing is common among physically, socially, or religiously isolated populations (e.g., the Amish community or Ashkenazi Jews).

There often is appreciable *variability among families with the same genetic disease.* The early discovery that sickle cell hemoglobin resulted from a point mutation leading to a single amino acid substitution in the beta chain of hemoglobin in every case of sickle cell disease encouraged geneticists to attribute specific gene disorders to identical changes in a single gene. It is now known that human genes are quite complex and that changes in different parts of the same gene can result in significant variation in the expression of a disease. It is probable that individuals homozygous for a recessive gene condition are actually heterozygous for specific alleles but that both alleles are abnormal. Data extracted from studies of families with hemophilia A (factor VIII deficiency) indicate that most families have gene alterations specific only to that family. It is probable that inherited conditions will display many kinds of gene changes. Some changes will be quite specific and common to many families (as with the sickle cell point mutation), but differences in disease expression may depend on the modulating effects from other components of the genome (hereditary persistence of fetal hemoglobin attenuates sickle cell anemia). Other gene changes may be variable, because the gene is affected in different ways by a plethora of mutational mechanisms, duplications, deletions, and frame shifts. Mechanisms relating to expressivity always can be expected to alter the clinical condition.

Heterogeneity refers to the fact that a condition may have separate causes. The condition, disease, or phenotype may represent the final common pathway in an abnormal process. For example, if a patient is found to have a hemolytic anemia, there are numerous causes, some acquired and some inherited. Even if the cause of the hemolytic anemia is limited to an inherited hemoglobinopathy, numerous abnormalities of hemoglobin synthesis must still be considered. These abnormalities include thalassemia, hemoglobin SS, hemoglobin SC, and others. The concept of heterogeneity must be kept in mind in the practice of medicine and in the practice of genetics. In genetic heterogeneity, separate genetic mechanisms may produce the same phenotype.

Another important concept is *expressivity*, which refers to the extent to which an individual is phenotypically affected by a gene or genes. For example, in some patients sickle cell anemia has a mild clinical course, in part because of persistent production of fetal hemoglobin. *Penetrance* refers to the difference between the persons with a gene composition who exhibit the effects of the gene and those with the same gene composition who do not exhibit the effects. If a gene has a penetrance of 80%, 8 in 10 persons with the gene can be expected to exhibit some effects of the gene. This does not mean that a person with the gene will be 80% affected; a gene is either penetrant or not penetrant in an individual.

Pleiotropism means that one gene or pair of genes can have many effects on the individual. When the mechanism of action of the gene or genes is not known, it may be difficult to explain why a single gene pair can have so many different effects on the person. For example, if the molecular and cellular pathology of sickle cell disease were not known, the separate clinical manifestations of the condition would be difficult to explain on the basis of one homozygous gene pair because the effects seem so diverse. Persons with sickle cell disease would be described as having anemia, susceptibility to bacterial infections, renal disease, musculoskeletal pain, hand and foot swelling, and a predisposition to cerebrovascular accidents. When the molecular basis of the condition is understood, the multiple effects of the gene make more sense.

Evaluating an Infant with Unusual Physical Findings and Clinical Malformations (Dysmorphology)

The challenge in physical diagnosis of conditions in an infant or child with unusual findings is describing as clearly as possible, in nonjudgmental terms, what is observed in the patient. Human variation is extensive but occurs on a continuum, with significant overlaps between what is called normal and what is termed abnormal. The subset of genetics that deals with the study of structural defects that alter appearance is called *dysmorphology*.

During the evaluation of an infant with unusual physical findings, a careful history is important even if it proves to be negative. Measurements of height, weight, and head circumference are essential, as are careful observations, documented in detail, for syndrome identification. Judicious laboratory tests can identify metabolic acidosis, elevated levels of ammonia, and hypoglycemia quickly, and chromosome analysis may be helpful. Sonography, computed tomography (CT), and magnetic resonance imaging (MRI) can identify internal abnormalities.

Congenital malformations (anomalies) usually occur early in gestation during tissue embryogenesis (Table 4–6) and may result from a variety of causes (Table 4–7). Malformations may be isolated and affect one organ system (as in the case of spina bifida), or they may be multiple, affecting unrelated organs (as in the case of trisomy 21). A *malformation sequence* is caused by a single but localized abnormal tissue formation during development, which initiates a chain of subsequent defects. For example, the prechordal mesoderm gene defect in the holoprosencephaly sequence that is controlled by several different genes produces deficits of midfacial development resulting in varying degrees of forebrain, ocular (hypotelorism to cyclopia), and nasal malformations. The *DiGeorge sequence* is caused by a primary defect of the fourth branchial arch and derivatives of the third and fourth pharyngeal pouches and results in varying degrees of thymus and parathyroid gland

---

TABLE 4–6
Relative Timing and Developmental Pathology of Certain Malformations

Tissue	Malformation	Defect in	Causes Prior to	Comment
Central nervous system	Anencephaly	Closure of anterior neural tube	26 days	Subsequent degeneration of forebrain
	Meningomyelocele	Closure in a portion of the posterior neural tube	28 days	80% lumbosacral
Face	Cleft lip	Closure of lip	36 days	42% are associated with cleft palate
	Cleft maxillary palate	Fusion of maxillary palatal shelves	10 wk	
	Branchial sinus and/or cyst	Resolution of branchial cleft	8 wk	Preauricular and along the line anterior to sternocleidomastoid

TABLE 4–6
Relative Timing and Developmental Pathology of Certain Malformations—cont'd

Tissue	Malformation	Defect in	Causes Prior to	Comment
Gut	Esophageal atresia plus tracheoesophageal fistula	Lateral septation of foregut into trachea and foregut	30 days	
	Rectal atresia with fistula	Lateral septation of cloaca into rectum and urogenital sinus	6 wk	
	Duodenal atresia	Recanalization of duodenum	7–8 wk	
	Malrotation of gut	Rotation of intestinal loop so that cecum lies to the right	10 wk	Associated incomplete or aberrant mesenteric attachments
	Omphalocele	Return of midgut from yolk sac to abdomen	10 wk	
	Meckel diverticulum	Obliteration of vitelline duct	10 wk	May contain gastric or pancreatic tissue
	Diaphragmatic hernia	Closure of pleuroperitoneal canal	6 wk	
Genitourinary system	Exstrophy of bladder	Migration of infraumbilical mesenchyme	30 days	Associated müllerian and wolffian duct defects
	Bicornuate uterus	Fusion of lower portion of müllerian ducts	10 wk	
	Hypospadias	Fusion of urethral folds (labia minora)	12 wk	
	Cryptorchidism	Descent of testicle into scrotum	7–9 mo	
Heart	Transposition of great vessels	Directional development of bulbus cordis septum	34 days	
	Ventricular septal defect	Closure of ventricular septum	6 wk	
	Patent ductus arteriosus	Closure of ductus arteriosus	9–10 mo	
Limb	Aplasia of radius	Genesis of radial bone	38 days	Often accompanied by other defects of radial side of distal limb
	Severe syndactyly	Separation of digital rays	6 wk	
Complex	Cyclopia, holoprosencephaly	Prechordal mesoderm development	23 days	Secondary defects of midface and forebrain

Modified from Jones KL, editor: *Smith's recognizable patterns of human malformation*, ed 5, Philadelphia, 1997, WB Saunders.

TABLE 4–7
Causes of Congenital Malformations

Monogenic (7.5% of Serious Anomalies) X-linked hydrocephalus Achondroplasia Ectodermal dysplasia Apert disease Treacher Collins syndrome	**Environmental Agents (% Unknown)** Polychlorinated biphenyls Herbicides Mercury Alcohol
Chromosomal (6% of Serious Anomalies) Trisomies 21, 18, 13 XO, XXY Deletions 4p-, 5p-, 7q-, 13q-, 18p-, 18q-, 22q- Prader-Willi syndrome (50% have deletion of chromosome 15)	**Medications (% Unknown)** Thalidomide Diethylstilbestrol Phenytoin Warfarin Cytotoxic drugs Isotretinoin (vitamin A) D-penicillamine Valproic acid
Maternal Infection (2% of Serious Anomalies) Intrauterine infections (e.g., herpes simplex, CMV, varicella-zoster, rubella, and toxoplasmosis)	**Unknown Etiologies** *Polygenetic* Anencephaly/spina bifida Cleft lip/palate Pyloric stenosis
Maternal Illness (3.5% of Serious Anomalies) Diabetes mellitus Phenylketonuria Hyperthermia	Congenital heart disease *Sporadic Syndrome Complexes (Anomalads)* CHARGE syndrome VATER syndrome Pierre Robin syndrome Prune-belly syndrome
Uterine Environment (% Unknown) *Deformation* Uterine pressure, oligohydramnios: clubfoot, torticollis, congenital hip dislocation, pulmonary hypoplasia, 7th nerve palsy *Disruption* Amniotic bands, congenital amputations, gastroschisis, porencephaly, intestinal atresia *Twinning* Conjoined twins, intestinal atresia, porencephaly	**Nutritional** Low folic acid–neural tube defects

CMV, Cytomegalovirus; *HIV,* human immunodeficiency virus; *CHARGE, c*oloboma, *h*eart defects, *a*tresia choanae, *r*etarded growth, *g*enital anomalies, *e*ar anomalies (deafness); *VATER, v*ertebral defects, *a*nal atresia, *t*racheoesophageal fistula with *e*sophageal atresia, and *r*adial and renal anomalies.

hypoplasia, facial hypoplasia (micrognathia), and congenital heart disease (e.g., truncus arteriosus and interrupted aortic arch). Most patients with DiGeorge sequence have a partial monosomy of the proximal long arm of chromosome 22 or a microdeletion of 22q11.2. The recurrence rates for sequences are 1–5%.

A *malformation syndrome* is a nonsequential grouping of anomalies with multiple defects in more than one tissue. This type of syndrome is often the result of teratogens, chromosomal abnormalities, or genes operating in embryogenesis. A *malformation association* is a nonrandom grouping of abnormalities with a specific pattern of affected tissues. The *VATER* syndrome includes varying rates of tissue involvement with vertebral anomalies (70%), anal atresia (80%), tracheoesophageal fistula (70%), and radial bone (65%) and renal abnormalities (50%).

A *disruption sequence* often occurs later in gestation. An example is amniotic bands with distal extremity amputations or as constriction bands and

TABLE 4–8
A Glossary of Selected Terms Used in Dysmorphology

Terms Pertaining to the Face and Head

Brachycephaly: A condition in which head shape is shortened from front to back along the sagittal plane; the skull is rounder than normal

Canthus: The lateral or medial angle of the eye formed by the junction of the upper and lower lids

Columella: The fleshy tissue of the nose that separates the nostrils

Glabella: Bony midline prominence of the brows

Nasal alae: The lateral flaring of the nostrils

Nasolabial fold: Groove that extends from the margin of the nasal alae to the lateral aspects of the lips

Ocular hypertelorism: Increased distance between the pupils of the two eyes

Palpebral fissure: The shape of the eyes based on the outline of the eyelids

Philtrum: The vertical groove in the midline of the face between the nose and the upper lip

Plagiocephaly: A condition in which head shape is asymmetric in the sagittal or coronal planes; can result from asymmetry in suture closure or from asymmetry of brain growth

Scaphocephaly: A condition in which the head is elongated from front to back in the sagittal plane; most normal skulls are scaphocephalic

Terms Pertaining to the Face and Head—cont'd

Synophrys: Eyebrows that meet in the midline

Telecanthus: A wide space between the medial canthi

Terms Pertaining to the Extremities

Brachydactyly: A condition of having short digits

Camptodactyly: A condition in which a digit is bent or fixed in the direction of flexion (a "trigger finger"–type appearance)

Clinodactyly: A condition in which a digit is crooked and curves toward or away from adjacent digits

Hypoplastic nail: An unusually small nail on a digit

Melia: A suffix meaning "limb" (e.g., amelia—missing limb; brachymelia—short limb)

Polydactyly: The condition of having six or more digits on an extremity

Syndactyly: The condition of having two or more digits at least partially fused (can involve any degree of fusion, from webbing of skin to full bony fusion of adjacent digits)

---

pseudosyndactyly. Intrauterine infection or tissue infarction may also produce a disruption sequence.

A *dysplasia sequence* is caused by poor tissue organization or migration of precursor cells. Abnormal neural crest cell migration is one example and may result in the neurocutaneous melanosis sequence. Abnormal cell metabolism, such as in *Hurler syndrome,* may also result in dysplasia in multiple tissues (as exhibited by cloudy cornea, mitral regurgitation, stiff joints, mental retardation, and coarse facies).

A *deformation sequence* is secondary to abnormal mechanical forces that influence tissue growth, position, and shape, often after organogenesis is completed. Uterine compression caused by oligohydramnios secondary to renal agenesis produces the *Potter syndrome* (pulmonary hypoplasia, breech position, club feet, and flattened facies), whereas other causes of uterine constraint (e.g., bicornuate uterus, less severe degrees of oligohydramnios) may result in craniofacial (e.g., flat nose, crumpled ear, craniosynostosis, and craniotabes) and limb deformations (e.g., metatarsus adductus and congenital dislocated hip).

A variety of specific clinical terms are used to describe discrete features or structures; other, less clinical descriptions may also be used. For example, it may be said that the eyebrows meet in the midline or, alternatively, that *synophrys* is present. Table 4–8 lists a glossary of some additional terms used in clinical morphology. Syndromes are identified by the detailed description of unusual findings. If an infant's condition does not fit the description of any specific condition, the child can be observed over time for growth, development, and physical changes that eventually may define the condition. When the diagnosis is uncertain, photographs can help the physician discuss the child's condition with colleagues.

Throughout the physical examination, the taking of a family history, and each step of the evaluation, the physician should be compassionate, truthful, and respectful of patient, parents, and principles of the medical profession. Particularly, the physician should appreciate that diagnostic labels may produce untoward as well as beneficial effects on the family and, later, on the patient.

TABLE 4–9
Prenatal Diagnosis

DNA Analysis	Alpha$_1$-antitrypsin deficiency, thalassemia, sickle cell anemia, muscular dystrophy, hemophilia A, congenital adrenal hyperplasia, phenylketonuria, many others
Enzyme Assay	Tay-Sachs disease, galactosemia, Hunter syndrome, maple syrup urine disease, Wolman syndrome, Lesch-Nyhan syndrome, Gaucher disease, I-cell disease, Menkes disease
Chromosome Disorders	Trisomy 13, 18, 21; chromosome deletions; Turner syndrome; Klinefelter syndrome; fragile X
Alpha-Fetoprotein	
Elevated	Twins, neural tube defects, intestinal obstruction, congenital hepatitis, congenital nephrosis, impending fetal demise, omphalocele
Decreased	Trisomy 21 and possibly other chromosomal disorders
Chorionic Gonadotropin	
Elevated	Trisomy 21, triploidy
Decreased	Trisomy 13, trisomy 18
Unconjugated Estriol	
Decreased	Trisomy 21
Ultrasonography	Hydrops fetalis, hydronephrosis, neural tube defects, intestinal obstruction, congenital heart disease, diaphragmatic hernia, gastroschisis, omphalocele, limb reduction anomalies, assessment of growth
Cordocentesis	Fetal anemia, fetal acid-base and oxygenation disorders, fetal hypoalbuminemia, thrombocytopenia, thalassemia, cells for DNA
Fetal Skin Biopsy	Albinism, epidermolysis bullosa, xeroderma pigmentosum

PRENATAL DIAGNOSIS AND GENETICS

Prenatal diagnosis is a process for evaluating the health status of a fetus as early in gestation as possible. The process includes analysis of cells from the developing chorion frondosum, sampled at the 8th embryonic week (chorionic villus sampling [CVS]) maternal serum analysis for alpha-fetoprotein (MSAFP) or other substances of embryonic or fetal origin (e.g., chorionic gonadotropin and unconjugated estriol) after the 14th menstrual week; ultrasound examination of the fetus during gestation; and analysis of amniotic fluid and amniotic cells removed by amniocentesis or fetal blood removed by cordocentesis during the middle trimester of gestation (Table 4–9).

Genetic indications for prenatal diagnosis include parental age and the risk of a detectable genetic condition based on the history or a known carrier state (X-linked or autosomal recessive). Maternal serum triple screen testing (i.e., maternal alpha-fetoprotein [AFP], unconjugated estriols, and human chorionic gonadotropin [hCG]) is indicated for every pregnant woman. Chromosome analysis of amniotic fluid is virtually 100% accurate in detecting chromosomal abnormalities (Table 4–9). The combination of ultrasound, amniotic fluid AFP analysis, and amniotic fluid acetylcholinesterase measurement is capable of detecting 95–98% of all neural tube defects. Hemoglobinopathies and a number of other gene disorders can be detected by DNA analysis or gene product (hexosaminidase A) assay (Table 4-9). Many birth defects occur with no history in couples not at identifiable risk; therefore, it is unlikely that all major congenital malformations will be identified, even if all pregnant women receive antenatal ultrasonographic examinations.

ENVIRONMENTAL AGENTS CAPABLE OF PRODUCING BIRTH DEFECTS

Many environmental agents have been alleged to produce birth defects. It is best to consult the current literature and regional "hot lines" that are available for evaluating potential agents of embryonal and fetal injury. If an embryonic or fetal structure has formed before exposure to an agent, the agent cannot affect its formation. It is rare for an environmental agent to affect every exposed fetus, so most risks will be estimates of probable effects. Table 4–7 includes a list of some known environmental agents that present a risk to the developing fetus.

NEWBORN SCREENING

Newborn screening for PKU, which started in the mid-1960s, is now universal in the United States. Screening for other metabolic diseases has been added at the discretion of individual states. Testing for congenital hypothyroidism and hemoglobinopathies, especially those associated with sickling, is conducted in most states. General guidelines for newborn screening include a serious disease condition; a suitable test available, done preferably from a dried blood spot; few false positives; no false negatives; a treatment that can alter the outcome; and a system for following the infants detected in the screening.

REFERENCES

Behrman RE, Kliegman RM, Jenson HB, editors: *Nelson textbook of pediatrics*, ed 16, Philadelphia, 2000, WB Saunders, Chapters 75–80.
Friedman JM, Polifka JE: *Teratogenic effects of drugs: a resource for clinicians (TERIS)*, Baltimore, 1994, Johns Hopkins University Press.
Jones K: *Smith's recognizable patterns of human malformation*, ed 5, Philadelphia, 1997, WB Saunders.
McKusick VA: *Mendelian inheritance in man*, ed 12, Baltimore, 1998, Johns Hopkins University Press.
Rimoin DL, Connor JM, Pyeritz RE, editors: *Emery and Rimoin's principles and practice of medical genetics*, ed 3, New York, 1997, Churchill Livingstone.
Shepard TH: *Catalog of teratogenic agents*, ed 9, Baltimore, 1998, John Hopkins University Press.
Strachan T, Read AP: *Human molecular genetics*, ed 2, New York, 1999, Wiley-Liss.

CHAPTER 5

Inborn Errors of Metabolism

John F. Nicholson

Metabolic diseases are caused by a primary deficiency of an enzyme or transport protein or by lack of a stabilizing or activating factor necessary for enzyme action. Among the latter is faulty formation of biologic membranes. In general, failure of enzymatic function leads to the accumulation of a reactant, which may or may not have toxic effects (Table 5–1). The product of the blocked reaction, if not available otherwise, becomes deficient. Defects in transport can impair intestinal absorption of dietary constituents, renal tubular reabsorption of filtered compounds, and the disposition of compounds within the body and even within the cell. The other defects secondarily affect catalysis or transport (Table 5–2).

The molecular natures of the many defects are diverse, and inheritance, when evident, may be autosomal (dominant, recessive), X-linked, or mitochondrial. In some instances, therapeutic strategies can be developed to manage specific defects. For some disorders, the chemical problem is the failure of interaction between an enzyme and a cofactor, usually a vitamin, in which case provision of a large excess of the vitamin leads to chemical and clinical correction of the defect (e.g., cobalamin-responsive methylmalonic acidemia). Other strategies deal with basic pathogenetic mechanisms reducing the toxic reactant or providing the deficient product. In galactosemia, dietary elimination of galactose can be helpful. This can be done safely because galactose residues necessary for the formation of glycoproteins, polysaccharides, and complex lipids can be synthesized readily by humans. In contrast, treatment of phenylketonuria (PKU) requires reduction but not elimination of dietary phenylalanine because phenylalanine cannot be synthesized by humans. In biotinidase deficiency, which impairs the recycling of biotin, supplementation of the diet with biotin is curative. In some conditions (e.g., Gaucher

disease or alpha$_1$-antitrypsin deficiency) provision of the missing enzyme protein is beneficial.

GENERAL CONSIDERATIONS
Family History

Inherited metabolic disease frequently is discovered when the first affected child has distinct biochemical and clinical features or when the particular clinical disorder develops in the second child. Dominantly inherited diseases may be sporadic or evident in the family; X-linked disorders affect males, although some females may have mild symptoms, whereas mitochondrial gene mutations affect males and females but are passed through the mother. Consanguinity is common. When parents are closely related (e.g., first cousins), the possibility of two rare, inherited recessive disorders in a single child becomes significant. For a given gene defect there may be multiple abnormal alleles, which in part explains a wide range of clinical severity and age of onset for a particular metabolic defect. Carriers of recessive genes or X-linked genes (females) are usually asymptomatic except in a few conditions (Table 5–3).

Dominantly expressed disorders may be sporadic (new mutations) or familial. In autosomal recessive disorders, heterozygous expression of clinical traits is unusual, although there may be a risk factor for disease that is associated with the heterozygous state. X-linked disorders are expressed dominantly in males who have only one X-chromosome. Expression of X-linked disorders in females varies from purely recessive to apparent dominance because of random inactivation of one X-chromosome or the other in cell lines early in fetal development. In most X-linked disorders, the majority of heterozygous females are clinically unaffected. The inheritance of mitochondrial

TABLE 5–1
Pathogenesis of Enzymatic Disorders

| Enzymatic Disorder | Reactant | | Product | | Clinical Disease |
	Accumulated	Toxic?	Not Made	Deficient?	
Galactosemia	Galactose-1-phosphate	Yes	UDP-galactose	No	Yes
Biotinidase deficiency	Lysyl biotin	No	Biotin	Yes	Yes
Essential fructosuria	Fructose	No	Fructose-1-phosphate	No	No

UDP, Uridine diphosphate.

TABLE 5–2
Pathogenesis of Disorders of Transport

Disease	Transport System	Organs or Organelles Affected	Pathogenesis
Cystinuria	Cystine/arginine Lysine/ornithine	Kidney/intestine	Cystine stone formation
Hartnup disease	Monocarboxylic monoamino acids	Kidney/intestine	Tryptophan malabsorption
Glycogen storage disease Ib	Glucose-6-phosphate	Microsome	Hypoglycemia Excess glucose-6-phosphate

TABLE 5–3
Inheritance Patterns: Genotypes and Phenotypes

	Examples	Phenotypes	Clinical Problems
Autosomal Genes			
Dominant inheritance	Familial hyper-cholesterolemia	Heterozygous—afffected	Xanthomas and heart disease in adult life
		Homozygous—affected markedly by "gene dose effect"	Xanthomas and heart disease in childhood
Recessive inheritance	Phenylketonuria	Heterozygous—normal	Normal
		Homozygous—affected	Severe developmental delay
	Galactosemia	Heterozygous—risk factors	? Ovarian failure (adult) ? Cataracts (adult)
		Homozygous—affected	Neonatal liver failure, cataracts
X-Linked Genes	Ornithine trans-carbamylase deficiency	Male—affected	Severe infantile hyperammonemia
		Female—variably affected depending on X-chromosome inactivation	Normal phenotype, postpartum hyperammonemia, recurrent Reye syndrome, neonatal hyperammonemia
Mitochondrial Genes	Mutant leucine transfer RNA (A3243G)	Both sexes affected equally, but clinical manifestations variable among family members	Lactic acidosis, skeletal myopathy, cardiomyopathy, seizures, mental retardation, ataxia, deafness, etc. in various syndromic combinations

TABLE 5–4
Inborn Errors of Metabolism Presenting with Neurologic Signs in Infants <3 Months Old

Generalized Seizures	Encephalopathic Coma with or without Seizures
All disorders that cause hypoglycemia	Maple syrup urine disease
Most hepatic glycogen storage diseases	Nonketotic hyperglycinemia
Galactosemia, hereditary fructose intolerance	Diseases producing extreme hyperammonemia
Fructose-1,6-bisphosphatase deficiency	Disorders of the urea cycle
Disorders of the propionate pathway	Disorders of the propionate pathway
HMG-lyase deficiency	Disorders of beta oxidation
Disorders of beta oxidation	Congenital lactic acidosis (PCD)
Pyruvate carboxylase deficiency (PCD)	
Maple syrup urine disease	
Seizures and/or Posturing	
Nonketotic hyperglycinemia	
Maple syrup urine disease	

TABLE 5–5
Inborn Errors of Metabolism Presenting with Hepatomegaly or Hepatic Dysfunction in Infants

Hepatomegaly	Hepatic Failure	Jaundice
GSD I	Galactosemia	Galactosemia
GSD III	Hereditary fructose intolerance	Hereditary fructose intolerance
Mucopolysaccharidosis I and II	Infantile tyrosinemia (fumarylace-	Infantile tyrosinemia (fumarylace-
Gaucher and Niemann-Pick diseases	toacetate hydrolase deficiency)	toacetate hydrolase deficiency)
	GSD IV (slowly evolving)	Crigler-Najjar disease
		Rotor, Dubin-Johnson syndromes

GSD, Glycogen storage disease.

DNA (mtDNA) is maternal, and the clinical disorders produced by abnormalities of these maternal genes depend on the specific defects and the distribution of affected and normal mitochondria in tissues over time.

Clinical Patterns

Infants with inborn errors of metabolism frequently exhibit failure to thrive. Generally, metabolic defects severe enough to cause failure to thrive also produce readily recognizable chemical abnormalities. Additional clinical clues are recurrent emesis, lethargy, seizures, hypotonia, tachypnea, and unusual odors.

Neurologic complications are common and include seizures, hypotonia, varying degrees of de-

velopmental delay, microcephaly, macrocephaly and encephalopathic coma (Table 5–4). Intermittent, recurrent episodes of vomiting and lethargy or coma are highly suggestive of a metabolic disorder. In certain diseases (e.g., Krabbe disease or mitochondrial myopathies), the central and peripheral nervous systems and the skeletal muscles are involved.

Hepatic involvement may produce hepatomegaly from storage of macromolecules; chronic cholestasis; or a single or recurrent episode of acute fulminant hepatic insufficiency, with elevated serum liver enzyme levels and prolongation of the prothrombin time and hepatic coma (Table 5–5). Chronic liver disease may lead to cirrhosis and hepatomas.

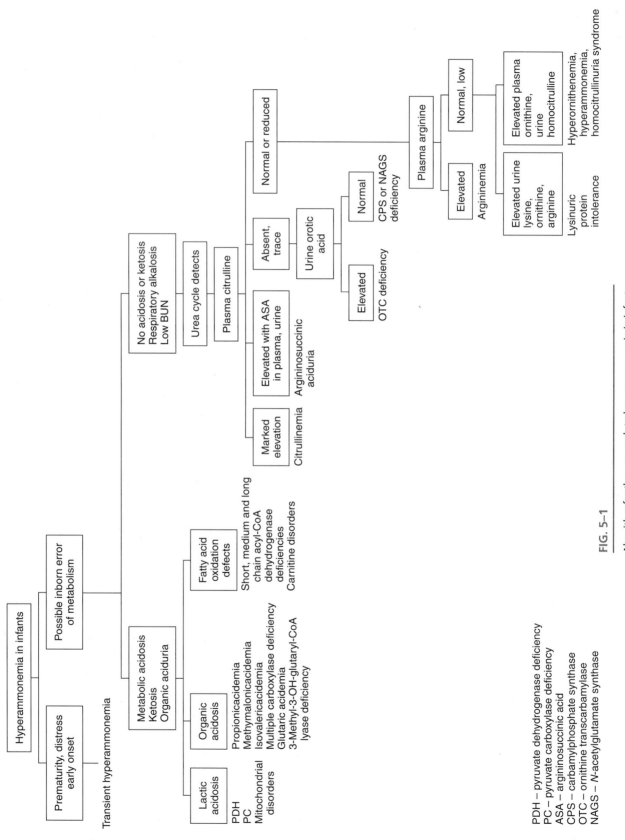

FIG. 5–1

Algorithm for the approach to hyperammonemia in infants.

PDH – pyruvate dehydrogenase deficiency
PC – pyruvate carboxylase deficiency
ASA – argininosuccinic acid
CPS – carbamylphosphate synthase
OTC – ornithine transcarbamylase
NAGS – N-acetylglutamate synthase

Laboratory Tests

Chemical clues to metabolic disease include hyperammonemia, hypoglycemia, acidosis, ketonuria, abnormalities in hepatic transaminases, and hyperbilirubinemia. The level of *plasma glucose* averages 80 mg/dL in the fasting state, with a range of 60–100 mg/dL. During acute illness with temporary starvation, the blood glucose level may fall below 60 mg/dL in normal individuals. It always is necessary to judge whether a given low value for blood glucose level represents an appropriate physiologic adaptation or a true disorder. Autonomic manifestations (e.g., pallor, sweating, tremor, and diplopia), seizures, and coma are clear manifestations of hypoglycemia as a disorder, whereas irritability and lethargy are defined as hypoglycemic in origin only when they respond dramatically to the administration of glucose. Hypoglycemia is an integral part of a number of metabolic diseases (see Chapter 17). In some of these diseases, acidosis or hyperammonemia may so dominate the clinical picture that the serious effects on glucose homeostasis are neglected.

Hypoglycemia secondary to an inborn error may or may not be associated with ketonuria.

Plasma ammonia is present in very small concentrations (10–50 μmol/L) in normal fasting individuals. Blood samples should be collected, placed on ice, and analyzed within ½ hour because ammonia levels spontaneously rise rapidly in shed blood. Hyperammonemia of hepatic origin gives rise to elevated levels of ammonia in both arterial and venous blood. Hyperammonemia of muscular origin elevates venous ammonia but not arterial ammonia. In general, elevations of less than twice the upper limit of normal in acutely ill patients do not indicate a significant disorder of nitrogen elimination. The differential diagnosis and approach to hyperammonemia are noted in Table 5–6 and Fig. 5–1.

In older infants and children, *ketonuria* is a normal response to starvation but not to a normal overnight fast. In the neonate, ketonuria is indicative of metabolic disease. A high anion gap metabolic acidosis with or without ketosis is also suggestive of a metabolic disorder (Tables 5–7 and 5–8).

TABLE 5–6
Etiologies of Hyperammonemia in Infants

Etiology of Hyperammonemia	Comments
Disorders of the urea cycle	Lethal hyperammonemia is common
Disorders of the propionate pathway	Severe hyperammonemia may precede acidosis
Disorders of fatty acid catabolism and of ketogenesis	Reye-like syndrome possible
Transient neonatal hyperammonemia	Idiopathic, self-limited
Portal-systemic shunting	Thrombosis of portal vein, cirrhosis, hepatitis
Idiopathic Reye syndrome	Uncommon
Drug intoxication: salicylate, valproic acid, acetaminophen	
Hyperinsulinism/hyperammonemia syndrome	Clinical hypoglycemia, subclinical hyperammonemia

---

TABLE 5–7
Etiologies of Metabolic Acidosis Caused by Inborn Errors of Metabolism in Infants

Disorder	Comment
Methymalonic acidemia (MMA)	Hyperammonemia, ketosis, neutropenia, thrombocytopenia
Propionic acidemia	Similar to MMA
Isovaleric acidemia	Similar to MMA
Pyruvate dehydrogenase deficiency	Lactic acidosis, hyperammonemia
Pyruvate carboxylase deficiency	Lactic acidosis, hypoglycemia, and ketosis

Continued

TABLE 5–7
Etiologies of Metabolic Acidosis Caused by Inborn Errors of Metabolism in Infants—cont'd

Disorder	Comment
Respiratory chain (mitochondrial) disorders	Lactic acidosis, ketosis
Medium-chain acyl-CoA dehydrogenase deficiency (MCAD)	Moderate acidosis, hypoglycemia, absent ketosis, possible hyperammonemia
Other fatty acid oxidation defects	Similar to MCAD
Galactosemia	Renal tubular acidosis, *E. coli* sepsis, hypoglycemia
3-Hyroxy-3-methyl-glutaryl-CoA lyase deficiency	Severe lactic acidosis, hyperammonemia, hypoglycemia
3-Methylcrotonyl-CoA carboxylase deficiency	Severe lactic acidosis, hyperammonemia, hypoglycemia, ketosis
Multiple acyl-CoA dehydrogenase deficiency (glutaric aciduria 2)	Lactic acidosis, hypoglycemia

TABLE 5–8
Initial Diagnostic Evaluation for a Suspected Inborn Error of Metabolism*

Blood and Plasma	Urine
Arterial blood gas	Glucose
Electrolytes—anion gap	pH
Glucose	Ketones
Ammonia	Reducing substances
Liver enzymes	Organic acids
Complete blood count, differential,† and platelet count	Acylcarnitine
Lactate, pyruvate	Orotic acid
Organic acids	
Amino acids	
Carnitine	

*Organ-specific evaluation is indicated for specific symptoms (e.g., cranial MRI for coma or seizures; echocardiography for cardiomyopathy; cerebrospinal fluid amino acids by column chromatography if nonketotic hyperglycemia is suspected).
†Thrombocytopenia and neutropenia are seen in organic acidosis; vacuolated lymphocytes and metachromatic granules are seen in lysosomal disorders.

Urine screening tests for metabolic disease include the ferric chloride test (for PKU, tyrosinosis, and other diseases), the dinitrophenylhydrazine test (for PKU and maple syrup urine disease [MSUD]), and the cyanide-nitroprusside test (for homocystinuria and cystinuria). When the clinical manifestations suggest the diagnosis, these tests can be used as a basis for initiating therapy, but they should never be considered definitive. Abnormalities in the concentrations of metabolites (amino acids and organic acids) in body fluids and urine can provide diagnoses that are sufficient for long-term management and genetic counseling, but definitive diagnosis is made only by demonstration of a specific enzymatic or transport deficiency.

DISORDERS OF METABOLISM FOR WHICH NEONATAL SCREENING IS PERFORMED

The purpose of neonatal screening is the early detection and rapid treatment of genetic diseases during their preclinical phases. The screening tests for inborn errors of metabolism have traditionally used microbiologic assays for single analytes. Tandem mass spectrometry of blood specimens allows rapid neonatal diagnosis of a great number of metabolic diseases. This technique is more effective in the management of galactosemia and MSUD, which tend not to remain subclinical for the time necessary to perform and report the microbiologic tests.

Phenylketonuria

PKU, an autosomal recessive disease, primarily affects the brain. It occurs in 1:10,000 persons. Classic PKU is the result of a defect in the hydroxylation of phenylalanine to form tyrosine (Fig. 5–2); the activity of phenylalanine hydroxylase in the liver is absent or greatly reduced. A small percentage of phenylke-

tonuric infants have a variant disorder, **malignant PKU**, that results from a defect in the synthesis or metabolism of tetrahydrobiopterin, the cofactor for phenylalanine hydroxylase and for other enzymes involved in the intermediary metabolism of aromatic amino acids.

Affected infants are normal at birth, and the only constant *clinical manifestation* of PKU is the evolution of severe mental retardation (an intelligence quotient <30). In addition, children may have blond hair, blue eyes, eczema, and mousy odor of the urine. In infants whose disease is caused by an error in the synthesis or metabolism of tetrahydrobiopterin (2% of PKU cases), a progressive, lethal central nervous system disease develops, reflecting abnormalities in other neural enzymatic reactions for which tetrahydrobiopterin is necessary.

In classic PKU, the *diagnosis* is made by demonstration of the following:
1. Hyperphenylalaninemia at a level of 1.2 mM (20 mg/dL) or higher (normal is ~0.06 mM, or 1 mg/dL) *and*
2. Normal or reduced plasma tyrosine (normal is ~0.06 mM, or 1 mg/dL).

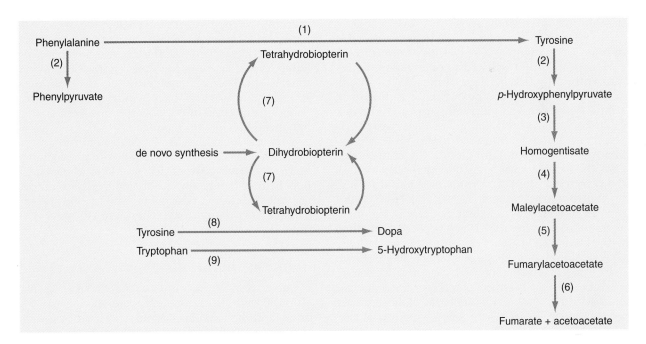

FIG. 5–2

Metabolism of aromatic amino acids: (1) phenylalanine hydroxylase, (2) transaminase, (3) *p*-hydroxyphenylpyruvate oxidase, (4) homogentisate oxidase, (5) maleylacetoacetate isomerase, (6) fumarylacetoacetate hydrolase, (7) dihydrobiopterin reductase, (8) tyrosine hydroxylase, (9) tryptophan hydroxylase.

The screening test for PKU usually measures whole-blood phenylalanine by a semiquantitative microbiologic assay; elevations should be confirmed by a more accurate assay (e.g., quantitative chromatography or tandem mass spectrometry). It is necessary to demonstrate normal (or lower) levels of tyrosine in blood. The pathway for phenylalanine metabolism develops late in gestation. A significant percentage of premature infants and a few full-term infants have transient elevations in both phenylalanine and tyrosine during the neonatal period. This condition, **transient tyrosinemia,** carries much less risk of permanent sequelae than does classic PKU.

Phenylpyruvic acid is present in the urine of phenylketonuric infants after the neonatal period; it can be detected by adding a few drops of 10% ferric chloride to freshly voided urine. In the presence of phenylpyruvic acid, a deep green color develops immediately.

Malignant PKU is diagnosed by measuring dihydrobiopterin reductase in erythrocytes and analyzing biopterin metabolites in urine. Screening for malignant PKU is carried out in all hyperphenylalaninemic infants because there is no other way to differentiate the hyperphenylalaninemia caused by deficiency of phenylalanine hydroxylase from that caused by a tetrahydrobiopterin deficiency.

Achievement of normal intelligence is possible in most infants with classic PKU by *treatment* with a diet specifically restricted in phenylalanine, begun within the first 10 days of life. Verbal intelligence quotient (IQ) can be normalized; however, subtle defects in spatial intelligence may be evident. For infants with malignant PKU, restriction of dietary phenylalanine reduces plasma phenylalanine but does not ameliorate the clinical disease; the disease must be treated by replacement of the cofactor if biopterin synthesis is impaired and by neuropharmacologic agents if tetrahydrobiopterin reductase is deficient. Success in the management of malignant PKU is less predictable than with classic PKU.

A significant percentage of infants who are shown to be hyperphenylalaninemic by neonatal screening do not satisfy the chemical criteria for the diagnosis of classic PKU and do not satisfy the clinical criteria for malignant PKU. These infants are defined as having **hyperphenylalaninemia.** In some infants, the level of plasma phenylalanine remains less than 0.6 mM (10 mg/dL) without therapeutic intervention; these infants need no treatment. For infants whose plasma phenylalanine level is ≥0.6 mM and for those with classic phenylketonuria, maintenance of the plasma phenylalanine level within the range of 0.12–0.36 mM (2–6 mg/dl) for the first 10 years of life is recommended.

Reversible cognitive dysfunction is associated with acute elevations of plasma phenylalanine in treated adults and children with phenylketonuria. In some instances in which the elevated level has been sustained, the dysfunction has become permanent. It is clear that control of the plasma phenylalanine level can be relaxed after the first 10 years; however, the optimum therapeutic level in older children and adults with PKU and alternative methods for normalizing amino acids in the brain are the subjects of continuing investigation. **Maternal hyperphenylalaninemia** is a major problem requiring rigorous management before conception and throughout pregnancy to prevent fetal brain damage and microcephaly in the fetus.

Related Disorders

Abnormalities in the catabolism of tyrosine can produce positive test findings for phenylketones in the urine, but not elevations in blood phenylalanine. Tyrosinemia can occur as a nonspecific consequence of severe liver disease; it is also the most striking finding in fumarylacetoacetate hydrolase deficiency (Fig. 5–2), a rare disease in which metabolites that accumulate as a result of the impaired reaction produce severe liver disease (e.g., bleeding disorder, hypoglycemia, hypoalbuminemia, elevated transaminases) and defects in renal tubular function. There are two clinical forms of the disease: *acute,* highly lethal liver disease in the first months of life, and *chronic* liver disease, frequently associated with rickets, that manifests itself later in infancy or childhood. A high proportion of patients develop hepatic malignancies in later childhood.

Treatment includes a low-phenylalanine, low-tyrosine diet, NTBC (an inhibitor of the oxidation of para-hydroxyphenylpyruvic acid), and liver transplantation. In more benign forms of hereditary tyrosinemia, enzymes catalyzing tyrosine transamination and the oxidation of *para*-hydroxyphenylpyruvate are specifically deficient.

Homocystinuria

Homocystinuria, an autosomal recessive disease (1:200,000 live births) involving connective tissue, the brain, and the vascular system, is caused by a deficiency of cystathionine beta-synthase. In the normal metabolism of the sulfur amino acids, methionine gives rise to cystine; homocysteine is a pivotal intermediate (Fig. 5–3). When cystathionine beta-synthase is deficient, homocysteine accumulates in the blood and appears in the urine. Another result is enhanced reconversion of homocysteine to methionine, result-

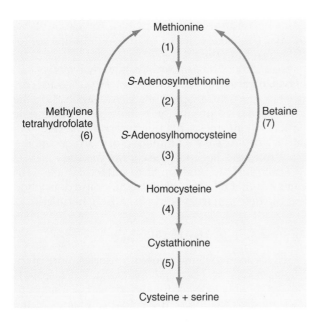

FIG. 5–3

Metabolism of methionine and homocysteine: (1) methionine adenosyltransferase, (2) *S*-methyltransferase, (3) *S*-adenosylhomocysteine hydrolase, (4) cystathionine beta-synthase, (5) cystathionase, (6) homocysteine methyltransferase, (7) betaine-homocysteine methyltransferase.

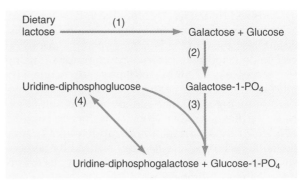

FIG. 5–4

Pathway of galactose metabolism: (1) lactase (intestinal), (2) galactokinase, (3) galactose-1-phosphate uridyltransferase, (4) uridine diphosphoglucose 4-epimerase.

ing in an increase in the level of methionine in the blood. The neonatal screening test most commonly used measures methionine in whole blood.

Through mechanisms not clearly understood, an excess of homocysteine produces a slowly evolving *clinical syndrome* that includes in its fully developed form dislocated lenses, the habitus of Marfan syndrome, malar flushing, and livedo reticularis. Arachnodactyly, scoliosis, pectus excavatum or carinatum, and genu valgum are skeletal features. Mental retardation, psychiatric illness, or both may be present. Major arterial or venous thromboses are a constant threat.

Homocystinuria has no neonatal manifestations. Confirmation of the *diagnosis* requires demonstration of gross elevation of homocysteine level in the blood.

Homocystinuria can sometimes be treated by giving, together with supplemental folate, large doses of pyridoxine (100–1000 mg/day) to provide a great excess of the cofactor for cystathionine beta-synthase. If pyridoxine therapy fails, the accumulation of homocysteine can be controlled with a diet restricted in methionine and supplemented with cystine and folate. The use of supplemental betaine to stimulate the alternative pathway for resynthesis

of methionine from homocysteine also appears to have a role in the management of pyridoxine-unresponsive patients. The prognosis is good for infants whose plasma homocysteine level is controlled.

Galactosemia

Galactosemia is an autosomal recessive disease (1:60,000 births) caused by an extreme deficiency of the enzyme galactose-1-phosphate uridyltransferase (Fig. 5–4). *Clinical manifestations* are most striking in the neonate who when fed milk generally exhibits evidence of liver failure (e.g., hyperbilirubinemia, disorders of coagulation, and hypoglycemia), disordered renal tubular function (e.g., acidosis, glycosuria, and aminoaciduria), and cataracts. The neonatal screening test has limited usefulness for severely affected infants because the infants may die before the test result is available. When neonatal manifestations are mild or nonexistent, failure to thrive may evolve. Major acute effects on liver and kidney function and the development of cataracts are limited to the first few years of life, but older children tend to have learning disorders. Ovarian failure is a late sequela that is not preventable by therapy. Pseudotumor cerebri is an additional complication.

Laboratory manifestations of galactosemia depend to a large extent on dietary galactose levels. When galactose is ingested (as lactose), levels of plasma galactose and erythrocyte galactose-1-phosphate are elevated. The levels of hepatocellular enzymes (alanine aminotransferase and aspartate aminotransferase) rapidly increase in plasma. Elevations of the levels of plasma conjugated and unconjugated bilirubin follow quickly, as do reductions in the levels of coagulation factors synthesized by the liver. Hypoglycemia is frequent, and albuminuria is present in infants with clinical disease. Galactose frequently is present in the urine and can be detected by a positive reaction for reducing substances (e.g., Clinitest tablets) and no reaction with glucose oxidase on urine strip tests. The absence of urinary reducing substance cannot be relied on to exclude the diagnosis. Renal tubular dysfunction may be evidenced by a normal anion gap hyperchloremic metabolic acidosis. The *diagnosis* is made by demonstrating extreme reduction in erythrocyte galactose-1-phosphate uridyltransferase.

Treatment by the elimination of dietary galactose results in rapid correction of abnormalities, but infants who are extremely ill before treatment may die before therapy is effective. Galactosemic infants are at increased risk for severe neonatal *Escherichia coli* sepsis.

It is possible to relax the dietary galactose restriction in later childhood. Congenital cataracts and mild brain damage have developed even when galactosemic infants are treated from birth. For this reason, dietary galactose is eliminated during pregnancy in mothers who have delivered galactosemic infants. Because the galactosemic fetus can synthesize galactose-1-phosphate, this therapeutic approach may have limited value.

Related Disorders

Galactokinase deficiency, an autosomal recessive disorder (1:250,000), also leads to the accumulation of galactose in body fluids (see Fig. 5–4), which results in the formation of galactitol (dulcitol) through the action of aldose reductase. Galactitol, acting as an osmotic agent, can be responsible for cataract formation and, rarely, for increased intracranial pressure. These are the only clinical manifestations. Persons homozygous for galactokinase deficiency develop cataracts in the neonatal period, whereas heterozy-

gous individuals may be at risk for cataracts as adults. *Treatment* consists of lifelong elimination of galactose from the diet.

Hereditary fructose intolerance in many ways is analogous to galactosemia. When fructose is ingested, deficiency of fructose-1-phosphate aldolase leads to the intracellular accumulation of fructose-1-phosphate with resultant emesis, hypoglycemia, and severe liver and kidney disease. Elimination of fructose and sucrose from the diet cures the clinical disease.

Fructosuria is analogous to galactokinase deficiency in that it is caused by fructokinase deficiency, but the defect in fructosuria is entirely harmless.

Maple Syrup Urine Disease

MSUD is an autosomal recessive disease, more properly named *branched-chain ketoaciduria*. The disease is caused by deficiency of the decarboxylase that initiates the degradation of the ketoacid analogs of the three branched-chain amino acids–leucine, isoleucine, and valine (Fig. 5–5). MSUD is rare (1:250,000) in the general population but much more common in some population isolates (e.g., among Pennsylvania Mennonites, 1:150). Neonatal screening programs commonly include MSUD.

Although MSUD does have intermittent and late-onset forms, clinical manifestations of the classic form typically begin within 1–4 weeks of birth. Poor feeding, vomiting, and tachypnea commonly are noted, but the hallmark of the disease is profound depression of the central nervous system, associated with alternating hypotonia and hypertonia (extensor spasms), opisthotonos, and seizures. The urine has the odor of maple syrup in most cases.

Laboratory manifestations of MSUD include hypoglycemia and a variable presence of metabolic acidosis with elevation of the undetermined anions; the acidosis is caused in part by plasma branched-chain

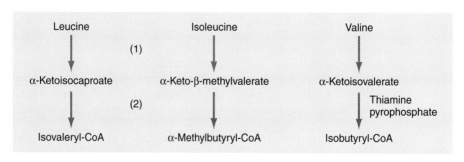

FIG. 5–5

Metabolism of the branched-chain amino acids: (1) aminotransferases, (2) alpha-ketoacid dehydrogenase complex.

organic acids and in part by the usual "ketone bodies," beta-hydroxybutyrate and acetoacetate. The branched-chain ketoacids (but not the beta-hydroxybutyrate nor the acetoacetate) react immediately with 2,4-dinitrophenylhydrazine to form a copious, white precipitate. This reaction is the basis for a urine screening test.

The definitive *diagnosis* of MSUD generally is made by demonstrating large increases in plasma leucine, isoleucine, and valine levels. Diagnosis by analysis of organic acids also is possible.

Treatment of MSUD consists of restricting the intake of branched-chain amino acids (all three are essential amino acids) to the amounts required for growth in severely affected infants. Hemodialysis, hemofiltration, or peritoneal dialysis can be lifesaving during acidotic crises. Treatment with special diets must be continued for life. Ordinary catabolic stresses, such as moderate infections, can precipitate clinical crises. Liver transplantation also effectively treats MSUD.

Testing for a *biotinidase deficiency* (discussed later in this chapter) also is included in some programs for neonatal screening.

INBORN ERRORS CAUSING CLINICAL DISEASE IN THE NEONATE

Most of the metabolic diseases that cause metabolic acidosis, hyperammonemia, or hypoglycemia can produce clinical manifestations in the neonate. The fetus can be considered as undergoing perpetual dialysis with an optimized nutrient solution; therefore, the newborn with an inborn error of metabolism seems normal at birth. As the infant adapts to extrauterine life and the oral intake of nutrients, chemical abnormalities appear and symptoms follow at an interval that reflects both the type and the severity of the inborn error. Clinical recognition can occur as early as the third day of life and generally is possible within the first week. Poor feeding, vomiting, tachypnea, lethargy, jaundice, and seizures are manifestations common to neonates with inborn errors of metabolism, but these also are manifestations of many other diseases, including neonatal septicemia. The most characteristic manifestation of metabolic disease is depression of the central nervous system exhibited by inattention to feedings, lethargy, unresponsiveness, and hypotonia, occurring in the absence of signs of disease of a specific organ or of neonatal septicemia. Laboratory evaluation of arterial blood gases, liver function, plasma glucose and ammonia levels and routine urinalysis, including a test for reducing substance, usually provides clues that lead to a diagnosis (Table 5–8).

Nonketotic Hyperglycinemia

Nonketotic hyperglycinemia, an autosomal recessive disease, is caused by a defect in the glycine cleavage system whereby glycine and serine are interconverted. The fetus is affected by this disorder; malformations of the brain (most notably agenesis of the corpus callosum) are common.

Clinically the disease produces profound deterioration in central nervous system function early in the neonatal period: alternating hypertonia and hypotonia, seizures, respiratory depression, inattentiveness, coma, and death within the first weeks of life. The P_{CO_2} may be increased as a result of respiratory depression, and hyperglycinemia may be present, but the *diagnosis* rests on the demonstration of greatly increased glycine level in cerebrospinal fluid and of an abnormal ratio of glycine in cerebrospinal fluid to glycine in plasma.

No effective *treatment* has been developed. However, sodium benzoate, which lowers plasma glycine levels, has some efficacy, as do agents (e.g., diazepam, strychnine, ketamine, and dextromethorphan) that antagonize glycine at receptors in the central nervous system. Although the genetic disease has a uniformly poor *prognosis,* there is a self-limited form of neonatal nonketotic hyperglycinemia that can mimic the genetic disease clinically and chemically but resolves spontaneously with no apparent residual effects.

Hyperammonemia

Hyperammonemia usually results from the failure of the liver to clear plasma ammonia. This failure can be caused mechanically by portal venous obstruction or chemically by the malfunction of an adequately perfused liver, as occurs in hepatitis with cellular necrosis, in Reye syndrome with generalized hepatocellular dysfunction, and in a number of inborn errors of metabolism involving the synthesis of urea and of glutamine (Fig. 5–1 and Table 5–6). Unusually, deamination of amino acids in muscle produces abnormally high levels of blood ammonia.

Clinical Manifestations

Symptoms and signs depend on the underlying cause of the hyperammonemia, the age at which it develops, and its degree.

Severe Neonatal Hyperammonemia. Infants with complete genetic defects in urea synthesis, infants with *transient neonatal hyperammonemia* (discussed later), and infants with interference in the synthesis of urea and glutamine secondary to genetic disorders of organic acid metabolism can have levels of blood ammonia 100 times normal (>1000 μmol/L) in the neonatal period. Poor feeding, hypotonia, apnea, hypothermia, and vomiting rapidly give way to coma and occasionally to intractable seizures. Death occurs within days if the condition remains untreated.

Moderate Neonatal Hyperammonemia. Moderate neonatal hyperammonemia, in the range of 200–400 μmol/L, is associated with depression of the central nervous system, poor feeding, and vomiting. Seizures are not characteristic. This type of hyperammonemia may be caused by partial blocks in urea synthesis and commonly is caused by disorders of organic acid metabolism that secondarily interfere with the elimination of nitrogen.

Clinical Hyperammonemia in Later Infancy and Childhood. Infants who are affected by defects in the urea cycle and who are not ill in the neonatal period may continue to do well while receiving the low-protein intake of breast milk, only to develop clinical hyperammonemia when dietary protein is increased or when catabolic stress occurs. The clinical presentation is dominated by vomiting and lethargy, which frequently progresses to coma. As protein intake is restricted by anorexia and vomiting, the sensorium clears and the infant recovers, only to develop symptoms again when the stimulus to hyperammonemia returns. Seizures are not typical of the disorder. During a crisis the plasma ammonia level is usually 200 to 500 μmol/L, but when dietary protein is restricted, the ammonia level decreases and may even become normal. If the manifestations are not striking (no coma), the condition may go unrecognized for years. When a crisis occurs during an epidemic of influenza, the child mistakenly may be thought to have Reye syndrome. Older children may have neuropsychiatric or behavioral abnormalities.

Subclinical Hyperammonemia. Infants and children with chronic elevations of plasma ammonia at the level of 100–200 μmol/L often do not have symptoms or signs of the derangement.

Transient Neonatal Hyperammonemia. Affected infants do not have a genetic disease, but striking hyperammonemia develops shortly after birth. Clinical manifestations (e.g., respiratory distress, apnea, and hypotonia) may be extreme. Exchange transfusion, hemofiltration, hemodialysis, or peritoneal dialysis may result in survival without neurologic sequelae. The etiology of this self-limited condition is unknown.

Defects in the Urea Cycle

Inherited enzymatic deficiencies have been described for each of the steps of urea synthesis (Fig. 5–6).

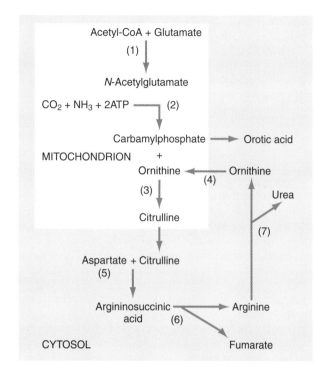

FIG. 5–6

The urea cycle: (1) *N*-acetylglutamate synthase, (2) carbamoylphosphate synthetase, (3) ornithine carbamoyltransferase (OCT), (4) ornithine translocator, (5) argininosuccinic acid synthetase, (6) argininosuccinic acid lyase, (7) arginase.

Ornithine Carbamoyltransferase Deficiency. Ornithine carbamoyltransferase (OCT) deficiency is unique among the defects in the urea cycle in that it is sex linked. The number of known genetic defects (polymorphisms) is quite large, and the affected enzyme may or may not have low-level activity. If the enzyme is nonfunctional, there is no OCT activity in the affected male, who is likely to die in the neonatal period if untreated. Affected females are heterozygous, with one affected cell line and one unaffected cell line; the relative preponderance of each line is randomly determined according to the Lyon hypothesis (see Chapter 4). Because the liver is a mosaic of affected and unaffected nests of cells, it is not possible to use needle biopsy to define the degree of enzymatic deficiency in clinically affected females; however, it seems likely that overall activity of OCT must be reduced to roughly 20% or less of the normal level in order to produce clinical disease. Thus *clinical manifestations* range from lethal disease in the male to clinical normalcy in a high percentage of females. Manifestations in clinically affected females include recurrent emesis, lethargy, mental retardation, and psychiatric problems.

The *diagnosis* relies on the fact that orotic acid, produced as a byproduct of carbamoyl phosphate, is excreted in greatly increased quantities in the urine (Figs. 5–1 and 5–6). The oroticaciduria, although it is much increased above normal, is not quantitatively significant for nitrogen excretion. Although some females heterozygous for the genetic defect excrete normal quantities of orotic acid, most affected females excrete excess orotic acid when given allopurinol.

Argininosuccinic Aciduria. Argininosuccinic acid lyase deficiency results in accumulation of argininosuccinic acid in tissues and blood; however, because the acid is cleared readily by the kidney, it is best identified in the urine, where it is found in gram quantities. Because the synthesis of argininosuccinic acid fixes ammonia nitrogen, hyperammonemia is not present at all times in all patients. However, the defect disrupts the urea cycle, and depletion of ornithine can lead to severe hyperammonemia. Death in the neonatal period has been reported, as has symptomatic hyperammonemia in later infancy and childhood. Failure to thrive, hepatomegaly, friable hair (trichorrhexis nodosa), slow motor and mental development, and seizures are characteristic features of the disease, with or without clinical hyperammonemia. Argininosuccinic aciduria is an autosomal recessive disease.

Treatment of Hyperammonemia. A reduction of dietary protein is the most important general treatment for hyperammonemia. During episodes of symptomatic hyperammonemia, protein intake is eliminated and intravenous glucose is given in sufficient quantity to suppress catabolism of endogenous protein. Because 20% of total urea production is accounted for by detoxification of ammonia generated by bacterial urease in the intestine, sterilization of the intestine can provide brief benefit during acute episodes of hyperammonemia. Long-term benefit is possible with lactulose, a disaccharide not digestible by humans, which is fermented to lactic acid by intestinal bacteria. The resultant reduction in pH inhibits the transluminal absorption of ammonia.

Other important acute and chronic treatment modalities include sodium benzoate and phenylacetic acid (or its precursor, phenylbutyric acid), which are excreted in the urine as conjugates of glycine and glutamine, respectively. It must also be noted that arginine is an essential amino acid when arginine synthesis via the urea cycle is grossly impaired. When hyperammonemia is extreme, direct removal of ammonia usually is carried out; for this purpose, hemodialysis or hemofiltration is more effective than exchange transfusion or peritoneal dialysis. Despite successful management of hyperammonemic crises, the long-term outcome for males with severe neonatal hyperammonemia is poor. Early liver transplantation may have some benefit.

Organic Acidoses

Metabolic acidosis is a state in which acid excretion in the urine is inadequate to remove the excessive production of abnormal acids and maintain a normal acid-base balance. *Renal tubular acidosis* frequently occurs in inborn errors of metabolism. It is caused by tubular injury and disordered acidification of urine, not by excessive acid production. Inborn errors of metabolism lead to metabolic acidosis by causing an overload of various metabolic acids to be excreted (Table 5–7). The latter condition is characterized by acidosis, acid urine, normal renal function, and an increase in circulating acids that is manifested by an abnormally large anion gap. In normal plasma, the **anion gap** as calculated by the formula ($Na - [Cl + HCO_3]$) is 10–15 mEq/L. The metabolic acidoses lead to values that are frequently 30 mEq/L or more as a result of the accumulation of organic acids. Both renal failure as a primary disorder and renal hypoperfusion associated with dehydration may increase the anion gap. Anion gaps exceeding 25 mEq/L usually do not occur in simple dehydration; however, for a particular child it may be necessary to defer evaluation of the anion gap until rehydration has been accomplished.

Starvation Ketosis and Ketotic Hypoglycemia

The most common circumstance in which acidosis is found in children is starvation associated with anorexia, vomiting, and diarrhea in the course of a viral illness. The *clinical manifestations* are those of the causative illness (see Chapters 2 and 11); the acidosis is mild, is associated with ketonuria, and promptly responds to the administration of carbohydrate. In this normal response to starvation, the blood glucose level is relatively low (generally 50–70 mg/dL, but occasionally lower), and no symptoms referable to hypoglycemia appear (see Chapter 17).

In contrast, *ketotic hypoglycemia* is a common but abnormal condition in which tolerance for fasting is impaired to the extent that symptomatic hypoglycemia with seizures or coma occurs when the child encounters a ketotic stress. The stress may be significant (e.g., viral infection with vomiting) or minor (e.g., a prolongation by several hours of the normal overnight fast). Ketotic hypoglycemia first appears in the second year of life. It occurs in otherwise healthy children and usually is treated by frequent snacks and the provision of glucose during periods of stress. *Clinical manifestations* typically are limited to the first 5–6 years of life. Carbohydrate tolerance, gluconeogenesis, and hormone responses characteristically are normal.

Lactic Acidosis

In most tissues glucose is oxidized to carbon dioxide and water, with pyruvate as an intermediate (Fig. 5–7). Interference with mitochondrial oxidative processes results in an accumulation of pyruvate. Because lactate dehydrogenase is ubiquitous and because the equilibrium catalyzed by this enzyme greatly favors lactate over pyruvate, the accumulation of pyruvate results in lactic acidosis. The most common interference with mitochondrial oxidation is oxygen deficiency caused by anoxia or poor perfusion, as seen in cardiac arrest, shock, severe cyanosis, and profound heart failure. Poisons, such as cyanide, sulfide, and carbon monoxide, that, like anoxia, block the terminal reaction of the mitochondrial respiratory chain, also produce lactic acidosis (see Chapter 16).

Defects of the mitochondria respiratory chain also can produce lactic acidosis. Given the complexity of the respiratory chain, it is not surprising that the defects described are varied as to cause, intensity, and tissues affected. Some show autosomal recessive inheritance; others, mitochondrial (maternal mtDNA)

inheritance; some appear to be sporadic. Myopathy is common, frequently showing ragged red fibers on muscle biopsy (Table 5–9). **Alpers syndrome** (cerebral degeneration and liver disease) and **Leigh disease** (subacute necrotizing encephalomyelopathy) show similar brain lesions but in distinctly different areas of the brain.

Lactic acidosis also occurs when specific reactions of pyruvate are impaired. Pyruvate has three major fates:
1. In muscle, transamination with glutamate, catalyzed by alanine aminotransferase, to form alanine, which can be used for protein synthesis or transported to the liver
2. Predominantly in the liver, carboxylation to form oxaloacetate; the reaction is catalyzed by pyruvate carboxylase (PC)
3. In many tissues, dehydrogenation and decarboxylation to form acetyl coenzyme A (CoA); the reaction is catalyzed by the pyruvate dehydrogenase complex (PDH)

Alanine, produced in muscle, is an important precursor to hepatic gluconeogenesis. The PC reaction initiates gluconeogenesis. The PDH reaction is the first step in pyruvate oxidation. Inborn defects in both PDH and PC have been described. For *PDH deficiency,* the spectrum of reported clinical disease ranges from intractable, lethal acidosis in the first months of life to episodes of ataxia that improve with substitution of fat for carbohydrate in the diet. PDH deficiency also has been noted in some cases of Leigh disease. *PC deficiency* can produce a rapidly lethal neonatal disease that has as one of its elements hyperammonemia secondary to a deficiency of aspartate, the product of transamination of oxaloacetate. Other infants with milder deficiencies exhibit metabolic acidosis and mental retardation. The initial clinical manifestations associated with lactic acidosis caused by inborn errors of metabolism frequently are nonspecific. Therefore, the evaluation of the patient must encompass a broad spectrum of both primary and secondary possibilities.

Treatment is limited for most mitochondrial defects. Disorders of gluconeogenesis may be treated with frequent carbohydrate feeding. Acidosis should be corrected (see Chapter 16).

Disorders of the Propionate Pathway

Propionyl-CoA, a major catabolic metabolite of amino acids and lipids, is converted to succinyl-CoA in a series of reactions called the propionate pathway (Fig. 5–8). A key step in the sequence is the formation of succinyl-CoA from methylmalonyl-CoA, the cofactor for which is adenosyl cobalamin; this cofactor is the product of a series of reactions involving

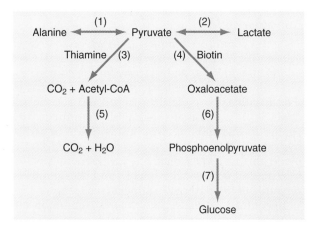

FIG. 5–7

Metabolism of pyruvate and lactate: (1) alanine aminotransferase, (2) lactate dehydrogenase, (3) pyruvate dehydrogenase, (4) pyruvate carboxylase, (5) Krebs cycle, (6) phosphoenolpyruvate carboxykinase, (7) reverse glycolysis. CoA, Coenzyme A.

TABLE 5–9
Some Disorders of the Respiratory Chain That Cause Lactic Acidosis

Disease	Inheritance	Clinical Picture
Myoclonic epilepsy with ragged red fibers (MERRF)	Maternal mtDNA	Lactic acidosis may be severe; variable clinical picture
Myopathy, encephalopathy, lactic acidosis, stroke-like episodes (MELAS)	Maternal mtDNA	Highly variable clinical picture, including type 2 diabetes mellitus
Pearson syndrome	Maternal mtDNA	Macrocytic anemia, sideroblasts, pancreatic insufficiency, etc.
Alpers syndrome	Unclear	Cerebral degeneration and liver disease
Leigh disease	Autosomal recessive in some and maternal mtDNA in others	Degenerative disease of thalamus, basal ganglia, and spinal cord

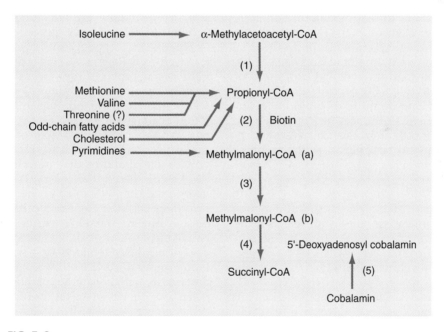

FIG. 5–8

The propionate pathway: (1) β-ketothiolase, (2) propionyl-CoA carboxylase, (3) methylmaloyl-CoA isomerase, (4) methylmalonyl-CoA mutase, (5) cobalamin metabolic pathway. *CoA*, Coenzyme A.

cobalamin (vitamin B_{12}). Defects in most steps of this pathway have been described, and all produce the ketotic hyperglycinemia syndrome. The specific entities are named for specific defects (e.g., propionicacidemia, methylmalonicacidemia, and beta-ketothiolase deficiency).

The *clinical manifestations* of ketotic hyperglycinemia, which can begin in the neonatal period, consist of intermittent ketoacidosis, hyperglycinemia, neutropenia, thrombocytopenia, hyperammonemia, and hypoglycemia. After the first months of life, mild to moderate metabolic acidosis generally occurs as a result of the accumulation of the acid whose metabolism is impaired. Crises involving the intermittent elements of the syndrome occur during periods of catabolic stress but also may occur without an apparent precipitating event. During periods of neutropenia, the risk of serious bacterial infection is increased. Failure to thrive and impaired development are common. The syndrome, caused by any of the reported defects, is inherited as an autosomal recessive trait.

Treatment with massive doses of vitamin B_{12} is helpful in some cases of methylmalonicacidemia. For the remainder of cases, management includes the restriction of dietary protein or of the specific amino acid precursors of propionyl-CoA (isoleucine, valine, methionine, and threonine). Carnitine supplementation is indicated. Because intestinal bacteria produce a significant quantity of propionate, antibacterial treatment to reduce the population of bacteria in the gut has some beneficial effect in propionic acidemia and vitamin B_{12}–unresponsive methylmalonicacidemia.

Isovalericacidemia

Isovalericacidemia is similar in its clinical manifestations to the disorders associated with defects in the propionate pathway; however, there are two significant differences:

1. Infants with isovalericacidemia have a "sweaty feet" odor.
2. Glycine therapy is beneficial through enhancement of the formation of isovalerylglycine, a relatively harmless conjugate of isovaleric acid (Fig. 5–9).

Defects in Beta-Oxidation

The catabolism of fatty acids (Fig. 5–10) proceeds through the serial, oxidative removal of acetyl groups (each as acetyl-CoA). The reactions are catalyzed by a group of enzymes that exhibit specificities related to the chain length and other properties of the fatty acids: for example, very-long-chain acyl-CoA dehydrogenase (VLCAD), long-chain acyl-CoA dehydrogenase (LCAD), medium-chain acyl-CoA dehydrogenase (MCAD), short-chain acyl-CoA dehydrogenase

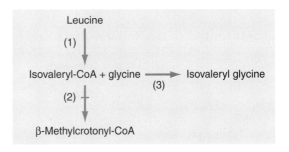

FIG. 5–9

Metabolism in isovalericacidemia: (1) leucine catabolic pathway (transamination and decarboxylation), (2) isovaleryl-CoA dehydrogenase, (3) glycine acyltransferase. *CoA*, Coenzyme A.

(SCAD), and 3-hydroxyacyl-CoA dehydrogenases for at least two chain lengths of fatty acids. *MCAD deficiency* is the most common inborn error of beta-oxidation. The deficiency prominently impairs hepatic adaptation to fasting. It involves failure of normal fatty acid oxidation and of ketone body production and thus a failure to spare glucose utilization.

Hypoketotic hypoglycemia is a common manifestation, as is **Reye syndrome** (encephalopathy and fatty degeneration of the viscera with severe liver dysfunction). Reye syndrome–like illnesses may be recurrent in the patient or the family. Rarely, **sudden infant death syndrome** (SIDS) may occur in infants with MCAD deficiency. Most of the other, much rarer, disorders of fatty acid oxidation tend to involve skeletal and cardiac muscle more than does MCAD (discussed under Type II Glutaric Aciduria later in the chapter). In all of the disorders of beta-oxidation, carnitine depletion can occur through excessive urinary excretion of carnitine and carnityl esters of incompletely oxidized fatty acids.

Hydroxymethylglutaryl-CoA lyase deficiency, although not a disorder of beta-oxidation, interferes profoundly with hepatic adaptation to fasting by impairing ketogenesis (see Fig. 5–10). The *clinical manifestations* are those of MCAD deficiency, except that carnitine depletion is less prominent than in MCAD deficiency because hydroxymethylglutaric acid does not form an ester with carnitine.

The *diagnosis* of disorders involving a deficiency of beta-oxidation is suggested by the clinical picture and by hypoketotic hypoglycemia. The definitive diagnosis is made by analysis of urinary organic acids, acylcarnitine pattern, and enzyme characterization.

Treatment consists of a high-carbohydrate diet, carnitine supplements, avoidance of fasting, and aggressive administration of dextrose during intercurrent stresses.

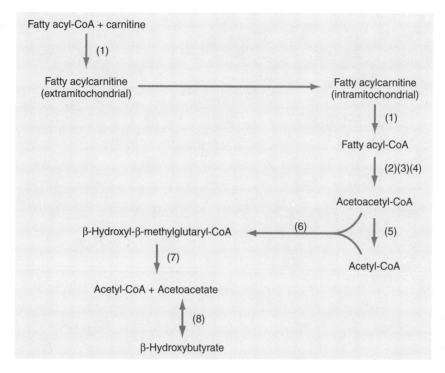

FIG. 5–10

Scheme of fatty acid catabolism and ketone body formation: (1) carnitine acyl-CoA dehydrogenases, (2) long-chain fatty acyl-CoA dehydrogenase, (3) medium-chain fatty acyl-CoA dehydrogenase, (4) short-chain fatty acyl-CoA dehydrogenase, (5) β-ketothiolase, (6) β-hydroxy-β-methylglutaryl-CoA synthase, (7) β-hydroxy-β-methylglutaryl-CoA lyase, (8) β-hydroxybutyrate dehydrogenase.

Carnitine Deficiency

Carnitine is a critically important cofactor in the transport of fatty acids across the mitochondrial inner membrane (Fig. 5–10). It is synthesized from lysine by humans and also is present in dietary red meat and dairy products. Carnitine deficiency is either primary (caused by failure of intake, synthesis, or transport to tissues of carnitine) or more likely secondary (caused by the excretion of excessive amounts of carnitine and carnityl esters in patients with other inborn errors of metabolism). Primary carnitine deficiency has not been defined completely, but there are numerous examples of secondary carnitine deficiency among the organic acidurias, most prominently in disorders of the propionate pathway and in disorders of the beta-oxidation of long- and medium-chain fatty acids.

Clinical manifestations of carnitine deficiency include failure to produce acetoacetic and beta-hydroxybutyric acids, hypoglycemia, lethargy, lassitude, muscle weakness, and cardiomyopathy.

Treatment with carnitine has been dramatically ef-fective in some cases and in general has facilitated the excretion of uncatabolizable organic acids and prevented carnitine depletion.

Biotinidase Deficiency, Beta-Methylcrotonylglycinuria, and Holocarboxylase Deficiency

Biotin is a ubiquitous vitamin that is covalently linked to a number of carboxylases by holocarboxylase synthetase in a variety of tissues. Normal turnover of the carboxylases is accompanied by the freeing of biotin for reuse through the action of biotinidase. Inherited biotinidase deficiency greatly increases the dietary requirement for biotin, with the result that affected individuals can become biotin deficient while consuming normal diets. Clinical disease can appear in the neonatal period or be delayed until later infancy.

The *clinical manifestations* of biotin deficiency vary greatly—seizures, hypotonia, alopecia, skin rash,

TABLE 5–10
Glycogen Storage Diseases

Disease	Affected Enzyme	Organs Affected	Clinical Syndrome	Neonatal Manifestations	Prognosis
Type I: von Gierke	Glucose-6-phosphatase	Liver, kidney, GI tract, platelets	Hypoglycemia, lactic acidosis, hepatomegaly, hypotonia, slow growth, diarrhea, bleeding disorder, gout, hypertriglyceridemia, xanthomas	Hypoglycemia, lactic acidemia, liver may not be enlarged	Early death from hypoglycemia, lactic acidosis; may do well with supportive management; hepatomas occur in late childhood
Type II: Pompe	Lysosomal alpha-glucosidase	All, notably striated muscle, nerve cells	Symmetric profound muscle weakness, cardiomegaly, heart failure, shortened PR interval	May have muscle weakness, cardiomegaly, or both	Very poor; death in the first year of life is usual; variants exist; experimental therapy with recombinant human alpha-glucosidase is promising
Type III: Forbes	Debranching enzyme	Liver, muscles	Early in course hypoglycemia, ketonuria, hepatomegaly that resolves with age; may show muscle fatigue	Usually none	Very good for hepatic disorder; if myopathy present, it tends to be like that of type V
Type IV: Andersen	Branching enzyme	Liver, other tissues	Hepatic cirrhosis beginning at several months of age; early liver failure	Usually none	Very poor; death from hepatic failure before age of 4 years
Type V: McArdle	Muscle phosphorylase	Muscle	Muscle fatigue beginning in adolescence	None	Good, with sedentary lifestyle
Type VI: Hers	Liver phosphorylase	Liver	Mild hypoglycemia with hepatomegaly, ketonuria	Usually none	Probably good
Type VII: Tarui	Muscle phosphofructokinase	Muscle	Clinical findings similar to type V	None	Similar to that of type V
Type VIII	Phosphorylase kinase	Liver	Clinical findings similar to type III, without myopathy	None	Good

GI, Gastrointestinal.
*Except for hepatic phosphorylase kinase, which is X-linked, these disorders are autosomal recessive.

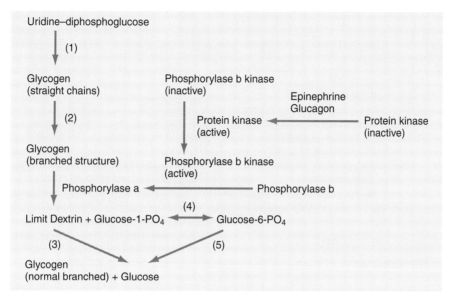

FIG. 5–11

Glycogen synthesis and degradation: (1) glycogen synthetase, (2) brancher enzyme, (3) debrancher enzyme, (4) phosphoglucomutase, (5) glucose-6-phosphatase.

metabolic acidosis, and immune deficits—and undoubtedly are dependent on which enzymes in which tissues bear the brunt of the biotin depletion. Carboxylation is a critical reaction in the metabolism of organic acids; most patients with biotinidase deficiency excrete abnormal amounts of several organic acids, among which beta-methylcrotonylglycine is prominent. In addition to biotinidase deficiency, an inherited deficiency of holocarboxylase synthetase gives rise to severe disease and to similar patterns of organic aciduria. Both conditions respond well to *treatment* with large (10–40 mg/day) doses of biotin.

Glycogen Storage Diseases

The glycogen storage diseases enter into the differential diagnoses of hypoglycemia and hepatomegaly (Table 5–10). Glycogen is the storage form of glucose. It is found most abundantly in the liver, where it serves to modulate blood glucose, and in muscles, where it facilitates anaerobic work.

Glycogen is synthesized from uridine diphosphoglucose through the concerted action of glycogen synthetase and brancher enzyme (Fig. 5–11). The accumulation of glycogen is stimulated by insulin. Glycogenolysis occurs through a cascade phenomenon. This phenomenon is initiated by epinephrine or glucagon. It culminates in rapid phosphorolysis of glycogen to yield glucose-1-phosphate, accompanied by a lesser degree of hydrolysis of glucose residues from the branch points in glycogen molecules (Fig.

5–11). In the liver and kidneys, glucose-1-phosphate can give rise to free glucose through the actions of phosphoglucomutase and glucose-6-phosphatase. The latter enzyme is not present in muscles.

Glycogen storage diseases fall into four categories:

1. Those that predominantly affect the liver and have a direct influence on blood glucose (types I, VI, and VIII)
2. Those that predominantly involve muscles and affect the ability to do anaerobic work (types V and VII)
3. Those that can affect both the liver and muscles and directly influence both blood glucose and muscle metabolism (type III)
4. Those that affect various tissues but have no direct effect on blood glucose or on the ability to do anaerobic work (types II and IV)

In general, the *diagnosis* of hepatic glycogen storage disease can be made noninvasively by testing the response of blood glucose and lactate to glucagon (type I shows no rise in glucose, but a striking increase in lactate), by assaying enzymes (debrancher and brancher enzymes, phosphorylase, and phosphorylase kinase) in white blood cells, and by analyzing the structure of glycogen in erythrocytes. Type IV is best diagnosed by liver biopsy. Glycogen storage disease involving muscles can be assessed by electromyography (pathognomonic changes in type II), by measurement of the response of blood lactate to ischemic exercise (little change in type V in contrast to the normal brisk rise), and by muscle biopsy.

Treatment of hepatic glycogen storage disease is aimed at maintaining satisfactory blood glucose levels. This usually is not difficult, except in glucose-6-phosphatase deficiency (type I), the treatment for which requires nocturnal intragastric feedings of glucose during the first year or two of life. Thereafter, snacks of uncooked cornstarch may be satisfactory, but hepatic tumors (sometimes malignant) are a threat in adolescence and adult life. No specific treatment exists for the diseases of muscle that impair ischemic exercise. Enzyme replacement has been attempted with some success for both of the lethal glycogenoses (types II and IV). Liver transplantation has been carried out successfully for severe hepatic glycogen storage disease.

Familial Hyperlipoproteinemia

Type I Hyperlipoproteinemia

In type I hyperlipoproteinemia (familial hypertriglyceridemia), autosomal recessive deficiency of lipoprotein lipase or of its cofactor, apolipoprotein C-II, leads to the accumulation of chylomicrons in serum. Serum cholesterol levels may exceed 1000 mg/dL, but low-density lipoprotein (LDL) cholesterol is actually low; serum is grossly milky, with an easily visible layer of chylomicrons. This condition is rarer than type II disease.

Clinical manifestations of type I disease include eruptive xanthomata and periodic episodes of severe abdominal pain (pancreatitis), which may begin in infancy as colic. A diet very low in fat may resolve the xanthomatosis and reduces the risk of the painful crises, which are sometimes fatal. Atherosclerotic disease does not occur.

Type II Hyperlipoproteinemia

In type II hyperlipoproteinemia (familial hypercholesterolemia), hepatic clearance of LDL cholesterol is impaired because of genetic defects related to the LDL receptor. This results in large elevations in the level of serum cholesterol (>500 mg/dL) in homozygous individuals and lesser elevations in heterozygous individuals.

The *clinical manifestations* of type II hyperlipoproteinemia include tendinous xanthomata and early atherosclerotic cardiovascular disease; angina pectoris and myocardial infarction may occur during late childhood and adolescence in homozygous individuals. The serum of affected subjects is clear. Liver transplantation is curative if it can be performed in early childhood.

Metabolic Diseases Associated with Dysmorphic Syndrome

Most children who have inborn errors of metabolism are not dysmorphic; conversely, most dysmorphic children do not have currently recognized inborn errors of metabolism. Exceptions include homocystinuria, which can produce Marfan syndrome (discussed earlier in this chapter); the glutaricacidurias; Zellweger syndrome; and the lysosomal storage diseases.

Type I Glutaricaciduria

Type I glutaricaciduria is an autosomal recessive disease produced by deficiency of glutaryl-CoA dehydrogenase activity (Fig. 5–12). *Clinical manifestations* include macrocephaly, which may be present at birth; dystonia, which characteristically develops after 6 months of age; and recurrent acute episodes of hepatic dysfunction, acidosis, hypoglycemia, and hyperammonemia (recurrent Reye syndrome). Intelligence is affected much less than motor function.

Treatment consisting of a low-protein diet, riboflavin, and agents (baclofen or valproic acid) that increase the concentration of gamma-amino butyric acid in the brain appears to be beneficial.

Type II Glutaricaciduria

Type II glutaricaciduria is a clinical disease produced by a defect in the transfer of electrons from flavine adenine nucleotides to the electron transport chain; this defect is caused by a deficiency of either electron transport flavoprotein or electron transfer flavoprotein-ubiquinone oxidoreductase (Fig. 5–12). When the enzyme essentially is nonfunctional, congenital anomalies are common: renal cysts, facial abnormalities, rocker-bottom feet, and hypospadias. Severely affected infants have hypoglycemia without ketosis, metabolic acidosis, and the odor of sweaty feet soon after birth; these infants may die within the neonatal period. Less severely affected infants may have a more episodic, Reye-like illness. Skeletal and cardiac myopathy can be prominent in this complex, pansystemic disease, the manifestations of which may be delayed until adulthood in some cases.

Treatment generally has not been effective in infants, but riboflavin in large doses (100–300 mg/day) has benefited some patients. Glutaricaciduria type II exhibits autosomal recessive inheritance.

Zellweger Syndrome

Zellweger syndrome, an autosomal recessive disease (1:100,000 births), is also known as *cerebrohepatorenal syndrome*. Peroxisomes are virtually absent, as are normal peroxisomal functions, which include the oxidation of very-long-chain fatty acids. Affected infants have high foreheads, flat orbital ridges, widely open fontanels, hepatomegaly, and hypotonia. Other anomalies are common. Failure to thrive, seizures, and nystagmus develop early, and death occurs within the first year. The disease is not

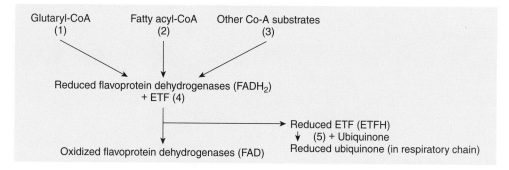

FIG. 5–12

Scheme of flavoprotein metabolism with reference to glutaricaciduria types I and II: (1) glutaryl-CoA dehydrogenase (deficient in glutaricaciduria type I), (2) fatty acyl-CoA dehydrogenases, (3) other flavoprotein dehydrogenases, (4) electron transfer flavoprotein (ETF) (deficiency results in glutaricaciduria type II), (5) ETF-ubiquinone oxidoreductase (deficiency results in glutaricaciduria type II). *CoA,* Coenzyme A.

treatable. *Neonatal adrenoleukodystrophy, infantile Refsum syndrome,* and *rhizomelic chondrodysplasia punctata* are related peroxisomal disorders.

Lysosomal Disorders

Lysosomes are ubiquitous cellular organelles that degrade various cellular constituents, including exogenous constituents, by hydrolysis, then return the products of hydrolysis (amino acids, sugars, and organic acids) to the cytoplasm for use in metabolism. The intralysosomal environment is acidic. The hydrolytic enzymes within are optimally active when the pH is at acid level. The breadth of activity of the enzymes includes virtually any macromolecule, even other enzymes.

Genetic error can occur in the formation of the lysosome and its hydrolytic enzymes, in the mechanisms that protect intralysosomal enzymes from hydrolytic destruction, and in the transport of materials into the lysosome and of metabolites out of the lysosome. The number of genetic errors is large. The clinical disorders are diverse, reflecting both tissue specificity of lysosomal function and the intrinsic turnover rates of the compounds whose cycling is affected. Some disorders affect many tissues but spare the brain, whereas others are apparent only during adult life.

Treatment is now available for some lysosomal disorders. For some individuals, bone marrow transplantation can provide clinically effective restoration of lysosomal function. For others, it is possible to replace a missing hydrolytic enzyme by systemic administration of the enzyme in a form that targets the enzyme for transport into the lysosome. For some diseases it is possible to inhibit synthesis of the moieties that are stored in excess. The diseases that can

be treated should be treated before clinical signs appear. Screening tests for this group of lysosomal disorders are now under investigation.

Some rules of thumb can help in the approach to a specific patient:
1. *Dysostosis multiplex* (gargoylism) is pathognomonic of mucopolysaccharide storage.
2. Macular cherry-red spots, seen on funduscopic examination, are pathognomonic of storage disease affecting the brain and specifically indicate lipid storage.
3. Rapid development of clinical manifestations over the first months of life often implies deficiency affecting more than one cellular constituent and may be associated with storage of both mucopolysaccharide and lipid.
4. Nonimmune hydrops fetalis occurs in several lysosomal disorders.

Table 5–11 presents information regarding some of the known storage diseases. Unless otherwise indicated, the disorder is an autosomal recessive trait.

CONGENITAL DISORDERS OF GLYCOSYLATION (CDG)

Extensive and complex reactions carry out posttranslational glycosylation of proteins and some subsequent modifications of the glycoproteins to produce functional molecules that can be secreted (transport proteins, hormones), components of membranes, or enzymes that must resist degradation. Because of the myriad functions of glycoproteins, disorders involving their synthesis and metabolism are clinically diverse. Their identification is greatly aided by the detection of abnormalities in the glycosylation of transferrin, revealed by isoelectric

TABLE 5–11
Lysosomal Storage Diseases

Disease (Eponym)	Enzyme Deficiency	Clinical Onset	Dysostosis Multiplex	Cornea	Retina
Mucopolysaccharidoses (MPS)					
MPS I (Hurler)	α-L-Iduronidase	~1 yr	Yes	Cloudy	—
MPS II (Hunter)	Iduronate-2-sulfatase	1–2 yr	Yes	Clear	Retinitis, papilledema
MPS III (Sanfilippo)	One of several degrading heparan SO$_4$s	2–6 yr	Mild	Clear	—
MPS IV (Morquio)	Galactose-6-sulfatase or beta-galactosidase	2 yr	No, dwarfism deformities	Faint clouding	—
MPS VI (Maroteaux-Lamy)	N-Acetylgalactosamine-4-sulfatase	2 yr	Yes	Cloudy	—
MPS VII (Sly)	Beta-glucuronidase	Variable neonatal	Yes	± Cloudy	—
Lipidoses					
Glucosylceramide lipidosis 1 (Gaucher 1)	Glucocerebrosidase	Any age	No	Clear	Normal
Glucosylceramide lipidosis 2 (Gaucher 2)	Glucocerebrosidase	Fetal life to 2nd year	No	Clear	Normal
Sphingomyelin lipidosis A (Niemann-Pick A)	Sphingomyelinase	1st mo	No	Clear	Cherry-red spots (50%)
Sphingomyelin lipidosis B (Niemann-Pick B)	Sphingomyelinase	1st mo or later	No	Clear	Normal
Niemann-Pick C	Unknown	Fetal life to adolescence	No	Clear	Normal
GM$_2$ gangliosidosis (Tay-Sachs)	Hexosaminidase A	3–6 mo	No	Clear	Cherry-red spots
Generalized gangliosidosis (infantile) (GM$_1$)	Beta-galactosidase	Neonatal to 1st mo	Yes	Clear	Cherry-red spots (50%)
Metachromatic leukodystrophy	Arylsulfatase A	1–2 yr	No	Clear	Normal
Fabry disease	Alpha-galactosidase A (cerebrosidase)	Childhood, adolescence	No	Cloudy by slit lamp	—
Galactosyl ceramide lipidosis (Krabbe)	Galactocerebroside beta-galactosidase	Early months	No	Clear	Optic atropy
Wolman disease	Acid lipase	Neonatal	No	Clear	Normal
Farber lipogranulomatosis	Acid ceramidase	1st 4 mo	No	Usually clear	Cherry-red spots (12%)

Liver, Spleen	CNS Findings	Stored Material in Urine	WBC/Bone Marrow	Comment	Multiple Forms
Both enlarged	Profound loss of function	Acid mucopoly-saccharide	Alder-Reilly bodies (WBC)	Kyphosis	Yes—Schei and compounds
Both enlarged	Slow loss of function	Acid muco-polysaccharide	Alder-Reilly bodies (WBC)	X-linked	Yes
Liver ± enlarged	Rapid loss of function	Acid muco-polysaccharide	Alder-Reilly bodies (WBC)	—	Several types biochemi-cally
—	Normal	Acid muco-polysaccharide	Alder-Reilly bodies (WBC)	—	Yes
Normal in size	Normal	Acid mucopoly-saccharide	Alder-Reilly bodies (WBC)	—	Yes
Both enlarged	± Affected	Acid mucopoly-saccharide	Alder-Reilly bodies (WBC)	Nonimmune hydrops	Yes
Both enlarged	Normal	No	Gaucher cells in marrow	Bone pain fractures	Variability is the rule
Both enlarged	Profound loss of function	No	Gaucher cells in marrow	—	Yes
Both enlarged	Profound loss of function	No	Foam cells in marrow	—	No
Both enlarged	Normal	No	Foam cells in marrow	—	Yes
Enlarged	Vertical ophthalmo-plegia, dystonia, cataplexy, seizures	No	Foam cells and sea-blue histiocytes in marrow	Pathogenesis not as for NP-A and NP-B	Lethal neona-tal to ado-lescent onset
Normal	Profound loss of function	No	Normal	Sandhoff disease related	Yes
Both enlarged	Profound loss of function	No	Inclusions in WBC	—	Yes
Normal	Profound loss of function	No	Normal	—	Yes
Liver may be large	Normal	No	Normal	X-linked	No
Normal	Profound loss of function	No	Normal	Storage not lysosomal	Yes
Both enlarged	Profound loss of function	No	Inclusions in WBC	—	Yes
May be enlarged	Normal or impaired	Usually not	—	Arthritis, nodules, hoarseness	Yes

Continued

TABLE 5–11
Lysosomal Storage Diseases—cont'd

Disease (Eponym)	Enzyme Deficiency	Clinical Onset	Dysostosis Multiplex	Cornea	Retina
Mucolipidoses (ML) and Clinically Related Disease					
Sialidosis II (formerly ML I)	Neuraminidase	Neonatal	Yes	Cloudy	Cherry-red spot
Sialidosis I (formerly ML I)	Neuraminidase	Usually second decade	No	Fine opacities	Cherry-red spot
Galactosialidosis	Absence of PP/CathA causes loss of neuraminidase and beta-galactosidase	Usually second decade	Frequent	Clouding	Cherry-red spot
ML II (I-cell disease)	Mannosyl phospho-transferase	Neonatal	Yes	Clouding	—
ML III (pseudo-Hurler polydystrophy)	Mannosyl phospho-transferase	2–4 yr	Yes	Late clouding	Normal
Multiple sulfatase deficiency	Many sulfatases	1–2 yr	Yes	Usually clear	Usually normal
Aspartylglycosaminuria	Aspartylglucos-aminidase	6 mo	Mild	Clear	Normal
Mannosidosis	Alpha-mannosidase	1st mo	Yes	Cloudy	—
Fucosidosis	Alpha-L-fucosidase	1st mo	Yes	Clear	May be pigmented
Storage Diseases Caused by Defects in Lysosomal Proteolysis					
Neuronal ceroid lipofuscinosis (NCL), Batten disease	Impaired lysosomal proteolysis—various specific etiologies	6 mo–10 yr, adult form	No	Normal	May have brown pigment
Storage Diseases Caused by Defective Synthesis of the Lysosomal Membrane					
Cardiomyopathy, myopathy, mental retardation, Danon disease	Lamp-2, a structural protein of lysosomes, is deficient	Usually 5–6 yr	No	Normal	Normal
Storage Diseases Caused by Dysfunction of Lysosomal Transport Proteins					
Nephropathic cystinosis	Defect in cystine transport from lysosome to cytoplasm	6 mo–1 yr	No	Cystine crystals	Pigmentary retinopathy
Salla disease	Defect in sialic acid transport from lysosome to cytoplasm	6–9 mo	No	Normal	Normal

Liver, Spleen	CNS Findings	Stored Material in Urine	WBC/Bone Marrow	Comment	Multiple Forms
Both enlarged	Yes	Oligosaccharides	Vacuolated lymphocytes	—	Yes (also see galactosiali-dosis)
Normal	Myoclonus, seizures	Oligosaccharides	Usually none	Cherry-red spot/ myoclonus syndrome	Severity varies
Occasionally enlarged	Myoclonus, seizures Mental retardation	Oligosaccharides	Foamy lymphocytes	Onset, from 1 yr to 40 yr	Congenital and infan-tile forms like sialido-sis 2
Liver often enlarged	Profound loss of function	Oligosaccharides	No	Gingival hyperplasia	No
Normal in size?	Modest loss of function	Oligosaccharides	No	—	No
Both enlarged	Profound loss of function	Acid mucopoly-saccharide	Alder-Reilly bodies (WBC)	Ichthyosis	Yes
Early, not late	Profound loss of function	Aspartylglu-cosamine	Inclusions in lymphocytes	Develop cataracts	No
Liver enlarged	Profound loss of function	Generally no	Inclusions in lymphocytes	Cataracts	Yes
Both enlarged commonly	Profound loss of function	Oligosaccharides	Inclusions in lymphocytes	—	Yes
Normal	Optic atrophy, seizures, dementia			Clinical picture consistent, time course variable	Etiologies dis-tinct for age-related forms
Hepatomegaly	Delayed develop-ment, seizures			X-linked; pedi-atric disease in males only	Variability in time course of signs
Hepatomegaly common	Normal CNS function	Generalized aminoaciduria	Elevated cystine in WBCs	Treatment with cysteamine is effective	Yes
Normal	Delayed development, ataxia, nystagmus, exotropia	Sialic aciduria	Vacuolated lym-phocytes may be found	Growth re-tarded in some	Lethal infan-tile form

TABLE 5–12
Congenital Disorders of Glycosylation

Name	Enzyme Deficient	Hypotonia and Mental Retardation	Cerebellar Hypoplasia	Strabismus	Retinitis Pigmentosa	Hepatomegaly	Renal Cysts	Failure to Thrive	Vomiting and Diarrhea, Enteropathy	Hypoglycemia	Facial Dysmorphism
CDG Ia neurologic	Phosphomannose mutase	++	++	++	++	+/−	+/−	−	−	−	+/− ears
CDG Ia neurovisceral	Phosphomannose mutase	++	+	+	+	++	++	+	+/−		+/− ears
CDG Ib*	Phosphomannose isomerase	−	−	−	−	++	−	++	+++	++	−
CDG IIa	N-Acetylglucosaminyl transferase II	+++	−	−	−	−	−	+	−	−	+++ (ears, nose, mouth)

CDG, Congenital disorders of glycosylation.
*Can be treated with mannose.

focusing (IEF). Specific mutations in enzymes have been identified in a few of the disorders. Mental retardation and hypotonia are common (Table 5–12).

REFERENCES

Behrman RE, Kliegman RM, Jenson HB, editors: *Nelson textbook of pediatrics*, ed 16, Philadelphia, 2000, WB Saunders, Part 10.

Burton BK: Inborn errors of metabolism in infancy: a guide to diagnosis, *Pediatrics* 102(6):E69, 1998.

Kakkis ED, Muenzer J, Tiller GE, et al: Enzyme-replacement therapy in mucopolysaccharidosis I, *N Engl J Med* 344(3):182–188, 2001.

Leonard JV, Morris AAM: Inborn errors of metabolism around time of birth, *Lancet* 356(9229):583–587, 2000.

Leonard JV, Schapira AHV: Mitochondrial respiratory chain disorders 1: mitochondrial DNA defects, *Lancet* 355(9200):299–304, 2000.

Maestri NE, Clissold D, Bruislow SW: Neonatal onset ornithine transcarbamylase deficiency: a retrospective analysis, *J Pediatr* 134(3):268–272, 1999.

National Institutes of Health Consensus Development Conference Statement: *Phenylketonuria: screening and management*, October 16-18, 2000. Available on-line at http://odp.od.nih.gov/consensus/cons/113/113intro.htm.

Norrgard KJ, Pomponio RJ, Hymes J, et al: Mutations causing profound biotinidase deficiency in children ascertained by newborn screening in the United States occur at different frequencies than in symptomatic children, *Pediatr Res* 46(1):20–27, 1999.

Nyhan WL, Rice-Kelts M, Klein J, et al: Treatment of the acute crisis in maple syrup urine disease, *Arch Pediatr Adolesc Med* 152(6):593–598, 1998.

Scriver CR, Beaudet AL, Sly WS, et al, editors: *The metabolic and molecular bases of inherited disease*, ed 8, New York, 2001, McGraw-Hill.

Summar M, Tuchman M: Proceedings of a consensus conference for the management of patients with urea cycle disorders, *J Pediatr* 138(1 Suppl):S6–S10, 2001.

Tegtmeyer-Metzdorf H, Roth B, Günther M, et al: Ketamine and strychnine treatment of an infant with nonketotic hyperglycinemia, *Eur J Pediatr* 154(8):649–653, 1995.

Van Ommen CH, Peters M, Barth PG, et al: Carbohydrate-deficient glycoprotein syndrome type 1a: a variant phenotype with borderline cognitive dysfunction, cerebellar hypoplasia, and coagulation disturbances, *J Pediatr* 136(3):400–403, 2000.

Walter JH, Collins JE, Leonard JV: Recommendations for the management of galactosemia, *Arch Dis Child* 80(1):93–96, 1999.

Wilson CJ, Champion MP, Collins JE, et al: Outcome of medium chain acyl-CoA dehydrogenase deficiency after diagnosis, *Arch Dis Child* 80(5):459–462, 1999.

Winchester B, Vellodi A, Young E: The molecular basis of lysosomal storage diseases and their treatment, *Biochem Soc Trans* 28(2):150–154, 2000.

CHAPTER 6

Fetal and Neonatal Medicine

Robert M. Kliegman

The optimal care of low-risk and high-risk newborn infants requires knowledge of the family history, the history of prior and current pregnancies, and the events of labor and delivery. Thus neonatal medicine, although focused on the care of the infant after birth, requires a comprehensive understanding of the physiology of normal pregnancy; placental and fetal growth, function, and maturity; and any extrauterine or intrauterine pathologic events that affect the mother, placenta, or fetus. These latter adverse effects often are interrelated and may result in an untoward neonatal outcome. They include such significant influences as poor maternal nutrition, poverty, physical or psychologic stresses, extremes of maternal age (<16 years, >35 years), black race, medical illness present prior to pregnancy, obstetric complications during the antepartum and intrapartum periods, perinatal infections, exposure to toxins, and the inherent genetic predisposition of the fetus.

The late fetal–early neonatal period is the time of life with the highest mortality rate of any age interval. *Perinatal mortality* refers to fetal deaths occurring from the twentieth week of gestation until the seventh (or twenty-eighth) day after birth and is expressed as number of deaths per 1000 live births. Intrauterine fetal death represents 40–50% of the perinatal mortality rate. Such infants, defined as *stillborn*, are born without a heart rate and are apneic, limp, pale, and cyanotic. Many exhibit evidence of maceration; pale, peeling skin; corneal opacification; and very soft cranial contents.

The *neonatal mortality rate* includes all infants dying during the period that begins after birth and continues up to the first 28 days of life. This rate also is expressed as number of deaths per 1000 live births. Modern neonatal intensive care has delayed the mortality of many newborn infants who have life-threatening diseases, so that they survive the neonatal period, only to die of their original diseases or of complications of therapy sometime after the twenty-eighth day of life. This delayed mortality, as well as mortality caused by acquired illnesses, occurs during the *postneonatal period*, which begins after 28 days of life and extends to the end of the first year of life.

The *infant mortality rate* encompasses both the neonatal and the postneonatal periods and also is expressed as number of deaths per 1000 live births. The infant mortality rate in the United States declined in 1998 to 7.2:1000; the rate for black infants was approximately 14.3:1000.

The most common causes of perinatal and neonatal death are recorded in Table 6–1. Overall, congenital anomalies and diseases of the premature infant are the most significant causes of neonatal mortality.

Low-birth-weight (LBW) infants, defined as those having birth weights of less than 2500 g, represent a disproportionately large component of the neonatal and infant mortality rates. Although these low-weight births make up only about 6–7% of all births, they account for two thirds of all neonatal deaths.

Very-low-birth-weight (VLBW) infants, weighing less than 1500 g at birth, represent only about 1% of all births but account for 50% of neonatal deaths. In comparison with infants weighing 2500 g or more, LBW infants are 40 times more likely to die in the neonatal period, and VLBW infants have a 200-fold higher risk of neonatal death. In contrast to improvements in the infant mortality rate, there has been no recent improvement in the LBW rate. The LBW rate is one of the major reasons that the infant mortality rate in the United States is high compared with that of other large, modern, industrialized countries. If birth weight–specific mortality rates are calculated, the United States has one of the highest survival rates; because of the large number of LBW infants, the total infant mortality rate remains relatively high.

TABLE 6–1
Major Causes of Perinatal and Neonatal Mortality

Fetus
Placental insufficiency
Intrauterine infection
Severe congenital malformations
Umbilical cord accident
Abruptio placentae
Hydrops fetalis
Multiple gestation

Preterm Infant
Respiratory distress syndrome/bronchopulmonary
  dysplasia*
Severe immaturity
Intraventricular hemorrhage
Congenital anomalies
Infection
Necrotizing entercolitis

Full-Term Infant
Congenital anomalies
Birth asphyxia
Infection
Meconium aspiration pneumonia
Persistent fetal circulation

*Bronchopulmonary dysplasia is also called chronic lung disease.

TABLE 6–2
Identifiable Causes of Preterm Birth

Fetal
Fetal distress
Multiple gestation
Erythroblastosis
Nonimmune hydrops fetalis
Congenital anomalies

Placental
Placenta previa
Abruptio placentae

Uterine
Bicornuate uterus
Incompetent cervix (premature dilation)
Short cervix

Maternal
Preeclampsia
Chronic medical illness (e.g., chronic hypertension or
  cyanotic heart disease)
Infection (e.g., group B streptococcal, herpes simplex,
  syphilis, bacterial vaginosis, genital mycoplasmal,
  and chorioamnionitis)
Drug use (e.g., cocaine)

Other
Premature rupture of membranes
Hydramnios
Iatrogenic (e.g., cesarean section)
Trauma/surgery

Chorioamnionitis is probably a fetal infection too. It is associated with increased risk of neonatal sepsis, respiratory distress syndrome, seizures, intraventricular hemorrhage, periventricular leukomalacia, and cerebral palsy.

Maternal factors associated with a low-weight birth caused by premature birth or intrauterine growth retardation include a previous LBW birth, low socioeconomic status, low level of maternal educational achievement, no antenatal care, maternal age younger than 16 years or older than 35 years, short interval between pregnancies, cigarette smoking, alcohol and illicit drug use, physical (e.g., excessive standing or walking) or psychologic stresses (little social support), unmarried status, low prepregnancy weight (<45 kg or 100 lb) and poor weight gain during pregnancy (<10 lb), and black race. Race is especially significant because LBW and VLBW rates for black women are twice those for white women. In addition, the neonatal and infant mortality rates are twofold higher among black infants. These racial differences are only partly explained by poverty.

In addition to the sociodemographic variables associated with LBW, there are specific, identifiable medical causes of preterm birth (Table 6–2). Factors such as uterine anomalies, hydrops fetalis, and most medical illnesses are not seen more frequently in blacks or in patients of lower socioeconomic status. Prematurity may be caused by spontaneous labor (in 50% of cases), spontaneous rupture of membranes (25%), or premature delivery for maternal or fetal indications (25%).

A comprehensive and multidisciplinary approach is required to identify and care for the high-risk pregnancy and to achieve the optimal neonatal outcome. Appropriate communication between the perinatal obstetrician and the pediatrician is essential. Additionally, the pediatrician must have a detailed, up-to-date understanding of relevant perinatal obstetrics.

REFERENCES

Adams MM, Elam-Evans LD, Wilson HG, et al: Rates of and factors associated with recurrence of preterm delivery, *JAMA* 283(12):1591–1596, 2000.

Barfield WD, Wise PH, Rust FP, et al: Racial disparities in outcomes of military and civilian births in California, *Arch Pediatr Adolesc Med* 150(10):1062–1067, 1996.

Behrman RE, Kliegman RM, Jenson HB, editors: *Nelson textbook of pediatrics,* ed 16, Philadelphia, 2000, WB Saunders, Chapter 89.

Guyer B, Freedman MA, Strobino DM, et al: Annual summary of vital statistics: trends in the health of Americans during the 20th century, *Pediatrics* 106(6):1307–1317.

Sumits T, Bennett R, Gould J: Maternal risks for very low birth weight infant mortality, *Pediatrics* 98(2 pt 1):236–241, 1996.

PERINATAL OBSTETRICS

Risk Assessment

Pregnancies associated with perinatal morbidity or mortality are those considered high risk, and their identification is an essential component of perinatal care. High-risk pregnancies may result in intrauterine fetal death; intrauterine growth retardation; congenital anomalies; excessive fetal growth; birth asphyxia and trauma; prematurity (birth before 38 weeks) or postmaturity (birth at 42 weeks or more); neonatal disease; or the long-term risks of cerebral palsy, mental retardation, and chronic sequelae of neonatal intensive care (Table 6–3). Between 10% and 20% of women can be considered at high risk at some time during their pregnancy. Although some obstetric complications are first seen during labor and delivery and cannot be predicted prior to parturition, many problems are present before labor and delivery. Overall, 50% of perinatal mortality and morbidity results from pregnancies identified before delivery as high risk. After a high-risk pregnancy is identified, measures can be instituted to prevent complications, provide intensive fetal surveillance, and initiate appropriate treatments of the mother and fetus.

Maternal factors associated with high-risk status include the previously mentioned factors associated with LBW births. Additional maternal factors may be identified from past pregnancies. A history of premature birth, intrauterine fetal death, multiple gestation, intrauterine growth retardation, congenital malformation, explained or unexplained neonatal death, birth trauma, preeclampsia, gestational diabetes, grand multipara status (five or more pregnancies), or cesarean section is associated with additional risk for the subsequent pregnancy.

Pregnancy complications during the current gestation that increase risk include placenta previa; abruptio placentae; preeclampsia; diabetes; oligohydramnios or polyhydramnios; multiple gestation; blood group sensitization; abnormal levels of unconjugated estriols, chorionic gonadotropin, or alpha-fetoprotein; abnormal fetal ultrasonography; hydrops fetalis; trauma or surgery; abnormal fetal presentation (breech); exposure to prescribed or illicit drugs; prolonged labor; cephalopelvic disproportion; prolapsed cord; fetal distress; prolonged or premature rupture of membranes; a cervical length <25 mm and the presence of fetal fibronecten in cervical secretions at <35 weeks' gestation; cervical infections and vaginosis; and exposure to rubella, cytomegalovirus, herpes simplex, human immunodeficiency virus (HIV), toxoplasmosis, syphilis, or gonorrhea.

Medical complications associated with increased risk of maternal and fetal morbidity and mortality include maternal diabetes; chronic hypertension; congenital heart disease (especially with right-to-left shunting or Eisenmenger complex); glomerulonephritis; collagen-vascular disease (especially systemic lupus erythematosus with or without antiphospholipid antibodies); lung disease, such as cystic fibrosis; severe anemia, such as sickle cell anemia; hyperthyroidism; myasthenia gravis; idiopathic thrombocytopenic purpura; inborn errors of metabolism, such as maternal phenylketonuria; and malignancy. Furthermore, inheritance of maternal autosomal recessive genes, such as those for cystic fibrosis, galactosemia, and sickle cell anemia, places the newborn infant at increased risk for complications of these diseases; complications may become manifest in utero, in the newborn, or in the older infant.

Obstetric Complications Associated with Fetal or Neonatal Risk

Vaginal bleeding in the first or early second trimester may be caused by a threatened or actual spontaneous abortion. If pregnancy continues, the fetus may be at increased risk for congenital malformations or chromosomal disorders. Vaginal bleeding that is painless, is not associated with labor, and occurs in the late second or (more likely) in the third trimester often is the result of placenta previa. Bleeding develops when the placental mass overlies the internal cervical os; this may produce maternal hemorrhagic shock, necessitating transfusions. The bleeding also may result in premature delivery. Painful vaginal bleeding is often the result of retroplacental hemorrhage and separation of an abruptio placentae. Associated findings may be polyhydramnios, twin gestation, and preeclampsia. Fetal asphyxia will ensue as the retroplacental hematoma causes placental separation that interferes with fetal

TABLE 6-3
Morbidities and Sequelae of Perinatal and Neonatal Illness

Morbidities	Examples
Central Nervous System	
Spastic diplegic-quadriplegic cerebral palsy	Hypoxic-ischemic encephalopathy, perivantricular leukomalacia, undetermined antenatal factors
Choreoathetotic cerebral palsy	Bilirubin encephalopathy (kernicterus)
Microcephaly	Hypoxic-ischemic encephalopathy, intrauterine infection (rubella, CMV)
Communicating hydrocephalus	Intraventricular hemorrhage, meningitis
Seizures	Hypoxic-ischemic encephalopathy, hypoglycemia
Encephalopathy	Congenital infections (rubella, CMV, human immunodeficiency virus, toxoplasmosis)
Educational failure	Immaturity, hypoxia, low socioeconomic status
Mental retardation	Hypoxia, hypoglycemia, cerebral palsy, intraventricular hemorrhage
Sensation-Peripheral Nerves	
Reduced visual acuity (blindness)	Retinopathy of prematurity (ROP)
Strabismus	Undetermined
Hearing impairment (deafness)	Drug toxicity (furosemide, aminoglycosides), bilirubin encephalopathy, hypoxia ± hyperventilation
Poor speech	Immaturity, chronic illness, hypoxia, prolonged endotracheal intubation, hearing deficit
Paralysis-paresis	Birth trauma—brachial plexus, phrenic nerve, spinal cord
Respiratory	
Chronic lung disease (CLD)	Oxygen toxicity, barotrauma
Subglottic stenosis	Endotracheal tube injury
Sudden infant death syndrome	Prematurity, BPD, infant of illicit drug user
Choanal stenosis, nasal septum destruction	Nasotracheal intubation
Cardiovascular	
Cyanosis	Precorrective palliative care of congenital cyanotic heart disease, cor pulmonale from BPD, reactive airway disease
Heart failure	Precorrective palliative care of complex congenital heart disease, BPD, ventricular septal defect
Gastrointestinal	
Short gut syndrome	Necrotizing enterocolitis, gastroschisis, malrotation-volvulus, cystic fibrosis, intestinal atresias
Cholestatic liver disease (cirrhosis, hepatic failure)	Hyperalimentation toxicity, sepsis, short gut syndrome
Failure to thrive	Short gut syndrome, cholestasis, BPD, cerebral palsy, severe congenital heart disease
Inguinal hernia	Unknown
Miscellaneous	
Cutaneous scars	Chest tube or IV placement; hyperalimentation subcutaneous infiltration; fetal puncture; intrauterine varicella; aplasia cutis
Absent radial artery pulse	Frequent arterial punctures
Hypertension	Renal thrombi: repair of coarctation of aorta

From Stoll BJ, Kliegman RM: The fetus and neonatal infant. In Berhman RE, Kliegman RM, Jenson HB, editors: *Nelson textbook of pediatrics,* ed 16, Philadelphia, 2000, WB Saunders.
BPD, Bronchopulmonary dysplasia; *CMV,* cytomegalovirus.

oxygenation. Both types of bleeding are associated with fetal blood loss. Neonatal anemia may be more common with placenta previa.

Abnormalities in the volume of amniotic fluid, resulting in oligohydramnios or polyhydramnios, are associated with increased fetal and neonatal risk. **Oligohydramnios** (amniotic ultrasound fluid index ≤2 cm) is associated with intrauterine growth retardation and major congenital anomalies, particularly of the fetal kidneys. It is also associated with chromosomal syndromes. Bilateral renal agenesis results in diminished production of amniotic fluid. It also results in a specific deformation syndrome **(Potter syndrome)** that is indicated by clubfeet, characteristic compressed facies, low-set ears, scaphoid abdomen, and diminished chest wall size that is accompanied by pulmonary hypoplasia and often by pneumothorax. Uterine compression in the absence of amniotic fluid retards lung growth, and patients with this condition die of respiratory failure rather than because of renal insufficiency. Twin-twin transfusion syndrome (donor) and complications from amniotic fluid leakage also are associated with oligohydramnios. Oligohydramnios increases the risk of fetal distress during labor (because of meconium-stained fluid and variable decelerations); the risk may be reduced by saline amnioinfusion during labor.

Polyhydramnios may be acute and may be associated with premature labor, maternal discomfort, and respiratory compromise. More often, polyhydramnios is chronic and is associated with diabetes, immune or nonimmune hydrops fetalis, multiple gestation, trisomy 18 or 21, and major congenital anomalies. Anencephaly, hydrocephaly, and meningomyelocele are neurologic problems associated with reduced fetal swallowing. Esophageal and duodenal atresia and cleft palate interfere with swallowing and gastrointestinal fluid dynamics. Additional causes of polyhydramnios include Werdnig-Hoffmann and Beckwith-Wiedemann syndromes, conjoined twins, chylothorax, cystic adenomatoid lung malformation, diaphragmatic hernia, gastroschisis, sacral teratoma, placental chorioangioma, and myotonic dystrophy. **Hydrops fetalis** may be a result of Rh or other blood group incompatibilities and anemia caused by intrauterine hemolysis of fetal erythrocytes by maternal immunoglobulin G (IgG)–sensitized antibodies crossing the placenta. Hydrops is characterized by fetal edema, ascites, hypoalbuminemia, and congestive heart failure. Causes of **nonimmune hydrops** include fetal supraventricular tachycardia, fetal anemia (resulting from bone marrow suppression, nonimmune hemolysis, or twin-twin transfusion), severe congenital malformation, intrauterine infections, congenital neuroblastoma, inborn errors of metabolism (storage diseases), fetal hepatitis, nephrotic syndrome, and pulmonary lymphangiectasia. Twin-twin transfusion syndrome (recipient) also may be associated with polyhydramnios. Polyhydramnios is often the result of unknown causes. If severe, polyhydramnios may be managed with bed rest, indomethacin, or serial amniocenteses.

Premature rupture of the membranes, which occurs in the absence of labor, and *prolonged rupture of the membranes* for more than 24 hours are both associated with an increased risk of maternal or fetal infection (chorioamnionitis) and preterm birth. Typically, group B streptococcus, *Escherichia coli,* and *Listeria monocytogenes* are associated with fetal infection, although *Mycoplasma hominis, Ureaplasma urealyticum, Chlamydia trachomatis,* and anaerobic bacteria of the vaginal flora also have been implicated in infection of the amniotic fluid. The risk of serious fetal infection increases as the length of time between rupture and labor (latent period) increases, especially if the period is greater than 24 hours. Antibiotic therapy increases the latency period to delivery and decreases the risks of neonatal sepsis and respiratory distress syndrome (RDS).

Multiple gestation is associated with increased risk resulting from polyhydramnios, premature birth, intrauterine growth retardation, abnormal presentation (breech), congenital anomalies (such as intestinal atresia, porencephaly, and single umbilical artery), intrauterine fetal demise, birth asphyxia, and the **twin-twin transfusion syndrome.** Twin-twin transfusion syndrome is associated with a high mortality and is seen only in monozygotic twins who share a common placenta and demonstrate an arteriovenous connection between their circulations. The fetus on the arterial side of the shunt serves as the blood donor, which results in its fetal anemia, growth retardation, and oligohydramnios. The recipient, or venous-side twin, is larger, or discordant in size; is plethoric and polycythemic; and may demonstrate polyhydramnios. Weight differences of 20% and hemoglobin differences of 5 g/dL suggest the diagnosis. Ultrasonography in the second trimester reveals discordant amniotic fluid volume with oliguria-oligohydramnios (stuck twin syndrome, against the uterine wall) and hypervolemia-polyuria-polyhydramnios with a distended bladder, with or without hydrops and heart failure. Mortality is high if presentation occurs in the second trimester; however, most monochorionic twins have bidirectional balanced shunts and are not affected. Treatment includes amniocentesis and attempts to ablate the arteriovenous connection (using a laser). In addition to the twin-twin transfusion syndrome, the birth order of twins also affects morbidity by increasing the risk of the second-born twin for breech position, birth asphyxia, birth trauma, and RDS.

Overall, twinning is observed in 1:80 pregnancies, and 80% of all twin gestations are dizygotic twins. The diagnosis of the type of twins can be determined by placentation, sex, fetal membrane structure, and, if necessary, tissue and blood group typing.

Toxemia of pregnancy, or preeclampsia-eclampsia, is a disorder of unknown but probably vascular etiology that may lead to maternal hypertension, uteroplacental insufficiency, intrauterine growth retardation, intrauterine asphyxia, maternal seizures, and maternal death. Toxemia is more common in nulliparous women and in women with twin gestation, chronic hypertension, obesity, renal disease, a positive family history of toxemia, or diabetes mellitus. A subcategory of preeclampsia, the HELLP syndrome (*h*emolysis, *e*levated *l*iver enzyme levels, *l*ow *p*latelets) is more severe and is often associated with a fetal inborn error of fatty acid oxidation (long-chain hydroxyacyl-CoA dehydrogenase of the trifunctional protein complex).

Medical Problems During Pregnancy Associated with Fetal or Neonatal Risk

Diseases presenting during pregnancy can affect the fetus directly or indirectly (Table 6–4). Various immunologically mediated diseases affecting maternal

---

TABLE 6–4
Maternal Disease Affecting the Fetus or Neonate

Disorder	Effects	Mechanism
Cyanotic heart disease	Intrauterine growth retardation	Low fetal oxygen delivery
Diabetes mellitus		
Mild	Large for gestational age, hypoglycemia	Fetal hyperglycemia—produces hyperinsulinemia; insulin promotes growth
Severe	Growth retardation	Vascular disease, placental insufficiency
Drug addiction	Intrauterine growth retardation, neonatal withdrawal	Direct drug effect, plus poor diet
Endemic goiter	Hypothyroidism	Iodine deficiency
Graves disease	Transient thyrotoxicosis	Placental immunoglobulin passage of thyrotropin receptor antibody
Hyperparathyroidism	Hypocalcemia	Maternal calcium crosses to fetus and suppresses fetal parathyroid gland
Hypertension	Intrauterine growth retardation, intrauterine fetal demise	Placental insufficiency, fetal hypoxia
Idiopathic thrombocytopenia	Thrombocytopenia	Nonspecific platelet antibodies cross placenta
Infection	See Table 6–28	
Isoimmune neutropenia or thrombocytopenia	Neutropenia or thrombocytopenia	Specific antifetal neutrophil or platelet antibody crosses placenta following sensitization of mother
Malignant melanoma	Placental or fetal tumor	Metastasis
Myasthenia gravis	Transient neonatal myasthenia	Immunoglobulin to acetylcholine receptor crosses the placenta
Myotonic dystrophy	Neonatal myotonic dystrophy	Autosomal dominant with genetic anticipation
Phenylketonuria	Microcephaly, retardation, ventricular septal defect	Elevated fetal phenylalanine levels
Rh or other blood group sensitization	Fetal anemia, hypoalbuminemia, hydrops, neonatal jaundice	Antibody crosses placenta directed at fetal cells with antigen
Systemic lupus erythematosus	Congenital heart block, rash, anemia, thrombocytopenia, neutropenia, cardiomyopathy, stillbirth	Antibody directed at fetal heart, red and white blood cells, and platelets; lupus anticoagulant

From Stoll BJ, Kliegman RM: The fetus and neonatal infant. In Berhman RE, Kliegman RM, Jenson HB, editors: *Nelson textbook of pediatrics*, ed 16, Philadelphia, 2000, WB Saunders.

tissues are caused by autoantibodies; such antibodies also may cross the placenta. Because IgG immunoglobulins are transported actively across the placenta during the second half of the third trimester, all IgG class antibodies will be present in the fetus. Pathologic antibodies can affect the same tissue in the fetus as in the mother. Other maternal illnesses, such as severe pulmonary disease (cystic fibrosis), cyanotic heart disease, and sickle cell anemia, may reduce oxygen availability to the fetus. Severe hypertensive or diabetic vasculopathy can result in uteroplacental insufficiency.

Diabetes mellitus that develops during pregnancy (gestational diabetes is noted in about 5% of women) or diabetes that is present before pregnancy adversely influences fetal and neonatal well-being (Fig. 6–1). The effect of the diabetes on the fetus depends in part on the severity of the diabetic state: age of onset of diabetes, duration of treatment with insulin, and the presence of arterial disease. Poorly controlled maternal diabetes leads to maternal hyperglycemia, which in turn, because glucose levels in the fetus are slightly lower than but directly proportional to maternal glucose values, produces fetal hyperglycemia that stimulates the fetal pancreas, resulting in hyperplasia of the islets of Langerhans. Fetal hyperinsulinemia, which acts as a fetal growth hormone in the last trimester, results in increased fat and protein synthesis and fetal macrosomia, producing a fetus that is large for gestational age. After birth, hyperinsulinemia persists, resulting in fasting neonatal hypoglycemia. Strictly controlling maternal diabetes during pregnancy and preventing hyperglycemia during labor and delivery prevent macrosomic fetal growth and neonatal hypoglycemia, respectively. Additional problems of the diabetic mother and her fetus and newborn are noted in Table 6–5.

In addition to the fact that the fetus is directly affected by maternal illnesses, both the fetus and the newborn may be adversely affected by the medications used to treat those maternal illnesses. These effects may appear as teratogenesis (Table 6–6) or as an adverse metabolic, neurologic, or cardiopulmonary adaptation to extrauterine life (Table 6–7).

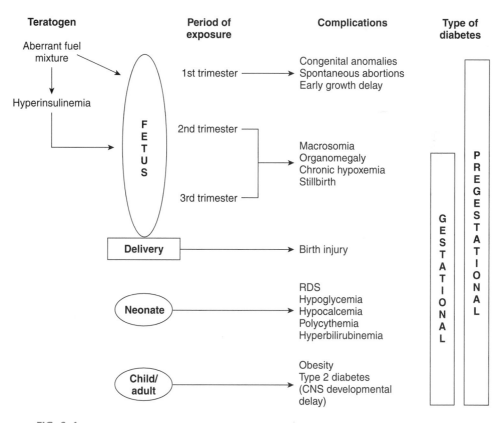

FIG. 6–1

Diagrammatic representation of the multiple deleterious effects of the pregnancy of a diabetic patient on the offspring, during various periods of fetal and postnatal life. *CNS,* Central nervous system; *RDS,* respiratory distress syndrome. (From Inzucchi SE: Diabetes in pregnancy. In Burrow GN, Duffy TP, editors: *Medical complications during pregnancy,* ed 5, Philadelphia, 1999, WB Saunders.)

TABLE 6–5
Problems of the Diabetic Pregnancy

Maternal	Neonatal—cont'd
Ketoacidosis	Transient tachypnea of newborn
Hypoglycemia	Hypoglycemia
Preeclampsia	Hypocalcemia
Polyhydramnios	Polycythemia
Retinopathy	Unconjugated hyperbilirubinemia
	Congenital malformations (heart, sacrum)
Neonatal	Cardiac septal hypertrophy (hypertrophic
Prematurity	cardiomyopathy)
Macrosomia and birth trauma	Small left colon syndrome
Birth asphyxia	Renal vein thrombosis
Respiratory distress syndrome	Intrauterine fetal death

TABLE 6–6
Common Teratogenic Drugs

Drug	Results
Alcohol	Fetal alcohol syndrome, microcephaly, congenital heart disease
Aminopterin	Mesomelia, cranial dysplasia
Coumarin	Hypoplastic nasal bridge, chondrodysplasia punctata
Fluoxetine	Minor malformations, low birth weight, poor neonatal adaptation
Folic acid antagonists*	Neural tube, cardiovascular, renal, and oral cleft defects
Isotretinoin (Accutane) and vitamin A	Facial and ear anomalies, congenital heart disease
Lithium	Ebstein anomaly
Methyl mercury	Microcephaly, blindness, deafness, retardation (Minimata disease)
Misoprostol	Arthrogryposis
Penicillamine	Cutis laxa syndrome
Phenytoin (Dilantin)	Hypoplastic nails, intrauterine growth retardation, typical facies
Radioactive iodine	Fetal hypothyroidism
Radiation	Microcephaly
Stilbestrol (DES)	Vaginal adenocarcinoma during adolescence
Streptomycin	Deafness
Testosterone-like drugs	Virilization of female
Tetracycline	Enamel hypoplasia
Thalidomide	Phocomelia
Toluene (solvent abuse)	Fetal alcohol–like syndrome, preterm labor
Trimethadione	Congenital anomalies, typical facies
Valproate	Spina bifida
Vitamin D	Supravalvular aortic stenosis

*Trimethoprim, triamterene, phenytoin, primidone, phenobarbitol, carbamazepine.

Acquired infectious diseases of the mother also may affect the fetus or newborn adversely (Table 6–30).

Assessment of Fetal Well-Being and Maturity

Fetal Growth

Fetal growth can be assessed clinically by determining the fundal height of the uterus through bimanual examination of the gravid abdomen. In addition, ultrasonographic measurement of the fetal biparietal diameter, femur length, and abdominal circumference all have been used to estimate fetal growth. A combination of these measurements predicts fetal weight. Deviations from the normal fetal growth curve are associated with high-risk conditions.

Intrauterine growth retardation is present when fetal growth stops and, over time, falls below the 5th percentile of growth for gestational age or when growth proceeds slowly but absolute size remains below the 5th percentile (Fig. 6–2). Growth retardation may result from fetal conditions that reduce the innate growth potential, such as fetal rubella infection, primordial dwarfing syndromes, chromosomal

---

TABLE 6–7
Agents Acting on Pregnant Women That May Adversely Affect the Newborn Infant

Agent	Potential Condition(s)
Acebutolol	IUGR, hypotension, bradycardia
Acetazolamide	Metabolic acidosis
Adrenal corticosteroids	Adrenocortical failure (rare)
Amiodarone	Bradycardia, hypothyroidism
Ammonium chloride	Acidosis (clinically inapparent)
Anesthetic agents (volatile)	CNS depression
Aspirin	Neonatal bleeding, prolonged gestation
Atenolol	IUGR, hypoglycemia
Blue cohosh herbal tea	Neonatal heart failure
Bromides	Rash, CNS depression, IUGR
Captopril, enalopril	Transient anuric renal failure, oligohydramnios
Caudal-paracervical anesthesia with mepivacaine (accidental introduction of anesthetic into scalp of baby)	Bradypnea, apnea, bradycardia, convulsions
Cholinergic agents (edrophonium, pyridostigmine)	Transient muscle weakness
CNS depressants (narcotics, barbiturates, benzodiazepines) during labor	CNS depression, hypotonia
Cephalothin	Positive direct Coombs test reaction
Fluoxetine	Possible transient neonatal withdrawal, hypertonicity, minor anomalies
Haloperidol	Withdrawal
Hexamethonium bromide	Paralytic ileus
Ibuprofen	Oligohydramnios, PFC
Imipramine	Withdrawal
Indomethacin	Oliguria, oligohydramnios, intestinal perforation, PFC
Intravenous fluids during labor (e.g., salt-free solutions)	Electrolyte disturbances, hyponatremia, hypoglycemia
Iodide (radioactive)	Goiter
Iodides	Neonatal goiter

From Stoll BJ, Kliegman RM: The fetus and neonatal infant. In Berhman RE, Kliegman RM, Jenson HB, editors: *Nelson textbook of pediatrics,* ed 16, Philadelphia, 2000, WB Saunders.
CNS, Central nervous system; *G6PD,* glucose-6-phosphate dehydrogenase; *IUGR,* intrauterine growth retardation; *PFC,* persistent fetal circulation.

Continued

TABLE 6–7
Agents Acting on Pregnant Women that May Adversely Affect the Newborn Infant—cont'd

Agent	Potential Condition(s)
Isoxsuprine	Ileus, hypocalcemia, hypoglycemia, hypotension
Lead	Reduced intellectual function
Magnesium sulfate	Respiratory depression, meconium plug, hypotonia
Methimazole	Goiter, hypothyroidism
Morphine and its derivatives (addiction)	Withdrawal symptoms (poor feeding, vomiting, diarrhea, restlessness, yawning and stretching, dyspnea and cyanosis, fever and sweating, pallor, tremors, convulsions)
Naphthalene	Hemolytic anemia (in G6PD-deficient infants)
Nitrofurantoin	Hemolytic anemia (in G6PD-deficient infants)
Oxytocin	Hyperbilirubinemia, hyponatremia
Phenobarbital	Bleeding diathesis (vitamin K deficiency), possible long-term reduction in IQ, sedation
Primaquine	Hemolytic anemia (in G6PD-deficient infants)
Propranolol	Hypoglycemia, bradycardia, apnea
Propylthiouracil (PTU)	Goiter, hypothyrodism
Pyridoxine	Seizures
Reserpine	Drowsiness, nasal congestion, poor temperature stability
Silicone breast implants	Possible esophageal dysmotility in breast-fed infants
Sulfonamides	Interfere with protein binding of bilirubin; kernicterus at low levels of serum bilirubin, hemolysis with G6PD deficiency
Sulfonylurea	Refractory hypoglycemia
Sympathomimetic (tocolytic-β agonist) agents	Tachycardia
Thiazides	Neonatal thrombocytopenia (rare)

From Stoll BJ, Kliegman RM: The fetus and neonatal infant. In Berhman RE, Kliegman RM, Jenson HB, editors: *Nelson textbook of pediatrics*, ed 16, Philadelphia, 2000, WB Saunders.
CNS, Central nervous system; *G6PD*, glucose-6-phosphate dehydrogenase; *IUGR* intrauterine growth retardation.

TABLE 6–8
Problems of Intrauterine Growth Retardation (Small for Gestational Age)

Problem*	Pathogenesis
Intrauterine fetal demise	Hypoxia, acidosis, infection, lethal anomaly
Perinatal asphyxia	↓ Uteroplacental perfusion during labor ± chronic fetal hypoxia-acidosis; meconium aspiration syndrome
Hypoglycemia	↓ Tissue glycogen stores, ↓ gluconeogenesis, hyperinsulinism, ↑ glucose needs of hypoxia, hypothermia, large brain
Polycythemia-hyperviscosity	Fetal hypoxia with ↑ erythropoietin production
Reduced oxygen consumption/hypothermia	Hypoxia, hypoglycemia, starvation effect, poor subcutaneous fat stores
Dysmorphology	Syndrome anomalads, chromosomal-genetic disorders, oligohydramnios-induced deformations, TORCH infection

Modified from Stoll BJ, Kliegman RM: The high-risk infant. In Behrman RE, Kliegman RM, Jenson HB, editors: *Nelson textbook of pediatrics*, ed 16, Philadelphia, 2000, WB Saunders.
TORCH, Toxoplasmosis, other (syphilis, hepatitis, zoster), rubella, cytomegalovirus, and herpes simplex.
*Other problems include pulmonary hemorrhage and those common to the gestational age–related risks of prematurity if born before 37 weeks.

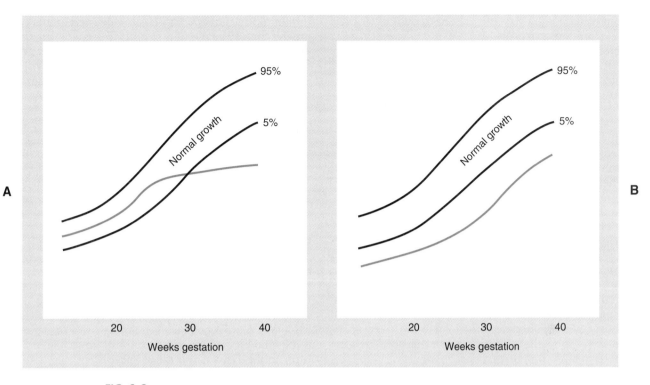

FIG. 6–2

Hypothetical fetal growth curves depicting two patterns of intrauterine growth retardation. **A,** In this pattern, there is normal fetal growth during the 20th to 30th week of gestation. Thereafter, fetal growth stops and the fetal growth parameter (biparietal diameter, abdominal circumference, and femur length) falls below 5%. In contrast to weight, head growth is usually spared and less severely affected. This "late flattening" pattern is noted in the donor twin involved in a twin-twin transfusion syndrome, in a fetus supplied by poor maternal nutrition, and in those growing within an environment of maternal preeclampsia. Catch-up growth is common after delivery from the adverse in utero environment. **B,** Fetal growth parameters are persistently below 5%. These fetuses demonstrate continued growth, albeit at a reduced rate. Fetuses with this "low-profile" pattern may have reduced growth potential, as noted in those with intrauterine viral infections, chromosome disorders, or malformation syndromes. Fetuses born to mothers who themselves were small for gestational age and who demonstrate reduced prepregnancy weight often have this characteristic growth profile. Some of these fetuses are normal in all other parameters except that they exhibit reduced intrauterine growth.

abnormalities, and congenital malformation syndromes. Reduced fetal production of insulin and insulin-like growth factor I (IGF-I) is associated with fetal growth retardation. Placental causes of intrauterine growth retardation include villitis (congenital infections), placental tumors, chronic abruptio placentae, twin-twin transfusions, and placental insufficiency. Maternal causes include severe peripheral vascular diseases that reduce uterine blood flow, such as chronic hypertension, diabetic vasculopathy, and preeclampsia-eclampsia. Additional maternal causes include reduced nutritional intake; alcohol or drug abuse; cigarette smoking; and uterine constraint, noted predominantly in mothers of small stature with a low prepregnancy weight and reduced weight gain during pregnancy. The outcome of intrauterine growth retardation of the fetus or newborn depends on the cause of the reduced fetal growth and the associated complications after birth (Table 6–8). Fetuses subjected to chronic intrauterine hypoxia as a result of uteroplacental insufficiency are at an increased risk for the comorbidities of birth asphyxia, polycythemia, and hypoglycemia. Fetuses with reduced tissue mass resulting from chromosomal, metabolic, or multiple congenital anomaly syndromes have poor outcomes based on the prognosis for the particular syndrome. Fetuses born to small mothers and fetuses with poor nutritional intake usually do well and demonstrate catch-up growth after birth.

Fetal Maturity

Fetal size can be accurately determined by means of ultrasonographic techniques. Unfortunately, fetal size does not always correlate with functional or structural maturity. Determining maturity is critical when a decision has been made to deliver a fetus because of fetal distress or severe maternal preeclampsia. Fetal gestational age may be determined accurately on the basis of a correct estimate of the last menstrual period. Furthermore, clinically relevant landmark dates can be used to determine gestational age; the first audible heart tones by fetoscope are detected at 18–20 weeks (12–14 weeks by Doppler methods), and quickening of fetal movements is usually perceived at 18–20 weeks. However, it is not always possible to determine fetal maturity by such dating, especially in a high-risk situation such as preterm labor or a diabetic pregnancy.

Fetal pulmonary maturity may be determined through examination of the profile of phospholipids present in the amniotic fluid. Surfactant, a combination of surface active phospholipids and proteins, is produced by the maturing fetal lung and eventually is secreted into the amniotic fluid. The amount of surfactant in amniotic fluid is a direct reflection of surface active material in the fetal lung and can be used to predict the presence or absence of pulmonary maturity. Because dipalmityl phosphatidylcholine, or lecithin, is a principal component of surfactant, the determination of lecithin in amniotic fluid is used to predict a mature fetus. Lecithin concentration increases with increasing gestational age, commencing at 32–34 weeks. This is discussed further under Lung Development in the Respiratory Distress Syndrome section later in this chapter.

Assessment of Fetal Well-Being

Methods used to assess fetal well-being before the onset of labor are focused on identifying the fetus at risk for asphyxia or the fetus who has hypoxia and is already compromised by uteroplacental insufficiency. The *oxytocin challenge test* simulates uterine contractions through an infusion of oxytocin sufficient to produce three contractions in a 10-minute period. The development of periodic fetal bradycardia out of phase with uterine contractions (late deceleration) is a positive test result and predicts the fetus at risk.

The *nonstress test* examines the heart rate response to fetal body movements. Heart rate increments of greater than 15 beats/min, lasting 15 seconds, are reassuring. If two such episodes occur in 30 minutes, the test result is considered reactive (versus nonreactive) and the fetus is not at risk. Additional signs of fetal well-being are fetal breathing movements, gross body movements, fetal tone, and the presence of amniotic fluid pockets of greater than 2 cm, as noted by ultrasound. The *biophysical profile* combines the nonstress test with these four parameters and offers the most accurate fetal assessment.

Doppler examination of the fetal aorta or umbilical arteries can permit identification of decreased or reversed diastolic blood flow, which is associated with increased peripheral vascular resistance, fetal hypoxia with acidosis, and placental insufficiency. *Cordocentesis* (percutaneous umbilical blood sampling) can provide fetal blood for PO_2, pH, lactate, and hemoglobin measurements. These values can be used to identify the hypoxic, acidotic, or anemic fetus who is at risk for intrauterine fetal demise or birth asphyxia. Cordocentesis also can be used to determine fetal blood type, platelet count, microbial culture, antibody titer, and rapid karyotype.

In the high-risk pregnancy, the fetal heart rate should be monitored continuously, as should uterine contractions during labor. Fetal heart rate abnormalities may indicate baseline tachycardia (>160 beats/min as a result of anemia, beta-sympathomimetic drugs, maternal fever, hyperthyroidism, arrhythmia, or fetal distress); baseline bradycardia (<120 beats/min as a result of fetal distress, complete heart block, or local anesthetics); or reduced beat-to-beat variability (flattened tracing resulting from fetal sleep, tachycardia, atropine, sedatives, prematurity, or fetal distress). In addition, periodic changes of the heart rate relative to the tracing of uterine pressure help determine the presence of hypoxia and acidosis caused by uteroplacental insufficiency or maternal hypotension (late or type II decelerations) or by umbilical cord compression (variable decelerations). In the presence of severe decelerations (any late or repeated prolonged variable), a fetal scalp blood-gas level should be obtained to assess fetal acidosis. A scalp pH of less than 7.20 indicates fetal hypoxic compromise. A pH between 7.20 and 7.25 is in a borderline zone and warrants repeating the test.

Fetal anomalies may be detected by ultrasonography; emphasis should be placed on visualization of the genitourinary tract; the head (for anencephaly or hydrocephaly), neck (for thickened nuchal translucency), and back (for spina bifida); the skeleton; the gastrointestinal tract; and the heart. Four-chamber and great artery views are required for detection of heart anomalies. *Chromosomal anomaly syndromes* may reveal choroid cysts, hypoplasia of the middle phalanx of the fifth digit, nuchal fluid, retrognathism, and low-set ears. In addition, chromosomal syndromes are often associated with an abnormal "triple test" (low estriols, low maternal serum alpha-fetoprotein levels, and elevated placental chorionic gonadotropin levels).

If a fetal abnormality is detected, fetal therapy (Table 6–9) or delivery with therapy in the neonatal intensive care unit may be lifesaving.

Delivery Room Care: Resuscitation

The approach to the birth of an infant, just as with the approach to any other medical situation, requires a detailed history (Table 6–10). Knowing the mother's risk factors (e.g., demographic risks and past and present medical illnesses, including a drug history, the prior pregnancy, and the problems of the current pregnancy) enables the delivery room team to anticipate problems that may occur after birth.

TABLE 6–9
Fetal Therapy

Disorder	Possible Treatment
Hematology	
Anemia with hydrops (erythroblastosis fetalis)	Umbilical vein packed red blood cell transfusion
Thalassemia	Fetal stem cell transplantation
Thrombocytopenia	
Isoimmune	Umbilical vein platelet transfusion, maternal intravenous immunoglobulin
Autoimmune (ITP)	Maternal steroids and intravenous immunoglobulin
Chronic granulomatous disease	Fetal stem cell transplantation
Metabolic-Endocrine	
Maternal PKU	Phenylaline restriction
Fetal galactosemia	Galactose-free diet (?)
Multiple carboxylase deficiency	Biotin if responsive
Methylmalonic acidemia	Vitamin B_{12} if responsive
21-Hydroxylase deficiency	Dexamethasone
Maternal diabetes mellitus	Tight insulin control during pregnancy, labor, and delivery
Fetal goiter	Maternal hyperthyroidism—maternal propylthiouracil
	Fetal hypothyroidism—intraamniotic T_4
Fetal Distress	
Hypoxia	Maternal oxygen, position
Intrauterine growth retardation	Maternal oxygen, position, improve nutrition if deficient
Oligohydramnios, premature rupture of membranes with variable deceleration	Amnioinfusion (antepartum and intrapartum)
Polyhydramnios	Amnioreduction (serial), indomethacin (if due to ↑ urine output) if indicated
Supraventricular tachycardia	Maternal digoxin,* flecainide, procainamide, amiodarone, quinidine
Lupus anticoagulant	Maternal aspirin, prednisone
Meconium-stained fluid	Amnioinfusion
Congenital heart block	Dexamethasone, pacemaker (with hydrops)
Premature labor	Sympathomimetics, magnesium sulfate, antibiotics

From Stoll BJ, Kliegman RM: The fetus. In Berhman RE, Kliegman RM, Jenson HB, editors: *Nelson textbook of pediatrics,* ed 16, Philadelphia, 2000, WB Saunders.
(?) denotes possible but not proved efficacy.
*Drug of choice (may require percutaneous umbilical cord sampling and umbilical vein administration if hydrops is present). Most drug therapy is given to the mother, with subsequent placental passage to the fetus.

Continued

TABLE 6–9
Fetal Therapy—cont'd

Disorder	Possible Treatment
Respiratory	
Pulmonary immaturity	Dexamethasone, betamethasone
Bilateral chylothorax–pleural effusions	Thoracentesis, pleuroamniotic shunt
Congenital Abnormalities†	
Neural tube defects	Folate, vitamins (preventions)
Diaphragmatic hernia	Surgery (correction or tracheal plug therapy) (?)
Obstructive uropathy (with oligohydramnios without renal dysplasia)	>24 wk <32 wk, vesicoamniotic shunt plus amniofusion, ablation of posterior urethral valve
Cystic adenomatoid malformation (with hydrops)	Pleuroamniotic shunt or resection
Infectious Disease	
Group B streptococcus	Ampicillin, penicillin
Chorioamnionitis	Antibiotics
Toxoplasmosis	Spiramycin, pyrimethamine, sulfadiazine, and folic acid
Syphilis	Penicillin
Tuberculosis	Antituberculosis drugs
Lyme disease	Penicillin, ceftriaxone
Parvovirus	Intrauterine red blood cell transfusion for hydrops, severe anemia
Chlamydia trachomatis	Erythromycin
HIV-AIDS	Zidovudine (AZT) plus protease inhibitors
Cytomegalovirus	Ganciclovir by umbilical vein
Other	
Nonimmune hydrops (anemia)	Umbilical vein packed red blood cell transfusion
Narcotic abstinence (withdrawal)	Maternal low-dose methadone
Severe combined immunodeficiency disease	Fetal stem cell transplantation
Sacrococcygeal teratoma (with hydrops)	In utero resection, or vessel obliteration
Twin-twin transfusion syndrome	Repeated amniocentesis, YAG-laser photocoagulation of shared vessels
Twin reversed arterial perfusion syndrome (TRAP)	Digoxin, indomethacin, cord occlusion
Multifetal gestation	Selective reduction

From Stoll BJ, Kliegman RM: The fetus. In Berhman RE, Kliegman RM, Jenson HB, editors: *Nelson textbook of pediatrics*, ed 16, Philadelphia, 2000, WB Saunders.
†Detailed fetal ultrasonography is needed to detect other anomalies; karyotype is also indicated.

TABLE 6–10
Components of the Perinatal History

Demographic Social Information
Age
Race
Sexually transmitted diseases, hepatitis, AIDS
Illicit drugs, cigarettes, ethanol, cocaine, abuse
Immune status (syphilis, rubella, hepatitis B, blood group)
Occupational exposure

Past Medical Diseases
Chronic hypertension
Heart disease
Diabetes mellitus
Thyroid disorders
Hematologic/malignancy
Collagen-vascular disease (SLE)
Genetic history—inborn errors of metabolism, bleeding, jaundice
Drug therapy

Prior Pregnancy
Abortion
Intrauterine fetal demise
Congenital malformation
Incompetent cervix
Birth weight
Prematurity
Twins
Blood group sensitization/neonatal jaundice
Hydrops
Infertility

Present Pregnancy
Current gestational age
Method of assessing gestational age

Present Pregnancy—cont'd
Fetal surveillance (OCT, NST, biophysical profile)
Ultrasonography (anomalies, hydrops)
Amniotic fluid analysis (L/S ratio)
Oligohydramnios-polyhydramnios
Vaginal bleeding
Preterm labor
Premature (prolonged) rupture of membranes (duration)
Preeclampsia
Urinary tract infection
Colonization status (herpes simplex, group B streptococcus)
Medications-drugs
Acute medical illness/exposure to infectious agents
Fetal therapy

Labor and Delivery
Duration of labor
Presentation—vertex, breech
Vaginal versus cesarean section
Spontaneous labor versus augmented or induced with oxytocin (Pitocin)
Forceps delivery
Presence of meconium-stained fluid
Maternal fever/amnionitis
Fetal heart rate patterns (distress)
Scalp pH
Maternal analgesia, anesthesia
Nuchal cord
Apgar score/methods of resuscitation
Gestational age assessment
Growth status (AGA, LGA, SGA)

AGA, Average for gestational age; *AIDS,* acquired immunodeficiency syndrome; *LGA,* large for gestational age; *L/S,* lecithin/sphingomyelin ratio; *NST,* nonstress test; *OCT,* oxytocin challenge test; *SGA,* small for gestational age; *SLE,* systemic lupus erythematosus.

Furthermore, the history of a woman's labor and delivery can reveal events that might lead to complications adversely affecting either the mother or neonate, even when the pregnancy was previously considered low risk. Anticipating the need to resuscitate a newborn as a result of its fetal distress increases the likelihood of successful resuscitation.

Transition from Fetal to Neonatal Physiology

Oxygen transport across the human placenta results in a gradient between the maternal and the fetal PaO_2. Although fetal oxygenated blood has a low PaO_2 level compared with that of adults and infants, the fetus is not anaerobic. Fetal oxygen uptake and consumption are similar to neonatal rates of oxygen use, even though the thermal environments and activity levels of fetuses and neonates differ significantly. Furthermore, the oxygen content of fetal blood is almost equal to that in older infants and children because fetal blood has a much higher concentration of hemoglobin.

Fetal hemoglobin (two alpha and two gamma chains) has a higher affinity for oxygen than adult hemoglobin does, thus facilitating oxygen transfer across the placenta. The fetal hemoglobin-oxygen dissociation curve thus is shifted to the left of the adult curve (Fig. 6–3); at the same PaO_2 level, fetal hemoglobin will be more saturated than adult hemoglobin. However, because fetal hemoglobin functions on the steep, lower end of the oxygen saturation curve (PaO_2 20–30 mm Hg), oxygen unloading to the tissue is not deficient. In contrast, at the higher oxygen concentrations present in the placenta, oxygen loading is enhanced. In the last trimester fetal hemoglobin production begins to decrease and adult hemoglobin production begins to increase, becoming the only hemoglobin available to the newborn by 3–6 months of life. At this time, the fetal hemoglobin dissociation curve has shifted to the adult position (Fig. 6–3).

A portion of the well-oxygenated umbilical venous blood returning to the heart from the placenta perfuses the liver. The remainder bypasses the liver through a shunt (the ductus venosus) and enters the interior vena cava. This oxygenated blood in the vena cava constitutes 65–70% of venous return to the right atrium. The crista dividens in the right atrium directs one third of this vena caval blood across the patent foramen ovale to the left atrium, where it is subsequently pumped to the coronary, cerebral, and upper extremity circulations by the left ventricle. Venous return from the upper body combines with the remaining two thirds of the vena caval blood in the right atrium and is then directed to the right ventricle. This mixture of venous low-oxygenated blood from the upper and lower body enters the pulmonary artery, from which only 8–10% of it is pumped to the pulmonary circuit. The remaining 80–92% of the right ventricular output bypasses the lungs through a patent ductus arteriosus (PDA) and enters the descending aorta. The amount of blood (8–10%) flowing to the pulmonary system is low because vasoconstriction produced by medial muscle hypertrophy of the small pulmonary arterioles and fluid in the fetal lung increases vascular resistance to blood flow. Pulmonary artery tone also responds to hypoxia, hypercapnia, and acidosis, with vasoconstriction, a response that may further increase pulmonary vascular resistance.

The ductus arteriosus remains patent in the fetus because of low PaO_2 levels and dilating prostaglandins (i.e., PGE_2). In utero the right ventricle is the dominant ventricle, pumping 65% of the combined ventricular output, which is a very high volume (450 mL/kg/min) compared with that pumped by the older infant's right ventricle (200 mL/kg/min).

The transition of the circulation occurring between the fetal and neonatal periods involves the removal of the low-resistance circulation of the placenta, the onset of air respiration and reduction of the pulmonary arterial resistance, and the closure of shunts that were used in utero. When the umbilical

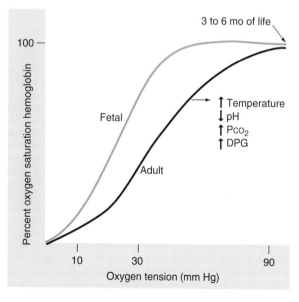

FIG. 6–3

Hemoglobin-oxygen dissociation curves. The position of the adult curve depends on the binding of adult hemoglobin to 2,3-diphosphoglycerate (DPG), temperature, carbon dioxide tension (Pco_2), and hydrogen ion concentration (pH).

cord is clamped, the low-pressure system of the placenta is eliminated, increasing systemic blood pressure. Venous return from the placenta is reduced, also decreasing right atrial pressure. When the breathing process begins, air replaces lung fluid, maintaining the functional residual capacity. Fluid leaves the lung, in part, through the trachea and is either swallowed or squeezed out during vaginal delivery. The pulmonary lymphatic and venous systems reabsorb the remaining fluid.

Most normal infants require very little pressure to "open" the lungs after birth (5–10 cm H_2O). A few infants require greater opening pressures (20–30 cm H_2O). With the onset of breathing, pulmonary vascular resistance falls, in part a result of the mechanics of breathing and in part a result of the elevated arterial oxygen tensions. The increased blood flow to the lungs results in a greater quantity of pulmonary venous blood returning to the left atrium; left atrial pressure now exceeds right atrial pressure, and the foramen ovale closes. As the flow through the pulmonary circulation increases and the arterial oxygen tensions become elevated, the ductus arteriosus begins to constrict. In the term infant, this constriction functionally closes the ductus arteriosus within 1 day after birth. A permanent closure requires thrombosis and fibrosis, a process that may take several weeks. In the premature infant, the ductus arteriosus is less sensitive to the effects of oxygen; if circulating levels of vasodilating prostaglandins are elevated, the ductus arteriosus may remain patent. This patency is a common problem in the premature infant who is exhibiting RDS.

Ventilation, oxygenation, and normal pH and PCO_2 levels immediately reduce pulmonary artery vasoconstriction by causing smooth muscle relaxation. Remodeling of the medial muscle hypertrophy begins at birth and continues for the next 3 months, resulting in a further reduction of pulmonary vascular resistance and a further increase of pulmonary blood flow. In infants with a ventricular septal defect (VSD), a significant left-to-right shunt and heart failure usually do not develop until pulmonary vascular resistance declines. Thus term infants with a VSD may become ill between 2 and 3 months of age. A full complement of pulmonary arteriole medial muscle has not developed in premature infants, and thus these infants have a more rapid decline of the pulmonary vascular resistance. Because of a more rapid decline of pulmonary artery pressure, the preterm infant with a VSD has left-to-right shunting and symptoms sooner than the term infant does, often before discharge from the nursery. Persistence or aggravation of pulmonary vasoconstriction caused by acidosis, hypoxia, hypercapnia, hypothermia, polycythemia, asphyxia, shunting of blood from the lungs, or pulmonary parenchymal hypoplasia results in persistent pulmonary hypertension or a persistent fetal circulation. This is discussed under Primary Pulmonary Hypertension of the Newborn (PPHN). Failure to replace pulmonary alveolar fluid completely with air can lead to respiratory distress. This is discussed further in Transient Tachypnea of the Newborn later in this chapter.

Asphyxia: Resuscitation

(See Hypoxic-Ischemic Encephalopathy)

Fetal or neonatal hypoxia, hypercapnia, poor cardiac output, and a metabolic acidosis can result from one or a number of many conditions affecting the fetus, the placenta, or the mother. Whether in utero or after birth, asphyxia-caused hypoxic-ischemic brain injury is the result of reduced gaseous exchange through the placenta or through the lungs, respectively. Asphyxia associated with severe bradycardia or cardiac insufficiency reduces or eliminates tissue blood flow, resulting in ischemia. The fetal and neonatal circulatory systems respond to reduced oxygen availability by shunting the blood preferentially to the brain, heart, and adrenal glands and away from the intestine, kidney, lung, and skin. When severe hypoxia and hypercapnia occur in utero, placental blood flow also is reduced.

The response to asphyxia also is characterized by the following:

1. Release of catecholamines (predominantly norepinephrine) from the adrenal glands
2. Transient hypertension and tachycardia followed by bradycardia and shock, which are both mediated in part from the chemoreceptors and baroreceptors
3. Production of a mixture of respiratory and metabolic acidosis
4. Hypoxemia

The metabolic acidosis is caused by the combined effects of poor cardiac output secondary to hypoxic depression of myocardial function, systemic hypoxia, and tissue anaerobic metabolism. With severe or prolonged intrauterine or neonatal asphyxia, multiple vital organs will be affected (Table 6–11).

Many conditions that contribute to fetal or neonatal asphyxia are the same medical or obstetric problems associated with the high-risk pregnancy (Table 6–12). Maternal diseases that interfere with uteroplacental perfusion, such as chronic hypertension, preeclampsia, and diabetes mellitus, place the fetus at risk for intrauterine asphyxia. Both maternal epidural anesthesia and the development of the vena caval compression syndrome may produce maternal hypotension, which decreases uterine perfusion. Maternal medications given to relieve pain during labor

TABLE 6–11
Effects of Asphyxia

System	Effect
Central nervous	Hypoxic-ischemic encephalopathy, IVH, PVL, cerebral edema, seizures, hypotonia, hypertonia
Cardiovascular	Myocardial ischemia, poor contractility, tricuspid insufficiency, hypotension
Pulmonary	Persistent fetal circulation, respiratory distress syndrome
Renal	Acute tubular or cortical necrosis
Adrenal	Adrenal hemorrhage
Gastrointestinal	Perforation, ulceration, necrosis
Metabolic	Inappropriate ADH, hyponatremia, hypoglycemia, hypocalcemia, myoglobinuria
Integument	Subcutaneous fat necrosis
Hematology	Disseminated intravascular coagulation

ADH, Antidiuretic hormone; *IVH,* intraventricular hemorrhage; *PVL,* periventricular leukomalacia.

TABLE 6–12
Etiology of Birth Asphyxia

Type	Example
Intrauterine	
Hypoxia-ischemia	Uteroplacental insufficiency, abruptio placentae, prolapsed cord, maternal hypotension, unknown
Anemia-shock	Vasa previa, placenta previa, fetomaternal hemorrhage, erythroblastosis
Intrapartum	
Birth trauma	Cephalopelvic disproportion, shoulder dystocia, breech presentation, spinal cord transection
Hypoxia-ischemia	Umbilical cord compression, tetanic contraction, abruptio placentae
Postpartum	
Central nervous system	Maternal medication, trauma, previous episodes of fetal hypoxia–acidosis
Congenital neuromuscular disease	Congenital myasthenia gravis, myopathy, myotonic dystrophy
Infection	Consolidated pneumonia, shock
Airway disorder	Choanal atresia, severe obstructing goiter, laryngeal webs
Pulmonary disorder	Severe immaturity, pneumothorax, pleural effusion, diaphragmatic hernia, pulmonary hypoplasia
Renal disorder	Pulmonary hypoplasia, pneumothorax

may cross the placenta and depress the infant's respiratory center, resulting in apnea at the time of birth.

Fetal conditions associated with asphyxia usually do not become manifest until delivery, when the infant must initiate and sustain ventilation, which requires an intact respiratory drive from the centers for respiration in the medulla. In addition, the upper and lower airways must be patent and unobstructed. The alveolus must be free from foreign material, such as meconium, amniotic fluid debris, and infectious exudate, that increases airway resistance, reduces lung compliance, and leads to respiratory distress and hypoxia (Table 6–12). Some very immature infants weighing less than 1000 g at birth may be un-

TABLE 6–13
Apgar Score

Signs	Points		
	0	1	2
Heart rate	0	<100/min	>100/min
Respiration	None	Weak cry	Vigorous cry
Muscle tone	None	Some extremity flexion	Arms, legs well flexed
Reflex irritability	None	Some motion	Cry, withdrawal
Color of body	Blue	Pink body, blue extremities	Pink all over

able to expand their lungs, even in the absence of pneumonia or other obvious signs of central nervous system dysfunction. Their compliant chest wall and surfactant deficiency may result in poor air exchange at birth, retractions, hypoxia, and apnea. Usually, more mature newborn infants do not manifest apnea in the delivery room as a sign of the respiratory distress syndrome.

Any condition leading to hypoxia in the delivery room may cause apnea because the newborn infant (particularly the preterm infant) responds paradoxically to hypoxia, with apnea rather than tachypnea, as occurs among adults. Episodes of intrauterine asphyxia also may depress the neonatal central nervous system. If recovery of the fetal heart rate occurs as a result of improved uteroplacental perfusion, fetal hypoxia and acidosis may resolve. Nonetheless, if the effect on the respiratory center is more severe, the newborn infant may not initiate an adequate ventilatory response at birth and thus may undergo another episode of asphyxia.

The *Apgar examination,* a rapid scoring system based on physiologic responses to the birth process, is a very good method for assessing the need to resuscitate a newborn infant (Table 6–13). At intervals of 1 minute and 5 minutes after birth, each of the five physiologic parameters is observed or elicited by a qualified examiner. Full-term infants with a normal cardiopulmonary adaptation should score 8–9 at 1 and 5 minutes. Apgar scores of 4–7 warrant close attention to determine whether the infant's status will improve and to ascertain whether any pathologic condition resulting from labor or delivery or residing within the newborn is contributing to the low Apgar score.

By definition, an Apgar score of 0–3 represents either a cardiopulmonary arrest or a condition caused by severe bradycardia, hypoventilation, or central nervous system depression. Most low Apgar scores are caused by difficulty in establishing adequate ventilation and not by primary cardiac pathology.

Infants with the most severe types of complex congenital heart disease (such as lethal hypoplastic left heart syndrome) do not have low Apgar scores because of the cardiac lesion. In addition to an Apgar score of 0–3, most infants with asphyxia severe enough to cause neurologic injury also manifest fetal acidosis (pH <7); seizures, coma, or hypotonia; and multiorgan dysfunction (Table 6–11). Low Apgar scores may be caused by fetal hypoxia or other factors listed in Table 6–12. Most infants with low Apgar scores respond to assisted ventilation by face mask or by endotracheal intubation and usually do not need emergency medication.

Resuscitation of the newborn infant having a low Apgar score follows the same systematic sequence (see Cardiopulmonary Resuscitation in Chapter 3) as that for resuscitation of older patients, but in the newborn period this simplified "ABCD" approach requires some qualification (Fig. 6–4).

In the ABCD approach, "A" stands for securing a patent airway by clearing amniotic fluid or meconium by suctioning; however, "A" should also remind us about "anticipation" and the need for knowing the events of pregnancy, labor, and delivery. This history also should include knowledge of fetal distress, fetal heart rate and acid-base status, abnormal position, vaginal bleeding, blood group sensitization, and ultrasonographic evidence of hydrops or congenital malformations; such knowledge may modify the approach to the airway. For example, evidence of a diaphragmatic hernia and a low Apgar score indicate that immediate endotracheal intubation is required. If a mask and bag are used, gas will enter both the lung and the stomach, and the latter may act as an expanding mass in the chest that compromises respiration. Knowing the blood group sensitization and that fetal hydrops has occurred with pleural effusions may indicate the need for bilateral thoracentesis to evacuate the pleural effusions, so that adequate ventilation can be established.

"B" represents breathing. If the patient is apneic or hypoventilates and remains cyanotic, artificial

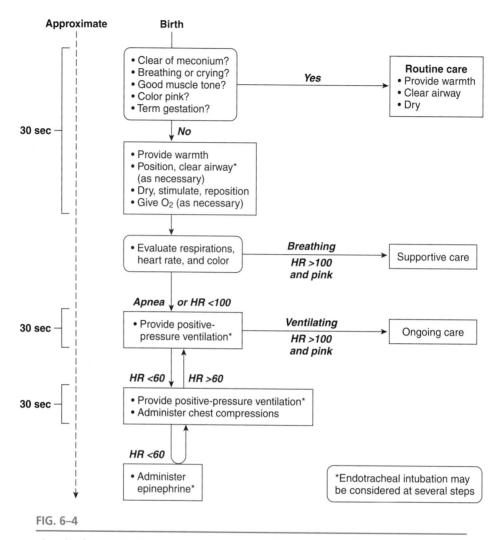

FIG. 6–4

Algorithm for resuscitation of the newly born infant. (From National guidelines for neonatal resuscitation, *Pediatrics* 106:E29, 2000.)

ventilation should be initiated. Ventilation should be performed with a well-fitted mask that is attached to an anesthesia bag and a manometer to prevent very high pressures from being given to the newborn infant. One-hundred-percent oxygen should be given through the mask. If the infant does not revive, an endotracheal tube should be placed through the vocal cords and then attached to the anesthesia bag and manometer, and 100% oxygen should be administered. The pressure generated should begin at 20–25 cm H_2O, with a rate of 40–60 breaths/min. An adequate response to ventilation is indicated by good chest rise, return of breath sounds, well-oxygenated color, heart rate returning to the normal range (120–160 beats/min), normal end-tidal CO_2, and later by increased muscle activity and wakefulness. The usual recovery after a cardiac arrest first involves a return to a normal heart rate. After that, cyanosis disappears and the infant will appear well perfused. An infant may remain limp and may be apneic for a prolonged time after return of cardiac output and correction of acidosis.

For the asphyxiated newborn infant, breathing should initially be briefly delayed if meconium-stained amniotic fluid is present. If the meconium is not cleared from the oropharyngeal and tracheal airways, it may be disseminated into the lungs, producing a severe aspiration pneumonia. If meconium is noted in the amniotic fluid, the oropharynx should be suctioned by the birth attendant once the head is delivered. After the birth of the depressed infant, the oral cavity should be suctioned again; the vocal cords then should be visualized with a laryngoscope and the infant intubated, with suction applied while the tube is below the vocal cords. If meconium is noted below the cords, intubation should be repeated quickly to clear the remaining meconium. During this time, the infant should not be stimulated to breathe, and positive-pressure ventilation should not be applied.

"C" represents circulation and external cardiac massage. If artificial ventilation does not improve the bradycardia, if asystole is present, or if peripheral pulses cannot be palpated, external cardiac massage should be performed at a rate of 90 compressions per minute with intervening 30 breaths per minute. External cardiac massage usually is not needed because most infants in the delivery room respond to ventilation.

"D" represents the administration of drugs. If bradycardia that is unresponsive to ventilation persists or if asystole is present, drugs should be added to the process of resuscitation. Intravenous epinephrine (1:10,000, 0.1–0.3 mL/kg) should be given through an umbilical venous line or may be injected into the endotracheal tube. If this dose is ineffective, 10 times the dose of epinephrine (1:1000) may be used. Additional medications for resuscitation may include 1–2 mEq/kg of sodium bicarbonate (0.5 mEq/mL) if acidosis is prolonged; calcium gluconate (2–4 mL/kg of 10% solution) if there is evidence of hypocalcemia; or a rapid infusion of fluids (normal saline, or O-negative red blood cells if anemia is present) if poor perfusion suggests hypovolemia. Before medications are administered in the presence of electrical cardiac activity with poor pulses, it is important to determine whether there is a pneumothorax. Transillumination of the thorax, involving the use of a bright light through each of the two sides of the thorax and over the sternum, may suggest pneumothorax if one side transmits more light than the other. Breath sounds are also decreased over a pneumothorax. There is a shift of the heart tones away from the side of a tension pneumothorax.

If central nervous system depression in the infant is thought to be caused by an analgesic medication, such as meperidine, that was given to the mother, naloxone (Narcan) can be given to the infant as a specific antidote. Before this drug is administered, however, the ABCs should be followed carefully, and naloxone should be given only after full resuscitation has been completed.

Other Neonatal Emergencies in the Delivery Room

Cyanosis

Acrocyanosis (blue color of the hands and feet with pink color of the rest of the body) is common in the delivery room and is usually normal. *Central cyanosis* of the trunk, mucosal membranes, and tongue can occur in the delivery room or at any time after birth and is always a manifestation of a serious underlying condition. Cyanosis is noted with 4–5 g/dL of deoxygenated hemoglobin. Central cyanosis can be caused by problems in many different organ systems, although cardiopulmonary diseases are the most common (Table 6–14). RDS, sepsis, and cyanotic heart disease are the three most common causes of cyanosis among infants admitted to a neonatal intensive care unit (NICU). A systematic evaluation of these and other causes of cyanosis is required for every cyanotic infant after prompt administration of oxygen, with or without assisted ventilation as indicated.

Life-Threatening Congenital Malformations

(Table 6–15)

Various congenital anomalies can interfere with vital organ function after birth. Some malformations, such as choanal atresia and other lesions obstructing the airway, may prevent ventilation. Intrathoracic lesions, such as cysts or bowel that has herniated into the chest, also interfere with respiration. Other malformations that obstruct the gastrointestinal system at the level of the esophagus, duodenum, ileum, or colon may lead to aspiration pneumonia, intestinal perforation, or gangrene. Gastroschisis and omphalocele both are associated with exposed bowel on the abdominal wall. Omphalocele also is associated with other malformations, whereas intestinal necrosis is more common in gastroschisis.

Many congenital malformations are obvious in the delivery room. By using fetal ultrasonography, the obstetrician is able to detect many serious congenital anomalies in utero. Immediate palliative medical or surgical treatment or corrective surgery must be planned for most infants with major congenital malformations. Prompt stabilization, as noted for the asphyxiated infant, is essential. In addition, specific attention must be given to the particular problems associated with the malformation.

Shock

Shock in the delivery room is manifested by cyanosis, pallor, poor capillary refill time, unpalpable pulses, hypotonia, and, eventually, cardiopulmonary arrest. Cyanosis in the presence of pallor, with or

TABLE 6–14
Differential Diagnosis of Neonatal Cyanosis

System/Disease	Mechanism
Pulmonary	
Respiratory distress syndrome	Surfactant deficiency
Sepsis, pneumonia	Inflammation, pulmonary hypertension, ARDS
Meconium aspiration pneumonia	Mechanical obstruction, inflammation, pulmonary hypertension
Persistent fetal circulation	Pulmonary hypertension
Diaphragmatic hernia	Pulmonary hypoplasia, pulmonary hypertension
Transient tachypnea	Retained lung fluid
Cardiovascular	
Cyanotic heart disease with decreased pulmonary blood flow	Right-to-left shunt as in pulmonary atresia, tetralogy of Fallot
Cyanotic heart disease with increased pulmonary blood flow	Right-to-left shunt as in d-transposition, truncus arteriosus
Cyanotic heart disease with congestive heart failure	Right-to-left shunt with pulmonary edema and poor cardiac output as in hypoplastic left heart and coarctation of aorta
Heart failure alone	Pulmonary edema and poor cardiac contractility as in sepsis, myocarditis, supraventricular tachycardia, or complete heart block; high-output failure as in PDA or vein of Galen or other arteriovenous malformation
Central Nervous System	
Maternal sedative drugs	Hypoventilation, apnea
Asphyxia	CNS depression
Intracranial hemorrhage	CNS depression, seizure
Neuromuscular disease	Hypotonia, hypoventilation, pulmonary hypoplasia
Hematologic	
Acute blood loss	Shock
Chronic blood loss	Congestive heart failure
Polycythemia	Pulmonary hypertension
Methemoglobinemia	Low-affinity hemoglobin or red blood cell enzyme defect
Metabolic	
Hypoglycemia	CNS depression, congestive heart failure
Adrenogenital syndrome	Shock (salt-losing)

ARDS, Acute respiratory distress syndrome; *CNS,* central nervous system; *PDA,* patent ductus arteriosus.

without mottling and ecchymosis, is highly suggestive of shock. Blood loss before or during labor and delivery is a common cause of shock in the delivery room. Blood loss may be caused by a fetal-maternal hemorrhage; placenta previa; vasa previa; a twin-twin transfusion; or displacement of blood from the fetus to the placenta, as during asphyxia (hence the term *asphyxia pallida*). Hemorrhage into a viscus such as the liver or spleen may be noted in macrosomic in-

fants, and hemorrhage into the cerebral ventricles may produce shock and apnea in preterm infants. Finally, anemia, hypoalbuminemia, hypovolemia, and shock at birth are common manifestations of Rh immune hydrops. Diseases causing nonimmune hydrops also can lead to fetal anemia and hypovolemia.

Severe intrauterine bacterial sepsis may present with septicemic shock in the delivery room or immediately after the infant is transferred to the

TABLE 6-15
Life-Threatening Congenital Anomalies

Name	Manifestations
Choanal atresia	Respiratory distress in delivery room, apnea, unable to pass nasogastric tube through nares
Pierre Robin syndrome	Micrognathia, cleft palate, airway obstruction
Diaphragmatic hernia	Scaphoid abdomen, bowel sounds present in left chest, heart shifted to right, respiratory distress, polyhydramnios
Tracheoesophageal fistula	Polyhydramnios, aspiration pneumonia, excessive salivation, unable to place nasogastric tube in stomach
Intestinal obstruction: volvulus, duodenal atresia, ileal atresia	Polyhydramnios, bile-stained emesis, abdominal distention
Gastroschisis/omphalocele	Polyhydramnios; intestinal obstruction
Renal agenesis/Potter syndrome	Oligohydramnios, anuria, pulmonary hypoplasia, pneumothorax
Hydronephrosis	Abdominal masses
Neural tube defects: anencephalus, meningomyelocele	Polyhydramnios, elevated alpha-fetoprotein; decreased fetal activity
Down syndrome (trisomy 21)	Hypotonia, congenital heart disease, duodenal atresia
Ductal-dependent congenital heart disease	Cyanosis, murmur, shock

nursery. Typically these infants are mottled, hypotonic, and cyanotic and have diminished peripheral pulses. They have a normal hemoglobin concentration but may manifest neutropenia, thrombocytopenia, and disseminated intravascular coagulation (DIC). Peripheral symmetric gangrene (purpuric rash) often is a sign of hypotensive shock among infants with severe congenital bacterial infections.

Congenital left ventricular cardiac obstruction (e.g., critical aortic stenosis or hypoplastic left heart syndrome) also produces shock, although not usually in the delivery room.

Treatment of newborn infants with shock should involve the management approaches used for the sick infant (discussed under Asphyxia: Resuscitation earlier in this chapter). Problems may be anticipated through knowledge of the infant's immune status, evidence of hydrops, or suspicion of intrauterine infection or anomalies. Stabilization of the airway, institution of respiratory support, and external cardiac massage are essential. Hypovolemic shock should be managed with repeated boluses of 10–15 mL/kg of normal saline or lactated Ringer's solution. If severe immune hemolysis is predicted, blood typed against the mother's blood should be available in the delivery room and should be given to the newborn infant if signs of anemia and shock are present. Thereafter, all blood should be cross-matched with both the in-

fant's and mother's blood before transfusion. Vasoactive drugs, such as dopamine, dobutamine, and epinephrine, may improve cardiac output and tissue perfusion.

Birth Injury

Birth injury refers to both avoidable and unavoidable injury to the fetus during the birth process.

Caput succedaneum is a diffuse, edematous, often dark swelling of the soft tissue of the scalp that extends across the midline and suture lines. In infants delivered from a face presentation, soft tissue edema of the eyelids and face is an equivalent phenomenon. Caput succedaneum may be seen after prolonged labor in both full-term and premature infants. Molding of the head often is associated with caput succedaneum and is the result of pressure that is induced from overriding the parietal and frontal bones against their respective sutures.

A *cephalhematoma* is a subperiosteal hemorrhage that does not cross the suture lines surrounding the respective bones. A linear skull fracture rarely may be seen underlying a cephalhematoma. With time, the cephalhematoma may organize, calcify, and form a central depression.

Infants with cephalhematoma and caput succedaneum require no specific treatment. Occasionally a premature infant may develop a massive scalp hemorrhage. This *subgaleal bleeding* and the bleeding noted from a cephalhematoma may cause indirect hyperbilirubinemia that requires treatment with phototherapy.

Retinal and *subconjunctival hemorrhages* are common but usually are small and insignificant. No treatment is necessary.

Spinal cord or *spine injuries* may occur in the fetus as a result of the hyperextended "star gazing" posture. They may also occur in infants after excessive rotational (at C3–4) or longitudinal (at C7–T1) force is transmitted to the neck during vertex or breech delivery. Fractures of vertebrae are rarer and may cause direct damage to the spinal cord, leading to transection and permanent sequelae or hemorrhage, edema, and neurologic signs. Rarely, a snapping sound indicative of cord transection rather than vertebral displacement is heard at the time of delivery. Neurologic dysfunction usually involves complete flaccid paralysis, absence of deep tendon reflexes, and absence of responses to painful stimuli below the lesion. Painful stimuli may elicit reflex flexion of the legs. Infants with spinal cord injury often are flaccid, apneic, and asphyxiated, all of which may mask the underlying spinal cord transection. With time, these infants will experience bowel and bladder problems, spasticity, and hyperreflexia.

Injury to the nerves of the *brachial plexus* may result from excessive traction on the neck, producing paresis or complete paralysis. The mildest injury (neurapraxia) is edema; axonotmesis is more severe and consists of disrupted nerve fibers with an intact myelin sheath; neurotmesis, or complete nerve disruption or root avulsion, is most severe. **Erb-Duchenne paralysis** involves the fifth and sixth cervical nerves and is the most common and usually mildest injury. The infant cannot abduct the arm at the shoulder, externally rotate the arm, or supinate the forearm. The usual picture is one of painless adduction, internal rotation of the arm, and pronation of the forearm. The **Moro reflex** is absent on the involved side, and the hand grasp is intact. A **phrenic nerve palsy** (C3, 4, and 5) may lead to diaphragmatic paralysis and respiratory distress. Elevation of the diaphragm caused by nerve injury must be differentiated from elevation caused by eventration resulting from congenital weakness or absence of diaphragm muscle. **Klumpke paralysis** is caused by injury to the seventh and eighth cervical nerves and the first thoracic nerve, resulting in a paralyzed hand and if the sympathetic nerves are injured, an ipsilateral *Horner syndrome* (ptosis, miosis). Complete arm and hand paralysis is noted with the severest form of damage to C5, 6, 7, and 8 and T1. *Treatment* of brachial plexus injury is supportive and includes positioning to avoid contractures. Active and passive range-of-motion exercises also may be of benefit. If the deficit persists, nerve grafting may be beneficial.

Facial nerve injury may be the result of compression of the seventh nerve between the facial bone and the mother's pelvic bones or the physician's forceps. This peripheral nerve injury is characterized by an asymmetric, crying face whose normal side, including the forehead, moves in a regular manner. The affected side is flaccid, the eye does not close, the nasolabial fold is absent, and the side of the mouth droops at rest. If there is a central injury to the facial nerve, only the lower two thirds of the face (not the forehead) is involved. Complete agenesis of the facial nucleus results in a central facial paralysis; when this is bilateral, as in **Möbius syndrome,** the face appears expressionless.

Fractures of the cranium are rare, are usually linear, and require no treatment other than observation for very rare, delayed (1–3 mo) complications (e.g., leptomeningeal cyst). Depressed **skull** fractures are unusual but may be seen with complicated forceps delivery; they may need surgical elevation. Fractures of the **clavicle** usually are unilateral and are noted in macrosomic infants after shoulder dystocia. Often a snap is heard after a difficult delivery, and the infant exhibits an asymmetric Moro response and decreased movement of the affected side. The prognosis is excellent; many infants require no treatment or a simple figure-of-eight bandage to immobilize the bone.

Extremity fractures are less common than those of the clavicle and involve the humerus more often than the femur. *Treatment* involves immobilization and a triangular splint bandage for the humerus and traction suspension of the legs for femoral fractures. The *prognosis* is excellent.

Fractures of the **facial bones** are rare, but dislocation of the cartilaginous part of the nasal septum out of the vomeral groove and columella is common. *Clinical manifestations* include feeding difficulty, respiratory distress, asymmetric nares, and a flattened, laterally displaced nose. *Treatment* reduces the dislocation by elevating the cartilage back into the vomeral groove.

Visceral trauma to the liver, spleen, or adrenal gland is noted in macrosomic infants and in very premature infants, with or without breech or vaginal delivery. Rupture of the liver with subcapsular hematoma formation may lead to anemia, hypovolemia, shock, hemoperitoneum, and DIC. Infants with anemia and shock who are suspected of having an intraventricular hemorrhage but who have normal findings with head ultrasound examination should be evaluated for hepatic or splenic rupture. Adrenal hemorrhage may be asymptomatic, as noted by a high incidence of normal infants with calcified adrenal glands. Nonetheless, infants with severe adrenal hemorrhage may exhibit a flank mass, jaundice, and hematuria, with or without shock.

Temperature Regulation

In utero thermoregulation of the fetus is performed by the placenta, which acts as an efficient heat exchanger. Fetal temperature is nonetheless higher than the mother's temperature. If maternal temperature becomes elevated during a febrile illness or on exposure to environmental heat, fetal temperature will increase further. Thus the immediate temperature at birth of an infant born to a febrile mother with chorioamnionitis will be elevated regardless of the presence of infection in the infant, unless the infant has cooled in the delivery room.

After birth, the newborn infant begins life covered by amniotic fluid and situated in a cold environment (20–25° C). An infant's skin temperature may fall 0.3° C/min, and the core temperature may decline 0.1° C/min in the delivery room. In the absence of an external heat source, the infant must increase metabolism substantially to maintain body temperature.

Heat loss occurs through four basic mechanisms. In the cold delivery room the wet infant loses heat predominantly by *evaporation* (cutaneous and respiratory loss when wet or in low humidity), *radiation* (loss to nearby cold, solid surfaces), and *convection* (loss to air current). Once the infant is dry, radiation, convection, and *conduction* (loss to object in direct contact with infant) are important causes of heat loss. After birth, all high-risk infants should be dried immediately to eliminate evaporative heat losses (Table 6–16). Furthermore, a radiant or convective heat source should be provided for these high-risk infants. Normal term infants should be dried and wrapped in a blanket.

The ideal environmental temperature is the *neutral thermal environment*, the ambient temperature that results in the lowest rate of heat being produced by the infant and maintains normal body temperature. The neutral thermal environmental temperature decreases with increasing gestational age and increasing postnatal age. Ambient temperatures below the neutral thermal environment first result in increasing rates of oxygen consumption for heat production, which is designed to maintain normal body temperature. If the ambient temperature falls further or if oxygen consumption cannot increase sufficiently (as a result of hypoxia, hypoglycemia, or drugs), the core body temperature falls.

Heat production by the newborn infant is created predominantly by *nonshivering thermogenesis* from chemical reactions of adenosine triphosphate (ATP) hydrolysis in specialized areas of tissue containing brown adipose tissue. Brown fat is highly vascular, contains many mitochondria per cell, and is situated around large blood vessels, resulting in rapid heat transfer to the circulation. The vessels of the neck, thorax, and interscapular region are common locations of brown fat. These tissues also are innervated by the sympathetic nervous system, which serves as a primary stimulus for heat production by brown adipose cells. Shivering does not occur in newborn infants.

Severe *cold injury* in the infant is manifested by acidosis, hypoxia, hypoglycemia, apnea, bradycardia, pulmonary hemorrhage and a pink skin color. The color is caused not by adequate oxygenation, but rather by trapping of oxygenated hemoglobin in the cutaneous capillaries. Many of these infants appear dead, but most respond to treatment and recover. Milder degrees of cold injury in the delivery room may contribute to metabolic acidosis and hypoxia after birth. Conversely, hypoxia delays heat generation in cold-stressed infants.

Treatment of severe hypothermia should involve resuscitation and rapid warming of both core (e.g.,

---

TABLE 6–16
General Management Strategies for Sick Newborns

Procedure	Rationale
Warmth in a neutral thermal environment	Avoids cold stress, minimizes oxygen consumption
Humidification	Reduces insensible water losses
Intravenous fluids and glucose	Maintains fluid balance, avoids dehydration, prevents hyperbilirubinemia, prevents prerenal azotemia, prevents hypoglycemia, provides supplemental calories to support oxygen consumption
Oxygen	Treats hypoxia, supports oxygen consumption, prevents cell injury and death
Monitor blood gases and arterial oxygen saturation	Avoids hyperoxic retinal injury and hypoxic brain injury, guides treatment with mechanical ventilation

lung and stomach) and external surfaces. Fluid resuscitation also is needed to treat the hypovolemia seen in many of these infants. Reduced core temperature (32–35° C) in the immediate newborn period often requires only external warming with a radiant warmer, incubator, or both.

Elevated Temperature. Exposure to ambient temperatures above the neutral thermal environment results in *heat stress* and an elevated core temperature. Sweating is uncommon in newborn infants and may be noted only on the forehead. However, in response to moderate heat stress, infants may increase their respiratory rate to dissipate heat. Excessive environmental temperatures may result in heat stroke or in the hemorrhagic shock encephalopathy syndrome.

Routine Delivery Room Care

Once the cardiopulmonary transition from fetal to newborn life has successfully occurred and no acute life-threatening conditions exist, routine delivery room or postpartum room care should be provided. Silver nitrate (1%) instilled into both eyes without being washed out is an indicated effective therapy for the prevention of neonatal gonococcal ophthalmia, which can result in severe panophthalmitis and subsequent blindness. Silver nitrate may produce a chemical conjunctivitis with a mucopurulent discharge and is not effective against *Chlamydia trachomatis.* Therefore, many hospitals use erythromycin drops to prevent neonatal gonococcal and chlamydial eye disease.

Bacterial colonization of the newborn may begin in utero if the fetal membranes have been ruptured before or during labor. Most infants undergo colonization after birth and acquire the bacteria present in the mother's genitourinary system, such as group B streptococcus, staphylococci, *Escherichia coli,* and clostridial species. Colonization is common at the umbilicus, skin, nasopharynx, and intestine. Antiseptic skin or cord care is routine in most nurseries to prevent the spread of pathologic bacteria from one infant to another and to prevent disease in the individual infant. Staphylococcal bullous impetigo, omphalitis, diarrhea, and systemic disease may result from colonization with virulent *Staphylococcus aureus.* For term infants, washing of the skin with 3% hexachlorophene is not routinely recommended but may prevent serious staphylococcal disease; preterm infants may absorb hexachlorophene, and neurotoxicity may develop. Triple dye or bacitracin may be applied to the umbilical cord to effectively reduce its colonization with gram-positive bacteria. Epidemics of *S. aureus* nursery infections are managed with strict infectious disease control measures (e.g., cohorting, hand washing, and monitoring for colonization).

Vitamin K prophylaxis (IM) should be given to all infants to prevent hemorrhagic disease of the newborn. Before discharge, infants should receive the hepatitis B vaccine and be screened for various diseases (Tables 16–17 and 6–18).

TABLE 6–17

Approximate Frequencies in the United States of Disorders Included in or Considered for Newborn Screening

Disorder	Estimated Frequency	Disorder	Estimated Frequency
Congenital hypothyroidism	1:4000	Sickle cell disease	1:4000
Phenylketonuria	1:12,000	Cystic fibrosis	1:4000
Medium chain acyl-CoA dehydrogenase	1:10,000	Duchenne muscular dystrophy	1:8000*
Galactosemia	1:60,000	Congenital toxoplasmosis	1:10,000
Maple syrup urine disease	1:200,000	Hyperlipidemia	1:500
Homocystinuria	1:200,000	Alpha$_1$-antitrypsin deficiency	1:8000
Biotinidase deficiency	1:70,000	Neuroblastoma	1:4000
Congenital adrenal hyperplasia	1:19,000		

From Kim SZ, Levy HL: Newborn screening. In Taeusch HW, Ballard RA, editors: *Avery's diseases of the newborn,* ed 7, Philadelphia, 1998, WB Saunders.
*For males, 1:4000.

TABLE 6–18
Abnormal Newborn Screening Results: Possible Implications and Initial Action to Be Taken

Newborn Screening Finding	Differential Diagnosis	Initial Action
↑ Phenylalanine	PKU, non-PKU hyperphenylalaninemia, pterin defect, galactosemia, transient hyperphenylalaninemia	Repeat blood specimen
↓ T$_4$, ↑ TSH	Congenital hypothyroidism, iodine exposure	Repeat blood specimen or thyroid function testing, begin thyroxine treatment
↓ T$_4$, normal TSH	Maternal hyperthyroidism, thyroxine-binding globulin deficiency, secondary hypothyroidism, congenital hypothyroidism with delayed TSH elevation	Repeat blood specimen
↑ Galactose (1-P)	Galactosemia, liver disease, portosystemic shunt, transferase deficiency variant (Duarte), transient	Clinical evaluation, urine for reducing substance, repeat blood specimen. If reducing substance positive, begin lactose-free formula
↓ Galactose-1-phosphate uridyltransferase	Galactosemia, transferase deficiency variant (Duarte), transient	Clinical evaluation, urine for reducing substance, repeat blood specimen. If reducing substance positive, begin lactose-free formula
↑ Methionine	Homocystinuria, isolated hypermethioninemia, liver dysfunction, tyrosinemia type I, transient hypermethioninemia	Repeat blood and urine specimen
↑ Leucine	Maple syrup urine disease, transient elevation	Clinical evaluation including urine for ketones, acid-base status, amino acid studies, immediate neonatal intensive care unit care if urine ketones positive
↑ Tyrosine	Tyrosinemia type I or type II, transient tyrosinemia, liver disease	Repeat blood specimen
↑ 17 alpha-hydroxyprogesterone	Congenital adrenal hyperplasia, prematurity, transient (residual fetal adrenal cortex), stress in neonatal period, early specimen collection	Clinical evaluation including genital examination, serum electrolytes, repeat blood specimen
S-hemoglobin	Sickle cell disease, sickle cell trait	Hemoglobin electrophoresis
↑ Trypsinogen	Cystic fibrosis, transient, intestinal anomalies, perinatal stress, trisomies 13 and 18, renal failure	Repeat blood specimen, possible sweat test and DNA testing
↑ Creatinine phosphokinase	Duchenne muscular dystrophy, other type of muscular dystrophy, birth trauma, invasive procedure	Repeat blood test

From Kim SZ, Levy HL: Newborn screening. In Taeusch HW, Ballard RA, editors: *Avery's diseases of the newborn,* ed 7, Philadelphia, 1998, WB Saunders.

Continued

TABLE 6–18
Abnormal Newborn Screening Results: Possible Implications and Initial Action to Be Taken—cont'd

Newborn Screening Finding	Differential Diagnosis	Initial Action
↓ Biotinidase	Biotinidase deficiency	Serum biotinidase assay, biotin therapy
↓ G-6-PD	G-6-PD deficiency	Complete blood count, bilirubin determination
↓ Alpha₁-antitrypsin	Alpha₁-antitrypsin deficiency	Confirmatory test
Toxoplasma antibody (IgM)	Congenital toxoplasmosis	Infectious disease consultation
HIV antibody (IgG)	Maternally transmitted HIV, possible AIDS	Infectious disease consultation
↑ Urine vanillylmandelic acid, homovanillic acid	Neuroblastoma, other catecholamine-secreting tumors, transient elevation	Repeat urine test
↑ Organic acids	Fatty acid oxidation defects (medium chain acyl-CoA dehydrogenase deficiency)	Perform specific assay (tandem mass spectroscopy); frequent feeds

From Kim SZ, Levy HL: Newborn screening. In Taeusch HW, Ballard RA, editors: *Avery's diseases of the newborn*, ed 7, Philadelphia, 1998, WB Saunders.

REFERENCES

Behrman RE, Kliegman RM, Jenson HB, editors: *Nelson textbook of pediatrics,* ed 16, Philadelphia, 2000, WB Saunders, Chapters 90–96.

Carrero J, Torrents M, Mortera C, et al: Routine prenatal ultrasound screening for fetal abnormalities: 22 years experience, *Ultrasound Obstet Gynecol* 5(3):174–179, 1995.

Committee on Fetus and Newborn, American Academy of Pediatrics, and Committee on Obstetric Practice, American College of Obstetricians and Gynecologists: Use and abuse of Apgar score, *Pediatrics* 98(1):141–142, 1996.

Chiswick M: Assessing outcomes in twin-twin transfusion syndrome, *Arch Dis Child Fetal Neonatal Ed* 83(3):F165–F167, 2000.

Hernandez-Diaz S, Werler MM, Walker AM, et al: Folic acid antagonists during pregnancy and the risk of birth defects, *N Engl J Med* 343(22):1608–1614, 2000.

Hickok DE, Mills M, Western Collaborative Perinatal Group: Percutaneous umbilical blood sampling: results from a multicenter collaborative registry, *Am J Obstet Gynecol* 166(6 Pt 1):1614–1617, 1992.

Ibdah JA, Bennett MJ, Rinaldo R, et al: A fetal fatty-acid oxidation disorder a a cause of liver disease in pregnant women, *N Engl J Med* 340(22):1723–1731, 1999.

International guidelines for neonatal resuscitation: an excerpt from the guidelines 2000 for cardiopulmonary resuscitation and emergency cardiovascular care: international consensus on science, *Pediatrics* 106(3):E29, 2000.

Martin-Ancel A, Garcia-Alix A, Gaya F, et al: Multiple organ involvement in perinatal asphyxia, *J Pediatr* 127:786, 1995.

Mello G, Parretti E, Mecacci F, et al: What degree of maternal metabolic control in women with type 1 diabetes is associated with normal body size and proportions in full-term infants? *Diabetes Care* 23(10):1494–1498, 2000.

Strombeck C, Krumlinde-Sundholm L, Forssberg H: Functional outcome at 5 years in children with obstetrical brachial plexus palsy with and without microsurgical reconstruction, *Dev Med Child Neurol* 42(3):148–157, 2000.

PHYSICAL EXAMINATION AND GESTATIONAL AGE ASSESSMENT

The first physical examination of the newborn infant serves many important purposes. It may be a general physical examination of a well baby or an examination to confirm fetal diagnoses or determine the cause of various manifestations of neonatal diseases. Because the transition from fetal to neonatal life requires significant cardiopulmonary adjustments, problems in this transition may be detectable immediately in the delivery room or during the first day of life. Physical examination may also reveal effects of the labor and delivery resulting from asphyxia, drugs, or birth trauma. Furthermore, the first newborn examination is an important way to detect congenital malformations or deformations (Table 6–15). Congenital malformations are the result of many different causes—for example, chromosomal trisomies, teratogens, or recognizable syndromes without identifiable causes. Significant congenital malformations may be present in as many as 1–3% of all births (see Chapter 4). Congenital deformations are caused by compression of fetal parts by the uterus, usually in the absence of amniotic fluid. Thus some cases of clubfoot are a result of compression of the fetal foot by the uterine wall (see Chapter 19).

Appearance

The general appearance of the infant should be evaluated first. Signs such as cyanosis, nasal flaring, in-

Physical maturity	−1	0	1	2	3	4	5
Skin	Sticky, friable, transparent	Gelatinous, red, translucent	Smooth, pink, visible veins	Superficial peeling or rash, few veins	Cracking, pale areas, rare veins	Parchment, deep cracking, no vessels	Leathery, cracked, wrinkled
Lanugo	None	Sparse	Abundant	Thinning	Bald areas	Mostly bald	
Plantar surface	Heel–toe 40–50 mm: −1 Less than 40 mm: −2	<50 mm, no crease	Faint red marks	Anterior transverse crease only	Creases on anterior 2/3	Creases over entire sole	
Breast	Impercep-tible	Barely perceptible	Flat areola–no bud	Stripped areola, 1–2 mm bud	Raised areola, 3–4 mm bud	Full areola, 5–10 mm bud	
Eye/ear	Lids fused, loosely (−1), tightly (−2)	Lids open, pinna flat, stays folded	Slightly curved pinna; soft: slow recoil	Well-curved pinna, soft but ready recoil	Formed and firm; instant recoil	Thick cartilage, ear stiff	
Genitals male	Scrotum flat, smooth	Scrotum empty, faint rugae	Testes in upper canal, rare rugae	Testes descending, few rugae	Testes down, good rugae	Testes pendulous, deep rugae	
Genitals (female)	Clitoris prominent, labia flat	Prominent clitoris, small labia minora	Prominent clitoris, enlarging minora	Majora and minora equally prominent	Majora large, minora small	Majora cover clitoris and minora	

FIG. 6–5

Physical criteria for assessment of maturity and gestational age. Expanded New Ballard Score (NBS) includes extremely premature infants and has been refined to improve accuracy in more mature infants. (From Ballard JL et al: *J Pediatr* 119:417, 1991.)

tercostal retractions, and grunting suggest pulmonary disease. Meconium staining of the umbilical cord, nails, and skin suggests fetal distress and the possibility of aspiration pneumonia (discussed in the following sections). The level of spontaneous activity, passive muscle tone, the quality of the cry, and apnea are useful screening signs to evaluate the state of the nervous system initially.

Vital Signs

After the general appearance of the infant is evaluated, the examination should proceed with an assessment of vital signs, particularly heart rate (a normal rate is 120–160 beats/min), respiratory rate (normal rate is 30–60 breaths/min), temperature (usually done initially per rectum and later as an axillary measure-

ment), and blood pressure (often reserved for sick infants). In addition, length, weight, and head circumference should be measured and plotted on growth curves to determine whether growth is normal, accelerated, or retarded for the specific gestational age.

Gestational Age

Gestational age is determined by an assessment of various physical signs (Fig. 6–5) and neurologic characteristics (Fig. 6–6) that vary according to fetal age and maturity. Physical criteria are features that mature with advancing fetal age, including increasing firmness of the pinna of the ear; increasing size of the breast tissue; decreasing fine, immature lanugo hair over the back; and decreasing opacity of the skin. Neurologic criteria are feaures that mature with

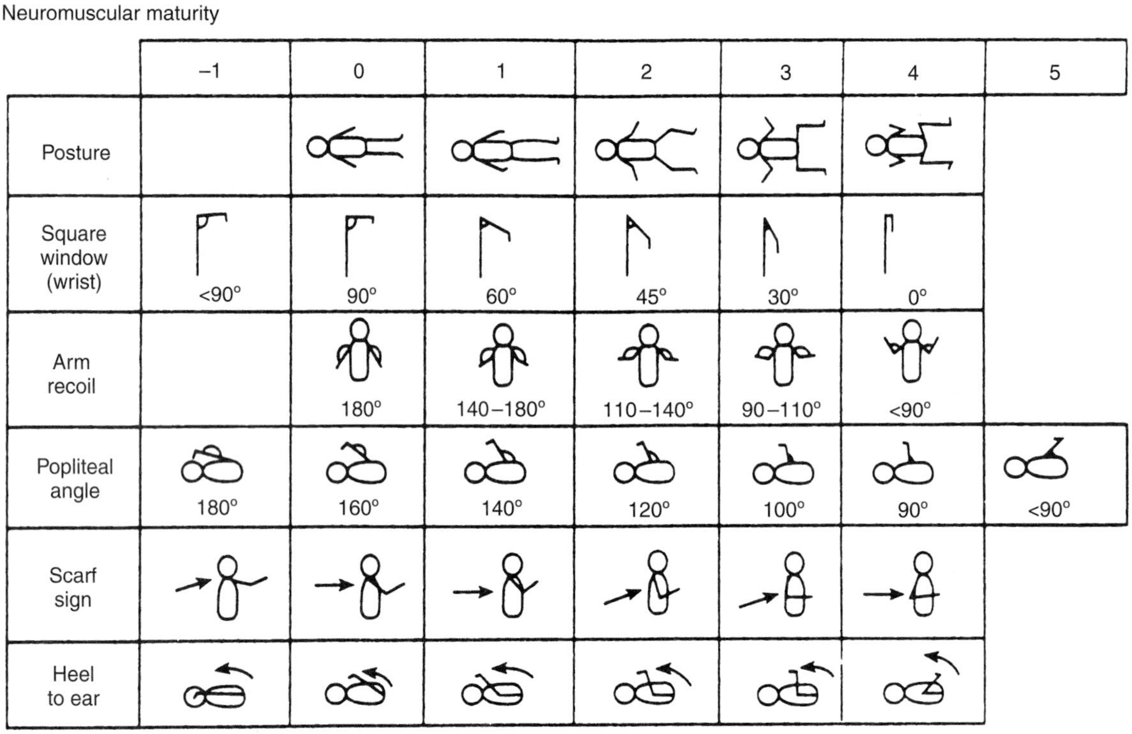

Neuromuscular maturity

	−1	0	1	2	3	4	5
Posture							
Square window (wrist)	<90°	90°	60°	45°	30°	0°	
Arm recoil		180°	140–180°	110–140°	90–110°	<90°	
Popliteal angle	180°	160°	140°	120°	100°	90°	<90°
Scarf sign							
Heel to ear							

FIG. 6–6

Neuromuscular criteria for assessment of maturity and gestational age. Expanded New Ballard Score includes extremely premature infants and has been refined to improve accuracy in more mature infants. (From Ballard JL et al: *J Pediatr* 119:417, 1991.)

gestational age, including increasing flexion of the legs, hips, and arms; increasing tone of the flexor muscles of the neck; and decreasing laxity of the joints. These signs are determined during the first day of life and are assigned scores. The cumulative score is correlated with a gestational age, which is usually accurate to within 2 weeks (Fig. 6–7).

Gestational age assessment permits the detection of abnormal fetal growth patterns, thus aiding in predicting the neonatal complications of largeness or smallness for gestational age (Fig. 6–8). Infants born at a weight greater than the 90th percentile for their age are considered **large for gestational age** (LGA). Among the risks associated with being LGA are all the risks of the infant of a diabetic mother (Table 6–5) and risks associated with postmaturity. Infants born at a weight less than the 10th percentile for their age (some growth curves use less than two standard deviations or the 5th percentile) are **small for gestational age** (SGA) and have intrauterine growth retardation. Problems associated with the SGA infant include congenital malformations, in addition to the problems listed in Table 6–8.

Skin

The skin should be evaluated for pallor, plethora, jaundice, cyanosis, meconium staining, petechiae, ecchymoses, congenital nevi, and neonatal rashes. Vasomotor instability with cutis marmorata, telangiectasia, phlebectasia (intermittent mottling with venous prominence), and acrocyanosis (feet and hands) is normal in the premature infant. Acrocyanosis also may be noted in the healthy term infant in the first days after birth. The **harlequin color change** is a striking, transient, but normal sign of vasomotor instability and divides the body from head to pubis, through the midline, into equal halves of pink and pale color.

The skin is covered with lanugo hair, which disappears by term gestation. **Hair tufts** over the lumbosacral spine suggest a spinal cord defect. **Vernix caseosa,** a soft, white, creamy layer covering the skin in preterm infants, disappears by term. Postterm infants often have peeling, parchment-like skin. **Mongolian spots** are transient, dark blue to black pigmented macules seen over the lower back and buttock in 90% of black, Indian, and Asian infants.

Maturity rating

Score	Weeks
−10	20
−5	22
0	24
5	26
10	28
15	30
20	32
25	34
30	36
35	38
40	40
45	42
50	44

FIG. 6–7

Maturity rating as calculated by adding the physical and neurologic score, thus calculating the gestational age. (From Ballard JL et al: *J Pediatr* 119:417, 1991.)

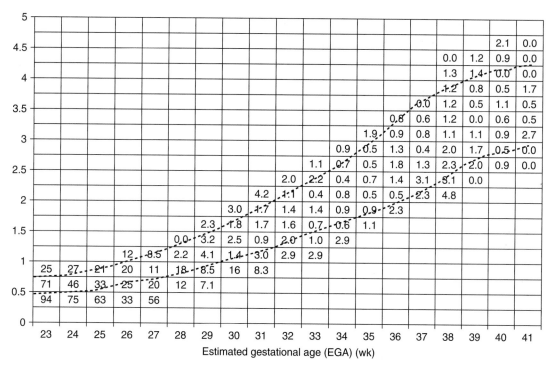

FIG. 6–8

Birth weight– and EGA-specific mortality rates. The dashed lines of the figure represent the 10th and 90th percentile weights. The grid lines are plotted by each gestational age and in 250-g weight increments. Each number in the box is the percent mortality rate for the grid defined by gestational age and birth weight range. (From Thomas P, Peabody J, Turnier V, et al: *Pediatrics* 106:E21, 2000.)

Nevus simplex (salmon patch), or pink macular hemangiomas, is common, usually transient, and noted on the back of the neck, eyelids, and forehead. **Nevus flammeus**, or the **port-wine stain**, commonly is seen on the face and should cause the examiner to consider the Sturge-Weber syndrome (trigeminal angiomatosis, convulsions, and ipsilateral intracranial "tram-line" calcifications).

Congenital melanocytic nevi are pigmented lesions of varying size noted in 1% of neonates. **Giant pigmented nevi** are uncommon but have malignant potential. **Capillary hemangiomas** are raised, red lesions, whereas **cavernous hemangiomas** are deeper, blue masses. Both increase in size after birth, only to resolve when the infant is 1–4 years of age. When enlarged, these hemangiomas may produce high-output heart failure or platelet trapping and hemorrhage. **Erythema toxicum** is an erythematous, papular-vesicular rash common in neonates that develops after birth and involves eosinophils in the vesicular fluid. **Pustular melanosis,** more common in black infants, may be seen at birth and consists of a small, dry vesicle on a pigmented brown macular base. Both erythema toxicum and pustular melanosis are benign lesions but may mimic more serious conditions, such as the vesicular rash of disseminated herpes simplex or the bullous eruption of *Staphylococcus aureus* impetigo. Tzanck smear, Gram stain, Wright stain, direct fluorescent antibody stain, polymerase chain reaction (PCR) for herpes deoxyribonucleic acid (DNA), and appropriate cultures may be needed to distinguish these rashes. Other common characteristic rashes are **milia** (yellow-white epidermal cysts of the pilosebaceous follicles that are noted on the nose) and **miliaria** (prickly heat), which is caused by obstructed sweat glands. **Edema** may be present in preterm infants but also suggests hydrops fetalis, sepsis, or lymphatic disorders.

Skull

The skull may be elongated and molded after a prolonged labor, but this resolves 2–3 days after birth. The sutures should be palpated to determine the width and the presence of premature fusion, or **cranial synostosis.** The anterior and posterior fontanels should be soft and nonbulging, with the anterior larger than the posterior. A **large fontanel** is associated with hydrocephalus, hypothyroidism, rickets, and other disorders. Soft areas away from the fontanel are **craniotabes;** these lesions feel like a ping-pong ball when they are palpated. They may be a result of in utero compression. The skull should be examined carefully for signs of trauma or lacerations from internal fetal electrode sites or fetal scalp pH sampling; abscess formation may develop in these areas. **Caput succedaneum** and **subgaleal hemorrhage** are discussed under Birth Injury earlier in this chapter.

Face, Eyes, Mouth

The face should be inspected for dysmorphic features such as epicanthal folds, hypertelorism, preauricular tags or sinuses, low-set ears, long philtrum, and cleft lip or palate. Facial asymmetry may be a result of seventh nerve palsy; head tilt may be caused by torticollis.

The eyes should open spontaneously, especially in an upright position. Before 28 weeks' gestational age, the eyelids may be fused. Coloboma, megalocornea, and microphthalmia suggest other malformations or intrauterine infections. A cloudy cornea greater than 1 cm in diameter also may be seen in congenital glaucoma, uveal tract dysgenesis, and storage diseases. Conjunctival and retinal hemorrhages are common and usually of no significance. The pupillary response to light is present at 28 weeks of gestation, and the **red reflex** of the retina is demonstrated easily. A white reflex, or **leukokoria,** is abnormal and may be the result of cataracts, ocular tumor, severe chorioretinitis, persistent hyperplastic primary vitreous, or retinopathy of prematurity.

The mouth should be inspected for the presence of natal teeth, clefts of the soft and hard palate and uvula, and micrognathia. A bifid uvula suggests a submucosal cleft. White, shiny, multiple transient epidermal inclusion cysts (Epstein pearls) on the hard palate are normal. Hard, marble-sized masses in the buccal mucosa are usually transient idiopathic fat necrosis. The *tympanic membranes* are dull, gray, opaque, and immobile. These findings may persist for 1–4 weeks and should not be confused with otitis media.

Neck and Chest

The neck appears short and symmetric. Abnormalities include midline clefts or masses caused by thyroglossal duct cysts or by goiter and lateral neck masses (or sinuses), which are, in turn, the result of branchial clefts. Cystic hygromas and hemangiomas are other masses that may be present. Shortening of the sternocleidomastoid muscle with a fibrous "tumor" over the muscle produces head tilt and asymmetric facies **(neonatal torticollis).** The Arnold-Chiari malformation and cervical spine lesions also produce torticollis. Edema and webbing of the neck suggest *Turner syndrome.* Both clavicles should be palpated for fractures.

Examination of the *chest* includes inspection of the chest wall to identify asymmetry resulting from absence of the pectoralis muscle and inspection of the breast tissue to determine gestational age and detect a breast abscess. Both boys and girls may have breast engorgement and produce milk; milk expression should not be attempted. **Supernumerary nipples** may be bilateral and occasionally are associated with renal anomalies.

Lungs

Examination of the lungs includes observations of the rate, depth, and nature of intercostal or sternal retractions. Breath sounds should be equal on both sides of the chest, and rales should not be heard after the first 1–2 hours of life. Diminished or absent breath sounds on one side suggest **pneumothorax,** collapsed lung, pleural effusion, or diaphragmatic hernia. Shift of the cardiac impulse away from a tension pneumothorax and diaphragmatic hernia and toward the collapsed lung is a helpful physical finding for differentiating these disorders. **Subcutaneous emphysema** of the neck or chest also suggests a pneumothorax, whereas bowel sounds auscultated in the chest in the presence of a scaphoid abdomen suggest a diaphragmatic hernia.

Heart

The position of the heart in infants is more midline than in older children. The first heart sound is normal, whereas the second heart sound may not be split in the first day of life. Decreased splitting of the second heart sound is noted in primary pulmonary hypertension (PPHN) (also known as persistent fetal circulation [PFC]), transposition of the great vessels, and pulmonary atresia. **Heart murmurs** in the newborn are common in the delivery room and during the first day of life. Most of these murmurs are transient and are a result of closure of the ductus arteriosus, peripheral pulmonary artery stenosis, or a small VSD. Pulses should be palpated in the upper and lower extremities, usually over the brachial and femoral arteries. Blood pressure in the upper and lower extremities should be measured in all patients with a murmur or heart failure. An upper-to-lower extremity gradient of more than 10–20 mm Hg suggests coarctation of the aorta.

Abdomen

In the abdomen the liver may be palpable 2 cm below the right costal margin. The spleen tip is less likely to be palpable. A left-sided liver suggests situs inversus and the asplenia syndrome. Both kidneys should be palpable in the first day of life with gentle, deep palpation. The first urination occurs during the first day of life in over 95% of normal term infants.

Abdominal masses usually represent hydronephrosis or dysplastic-multicystic kidney disease. Less often they indicate ovarian cysts, intestinal duplication, neuroblastoma, or mesoblastic nephroma. Masses should be evaluated immediately with ultrasound. Abdominal distention may be caused by intestinal obstructions such as ileal atresia, meconium ileus, midgut volvulus, imperforate anus, or Hirschsprung disease. Meconium stool is passed normally within 48 hours of birth in 99% of term infants. The anus should be patent. An imperforate anus is not always visible; therefore, the first temperature taken with a rectal thermometer should be taken carefully. The abdominal wall musculature may be absent, as in prune-belly syndrome, or weak, resulting in diastasis recti. **Umbilical hernias** are common among black infants. The umbilical cord should be inspected to determine the presence of two arteries and one vein and the absence of a urachus or a herniation of abdominal contents, as occurs with an **omphalocele.** The latter is associated with extraintestinal problems such as genetic trisomies and hypoglycemia *(Beckwith-Wiedemann syndrome)*. Bleeding from the cord suggests a coagulation disorder, and a chronic discharge may be a granuloma of the umbilical stump or less frequently a draining omphalomesenteric cyst. Erythema around the umbilicus is **omphalitis** and may cause portal vein phlebitis and subsequent extrahepatic portal hypertension. The herniation of bowel through the abdominal wall 2–3 cm lateral to the umbilicus is a **gastroschisis.**

Genitalia

The appearance of the genitalia varies with gestational age. At term, the testes should be descended into a well-formed pigmented and rugated scrotum. The testes occasionally are in the inguinal canal; this is more common among preterm infants, as is **cryptorchidism.** Scrotal swelling may represent a hernia, transient hydrocele, in utero torsion of the testes, or, rarely, dissected meconium from meconium ileus and peritonitis. Hydroceles are clear and readily seen by transillumination, whereas testicular torsion in the newborn may present as a painless, dark swelling. The urethral opening should be at the end of the penis. Epispadias or hypospadias alone should not raise concern about pseudohermaphroditism. However, if no testes are present in the scrotum and hypospadias is present, problems of sexual development should be suspected. Circumcision should be deferred with hypospadias because the foreskin is needed for the repair. The normal prepuce is often too tight to retract in the neonatal period.

The female genitalia normally may reveal a milky white or blood-streaked vaginal discharge as a result of maternal hormone withdrawal. Mucosal tags of the labia majora are common. Distention of an **imperforate hymen** may produce **hydrometrocolpos** and a lower midline abdominal mass as a result of an enlarged uterus. Clitoral enlargement with fusion of the labial-scrotal folds (labia majora) suggests adrenogenital syndrome or exposure to masculinizing maternal hormones.

Extremities

Examination of the *extremities* should involve assessment of length, symmetry, and presence of hemihypertrophy; atrophy; polydactyly; syndactyly; simian creases; absent fingers; overlapping fingers; rocker-bottom feet; clubfoot; congenital bands; fractures; and amputations.

Spine

The spine should be examined for evidence of sacral hair tufts, a dermal sinus tract above the gluteal folds, congenital scoliosis (a result of hemivertebra), and soft tissue masses such as lipomas or meningomyeloceles.

Hips

The hips should be examined for congenital dysplasia (dislocation). Gluteal fold asymmetry or leg length discrepancy is a suggestive sign of dysplasia, but the examiner should perform the **Barlow test** and the **Ortolani maneuver** to evaluate the stability of the hip joint. These tests determine whether the femoral head can be displaced from the acetabulum (Barlow test) and then replaced (Ortolani maneuver). The examiner's long finger is placed over the greater trochanter, and the thumb is placed medially, just distal to the long finger. With the thighs held in midabduction, the examiner attempts to pull the femoral head gently out of the acetabulum with lateral pressure of the thumb and by rocking the knee medially. The reverse maneuver is performed by pressing the long finger on the greater trochanter and rocking the knee laterally. A "clunking" sensation is palpated when the femoral head leaves and returns to the acetabulum.

Neurologic Assessment

The neurologic examination should include assessment of active and passive tone, level of alertness, primary neonatal (primitive) reflexes, deep tendon reflexes, spontaneous motor activity, and cranial nerves (involving retinal examination, extraocular muscle movement, masseter power as in sucking, facial motility, hearing, and tongue function). The **Moro reflex** is one of the primary newborn reflexes. This reflex is present at birth and gone in 3–6 months. It is elicited by sudden, slight dropping of the supported head from a slightly raised supine position. This slight drop should elicit opening of the hands and extension and abduction of the arms, followed by upper extremity flexion and a cry. The **palmar grasp** is present as early as 28 weeks of age and gone by 4 months of age. **Deep tendon reflexes** may be brisk in the normal newborn; 5–10 beats of ankle clonus are normal. The **Babinski sign** is extensor or upgoing. The sensory examination can be evaluated by withdrawal of an extremity, grimace, and cry in response to painful stimuli. The **rooting reflex,** or the turning of the head toward light tactile stimulation of the perioral area, is present as early as 32 weeks of age.

REFERENCES

Behrman RE, Kliegman RM, Jenson HB, editors: *Nelson textbook of pediatrics*, ed 16, Philadelphia, 2000, WB Saunders, Chapters 90, 93, 95.

Illingworth R: *The normal child*, ed 10, Edinburgh, 1991, Churchill Livingstone.

Leppig K, Werler M, Cann C, et al: Predictive value of minor anomalies. I. Association with major malformations, *J Pediatr* 110(4):530-537, 1987.

RESPIRATORY DISORDERS
Approach to the Patient

Respiratory distress that becomes manifest by tachypnea, intercostal retractions, reduced air exchange, cyanosis, expiratory grunting, and flaring of the ala nasi is a nonspecific response to serious illness. Not all of the disorders producing neonatal respiratory distress are primary diseases of the lungs. The differential diagnosis of respiratory distress includes pulmonary, cardiac, hematologic, infectious, anatomic, and metabolic disorders that may directly or indirectly involve the lungs (Tables 6–14 and 6–19). Surfactant deficiency causes *respiratory distress syndrome* (RSD), resulting in cyanosis and tachypnea; *infection* produces pneumonia, demonstrated by interstitial or lobar infiltrates; *meconium aspiration* results in chemical pneumonitis with pulmonary hypertension; *hydrops fetalis* causes anemia and hypoalbuminemia with high-output heart failure and pulmonary edema; and congenital or acquired *pulmonary hypoplasia* causes pulmonary hypertension and pulmonary insufficiency. It also is useful to differentiate the common causes of respiratory distress according to gestational age (Table 6–19).

TABLE 6–19
Etiology of Respiratory Distress

Preterm Infant	Preterm and Full-Term Infant
Respiratory distress syndrome	Bacterial sepsis (GBS)
Erythroblastosis fetalis	Transient tachypnea
Nonimmune hydrops	Spontaneous pneumothorax
Pulmonary hemorrhage	Congenital anomalies (e.g., congenital lobar emphysema, cystic adenomatoid malformation, diphragmatic hernia)
Full-Term Infant	Congenital heart disease
Meconium aspiration pneumonia	Pulmonary hypoplasia
Polycythemia	Viral infection (e.g., herpes simplex, CMV)
Amniotic fluid aspiration	Inborn metabolic errors
Primary pulmonary hypertension of the neonate	

CMV, Cytomegalovirus; *GBS,* group B streptococcus.

TABLE 6–20
Initial Laboratory Evaluation of Respiratory Distress

Test	Rationale
Chest roentgenogram	To determine reticular granular pattern of RDS; to determine presence of pneumothorax, cardiomegaly, life-threatening congenital anomalies
Arterial blood gas	To determine severity of respiratory compromise, hypoxemia, and hypercapnia and type of acidosis; the severity determines treatment strategy
Complete blood count	Hemoglobin/hematocrit to determine anemia and polycythemia; white blood cell count to determine neutropenia/sepsis; platelet count and smear to determine DIC
Blood culture	To recover potential pathogen
Blood glucose	To determine presence of hypoglycemia, which may produce or occur simultaneously with respiratory distress; to determine stress hyperglycemia
Echocardiogram, electrocardiogram	In the presence of a murmur, cardiomegaly, or refractory hypoxia; to determine structural heart disease or PPHN

DIC, Disseminated intravascular coagulation; *PPHN,* primary pulmonary hypertension of the neonate; *RDS,* respiratory distress syndrome.

In addition to the specific therapy for the individual disorder, the supportive care and evaluation of the infant with respiratory distress can be applied to all the problems mentioned earlier (Tables 6–16 and 6–20). Blood gas monitoring and interpretation are key components of general respiratory care.

Treatment of hypoxemia requires knowledge of normal values. In term infants the arterial PaO_2 level is 55–60 mm Hg at 30 minutes of life, 75 mm Hg at 4 hours, and 90 mm Hg by 24 hours. Preterm infants have slightly lower values. $PaCO_2$ levels should be between 35 and 40 mm Hg, and the pH should be 7.35–7.40. It is imperative that arterial blood gas analysis be performed in all infants with significant respiratory distress, whether or not cyanosis is perceived. Cyanosis becomes evident when there are 5 g of unsaturated hemoglobin; therefore, anemia may interfere with the perception of cyanosis. Jaundice also may interfere with the appearance of cyanosis. Capillary blood gas determinations are useful in determining blood pH and the P_{CO_2} level. Because of the nature of the heel-stick capillary blood gas technique, venous blood may mix with arterial blood, resulting in falsely low blood Pa_{O_2} readings. Serial blood gas levels may be monitored by an indwelling arterial catheter placed in a peripheral artery or through the umbilical artery to the aorta at the level of the T6-10 or the L4-5 vertebrae. This placement avoids catheter occlusion of the celiac (T12), superior mesenteric (T12-L1), renal (L1-2), and inferior mesenteric (L2-3) arteries. Another method for monitoring blood gas levels is to combine capillary blood gas techniques with noninvasive methods used to monitor oxygen (e.g., pulse oximetry or transcutaneous oxygen diffusion [TcP_{O_2}]).

Metabolic acidosis, defined as a reduced pH (<7.25) and bicarbonate concentration (<18) accompanied by a normal or low P_{CO_2} level, may be caused by hypoxia or by insufficient tissue perfusion; the origin of the disorder may be pulmonary, cardiac, infectious, renal, hematologic, nutritional, metabolic, or iatrogenic. The initial approach to metabolic acidosis is to determine the cause and treat the pathophysiologic problem. This approach may include, as in the sequence of therapy for hypoxia, increasing the inspired oxygen concentration; applying continuous positive airway pressure nasally, using oxygen as the gas; or initiating mechanical ventilation using positive end-expiratory pressure and oxygen. Patients with hypotension produced by hypovolemia require fluids and may need inotropic or vasoactive drug support. If metabolic acidosis persists despite specific therapy, sodium bicarbonate (1 mEq/kg/dose) may be given by slow intravenous infusion.

Respiratory acidosis, defined as an elevated P_{CO_2} level and reduced pH without a reduction in the bicarbonate concentration, may be caused by pulmonary insufficiency or central hypoventilation. Most disorders producing respiratory distress can lead to hypercapnia. *Treatment* involves assisted ventilation but *not* sodium bicarbonate. If central nervous system depression of respirations is caused by placental passage of narcotic analgesics, assisted ventilation is instituted first, and then the central nervous system depression is reversed by naloxone.

Mixed metabolic/respiratory acidosis is common and requires combined therapy. Other acid-base disturbances such as metabolic alkalosis and respiratory alkalosis are uncommon in the neonatal period, unless caused by chronic use of diuretics or by ventilator-induced hyperventilation, respectively.

Respiratory Distress Syndrome (Hyaline Membrane Disease)

Lung Development

An appreciation of lung development is basic to understanding the pathophysiology of RDS. The lining of the alveolus consists of 90% type I cells and 10% type II cells. After 20 weeks of gestation, the type II cells contain vacuolated, osmophilic, lamellar inclusion bodies, which are packages of surface-active material (Fig. 6–9). This lipoprotein *surfactant* is 90% lipid and is composed predominantly of saturated phosphatidylcholine (dipalmityl phosphatidylcholine, or lecithin) but also contains phosphatidylglycerol, other phospholipids, and neutral lipids. The surfactant proteins SP-A, SP-B, SP-C, and SP-D are packaged into the lamellar body and contribute to surface-active properties and recycling of surfactant. Surfactant prevents atelectasis by reducing surface tension at low lung volumes when it is concentrated at end-expiration as the alveolar radius decreases; surfactant contributes to lung recoil by increasing surface tension at larger lung volumes when it is diluted during inspiration as the alveolar radius increases. Without surfactant, surface tension forces are not reduced and atelectasis develops during end-expiration as the alveolus collapses.

The timing of surfactant (lecithin) production in quantities sufficient to prevent atelectasis depends on an increase in fetal cortisol levels that begins between 32 and 34 weeks of gestation. Between 34 and 36 weeks, sufficient surface-active material is produced by the type II cells in the lung, is secreted into the alveolar lumen, and is excreted into the amniotic fluid. Thus the concentration of lecithin in amniotic fluid indicates fetal pulmonary maturity. Because the amount of lecithin is difficult to quantify, the ratio of lecithin (which increases with maturity) to sphingomyelin (which remains constant during gestation) (L/S ratio) is determined. A ratio of 2:1 usually indicates pulmonary maturity. The presence of minor phospholipids such as phosphatidylglycerol also is indicative of fetal lung maturity and may be useful in situations in which the L/S ratio is borderline or possibly affected by maternal diabetes, which reduces lung maturity.

Clinical Manifestations

Respiratory distress syndrome is caused by a deficiency of pulmonary surfactant that results in atelectasis, a decreased functional residual capacity, arterial hypoxemia, and respiratory distress. In addition to the developmental deficiency, surfactant synthesis may be reduced as a result of hypovolemia, hypothermia, acidosis, hypoxemia, and rare genetic dis-

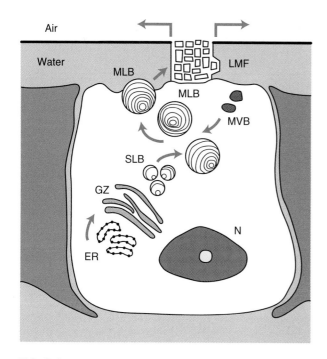

Air

Water

MLB

LMF

MLB

MVB

SLB

GZ

N

ER

FIG. 6–9

Proposed pathway of synthesis, transport, secretion, and reuptake of surfactant in the type II alveolar cell. Phospholipids are synthesized in the smooth endoplasmic reticulum (ER). The glucose/glycerol precursor may be derived from lung glycogen or circulating glucose. Phospholipids and surfactant proteins are packaged in the Golgi apparatus (GZ), emerge as small lamellar bodies (SLB), coalesce to mature lamellar bodies (MLB), migrate to the apical membrane, and are released by exocytosis into the liquid hypophase below the air-liquid interface. The tightly coiled lamellar body unravels to form the lattice (tubular) myelin figure (LMF), the immediate precursor to the phospholipid monolayer at the alveolar surface. Reuptake by endocytosis forms multivesicular bodies (MVB) that recycle surfactant. The enzymes, receptors, transporters, and surfactant proteins are controlled by regulatory processes at the transcriptional level in the nucleus (N). Corticosteroid and thyroid hormones are regulatory ligands that may accelerate surfactant synthesis. (From Hansen T, Corbet A: Lung development and function. In Taeusch HW, Ballard R, Avery ME, editors: *Diseases of the newborn*, ed 6, Philadelphia, 1991, WB Saunders.)

orders of surfactant synthesis. These factors also produce pulmonary artery vasospasm, which may contribute to RDS in larger premature infants who have developed sufficient pulmonary arteriole smooth muscle to produce vasoconstriction. Surfactant deficiency–induced atelectasis causes alveoli to be perfused but not ventilated, which results in a pulmonary shunt and hypoxemia. As atelectasis in-

creases, the lungs become increasingly difficult to expand, and lung compliance decreases. Because the chest wall of the premature infant is very compliant, the infant attempts to overcome decreased lung compliance with increasing inspiratory pressures, resulting in retractions of the chest wall. The sequence of decreased lung compliance and chest wall retractions leads to poor air exchange, an increased physiologic dead space, alveolar hypoventilation, and hypercapnia. A cycle of hypoxia, hypercapnia, and acidosis acts on type II cells to reduce surfactant synthesis and, in some infants, on the pulmonary arterioles to produce pulmonary hypertension.

Pathologic examination of the lung reveals atelectasis and acidophilic pink membranes (hyaline membranes) lining the air spaces. Hyaline membrane formation results from transudation of fluid through the capillary endothelium into the surfactant-deficient alveolus.

The infants at greatest risk for RDS are premature and have an immature L/S ratio. The incidence of RDS increases with decreasing gestational age. Nonetheless, RDS develops in only 30–60% of infants between 28 and 32 weeks of gestation. Other risk factors include delivery of a previous preterm infant with RDS, maternal diabetes, hypothermia, fetal distress, asphyxia, male sex, Caucasian race, being a second twin, and delivery by cesarean section without labor.

Signs of RDS may develop immediately in the delivery room in very immature infants at 26–30 weeks of gestation. However, some more mature infants (34 weeks of gestation) may not show signs of RDS until 3–4 hours after birth. Manifestations of RDS include cyanosis, tachypnea, nasal flaring, intercostal and sternal retractions, and a whining, crying, moaning sound called **grunting.** Grunting is a result of partial closure of the glottis during expiration, which leads to higher end-expiratory airway pressures that may ameliorate atelectasis. Atelectasis is well documented by radiographic examination of the chest, which demonstrates a ground-glass haze in the lung surrounding air-filled bronchi (the air bronchogram) (Fig. 6–10). Severe RDS may demonstrate an airless lung field or a "whiteout" on a roentgenogram, even obliterating the distinction between the atelectatic lungs and the heart.

During the first 72 hours, infants with RDS have increasing distress and hypoxemia. In infants with severe RDS, the development of edema, apnea, and respiratory failure necessitates mechanical ventilation. Thereafter, uncomplicated cases demonstrate a spontaneous improvement that often is heralded by diuresis and a marked resolution of edema. Complications include those noted in Table 6–21 and the

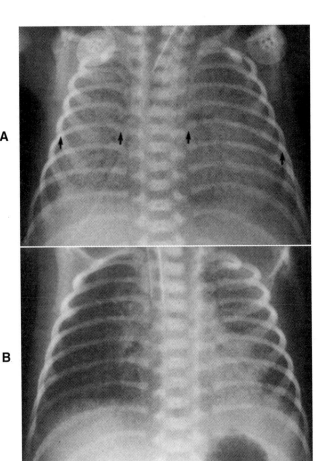

FIG. 6–10

Respiratory distress syndrome. The infant is intubated, and the lungs show a dense reticulonodular pattern with air bronchograms **(A)**. Note how to evaluate rotation on the frontal chest: the lengths of the posterior ribs are compared from left to right *(arrows)*. Because the infant is supine, the side of the longer ribs indicates to which side the thorax is rotated. In this case, the left ribs are longer and this radiograph is thus a left posterior oblique view. Surfactant was administered, resulting in significant improvement in the density of the lung **(B)**. The right lung is slightly better aerated than the left. Uneven distribution of clearing is common. (From Hilton S, Edwards D: *Practical pediatric radiology,* ed 2, Philadelphia, 1994, WB Saunders.)

TABLE 6–21
Acute Deterioration in Respiratory Distress Syndrome
Pneumothorax
Extubation
Endotracheal tube in right main stem bronchus
Mucous plug in endotracheal tube
Pulmonary hemorrhage
Intraventricular hemorrhage
Pneumopericardium
Sepsis
Intraabdominal hemorrhage (liver, spleen, adrenal gland)
Acute pulmonary hypertension (shunting)

sarean section or premature labor. In addition, prevention of cold stress, birth asphyxia, and hypovolemia reduces the risk of RDS and its severity. If premature delivery is unavoidable, the antenatal administration of corticosteroids (e.g., betamethasone) to the mother (and thus to the fetus) stimulates fetal lung production of surfactant; this approach requires multiple doses for at least 48 hours.

After birth, RDS may be prevented or its severity reduced by the intratracheal administration of synthetic or the more effective natural surfactants to premature infants with immature amniotic L/S ratios. Synthetic (e.g., lecithin, tyloxapol, and hexadecanol) or natural (e.g., lecithin-fortified extract of cow lungs) surfactant also can be administered repeatedly during the course of RDS in patients receiving endotracheal intubation, mechanical ventilation, and oxygen therapy. Additional management includes the general supportive and ventilation care presented in Tables 6–16, 6–20, and 6–22.

The PaO_2 level should be maintained between 60 and 70 mm Hg (O_2 saturation >90%), and the pH should be kept above 7.25. An increased concentration of warm and humidified inspired oxygen administered by an oxygen hood or nasal cannula may be all that is needed for larger premature infants. If hypoxemia (PaO_2 <50 mm Hg) is present and the needed inspired oxygen concentration is 70–100%, continuous positive airway pressure (nasal CPAP) should be added at a distending pressure of 8–10 cm H_2O. If respiratory failure ensues (PCO_2 >60 mm Hg, pH <7.20, and PaO_2 <50 mm Hg with 100% O_2), mechanical ventilation using a respirator is indicated. Conventional rate (25–60 breaths/min), high-frequency jet (150–600 breaths/min), and oscillator (900–3000 breaths/min) ventilators each have been

development of a PDA and bronchopulmonary dysplasia (BPD). The differential diagnosis of RDS includes diseases associated with cyanosis and respiratory distress (Tables 6–14 and 6–19).

Prevention and Treatment

Essential preventive measures for RDS include preventing premature birth from either elective ce-

TABLE 6–22
Ventilator Management of Respiratory Distress Syndrome

Setting	Result	Rationale	Risks
↑ FiO_2	↑ PO_2	↑ Alveolar O_2	Oxygen toxicity
↑ PIP	↑ PO_2	↑ $\overline{P}aw$	Pneumothorax, barotrauma, ↓ cardiac output?
	↓ PCO_2	↑ Tidal volume	
↑ PEEP	↑ PO_2	↑ $\overline{P}aw$	↑ PCO_2 by ↓ tidal volume
			↓ Cardiac output?
↑ Rate	↓ PCO_2	↑ Alveolar ventilation	↓ Expiratory time causes gas trapping
↑ I:E ratio	↑ PO_2	↑ $\overline{P}aw$	↓ Expiratory time causes gas trapping

FiO_2, Fraction of inspired oxygen; *I:E*, inspiratory to expiratory time ratio; $\overline{P}aw$, mean airway pressure; *PEEP*, positive end-expiratory pressure; *PIP*, peak inspiratory pressure.

successful in managing respiratory failure caused by severe RDS. Suggested starting settings on a conventional ventilator are: fraction of inspired oxygen (FiO_2), 60–100%; peak inspiratory pressure (PIP), 20–25 cm H_2O; positive end-expiratory pressure (PEEP), +5 cm H_2O; and a rate of 30–50 breaths/min. The inspiratory-to-expiratory time (I:E) ratio is 1:1.2 to 1:2.0.

In response to persistent hypercapnia, alveolar ventilation (tidal volume − dead space × rate) must be increased. Ventilation can be increased by an increase in the ventilator's rate or an increase in the tidal volume, which is the gradient between PIP and PEEP. In response to hypoxia the inspired oxygen content may be increased. Alternatively, the degree of oxygenation is dependent on the mean airway pressure ($\overline{P}aw$). $\overline{P}aw$ is directly related to PIP, PEEP, flow, and I:E ratio. Increased $\overline{P}aw$ may improve oxygenation by improving lung volume, thus enhancing ventilation-perfusion matching (Table 6–22).

Because of the difficulty in distinguishing sepsis and pneumonia from RDS, broad-spectrum parenteral antibiotics (e.g., ampicillin and gentamicin) are administered for 72 hours, pending the recovery of an organism from a previously obtained blood culture.

Complications

Patent Ductus Arteriosus. The ductus arteriosus constricts after birth in normal term infants in response to an elevated PaO_2 level. The ductus arteriosus in the preterm infant is less responsive to vasoconstrictive stimuli, in part as a result of the persistent vasodilatory effect of PGE_2. This decreased vasoconstriction response, combined with hypoxemia during RDS, may lead to a persistent PDA that creates a shunt between the pulmonary and systemic circulations.

During the acute phase of RDS, hypoxia, hypercapnia, and acidosis lead to pulmonary arterial vasoconstriction and increased pressure. Therefore, the pulmonary and systemic pressures may be equal, and flow through the ductus may be small or bidirectional. When RDS improves and pulmonary vascular resistance declines, flow through the ductus arteriosus increases in a left-to-right direction. Significant systemic-to-pulmonary shunting may lead to heart failure and pulmonary edema. Excessive intravenous fluid administration may increase the incidence of symptomatic PDA. The infant's respiratory status deteriorates because of increased lung fluid, hypercapnia, and hypoxemia. In response to poor blood gas levels, the infant is subjected to higher inspired oxygen concentrations and higher peak inspiratory ventilator pressures, both of which damage the lung. This is discussed under Bronchopulmonary Dysplasia.

Clinical manifestations of a PDA usually become apparent on the second to fourth day of life. Because the left-to-right shunt directs flow to a low-pressure circulation from one of high pressure, the pulse pressure widens; a previously inactive precordium now demonstrates a very active precordial impulse, and the peripheral pulses become easily palpable and bounding. The murmur of a PDA may be continuous in systole and diastole, but usually only the systolic component is auscultated. Heart failure and pulmonary edema result in rales and hepatomegaly. A chest roentgenogram demonstrates cardiomegaly and pulmonary edema; a two-dimensional echocardiogram demonstrates patency, whereas Doppler studies demonstrate markedly increased left-to-right flow through the ductus.

Treatment of a PDA during RDS involves an initial period of fluid restriction and diuretic administration. If there is no improvement after 24–48 hours, indomethacin, a prostaglandin synthetase inhibitor, is administered (0.2 mg/kg) intravenously every 12 hours for three doses. Thereafter the drug is administered at 0.1–0.2 mg/kg every 24 hours for 5 days. This has been most successful in closing the PDA among premature infants in the first 2 weeks of life, when prostaglandins may still be playing a significant role in maintaining ductal patency. Contraindications to using indomethacin include thrombocytopenia (platelets <50,000), bleeding, serum creatinine measuring more than 1.8 mg/dL, and oliguria. Because 20–30% of infants do not respond initially to indomethacin and because the PDA reopens in 10% of those who do, a repeated course of indomethacin or surgical ligation is required in a significant number of patients. Ibuprofen may be as effective as indomethacin, with fewer side effects.

Pulmonary Air Leaks. High PIPs and PEEPs may cause overdistention of alveoli in localized areas of the lung. Rupture of the alveolar epithelial lining may produce **pulmonary interstitial emphysema** (PIE) as gas dissects along the interstitial space and the peribronchial lymphatics. Extravasation of gas into the parenchyma reduces lung compliance and worsens respiratory failure. Gas dissection into the mediastinal space produces a **pneumomediastinum,** occasionally with gas dissecting into the subcutaneous tissues around the neck, causing **subcutaneous emphysema.**

Alveolar rupture adjacent to the pleural space produces a **pneumothorax** (this is discussed further in this chapter under Physical Examination and Gestational Age Assessment). If the gas is under tension, the pneumothorax shifts the mediastinum to the opposite side of the chest, producing hypotension, hypoxia, and hypercapnia. The diagnosis of a pneumothorax may be based on unequal transillumination of the chest and may be confirmed by chest roentgenogram (Fig. 6–11). *Treatment* of a symptomatic pneumothorax requires insertion of a pleural chest tube connected to negative pressure or to an underwater drain. Prophylactic or therapeutic use of exogenous surfactant has reduced the incidence of pulmonary air leaks.

Pneumothorax also is observed following vigorous resuscitation, meconium aspiration pneumonia, pulmonary hypoplasia, and diaphragmatic hernia. Spontaneous pneumothorax is seen in fewer than 1% of deliveries and may be associated with renal malformations.

Pneumopericardium is a severe life-threatening condition that may cause cardiac tamponade. Sys-

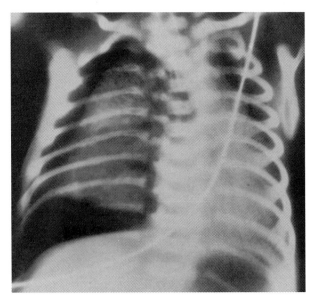

FIG. 6–11

Pneumothorax. Right-sided hyperlucent pleural air is obvious. The findings of linear interstitial air and the resultant noncompliant but collapsed right lung are also noted. (From Heller R, Kirchner S: *Advanced exercises in diagnostic radiology: the newborn,* Philadelphia, 1979, WB Saunders.)

temic gas embolism is a rare but lethal complication of mechanical ventilation.

Bronchopulmonary Dysplasia (Chronic Lung Disease). Oxygen concentrations above 40% are toxic to the neonatal lung. Oxygen-mediated lung injury results from the generation of superoxides, hydrogen peroxide (H_2O_2), and oxygen free radicals, which disrupt membrane lipids. Mechanical ventilation with high peak pressures produces barotrauma, compounding the damaging effects of high inspired oxygen levels. In most patients, BPD develops following ventilation for RDS that may have been complicated by PDA or PIE. Failure of RDS to improve after 2 weeks, the need for prolonged mechanical ventilation, and oxygen therapy required at 36 weeks postconception age are characteristic of patients with RDS in whom BPD develops. BPD may also develop in infants weighing less than 1000 g who require mechanical ventilation for poor respiratory drive in the absence of RDS. Fifty percent of infants of 24–26 weeks' gestational age require oxygen at 36 weeks corrected age.

The roentgenographic appearance of BPD may involve phases that are characterized initially by lung opacification and, subsequently, by development of cysts accompanied by areas of overdistention and atelectasis, giving the lung a sponge-like appearance.

The histopathology of BPD reveals interstitial edema, atelectasis, mucosal metaplasia, interstitial fibrosis, necrotizing obliterative bronchiolitis, and overdistended alveoli.

The *clinical manifestations* of BPD are oxygen dependence, hypercapnia, compensatory metabolic alkalosis, pulmonary hypertension, poor growth, and the development of right-sided heart failure. Increased airway resistance with reactive airway bronchoconstriction is also noted and is treated with bronchodilating agents. Severe chest retractions produce very negative interstitial pressure that draws fluid into the interstitial space. Together with cor pulmonale, these chest retractions cause fluid retention, necessitating fluid restriction and the administration of diuretics.

Patients with severe BPD may need *treatment* with mechanical ventilation for many months. To reduce the risk of subglottic stenosis, a tracheotomy may be indicated. To reduce oxygen toxicity and barotrauma, ventilator settings are reduced to maintain blood gases with slightly lower PaO_2 (50 mm Hg) and higher $PaCO_2$ (50–75 mm Hg) levels than for infants during the acute phase of RDS. Dexamethasone therapy may reduce inflammation, improve pulmonary function, and enhance weaning of patients from mechanical ventilation. Dexamethasone may increase neurodevelopmental morbidities. Older survivors of BPD have hyperinflation, reactive airways, and developmental delay. They are at risk for severe RSV pneumonia and as infants should receive prophylaxis against RSV.

Retinopathy of Prematurity (Retrolental Fibroplasia). Retinopathy of prematurity (ROP) is caused by the acute and chronic effects of oxygen toxicity on the developing blood vessels of the premature infant's retina. The completely vascularized retina of the term infant is not susceptible to ROP. ROP is a leading cause of blindness for VLBW infants (<1500 g). Excessive arterial oxygen tensions produce vasoconstriction of the immature retinal vasculature in the first stage of this disease. The vasoconstriction is followed by vasoobliteration if the duration and extent of hyperoxia are prolonged beyond the time when vasoconstriction is reversible. Hypercarbia and hypoxia may contribute to ROP. The subsequent proliferative stages are characterized by extraretinal fibrovascular proliferation, forming a ridge between the vascular and avascular portions of the retina, and by the development of neovascular tufts. In mild cases, vasoproliferation is noted at the periphery of the retina. Severe cases may have neovascularization involving the entire retina, retinal detachment resulting from traction on vessels as they leave the optic disc, fibrous proliferation behind the lens producing leukokoria, and synechiae displacing the lens forward and leading to glaucoma. Both eyes usually are involved, but severity may be asymmetric.

The incidence of ROP may be reduced by careful monitoring of arterial blood gas levels in all patients receiving oxygen. Although there is no absolutely safe PaO_2 level, it is wise to keep the arterial O_2 level between 50 and 70 torr in premature infants. Infants who weigh less than 1500 g or who are born before 28 weeks gestational age (some say 32 weeks) should be screened when they are older than 7 weeks old or more than 34 weeks corrected gestational age, whichever comes first. Laser therapy or (less often) cryotherapy may be used for vitreous hemorrhage or for severe, progressive vasoproliferation. Surgery is indicated for retinal detachment. Less severe stages of ROP resolve spontaneously and without visual impairment in the majority of patients.

Transient Tachypnea of the Newborn

Transient tachypnea of the newborn (TTN) is a self-limited condition characterized by tachypnea, mild retractions, and occasional grunting, usually without signs of severe respiratory distress. Cyanosis, when present, usually requires no more than 30–40% O_2. TTN usually is noted in larger premature infants and in term infants born by cesarean section without prior labor. The infant of a diabetic mother and the infant with poor respiratory drive as a result of placental passage of analgesic drugs are also at risk. Chest roentgenograms show prominent central vascular markings, fluid in the lung fissures, overaeration, and occasionally a small pleural effusion. Air bronchograms and a reticulogranular pattern are not seen in TTN, and their presence suggests another pulmonary process such as RDS or pneumonia. TTN may be caused by retained lung fluid or slow resorption of lung fluid.

Meconium Aspiration Syndrome

Meconium-stained amniotic fluid is seen in 10% of predominantly term, growth-retarded, and postterm deliveries. Although the passage of meconium into amniotic fluid is quite common among infants born in the breech presentation, meconium-stained fluid should be considered a sign of fetal distress for infants born in all presentations. Fetal scalp pH should be determined, and biophysical evaluation should be performed to assess the well-being of the fetus. The presence of meconium in the amniotic fluid suggests in utero asphyxia, hypoxia, and acidosis.

Aspiration of amniotic fluid contaminated with particulate meconium is an additional risk. Aspiration may occur in utero in a distressed, gasping fetus; more often, meconium is aspirated into the lung immediately after delivery. Affected infants have abnormal chest roentgenograms, demonstrating a high incidence of pneumonia and pneumothoraces.

Meconium aspiration pneumonia is characterized by tachypnea, hypoxia, hypercapnia, and small airway obstruction that produces a ball-valve effect, leading to air trapping, overdistention, and extraalveolar air leaks. Complete small airway obstruction produces atelectasis. Within 24–48 hours, a chemical pneumonia develops in addition to the mechanical effects of airway obstruction. The chest roentgenogram reveals patchy infiltrates, overdistention, flattening of the diaphragm, increased anteroposterior diameter, and a very high incidence of pneumomediastinum and pneumothoraces. Quite unexpectedly, many symptomatic infants with severe hypoxia appear completely normal on chest films. The condition of these infants with severe pulmonary hypertension is quite similar to that of infants with PPHN (PFC). Comorbid diseases include those associated with in utero asphyxia that initiated the passage of meconium (Table 6–11).

Treatment of meconium aspiration includes general supportive care and mechanical ventilation. Infants with a PPHN-like presentation should be treated for PPHN. If severe hypoxia does not subside with conventional or high-frequency ventilation, surfactant therapy and then inhaled nitric oxide (NO) followed by extracorporeal membrane oxygenation (ECMO) may be beneficial.

Prevention of meconium aspiration syndrome involves careful in utero monitoring to prevent asphyxia. When meconium-stained fluid is observed, the obstetrician should suction the infant's oropharynx before delivering the rest of the infant's body. After birth the depressed or distressed infant's oropharynx should be suctioned, the vocal cords visualized, and the area below the vocal cords suctioned to remove meconium from the trachea. This procedure can be repeated two to three times as long as meconium is present, before either stimulating the infant to breathe or initiating artificial ventilation (this is further discussed in this chapter under Resuscitation in the section on Asphyxia). Saline intrauterine amnioinfusion during labor may reduce the incidence of aspiration and pneumonia.

Primary Pulmonary Hypertension of the Newborn

(Persistent fetal circulation)

PPHN is characterized by severe hypoxemia, without evidence of parenchymal lung or structural heart disease that also may cause right-to-left shunting. The disorder is often seen in term or postterm infants who are asphyxiated or who have had meconium-stained fluid. The chest roentgenogram usually reveals normal lung fields rather than the expected infiltrates and hyperinflation that may accompany massive meconium aspiration pneumonia. Additional problems that may lead to PPHN are congenital pneumonia, hyperviscosity-polycythemia, congenital diaphragmatic hernia, pulmonary hypoplasia, hypoglycemia, and hypothermia. Total anomalous venous return associated with obstruction of blood flow may produce a clinical picture that involves severe hypoxia and that is indistinguishable from PPHN; a chest roentgenogram, however, reveals severe pulmonary venous engorgement and a small heart. Echocardiography or (rarely) cardiac catheterization will confirm the diagnosis.

Significant right-to-left shunting through a patent foramen ovale, through a PDA, and through intrapulmonary channels is also characteristic of PPHN. The pulmonary vasculature often demonstrates hypertrophied arterial wall smooth muscle, suggesting that the process of or predisposition to PPHN began in utero as a result of previous periods of fetal hypoxia. After birth, hypoxia, hypercapnia, and acidosis exacerbate pulmonary artery vasoconstriction, leading to further hypoxia and acidosis. In addition to pulmonary hypertension, some infants with PPHN have extrapulmonary manifestations as a result of asphyxia (Table 6–11). Myocardial injuries include heart failure, transient mitral insufficiency, and papillary muscle or myocardial infarction. Thrombocytopenia, right atrial thrombi, and pulmonary embolism also may be noted.

The *diagnosis* may be confirmed by echocardiographic examination, which demonstrates elevated pulmonary artery pressures and sites of right-to-left shunting. Echocardiography also is helpful to rule out structural congenital heart disease and transient myocardial dysfunction.

Treatment involves general supportive care; correction of hypotension, anemia, and acidosis; and the management of complications associated with asphyxia. If myocardial dysfunction is present, dopamine or dobutamine is needed. The most important therapy for PPHN is mechanical ventilation. Reversible mild pulmonary hypertension may respond to conventional ventilator settings (Table 6–22). However, patients with severe PPHN do not always respond to conventional therapy; some clinicians try hyperventilation to reverse pulmonary vasoconstriction by reducing P_{CO_2} to 20 mm Hg and increasing pH to 7.5–7.6. Paralysis with pancuronium may be needed to assist such vigorous ventilation. If mechanical ventilation and supportive care are unsuccessful in improving oxygenation, inhaled nitric oxide, a selective pulmonary artery vasodilating agent, should be administered. If hypoxia persists, the patient may be a candidate for ECMO. Infants who require very high ventilator settings, marked by an alveolar-to-arterial oxygen gradient greater than 620 mm Hg, have a high mortality rate and benefit from ECMO if they do not respond to nitric oxide.

Apnea

Apnea is defined as the cessation of pulmonary airflow for a specific time interval, usually longer than 10–20 seconds. Bradycardia often accompanies prolonged apnea. **Central apnea** refers to a complete cessation of airflow and respiratory efforts with no chest wall movement; in **obstructive apnea** no airflow is exhibited, but the chest wall movements continue. A combination of these two events, **mixed apnea,** is the most frequent type. It may begin as a brief episode of obstruction followed by a central apnea. Alternatively, central apnea may produce upper airway closure (passive pharyngeal hypotonia), resulting in mixed apnea.

A careful *evaluation* to determine the cause of apnea should be performed immediately in any infant with apnea (Table 6–23). The incidence of apnea increases as gestational age decreases. Idiopathic apnea, a disease of premature infants, appears in the absence of any other identifiable disease states during the first week of life and resolves by 36 weeks of postconceptional age (gestational age at birth + postnatal age). The premature infant's process of regulating respiration is especially vulnerable to apnea. For example, preterm infants respond paradoxically to hypoxia by developing apnea rather than by increasing respirations as mature infants do. Poor tone of the laryngeal muscles also may lead to collapse of the upper airway, causing obstruction. Isolated obstructive apnea also may occur as a result of flexion or extreme lateral positioning of the premature infant's head, which obstructs the soft trachea.

Treatment of apnea of prematurity involves administration of oxygen to hypoxic infants, transfusion of anemic infants, and physical cutaneous stimulation for infants with mild apnea. Persistent apnea with bradycardia can be treated with methylxanthines (caffeine or theophylline). Theophylline decreases the incidence of apnea by acting as a central nervous system stimulant. Loading doses of 5 mg/kg followed by 1–2 mg/kg every 8–12 hours are sufficient. Elimination of theophylline is prolonged in preterm infants, and serum levels should be carefully monitored and maintained between 5 and 10 μg/mL. In the newborn infant, theophylline also is converted to caffeine, thus increasing its efficacy. Nasal CPAP of 3–5 cm H_2O also is an effective method of treating obstructive or mixed apneas; it may work by splinting the upper airway.

Miscellaneous Respiratory Disorders

Pulmonary hypoplasia becomes manifest as severe respiratory distress in the delivery room that progresses rapidly to pulmonary insufficiency. The lungs, which are very small, develop pneumothoraces with normal resuscitative efforts. A small chest size roentgenographically, joint contractures, and early onset of pneumothoraces (often bilateral) are early clues to the diagnosis. Pulmonary hypertension results from the decreased lung mass and hypertrophy of pulmonary arteriole muscle.

Pulmonary hypoplasia may be a result of asphyxiating thoracic dystrophies (a small chest wall) or of decreased amniotic fluid volume that causes uterine compression of the developing chest wall,

---

TABLE 6–23
Potential Causes of Neonatal Apnea

CNS	IVH, drugs, seizures, hypoxic injury
Respiratory	Pneumonia, obstructive airway lesions, atelectasis, extreme prematurity (<1000 g), laryngeal reflex, phrenic nerve paralysis, severe RDS, pneumothorax
Infectious	Sepsis, necrotizing enterocolitis, meningitis (bacterial, fungal, viral)
Gastrointestinal	Oral feeding, bowel movement, gastroesophageal reflux, esophagitis, intestinal perforation
Metabolic	$\downarrow$ Glucose, $\downarrow$ calcium, $\downarrow$ PO$_2$, $\downarrow$$\uparrow$ sodium, $\uparrow$ ammonia, $\uparrow$ organic acids, $\uparrow$ ambient temperature, hypothermia
Cardiovascular	Hypotension, hypertension, heart failure, anemia, hypovolemia, change in vagal tone
Idiopathic	Immaturity of respiratory center, sleep state, upper airway collapse

CNS, Central nervous system; *IVH,* intraventricular hemorrhage; *RDS,* respiratory distress syndrome.

thus inhibiting lung growth. The latter failure of lung development may be associated with renal agenesis (Potter syndrome) or with a chronic leak of amniotic fluid from ruptured membranes. Isolated agenesis of one lung (usually the left lung) often is asymptomatic and familial. In contrast, serious pulmonary hypoplasia is noted in patients with a **diaphragmatic hernia.** Herniated bowel interferes with lung growth and also leads to hypertrophy of the muscle layers of small pulmonary arteries, producing pulmonary hypertension. Pneumothoraces are common.

Treatment of a diaphragmatic hernia involves surgical evacuation of the chest and repair of the diaphragmatic defect after the pulmonary hypertension is treated. Respiratory care is similar to that for patients with PPHN.

Neuromuscular diseases that interfere with fetal breathing movements also may produce pulmonary hypoplasia (e.g., congenital anterior horn cell disease **[Werdnig-Hoffmann syndrome]**).

Another cause of bilateral pulmonary hypoplasia is **hydrops fetalis** (discussed under Obstetric Complications Associated with Fetal or Neonatal Risk earlier in this chapter). Hydrops from any cause is characterized by anasarca, ascites, and pleural and pericardial effusions. Bilateral pleural effusions act as space-occupying masses that interfere with lung growth, resulting in pulmonary hypoplasia.

REFERENCES

Behrman RE, Kliegman RM, Jenson HB, editors: *Nelson textbook of pediatrics*, ed 16, Philadelphia, 2000, WB Saunders, Chapter 97.

Committee on Fetus and Newborn: Use of inhaled nitric oxide, *Pediatrics* 106(2 Pt 1):344–345, 2000.

Davis P, Turner-Gomes S, Cunningham K, et al: Precision and accuracy of clinical and radiological signs in premature infants at risk of patent ductus arteriosus, *Arch Pediatr Adolesc Med* 149(10):1136–1141, 1995.

Jobe AH: Glucocorticoids in perinatal medicine: misguided rockets? *J Pediatr* 137(1):1–3, 2000.

Jobe AH: Which surfactant for treatment of respiratory distress syndrome, *Lancet* 355(9213):1380–1381, 2000.

Le Souef PN: Persistent tachypnoea in neonates, *BMJ* 312(7039): 1113–1114, 1996.

McIntosh N, Becher JC, Cunningham S, et al: Clinical diagnosis of pneumothorax is late: use of trend data and decision support might allow preclinical detection, *Pediatr Res* 48(3):408–415, 2000.

O'Brien LM, Stebbens VA, Poets CF, et al: Oxygen saturation during the first 24 hours of life, *Arch Dis Child Fetal Neonatal Ed* 83(1):F35–F38, 2000.

Shinwell ES, Karplus M, Reich D, et al: Early postnatal dexamethasone treatment and increased incidence of cerebral palsy, *Arch Dis Child Fetal Neonatal Ed* 83(3):F177–F181, 2000.

UK Collaborative ECMO Trial Group: UK collaborative randomised trial of neonatal extracorporeal membrane oxygenation, *Lancet* 348(9020):75–82, 1996.

Upton CJ, Milner AD, Stokes GM: Upper airway patency during apnea of prematurity, *Arch Dis Child* 67(4 Spec No):419–424, 1992.

Van Overmeire B, Smets K, Lecoutere D, et al: A comparison of ibuprofen and indomethacin for closure of patent ductus arteriosus, *N Engl J Med* 343(10):674–681, 2000.

Wiswell TE, Henley MA: Intratracheal suctioning, systemic infection and the meconium aspiration syndrome, *Pediatrics* 89(2): 203–206, 1992.

HEMATOLOGIC DISORDERS
Anemia

Embryonic hematopoiesis begins by the twentieth day of gestation and is evidenced as blood islands in the yolk sac. In midgestation, erythropoiesis occurs in the liver and spleen; the bone marrow becomes the predominant site in the last trimester. Hemoglobin concentration increases from 8–10 g/dL at 12 weeks to 16.5–18.0 g/dL at 40 weeks. Fetal red blood cell production is responsive to erythropoietin, and the concentration of this hormone increases with fetal hypoxia and anemia.

After birth, hemoglobin levels increase transiently at 6–12 hours and then decline to 11 g/dL at 3–6 months. The prematurely born infant, who is less than 32 weeks of gestational age, has a lower hemoglobin concentration and a more rapid postnatal decline of hemoglobin level, which achieves a nadir 1–2 months after birth. Fetal and neonatal red blood cells have a shorter life span (70–90 days) and a higher mean corpuscular volume (110–120 fL) than adult cells. Infants demonstrate a reticulocytosis of between 5% and 10% during the first day of life. Hemoglobin and hematocrit levels are higher in neonatal capillary samples obtained by skin pricks than they are in central venous or arterial samples.

In the fetus, *hemoglobin synthesis* in the last two trimesters of pregnancy produces fetal hemoglobin (hemoglobin F), composed of two alpha chains and two gamma chains. Immediately before term, the infant begins to synthesize beta-hemoglobin chains; thus the term infant should have some adult hemoglobin (two alpha chains and two beta chains). Fetal hemoglobin represents 60–90% of hemoglobin at birth, and the levels decline to adult levels of less than 5% by 4 months of age.

The time of presentation of hemoglobinopathy depends on the timing of chain synthesis. Thus, α-thalassemia caused by a four-gene defect produces no alpha chains and presents as severe anemia and hydrops (Bart hemoglobin, composed of four gamma chains). Hemoglobin H is caused by a thalassemia three-gene defect resulting in four beta chains, and appears with hemolysis and anemia in the infant. In contrast, infants with beta-chain abnormalities, such as Cooley anemia (β-thalassemia major) and sickle cell anemia, do not manifest anemia in the neonatal period.

The *blood volume* of the term infant is between 72–93 mL/kg. The placenta and umbilical vessels contain approximately 20–30 mL/kg of additional blood that can transiently increase neonatal blood volume and hemoglobin levels for the first 3 days of life if clamping or milking ("stripping") of the umbilical cord is delayed at birth. Delayed clamping increases the risk for polycythemia, increased pulmonary vascular resistance, hypoxia, and jaundice but improves glomerular filtration. Early clamping may lead to anemia, a cardiac murmur, poor peripheral perfusion but lower pulmonary vascular pressures, and less tachypnea. To prevent both situations, the cord should be clamped at approximately 30 seconds after birth. Hydrostatic pressure affects blood transfer between the placenta and the infant at birth, and an undesired fetal-to-placental transfusion will occur if the infant is situated above the level of the placenta.

The *physiologic anemia* noted at 2–3 months of age in term infants and at 1–2 months of age in preterm infants is associated with undetectable erythropoietin levels. Although hemoglobin levels decline during this period, an increased amount of tissue oxygen becomes available as a result of the production of hemoglobin A, which releases oxygen to the tissues (hemoglobin A becomes unsaturated) at a higher PO_2 level than does hemoglobin F. This is described with the oxygen dissociation curve of hemoglobin A in Fig. 6–3 and further discussed under Transition from Fetal to Neonatal Physiology earlier in this chapter.

Etiology

Symptomatic anemia in the newborn period (Fig. 6–12) may be caused by the following:
1. Blood loss
2. Decreased red blood cell production
3. Hemolysis

Blood Loss. Anemia from blood loss at birth is manifested by two patterns of presentation, depending on the rapidity of blood loss. Acute blood loss following fetomaternal hemorrhage, rupture of the umbilical cord, placenta previa, and internal hemorrhage (hepatic or splenic hematoma; retroperitoneal) is characterized by pallor, diminished peripheral pulses, and shock. There are no signs of extramedullary hematopoiesis and no hepatosplenomegaly. The hemoglobin content and serum iron levels initially are normal, but the hemoglobin levels decline during the subsequent 24 hours. Chronic blood loss caused by chronic fetomaternal hemorrhage or a twin-twin transfusion presents with marked pallor, heart failure, hepatosplenomegaly with or without hydrops, a low hemoglobin level at birth, a hypochromic microcytic blood smear, and

decreased serum iron stores. Fetomaternal bleeding occurs in 50–75% of all pregnancies, with fetal blood losses ranging between 1 and 50 mL; most blood losses are ≤1 ml, 1 in 400 are ~30 mL, and 1 in 2000 are ~100 mL.

The *diagnosis* of fetomaternal hemorrhage is confirmed by the acid elution test of Kleihauer and Betke; pink fetal red blood cells are observed and counted in the mother's peripheral blood smear because fetal hemoglobin is resistant to acid elution; adult hemoglobin is eluted, leaving discolored maternal cells (patients with sickle cell anemia or hereditary persistence of fetal hemoglobin may have a false positive result, and ABO incompatability may produce a false negative result).

Decreased Red Blood Cell Production. Anemia caused by decreased production of red blood cells appears at birth with pallor, a low reticulocyte count, and absence of erythroid precursors in the bone marrow. There may be associated physical anomalies (see Chapter 14). Potential causes include congenital infections, Diamond-Blackfan syndrome, parvovirus, osteopetrosis, congenital malignancies (e.g., leukemia and neuroblastoma), histiocytic disorders, sideroblasic anemia, and intrauterine transfusion.

Hemolysis. Immunologically mediated hemolysis in utero may lead to **erythroblastosis fetalis,** or the fetus may be spared and **hemolytic disease** may appear in the newborn infant. Hemolysis of fetal erythrocytes is a result of blood group differences between the sensitized mother and fetus, which causes production of maternal IgG antibodies directed against an antigen on fetal cells.

ABO blood group incompatibility with neonatal hemolysis develops only if the mother has IgG antibodies from a previous exposure to A or B antigens. These IgG antibodies cross the placenta by active transport and affect the fetus or newborn. Sensitization of the mother to fetal antigens may have occurred by previous transfusions or by conditions of pregnancy that result in transfer of fetal erythrocytes into the maternal circulation, such as first-trimester abortion, an ectopic pregnancy, amniocentesis, or even a normal pregnancy. The risk of fetomaternal transfusion is increased by manual extraction of the placenta and by version (external or internal) procedures.

ABO incompatibility with sensitization usually does not cause fetal disease other than very mild anemia. However, it may produce **hemolytic disease of the newborn** that is manifested as significant anemia and hyperbilirubinemia (discussed later). Because many mothers who have blood group O have IgG antibodies to A and B before pregnancy, the firstborn infant of A or B blood type may be affected. In contrast to Rh disease, ABO hemolytic disease does not become more severe with subsequent pregnancies.

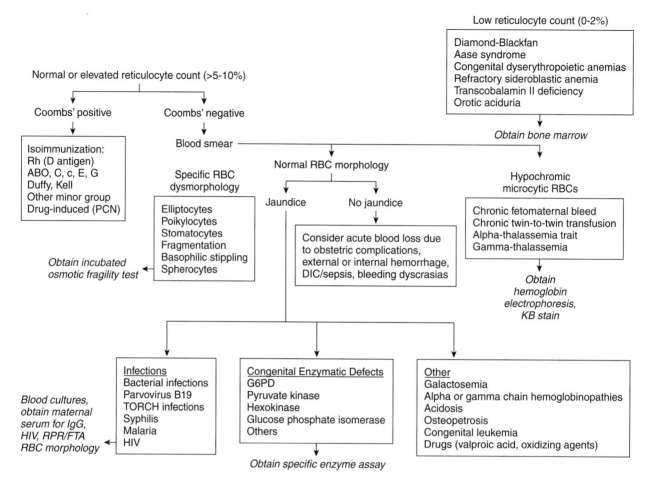

FIG. 6–12

Differential diagnosis of neonatal anemia. The physician obtains information from the family, maternal, and labor and delivery histories and then laboratory tests: hemoglobin, reticulocyte (retic) count, blood type, direct Coombs test, peripheral smear, red blood cell (RBC) indices, and bilirubin concentration. *DIC,* Disseminated intravascular coagulation; *HIV,* human immunodeficiency virus; *PCN,* penicillin; *RPR,* rapid plasma reagin tests; *FTA,* fluorescent treponemal antibody test; *G6PD,* glucose-6-phosphate dehydrogenase. *ATR-X, ATR-16,* X-linked α-thalassemia mental retardation syndromes. (From Ohls RK. In Christensen RD, editor: *Hematologic problems of the neonate,* Philadelphia, 2000, WB Saunders.)

Hemolysis with ABO incompatibility is less severe than hemolysis in Rh-sensitized pregnancy, either because the anti-A or anti-B antibody may bind to nonerythrocytic cells that contain A or B antigen or because fetal erythrocytes have fewer A or B antigenic determinants than they have Rh sites. ABO incompatibility is the most common cause of isoimmune hemolysis of the newborn infant.

Erythroblastosis fetalis classically is caused by Rh blood group incompatibility. Rh-negative women do not develop natural IgM antibodies, and most Rh-negative women have no anti-Rh antibodies at the time of their first pregnancy. The Rh antigen system consists of five antigens: C, D, E, c, and e; the d type is not antigenic. In the majority of Rh-sensitized cases, the D antigen of the fetus sensitizes the Rh-negative (d) mother, resulting in IgG antibody production during the first pregnancy.

Because most mothers are not sensitized to Rh antigens at the start of pregnancy, Rh erythroblastosis fetalis is usually a disease of the second and subsequent pregnancies. The first affected pregnancy results in an antibody response in the mother, which may be detected during antenatal screening with the Coombs test and determined to be anti-D antibody. The first affected newborn may demonstrate no serious fetal disease and may manifest hemolytic disease of the newborn only by the development of anemia and hyperbilirubinemia (discussed later). Subsequent pregnancies result in an increasing severity of response because of an earlier onset of hemolysis in utero. Fetal anemia, heart failure, elevated venous pressure, portal vein obstruction, and hypoalbuminemia result in **fetal hydrops**, which is characterized by ascites, pleural and pericardial effusions, and anasarca. The risk of fetal death is high.

The *management* of the pregnancy complicated by Rh sensitization depends on the severity of hemolysis, its effects on the fetus, and the maturity of the fetus at the time it becomes affected. The severity of the hemolysis can be assessed by the quantity of bilirubin transferred from the fetus to the amniotic fluid, quantified by spectrophotometric analysis of the optical density (at 450 nm) of amniotic fluid. Bilirubin levels in normal pregnancies are higher at earlier gestational ages and decrease as the fetus matures.

Three zones of optical densities with decreasing slopes toward term gestation have been developed to predict the severity of the illness. The high-optical-density zone 3 is associated with severe hemolysis; fetuses in the lower zones probably are not affected. If a fetus's optical density measurement for bilirubin falls into zone 3 and the fetus has pulmonary maturity as determined by the L/S ratio, it should be delivered and treated in the NICU. If the lungs are immature and the fetus is between 22 and 33 weeks of gestational age, an ultrasound-guided intrauterine transfusion with O-negative blood into the umbilical vein is indicated and may have to be repeated until pulmonary maturity is reached or fetal distress is detected. Indications for fetal intravascular transfusion in sensitized fetuses between 22 and 32 weeks of gestational age include a fetal hematocrit of less than 25–30%, fetal hydrops, and fetal distress too early in gestation for delivery and successful management with neonatal intensive care. Intravascular intrauterine transfusion corrects fetal anemia, improves the outcome of severe hydrops, and reduces the need for postnatal exchange transfusion but is associated with neonatal anemia as a result of continued hemolysis plus suppressed erythropoiesis.

Prevention of sensitization of the mother carrying an Rh-positive fetus is possible by treating the mother during gestation (after 28 weeks) and within 72 hours after birth with anti-Rh-positive immune globulin (RhoGAM). The dose of RhoGAM (300 μg) is based on the ability of this amount of anti–Rh-positive antibody to bind all the possible fetal Rh-positive erythrocytes entering the maternal circulation during the fetal-to-maternal transfusion at birth (~30 mL). RhoGAM may bind Rh-positive fetal erythrocytes or interfere with maternal anti–Rh-positive antibody production by another, unknown mechanism. RhoGAM is effective only in preventing sensitization to the D antigen. Other blood group antigens that can cause immune hydrops and erythroblastosis include Rh C, E, Kell, and Duffy. Anti-Kell alloimmunity produces lower amniotic bilirubin levels and a lower reticulocyte count because in addition to hemolysis it inhibits erythropoiesis.

Nonimmune causes of hemolysis in the newborn include *red cell enzyme deficiencies* of the Embden-Meyerhof pathway, such as pyruvate kinase or glucose-6-phosphate dehydrogenase deficiency. *Red cell membrane disorders* are another cause of nonimmune hemolysis. Hereditary spherocytosis is inherited as a severe autosomal recessive form or less severe autosomal dominant form and is the result of a deficiency of spectrin, a protein of the red blood cell membrane.

Hemoglobinopathies such as thalassemia are another cause of nonimmunologically mediated hemolysis.

Diagnosis and Management

Hemolysis in utero resulting from any cause may produce a spectrum of *clinical manifestations* at birth. Severe hydrops with anasarca, heart failure, and pulmonary edema may prevent adequate ventilation at birth, resulting in asphyxia. Infants affected with hemolysis in utero have hepatosplenomegaly and pallor and become jaundiced within the first 24 hours after birth. Less severely affected infants manifest pallor and hepatosplenomegaly at birth and become jaundiced subsequently. Patients with ABO incompatibility often are asymptomatic and without physical signs at birth; mild anemia with jaundice develops during the first 24–72 hours of life.

Because hydrops, anemia, or jaundice is secondary to many diverse causes of hemolysis, *a laboratory evaluation is needed in all patients with suspected hemolysis.* A complete blood count, blood smear, reticulocyte count, blood type, and direct Coombs test (to determine the presence of antibody-coated red blood cells) should be performed in the initial evaluation of all infants with hemolysis. Reduced hemoglobin levels, reticulocytosis, and a blood smear characterized by polychromasia and anisocytosis are expected with isoimmune hemolysis. Spherocytes are commonly observed in ABO incompatibility. The determination of the blood type and the Coombs test identify the responsible antigen and antibody in immunologically mediated hemolysis.

In the absence of a positive Coombs test and blood group differences between the mother and fetus, other causes of nonimmune hemolysis must be considered. Red cell enzyme assays, hemoglobin electrophoresis, or red cell membrane tests (e.g., osmotic fragility; spectrin assay) should be performed. Internal hemorrhage also may be associated with anemia, reticulocytosis, and jaundice when the hemorrhage reabsorbs; ultrasonographic evaluation of the brain, liver, spleen, or adrenal gland may be indicated when nonimmune hemolysis is suspected. Shock is more typical in patients with internal hemorrhage, whereas in hemolytic diseases heart failure may be seen with severe anemia. Evaluation of a possible fetomaternal hemorrhage should include the Kleihauer-Betke test.

The *treatment* of *symptomatic* neonatal anemia is transfusion of cross-matched packed red blood cells. If immune hemolysis is present, the cells to be transfused must be cross-matched against both maternal and neonatal plasma. Acute volume loss may necessitate resuscitation with nonblood products such as saline if blood is not available; packed red blood cells can be given subsequently. Ten to 15 mL/kg of packed red blood cells should be sufficient to correct anemia and any remaining blood volume deficit. Cytomegalovirus (CMV)-seronegative blood should be given to CMV-seronegative infants, and all blood products should be irradiated to reduce the risk of graft-versus-host disease; blood should be screened for HIV, hepatitis B and C, and syphilis. Recombinant erythropoietin may improve the hematocrit in infants with a hyporegenerative anemia following in utero transfusion.

Hyperbilirubinemia

Hemolytic disease of the newborn is a common cause of neonatal jaundice. Nonetheless, because of the immaturity of the pathways of bilirubin metabolism, many newborn infants without evidence of hemolysis become jaundiced.

Bilirubin is produced by the catabolism of hemoglobin in the reticuloendothelial system. The tetrapyrrole ring of heme is cleaved by heme oxygenase to form equivalent quantities of biliverdin and carbon monoxide. Because no other biologic source of carbon monoxide exists, the excretion of this gas is stoichiometrically identical to the production of bilirubin. Biliverdin is converted to bilirubin by biliverdin reductase. One gram of hemoglobin produces 35 mg of bilirubin. Sources of bilirubin other than circulating hemoglobin represent 20% of bilirubin production; these sources include inefficient (shunt) hemoglobin production and lysis of precursor cells in bone marrow. Compared with adults, newborn infants have a twofold to threefold greater rate of bilirubin produc-

tion (6–10 mg/kg/24 hr versus 3 mg/kg/24 hr). This is caused in part by an increased red blood cell mass (higher hematocrit) and a shortened erythrocyte life span of 70–90 days, compared with the 120-day erythrocyte life span in adults.

Bilirubin produced following hemoglobin catabolism is lipid soluble and unconjugated and reacts as an indirect reagent in the van den Bergh test. Indirect-reacting, unconjugated bilirubin is toxic to the central nervous system and is insoluble in water, thus limiting its excretion. Unconjugated bilirubin binds to albumin on specific bilirubin binding sites; 1 g of albumin binds 8.5 mg of bilirubin in the newborn. If the binding sites become saturated or if a competitive compound binds at the site, displacing bound bilirubin, free bilirubin becomes available to enter the central nervous system. Organic acids such as free fatty acids and drugs such as sulfisoxazole can displace bilirubin from its binding site on albumin.

Bilirubin dissociates from albumin at the hepatocyte and becomes bound to a cytoplasmic liver protein "Y" (ligandin). Hepatic conjugation results in the production of bilirubin diglucuronide, which is water soluble and capable of biliary and renal excretion. The enzyme UDP-glucuronyl transferase represents the rate-limiting step of bilirubin conjugation. The concentrations of ligandin and glucuronyl transferase are lower in the newborn infant, particularly in the premature infant, than in the older child.

Conjugated bilirubin gives a direct reaction in the van den Bergh test. Most conjugated bilirubin is excreted through the bile into the small intestine and eliminated in the stool. However, some bilirubin may undergo hydrolysis back to the unconjugated fraction by intestinal glucuronidase and then may be reabsorbed (enterohepatic recirculation). In addition, bacteria in the neonatal intestine convert bilirubin to urobilinogen or stercobilinogen, which are excreted in urine and stool, respectively, and usually limit bilirubin reabsorption. Delayed passage of meconium, which contains bilirubin, also may contribute to the enterohepatic recirculation of bilirubin.

Bilirubin is produced in utero by the normal fetus and by the fetus affected by erythroblastosis fetalis. Indirect, unconjugated, lipid-soluble fetal bilirubin is transferred across the placenta and subsequently becomes conjugated by maternal hepatic enzymes. The placenta is impermeable to conjugated water-soluble bilirubin. Fetal bilirubin levels become only mildly elevated in the presence of severe hemolysis but may increase when hemolysis produces fetal hepatic inspissated bile stasis and conjugated hyperbilirubinemia. Maternal indirect (but not direct) hyperbilirubinemia also may increase fetal bilirubin levels.

Etiology of Indirect Unconjugated Hyperbilirubinemia

(Table 6–24)

Physiologic jaundice is a common cause of hyperbilirubinemia among newborn infants. It is a diagnosis of exclusion, made after careful evaluation has ruled out more serious causes of jaundice such as hemolysis, infection, and metabolic diseases. Physiologic jaundice is the result of many factors that are normal physiologic characteristics of the newborn infant: increased bilirubin production resulting from an increased red blood cell mass, shortened red blood cell life span, and hepatic immaturity of ligandin and glucuronyl transferase. Physiologic jaundice may be exaggerated among infants of Greek and Asian ancestry.

The clinical pattern of physiologic jaundice in term infants includes a peak indirect-reacting bilirubin level of no more than 12 mg/dL on the third day of life. In premature infants the peak is higher (15 mg/dL) and occurs later (fifth day).

The peak level of indirect bilirubin during physiologic jaundice may be higher in breast milk–fed infants than in non-breast milk–fed infants (15–17 mg/dL versus 12 mg/dL). This may be in part a result of the decreased fluid intake of the infants fed breast milk. Jaundice is unphysiologic or pathologic if it is evident on the first day of life, if the bilirubin level increases more than 0.5 mg/dL/hr, if the peak bilirubin is greater than 13 mg/dL in term infants, if the direct bilirubin fraction is greater than 1.5 mg/dL, or if hepatosplenomegaly and anemia are present.

Crigler-Najjar syndrome is a serious, rare, permanent deficiency of UDP-glucuronyl transferase that results in severe indirect hyperbilirubinemia. The autosomal dominant variety responds to enzyme induction by phenobarbital, producing an increase in enzyme activity and a reduction of bilirubin levels.

The autosomal recessive form does not respond to phenobarbital and manifests as persistent indirect hyperbilirubinemia, often leading to kernicterus (discussed later). Gilbert disease is caused by a mutation of the promotor region of the UDP-glucuronyl transferase and results in a mild indirect hyperbilirubinemia. In the presence of another icterogenic factor (hemolysis), more severe jaundice may develop.

Breast milk feeding may be associated with unconjugated hyperbilirubinemia without evidence of hemolysis during the first to second week of life. Bilirubin levels rarely increase above 20 mg/dL. Interruption of breast-feeding for 1–2 days results in a rapid decline of bilirubin levels, which do not increase significantly after breast-feeding resumes. Breast milk may contain an inhibitor of bilirubin conjugation or may increase the enterohepatic recirculation of bilirubin because of breast milk glucuronidase.

Jaundice on the first day of life is always pathologic, and immediate attention is needed to establish the cause. Early onset often is a result of hemolysis, internal hemorrhage (e.g., cephalhematoma, hepatic or splenic hematoma), or infection (Table 6–24). Infection also is often associated with direct-reacting bilirubin (discussed later) resulting from perinatal congenital infections or from bacterial sepsis.

Physical evidence of jaundice is observable in infants when the bilirubin levels reach 5–10 mg/dL, versus only 2 mg/dL in adults. Once jaundice is observed, the laboratory evaluation for hyperbilirubinemia should include a total bilirubin measurement to determine the magnitude of hyperbilirubinemia. Bilirubin levels in excess of 5 mg/dL on the first day of life or in excess of 13 mg/dL thereafter in term infants should be evaluated further with measurement of indirect and direct bilirubin levels, blood typing, a Coombs test, a complete blood

---

TABLE 6–24
Etiology of Unconjugated Hyperbilirubinemia

	Hemolysis Present	Hemolysis Absent
Common	*Blood group incompatibility:* ABO, Rh, Kell, Duffy *Infection*	Physiologic jaundice, breast milk jaundice, internal hemorrhage, polycythemia, infant of diabetic mother
Rare	*Red cell enzyme defects:* glucose-6-phosphate dehydrogenase, pyruvate kinase *Red cell membrane disorders:* spherocytosis, ovalocytosis *Hemoglobinopathy:* thalassemia	Mutations of glucuronyl transferase enzyme (Crigler-Najjar syndrome, Gilbert disease), pyloric stenosis, hypothyroidism, immune thrombocytopenia

count, a blood smear, and a reticulocyte count. These tests must be performed before the treatment of hyperbilirubinemia with phototherapy or exchange transfusion. In the absence of hemolysis or evidence for either the common or the rare causes of nonhemolytic indirect hyperbilirubinemia, the diagnosis is either physiologic or breast milk jaundice. Jaundice present after 2 weeks of age is pathologic and suggests a direct-reacting hyperbilirubinemia.

Etiology of Direct Conjugated Hyperbilirubinemia

Direct-reacting hyperbilirubinemia should be evaluated according to the diagnostic categories noted in Table 6–25. Direct-reacting bilirubin (composed mostly of conjugated bilirubin) is not neurotoxic to the infant but signifies a serious underlying disorder involving cholestasis or hepatocellular injury. The diagnostic evaluation of patients with direct-reacting hyperbilirubinemia involves the determination of the levels of liver enzyme (aspartate aminotransferase [AST], alkaline phosphatase, alanine aminotransferase [ALT], and gamma-glutamyltranspeptidase), bacterial and viral cultures, metabolic screening tests, hepatic ultrasonography, a sweat chloride test,

---

TABLE 6–25
Etiology of Conjugated Hyperbilirubinemia

Common
Hyperalimentation cholestasis
CMV infection
Other perinatal congenital infections (TORCH)
Inspissated bile from prolonged hemolysis
Neonatal hepatitis
Sepsis

Uncommon
Hepatic infarction
Inborn errors of metabolism (galactosemia, tyrosinosis)
Cystic fibrosis
Biliary atresia
Choledochal cyst
Alpha₁-antitrypsin deficiency
Neonatal iron storage disease
Alagille syndrome (arteriohepatic dysplasia)
Byler disease

CMV, Cytomegalovirus; *TORCH,* toxoplasmosis, other, rubella, cytomegalovirus, herpes simplex.

---

and, occasionally, liver biopsy. Additionally, the presence of dark urine and gray-white (acholic) stools with jaundice after the second week of life strongly suggests biliary atresia. The *treatment* of disorders manifested by direct bilirubinemia is specific for those diseases that are noted in Table 6–25 (see Chapter 11). These diseases do not respond to phototherapy or exchange transfusion.

Kernicterus (Bilirubin Encephalopathy)

Lipid-soluble, unconjugated, indirect bilirubin fraction is toxic to the developing central nervous system, especially when indirect bilirubin concentrations are high and exceed the binding capacity of albumin. Kernicterus results when indirect bilirubin is deposited in brain cells and disrupts neuronal metabolism and function, especially in the basal ganglia. Indirect bilirubin may cross the blood-brain barrier because of its lipid solubility; other theories propose that a disruption of the blood-brain barrier permits entry of a bilirubin-albumin or free bilirubin–fatty acid complex.

Kernicterus usually is noted when the bilirubin level is excessively high for gestational age. Kernicterus does not usually develop in term infants when bilirubin levels are below 20–25 mg/dL. The incidence of kernicterus increases as serum bilirubin levels increase above 25 mg/dL. Kernicterus may be noted at bilirubin levels below 20 mg/dL in the presence of sepsis, meningitis, hemolysis, asphyxia, hypoxia, hypothermia, hypoglycemia, bilirubin-displacing drugs, and prematurity. Other risks for kernicterus in term infants are hemolysis, jaundice noted within 24 hours of birth, and delayed diagnosis of hyperbilirubinemia. Kernicterus has developed in very immature infants weighing less than 1000 g when bilirubin levels are less than 10 mg/dL.

The earliest *clinical manifestations* of kernicterus are lethargy, hypotonia irritability, poor Moro response, and poor feeding. A high-pitched cry and emesis also may be present. Early signs are noted after the fourth day of life. Later signs include bulging fontanel, opisthotonic posturing, pulmonary hemorrhage, fever, hypertonicity, paralysis of upward gaze, and seizures. Infants with severe cases of kernicterus die in the neonatal period. Spasticity resolves in surviving infants, who may later manifest nerve deafness, choreoathetoid cerebral palsy, mental retardation, enamel dysplasia, and discoloration of teeth as permanent sequelae. Kernicterus may be *prevented* by avoiding excessively high indirect bilirubin levels and by avoiding conditions or drugs that may displace bilirubin from albumin. Very early signs of kernicterus occasionally may be reversed by immediately instituting an exchange transfusion (discussed later).

Therapy of Indirect Hyperbilirubinemia

Phototherapy is an effective and relatively safe method for reducing indirect bilirubin levels, particularly when initiated before serum bilirubin increases to levels associated with kernicterus. In term infants phototherapy is begun when indirect bilirubin levels are between 16 and 18 mg/dL. Phototherapy is initiated in premature infants when bilirubin is at lower levels, to prevent bilirubin from reaching the high concentrations necessitating exchange transfusion. Both blue lights and white lights are effective in reducing bilirubin levels.

Phototherapy acts by producing nontoxic photoisomers from the native bilirubin deposited in the skin. Unconjugated bilirubin (IX) is in the 4Z,15Z configuration (referring to the arrangement of atoms around the respective double bonds). Phototherapy causes a photochemical reaction producing the reversible, more water-soluble isomer 4Z,15E bilirubin IX. This configurational isomer is excreted readily in an unconjugated form in bile and is one of the mechanisms of the action of phototherapy. Another photochemical reaction results in the rapid production of lumirubin, a more water-soluble isomer than the aforementioned isomer, that does not spontaneously revert to unconjugated native bilirubin and also can be excreted in urine.

Complications of phototherapy include an increased insensible water loss, diarrhea, and dehydration. Additional problems are macular-papular red skin rash, lethargy, masking of cyanosis, nasal obstruction by eye pads, and the potential for retinal damage. Skin bronzing may be noted in infants with direct-reacting hyperbilirubinemia. Infants with mild hemolytic disease of the newborn occasionally may be successfully managed with phototherapy for hyperbilirubinemia, but care must be taken to follow these infants for the late occurrence of anemia from continued hemolysis.

Exchange transfusion usually is reserved for infants with dangerously high indirect bilirubin levels who are at risk for kernicterus. As a rule of thumb, a level of 20 mg/dL for indirect-reacting bilirubin is the "exchange number" for infants with hemolysis who weigh over 2000 g. Asymptomatic infants with physiologic or breast milk jaundice may not require exchange transfusion unless the indirect bilirubin level exceeds 25 mg/dL. The exchangeable level of indirect bilirubin for other infants may be estimated by calculating 10% of the birth weight in grams; thus the level in an infant weighing 1500 g would be 15 mg/dL. Infants weighing less than 1000 g usually do not require an exchange transfusion until the bilirubin level exceeds 10 mg/dL.

Small infusions of whole blood cross-matched with that of the mother and infant are alternated with withdrawals of an equivalent quantity of the infant's blood, which is discarded. Depending on the size of the infant, aliquots of 5–20 mL per cycle are withdrawn and infused, with the total procedure lasting 45–90 minutes. The total amount of blood exchanged is equal to twice the infant's blood volume, calculated as:

$$\text{Weight (kg)} \times 85 \text{ mL/kg} \times 2$$

This volume should remove 85% of the infant's red blood cells (the source of bilirubin), maternal antibodies, and exchangeable tissue indirect bilirubin. The exchange transfusion usually is performed through an umbilical venous catheter placed in the inferior vena cava or, if free flow is obtained, at the confluence of the umbilical vein and the portal system. The level of serum bilirubin immediately after the exchange transfusion declines to levels that are about half of those before the exchange; levels rebound 6–8 hours later as a result of continued hemolysis and redistribution of bilirubin from tissue stores.

Complications of exchange transfusion include problems related to the blood (e.g., transfusion reaction, metabolic instability, or infection), the catheter (e.g., vessel perforation or hemorrhage), or the procedure (e.g., hypotension or necrotizing enterocolitis). Unusual complications include thrombocytopenia and graft-versus-host disease. Continuation of phototherapy may reduce the necessity for subsequent exchange transfusions.

Heme oxygenase inhibitors (e.g., tin mesoporphyrin) administered systemically may attenuate hyperbilirubinemia. The level of indirect bilirubin and the need for phototherapy are reduced.

Polycythemia

(Hyperviscosity syndrome)

Polycythemia is an excessively high hematocrit (65% or more) and leads to hyperviscosity that produces symptoms related to vascular stasis, hypoperfusion, and ischemia. As the hematocrit increases from 40% to 60%, there is a very small increase in blood viscosity. Once the central hematocrit increases above 65%, the blood viscosity begins to increase markedly and symptoms may appear. Neonatal erythrocytes are less filterable or deformable than adult erythrocytes, which further contributes to hyperviscosity. A central venous hematocrit of 65% or more is noted in 3–5% of infants. Infants at special risk for polycythemia are term and postterm SGA infants, infants of diabetic mothers, infants with delayed cord clamping, and infants with neonatal hyperthyroidism, adrenogenital syndrome, trisomy 13, 18, or 21, twin-twin transfusion syndrome (recipient), and

Beckwith-Wiedemann syndrome. In some infants, polycythemia may reflect a compensation for prolonged periods of fetal hypoxia caused by placental insufficiency; these infants have increased erythropoietin levels at birth.

Polycythemic patients appear plethoric or ruddy and may develop acrocyanosis. Symptoms are a result of the increased red cell mass and of vascular compromise. Thus seizures, lethargy, and irritability reflect abnormalities of microcirculation of the brain, whereas hyperbilirubinemia may reflect the poor hepatic circulation or the increased amount of hemoglobin that is being broken down into bilirubin. Additional problems include respiratory distress and PPHN that result in part from elevated pulmonary vascular resistance. The chest roentgenogram often reveals cardiomegaly, increased vascular markings, pleural effusions, and interstitial edema. Other problems are necrotizing enterocolitis, hypoglycemia, thrombocytopenia, priapism, testicular infarction, hemiplegic stroke, and feeding intolerance. Many of these complications also are related to the primary condition associated with polycythemia (e.g., SGA infants are at risk for hypoglycemia and PPHN following periods of hypoxia in utero).

Long-term sequelae of neonatal polycythemia relate to neurodevelopmental abnormalities that may be prevented by treatment of symptomatic infants with partial-exchange transfusion after birth. A partial-exchange transfusion removes whole blood and replaces it with normal saline. The equation used to calculate the volume exchanged is based on the central venous hematocrit (Hct), because peripheral hematocrits may be falsely elevated:

$$\text{Volume to exchange (mL)} = \frac{\text{Blood volume} \times (\text{Observed Hct} - \text{Desired Hct})}{\text{Observed Hct}}$$

The desired hematocrit is 50%, and the blood volume 85 mL/kg.

Coagulation Disorders

(Also see Chapter 14)

Disorders of coagulation are quite common in the neonatal period. Hemorrhage during this time may be a result of trauma, inherited permanent deficiency of coagulation factors, transient deficiencies of vitamin K–dependent factors, disorders of platelets, and DIC seen in sick newborn patients with shock or hypoxia. Thrombosis is also a potential problem in the newborn because of developmentally lower circulating levels of antithrombin III, protein C (a vitamin K–dependent protein that inhibits factors VIII and V), and the fibrinolytic system.

Coagulation factors do not pass through the placenta to the fetus, and and newborn infants have relatively low levels of the vitamin K–dependent factors II, VII, IX, and X. Contact factors XI and XII, prekallikrein, and kininogen also are lower in newborn infants than in adults. Fibrinogen (factor I); plasma levels of factors V, VIII, and XIII; and platelet count are within the adult normal range.

Because of the transient, relative deficiencies of the contact and the vitamin K–dependent factors, the *partial thromboplastin time* (PTT), which is dependent on factors XII, IX, VIII, X, V, II, and I, is prolonged in the newborn period. Preterm infants have the most marked prolongation of the PTT (50–80 seconds) compared with term infants (35–50 seconds) and older, more mature infants (25–35 seconds). The administration of heparin and the presence of DIC, hemophilia, and severe vitamin K deficiency prolong the PTT.

The *prothrombin time* (PT), which is dependent on factors VII, X, V, II, and I, is a more sensitive test for vitamin K deficiency. The PT is only slightly prolonged in the term infant (13–20 seconds) as compared with the preterm infant (13–21 seconds) and the more mature patient (12–14 seconds). Abnormal prolongations of the PT occur with vitamin K deficiency, hepatic injury, and DIC. Levels of *fibrinogen* and *fibrin degradation products* are similar in infants and adults. The *bleeding time,* which reflects platelet function and number, is normal during the newborn period in the absence of maternal salicylate therapy.

Vitamin K is a necessary cofactor for the carboxylation of glutamate on precursor proteins, converting them into the more active coagulation factors II, VII, IX, and X; gamma-carboxyglutamic acid binds calcium, which is required for the immediate activation of factors during hemorrhage. There is no congenital deficiency of hepatic synthesis of these precursor proteins, but in the absence of vitamin K their conversion to the active factor is not possible. PIVKA (protein induced by vitamin K absence) levels increase in vitamin K deficiency and are helpful diagnostic markers; vitamin K administration rapidly corrects the coagulation defects, reducing PIVKA to undetectable levels.

Although most newborn infants are born with reduced levels of vitamin K–dependent factors, hemorrhagic complications develop only rarely. Infants at risk for **hemorrhagic disease of the newborn** have the most profound deficiency of vitamin K–dependent factors, and these factors decline further after birth. Because breast milk is a poor source of vitamin K, infants fed breast milk are also at increased risk for hemorrhage that usually occurs between the third and seventh days of life. Bleeding usually ensues from the umbilical cord, circumcision site, intestines, scalp, mucosa, and skin, but internal hemorrhage places the infant at risk for fatal complications, such as intracranial bleeding.

Hemorrhage on the first day of life resulting from a deficiency of the vitamin K–dependent factors often is associated with administration to the mother of drugs that affect vitamin K metabolism in the infant. This early pattern of hemorrhage has been seen with maternal warfarin or antibiotic (e.g., isoniazid or rifampin) therapy and in infants of mothers receiving phenobarbital and phenytoin. Bleeding also may occur as late as 1–3 months after birth, particularly among breast-fed infants. Vitamin K deficiency in breast-fed infants should also raise suspicion about the possibility of vitamin K malabsorption resulting from cystic fibrosis, biliary atresia, hepatitis, or antibiotic suppression of the colonic bacteria that produce vitamin K.

Bleeding associated with vitamin K deficiency may be *prevented* by administration of vitamin K to all infants at birth. Before routine administration of vitamin K, 1–2% of all newborn infants have hemorrhagic disease of the newborn. One intramuscular dose (1 mg) of vitamin K prevents vitamin K–deficiency bleeding.

Treatment of bleeding resulting from vitamin K deficiency involves intravenous administration of 1 mg of vitamin K. If severe, life-threatening hemorrhage is present, fresh frozen plasma should also be given. Unusually high doses of vitamin K may be needed for hepatic disease and for maternal warfarin or anticonvulsant therapy.

Clinical Manifestations and Differential Diagnoses of Bleeding Disorders

Bleeding disorders in the newborn may be associated with cutaneous bleeding such as cephalhematoma, subgaleal hemorrhage, ecchymosis, and petechiae. Facial petechiae are common in infants born by vertex presentation, with or without a nuchal cord, and usually are insignificant. Mucosal bleeding may appear as hematemesis, melena, or epistaxis. Internal hemorrhage results in organ-specific dysfunction such as seizures accompanied by intracranial hemorrhage. Bleeding from venipuncture or heel stick sites, circumcision sites, or the umbilical cord also is common.

The *differential diagnosis* depends in part on the clinical circumstances associated with the hemorrhage. In the **sick newborn** the differential diagnosis should include DIC, hepatic failure, and thrombocytopenia. Thrombocytopenia in an ill neonate may be secondary to consumption by trapping of platelets in a hemangioma **(Kasabach-Merritt syndrome)** or may be associated with perinatal, congenital, or bacterial infections; necrotizing enterocolitis (NEC); thrombotic endocarditis; PPHN; organic acidemia;

maternal preeclampsia; or asphyxia. Thrombocytopenia also may the result of peripheral washout of platelets following an exchange transfusion. *Treatment* of the sick infant with thrombocytopenia should be directed at the underlying disorder, supplemented by infusions of platelets, blood, or both.

The etiology of DIC in the newborn infant includes hypoxia, hypotension, asphyxia, bacterial or viral sepsis, NEC, death of a twin while in utero, cavernous hemangioma, nonimmune hydrops, neonatal cold injury, neonatal neoplasm, and hepatic disease. The *treatment* of DIC should be focused primarily on therapy for the initiating or underlying disorder. Supportive management of consumptive coagulopathy involves platelet transfusions and factor replacement with fresh frozen plasma. Heparin and factor C concentrate should be reserved for those infants with DIC who also demonstrate thrombosis.

Disorders of hemostasis in the well child are not associated with systemic disease in the newborn but reflect coagulation factor or platelet deficiency. *Hemophilia* initially is associated with cutaneous or mucosal bleeding and no systemic illness. If bleeding continues, hypovolemic shock may develop. Bleeding into the brain, liver, or spleen may result in organ-specific signs and shock.

In the **well child,** *thrombocytopenia* may be part of a syndrome such as Fanconi anemia syndrome (involving hypoplasia and aplasia of the thumb), the radial aplasia–thrombocytopenia (TAR) syndrome (thumbs present), or Wiskott-Aldrich syndrome. Various maternal drugs also may reduce the neonatal platelet count without producing other adverse effects. These drugs include sulfonamides, quinidine, quinine, and thiazide diuretics.

The most common causes of thrombocytopenia in well newborn infants are transient isoimmune thrombocytopenia and transient neonatal thrombocytopenia in well infants born to mothers with idiopathic thrombocytopenic purpura (ITP). **Isoimmune thrombocytopenia** is caused by antiplatelet antibodies produced by the HPLA1-negative mother after her sensitization to specific paternal platelet antigen (HPA-1a and HPA-5b represent 85% and 10% of cases, respectively) expressed on the fetal platelet. The incidence is 1:1000–1:2000 births. This response to maternal-sensitized antibodies that produce isoimmune thrombocytopenia is analogous to the response that produces erythroblastosis fetalis. The maternal antiplatelet antibody does not produce maternal thrombocytopenia, but after crossing the placenta this IgG antibody binds to fetal platelets that are trapped by the reticuloendothelial tissue, resulting in thrombocytopenia. Infants with thrombocytopenia produced in this manner are at risk for development of petechiae, purpura, and intracranial hemorrhage (an incidence of 10–15%) before or after birth. Vaginal delivery may increase the risk for neonatal bleeding; thus cesarean section may be indicated.

Specific *treatment* for severe thrombocytopenia (<20,000 platelets/mm^3) or significant bleeding is transfusion of ABO- and RhD-compatible, HPA-1a– and HPA-5b–negative maternal platelets. Because the antibody in isoimmune thrombocytopenia is directed against the fetal rather than the maternal platelet, plateletpheresis of the mother yields sufficient platelets for carrying out a platelet transfusion to treat the affected infant. After one platelet transfusion, the infant's platelet count dramatically increases and usually remains in a safe range. Without treatment, thrombocytopenia resolves during the first month of life as the maternal antibody level declines. *Treatment* of the mother with intravenous immunoglobulin or the thrombocytopenic fetus with intravascular platelet transfusion (cordocentesis) is also effective. Cesarean section reduces the risk of intracranial hemorrhage.

Neonatal thrombocytopenia in infants born to women with ITP also is a result of placental transfer of maternal IgG antibodies. In ITP these autoantibodies are directed against all platelet antigens, and thus both mother and newborn may have low platelet counts. The risks of hemorrhage in the infant born to the woman with ITP may be lessened by cesarean section and by treatment of the mother with corticosteroids.

Treatment of the affected infant born to the woman with ITP may involve prednisone and intravenous immunoglobulin. In an emergency, random donor platelets may be used and may produce a transient rise in the infant's platelet count. Thrombocytopenia will resolve spontaneously during the first month of life as maternal-derived antibody levels decline. Elevated levels of platelet-associated antibodies also have been noted in thrombocytopenic infants with sepsis and thrombocytopenia of unknown cause who were born to mothers without demonstrable platelet antibodies.

The *laboratory evaluation* of an infant (well or sick) with bleeding must include a platelet count, blood smear, and evaluation of PTT and PT. Isolated thrombocytopenia in a well infant suggests immune thrombocytopenia. Laboratory evidence of DIC includes a markedly prolonged PTT and PT (minutes rather than seconds), thrombocytopenia, and a blood smear suggestive of a microangiopathic hemolytic anemia (burr or fragmented blood cells). Further evaluation reveals very low levels of fibrinogen (below 100 mg/dL) and elevated levels of fibrin degradation products. Vitamin K deficiency prolongs the PT more than the PTT, whereas hemophilia result-

ing from factors VIII and IX deficiency prolongs only the PTT. Specific factor levels confirm the *diagnosis* of hemophilia.

REFERENCES

Behrman RE, Kliegman RM, Jenson HB, editors: *Nelson textbook of pediatrics*, ed 16, Philadelphia, 2000, WB Saunders, Chapters 98, 99.

Kaplan M, Hammerman C, Renbaum P, et al: Gilbert's syndrome and hyperbilirubinaemia in AB-incompatible neonates, *Lancet* 356(9230):652–653, 2000.

Maisels MJ, Newman TB: Kernicterus in otherwise healthy, breast-fed term newborns, *Pediatrics* 96(4 Pt 1):730–733, 1995.

Mari G: Noninvasive diagnosis by Doppler ultrasonography of the fetal anemia due to maternal red-cell alloimmunization, *N Engl J Med* 342(1):9–14, 2000.

Newman TB, Xion B, Gonzales VM, et al: Prediction and prevention of extreme neonatal hyperbilirubinemia in a mature health maintenance organization, *Arch Pediatr Adolesc Med* 154(11):1140–1147, 2000.

Obladen M, Diepold K, Maier RF, et al: Venous and arterial hematologic profiles of very low birth weight infants, *Pediatrics* 06(4):707–711, 2000.

Ouwehand WH, Smith G, Ranasinghe E: Management of severe alloimmune thrombocytopenia in the newborn, *Arch Dis Child Fetal Neonatal Ed* 82(3):F173–F175, 2000.

Zipursky A: Vitamin K at birth, *BMJ* 313(7051):179–180, 1996.

NUTRITION AND GASTROINTESTINAL DISORDERS
Nutrition and Feeding

All newborn infants require water and a source of calories during the first day of life. In healthy, full-term infants, breast milk, formula, or both are given on the first day of life as the source of fluid and nutrients during enteric alimentation; sick and very premature infants usually are managed with intravenous alimentation. Enteric alimentation of sick infants often is delayed until after the acute illnesses have resolved because of the risk of abdominal distention or ileus, either of which may lead to regurgitation and subsequent aspiration pneumonia, and because of the risk of the development of NEC. Delay in the onset of intravenous and enteric alimentation may be associated with fluid and electrolyte abnormalities such as hypernatremia, azotemia, dehydration, oliguria, fever, hypoglycemia, and hyperbilirubinemia.

Full-term infants usually are breast-fed or are fed formula by mouth during the first few hours after birth. Because premature infants before 32–34 weeks of gestational age may not be able to coordinate the mechanisms for sufficient oral feeding, they usually are fed through a nasal or oral gastric tube. Such "gavage feedings" may be given continuously or intermittently by gravity drip every 1–3 hours. Subsequently, oral feedings are started when the infant can coordinate sucking, cheek and tongue movement, uvula closure of the nasopharynx, and epiglottal closure of the larynx; has acquired the esophageal motility to propel the milk feeding to the stomach; and has developed a gag reflex.

Problems of enteric alimentation are common in premature infants; these problems are caused by immaturity of the gastrointestinal tract and by systemic diseases that alter gastrointestinal function. The causes include gastroesophageal reflux, gastric stasis and retention of formula, abdominal distention and ileus, failure to defecate, and a variety of abnormalities related to the composition of milk. Premature infants also may have bradycardia during enteral feedings, in part because of a reduced arterial oxygen content and gastric distention. Reflux of gastric contents may cause laryngospasm or aspiration pneumonia; both are associated with hypoxia, apnea, and bradycardia. Rapid feeding with excessively large volumes of formula over a short time has been associated with the development of NEC. Problems associated with feeding tubes include erosive esophagitis, bowel perforation, fat malabsorption, and abnormal bacterial colonization of the upper intestine. If gavage or intravenous feeding is of long duration, the ability to feed directly by mouth may be temporarily lost.

The composition of commonly used formulas and the indications for the initiation of *special infant formulas* are presented in Table 6–26. Breast milk is often the standard milk fed to newborn infants and serves as a nutritional reference point for comparison with other infant formulas. Breast milk is often supplemented when fed to VLBW infants; additions include calories, protein, sodium, and calcium.

The caloric requirements of the newborn infant include energy for growth, for regulation of body temperature, and for maintenance (replacement and turnover) of body macromolecules (Table 6–27). When fed 100–120 kcal/kg/24 hr, the infant should gain 10–30 g/24 hr. In term infants between 0 and 3 months old, weight gain is 25–35 g/24 hr; between 3 and 6 months of life, weight gain declines to 12–21 g/24 hr. The energy required for tissue synthesis is a small proportion, and that required for storage as macromolecules is a large proportion, of the energy required for growth. Energy partitioning for synthesis and storage depends on the composition of the new tissue; more calories are required for fat synthesis than for protein synthesis. Net deposition of new tissue macromolecules (depositing 20–30% fat and 10–12% protein) requires 4–6 kcal/g tissue. Energy requirements may be spared for tissue synthesis if the infant is kept warm in a neutral thermal environment to avoid cold stress–induced energy utilization.

The *protein* requirement of the breast-fed, full-term infant may be as little as 1.5–2.0 g/kg/24 hr. Colostrum has a higher protein content than breast milk, which may contain as little as 0.9 g/dL. Standard formula for older premature infants and for full-term infants provides more protein than breast milk (Table 6–26); growing infants consuming 150 mL/kg/24 hr have a protein intake of 2.25 g/kg/24 hr. Preterm infants may have an increased requirement for protein to support growth but may develop an elevated blood urea nitrogen (BUN) level, hyperaminoacidemia, hyperammonemia, and metabolic acidosis when fed casein-predominant (80%) formula or when fed greater than 4.5 g/kg/24 hr total proteins. The **late metabolic acidosis of prematurity** probably is caused in part by increased endogenous acid production from casein-containing formula (i.e., formula high in sulfur and acidic amino acids). This disorder is characterized by metabolic acidosis and reduced weight gain in VLBW infants. *Treatment* includes substitution of a "humanized" whey-predominant formula and oral sodium bicarbonate.

All infants have an absolute requirement for the essential amino acids. Preterm infants also have an additional requirement for cystine and tyrosine because of immaturity of the enzymes required to convert cystathionine and phenylalanine to these amino acids. In addition, histidine and taurine may be essential for the premature infant. Recommended protein intakes for the VLBW infant are 3.0–4.0 g/kg/24 hr of whey-predominant formula for infants fed enterally and 2.5–3.5 g/kg/24 hr of crystalline amino acids for intravenously fed infants.

Fat absorption by the newborn infant may be reduced as a result of a small bile salt pool and a low level of pancreatic lipase activity. The latter may be compensated for by breast milk and lingual and gastric lipase activities. Reduced bile salt concentrations will be exacerbated by cholestatic jaundice. With the exception of human milk fat, animal fats are not well absorbed. Corn or soy oils are better tolerated, as are medium-chain triglycerides that do not require bile salts for absorption. Of the total calories, 3–5% should be in the form of essential fatty acids. Provision of linolenic and linoleic acids (unsaturated fatty acids) provides precursors for arachidonic acid, membrane phospholipids, and prostaglandin synthesis, thus avoiding **essential fatty acid deficiency.** This deficiency is characterized by growth failure, dermatitis, reduced pigmentation, and hypotonia. Poor intake of linolenic acid may impair visual function and neurodevelopment in VLBW infants. Excessive intake of polyunsaturated fatty acids may produce hemolysis by overcoming the antioxidant mechanisms of the erythrocyte. The provision of additional vitamin E may prevent this hemolysis.

TABLE 6–26
Composition of Breast Milk and Infant Formulas

	Breast Milk (per dL)	Standard Formula (per dL)	Premature Formula (per dL)	Soy Formula (per dL)	Nutramigen (per dL)	Pregestimil (per dL)
Calories (kcal)	67	67	67–81	67	67	67
Protein (g)	1.1	1.5	2.0–2.4	1.7	1.9	1.9
(% calories)	(6%)	(9%)	(12%)	(10%)	(11%)	(11%)
Whey/casein protein ratio	80/20	60/40, 18/82	60/40	Soy protein, methionine	Casein hydrolysate plus L-cystine, L-tyrosine, and L-tryptophan	Casein hydrolysate plus L-cystine, L-tyrosine, and L-tryptophan
Fat (g)	4.0	3.6	3.4–4.4	3.6	3.3	3.8
(% calories)	(55%)	(50%)	(45%)	(48%)	(45%)	(48%)
MCT (%)	0	0	40–50	0	0	55
Carbohydrate	7.2	6.9–7.2	8.5–8.9	6.8	7.3	6.9
(% calories)	40	41	42	40	44	41
Source	Lactose	Lactose	Lactose, corn syrup	Corn syrup, sucrose	Corn, syrup solids, cornstarch	Corn syrup solids, cornstarch, dextrose
Minerals (per L)						
Calcium (mg)	290	420–550	1115–1452	700	635	777
Phosphorus (mg)	140	280–390	561–806	500	420	500
Sodium (mEq)	8.0	6.5–8.3	11–15	13	14	14
Vitamin D	Variable	400	1000–1800	400	400	400
Osmolality (mOsm/L)	253	270	230–270	200–220	290	290
Renal solute load (mOsm/L)	75	100–126	175–213	126–150	175	125
Comments	Reference standard, deficient in vitamin K; may be deficient in Na$^+$, Ca^{2+}, protein, vitamin D for VLBW infants	Risk of milk protein intolerance—gastrointestinal bleeding, anemia, wheezing, eczema	Specifically fortified with additional protein, Ca^{2+}, P, Na$^+$, vitamin D, and MCT oil	Useful for lactose and milk protein intolerance; may lead to soy protein intolerance; rickets develops in VLBW infants	Useful for lactose and milk protein intolerance (allergy)	Useful for malabsorption states, lactose and milk protein intolerance (allergy)

TABLE 6–27
Neonatal Caloric Requirements

Source	kcal/kg/24 hr
Maintenance	50
Growth	25–35
Activity	0–15
Cold stress	0–10
Specific dynamic action (caloric cost of food)	10
Nutrient losses (stool)	10–20
TOTAL	95–120

Of milk calories, 40% are derived from *carbohydrates* (Table 6–26). There is no absolute requirement for specific carbohydrates; however, both glucose and galactose can produce glycogen and prevent hypoglycemia. Lactose, a disaccharide of glucose and galactose, is the natural carbohydrate of human milk and of most formulas. Preterm infants have not developed normal full-term levels of the intestinal mucosal enzyme lactase, which is necessary to digest lactose. Malabsorption of lactose may result in watery, acidic stools from the production of organic acids by colonic bacteria. These organic acids may be absorbed and may contribute to the development of late metabolic acidosis of prematurity. Newborn infants with gastrointestinal injury frequently become lactose intolerant and require lactose-free formula. Because of the developmental immaturity of lactase activity, formulas for premature infants usually contain glucose polymers that will be digested by pancreatic amylase.

Vitamin deficiency is rare in the immediate newborn period; however, in breast-fed infants of strict vegan mothers vitamin B_{12} deficiency may develop, and infants fed goat's milk may become folate deficient. Vitamin D deficiency may be seen in infants of mothers with osteomalacia and in infants with cholestatic jaundice. Vitamin D deficiency occurs rarely in the breast-fed infant and occasionally is a contributing factor to osteopenia of prematurity (discussed later). Preterm infants may need more vitamin C to improve tyrosine metabolism.

Vitamin E deficiency in the immediate newborn period may be the result of an excess of oxidants, such as iron, and an abundance of oxidizable polyunsaturated fatty acids. Vitamin E deficiency of the premature infant may lead to edema, anemia, reticulocytosis, and thrombocytosis.

Vitamin K deficiency is discussed under Coagulation Disorders earlier in this chapter.

Trace element deficiency is unusual in formula-fed infants. It usually occurs during unsupplemented total parenteral alimentation. *Copper deficiency,* once common before the addition of trace elements to total intravenous alimentation solutions, manifests as anemia, neutropenia, and periosteal bone formation.

Zinc deficiency may be noted during total intravenous alimentation or among breast-fed infants whose mothers have low zinc levels in their milk. These infants have alopecia, growth failure, and dermatitis around the anus and on the hands and feet.

Iron deficiency rarely is manifested during the first month of life. Prophylactic iron therapy should be started in preterm infants when they double their birth weight and in term infants after the sixth month of life or at any age during treatment with erythropoietin; therapy for both should be in the form of iron-fortified formula and cereal or ferrous sulfate solution.

Fluid Requirements

Fluid balance in the normal, growing infant is always positive because of the high water content present during cellular growth. Oral feedings, intravenous solutions, or a combination of the two is the usual source of fluid intake. Water from oxidation is an additional internal source of small quantities of water (10 mL/kg/24 hr). Fluid intake is required because of continuous insensible, urine, and stool water losses (Table 6–28). Excessive fluid intake may predispose the premature infant to a PDA, congestive heart failure, BPD, NEC, hyponatremia, and edema. Insufficient fluid intake results in dehydration, azotemia, hyperbilirubinemia, and hypernatremia.

The correct amount of fluid intake depends on the size of the infant, the postnatal age, and coexistent diseases affecting fluid balance. On the first day of life, most infants should receive 60–80 mL/kg/24 hr of fluid. On subsequent days this amount should be increased to 100–140 mL/kg/24 hr. Fluid intake greater than 150–160 mL/kg/24 hr has been associated with PDA, BPD, and NEC and should be avoided unless there are excessive free water needs as a result of large insensible water losses. Hydration can be assessed by monitoring serum BUN, Na^+, urine output, and urine specific gravity (discussed later). Rising serum Na^+, BUN, and urine specific gravity with weight loss suggest dehydration and a free water deficit.

Fluid balance in the newborn infant is tenuous because of very high rates of insensible water losses and immature renal function. Before 34 weeks of gestation, the premature infant has a greatly reduced glomerular filtration rate (GFR). Although the GFR

TABLE 6–28
Components of Fluid Losses

Source	Significance
Insensible water loss (IWL)	Varies with gestational and postnatal age; greatest in youngest, most immature (2–3 mL/kg/hr) versus term (0.5–0.8 mL/kg/hr); phototherapy, radiant warmer, low humidity increase IWL; ventilation, humidity, inner-plastic warmer shield decrease IWL
Urine output	Necessary to excrete obligate renal solute load; renal solute increases with fasting or a high-protein, high-electrolyte–containing formula; neonate has narrow range of urine concentration of diluting ability
Sweat	Uncommon in newborn; term infants sweat if overheated, with visible perspiration on forehead
Stool loss	Not a variable when on total parenteral alimentation; increased stool water loss with phototherapy and diarrhea

increases after 34 weeks of age, the rate of filtration is still below adult values, even in full-term infants. Sodium reabsorption is reduced in the full-term infant and even more reduced in the preterm infant. Because of this, the fractional excretion of sodium is higher in the VLBW infant (up to 6–12%) than in the full-term infant or older child (<2%). Thus although the required sodium intake in the term infant is 1–3 mEq/kg/24 hr, the VLBW term infant may require 3–5 mEq/kg/24 hr to prevent sodium wasting and hyponatremia. The newborn infant also has a limited ability to excrete a diluted or a concentrated urine. Maximum urinary concentrating ability of the newborn is 600–700 mOsm/L, compared with 1200–1400 mOsm/L in the adult. Urine osmolality should be maintained between 50 and 300 mOsm/L, which corresponds to a urine specific gravity of 1.003–1.012; overhydration is a risk when urine osmolality is below 20–30 mOsm/L. The immature kidney also is limited in its capacity to excrete excessive solute, which may result in diminished excretion of sodium and other components of the renal solute load (also known as ash components of formula). Additional signs of immaturity of renal function in the newborn include reduced sodium bicarbonate reabsorption, diminished capacity to acidify the urine, and reduced excretion of drugs such as the aminoglycosides.

Parenteral Alimentation

See Chapter 2.

Gastrointestinal Diseases

For a discussion of obstruction and hemorrhage, see Chapter 11.

Gastrointestinal Perforation

Perforation of the small intestine associated with ileal atresia and cystic fibrosis results in sterile peritonitis in utero (*meconium peritonitis*). After birth, bacterial colonization of the intestines leads to a combined bacterial and chemical peritonitis following a postnatal perforation. Neonatal intestinal perforation may be traumatic (iatrogenic), idiopathic (stomach), stress related, drug induced (e.g., dexamethasone or indomethacin), or associated with gastrointestinal obstruction.

Necrotizing enterocolitis is a common cause of intestinal perforation during the neonatal period, but not all cases of NEC result in perforation. Patients with NEC are usually premature infants (10% are term infants with other diseases such as congenital heart disease) who are receiving oral feedings and have recovered from previous diseases of prematurity. The onset of symptoms is usually in the first week of life but may be delayed 1–2 months after birth.

The *clinical manifestations* of NEC include abdominal distention and tenderness, rectal bleeding, and a septic shock–like appearance. Abdominal roentgenograms reveal pneumatosis intestinalis and intrahepatic venous gas; pneumoperitoneum is noted with perforation.

Because epidemics of NEC are common and blood cultures demonstrate positive results in 30% of patients, the *treatment* of NEC includes the initiation of broad-spectrum antibiotics and gastrointestinal decompression with a nasogastric tube and parenteral alimentation to put the bowel at rest. All newborn patients with evidence of intestinal perforation, such as pneumoperitoneum, require exploratory laparotomy.

TABLE 6–29
Risk Factors for Neonatal Hypoglycemia

Factors	Mechanism
Common	
Prematurity	Limited glycogen stores, fasting
Infant of a diabetic mother	Hyperinsulinism
Intrauterine growth retardation	Limited glycogen stores, hyperinsulinism, fasting
Asphyxia–perinatal stress	Depleted glycogen stores, anaerobic metabolism
Hypothermia	Increased glucose utilization
Fasting	Depleted glycogen stores
Large for gestational age	Possible hyperinsulinism
Maternal medications (tocolytics, propranolol, chlorpropamide, high-glucose infusion in labor)	Possible hyperinsulinism
Uncommon	
Erythroblastosis fetalis	Hyperinsulinism
Beckwith-Wiedemann syndrome	Hyperinsulinism
Islet cell adenoma	Hyperinsulinism
Familial and nonfamilial hyperinsulinism	Hyperinsulinism
Polycythemia	Increased glucose utilization/decreased production
Sepsis	Increased glucose utilization
Inborn errors of metabolism	Decreased glycogenolysis, gluconeogenesis, or utilization of alternate fuels (fatty acids)
Growth hormone deficiency	Increased glucose utilization, decreased gluconeogenesis
Adrenal insufficiency	Decreased glucose production (gluconeogenesis)

REFERENCES

Behrman RE, Kliegman RM, Jenson HB, editors: *Nelson textbook of pediatrics,* ed 16, Philadelphia, 2000, WB Saunders, Chapters 93, 98.

Cooke RJ, Embleton ND: Feeding issues in preterm infants, *Arch Dis Child Fetal Neonatal Ed* 83(3):F215–F218, 2000.

Kavvadia V, Greenough A, Dimitriou G, et al: Randomized trial of fluid restriction in ventilated very low birthweight infants, *Arch Dis Child Fetal Neonatal Ed* 83(2):F91–F96, 2000.

McElhinney DB, Hedrick HL, Bush DM, et al: Necrotizing enterocolitis in neonates with congenital heart disease: risk factors and outcomes, *Pediatrics* 106:1080, 2000.

Reis BB, Hall RT, Schanler RJ, et al: Enhanced growth of preterm infants fed a new powdered human milk fortifier: a randomized, controlled study, *Pediatrics* 106(3):581–588, 2000.

METABOLIC DISORDERS
Hypoglycemia

Hypoglycemia is common during the neonatal period. Infants in many categories are at risk for neonatal hypoglycemia (Table 6–29). Serum glucose levels in healthy term infants are rarely less than 40 mg/dL between 1 and 3 hours of age, less than 45 mg/dL between 3 and 24 hours of age, or less than 50 mg/dL thereafter. Lower glucose levels among term or preterm infants suggest hypoglycemia. Alternatively, an infant with higher glucose levels is still considered to have hypoglycemia if the infant has symptoms compatible with hypoglycemia that respond to glucose infusions.

Hypoglycemia in the **infant of a diabetic mother** is the result of persistent hyperinsulinemia and a decreased ability to produce glucose (from glycogen) during neonatal fasting (this is discussed under Medical Problems During Pregnancy Associated with Fetal or Neonatal Risk earlier in this chapter, in Table 6–5, and in Fig. 6–1). Poorly controlled maternal diabetes produces maternal and hence fetal hyperglycemia, which stimulates the fetal beta cells of the pancreas to produce large quantities of insulin. After birth, hyperinsulinemia persists, suppressing fasting hepatic glucose production (from glycogenolysis). Hyperinsulinemia also suppresses lipolysis and reduces levels of free fatty acids and ketones. Oxidation of fatty acids is an important source of energy after birth, as noted by a decline of the respiratory quotient from 1 at birth to 0.8 at 2–3 hours after birth. If free fatty acid mobilization is reduced, there is less alternative fuel available for oxidation. In normal infants, free fatty acid metabolism spares glucose utilization and helps prevent hypoglycemia.

In infants with **intrauterine growth retardation,** hypoglycemia occurs as a result of reduced tissue stores of glycogen and fat. Thus glucose availability and fatty acid oxidation may be attenuated, resulting in a reduced total body energy production. The level of oxygen consumption increases markedly with the provision of exogenous fuels during enteric feedings.

The *clinical manifestations* of neonatal hypoglycemia usually are noted on the first or second day of life and vary from an asymptomatic state to central nervous system and cardiopulmonary disturbances. Hypotonia, lethargy, apathy, poor feeding, jitteriness, and seizures are common. Congestive heart failure, tachycardia, cyanosis, pallor, diaphoresis, apnea, and hypothermia are additional manifestations. Because many of these symptoms and signs are not specific for hypoglycemia, systemic (e.g., congenital heart disease, sepsis, and intraventricular hemorrhage) or other metabolic (e.g., hypocalcemia, hypomagnesemia, inborn errors of metabolism, and narcotic withdrawal) disorders must be considered. Hypoglycemia also may be seen in association with other diseases such as complex cyanotic heart disease and asphyxia.

The occurrence of hypoglycemia can be anticipated and may be *prevented* by identification of a high-risk population (Table 6–29). Newborn infants who are at risk but who are asymptomatic and have no contraindications for oral feeding should be breast-fed or given formula within the first few hours of birth. When early feedings are not possible because of concomitant cardiopulmonary disease, 10% glucose should be given intravenously. All asymptomatic newborn infants who are at risk should be monitored, with serial capillary blood glucose levels measured during the first day of life; a low glucose value on the Chemstrip should be confirmed by serum glucose determination.

Treatment of hypoglycemia requires an initial intravenous bolus infusion of 200–400 mg/kg (2–4 mL/kg) of 10% glucose solution that rapidly raises the blood glucose level to the physiologic range. This should be followed immediately by a continuous infusion of 6–8 mg/kg/min of glucose. If hypoglycemia recurs, the bolus is repeated and the glucose infusion rate is incrementally increased to maintain physiologic glucose concentrations. Persistent hypoglycemic requiring >8 mg/kg/min of a glucose infusion is suggestive of hyperinsulinism, especially if the infant is LGA.

The *prognosis* of symptomatic neonatal hypoglycemia with seizures is poor and is associated with abnormal neurointellectual development. The prognosis for other forms of hypoglycemia is better. Infants with hyperinsulinemia or hypoglycemia often require surgical resection of most of the pancreas if medical management with diazoxide, nifedipine, or somatostatin fails.

Hypocalcemia

Hypocalcemia is common among sick and premature newborn infants. Most infants are born with calcium levels that are higher in cord blood than in maternal blood because of active placental transfer of calcium to the fetus. Fetal calcium accretion in the third trimester approaches 150 mg/kg/24 hr, and fetal bone mineral content doubles between 30 and 40 weeks of gestation. All infants show a slight decline of serum calcium levels after birth; the decline reaches trough levels at 24–48 hours, the point at which hypocalcemia usually occurs. Total serum calcium levels of less than 7 mg/dL and ionized calcium levels of less than 3.0–3.5 mg/dL are considered hypocalcemic.

The *etiology* of hypocalcemia varies with the time of onset and the associated illnesses of the child. **Early neonatal hypocalcemia** occurs in the first 3 days of life and is often asymptomatic. Transient hypoparathyroidism and a reduced parathyroid response to the usual postnatal decline of serum calcium levels may be responsible for hypocalcemia among premature infants and infants of diabetic mothers. Congenital absence of the parathyroid gland and DiGeorge syndrome also have been associated with hypocalcemia. *Hypomagnesemia* (<1.5 mg/dL) may be seen simultaneously with hypocalcemia, especially in infants of diabetic mothers. Treatment with calcium alone does not relieve symptoms or increase serum calcium levels; for this to occur, the hypomagnesemia also must treated. Sodium bicarbonate therapy, phosphate release from cell necrosis, transient hypoparathyroidism, and hypercalcitoninemia may be responsible for early neonatal hypocalcemia associated with asphyxia. Early-onset hypocalcemia associated with asphyxia often occurs with seizures as a result of the hypoxic-ischemic encephalopathy or hypocalcemia. **Late neonatal hypocalcemia,** or **neonatal tetany,** often is the result of ingestion of high-phosphate–containing milk or of the inability to excrete the usual phosphorus in commercial infant formula. Hyperphosphatemia (>8 mg/dL) usually occurs in infants with hypocalcemia after the first week of life. Vitamin D deficiency states and malabsorption also have been associated with late-onset hypocalcemia.

The *clinical manifestations* of hypocalcemia and hypomagnesemia include apnea, muscle twitching, seizures, laryngospasm, **Chvostek sign** (facial muscle spasm when the side of the face over the 7th nerve is tapped), and **Trousseau sign** (carpopedal spasm induced by partial inflation of a blood pressure cuff). The latter two signs are rare in the immediate newborn period. On occasion, heart failure has been associated with hypocalcemia.

Neonatal hypocalcemia may be *prevented* by administration of intravenous or oral calcium supplementation at a rate of 25–75 mg/kg/24 hr. Early asymptomatic hypocalcemia of preterm infants and infants of diabetic mothers often resolves spontaneously. Symptomatic hypocalcemia should be treated with 2–4 mL/kg of 10% calcium gluconate given intravenously and slowly over 10–15 minutes; a continuous infusion of 75 mg/kg/24 hr of elemental calcium should then be administered. If hypomagnesemia is associated with hypocalcemia, 50% magnesium sulfate, 0.1 mL/kg, should be given by intramuscular injection and repeated every 8–12 hours.

The *treatment* of late hypocalcemia includes immediate management, as in early hypocalcemia, plus the initiation of feedings with formula containing low phosphate levels. Subcutaneous infiltration of intravenous calcium salts can cause tissue necrosis; oral supplements are hypertonic and may irritate the intestinal mucosa.

Osteopenia or Metabolic Bone Disease of Prematurity

The rate of fetal bone mineralization is not always maintained by the prematurely born infant fed breast milk or standard formula. Bone undermineralization or frank rickets may develop and result in pathologic fractures, altered growth, and respiratory insufficiency. Osteopenia predominantly is noted in infants weighing less than 1000 g and in infants with chronic diseases of prematurity, such as BPD, after the first 2–3 months of life. Roentgenographic signs include bone demineralization and fractures. Serum alkaline phosphatase levels always are elevated, sometimes at two to three times the normal level. The cause most probably is dietary deficiency of calcium and phosphate. Vitamin D deficiency, copper deficiency, aluminum toxicity, diuretic-induced hypercalciuria, cholestatic jaundice–induced malabsorption of calcium, and altered metabolism of vitamin D are less likely causes or contributing factors.

Prevention may be possible with a formula containing higher concentrations of calcium, phosphate, and vitamin D (Table 6–26). *Treatment* consists of dietary supplementation with calcium, phosphate, and vitamin D if indicated.

Neonatal Drug Addiction and Withdrawal

Infants may become passively and physiologically addicted to medications or to drugs of abuse (e.g., heroin, methadone, barbiturates, tranquilizers, and amphetamines) taken by the mother during pregnancy; these infants subsequently may have signs and symptoms of drug withdrawal. Many of these pregnancies are at high risk for other complications related to intravenous drug abuse, such as hepatitis, acquired immunodeficiency syndrome (AIDS), and syphilis. In addition, the LBW rate and the long-term risk for sudden infant death syndrome (SIDS) are higher in the infants of these high-risk women.

Heroin and Opiates

Neonatal withdrawal signs and symptoms usually begin at 1–5 days of life with maternal heroin use and at 1–4 weeks with maternal methadone addiction. *Clinical manifestations* of withdrawal include sneezing, yawning, ravenous appetite, emesis, diarrhea, fever, diaphoresis, tachypnea, high-pitched cry, tremors, jitteriness, poor sleep, poor feeding, and seizures. The illness tends to be more severe during methadone withdrawal. The initial *treatment* includes swaddling in blankets in a quiet, dark room. When hyperactivity is constant and irritability interferes with sleeping and feeding or when diarrhea or seizures are present, pharmacologic treatment is indicated. Seizures usually are treated with phenobarbital. The other symptoms may be managed with replacement doses of a narcotic (usually tincture of opium) to calm the infant; weaning from narcotics may be prolonged over 1–2 months.

Cocaine

Cocaine use during pregnancy is associated with preterm labor, abruptio placentae, neonatal irritability, and decreased attentiveness. Infants may be SGA and have small head circumferences. Usually no treatment is needed.

REFERENCES

Bateman DA, Chiriboga CA: Dose-response effects of cocaine on newborn head circumference, *Pediatrics* 106(3):E33, 2000.

Behrman RE, Kliegman RM, Jenson HB, editors: *Nelson textbook of pediatrics*, ed 16, Philadelphia, 2000, WB Saunders, Chapters 102, 103.

Burton BK: Inborn errors of metabolism: the clinical diagnosis in early infancy, *Pediatrics* 79(3):359–369, 1987.

de Lonlay-Debeney P, Poggi-Travert F, Fournet JC, et al: Clinical features of 52 neonates with hyperinsulinism, *N Engl J Med* 340(15):1169–1175, 1999.

Rivers RPA: Neonatal opiate withdrawal, *Arch Dis Child* 61(12): 1236–1239, 1986.

Ryan S: Nutritional aspects of metabolic bone disease in the new-born, *Arch Dis Child Fetal Neonatal Ed* 74(2):F145–F148, 1996.

NEONATAL INFECTIOUS DISEASE

(See Chapter 10 and Appendices)

Systemic and local infections (e.g., lung, cutaneous, ocular, umbilical, kidney, bone-joint, and meningeal infections) are common in the newborn period. Infection may be acquired in utero through the transplacental or transcervical routes and during and after birth. Ascending infection through the cervix, with or without rupture of the amniotic fluid membranes, may result in amnionitis, funisitis (infection of the umbilical cord), congenital pneumonia, and sepsis. The bacteria responsible for ascending infection of the fetus are common bacterial organisms of the maternal genitourinary tract such as group B streptococcus, *E. coli*, *Haemophilus influenzae*, and *Klebsiella*. Herpes simplex virus (HSV)-1 or more often HSV-2 also causes ascending infection that at times may be indistinguishable from bacterial sepsis. Syphilis and *Listeria monocytogenes* are acquired by transplacental infection.

Maternal humoral immunity may protect the fetus against some neonatal pathogens, such as group B streptococcus and HSV. Nonetheless, various deficiencies of the neonatal antimicrobial defense mechanism probably are more important than maternal immune status as a contributing factor for neonatal infection, especially in the LBW infant. The incidence of sepsis is approximately 1:1500 in full-term infants and 1:250 in preterm infants. The six-fold-higher rate of sepsis among preterm infants compared with term infants relates both to the preterm infants' more immature immunologic systems and to their prolonged periods of hospitalization, which hold the added risk of nosocomially acquired infectious diseases.

Preterm infants before 32 weeks of gestational age have not received the full complement of maternal antibodies (IgG), which cross the placenta by active transport predominantly in the latter half of the third trimester. In addition, although LBW infants may generate IgM antibodies, their own IgG response to infection is reduced. These infants also have deficiencies of the alternate and, to a smaller degree, the classic complement activation pathways, which results in diminished complement-mediated opsonization. Newborn infants also demonstrate a deficit in phagocytic migration to the site of infection (e.g., to the lung) and in the bone marrow reserve pool of leukocytes. In addition, in the presence of suboptimal activation of complement, neonatal neutrophils ingest and kill bacteria less effectively than adult neutrophils do. Furthermore, neutrophils from sick infants seem to have an even greater deficit in bacterial killing capacity compared with phagocytic cells from normal neonates.

Defense mechanisms against viral pathogens also may be deficient in the newborn infant. Neonatal antibody-dependent, cell-mediated immunity by the natural killer lymphocytes is deficient in the absence of maternal antibodies and in the presence of reduced interferon production; reduced antibody levels occur in premature infants and in infants born during a primary viral infection of the mother, such as with HSV-2 or cytomegalovirus. In addition, antibody-independent cytotoxicity may be reduced in lymphocytes of newborn infants.

Neonatal Sepsis

Neonatal sepsis presents during three periods. **Early-onset sepsis** often begins in utero and usually is a result of infection caused by the bacteria in the mother's genitourinary tract. Organisms related to this sepsis include group B streptococcus, *E. coli*, *Klebsiella*, *L. monocytogenes*, and nontypable *H. influenzae*. Most infected infants are premature and show nonspecific cardiorespiratory signs such as grunting, tachypnea, and cyanosis at birth. Risk factors for early-onset sepsis include vaginal colonization with group B streptococcus, prolonged rupture of the membranes (>24 hr), amnionitis, maternal fever or leukocytosis, fetal tachycardia, and preterm birth. Black race and male sex are unexplained additional risk factors for neonatal sepsis.

Early-onset sepsis (birth to 7 days) is an overwhelming multi-organ-system disease frequently manifested as respiratory failure, shock, meningitis (in 30% of cases), DIC, acute tubular necrosis, and symmetric peripheral gangrene. Early manifestations—grunting, poor feeding, pallor, apnea, lethargy, hypothermia, or an abnormal cry—may be nonspecific. Profound neutropenia, hypoxia, and hypotension may be refractory to treatment with broad-spectrum antibiotics, mechanical ventilation, and vasopressors such as dopamine and dobutamine. In the initial stages of early-onset septicemia in the preterm infant, it is often quite difficult to differentiate sepsis from RDS. Because of this difficulty, most premature infants with RDS receive broad-spectrum antibiotics.

Infants with early-onset sepsis should be *evaluated* by blood and cerebrospinal fluid (CSF) cultures, by CSF Gram stain, cell count, and protein and glucose levels. Buffy coat Gram stain or methylene blue stain also may help identify bacteria. Normal newborn infants generally have an elevated CSF protein content (100–150 mg/dL) and may have as many as 25 white blood cells (mean, 9/mm³), which are 75% lymphocytes in the absence of infection. Some infants with neonatal meningitis caused by group B steptococcus do not have an elevated CSF leukocyte count but are seen to have microorganisms in the spinal fluid when a Gram stain. In addition to culture, other methods of identifying the pathogenic bacteria are the determination of bacterial antigen in samples of blood, urine, or spinal fluid by methods such as counterimmunoelectrophoresis or latex agglutination. Serial complete blood counts should be performed to identify neutropenia, an increased number of immature neutrophils (bands), and thrombocytopenia. C-reactive protein levels are often elevated in neonatal patients with bacterial sepsis.

A chest roentgenogram also should be obtained to determine the presence of pneumonia. In addition to the traditional neonatal pathogens, pneumonia in VLBW infants may be the result of acquisition of maternal genital mycoplasmal agent (e.g., *U. urealyticum* or *M. hominis*). Arterial blood gases should be monitored to detect hypoxemia and metabolic acidosis that may be caused by hypoxia, shock, or both. Blood pressure, urine output, and peripheral perfusion should be monitored to determine the need to treat septic shock with fluids and vasopressor agents.

A combination of ampicillin and gentamicin for 10–14 days is effective *treatment* against most organisms responsible for early-onset sepsis. If meningitis is present, the treatment is extended to 21 days, or 14 days after a negative result from a CSF culture. Persistently positive results from CSF cultures are common with neonatal meningitis caused by gram-negative organisms, even with appropriate antibiotic treatment, and may be present for 2–3 days after antibiotic therapy. If gram-negative meningitis is present, some authorities continue to treat with an effective penicillin derivative combined with an aminoglycoside, whereas most change to a third-generation cephalosporin. High-dose penicillin (250,000 U/kg/24 hr) is appropriate for group B streptococcus meningitis. Inhaled nitric oxide, ECMO (in term infants), or both may improve the outcome of sepsis-related pulmonary hypertension. Intratracheal surfactant may reverse resiratory failure.

Intrapartum penicillin empiric prophylaxis for group B streptococcal colonized mothers or those with risk factors (e.g., fever, preterm labor, previous infant with group B streptococcus, and amnionitis) has reduced the rate of early-onset infection. The approach to the infant after prophylaxis is noted in Fig. 6–13.

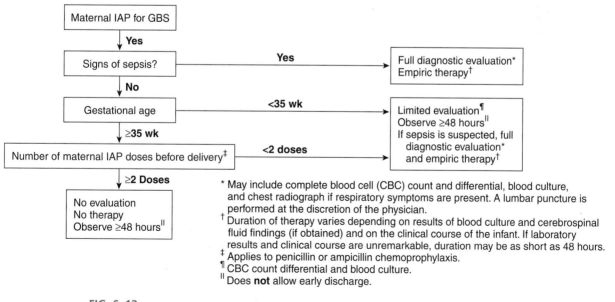

Empiric management of a neonate born to a mother who received intrapartum antimicrobial prophylaxis (IAP) for prevention of early-onset group B streptococcal (GBS) disease.

This algorithm is a suggested but is not an exclusive approach to management.

* May include complete blood cell (CBC) count and differential, blood culture, and chest radiograph if respiratory symptoms are present. A lumbar puncture is performed at the discretion of the physician.
† Duration of therapy varies depending on results of blood culture and cerebrospinal fluid findings (if obtained) and on the clinical course of the infant. If laboratory results and clinical course are unremarkable, duration may be as short as 48 hours.
‡ Applies to penicillin or ampicillin chemoprophylaxis.
¶ CBC count differential and blood culture.
‖ Does **not** allow early discharge.

FIG. 6–13

Suggested empiric management of a neonate following maternal antimicrobial prophylaxis for group B streptococcus. (From American Academy of Pediatrics: *Red book 2000*, ed 25, Chicago, 2000, The Academy.)

Late-onset sepsis (8–28 days) usually occurs in the healthy full-term infant who was discharged in good health from the normal newborn nursery. *Clinical manifestations* may include lethargy, poor feeding, hypotonia, apathy, seizures, bulging fontanel, fever, and direct-reacting hyperbilirubinemia. In addition to bacteremia, hematogenous seeding may result in focal infections such as meningitis (in 75% of cases), osteomyelitis (group B streptococcus, *Staphylococcus aureus*), arthritis (gonococcus, *S. aureus, Candida albicans*, gram-negative bacteria), and urinary tract infection (gram-negative bacteria).

The *evaluation* of infants with late-onset sepsis is similar to that for those with early-onset sepsis, with special attention given to a careful physical examination of the bones (infants with osteomyelitis may exhibit pseudoparalysis) and to the laboratory examination and culture of urine obtained by sterile suprapubic aspiration or urethral catheterization. Late-onset sepsis may be caused by the same pathogens as early-onset sepsis, but those infants exhibiting sepsis late in the neonatal period also may have infections caused by the pathogens usually found in older infants (*H. influenzae, Streptococcus pneumoniae,* and *Neisseria meningitidis*). In addition, viral agents (HSV cytomegalovirus [CMV], or enteroviruses) may present with a late-onset, sepsis-like picture.

Because of the increased rate of resistance of *H. influenzae* pneumococcus to ampicillin, some centers begin treatment with ampicillin and a third-generation cephalosporin (and vancomycin if meningitis is present) when sepsis occurs in the last week of the first month of life. The treatment of late-onset neonatal sepsis and meningitis is the same as that for early-onset sepsis.

Nosocomially acquired sepsis (8 days to discharge) occurs predominantly among premature infants in the NICU; many of these infants have been colonized with the multi-drug-resistant bacteria indigenous to the NICU. The risk of such serious bacterial infection is increased by frequent treatment with broad-spectrum antibiotics for sepsis and by the presence of central venous indwelling catheters, endotracheal tubes, umbilical vessel catheters, and electronic monitoring devices. Epidemics of bacterial or viral sepsis, bacterial or aseptic meningitis, staphylococcal bullous skin infections, cellulitis, pneumonia (bacterial or caused by adenovirus or respiratory syncytial virus), omphalitis (caused by *S. aureus* or gram-negative bacilli), and diarrhea (staphylococcal, enteroviral, or caused by rotavirus or enteropathogenic *E. coli*) are not uncommon in the NICU or even in the nursery for well babies.

The initial *clinical manifestations* of nosocomial infection in the premature infant may be subtle and include apnea and bradycardia, temperature instability, abdominal distention, and poor feeding. In the later stages, signs of infection are shock, DIC, worsening respiratory status, and local reactions such as omphalitis, eye discharge, diarrhea, and bullous impetigo.

The *treatment* of nosocomially acquired sepsis depends on the indigenous microbiologic flora of the particular hospital and their antibiotic sensitivities. Because *S. aureus* (occasionally methicillin-resistant), *Staphylococcus epidermidis* (usually methicillin-resistant), and gram-negative pathogens are common nosocomial bacterial agents in many nurseries, a combination of vancomycin or nafcillin (some use ampicillin) with gentamicin is appropriate. The dose and interval for administering all aminoglycosides, such as gentamicin, vary with postnatal age and birth weight. In addition, treatment with aminoglycosides for more than 3 days necessitates monitoring of the serum peak and trough concentrations to optimize therapy and to avoid ototoxicity and nephrotoxicity. Persistent signs of infection despite antibacterial treatment suggest candidal or viral sepsis.

Perinatal Congenital (Torch) Infections

The acronym "TORCH" represents a generic group of parasitic, bacterial, and viral pathogens that produce congenital or perinatally acquired infections: *t*oxoplasmosis, *o*ther, *r*ubella, *c*ytomegalovirus, and *h*erpes simplex. The "other" is an increasing number of agents responsible for fetal infection, such as syphilis, varicella-zoster, parvovirus, HIV, malaria, enteroviruses, *Borrelia burgdorferi*, and hepatitis B, C, or G.

Many of the *clinical manifestations* of TORCH infections are similar, including intrauterine growth retardation, nonimmune hydrops, anemia, thrombocytopenia, jaundice, hepatosplenomegaly, chorioretinitis, and congenital malformations. Some of the unique manifestations and epidemiologic characteristics of these infections are noted in Table 6–30.

Evaluation of patients thought to have TORCH infections should include attempts to isolate the organism by culture (for rubella, CMV, HSV, gonorrhea, and *Mycobacterium tuberculosis*); to identify the antigen of the pathogen (for hepatitis B and *Chlamydia trachomatis*); to identify the pathogen's genome with the polymerase chain reaction; and to identify specific fetal production of antibodies (IgM or increasing titer of IgG for *Toxoplasma*, syphilis, parvovirus, HIV, or *Borrelia*).

Treatment is not always available, specific, or effective. Nonetheless, some encouraging results have been reported for preventing the disease and for specifically treating the infant once the correct diagnosis is made (Table 6–30).

TABLE 6–30
Perinatal Congenital Infections (TORCH)

Agent	Maternal Epidemiology	Neonatal Features
Toxoplasma gondii	Heterophil-negative mononucleosis Exposure to cats or raw meat or immunosuppression High-risk exposure at 10–24 wk gestation	Hydrocephalus, abnormal spinal fluid, intracranial calcifications, chorioretinitis, jaundice, hepatosplenomegaly, fever Many infants asymptomatic at birth *Treatment:* pyrimethamine plus sulfadiazine
Rubella virus	Unimmunized seronegative mother; fever ± rash Detectable defects with infection: by 8 wk, 85% 9–12 wk, 50% 13–20 wk, 16% Virus may be present in infant's throat for 1 yr *Prevention:* vaccine	Intrauterine growth retardation, microcephaly, microphthalmia, cataracts, glaucoma, "salt and pepper" chorioretinitis, hepatosplenomegaly, jaundice, PDA, deafness, blueberry muffin rash, anemia, thrombocytopenia, leukopenia, metaphyseal lucencies, B-cell and T-cell deficiency Infant may be asymptomatic at birth
Cytomegalovirus	Sexually transmitted disease: primary genital infection may be asymptomatic Heterophil-negative mononucleosis; infant may have viruria for 1–6 yr	Sepsis, intrauterine growth retardation, chorioretinitis, microcephaly, periventricular calcifications, blueberry muffin rash, anemia, thrombocytopenia, neutropenia, hepatosplenomegaly, jaundice, deafness, pneumonia Many asymptomatic at birth *Prevention:* CMV-negative blood products *Possible treatment:* ganciclovir?
Herpes simplex type 2 or 1 virus	Sexually transmitted disease: primary genital infection may be asymptomatic; intrauterine infection rare, acquisition at time of birth more common	*Intrauterine infection:* chorioretinitis, skin lesions, microcephaly *Postnatal:* encephalitis, localized or disseminated disease, skin vesicles, keratoconjunctivitis *Treatment:* acyclovir
Varicella-zoster virus	Intrauterine infection with chickenpox during first trimester Infant develops severe neonatal varicella with maternal illness 5 days prior to or 2 days after delivery	Microphthalmia, cataracts, chorioretinitis, cutaneous and bony aplasia/hypoplasia/atrophy, cutaneous scars Zoster as in older child *Prevention of neonatal* condition with VZIG *Treatment of ill neonate:* acyclovir
Treponema pallidum (syphilis)	Sexually transmitted disease Maternal primary asymptomatic: painless "hidden" chancre Penicillin, not erythromycin, prevents fetal infection	Presentation *at birth* as nonimmune hydrops, prematurity, anemia, neutropenia, thrombocytopenia, pneumonia, hepatosplenomegaly *Late neonatal* as snuffles (rhinitis), rash, hepatosplenomegaly, condylomata lata, metaphysitis, cerebrospinal fluid pleocytosis, keratitis, periosteal new bone, lymphocytosis, hepatitis *Late onset:* teeth, eye, bone, skin, CNS, ear *Treatment:* penicillin

AIDS, Acquired immunodeficiency syndrome; *AZT,* zidovudine (azidothymidine); *BCG,* bacille Calmette-Guérin; *CMV,* cytomegalovirus; *CNS,* central nervous system; *HBIG,* hepatitis B immune globulin; *INH,* isoniazid; *PDA,* patent ductus arteriosus; *PPD,* purified protein derivative; *TB,* tuberculosis; *VZIG,* varicella-zoster immune globulin.

Continued

TABLE 6–30
Perinatal Congenital Infections (TORCH)—cont'd

Agent	Maternal Epidemiology	Neonatal Features
Parvovirus	Etiology of fifth disease; fever, rash, arthralgia in adults	Nonimmune hydrops, fetal anemia *Treatment:* in utero transfusion
Human immuno-deficiency virus (HIV)	AIDS; most mothers are asympto-matic and HIV positive; high-risk history; prostitute, drug abuse, married to bisexual, or hemophiliac	AIDS symptoms develop between 3 and 6 mo of age in 10–25%; failure to thrive, recurrent infection, hepa-tosplenomegaly, neurologic abnormalities *Management:* trimethoprim/sulfamethoxazole, AZT, other antiretroviral agents *Prevention:* prenatal, intrapartum, postpartum AZT; avoid breast feeding
Hepatitis B virus	Vertical transmission common; may result in cirrhosis, hepatocellular carcinoma	Acute neonatal hepatitis; many become asymptomatic carriers *Prevention:* HBIG, vaccine
Neisseria gonorrhoeae	Sexually transmitted disease, infant acquires at birth *Treatment:* cefotaxime, ceftriaxone	Gonococcal ophthalmia, sepsis, meningitis *Prevention:* silver nitrate, erythromycin eye drops *Treatment:* intravenous ceftriaxone
Chlamydia trachomatis	Sexually transmitted disease, infant acquires at birth *Treatment:* oral erythromycin	Conjunctivitis, pneumonia *Prevention:* erythromycin eye drops *Treatment:* oral erythromycin
Mycobacterium tuberculosis	Positive PPD skin test, recent con-verter, positive chest roentgenogram, positive family member *Treatment:* INH and rifampin ± ethambutol	Congenital rare septic pneumonia; acquired primary pulmonary TB; asymptomatic, follow PPD *Prevention:* INH, BCG, separation *Treatment:* INH, rifampin, pyrazinamide
Trypanosoma cruzi (Chagas disease)	Central South American native, immigrant, travel Chronic disease in mother	Failure to thrive, heart failure, achalasia *Treatment:* nifurtimox

AIDS, Acquired immunodeficiency syndrome; *AZT,* zidovudine (azidothymidine); *BCG,* bacille Calmette-Guérin; *CMV,* cy-tomegalovirus; *CNS,* central nervous system; *HBIG,* hepatitis B immune globulin; *INH,* isoniazid; *PDA,* patent ductus arteriosus; *PPD,* purified protein derivative; *TB,* tuberculosis; *VZIG,* varicella-zoster immune globulin.

REFERENCES

Behrman RE, Kliegman RM, Jenson HB, editors: *Nelson textbook of pediatrics,* ed 16, Philadelphia, 2000, WB Saunders, Chapters 105, 106.

Best J, Sutherland S: Diagnosis and prevention of congenital and perinatal infections: TORCH screening should be discouraged, *BMJ* 301(6757):888–889, 1990.

Escobar GJ, Li D, Armstrong MA, et al: Neonatal sepsis workups in infants ≥2000 grams at birth: a population-based study, *Pediatrics* 106(2 Pt 1):256–263, 2000.

Jobe AH: Commentary on surfactant treatment of neonates with respiratory failure and group B streptococcal infection, *Pediatrics* 106(5):1135, 2000.

Klinger G, Chin CN, Beyene J, et al: Predicting the outcome of neonatal bacterial meningitis, *Pediatrics* 106(3):477–482, 2000.

Lazzaroto T, Varani S, Guerra B, et al: Prenatal indicators of congenital cytomegalovirus infection, *J Pediatr* 137(1):90–95, 2000.

Modi N, Carr R: Promising stratagems for reducing the burden of neonatal sepsis, *Arch Dis Child Fetal Neonatal Ed* 83(2): F150–F153, 2000.

Risser WL, Hwang L-Y: Problems in the current case definitions of congenital syphilis, *J Pediatr* 129(4):499–505, 1996.

White K, Rainbow J, Johnson S, et al: Early onset group B strep-tococcal disease—United States, 1998-1999, *MMWR* 49(35): 793–796, 2000.

NEONATAL NEUROLOGY AND OUTCOME

The neonatal central nervous system is anatomically and functionally immature. Although division of cerebral cortical neuronal cells stops during the sec-ond trimester of pregnancy, glial cell growth, dendritic arborization, myelination, and cerebellar neuronal cell number continue to increase beyond term gestation and into infancy. At birth, the human newborn spends more time asleep (predominantly in rapid eye movement [REM] or active sleep) than in a wakeful state and is totally dependent on adults. Primitive reflexes such as the Moro, grasp, stepping, rooting, sucking, and crossed extensor reflexes are readily elicited and are normal for this age. In addition, the newborn infant has a wealth of cortical functions that are less easily demonstrated (e.g., the ability to extinguish repetitive or painful stimuli and to show visual preference for new or novel objects). The newborn also has the capacity for attentive eye fixation and differential responses to the mother's voice.

During the perinatal period, many pathophysiologic mechanisms can adversely and permanently affect the developing brain. These include prenatal events such as hypoxia, ischemia, infections, inflammation, malformations, maternal drugs, and coagulation disorders, and postnatal events such as birth trauma, hypoxia-ischemia, inborn errors of metabolism, hypoglycemia, hypothyroidism, hyperthyroidism, polycythemia, hemorrhage, and meningitis.

Neonatal Seizures

Seizures during the neonatal period may be the result of multiple causes, with characteristic historical and clinical manifestations. Seizures caused by **hypoxic-ischemic encephalopathy** (postasphyxial seizures), a common cause of seizures in the full-term infant, usually occur 12–24 hours after a history of birth asphyxia and often are refractory to conventional doses of anticonvulsant medications. Postasphyxial seizures also may be caused by metabolic disorders associated with neonatal asphyxia, such as hypoglycemia and hypocalcemia. **Intraventricular hemorrhage** (IVH) is a common cause of seizures in premature infants and often occurs between 1 and 3 days of age. Seizures with IVH are associated with a bulging fontanel, hemorrhagic spinal fluid, anemia, lethargy, and coma. Seizures caused by **hypoglycemia** often occur when blood glucose levels decline to the lowest postnatal value (e.g., at 1–2 hours of age or after 24–48 hours of poor nutritional intake) (Table 6–29). Seizures caused by **hypocalcemia** and **hypomagnesemia** develop among high-risk infants and respond well to therapy with calcium, magnesium, or both.

Seizures noted in the delivery room often are caused by direct *injection of local anesthetic agents* into the fetal scalp (associated with transient bradycardia and fixed dilated pupils), severe *anoxia*, or *congenital brain malformation*. Seizures after the first 5 days of life may be the result of *infection* or *drug withdrawal*.

Seizures associated with lethargy, acidosis, and a family history of infant deaths may be the result of an *inborn error of metabolism*. An infant whose parent has a history of a neonatal seizure also is at risk for *benign familial seizures*. In an infant who appears well, a sudden onset on days 1–3 of seizures that are of short duration and that do not recur may be the result of a *subarachnoid hemorrhage*. Focal seizures often are the result of local cerebral infarction.

Seizures may be difficult to differentiate from benign jitteriness or from tremulousness in infants of diabetic mothers, in infants with narcotic withdrawal syndrome, and in any infants after an episode of asphyxia. In contrast to seizures, jitteriness and tremors are sensory dependent, elicited by stimuli, and interrupted by holding the extremity. Seizure activity becomes manifest as coarse, fast and slow clonic activity, whereas jitteriness is characterized by fine, rapid movement. Seizures may be associated with abnormal eye movements, such as tonic deviation to one side. The electroencephalogram (EEG) often demonstrates seizure activity when the clinical diagnosis is uncertain. Identifying seizures in the newborn period is often difficult because the infant, especially the LBW infant, usually does not demonstrate the tonic-clonic major motor activity typical of the older child (Table 6–31). Subtle seizures are quite a common manifestation among newborn infants. The subtle signs of seizure activity include apnea, eye deviation, tongue thrusting, eye blinking, fluctuation of vital signs, and staring. Continuous bedside EEG monitoring can help identify subtle seizures.

The *diagnostic evaluation* of infants with seizures should involve an immediate determination of capillary blood glucose levels with a Chemstrip. In addition, blood concentrations of sodium, calcium, glucose, and bilirubin should be determined. When infection is suspected, CSF and blood specimens should be obtained for culture. After the seizure has stopped, a careful examination should be done to identify signs of increased intracranial pressure, congenital malformations, and systemic illness. If signs of elevated intracranial pressure are absent, a lumbar puncture should be performed. If the diagnosis is not apparent at this point, further evaluation should involve magnetic resonance imaging (MRI), computed tomography (CT), or cerebral ultrasonography and tests to determine the presence of an inborn error of metabolism. Determinations of inborn errors of metabolism are especially important in infants with unexplained lethargy, coma, acidosis, ketonuria, or respiratory alkalosis.

The *treatment* of neonatal seizures may be specific, such as treatment of meningitis or the correction of hypoglycemia, hypocalcemia, hypomagnesemia,

TABLE 6–31
Clinical Characteristics of Neonatal Seizures

Designation	Characterization
Focal clonic	Repetitive, rhythmic contractions of muscle groups of the limbs, face, or trunk
	May be unilateral or multifocal
	May appear synchronously or asynchronously in various body regions
	Cannot be suppressed by restraint
Focal tonic	Sustained posturing of single limbs
	Sustained asymmetric posturing of the trunk
	Sustained eye deviation
	Cannot be provoked by stimulation or suppressed by restraint
Myoclonic	Arrhythmic contractions of muscle groups of the limbs, face, or trunk
	Typically not repetitive or may recur at a slow rate
	May be generalized, focal, or fragmentary
	May be provoked by stimulation
Generalized tonic	Sustained symmetric posturing of limbs, trunk, and neck
	May be flexor, extensor, or mixed extensor/flexor
	May be provoked by stimulation
	May be suppressed by restraint or repositioning
Ocular signs	Random and roving eye movements or nystagmus
	Distinct from tonic eye deviation
Orobuccolingual movements	Sucking, chewing, tongue protrusions
	May be provoked by stimulation
Progression movements	Rowing or swimming movements of the arms
	Pedaling or bicycling movements of the legs
	May be provoked by stimulation
	May be suppressed by restraint or repositioning

From Mizrahi EM: Neonatal seizures. In Shinnar S, Branski D, editors: *Pediatric and adolescent medicine. vol 6. Childhood seizures,* Basel, 1995, S. Karger.

hyponatremia, or vitamin B_6 deficiency or dependency. In the absence of an identifiable cause, therapy should involve an anticonvulsant agent, such as 20–40 mg/kg of phenobarbital, 10–20 mg/kg of phenytoin (Dilantin), or 0.1–0.3 mg/kg of diazepam (Valium), followed by one of the two longer-acting drugs. Treatment of status epilepticus requires repeated doses of phenobarbital and may also require diazepam or midazolam, titrated to clinical signs.

The long-term outcome for neonatal seizures usually is related to the underlying cause and to the primary pathology, such as hypoxic-ischemic encephalopathy, meningitis, drug withdrawal, stroke, or hemorrhage.

Intracranial Hemorrhage

Intracranial hemorrhage may be confined to one anatomic area of the brain, such as the subdural, subarachnoid, periventricular, intraventricular, intraparenchymal, or cerebellar region. **Subdural hemorrhages** are seen in association with birth trauma, cephalopelvic disproportion, forceps delivery, LGA infants, skull fractures, and postnatal head trauma. The subdural hematoma does not always cause symptoms immediately after birth; with time, however, the red blood cells undergo hemolysis and water is drawn into the hemorrhage because of the high oncotic pressure of protein, resulting in an expanding symptomatic lesion. Anemia, vomiting, seizures, and macrocephaly may occur in the infant who is 1–2 months old and has a subdural hematoma. *Child abuse* must also be suspected, and appropriate diagnostic evaluation must be undertaken to identify other possible signs of skeletal, ocular, or soft tissue injury. Occasionally a massive subdural hemorrhage in the neonatal period is caused by rupture of the vein of Galen or by an inherited coagulation disorder such as hemophilia. Infants with these conditions exhibit shock, seizures, and coma. The **treat-**

ment of all symptomatic subdural hematomas is surgical evacuation.

Subarachnoid hemorrhages may be spontaneous, associated with hypoxia or caused by bleeding from a cerebral arteriovenous malformation. Seizures are a common presenting manifestation, and the *prognosis* depends on the underlying injury. *Treatment* is directed at the seizure and the rare occurrence of posthemorrhagic hydrocephalus.

Periventricular hemorrhage and **IVH** are common among VLBW infants, and the risk decreases with increasing gestational age. Up to 50% of infants under 1500 g have evidence of intracranial bleeding. The *pathogenesis* for these hemorrhages is unknown (they usually are not caused by coagulation disorders), but the initial site of bleeding may be the weak blood vessels in the periventricular germinal matrix. The vessels in this area have poor structural support. These vessels may rupture and hemorrhage because of passive changes in cerebral blood flow occurring with the variations of blood pressure that sick premature infants often exhibit (failure of autoregulation). In some sick infants these blood pressure variations are the only identifiable etiologic factors. In others, the disorders that may cause the elevation or depression of blood pressure or that interfere with venous return from the head (venous stasis) increase the risk of IVH; these disorders include asphyxia, pneumothorax, mechanical ventilation, hypercapnia, hypoxemia, prolonged labor, breech delivery, PDA, heart failure, intravenous therapy with blood volume–expanding agents such as albumin, and therapy with hypertonic solutions such as sodium bicarbonate.

Most periventricular and intraventricular hemorrhages occur in the first 3 days of life. It is unusual for IVH to occur after the fifth day of life. The *clinical manifestations* of IVH include seizures, apnea, bradycardia, lethargy, coma, hypotension, metabolic acidosis, anemia not corrected by blood transfusion, bulging fontanel, and cutaneous mottling. Many infants with small hemorrhages (grade 1 or 2) are asymptomatic; those with larger hemorrhages (grade 4) often have a catastrophic event that rapidly progresses to shock and coma.

The *diagnosis* of IVH is confirmed and the severity graded by ultrasonographic or CT examination through the anterior fontanel. Grade 1 IVH is confined to the germinal matrix; grade 2 is an extension of grade 1, with blood noted in the ventricle without ventricular enlargement; grade 3 is an extension of grade 2 with ventricular dilation; and grade 4 has blood in dilated ventricles and in the cerebral cortex, either contiguous with or distant from the ventricle. Grade 4 hemorrhage carries a poor prognosis, as does the development of periventricular, small,

echolucent cystic lesions, with or without porencephalic cysts and posthemorrhagic hydrocephalus. Periventricular cysts often are noted after the resolution of echodense areas in the periventricular white matter. The cysts may correspond to the development of periventricular leukomalacia, which may be a precursor to cerebral palsy. Extensive intraparenchymal echodensities represent hemorrhagic necrosis. They are associated with a high mortality rate and have a poor neurodevelopmental prognosis for survivors.

Treatment of the acute hemorrhage involves standard supportive care, including ventilation for apnea and blood transfusion for shock. Posthemorrhagic hydrocephalus may be managed with serial daily lumbar punctures, an external ventriculostomy tube, or a permanent ventricular-peritoneal shunt. Implementation of the shunt often is delayed because of the high protein content of the hemorrhagic ventricular fluid.

Hypoxic-Ischemic Encephalopathy

(See also the section on Asphyxia: Resuscitation in this chapter)

Conditions known to reduce uteroplacental blood flow or to interfere with spontaneous respiration lead to perinatal hypoxia; to lactic acidosis; and if severe enough to reduce cardiac output or cause cardiac arrest, to ischemia. The combination of the reduced availability of oxygen for the brain that is a result of hypoxia and the diminished or absent blood flow to the brain that is a result of ischemia leads to reduced glucose for metabolism and to an accumulation of lactate that produces local tissue acidosis. After reperfusion, hypoxic-ischemic injury also may be complicated by cell necrosis and vascular endothelial edema, reducing blood flow distal to the involved vessel. Typically, hypoxic-ischemic encephalopathy in the term infant is characterized by cerebral edema, cortical necrosis, and involvement of the basal ganglia, whereas in the preterm infant it is characterized by periventricular leukomalacia. Both lesions may result in cortical atrophy, mental retardation, and spastic quadriplegia or diplegia.

The *clinical manifestations* and characteristic course of hypoxic-ischemic encephalopathy vary according to the severity of the injury (Table 6–32). Infants with severe stage 3 hypoxic-ischemic encephalopathy are usually hypotonic, although occasionally they initially appear hypertonic and hyperalert at birth. As cerebral edema develops, brain functions are affected in a descending order; cortical depression produces coma, and brainstem depression results in apnea. As cerebral edema progresses, refractory seizures begin between 12 and 24 hours after birth.

TABLE 6–32
Hypoxic-Ischemic Encephalopathy in Term Infants

Signs	Stage 1	Stage 2	Stage 3
Level of consciousness	Hyperalert	Lethargic	Stuporous
Muscle tone	Normal	Hypotonic	Flaccid
Tendon reflexes/clonus	Hyperactive	Hyperactive	Absent
Moro reflex	Strong	Weak	Absent
Pupils	Mydriasis	Miosis	Unequal, poor light reflex
Seizures	None	Common	Decerebration
Electroencephalographic	Normal	Low voltage changing to seizure activity	Burst suppression to isoelectric
Duration	More than 24 hr if progresses, otherwise may remain normal	24 hr to 14 days	Days to weeks

Modified from Sarnat HB, Sarnat MS: *Arch Neurol* 33:696, 1976.

At this time the infant has no signs of spontaneous respirations, is hypotonic, and has diminished or absent deep tendon reflexes.

Survivors of stage 3 hypoxic-ischemic encephalopathy have a high incidence of seizures and serious neurodevelopmental handicaps. The prognosis of severe asphyxia also depends on other organ system injury (Table 6–11). Another indicator of poor prognosis is time of onset of spontaneous respiration as estimated by Apgar score. Infants with Apgar scores of 0–3 at 10 minutes have a 20% mortality and a 5% incidence of cerebral palsy; if the score remains this low by 20 minutes, the mortality increases to 60% and the incidence of cerebral palsy rises to 57%.

Neonatal Hypotonia

Decreased tone, floppiness, or hypotonia in the newborn infant may be transient and resolve without future problems or may be caused by serious, permanent disease originating in the central nervous system, spinal cord, anterior horn cell, neuromuscular junction, or muscle. **Diseases of the brain** that produce hypotonia may be caused by hypoxic-ischemic encephalopathy, IVH, meningitis, metabolic toxins from inborn errors of metabolism (e.g., organic acids and ammonia), or centrally acting drugs. The infant does not appear alert and has a weak cry, seizures, normal deep tendon reflexes, and an abnormal EEG.

Spinal cord lesions often are the result of trauma or malformation. Lesions present in an alert-looking child as a strong cry, decreased deep tendon reflexes, reduced spontaneous movement below the cord lesions, and a normal EEG. *Anterior horn cell disease,* such as Werdnig-Hoffmann disease, is indicated by an alert-appearing infant with hypotonia, tongue fasciculations, absent deep tendon reflexes, and reduced muscle mass; diagnosis is based on results of a neurogenic electromyogram (EMG) and muscle biopsy.

Neuromuscular junction disease, such as neonatal transient myasthenia gravis (in a child born to a woman with myasthenia gravis), is indicated by an alert infant with a weak cry, ophthalmoplegia, ptosis, normal deep tendon reflexes, an abnormal EMG, and a positive result from a physostigmine test.

Muscle disease may have an onset before or immediately after birth and may be a result of congenital muscular dystrophy, myotonic dystrophy, congenital myotonia, glycogen storage disease, mitochondrial defects, congenital lactic acidosis, or other myopathies. The infant with muscle disease is alert and has a good cry but also displays decreased muscle mass, contractures, a myopathic EMG, characteristic muscle biopsy, and an elevated level of serum creatine phosphokinase (CPK), with or without diminished deep tendon reflexes.

Respiratory difficulty is present in many conditions related to neonatal hypotonia; affected infants have difficulty swallowing secretions, which they may aspirate. Respiratory failure also may occur as a result of weakness of the respiratory muscles. The evaluation of infants with hypotonia should involve a family history of myasthenia gravis, myotonic dystrophy, muscular dystrophy, inheritable myopathies, and the existence of other infants with metabolic diseases.

Laboratory evaluation depends on the history and physical examination and may involve metabolic tests for organic acids and carnitine, muscle and head ultrasound examination, nerve conduction, an EMG, measurement of the level of serum CPK, a physostigmine test, and muscle biopsy, with specific attention to electron microscopy. Chromosomal analysis also is helpful for diagnosing hypotonia and Prader-Willi syndrome, which has a deletion of the long arm of chromosome 15.

REFERENCES

Adamson S, Alessandi L, Badawi N, et al: Predictors of neonatal encephalopathy in full term infants, *BMJ* 311(7005):598–602, 1995.

Azzopardi D, Robertson NJ, Cowan FM, et al: Pilot study of treatment with whole body hypothermia for neonatal encephalopathy, *Pediatrics* 106(4):684–694, 2000.

Bada HS, Korones SB, Perry EH, et al: Mean arterial blood pressure changes in premature infants and those at risk for intraventricular hemorrhage, *J Pediatr* 117(4):607–614, 1990.

Behrman RE, Kliegman RM, Jenson HB, editors: *Nelson textbook of pediatrics,* ed 16, Philadelphia, 2000, WB Saunders, Chapters 64, 95, 615.

Dammann O, Leviton A: Brain damage in preterm newborns: biological response modification as a strategy to reduce disabilities, *J Pediatr* 136(4):433–438, 2000.

Mercuri E, Ricci D, Cowan FM, et al: Head growth in infants with hypoxic-ischemic encephalopathy: correlation with neonatal magnetic resonance imaging, *Pediatrics* 106(2 Pt 1):235–243, 2000.

OUTCOME AND FOLLOW-UP OF LOW-BIRTH-WEIGHT OR PREMATURE INFANTS

Most LBW infants survive neonatal illnesses without long-term sequelae. More than 90% of infants weighing more than 1500 g survive, and as many as 50% of infants weighing as little as 750 g survive. Between 10% and 25% of LBW survivors have mild developmental problems, and 5–10% have severe developmental problems; the smallest at birth are at greatest risk. Long-term sequelae include retinopathy of prematurity with blindness, hearing loss, hydrocephalus, microcephaly, mental retardation, cerebral palsy (spastic diplegia), chronic pulmonary insufficiency (BPD), short bowel syndrome (post-NEC), and growth failure.

Many infants demonstrate transient neonatal hypotonia, which resolves by 8 months "corrected age" and is not associated with future problems. However, diagnosing cerebral palsy before this age is difficult, and all hypotonic infants should be considered at high risk until proven otherwise. Additionally, many VLBW infants have functional limitations (e.g., vision, hearing, motor, and learning) that may result in poor performance or failure in school. Although the intelligence quotient (IQ) often relates to adverse events affecting the central nervous system during the neonatal period, the intelligence of premature infants also is influenced directly by maternal socioeconomic status.

Most infants with cerebral palsy are not preterm infants or term infants with birth asphyxia. Perinatal causes account for fewer than 10% of older infants who have severe mental retardation. Furthermore, although 10–25% of VLBW infants demonstrate some handicap, the vast majority of these infants are functional and able to attend regular schools.

REFERENCES

Behrman RE, Kliegman RM, Jenson HB, editors: *Nelson textbook of pediatrics,* ed 16, Philadelphia, 2000, WB Saunders.

Colver AF, Gibson M, Hen EN, et al: Increasing rates of cerebral palsy across the severity spectrum in northeast England 1964-1993, *Arch Dis Child Fetal Neonatal Ed* 83(1):F7–F12, 2000.

Hack M, Taylor HG, Klein N, et al: Functional limitations and special health care needs of 10- to 14-year-old children weighing less than 750 grams at birth, *Pediatrics* 106(3):554–560, 2000.

Maas YG, Mirmiran M, Hart AA, et al: Predictive value of neonatal neurological tests for developmental outcome of preterm infants, *J Pediatr* 137(1):100–106, 2000.

Perlman JM, Risser R, Broyles RS: Bilateral cystic periventricular leukomalacia in the premature infant: associated risk factors, *Pediatrics* 97(6 Pt 1):822–827, 1996.

Peterson BS, Vohr B, Staib LH, et al: Regional brain volume abnormalities and long-term cognitive outcome in preterm infants, *JAMA* 284(15):1939–1947, 2000.

Vohr BR, Wright LL, Dusick AM, et al: Neurodevelopment and functional outcomes of extremely low birth weight infants in the national institute of child health and human development neonatal research network, 1993-1994, *Pediatrics* 105(6): 1216–1226, 2000.

Wu YW, Colford JM Jr: Chorioamnionitis as a risk factor for cerebral palsy, *JAMA* 284(11):1417–1424, 2000.

CHAPTER 7

Adolescent Medicine

Richard E. Kreipe ▼ Cheryl M. Kodjo

ADOLESCENT GROWTH AND DEVELOPMENT

Adolescence refers to the passage from childhood to adulthood, whereas *puberty* refers to those biologic changes that lead to reproductive capacity. The events of puberty occur in a predictable sequence, but the timing of the initiation and the velocity of these changes are highly variable among individuals. The integration of pubertal changes into the adolescent's self-concept is crucial to normal adolescence.

Even "normal" conditions such as acne or dysmenorrhea deserve attention because they may seriously affect daily life. Providers of adolescent health care must be familiar with adolescent growth and development, the specific context in which these changes are occurring, health promotion strategies, and the manifestations of disease during adolescence.

Physical Growth and Development of Adolescents

Girls

Soon after adipose deposition and changes in the bony pelvis widen the contour of the hips, females experience breast budding immediately under the areola *(thelarche)* and the appearance of fine, dark, straight pubic hair over the mons veneris *(adrenarche* or *pubarche)* (Fig. 7–1). These latter two changes, occurring at about 11 years of age (a range of 8–13 years), mark the sexual maturity rating (SMR, also known as Tanner) stage II of pubertal development. These events appear to be occurring earlier than in previous generations, especially for black adolescents. A large, nationally representative study of girls in the United States revealed that the mean age of menarche and adrenarche now is approximately 9 years of age for black girls and 10 years of age for white girls; the mean age of menarche (12.2 and 12.9 years of age for black and white girls, respectively)

has not decreased appreciably over time. Thus the duration of puberty may be lengthening for girls.

Breast development proceeds to the SMR V (adult) stage over approximately 4 years; however, these changes can occur during a period as short as 18 months or may take as long as 9 years. The progression of the growth of pubic hair to the SMR V (adult) stage takes about 2½ years on average, with a range of 1½–3½ years. About 1 year after the initiation of breast development, during the SMR III stage, girls have a very rapid increase in height (Fig. 7–2). The peak of this growth spurt (peak height velocity [PHV]) should precede the onset of menstruation *(menarche)* in normal individuals. Thus menarche is a relatively late pubertal event, usually occurring approximately 6 months after the growth spurt, during or just before the SMR IV stage of breast development. Girls grow only 1–2 inches in height after menarche.

Boys

Boys also have a regular sequence of physical changes during puberty but lack any milestone as obvious as breast development or menarche. Nocturnal emissions (wet dreams) can be considered the male counterpart of menstruation, first appearing during the SMR III stage, but they are not as regular as the menses. From 11–13 years of age, the average boy is shorter than the average girl because the PHV occurs later in the male pubertal sequence, in contrast to the relatively early female growth spurt (Fig. 7–3).

Testicular enlargement (long axis of testes >2.5 cm) indicates a transition from the SMR I to the SMR II stage (Fig. 7–4). It begins at about 11½ years of age (ranging from 9½–13½ years). Within a year of testicular enlargement, penile enlargement commences, marking the SMR III stage. This is usually preceded by the appearance of pubic hair at the base of the penis *(adrenarche)*, followed by growth of axillary hair. Completion of testicular growth can occur any time

Pubertal Development in Size of Female Breasts

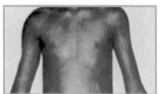 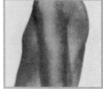

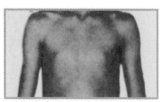 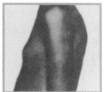

Stage 1 The breasts are preadolescent. There is elevation of the papilla only.

Stage 2 Breast bud stage. A small mound is formed by the elevation of the breast and papilla. The areolar diameter enlarges.

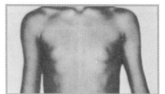 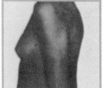

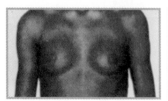 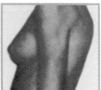

Stage 3 There is further enlargement of breast and areola with no separation of their contours.

Stage 4 There is a projection of the areola and papilla to form a secondary mound above the level of the breast.

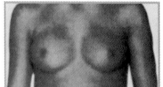 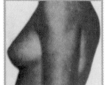

Stage 5 The breasts resemble those of a mature female as the areola has recessed to the general contour of the breast.

Pubertal Development of Female Pubic Hair
Stage 1 There is no pubic hair.

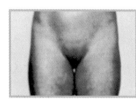 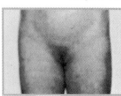 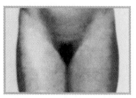 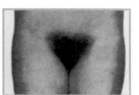

Stage 2 There is sparse growth of long, slightly pigmented, downy hair, straight or only slightly curled, primarily along the labia.

Stage 3 The hair is considerably darker, coarser, and more curled. The hair spreads sparsely over the junction of the pubes.

Stage 4 The hair, now adult in type, covers a smaller area than in the adult and does not extend onto the thighs.

Stage 5 The hair is adult in quantity and type, with extension onto the thighs.

FIG. 7–1

Typical progression of female pubertal development. (Adapted from Tanner JM: *Growth at adolescence,* ed 2, Oxford, 1962, Blackwell Scientific Publications. Reprinted from *Assessment of pubertal development,* Columbus, Ohio, 1986, Ross Laboratories.)

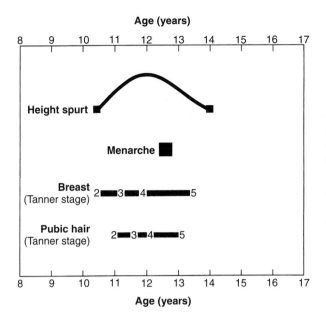

FIG. 7–2

Sequence of pubertal events in the average American female. Recent studies suggest that onset of breast development may be as early as 9 years of age for black girls and 10 years of age for white girls. (Adapted from Brookman RR, Rauh JL, Morrison JA, et al: *The Princeton maturation study,* 1976, unpublished data for adolescents in Cincinnati, Ohio. Reprinted from *Assessment of pubertal development,* Columbus, Ohio, 1986, Ross Laboratories.)

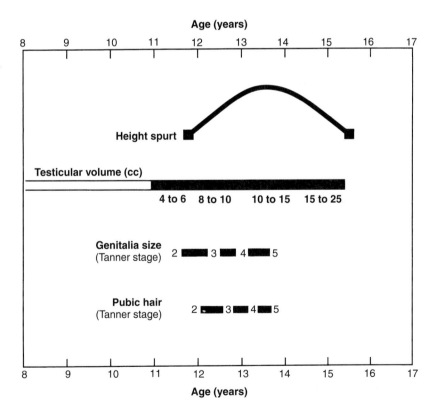

FIG. 7–3

Sequence of pubertal events in the average American male. Testicular volume less than 4 cc using orchidometer (Prader Beads) represents prepubertal stage. (Adapted from Brookman RR, Rauh JL, Morrison JA, et al: *The Princeton maturation study,* 1976, unpublished data for adolescents in Cincinnati, Ohio. Reprinted from *Assessment of pubertal development,* Columbus, Ohio, 1986, Ross Laboratories.)

Pubertal Development in Size of Male Genitalia

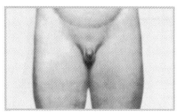 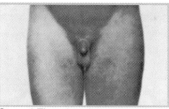 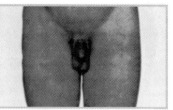

Stage 1 The penis, testes, and scrotum are of childhood size.

Stage 2 There is enlargement of the scrotum and testes, but the penis usually does not enlarge. The scrotal skin reddens.

Stage 3 There is further growth of the testes and scrotum and enlargement of the penis, mainly in length.

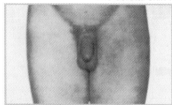 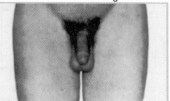

Stage 4 There is still further growth of the testes and scrotum and increased size of the penis, especially in breadth.

Stage 5 The genitalia are adult in size and shape.

Pubertal Development of Male Pubic Hair
Stage 1 There is no pubic hair.

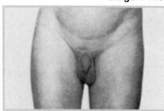 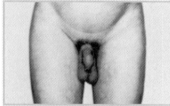

Stage 2 There is sparse growth of long, slightly pigmented, downy hair, straight or only slightly curled, primarily at the base of the penis.

Stage 3 The hair is considerably darker, coarser, and more curled. The hair spreads sparsely over the junction of the pubes.

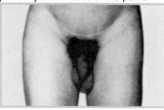 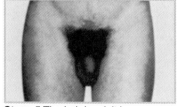

Stage 4 The hair, now adult in type, covers a smaller area than in the adult and does not extend onto the thighs.

Stage 5 The hair is adult in quantity and type, with extension onto the thighs.

FIG. 7–4

Typical progression of male pubertal development. (Adapted from Tanner JM: *Growth at adolescence,* ed 2, Oxford, 1962, Blackwell Scientific Publications. Reprinted from *Assessment of pubertal development,* Columbus, Ohio, 1986, Ross Laboratories.)

between 13½ and 17 years of age. Penile lengthening and widening begin normally between 10½ and 14½ years of age; development of the penis reaches the SMR V stage between 12½ and 16½ years of age. The growth spurt, as previously noted, is a relatively late event in boys but normally is initiated from 10½–16 years of age and is completed by 13½–17½ years of age, depending on the individual. Growth in boys continues at a slower pace for several years after the spurt and can continue into the third decade of life.

Reproductive Endocrinology

Puberty is initiated following the release from inhibition of the gonadotropin-releasing hormone (GnRH) that secretes medial-basal hypothalamic neurons. Decreased sensitivity to negative feedback by endogenous sex steroids results in pulsatile release of GnRH, which causes the pulsatile release of luteinizing hormone (LH) and follicle-stimulating

hormone (FSH) from the pituitary gland. Initially this occurs during sleep; later in puberty, it occurs throughout wakefulness. Pituitary secretion of gonadotropins initiates gonadal growth and maturation. Ovarian estradiol and testicular testosterone affect breast and penis growth, respectively. Both hormones augment linear growth. Adrenarche is mediated by adrenal androgens in both girls and boys; as puberty progresses in males, testosterone accounts for most sexual hair development.

Precocious Puberty

See Chapter 17.

Changes Associated with Physical Maturation

SMR is a marker of biologic maturation that can be related to both specific laboratory value changes and certain conditions (Tables 7–1 and 7–2). For example,

TABLE 7–1
Correlates of Female Pubertal Maturation

	Sexual Maturity Rating (Tanner Stage)				
	1	2	3	4	5
Hematocrit (%)					
White *mean*	39.1	39.2	39.6	39.2	39.2
White *range*	36.1–42.1	37.1–41.3	37.0–42.2	36.9–41.6	36.2–42.2
Black *mean*	37.3	38.9	39.0	38.4	38.7
Black *range*	34.6–39.9	35.7–42.1	35.2–42.6	34.9–42.8	35.9–41.5
Alkaline phosphatase (IU/L) (serum)					
White *mean*	70	89	76	33	38
White *range*	51–90	49–134	36–108	16–60	23–76
Black *mean*	84	95	86	44	31
Black *range*	69–108	65–138	26–148	18–144	13–70
Short female with growth potential		+		+	++
Short female with limited growth potential					
Slipped capital femoral epiphysis		+	++		
Acute worsening of scoliosis		+	+++		
Osgood-Schlatter disease		+	+		
Oral contraceptive prescription				+	++
Diaphragm prescription					+
Acute worsening of straight back syndrome		+	++	+	
Acne vulgaris		+	++	++	
Physiologic leukorrhea			+		
Gonococcal vaginitis	+				
Gonococcal cervicitis		+	+	+	+
Regression of virginal breast hypertrophy					+
Timing of breast reduction or rhinoplasty					+

Data from Copeland KC, Brookman RR, Rauh JL: *Assessment of pubertal development*, Columbus, Ohio, 1986, Ross Laboratories; Daniel WA: *Semin Adolesc Med* 1(1):15–24, 1985.
+, Possible; ++, more likely than +; +++, most likely.

TABLE 7–2
Correlates of Male Pubertal Maturation

	Sexual Maturity Rating (Tanner Stage)				
	1	2	3	4	5
Hematocrit (%)					
White *mean*	39.5	39.8	40.9	42.3	43.8
White *range*	37.1–41.8	36.7–42.8	38.2–43.5	39.7–44.8	41.1–46.4
Black *mean*	37.7	38.4	39.7	41.1	42.7
Black *range*	35.2–40.2	36.0–40.9	37.3–42.0	38.3–43.8	39.6–45.9
Alkaline phosphatase (IU/L) (serum)					
White *mean*	72	77	101	75	58
White *range*	54–110	42–106	53–141	41–158	21–120
Black *mean*	77	94	122	116	75
Black *range*	43–130	53–204	46–240	32–228	23–228
Short male with growth potential		+			
Short male with limited growth potential				+	++
Slipped capital femoral epiphysis		+	++		
Acute worsening of scoliosis		+	+++		
Osgood-Schlatter disease		+	+		
Acute worsening of straight back syndrome		+	++	+	
Gynecomastia		+	++		
Acne vulgaris		+	++	++	
Orchiopexy timing	+				
Timing of rhinoplasty					+

Data from Copeland KC, Brookman RR, Rauh JL: *Assessment of pubertal development,* Columbus, Ohio, 1986, Ross Laboratories; Daniel WA: *Semin Adolesc Med* 1(1):15–24, 1985.
+, Possible; ++ more likely than +; +++ most likely.

higher hematocrit values in adolescent males than in adolescent females are the result of greater androgenic stimulation of the bone marrow, not of loss through menstruation. Alkaline phosphatase levels in both boys and girls increase during puberty because of rapid bone turnover, especially during the growth spurt. Worsening of scoliosis is especially common in adolescent girls at the SMR II and III stages, during the growth spurt.

Psychologic Growth and Development of Adolescents

See Table 7–3 and Chapter 1.

REFERENCES

Behrman RE, Kliegman RM, Jenson HB: *Nelson textbook of pediatrics,* ed 16, Philadelphia, 2000, WB Saunders, Chapter 16.

Herman-Giddens ME, Slora EJ, Wasserman RC, et al: Secondary sexual characteristics and menses in young girls seen in office practice: a study from the Pediatric Research in Office Settings Network, *Pediatrics* 99(4):505–512, 1997.

McAnarney ER, Kreipe RE, Orr DP, et al, editors: *Textbook of adolescent medicine,* Philadelphia, 1992, WB Saunders, Secs. 2 and 3.

Root AW: Precocious puberty, *Pediatr Rev* 21(1):10–19, 2000.

ADOLESCENT HEALTH CARE
Overview

The leading causes of mortality (Table 7–4) and morbidity (Table 7–5) among adolescents in the United States relate to the following categories of health behavior: (1) behaviors that contribute to motor-vehicle crashes and other unintentional or intentional injuries (accounting for three fourths of all deaths, Table 7–4); (2) tobacco use; (3) alcohol and other drug use; (4) sex-

TABLE 7–3
Developmental Characteristics Related to Adolescent Health Care Needs

Task	Characteristics	Health Care Needs
10–14-Year-Olds		
Puberty	Wide variation in rapid physical changes; self-consciousness	Confidentiality; privacy
Independence	Ambivalence	Support for growing autonomy
Identity	Am I normal?; peer group	Reassurance and positive attitude
Thinking	Concrete operational; egocentric; imaginary audience; focus on present	Emphasis on immediate consequences of actions
15–17-Year-Olds		
Puberty	Females ahead of males; chronic illness may delay puberty	Emotional support for adolescents who vary from "normal"
Independence	Limit testing; noncompliance; "experimental" behaviors; dating	Consistency; limit setting
Identity	Who am I?; introspection; global issues	Nonjudgmental acceptance; gentle reality testing
Thinking	Concrete → formal operational; personal fable; experiments with ideas	Problem solving; decision making; education
18–21-Year-Olds		
Puberty	Adult appearance; slow change	Minimal needs except in chronic illness
Independence	Ambivalence about real independence, separation/individuation from family	Support
Identity	Who am I with respect to others, sexuality, education, job?	Encouragement of identity allowing maximal growth
Thinking	Formal operational; contemplation of future; introspection; commitments	Approach as adult, but recognize that adolescent still changing

TABLE 7–4
Leading Causes of Death in Adolescents

Rank	Cause	Rate (per 100,000)
1	Accidents and adverse affects	36.9
	Motor-vehicle accidents	28.3
	All other	8.6
2	Homicide and legal intervention	17.1
3	Suicide	11.6
4	Malignant neoplasms	4.5
5	Diseases of the heart	2.7
6	Congenital anomalies	1.0
7	Human immunodeficiency virus infection	0.8
All others	Pulmonary disease, pneumonia, cerebrovascular disease, etc.	12.7

From Anderson RN, Ventura SJ, Peters KD, et al: *Mon Vital Stat Rep* 46(12 Suppl 2):1–42, 1998.

TABLE 7–5
Prevalence of Common Chronic Illnesses of Children and Adolescents

Illness	Prevalence
Pulmonary	
Asthma	3–5%
Cystic fibrosis	1:2500 white, 1:17,000 black
Neuromuscular	
Cerebral palsy	2:1000
Mental retardation	3%
Seizure disorder	3:1000
Auditory-visual defects	10–30%
Traumatic paralysis	2:1000
Scoliosis	5% males, 10% females
Migraine	10%
Endocrine–Nutrition	
Diabetes mellitus	2:1000
Obesity	10–25%
Anorexia nervosa	0.5–1%
Bulimia	1% (young adolescence), 5–10% (19–20 yr)
Dysmenorrhea	10%
Acne	80%

Modified from Gortmaker S, Sappenfield W: *Pediatr Clin North Am* 31(1):3–18, 1984.

ual behaviors that contribute to unintended pregnancy and sexually transmitted diseases (STDs), including human immunodeficiency virus (HIV) infection; (5) unhealthy dietary behaviors; and (6) physical inactivity. These behaviors are frequently interrelated and often extend into adulthood.

Recent studies have shown that income, race, ethnicity, and family structure play a limited role in adolescent risk behaviors such as smoking, alcohol, violence, suicide, and sexual intercourse. Controlling for these demographic factors explains less than 10% of the variance in the adolescent risk behaviors. Differences do exist across groups, however; white youths are more likely to smoke cigarettes, drink alcohol, and attempt suicide in the younger years than are black and Hispanic youths; black adolescents are more likely to have sexual intercourse; both black and Hispanic youths are more likely than white teens to engage in violence. Although these generalizations exist, stereotyping any individual adolescent should be avoided, especially in a clinical setting.

Adolescents present many challenges to health care providers because their physical symptoms often are related to psychosocial rather than biologic disorders. Nonetheless, adolescents frequently have chronic medical illnesses (Table 7–5) and psychosocial problems. Nonadherence to medical regimens is common. Limit testing, resistance to authority figures, and requests for confidentiality can complicate clinical care. Adolescents and their families usually respond well to health care that is based on respect, with attention to the adolescent's individual developmental needs (Table 7–3).

Ideally, adolescent health care is provided in a setting where the self-conscious adolescent feels comfortable and welcome. Sufficient time and privacy should be allowed so that the adolescent and the clinician can adequately discuss sensitive topics, such as physical growth and development, medical and psychologic concerns, substance use, sexuality, and personal goals.

Interview

The successful interview of an adolescent resembles a conversation between two persons with a great many interests in common. Developmental principles are applied so that the interview of early adolescents is directed toward specific questions that concrete-thinking adolescents understand; the interview of older adolescents is directed toward open-ended questions that conceptually competent and rationalizing older adolescents understand (compared in Table 7–3, under the entry "Thinking").

Confidentiality

Confidentiality is a key element of the care of adolescents; it relates more to emerging autonomy and respect for privacy than to keeping secrets. Some issues cannot be kept confidential because of their serious adverse health consequences (e.g., suicidal ideation). Thus it is important that clinicians caring for adolescents follow certain guidelines regarding confidentiality (Table 7–6) and discuss the issue of confidentiality at the outset. As part of anticipatory guidance, clinicians can spend a few minutes alone with preadolescent patients to prepare them and their parents for increasingly private health care that will occur in adolescence.

Occasionally an adolescent insists on absolute confidentiality. The clinician's decision whether to agree to this depends on the reason for the request, the adolescent's developmental age, and whether this request is for one or several visits. Usually an

TABLE 7–6
Guidelines for Confidentiality in Adolescent Health Care

Based on principles of adolescent growth and development (Table 7–3)

Assumes a developing ability of the adolescent to take responsibility for his or her own health care that will culminate in full adult responsibility

Reflects mutual respect and trust between adolescent and health care provider

Extends to both the adolescent and the adolescent's parents (i.e., parental communication also is privileged)

Should be relative, with the scope determined by the individual situation

Should be discussed with patient and parents at the outset of adolescent health care

TABLE 7–7
Legal Rights of Minors

Age of majority (≥18 years of age in most states)

Exceptions in Which Health Care Services
Can Be Provided to a Minor*

Emergency care (e.g., life-threatening condition or condition in which a delay in treatment would significantly increase the likelihood of morbidity)

Diagnosis and treatment of sexuality-related health care

Diagnosis and treatment of drug-related health care

Emancipated minors (physically and financially independent of family; Armed Forces; married; childbirth)

Mature minors (able to comprehend the risks and benefits of evaluation and treatment)

All exceptions should be clearly documented in health record.

*Determined by individual state laws.

adolescent can be seen just once for exploration of a problem, but it should be made clear from the beginning, particularly for a younger adolescent who lives at home, that there may be a need to involve the parents.

Legal and Ethical Issues

Adolescent health care providers should know the laws of the state and the policies of the institution in which they practice. The law confers certain rights on adolescents, depending on the health condition and personal characteristics, allowing them to receive health services without parental permission (Table 7–7). As a general rule, adolescents can seek health care without parental consent for reproductive, mental, and emergency health services. In addition, emancipated adolescents and "mature minors" may be treated without parental consent; such status of the adolescent should be documented in the record. In addition to legal concerns, the physician should consider ethical considerations based in principles such as respect for autonomy, beneficence, and nonmaleficence.

Chaperons

It is often stated that a female chaperon should be present during the examination of a female by a male physician. In general, early adolescents may want a parent present, but middle adolescents and late adolescents usually prefer to be seen alone or with a chaperon of the same sex. A choice should be offered if one is available.

Well Adolescent Care

Guidelines for Adolescent Preventive Services (GAPS) and Bright Futures are recommendations for the organization and content of preventive services for individualized adolescent health supervision (Table 7–8). The focus of the visit is more on psychosocial evaluation than on physical examination. A common error is to interact with an adolescent based on his or her physical appearance; adolescents with early-developing sexual maturity are often still emotionally immature, and adolescents with chronic illness may appear younger than their chronologic age although they have achieved an advanced level of psychosocial maturity.

Early Adolescence (Ages 10–14 Years)

Rapid changes in physical appearance and behavior are the major characteristics of early adolescence, a substage of adolescence. The early adolescent has a great deal of self-consciousness and need for privacy. The history focuses on an overall appraisal of the early adolescent's physical and psychosocial health.

Middle Adolescence (Ages 15–17 Years)

Autonomy and a global sense of identity are the major characteristics of middle adolescence. The history

TABLE 7–8
Guidelines for Adolescent Health Supervision Visits

Early Adolescent (10–14 Years Old)	Middle Adolescent (15–17 Years Old)	Late Adolescent (18–21 Years Old)
Health Guidance		
Parenting concerns	Normal development review	Parents generally not interviewed unless specifically indicated
Normal development review	Discussing sexuality, drugs, and other topics	
Discussing sexuality, drugs, etc.	Healthy lifestyle role-modeling	
Healthy lifestyle role-modeling	Positive qualities, strengths of adolescent	
Positive qualities, strengths of adolescent		
Interview with Patient*		
Healthy lifestyles	Healthy lifestyles	Healthy lifestyles
Peer activities	Peer activities	Peer activities
High-risk behaviors (e.g., sexuality, drugs, smoking, violence, abuse)	High-risk behaviors (sexuality, drugs, smoking, violence, abuse)	High-risk behaviors (sexuality, drugs, smoking, violence, abuse)
Diet, fitness, exercise, body image	Diet, fitness, exercise, body image	Diet, fitness, exercise, body image
Safety (seat belt, helmet, guns)	Safety (seat belt, helmet, guns)	Safety (seat belt, helmet, guns)
Home and school	Home and school	Home and school
Self-esteem, positive qualities, and personal strengths	Self-esteem, positive qualities, and personal strengths	Self-esteem, positive qualities, and personal strengths
Physical Examination† (patient alone; chaperon may be indicated for patients requiring pelvic examination)		
Height/weight plotted on curve	Height/weight plotted on curve	Height/weight
Vision/hearing screening	Vision/hearing screening	Vision/hearing screening
Blood pressure	Blood pressure	Blood pressure
Tanner stage/external genital examination	Tanner stage/external genital examination	Tanner stage/external genital examination
Gynecomastia/breast asymmetry	Gynecomastia	Periodontal health
Scoliosis screen	Scoliosis screen	Skinfold thickness
Skinfold thickness, acne	Skinfold thickness, acne	Self-examination of breasts/testes
Self-examination of breast/testes, if mature	Self-examination of breast/testes	Pelvic examination
Pelvic examination if menstrual problem or sexually active	Pelvic examination if menstrual problem or sexually active	
Screening		
Hyperlipidemia (if family history)	Hypertension	Hyperlipidemia (once in decade)
Hypertension	Eating disorders, obesity	Hypertension
Eating disorders, obesity	Tobacco, alcohol, and drug use	Eating disorders, obesity
Tobacco, alcohol, and drug use	Sexual behavior, if sexually active	Tobacco, alcohol, and drug use
Sexual behavior, if sexually active	STDs, including HIV if high-risk	Sexual behavior; if sexually active

Adapted with permission from American Academy of Pediatrics: *Guidelines for health supervision III*, Elk Grove Village, Ill, 1997, The Academy.
Data from Green M, editor: *Bright futures: guidelines for health supervision of infants, children and adolescents*, Arlington, Va, 1994, National Center for Education in Maternal and Child Health; Elster AB, Kuznets NJ: *AMA guidelines for adolescent preventive services: recommendations and rationale*, Baltimore, 1994, Williams & Wilkins.
HIV, Human immunodeficiency virus; *Pap*, Papanicolaou; *STD*, sexually transmitted disease; *WBC*, white blood cell.
*Adolescents should be interviewed alone during talks about high-risk behaviors.
†Only three "routine" physical examinations are recommended during adolescence to allow time to address psychosocial issues.

TABLE 7–8
Guidelines for Adolescent Health Supervision Visits—cont'd

Early Adolescent (10–14 Years Old)	Middle Adolescent (15–17 Years Old)	Late Adolescent (18–21 Years Old)
Screening—cont'd		
STDs, including HIV if high-risk	Urine for WBCs (males)	STDS, including HIV if high-risk
Urine for WBCs (males)	Cervical cancer (Pap smear)	Urine for WBCs (males)
Cervical cancer (Pap smear)	Abuse (physical, sexual, emotional)	Cervical cancer (Pap smear)
Abuse (physical sexual, emotional)	Depression/suicide	Abuse (physical, sexual, emotional)
Depression/suicide	Learning problems	Depression/suicide
Learning problems	Tuberculin if indicated	Learning problems
Tuberculin if indicated		Tuberculin if indicated
Immunizations		
Check immunization status	Check immunization status	Check immunization status
Mumps, measles vaccine if none previously	Tetanus-diphtheria (Td) booster q 10 years	Td booster q 10 years
Rubella vaccine for nonimmune females if not pregnant	Mumps, measles vaccine if none previously	Mumps, measles vaccine if none previously
Hepatitis B vaccine, if not done previously	Rubella vaccine for nonimmune females if not pregnant	Rubella vaccine for nonimmune females if not pregnant
	Hepatitis B vaccine, if not done previously	Hepatitis B vaccine, if not done previously
		Meningococcal vaccine should be made available, especially for college students

HIV, Human immunodeficiency virus; *Pap,* Papanicolaou; *STD,* sexually transmitted disease; *WBC,* white blood cell.

focuses on the middle adolescent's interactions with family, school, and peers. High-risk behaviors as a result of experimentation are common. However, normal middle adolescence is not a time of "stress and storm."

Late Adolescence (Ages 18–21 Years)

Individuality and planning for the future are the major characteristics of late adolescence. The content of the visit is similar to that of the visit with the middle adolescent, but greater emphasis is placed on the late adolescent's responsibility for his or her health. Transfer of health care to a provider who cares for adults and the details of that transfer may be discussed during this visit.

Pelvic Examination

During a pelvic examination, the patient's comfort is maximized by using a padded examination table with stirrups, keeping the examination room and in-struments warm, and performing the examination in an unhurried but efficient manner. The patient is afforded control is by being allowed to choose a supine or partially sitting position, by maintaining eye contact with the examiner, by being told the importance of the examination, by being informed of all maneuvers before they are performed, by being informed of normal and abnormal findings, and by being encouraged to ask questions before, during, or after the examination.

Inspection of the genitalia includes evaluation of the pubic hair, labia majora and minora, clitoris, urethra, and hymenal ring. Bimanual palpation of the cervix, uterus, fallopian tubes, and ovaries should follow the speculum examination, because the lubricant used for bimanual evaluation interferes with samples obtained for microscopic and microbiologic evaluation. A Huffman (0.5 in × 4.5 in) or Pedersen (0.9 in × 4.5 in) speculum should be used with young virginal females; alternatively, a rectal examination can provide valuable information, since all of the midline internal genitalia are immediately anterior to the rectal wall. A nonvirginal introitus frequently admits a small- to medium-sized adult speculum. Visualization of the vaginal walls and cervical os allows for the collection of appropriate specimens for Papanicolaou (Pap) smear, culture, Gram stain, and saline wet mount.

REFERENCES

American Academy of Pediatrics: *Guidelines for health supervision: III*, Elk Grove Village, Ill, 1997, The Academy.

Anderson RN, Ventura SJ, Peters KD, et al: Births and deaths: United States, *Mon Vital Stat Rep* 46(11 Suppl 2):1–42, 1998.

Behrman RE, Kliegman RM, Jenson HB, editors: *Nelson textbook of pediatrics*, ed 16, Philadelphia, 2000, WB Saunders, Chapter 16.

Blum RW, Beuhring T, Shew ML, et al: The effects of race/ethnicity, income, and family structure on adolescent risk behaviors, *Am J Public Health* 90(12):1885–1891, 2000.

Braverman PK, Strasburger VC: Office-based adolescent health care: issues and solutions, *Adolesc Med* 8(1):1–14, 1997.

Centers for Disease Control and Prevention: CDC surveillance summaries. Youth risk behavior surveillance—United States, 1999, *MMWR* 49(SS05):1–96, 2000.

NORMAL VARIANTS OF PUBERTY
Breast Asymmetry and Masses

In normal females, one breast may develop before or more rapidly than the other, resulting in asymmetry. This can be a source of concern for the early adolescent. The patient should be reassured that the asymmetry should become less noticeable as maturation progresses. The physical examination reveals no masses or discharge, although tenderness can occur in the breast-bud stage. A true breast mass is most commonly a benign fibroadenoma or cyst; cancer is exceedingly rare at this age (Table 7–9). For imaging, ultrasonography is preferred to mammography because of the density of adolescent breast tissue.

Physiologic Leukorrhea

Endogenous estrogen production stimulates glandular proliferation of the endometrium; this often results in a vaginal discharge that usually occurs just before menarche, in SMR stage III. The discharge usually is scant, thin, mucoid, acidic, clear to milky, and neither pruritic nor foul-smelling. Characteristics other than these indicate the need for further evaluation. Physiologic leukorrhea is associated with low white blood cell count and microscopic evidence of the maturational effect of estrogen on the vaginal epithelium. Pathogens are not present in cultures. Physical examination reveals only the changes of midpuberty, without evidence of introital trauma or inflammation. Rubbing related to self-consciousness

TABLE 7–9
Etiology of Breast Masses in Adolescents
Classic or juvenile fibroadenoma (70%)
Fibrocystic disease
Breast cyst
Abscess/mastitis
Intraductal papilloma
Fat necrosis/lipoma
Cystosarcoma phyllodes (low-grade malignancy)
Adenomatous hyperplasia
Hemangioma, lymphangioma, lymphoma (rare)
Carcinoma (<1%)

or masturbation may result in mild erythema, but abrasions or tears should raise concern about sexual abuse. Unless specifically indicated, bimanual pelvic examination generally is not necessary.

Irregular Menses

In the year following menarche the menses often are irregular and anovulatory. Both the interval between periods and the duration of periods may vary as the hypothalamic-pituitary-ovarian system matures. On the average the first 12 menstrual periods are completed in 18 months. Anovulatory periods often are irregular, with prolonged heavy bleeding but without midcycle or menstrual pain. However, some adolescents ovulate with their first cycle, as indicated by the fact that pregnancy can occur before menarche. **Polycystic ovary syndrome** (PCOS) can cause irregular menses or absence of menses, in association with elevated LH levels, androgen excess, and weight gain. PCOS can usually be treated effectively with a combination of estrogen, progestin, spironolactone, and weight loss. The irregularity of early postmenarchal periods can be inconvenient, but treatment with birth control pills should be avoided unless there is some evidence of hormonal imbalance, such as in PCOS. Reassurance, education about menstrual physiology, and awaiting more regular periods usually suffice.

Gynecomastia

Breast enlargement in the male (gynecomastia) is usually a benign, self-limited condition. It is noted in 50–60% of boys during early adolescence. Gynecomastia is often idiopathic but may be noted in various conditions (Table 7–10). Typical findings include the appearance of a 1–3-cm, round, freely mobile, often tender, firm mass immediately beneath the are-

TABLE 7–10
Etiology of Gynecomastia

Idiopathic
Hypogonadism (primary or secondary)
Liver disease
Renal disease
Hyperthyroidism
Neoplasms
   Adrenal
   Ectopic human chorionic gonadotropin (hCG)
     secreting
   Testicular
Drugs
   Antiandrogens
   Antibiotics (isoniazid, ketoconazole, metronidazole)
   Antacids (H_2 blockers)
   Cancer chemotherapy (especially alkylating agents)
   Cardiovascular drugs
   Drugs of abuse
     Alcohol
     Amphetamines
     Heroin
     Marijuana
Hormones (for female sex)
Psychoactive agents (e.g., diazepam, phenothiazines,
   tricyclics)

ola during SMR stage III. Large, hard, or fixed enlargements and masses associated with any nipple discharge warrant further investigation. Reassurance that the condition is self-limited is usually the only treatment required. If the condition worsens and is associated with psychologic morbidity, it may be treated pharmacologically with bromocriptine. Surgical treatment with reduction mammoplasty can be helpful with massive hypertrophy.

Short Stature (Constitutionally Delayed Puberty)

See Chapter 17.

REFERENCES

Behrman RE, Kliegman RM, Jenson HB, editors: *Nelson textbook of pediatrics,* ed 16, Philadelphia, 2000, WB Saunders, Chapters 571, 572.

Coupey SM, editor: *Primary care of adolescent girls,* Philadelphia, 1999, Hanley & Belfus.

Templeman C, Hertweck SP: Breast disorders in the pediatric and adolescent patient, *Obstet Gynecol Clin North Am* 27(1):19-34, 2000.

MENSTRUAL DISORDERS

Lack of menstrual periods *(amenorrhea)* and irregularity of menstrual periods are among the most common complaints of early adolescents. As regular ovulatory cycles become established, pain with menstruation *(dysmenorrhea)* becomes more frequent. Abnormal uterine bleeding, sometimes called *dysfunctional uterine bleeding,* may be caused by physiologic hormonal imbalances or by pathologic conditions.

Amenorrhea

Primary amenorrhea refers to a lack of menstruation by age 16 years in the presence of breast development or by age 14 years in the absence of breast development. (Most girls have menarche within 2 years of breast development.) *Secondary amenorrhea* refers to the cessation of previously regular menstruation for more than 3 consecutive months, any time after menarche. Within the first year after menarche, such irregularity of menses is physiologic.

Amenorrhea may be a result of functional or anatomic abnormalities of the hypothalamus, pituitary gland, ovary, or uterus. It may be associated with inadequate hormonal stimulation of the endometrium, unresponsiveness of the endometrium to hormones, or obstruction of flow during endometrial shedding. The *differential diagnosis* of primary or secondary amenorrhea is broad (Tables 7–11 and 7–12). Physiologic immaturity, stress, exercise, and abnormal dietary patterns are the most common causes of amenorrhea. Pregnancy should be considered in all cases of secondary amenorrhea, even if the patient denies having had intercourse.

The history and physical examination (Tables 7–13 and 7–14) provide the most valuable information and should guide the laboratory evaluation of any abnormality of vaginal bleeding, including amenorrhea. Thus females with short stature and other stigmata of *Turner syndrome* (gonadal dysgenesis) should undergo chromosomal analysis, whereas those with signs of hypothyroidism, adrenogenital syndrome, or diabetes should be evaluated with specific tests for these diseases. If the patient with amenorrhea has normal secondary sex characteristics, a negative result on a pregnancy test, normal prolactin and thyroid levels, and no evidence of androgen excess (e.g., hirsutism or virilization) or uterine (imperforate hymen) pathology, the presence or absence of estrogen effect should be determined. If hirsutism or virilization is present, serum dihydroepiandrosterone sulfate (DHEA-S) and free and total testosterone should be measured to rule out ovarian or adrenal tumors or to prompt an evaluation for 21-α-hydroxylase deficiency.

Superficial vaginal epithelial cells representing greater than 10% of the cells on a smear obtained

Text continued on p. 268

TABLE 7-11
Differential Diagnosis of Primary Amenorrhea

Etiology	History	Breast Development	Female Genitalia	Karyotype	Follicle-Stimulating Hormone	Prolactin	Thyroid
Hypothalamic							
Physiologic delay	Positive family history of delayed puberty	Delayed	Normal	Normal (46,XX)	Low to normal	Normal	Normal
Nutritional	History of dietary restriction, severe systemic disease, or malabsorption	Delayed	Normal	Normal	Low to normal	Normal	Normal
Gonadotropin-releasing hormone (GnRH) deficiency	Anosmia (Kallmann syndrome); acquired or congenital anatomic lesions	Delayed	Normal	Normal	Low to normal	Normal	Normal
Pituitary							
Hypopituitarism	Other signs and symptoms of hypopituitarism	Variable	Normal	Normal	Low	Normal	Low to normal
Gonadal							
Chromosomally incompetent ovarian failure	Wide range of phenotypic expression of Turner syndrome	Delayed	Normal	45,XO or mosaic	High	Normal	Normal
Chromosomally competent ovarian failure	May be congenital or acquired	Delayed	Small uterus	Normal	High	Normal	Normal

Uterine

Condition							
Congenital absence of uterus (Rokitansky syndrome)	May have associated renal anomalies	Normal	Absent uterus + varying degrees of vaginal dysgenesis	Normal	Normal	Normal	Normal

Vaginal

Imperforate hymen	May have abdominal pain, pelvic "mass"	Normal	Bulging hymen	Normal	Normal	Normal	Normal

Biosynthetic/Hormone Defects

Hypothyroidism	May simulate pituitary tumor	Delayed	Normal	Normal	Low to normal	High	Low
Hyperprolactinemia	May not have galactorrhea	Normal	Normal	Normal	Low to normal	High	Normal
Hypercortisolism	Other signs and symptoms of Cushing syndrome	Normal	Normal	Normal	Low to normal	Normal	Normal
Androgen excess (polycystic ovarian disease)	Hirsutism, virilization	Minimal	Normal	Normal	LH high	Normal	Normal
Androgen resistance (testicular examination)	Male pseudohermaphroditism	Normal	Absent uterus, shallow vagina, no pubic hair	46,XY	Low to normal	Normal	Normal

LH, Luteinizing hormone.

TABLE 7–12
Differential Diagnosis of Secondary Amenorrhea

Etiology	History	Physical Examination	Galactorrhea	Pelvic Examination	Prolactin	Thyroid	Response to Progesterone Challenge	Gonadotropins
Hypothalamic								
Weight loss	Simple dieting; anorexia nervosa	Low weight, blood pressure, pulse, temperature	No	Normal	Normal	Normal	Bleeding	Low to normal
Weight gain	Overeating	Moderate to severe obesity	No	Normal	Normal	Normal	Bleeding	Low to normal
Exercise	Running >25 miles/week, ballet	Physically healthy if weight normal	No	Normal	Normal	Normal	Bleeding	Low to normal
Stress	Family, school, peer problems	Normal	No	Normal	Normal	Normal	Bleeding	Low to normal
Chronic illness	Severe systemic illness	Signs of chronic illness	No	Normal	Normal	Normal	Bleeding	Low to normal
Idiopathic	Negative	Normal	No	Normal	Normal	Normal	Bleeding	Low to normal
Medication	Phenothiazines; oral contraceptive	No distinctive physical findings	Often	Normal	Normal to high	Normal	Bleeding	Low to normal
Pituitary								
Destructive lesions	Symptoms of hypopituitarism	Signs of pituitary failure or tumor	No	Normal	Normal to high	Normal to low	No bleeding	Low

Gonadal

Disorder	History	Physical						
Ovarian failure	Radiation, surgery	Signs of estrogen deficiency	No	Normal	Normal	Normal	No bleeding	High FSH
Polycystic ovarian disease	May have oligomenorrhea	Obesity, hirsutism, and virilization	No	Enlarged ovaries	Normal	Normal	Bleeding	High LH

Uterine

Synechiae (Asherman syndrome)	Uterine curettage, endometritis	Normal	No	Normal	Normal	Normal	No bleeding	Normal

Hormonal/Metabolic

Pregnancy	Highly variable, may deny sexual intercourse	Breast engorgement, weight gain	No	Enlarged uterus; soft, cyanotic cervix	Normal	Normal	No bleeding	Low to normal
Hyperprolactinemia	Medications; may be negative	Usually normal physical examination	Often	Normal	High	High	Bleeding	Low to normal
Androgen excess	Concerns about virilization	Clitoromegaly	No	Clitoromegaly	Normal	Normal	Bleeding	Low to normal
Hypothyroidism	Symptoms of ↓ thyroid	May be normal	Often	Normal	Normal to high	Normal to high	Bleeding	Low to normal
Hypercortisolism	Symptoms of ↑ cortisol	Signs of Cushing syndrome	Often	Normal	Normal to high	Normal to high	Bleeding	Low to normal

FSH, Follicle-stimulating hormone; *LH*, luteinizing hormone.

TABLE 7–13
History and Review of Systems in Abnormal Vaginal Bleeding

History	
Bleeding	How long; how much (number of pads or tampons per day); color (bright red or brown): presence of clots or tissue; cramping; bleeding from other sites (nose, gingiva, after tooth extraction or surgery); relationship to intercourse?
Menstrual	Age of menarche; frequency, duration, amount; last menstrual period (dates of last three episodes of bleeding); dysmenorrhea, spotting, midcycle pain?
Sexual	Sexual activity; sexual abuse; masturbation with foreign objects; sexually transmitted diseases; pelvic surgery; previous pregnancies, abortions (spontaneous or terminated pregnancies), dyspareunia; sharp pain during intercourse?
Contraceptive use	What kind, how often, any used since last period; missed contraceptive pills?
Medications	All prescription or over-the-counter medications, drug abuse
Illnesses	Recent, chronic, bleeding disorders, cancers?
Family	Bleeding disorders, diethylstilbestrol (DES) exposure, thyroid disease?
Diet	Anorexia, bulimia, crash diets, diet medications?
Exercise	Amount, frequency, competition, kind?
Review of Systems	
General	Fatigue, weight loss, fever, chills, anorexia
Skin	Dry, ecchymosis, petechiae, acne
Hair	Dry, hair loss, brittle, hirsutism
Head/ENT	Visual changes, nosebleeds, gingival bleeding with flossing or brushing
Neck	Swelling or lumps, shoulder pain
Breasts	Soreness, enlargement, galactorrhea
Abdominal	Tenderness, swelling, waistband tight, pain
Genitourinary	Bleeding, dysuria, vaginal discharge, foreign body, trauma, abuse, hematuria, frequency, urgency
Gastrointestinal	Nausea, vomiting, diarrhea, rectal bleeding, mucus, cramps, tenesmus
CNS	Syncope or presyncope, headaches, fatigue
Endocrine	Weight change, nervousness, irritability, change in school performance, heat or cold intolerance

From Anderson MM, Irwin CE, Snyder DL: *Pediatr Ann* 15(10):697–707, 1986.
CNS, Central nervous system; *ENT*, ear-nose-throat.

from the lateral vaginal wall indicate the presence of estrogen, as does "ferning" of cervical mucus. Withdrawal bleeding 1–4 days after oral administration of 10 mg medroxyprogesterone, twice a day for 5 days (positive progesterone challenge), indicates estrogen priming of the endometrium and an intact hypothalamic-pituitary-ovarian axis. Withdrawal bleeding is reassuring and indicates that regular menses should begin soon. The absence of estrogen effects warrants further evaluation and determination of LH and FSH levels. In the absence of estrogen effects, low levels of LH and FSH indicate hypothalamic-pituitary pathology, such as a prolactin-secreting tumor. High gonadotropin levels indicate primary ovarian failure, such as in Turner syndrome.

Abnormal Uterine Bleeding

Normal periods are 28 ±7 days apart, measured from the first day of one to the first day of the next period. Some girls may have 45-day intermenstrual intervals soon after menarche. Flow does not usually last more than 7 days. Excessive flow may be quantified by the use of more than six pads or 10 tampons per day for more than 8 days; however, the fre-

---

TABLE 7–14
Physical Examination in the Evaluation of Abnormal Vaginal Bleeding

General Physical Examination	
Growth	Height, weight, obesity, overly thin
Vital signs	Heart rate and blood pressure changes with position, temperature
Skin	Ecchymosis, petechiae, pigmentation, pallor, sweating, capillary refill, striae, acne
Hair	Texture, amount, distribution, hirsutism, balding, low hairline
Eyes	Lid lag, proptosis, funduscopic examination (hemorrhages), visual fields
Nose/throat	Mucous membrane bleeding, petechiae, pallor
Neck	Enlarged thyroid, nodes, web neck
Breasts	Galactorrhea, Tanner stage
Cardiovascular	
Heart	Heart rate, murmurs
Pulses	Presence in extremities
Abdomen	Tenderness, masses, organomegaly, rebound
Rectal	Tone, blood, masses, fissures
Neurologic	Deep tendon reflexes, mental status, cranial nerves, visual fields
Nodes	Generalized lymphadenopathy
Pelvic Examination	
External examination	Tanner stage; male vs. female hair pattern; clitoromegaly, discharge, condyloma, lacerations, erythema
Speculum examination	
Vagina	Erythema, punctate hemorrhages, discharge; rotate speculum to look for lacerations, masses, condyloma
Cervix	Color, discharge, punctate hemorrhages, tissue, erosion, friability, condyloma, polyps, abnormal shape
Bimanual examination	Palpate vaginal wall for masses or lacerations; cervical motion tenderness; softening of the cervix or uterocervical junction; adnexal tenderness or masses; size and shape of ovaries; uterine size, shape, and position; uterine tenderness
Laboratory evaluation	Cervical cultures for gonorrhea and *Chlamydia,* cervical smear for Gram stain, vaginal smears for potassium hydroxide (yeast, whiff test), saline (clue cells, *Trichomonas*), vaginal pH, cervical cytology (Papanicolaou [Pap] smear)

From Anderson MM, Irwin CE, Snyder DL: *Pediatr Ann* 15(10):697–707, 1986.

---

quency of pad change varies greatly among women. Excessively heavy, prolonged, or frequent bleeding in the first year after menarche is often physiologic but may cause iron-deficiency anemia and, rarely, hypovolemia.

Dysfunctional uterine bleeding, one of the few conditions in adolescent health care that involves a diagnosis by exclusion, is any abnormal pattern of endometrial shedding not caused by an underlying pathologic process (Table 7–15). Anovulation occurs in 75% of cases. Without production of progesterone by the corpus luteum, unopposed estrogen produc-

tion can result in two abnormal patterns of bleeding: mild breakthrough bleeding caused by estrogen levels that are insufficient to support a proliferated endometrium, and heavy, prolonged, sometimes life-threatening menses resulting from lack of sufficient progesterone to stop menstrual flow by myometrial and vascular contractions. Once regular ovulatory cycles have continued for 1 year, irregular bleeding usually indicates an organic abnormality.

Because the diagnosis of dysfunctional uterine bleeding can be made only after underlying pathology is excluded (Table 7–16), caution must be used

TABLE 7–15
Abnormal Patterns of Menstrual Flow

Pattern	Regularity of Cycles	Interval Between Cycles	Flow		
			Amount	Duration	Timing
Amenorrhea			Absent >3 months		
Hypomenorrhea	Regular	28 ± 7 days	Decreased	Normal	Normal
Menorrhagia (hypermenorrhea)	Regular	28 ± 7 days	Increased	Normal	Normal
Metrorrhagia (spotting)	Irregular	Normal	Decreased	Decreased	Intermenstrual as well as menstrual
Menometrorrhagia	Irregular	Decreased	Increased	Increased	Variable
Oligomenorrhea	Regular	>35 days	Decreased	Decreased	Variable
Polymenorrhea	Regular	<21 days	Decreased	Decreased	Variable

in evaluating and treating this condition. A thorough history (using a menstrual calendar indicating the amount of flow and associated symptoms each day) and physical examination, including a pelvic examination, should be combined with a complete blood count and testing for pregnancy, genital infections, thyroid abnormality, and coagulation defect.

Approximately 20% of adolescents with heavy or prolonged menstrual bleeding, especially those who have reached menarche, have a coagulation disorder; an additional 10% of cases are related to other pathology. If underlying pathology is discovered, treatment should be directed at the primary disorder, as well as at the secondary menstrual dysfunction. Unpredictable, heavy, and prolonged menses may seriously impair an adolescent's ability to attend school and function socially. Thus the health care provider also must attend to these psychosocial dysfunctions.

Treatment of abnormal uterine bleeding is essential if menstrual periods are heavy. The aim is to normalize the imbalance between estrogen and progesterone. Birth control pills are effective and have a rapid onset. In rare instances of uncontrollable bleeding, hospital admission for intravenous fluids and estrogen is necessary. Uterine curettage is rarely indicated in adolescents. In the presence of a bleeding disorder (e.g., von Willebrand disease), estrogen may raise the level of factor VIII. Treatment with iron is also important for adolescents with continued excessive blood loss.

Dysmenorrhea

Dysmenorrhea refers to cramping, lower abdominal pains during the first 1–3 days of flow in a menstrual period. Painful uterine cramps are experienced by 65% of adolescent girls and are a leading cause of short-term school absenteeism. **Secondary dysmenorrhea** is pain associated with a pelvic pathologic condition, such as pelvic inflammatory disease, ectopic pregnancy, endometriosis, intrauterine device use, benign tumors, or anatomic abnormalities. **Primary dysmenorrhea** is more common and is not associated with a specific underlying structural problem. These two types of dysmenorrhea usually can be distinguished by history and physical examination (including pelvic examination), without the need for surgical or laboratory evaluation.

The *treatment* of dysmenorrhea is directed at the underlying pathology. **Endometriosis,** which is a common cause of secondary dysmenorrhea in adolescents, requires management with combined estrogen-progestin oral contraceptives, danazol (a weak synthetic male hormone), or gonadotropin-releasing hormone agonists such as nafarelin or leuprolide. Primary dysmenorrhea is associated with myometrial contractions related to local prostaglandin activity in the early phases of shedding of the endometrium. Because prostaglandin production is related to progesterone produced by the corpus luteum after ovulation, painful menstruation is associated with ovulatory cycles. Effective medical therapy is directed primarily at inhibiting the synthesis or action of prostaglandins (Table 7–17). Hormonal regulation with combined estrogen-progestin oral contraceptives can be added if these approaches are not beneficial. Failure to respond to these regimens increases the likelihood of unrecognized pelvic pathology.

TABLE 7–16
Differential Diagnosis of Abnormal Uterine Bleeding

Etiology	History	Pelvic Examination	Pregnancy Test	Coagulation Tests	Cervical Cultures
Complications of Pregnancy					
Threatened abortion	Abdominal cramps	Enlarged uterus	Positive	Normal	Negative
Ectopic pregnancy	Abdominal pain; syncope	Enlarged adnexa	Positive	Normal	Negative
Systemic Conditions					
Coagulation defects					
Secondary to liver disease	Chronic or severe acute liver disease	Normal	Negative	Abnormal	Negative
Secondary to blood dyscrasia	Leukemia	Normal	Negative	Thrombocytopenia	Negative
Primary coagulopathy	von Willebrand disease	Normal	Negative	Abnormal bleeding time	Negative
Hypothyroidism	Symptoms of ↓ thyroid; may be normal	Normal	Negative	Normal	Negative
Hypercortisolism or hypocortisolism	Symptoms of ↑ or ↓ cortisol	Normal	Negative	Normal	Negative
Medications					
Birth control pills	Low-dose estrogen; noncompliance	Normal	Negative	Normal	Negative
Aspirin	Aspirin ingestion	Normal	Negative	Abnormal bleeding time	Negative
Pelvic Lesions					
Ovarian cyst	Abdominal pain	Tender, enlarged ovary	Negative	Normal	Negative
Endometriosis	Dysmenorrhea	Tender uterus	Negative	Normal	May be + for STD
Foreign body (intra-uterine device [IUD], retained tampon)	May have forgotten to remove tampon	Signs of foreign body	Negative	Abnormal if associated with toxic shock syndrome	May be + for *Staphylococcus aureus*
Cervicitis	Sexually transmitted disease (STD) contact	Severe inflammation	Negative	Normal	May be + for STD
Trauma	External genitalia may be normal	Signs of trauma	Negative	Normal	Negative
Diethylstilbestrol (DES) exposure	Maternal DES during pregnancy	Vaginal adenosis	Negative	Normal	Negative
Tumor	Often asymptomatic	Mass	Negative	Normal	Negative
Hypothalamic					
Anovulatory cycles	Symptoms related to anovulation	Normal	Negative	Normal	Negative
Stress	Family, school, peer problems; abnormal body image	Normal	Negative	Normal	Negative

TABLE 7–17
Treatment of Primary Dysmenorrhea

Severity	Characteristics	Treatment
Mild	Mild cramps Little interference with daily activities No systemic symptoms	Ibuprofen, 400 mg PO qid *or* Naproxen sodium, 550 mg PO, then 275 mg qid; treatment most effective if initiated at least 24 hr before menses begin *or* Mefenamic acid 500 mg PO, then 250 mg qid
Moderate	Moderate cramps Interference with daily activities No systemic symptoms	Treatment of mild dysmenorrhea *and* Cyclic combination oral contraceptive pills
Severe	Severe cramps Restriction of activities for several days each month Systemic symptoms	Treatment for moderate dysmenorrhea *and* Reevaluation for organic pathology, such as benign tumors, endometriosis, or anatomic abnormalities

REFERENCES

Acquavella AP, Braverman P: Adolescent gynecology in the office setting, *Pediatr Clin North Am* 46(3):489–503, 1999.

Behrman RE, Kliegman RM, Jenson HB, editors: *Nelson textbook of pediatrics*, ed 16, Philadelphia, 2000, WB Saunders, Chapter 116.

Emans SJH, Laufer MR, Goldstein DP: *Pediatrics and adolescent gynecology*, ed 4, Philadelphia, 1998, Lippincott, Williams & Wilkins.

Minjarez DA, Bradshaw KD: Abnormal uterine bleeding in adolescents, *Obstet Gynecol Clin North Am* 27(1):63–78, 2000.

Mitan LAP, Slap GB: Adolescent menstrual disorders: update, *Med Clin North Am* 84(4):851–868, 2000.

Sanfilippo JS: *Pediatric and adolescent gynecology*, ed 2, Philadelphia, 2001, WB Saunders.

PREGNANCY

Since peak rates were reached in the early 1990s in the United States, the teenage pregnancy rates, birth rates, and abortion rates have fallen 17%, 12%, and 31%, respectively, resulting in 97 pregnancies, 54 births, and 29 abortions per 1000 females less than 20 years of age. It is estimated that roughly one fourth of the decline in teenage pregnancy resulted from increased abstinence and three fourths from decreased pregnancy rates in sexually active individuals who used effective birth control. Approximately 40% of 15-year-olds and 66% of 17-year-olds in America have had sexual intercourse, with black males reporting the highest rates and white females reporting the lowest rates in any age group. Early initiation of coitus in females is linked to forced sexual activity, often incestuous. Most adolescent pregnancies occur out of wedlock; about one third end in abortion. Adolescent pregnancy is associated with premature birth, increased postneonatal mortality, child abuse, subsequent maternal unemployment, and poor maternal educational achievement. Most adolescents should not be considered high biologic risks. With appropriate prenatal care, good nutrition, and social support and the absence of sexually transmitted diseases (STDs), the pregnant adolescent has the same chance of delivering a healthy full-term infant as does an adult woman of similar sociodemographic background.

Diagnosis

Adolescent pregnancy is associated with secondary amenorrhea. Loss of menstrual periods in adolescents should be presumed to be the result of pregnancy until proven otherwise because frequently, pregnant adolescents delay seeking a diagnosis until several periods have been missed. In addition, nonvirginal girls initially may deny having had intercourse. However, serious consequences may result from a delayed diagnosis. Pregnant girls in early adolescence often are seen with other symptoms, such as vomiting, vague pains, or deteriorating behavior. They may report normal periods. Pregnancy during early adolescence may result from rape or incest, and early-adolescent patients are more likely to deny ever having had intercourse than older adolescents. Because of the varied presentations of adolescent pregnancy, a thorough menstrual history should be obtained in all menstruating girls. Sensitive urine tests facilitate diagnosis approximately 7–10 days after conception.

Decision About Pregnancy

If pregnancy is confirmed, dating of the gestation should be done immediately. Most clinicians will not consider abortion after 20–24 weeks of gestation. Pregnancy options are continuation of the pregnancy (the patient either keeps the infant or surrenders it for adoption) and termination of the pregnancy. During early adolescence, the clinician should urge the girl to involve the family in the decision because the adolescent may not be mature enough to make the decision alone.

Continuation of the Pregnancy

Adolescents who desire to carry their pregnancies to term require early, consistent, and comprehensive prenatal care by professionals. Although fewer than 5% of adolescents who deliver decide to have their babies adopted, this option should be discussed. Pregnancy is the most common cause of dropping out of school for girls. Special attention should be given to keeping the adolescent in school, both during and after pregnancy.

Termination

If a pregnant adolescent chooses to terminate her pregnancy, she should be referred immediately to a setting in which abortion services are rendered. The choice of an abortion procedure depends on the gestational age of the fetus. The procedures include menstrual extraction, suction curettage, and intra-amniotic instillation of hypertonic saline or prostaglandin. Medical termination with oral mifepristone (RU-486) in combination with misoprostol is still being studied in the United States and appears to a safe and effective form of abortion, although few adolescents have been included in the clinical trials. Psychosocial support should be available for adolescents who choose abortion.

Prevention of Pregnancy

Sexual activity often is initiated without birth control. For the young person who initiates coitus, knowledge about and use of contraception is critical. Because unintended, unwanted pregnancy can be associated with significant psychosocial morbidity for the adolescent mother, the adolescent father, and the child, prevention should be a primary goal. Reliable methods are discussed in the following sections and summarized in Table 7–18.

Abstinence

Abstaining from sexual intercourse remains the most commonly used and most effective adolescent birth-control method. A degree of self-control, self-assuredness, and self-esteem is necessary; unfortunately, these qualities are not found in all adolescents. For those who choose to be sexually active, some form of birth control should be offered because there is a 70% chance that a regularly sexually active adolescent not using birth control will become pregnant within a year.

Birth-Control Pills

Birth-control pills are extremely effective if taken regularly. The combined estrogen-progesterone pill prevents the LH surge, thus inhibiting ovulation. Contraindications are listed in Table 7–18. Following a detailed history and physical examination, birth-control pills can be started on the first Sunday after the patient's next menstrual period. Condoms should be used both as a backup method and to prevent STDs. Pills containing 30–35 µg of ethinyl estradiol (or the equivalent) and progestin in packs of 28 pills are prescribed first.

Common side effects are nausea, breast tenderness, fluid retention, and breakthrough bleeding, especially if pills are missed. Some adolescents discontinue using the pill because they attribute normal weight gain to the contraceptive. If bleeding occurs in the early part of the cycle, it may be necessary to prescribe pills with increased estrogenic activity. If breakthrough bleeding occurs late in the cycle, a pill with more progestational activity can be prescribed. Before any change in pills, however, the physician should ask, "How often do you forget to take your pills?" If the adolescent has forgotten to take the pill for 1 day, two pills may be taken on the subsequent day. If 2 days were missed, two pills may be taken on the 2 subsequent days. If 2 or more days are missed, the adolescent should use another form of birth control for the rest of the current cycle and the next cycle, while resuming regular pill use.

Emergency (Postcoital) Contraception

Emergency postcoital contraception may be effective (2–3% failure rate) if used within 72 hours of intercourse. *Treatment* consists of 100 µg ethinyl estradiol and 1 mg norgestrel (e.g., two Ovral tablets) administered twice, 12 hours apart (a total of four pills), or use of an equivalent contraceptive. Treatment with progestin only (0.75 mg levonorgestrel ["Plan B"], also administered twice, 12 hours apart) is reported to have greater effectiveness and fewer side effects (e.g., nausea) and may even be effective beyond 72 hours. Regardless of which pills are used, they should be taken as soon as possible after unprotected intercourse.

Condoms and Foam

When the condom is used with spermicidal foam in a conscientious manner, its effectiveness as a means of birth control can approach that of oral contraceptives,

TABLE 7-18
Birth Control Methods for Adolescents

Method	Advantages	Product	Contraindications	Pregnancy Rate	Side Effects/Problems
Birth Control Pills	Used properly, optimum protection ↓ Dysmenorrhea ↓ Risk of fibrocystic breast disease, cystic ovarian disease ↓ Risk of pelvic inflammatory disease ↓ Risk of ovarian, endometrial cancer	Combined birth control pills: 30–35 μg of ethinyl estradiol or its equivalent (50 μg of mestranol and a progestin) Mini-pills: progestin only	*Absolute:* Pregnancy Active liver disease with abnormal liver function tests Thrombophlebitis/ thrombotic disease Undiagnosed uterine bleeding Breast, uterine cancer Congenital hyperlipidemia *Relative:* Hypertension Migraine headache Sickle cell disease Active gallbladder disease or mononucleosis	~1/100 women-years	*Common:* Noncompliance Nausea Weight gain Breast tenderness Fluid retention Breakthrough bleeding Postpill amenorrhea Acne No protection against AIDS *Uncommon, but serious and rare in adolescence:* Thromboembolic phenomena Cardiovascular sequelae (stroke, hypertension)
Hormonal Injections/Implants Medroxyprogesterone (Depo-Provera)	Compliance Effectiveness	150 mg IM q 3 mo	Breast tumors?	~0.2–0.6/ 100 women-years	Menstrual irregularity Amenorrhea IM injection

Method	Advantages (Compliance/Effectiveness)	Description	Contraindications	Failure rate	Disadvantages
Levonorgestrel (Norplant)	Compliance Effectiveness	Subcutaneous implants	Obesity	~0.4–0.6/100 women-years	Menstrual irregularity Amenorrhea, weight gain Minor surgery to place and to remove
Barrier Methods Condoms	Inexpensive, few side effects No prescription needed Male method Protection against sexually transmitted diseases (STDs), including AIDS (especially latex condoms)	Condom (used with vaginal foam or with spermicidal lubricant)	Inability of adolescent to plan ahead and use method effectively	~2–10/100 women-years	Interruption of coitus Proper use Motivation Allergy to rubber (latex) in condom Only water-based lubricants
Diaphragm	Safe and effective Cream, jelly available without prescription Protection against STDs Use only when needed	Arcing, coil, flat spring diaphragm fitted by health professional— used with contraceptive cream or jelly	Inability of adolescent to plan ahead and use method properly	~1.9–2.3/100 women-years	Preparation for coitus Proper use and motivation Toxic shock syndrome "Messiness" Recurrent cystitis
Intrauterine device (IUD)	Compliance not necessary Effectiveness	Progesterone- or copper-impregnated device placed by physician in uterine cavity	Multiple sexual partners History of pelvic inflammatory disease or infection Uterine abnormalities Pregnancy	~2/100 women-years	*High incidence of:* Pelvic inflammatory disease among nulliparous women Ectopic pregnancies Extrusion Heavy bleeding

Data from Greydanus DE, McAnarney Er: *Pediatrics* 65:1-2, 1980; *Med Lett* 34:111, 1992; *N Engl J Med* 328:1543, 1993; and Eman SJH, Goldstein DP: *Pediatric and adolescent gynecology*, ed 3, Boston, 1990, Little, Brown.
AIDS, Acquired immunodeficiency syndrome.

especially for adolescents who have intercourse infrequently. Advantages of this method are its availability without a prescription and the prevention of STDs, particularly HIV infections, if latex condoms are used regularly.

Hormonal Injections and Implants

Intramuscular injection of 150 mg of medroxyprogesterone acetate (Depo-Provera) every 3 months is an effective form of birth control. Subdermal implantation of capsules containing levonorgestrel (Norplant) provides effective contraception for adolescents for up to 5 years or until removal. These forms of pregnancy prevention offer the advantage of not requiring use at each sexual encounter, minimizing problems of noncompliance. The main side effects are irregular menses, amenorrhea, and decreased bone density (see Table 7–18).

Coitus Interruptus

Withdrawal is a common method of birth control used by sexually active adolescents, but it is ineffective because sperm often are released into the vagina before ejaculation and because withdrawal of the penis occurs after ejaculation.

Rhythm Method (Periodic Coital Abstinence)

Few data support the use of the rhythm method in adolescents, whose irregular menses and common misunderstanding of the timing of ovulation may not allow its optimal use.

Oral and Anal Sex

Some adolescents engage in oral or anal sex because they believe that it eliminates the need for contraception. In addition, many do not consider this activity to mean "having sex." Condoms are generally not used during oral or anal sex, but the risk of acquiring an STD is still present. Therefore, heterosexual adolescents who deny being sexually active should be asked specifically about nonvaginal forms of sexual activity, and those who engage in oral and anal sex require STD and HIV counseling and screening.

REFERENCES

Behrman RE, Kliegman RM, Jenson HB, editors: *Nelson textbook of pediatrics*, ed 16, Philadelphia, 2000, WB Saunders, Chapters 117, 118.
Hewitt G, Cromer B: Update on adolescent contraception, *Obstet Gynecol Clin North Am* 27(1):143–162, 2000.
The Emergency Contraception Website, http://ec.princeton.edu/.

SEXUALLY TRANSMITTED DISEASES

Adolescents have one of the highest rates of STDs. Compared with adults, sexually active adolescents are more likely to come into contact with an infected sexual partner. They are less likely to receive health care when an STD develops, more likely to believe that they cannot contract an STD, and less likely to be compliant with treatment once an STD is discovered. In addition, biologic factors may make adolescents more susceptible to certain STDs, such as *Chlamydia trachomatis*.

Although HIV infection is not discussed in this chapter, it is important to keep in mind that HIV acquisition is associated with behaviors in which other STDs are acquired. The presence of any STD increases the risk of HIV infection; HIV testing should be offered to any adolescent who has an STD.

STDs are associated with significant biologic and psychologic morbidity. Early diagnosis and treatment are important for preventing medical complications and infertility. Primary prevention of STDs should be a goal for all providers of health care for adolescents.

Differential Diagnosis

Numerous pathogens are capable of being sexually transmitted, often asymptomatically. However, the number of clinical presentations is limited (Tables 7–19 through 7–22). Genital ulcers occur with both syphilis and herpes simplex type 2. External and mucosal genital warts are caused by human papillomavirus. Vaginal discharge can be noted in infections with *Trichomonas vaginalis* and *Gardnerella vaginalis*. Urethritis in the male and cervicitis or pelvic inflammatory disease in the female can result from infection with *Neisseria gonorrhoeae*, *Chlamydia trachomatis*, or both.

Syphilis

Syphilis is caused by the spirochete *Treponema pallidum*. Infection progresses through several clinical stages if left untreated. Primary syphilis is associated with a painless genital ulcer. Secondary syphilis may occur a few weeks to months later, manifesting as disseminated illness, including fever, malaise, headache, adenopathy, body rash, and mucosal lesions. Tertiary syphilis involves the cardiovascular, neurologic, and musculoskeletal systems. Diagnosis is based on serologic testing. Routine screening tests used are the rapid plasma reagin test and the Venereal Disease Research Laboratory test; respective titers are followed after treatment.

The treatment of choice for syphilis is administration of penicillin. Doxycycline and tetracycline are alternative treatments for patients who have a penicillin allergy.

Herpes Infection

Primary genital *herpes simplex type 2* and occasionally type 1 often are associated with headache, fever, malaise, myalgia, painful genital lesions, regional lymphadenopathy, discharge, and dysuria. Some primary and many secondary lesions are asymptomatic (Table 7–19). The multiple vesicles are red and painful. Secondary, recurrent, or reactivation eruptions are not as dramatic. Viral cultures are positive in 24 hours, but an immediate diagnosis can be made with a Tzanck smear showing multinucleated giant cells. The Pap smear also demonstrates these cells. Latency develops as the virus becomes dormant in the sacral nerve ganglion. In primary herpes simplex infection, viral shedding lasts 10–14

TABLE 7–19
Features of Sexually Transmitted Diseases Characterized by Genital Ulcers in Adolescents

	Chancroid	Genital Herpes	Syphilis	Granuloma Inguinale (Donovanosis)
Agent	*Haemophilus ducreyi*	Herpes simplex virus (HSV) 1, 2	*Treponema pallidum*	*Calymmatobacterium granulomatis*
Incubation (days)	3–10	4–14	10–90	8–80
Systemic findings	None	Headache, fever, malaise, myalgia in ⅓ of cases	Fever, rash, malaise, anorexia, arthralgia, adenopathy	Local spread only
Inguinal lymphadenopathy	Early, rapid, tender, and unilateral Suppuration likely	Early, bilateral, tender, no suppuration	Late, bilateral, nontender, no suppuration	Lymphatic obstruction Pseudoadenopathy
Primary lesion	Papule to pustule	Vesicle	Papule	Papule
Ulcer characteristics				
Number	<3	Multiple	1 or more	1 or more, may coalesce
Edges	Ragged, undermined	Reddened, ragged	Distinct	Rolled, distinct
Depth	Deep	Shallow	Shallow	Raised
Base	Necrotic	Red, smooth	Red, smooth	Beefy red, clean
Secretion	Pus, blood	Serous	Serous	None
Induration	None	None	Firm	Firm
Pain	Often	Usual	None	None
Diagnosis				
Serology	None	Complement fixation Ab rise only in 1° HSV; enzyme immunoassay	VDRL, ART, RPR, FTA-ABS, MHTP, TPI	None
Isolation	Aspirate of node, swab of ulcer on selective medium	Viral culture + in 48 hr	No in vitro test; rabbit inoculation	None
Microscopic	Gram-negative pleomorphic rods	Pap smear; Tzanck smear; direct FA staining	Darkfield examination	Staining of ulcer biopsy material for "Donovan" bodies (Wright or Giemsa)

From Abramowicz M, editor: *Med Lett* 37:117, 1995; Centers for Disease Control and Prevention: *MMWR* 42(RR-14):1–102, 1993.
ART, Automated reagin test; *FA,* fluorescent antibody; *FTA-ABS,* fluorescent treponemal antibody absorption; *MHTP,* microhemagglutination antibodies to *Treponema pallidum; Pap,* Papanicolaou; *RPR,* rapid plasma reagin; *TMP/SMX,* trimethoprim/sulfamethoxazole; *TPI, Treponema pallidum* immobilization test; *VDRL,* Venereal Disease Research Laboratory.
*Contraindicated in pregnancy.

Continued

TABLE 7–19
Features of Sexually Transmitted Diseases Characterized by Genital Ulcers in Adolescents—cont'd

	Chancroid	Genital Herpes	Syphilis	Granuloma Inguinale (Donovanosis)
Treatment (Treat Sexual Partners)	Aspirate fluctuant nodes Incision and drainage of buboes >5 cm Erythromycin 500 mg PO qid × 7 days *or* Ceftriaxone 250 mg IM × 1 dose *or* Azithromycin 1 g PO × 1 dose Ciprofloxacin* 500 mg PO bid × 3 days (alternative)	Soaks to keep lesions clean and dry; no occlusive ointments Avoid contacting lesions: use hand washing, gloves, condoms Acyclovir 400 mg PO tid × 5 days If proctitis, 800 mg PO tid × 7–10 days	*Early:* Benzathine penicillin G, 2.4 million U IM × 1 *or* Doxycycline 100 mg PO bid × 14 days Repeat VDRL *Late:* (>1 yr duration) Benzathine penicillin G, 2.4 million U IM q7d × 3 *or* Doxycycline 100 mg PO bid × 4 weeks Avoid contact with lesions	Doxycycline 100 mg PO bid × 1–3 weeks *or* TMP/SMX 1 DS PO bid × 14 days

From Abramowicz M, editor: *Med Lett* 37:117, 1995; Centers for Disease Control and Prevention: *MMWR* 42(RR-14):1–102, 1993.
ART, Automated reagin test; *FA,* fluorescent antibody; *FTA-ABS,* fluorescent treponemal antibody absorption; *MHTP,* microhemagglutination antibodies to *Treponema pallidum; Pap,* Papanicolaou; *RPR,* rapid plasma reagin; *TMP/SMX,* trimethoprim/sulfamethoxazole; *TPI, Treponema pallidum* immobilization test; *VDRL,* Venereal Disease Research Laboratory.
*Contraindicated in pregnancy.

days and ulcer healing occurs in 16–20 days. In recurrent disease, often with several episodes annually, virus is shed for less than 7 days and vesicles resolve in 8–10 days. The time of healing is 8–10 days. Many patients experience 5–8 recurrences per year.

Oral acyclovir is effective in reducing the severity and duration of symptoms in primary cases and may reduce recurrences. Local hygiene and sitz baths may relieve some discomfort. Education of patients to use condoms and to avoid having sex with anyone who has genital ulcers can help prevent the spread of this disease.

Genital Warts

Genital warts can occur on the squamous epithelium or mucous membranes of the genital and perineal structures of both females and males (Table 7–20). The warts are usually multiple, firm, gray to pink excrescences. They can become tender if macerated or secondarily infected. On cornified skin, patient-applied therapies such as podofilox solution or gel or imiquimod cream can be used. Provider-applied therapies include cryotherapy with liquid nitrogen, cryoprobe, or topical podophyllin, all of which can be applied until the lesions regress. Warts on mucous membranes that are unresponsive to topical treatment or that occur during pregnancy can be treated with cryosurgery, laser ablation excision, or electrodesiccation, but not with topical medications. Recurrences after treatment are common. Human papillomavirus infection may be the most common STD. It is most commonly asymptomatic and has been associated with carcinoma of the cervix.

Trichomoniasis

Trichomoniasis is often associated with other STDs, such as gonorrhea and chlamydial infection (Table 7–21). Infected females have vaginitis and are more likely to be symptomatic than infected males. A thin, frothy vaginal discharge and cervical "strawberry hemorrhages" are characteristic of *Trichomonas* infection. Diagnosis is based on visualization of motile, flagellated protozoans in the urine or in a saline wet mount. Single-dose treatment of both sexual partners with 2 g of metronidazole is effective.

TABLE 7–20
Features of Sexually Transmitted Diseases Characterized by Nonulcerative External Genital Symptoms in Adolescents

	Genital Warts	Vulvovaginal Candidiasis	Pediculosis Pubis (Crabs)
Agent	Human papillomavirus	*Candida albicans*	*Phthirus pubis*
Incubation (days)	30–90	Uncommon sexual transmission	5–10
Presenting complaints	Genital warts are seen or felt	Vulvar itching, discharge	Pubic itching, lice may be seen; sexual partner has "crabs"
Signs	Firm, gray to pink, single or multiple, fimbriated, painless excrescences on vulva, introitus, vagina, cervix, perineum, anus	Inflammation of vulva, with thick, white, "cottage cheese" discharge, pH <5 Friable mucosa that easily bleeds	Eggs (nits) at base of pubic hairs, lice may be visible Excoriated, red skin secondary to infection
Clinical associations	Cervical neoplasia, dysplasia	BCPs, diabetes, antibiotics can lead to overgrowth	
Diagnosis	Clinical appearance; most infections asymptomatic; acetowhite changes on colposcopy Enlarged cells with perinuclear halo and hyperchromatic nuclei	KOH (10%): pseudohyphae Gram stain: gram (+) pseudohyphae Nickerson or Sabouraud medium for culture	History and clinical appearance
Treatment (may need to treat sexual partner)	Cryotherapy with liquid nitrogen or cryoprobe Podofilox 0.5% solution or gel applied tid × 3 days or imiquimod 5% cream applied qhs, 3 times/week for up to 16 weeks Electrodesiccation; electrocauterization; laser; loop electrosurgical excision for internal, massive, or unresponsive warts Intralesional alpha-interferon	Fluconazole 150 mg PO × 1 dose *or* Miconazole or clotrimazole cream intravaginally hs × 3–7 days Lowest dose estrogen BCPs, glucose control, stop systemic antibiotics if possible	5% permethrin or 1% pyrethrin *or* Pyrethrin/piperonyl shampoo, or lotion May need to repeat

Modified from Abramowicz M, editor: *Med Lett* 37:117, 1995; Centers for Disease Control and Prevention: *MMWR* 42(RR-14):1–102, 1993.
BCP, Birth control pill; *KOH,* potassium hydroxide.

Nonspecific Bacterial Vaginosis

Gardnerella vaginalis is not necessarily sexually transmitted, although there is evidence that sexually active women are more likely to carry the organism than women who are not sexually active. In postpubertal females who have a thin, gray, foul-smelling vaginal discharge and mild vaginitis, *G. vaginalis* often is found on culture of the discharge (Table 7–21).

In addition to *G. vaginalis,* anaerobic bacteria such as *Bacteroides, Mobiluncus,* and *Peptostreptococcus* are important in the pathogenesis. The pH of the discharge is greater than 4.5, and on microscopic examination the squamous epithelial cells are studded with rod-shaped organisms (clue cells). With the addition of potassium hydroxide (KOH) to the discharge, a characteristic fishy odor is evident because of the re-

TABLE 7–21
Features of Syndromes with Vaginal Symptoms in Adolescents

	Physiologic Leukorrhea (Normal)	Trichomoniasis	Nonspecific Bacterial Vaginosis (*Gardnerella vaginalis*–Associated Vaginitis)
Agent	Normal flora	*Trichomonas vaginalis*	*Gardnerella vaginalis* and anaerobes
Incubation (days)	—	3–28	Not necessarily sexually transmitted
Predominant Symptoms			
Itching	None	Mild to moderate	None to mild
Discharge	Minimal	Moderate to severe	Mild to moderate
Pain	None	Mild	Uncommon
Discharge			
Amount	Small	Profuse	Moderate
Color	Clear, milky	Yellow-green or gray	Gray
Consistency	Flocculent	Frothy	Homogeneous
Viscosity	Thin	Thin	Thin
Foul odor	None	None	Yes
Odor c̄/KOH	None	Possible	Characteristic fish odor (amine)
pH	<4.5	>5.0	>4.5
Vulvar			
Inflammation	None	Common	Uncommon
Vaginal			
Inflammation	None	Usual	None to mild
Discharge	Nonadherent	Nonadherent	Adherent, white to grey
Tenderness	None	Common	Minimal
Cervical	Normal	"Strawberry" hemorrhages	Normal
Bimanual Exam	Normal	Normal	Normal
Microscopic Findings			
Saline drop	Squamous and few white blood cells (WBCs)	Motile flagellates, slightly larger than WBCs, and WBCs	Squamous cells studded with bacteria ("clue cells") and WBCs
Gram stain	Gram-positive and -negative rods and cocci	*Trichomonas* killed	Predominance of gram-negative rods
Culture	Mixed flora with *Lactobacillus* predominant	Culture generally not indicated; antigen detection and antibody tests available	*Gardnerella vaginalis, Mobiluncus* anaerobes
Treatment	Reassurance	Metronidazole 2 g PO × 1 dose Avoid alcohol for 24 hr Treat sexual partner Clotrimazole 100 mg intra-vaginal at night × 7 days	*Intravaginal:* Metronidazole gel 0.75% bid × 5 days, *or* Clindamycin 2% cream hs × 7 days *Oral:* Metronidazole 2 g × 1 *or* Clindamycin 300 mg b.i.d. × 7 days Treat sexual partner only if recurrent

Modified from Abramowicz M, editor: *Med Lett* 37:117, 1995; Centers for Disease Control and Prevention: *MMWR* 42(RR-14):1–102, 1993.

lease of aromatic amines (referred to as the "whiff test"). The clinical significance of this nonspecific bacterial vaginosis is unclear, but treatment with intravaginal or oral metronidazole or clindamycin is usually effective.

Gonorrhea

Gonorrhea is one of the most commonly reported STDs among adolescents. The most rapid rise in incidence is seen in the 15–19-year-old age group, especially among girls. The gram-negative diplococcus gains entry via the urethra, periurethral Skene glands, labial Bartholin glands, cervix, anus, pharynx, or conjunctiva. Purulent extension to the endometrium, fallopian tubes, and peritoneum is called **pelvic inflammatory disease (PID). Fitz-Hugh-Curtis syndrome,** a complication of PID, is inflammation of the capsule of the liver.

The differential diagnosis of PID includes pyelonephritis or cystitis, ectopic pregnancy, ovarian torsion, appendicitis, and mesenteric adenitis. Tuboovarian abscess may complicate PID. Pelvic ultrasonography is the imaging study of choice for determining the presence of these other diagnoses.

In males the urethra, epididymis, and prostate can be affected. Dissemination to the joints, skin, meninges, and endocardium can occur via the hematogenous route.

A single 400-mg dose of cefixime can be used to treat uncomplicated gonorrhea infection. Other oral single-dose treatment options are ciprofloxacin 500 mg or ofloxacin 400 mg plus azithromycin 1 g. Doxycycline 100 mg is another oral therapy to be used BID for 7 days. A single dose of ceftriaxone 125 mg as an intramuscular (IM) injection is another treatment option that is often used for outpatient treatment of gonorrheal PID.

Chlamydia

At least 30% of patients with gonococcal cervicitis, urethritis, proctitis, or epididymitis have a concomitant infection with *Chlamydia trachomatis*. Serovar L1–3 produces lymphogranuloma venereum, whereas serovars B and D–K are associated with cervicitis and urethritis. *Chlamydia* is the most frequently diagnosed bacterial STD in adolescents. It is diagnosed with a 5:1 female-to-male ratio (Tables 7–19 and 7–22). *Chlamydia* accounts for most cases of non-

---

TABLE 7–22

Features of Syndromes Characterized by Mucopurulent Cervicitis, Urethritis, or Pelvic Inflammatory Disease

	Gonorrhea	Chlamydia
Agent	*Neisseria gonorrhoeae*	*Chlamydia trachomatis*
Incubation (Days)	3–14	5–12
Possible Presentations	The following possible presentations apply to both gonorrhea and chlamydiosis:	
	Female	*Male Partner*
	Asymptomatic	Asymptomatic
	Urethritis	Urethritis
	Skenitis/bartholinitis	Epididymo-orchitis
	Pelvic inflammatory disease	Proctitis
		Pharyngitis
	Anorectal/pharyngeal	
	Disseminated (arthritis, dermatitis, endocarditis, meningitis)	
Typical Findings in Mucopurulent Cervicitis or Urethritis	Cervical erythema, friability, ectopy, with thick, creamy discharge (penile discharge in males)	Cervical erythema, friability, ectopy, with thick creamy discharge (penile discharge in males)
	Mucopus >10 polymorphonuclear cells (PMNs) per high-power field (hpf)	Mucopus >10 PMNs/hpf
	Gram-negative intracellular diplococci	May coexist with gonorrhea
	Mild cervical tenderness	Mild cervical tenderness

Modified from Abramowicz M, editor: *Med Lett* 37:117, 1995; Centers for Disease Control and Prevention: *MMWR* 42(RR-14):1–102, 1993.

Continued

TABLE 7–22
Features of Syndromes Characterized by Mucopurulent Cervicitis, Urethritis, or Pelvic Inflammatory Disease—cont'd

	Gonorrhea	Chlamydia
Typical Findings in PID		Onset day 3–10 of menstrual period
		Lower abdominal pain (95%)
		Adnexal tenderness, mass (95%)
		Pain on cervical motion (95%)
		Fever (35%)
		Mucopurulent cervical discharge (variable)
		Menstrual irregularities (variable)
		Nausea, vomiting (variable)
		Weakness, syncope, dizziness (variable)
		Perihepatitis (5%) (may be seen without PID)
		Laparoscopy: Definitive diagnosis = salpingitis
		Pelvic ultrasound: Thickened adnexal structures
		↑ Sedimentation rate (65%)
		↑ WBC count (45%)
Important Differential Diagnoses for PID		Ectopic pregnancy
		Ovarian cyst (torsion, rupture)
		Septic abortion
		Urinary tract infection
		Appendicitis
		Mesenteric adenitis
		Inflammatory bowel disease
Laboratory Studies	Gram stain in cervicitis: 60% sensitivity, 95% specificity; diagnostic in males	Tissue culture
	Thayer-Martin selective medium	Antigen detection
	Antigen detection tests (LCR amplification)	(1) Fluorescent antibody
		(2) Enzyme-linked immunoassay
		(3) DNA probe
		(4) Amplification with PCR, TMA, or LCR
Treatment		
Uncomplicated cervicitis, urethritis, pharyngitis, proctitis	Ceftriaxone 125 mg IM × 1 dose *or* Cefixime 400 mg PO × 1 *plus* Doxycycline 100 mg PO bid × 7 days for *Chlamydia*	Doxycycline 100 mg PO bid × 7 days *or* Erythromycin 500 mg PO qid × 7 days *or* Azithromycin 1 g PO × 1 dose
PID		
Outpatient		Ceftriaxone, 250 mg IM × 1 dose *or* Cefoxitin, 2 g IM × 1, with probenecid, 1 g PO *plus* Doxycycline, 100 mg PO bid × 14 days

Modified from Abramowicz M, editor: *Med Lett* 37:117, 1995; Centers for Disease Control and Prevention: *MMWR* 42(RR-14):1–102, 1993.
LCR, Ligase chain reaction; *PCR*, polymerase chain reaction; *TMA*, transcription-mediated amplification; *WBC*, white blood cell.

TABLE 7–22
Features of Syndromes Characterized by Mucopurulent Cervicitis, Urethritis, or Pelvic Inflammatory Disease—cont'd

Gonorrhea	Chlamydia
PID—cont'd	
Inpatient	Cefoxitin 2 g IV q6h
	or
	Cefotetan 2 g IV q12h
	plus
	Doxycycline 100 mg IV q12h until improved
	followed by
	Doxycycline 100 mg PO bid, to complete 14 days of treatment
	Alternative (especially if anaerobic infection likely): clindamycin, 900 mg IV q8h
	plus
	Gentamicin 2 mg/kg IV × 1 dose
	followed by
	Gentamicin 1.5 mg/kg IV q8h until improved
	followed by
	Doxycycline 100 mg PO bid, to complete 14 days of treatment
Disseminated gonococcal infection	Ceftriaxone 1 g IV q24h until asymptomatic × 48 hr, then complete 1 wk of therapy with cefuroxime 0.5 g bid or amoxicillin 0.5 g tid with clavulanic acid
	Cefoxitin 1 g IV q8h
	Cefotaxime 1 g IV q8h

gonococcal mucopurulent cervicitis and urethritis. It is associated with severe sequlae, such as female infertility, PID, and **Reiter syndrome**. Reiter syndrome is associated with human leukocyte antigen HLA B27. The syndrome has several clinical manifestations: conjunctivitis, uveitis, urethritis, buccal ulceration, peripheral arthritis, sacroiliitis, and keratoderma blennorrhagicum.

Diagnosis of *Chlamydia* by culture, direct immunofluorescent antibody (enzyme-linked immunoassay), and radioimmunoassay is available. Newer, less invasive methods based on DNA amplification are also available. Ligase chain reaction and polymerase chain reaction amplification can be used on cervical, urethral, and first-voided urine specimens.

A single oral dose of azithromycin 1 g is effective therapy for uncomplicated *Chlamydia* infection. This can be combined with a single oral dose of cefixime 400 mg to treat concomitant gonorrhea infection. Erythromycin base 500 mg qid for 7 days or erythromycin ethylsuccinate 800 mg qid for 7 days is also effective but frequently causes gastric upset, resulting in noncompliance. Doxycycline 100 mg bid for 7 days is another treatment option but is teratogenic and should not be used in pregnant patients. Ofloxacin 300 mg bid for 7 days may also be used.

Pelvic Inflammatory Disease

Outpatient Treatment. Outpatient treatment has has been recommended for adolescents with PID since guidelines were issued in 1998 by the Centers for Disease Control and Prevention (CDC). However, many authorities recommend inpatient treatment because of issues with compliance. Mandatory criteria for a diagnosis of PID are lower abdominal tenderness, adnexal tenderness, and cervical motion tenderness. Additional criteria that lend support to the diagnosis are fever, vaginal discharge, elevated

C-reactive protein or ESR levels, and documented infection with gonorrhea or *Chlamydia*. Regimens for outpatient treatment of PID include (1) ofloxacin 400 mg bid for 14 days and metronidazole 500 mg bid for 14 days, and (2) doxycycline 100 mg bid for 14 days and either ceftriaxone 250 mg IM, another third-generation cephalosporin, or cefoxitin 2 g IM bid for 14 days. Patients should be seen within 2–3 days of initial diagnosis to monitor improvement. Sexual partners need to be notified and treated.

The following are criteria for hospitalization: fever, vomiting, severe abdominal pain consistent with appendicitis or tuboovarian abscess, pregnancy, HIV infection, and failure of outpatient therapy. A common parenteral treatment is doxycycline 100 mg IV q12hr and cefotetan 2 g IV q12hr or cefoxitin 2 g IV q6hr. There are several alternative treatment options.

REFERENCES

Behrman RE, Kliegman RM, Jenson HB, editors: *Nelson textbook of pediatrics*, ed 16, Philadelphia, 2000, WB Saunders, Chapter 119.
Braverman PK: Sexually transmitted diseases in adolescents, *Med Clin North Am* 84(4):869–889, 2000.
Centers for Disease Control and Prevention: 1998 STD treatment guidelines, *MMWR* 47(RR-1):1–11, 1998.
Gevelber MA, Biro FM: Adolescents and sexually transmitted diseases, *Pediatr Clin North Am* 46(4):747–766, 1999.

RAPE

Rape is a legal term for unlawful, nonconsensual intercourse. Almost one half of rape victims are adolescents. The attacker is known in 50% of cases. Although gathering historical and physical evidence that may be used in later criminal investigation is important, the physician's primary responsibility to an alleged rape victim is to provide medical examination and treatment in a supportive, nonjudgmental manner. The acute trauma of rape can result in physical injury and untoward psychologic responses, ranging from a state of panic to extreme withdrawal. The history is important and should include details of the sexual assault, whether the victim cleaned herself, the last menstrual period, and previous sexual activity, if any.

Specimens from body surfaces and from the mouth, vagina, and anus, as well as any photographs taken to document the extent of injuries, should be maintained in a "chain of evidence" that cannot be called into question in court. Specimens should be taken so that sperm can be identified by microscopy, agglutination, and the acid phosphatase content of the posterior vaginal fornix and other locations. Attempts to identify *N. gonorrhoeae, Chlamydia,* and *Trichomonas* also are indicated.

In addition to physical trauma, specific, immediate medical issues include prevention of pregnancy and prophylaxis for STDs. Although the risk of conception is less than 5%, pregnancy can be prevented reliably if treatment is instituted within 72 hours of intercourse (discussed in this chapter under Emergency Contraception). The risk of STDs is indeterminate, and the need for STD prophylaxis is controversial. A regimen to treat *Chlamydia,* gonorrhea, *Trichomonas,* and bacterial vaginosis can be administered once (ceftriaxone 125 mg IM, plus metronidazole 2 g PO, plus azithromycin 1 g PO, at the time of the initial evaluation). Doxycycline 100 mg PO for 7 days can be used instead of single-dose azithromycin. Whether antimicrobial treatment is initiated or not, follow-up cultures and wet mounts at 2 weeks are necessary; syphilis, hepatitis, and HIV studies are indicated 12 weeks after the rape. Long-term sequelae are common; patients should be offered immediate and ongoing psychologic support, such as that offered by local rape crisis services. These may be given in conjunction with the medical follow up.

REFERENCES

American Academy of Pediatrics Committee on Adolescence: *Sexual assault and the adolescent,* Pediatrics 94(5):761–765, 1994.
Centers for Disease Control and Prevention: 1998 STD treatment guidelines, *MMWR* 47(RR-1):1–11, 1998.

SKIN CONDITIONS
Acne

At least 85% of adolescents have some form of acne. This skin condition usually is not a serious medical problem, but it may have devastating effects on physical appearance, body image, and self-esteem. Effective treatment should be offered to any adolescent with acne, regardless of the extent of involvement, to avoid physical and psychologic scarring.

Many *pathogenic factors* cause acne. Androgenic stimulation of the sebaceous glands leads to an outpouring of lipid-rich sebum that lubricates the hair follicle. The epidermal cells lining the follicle canal obstruct the flow of sebum onto the surface of the skin. The retained material then acts as a medium for the growth of commensal bacteria such as *Propionibacterium acnes* and coagulase-negative staphylococci. These bacteria produce lipases that hydrolyze the triglycerides contained in sebum, releasing free fatty acids. Inflammation occurs because neutrophils summoned by bacterial chemotactic factors produce hydrolases that disrupt the walls of the pilosebaceous unit. Because the adolescent may apply manual pressure to such lesions, the inflammatory products are released into the dermis rather than onto the surface of the skin. Open comedones are the earliest lesions and are the result of dilation of the follicular canal from retained epidermal lining cells (blackheads). A whitehead, or closed comedo, is impaction of debris that leads to inflammation and bacterial digestion of lipids, which results in the formation of papules, pustules, nodules, and cysts.

Treatment includes comedolytics (e.g., topical benzoyl peroxide and retinoic acid), topical bacteriostatics (e.g., benzoyl peroxide, erythromycin, clindamycin, and tetracyline), oral bacteriostatics (e.g., tetracycline and erythromycin), oral contraceptives, and 13-*cis*-retinoic acid (Accutane). Accutane causes congenital anomalies and should not be given to pregnant adolescents.

Crab Lice

Predominantly sexually transmitted, the pubic crab louse *(Phthirus pubis)* lives out its life cycle on pubic hair; therefore, the characteristic intense pruritus, erythematous papules, and egg cases (nits) of "crabs" are not seen before puberty (Table 7–20). *Treatment* consists of education regarding personal and environmental hygiene and the application of an appropriate pediculicide, such as permethrin or pyrethrin.

Fungal Infections (Jock Itch, Athlete's Foot)

See Chapter 10.

EATING DISORDERS

See Chapters 1 and 2.

BEHAVIORAL PROBLEMS
Psychosocial Conditions
Normal and Abnormal Behaviors

Normal adolescents may intermittently defy parents, provoke their teachers, and challenge physicians. They may refuse to participate in family events and argue incessantly with siblings. It is sometimes difficult to know whether these behaviors are a part of normal adolescent autonomy and individuality struggles or are pathologic. Normal behavior can generally be distinguished from abnormal behavior by taking into account the degree of interference that a particular behavior produces with regard to four main areas: school, family life, activities with friends, and work. Longitudinal studies indicate that most adolescents make the passage from childhood to adulthood with relatively little strife. Difficulties that are persistent or that involve two or more of the four areas noted should not be ignored.

Depression

Younger depressed adolescents, whose cognitive development usually is *concrete operational,* may not be able to acknowledge their affective state; the condition may be indicated by boredom, restlessness, difficulty in concentrating or decreasing school performance, preoccupation with somatic complaints (e.g., fatigue or vague or localized pains), running away, fights with peers, flight to or from people, and other "acting-out" behaviors. Older adolescents, who generally are *formal operational* in their thinking, may be able to reflect on their feelings of depression and sadness. The mood disturbance in depression includes feeling sad or "blue" for more than 3 hours, more than three times a week. Other symptoms are early morning awakening or hypersomnia, changes in appetite, loss of sexual interest, psychomotor retardation or fatigue, inability to concentrate, and feelings of excessive guilt, worthlessness, self-reproach, or hopelessness.

Antidepressant medication may be useful in adolescents who have a family history of depression or alcoholism (discussed further under Suicide, in the next section, Violence). However, few clinical trials have shown any significant difference in response to medication compared with response to a placebo. Therefore, if an antidepressant, such as a selective serotonin reuptake inhibitor, is prescribed, it should be used only as part of a treatment regimen that includes ongoing mental health visits.

Violence

Violence, both unintentional and intentional, is a major and increasing health problem among contemporary adolescents. Unintentional accidents are the leading cause of death in adolescents, followed by suicide and homicide. Although adolescent mass homicides in suburban school settings in the United States have drawn much media attention recently, most adolescent homicides occur among urban, minority males. Prevention of violent and destructive adolescent behavior is an important goal. Identifying the high-risk antecedents of being abused, depression, attention-deficit/hyperactivity disorder, impulse control problems, risk-taking behavior, and substance abuse before accidents, homicides, or suicides is critical for prevention. In addition, recent studies demonstrating the effectiveness of *positive youth development* are encouraging preventive interventions. That is, when a community encourages young people to have a sense of personal meaning and value to others, as well as a perception of being connected to and being an important member of their community, the adolescents in that community appear to be more resistant to numerous problem behaviors, including violence.

Accidents, particularly motor-vehicle collisions, often result from risk-taking by adolescents; judgment impaired by alcohol or other drugs is frequently a contributing factor. Efforts have been made in many states to mandate seat-belt use and, in some states, to raise the legal drinking age to 21 years. Data indicate a decrease in deaths from motor vehicle accidents following the use of such measures. Education programs do not appear to be as effective in changing behavior as does legislation; nevertheless, physicians should educate their young adolescent patients about the hazards of drinking and driving.

Homicide is disturbingly common among young minority males of lower socioeconomic status living in crowded urban areas, even though the adolescent homicide rate decreased by more than one third in the 1990s. A possible response to this situation may be to institute, at the local and national level, a combination of social programs to provide perpetrators, potential perpetrators, and potential victims with alternatives to violent behavior and destructive modes of thinking and relating to others. Primary prevention efforts also focus on child abuse, a common predecessor to adolescent violence. Gun control, improvements in education and economic opportunities, and training in conflict resolution may lower the number of premature deaths.

Suicide is the second-leading cause of death among adolescents 15–24 years of age in the United States. Suicide and attempted suicide may result from despair over the breakup with a boyfriend or girlfriend, grief over the death of a loved one, or a chronic depression. Data suggest that adolescents are more likely to try to harm themselves after viewing programs depicting suicide or after friends or classmates commit suicide, resulting in so-called cluster suicides. Other risk factors include poor impulse control, psychosis, family history of suicide, or risk-taking by the adolescent. Attempts outnumber completed suicides by a ratio of at least 100:1, with girls accounting for more than 80% of attempts. Boys outnumber girls in completed suicides, however, because they are more likely to use a violent method such as guns or hanging rather than poisoning.

REFERENCES

American Academy of Pediatrics, Task Force on Adolescent Assault Victim Needs: Adolescent assault victim needs: a review of issues and a model protocol, *Pediatrics* 98(5):991–1001, 1996.
Behrman RE, Kliegman RM, Jenson HB, editors: *Nelson textbook of pediatrics*, ed 16, Philadelphia, 2000, WB Saunders, Chapters 109–111, 120.
Hughes CW, Emslie GJ, Crismon ML, et al: The Texas children's medication algorithm project: report of the Texas Consensus Conference Panel on Medication Treatment of Childhood Major Depressive Disorder, *J Am Acad Child Adolesc Psychiatry* 38(11): 1442–1454, 1999.
National Center for Injury Prevention and Control, Centers for Disease Control and Prevention, http://www.cdc.gov/ncipc/.
Weiner IB: Normality during adolescence. In McAnarney ER, Kreipe RE, Orr DP, et al, editors: *Textbook of adolescent medicine*, Philadelphia, 1992, WB Saunders.

Substance Abuse

Exploratory drug use may be seen as part of normal psychosocial development for the contemporary adolescent. Many adolescents abandon or lessen their drug use as they develop into adults. However, it is hazardous to adopt an "everybody's doing it" attitude, especially with the more vulnerable younger adolescent, for several reasons (Table 7–23). The use of drugs is often purposive, goal directed, and psychologically adaptive. For example, drug use may allow the adolescent to attain independence from parental control and regulation; to express opposition to social norms; to cope with anxiety, frustration, and depression; or to gain admission to a peer group. The adolescent may fail to develop healthy ways of dealing with these problems if drugs are used as a ready solution. In addition, word of the *purported benefits* of using a drug tends to spread much faster among adolescents, particularly with the widespread use of electronic media and the Internet, than does information about *perceived risks* or *adverse consequences* of using a drug. Therefore, when a new drug comes into use (e.g., drugs used at "raves"), there is often a sharp rise in use before a decrease.

The use of substances by young people also is linked systematically to a larger constellation of problem behaviors that are considered inappropriate by society, such as prostitution and stealing. Compared with nonusing peers, adolescents who abuse drugs have lower grades, higher truancy rates, and fewer plans to attend college; they work less, have less of a religious commitment, have more radical political views, spend less time at home, and spend more time dating.

The younger a person is when he or she begins using substances, the greater is the likelihood of continued use and abuse. In this context marijuana, alcohol, and tobacco are often "gateway drugs." When they provide a positive experience to a seventh-grader, their use can lead to experimentation with other psychoactive substances ("seeking the high") for which the risk of psychologic or physical addiction is great.

Epidemiology. Overall, substance use and abuse among adolescents have trended downward since

TABLE 7–23
Classification of Substance Use by Adolescents

Nonuse	Abstinence from psychoactive or addictive substances for personal, family, or religious reasons
Experimental use	Infrequent, episodic use of various drugs during contact with peers that does not interfere with activities at home, in school, or at work
Recreational use	Episodic use of tobacco, alcohol, or marijuana during social encounters with peers, intended to make one feel accepted or at ease
Circumstantial use	Repeated substance use because of a learned association between its use and decreased anxiety or stress, with drugs serving as a coping tool; depending on stressors, such use can quickly lead to physical or psychologic dependency
Habitual use	Substance(s) use involves most, if not all, areas of life, with the adolescent being psychologically and socially addicted; because everything in the adolescent's life revolves around obtaining and using substance(s), drug use becomes its own reward
Compulsive use	Physiologic addiction to substance(s) so that the adolescent is unable to help himself or herself stop using the drug; because habituation underlies such use, it is best treated in a conscientiously prescribed program of abstinence, change of friends, change of school, and change of all other patterns that were associated with the substance(s) use

From Obermeier G, Henry P: *Semin Adolesc Med* 1:293–301, 1985.

the early 1980s. However, of high school seniors in United States, 80% have tried alcohol, 50% have tried marijuana, and 30% have used some illicit drug other than marijuana. In addition, about 30% of high school seniors report binge drinking (more than five drinks in a row) in the previous 2 weeks, and almost one fourth smoke cigarettes daily. There is wide geographic and sociocultural variability in substance use. For example, among adolescents from upper income levels living in the Northeast and large cities across the United States, the use of "club drugs" at "raves," such as 3-4 methylenedioxymethamphetamine (MDMA or "ecstasy"), ketamine, and so-called date-rape drugs like γ-hydroxybutyrate (GHB) or flunitrazepam (rohypnol, or "roofies") has risen sharply. Anabolic steroid use is primarily limited to adolescent males seeking enhanced athletic performance. Therefore, in addition to knowing what drugs are available in a community, a clinician must determine the epidemiology of substance use for an individual adolescent as part of routine health care or whenever the adolescent is seen for any problem.

Clinical Manifestations. Important factors in the history include types, frequency, timing, setting, circumstances, and outcomes of substance use. Although alcohol use may be considered statistically normative, adolescent alcohol abuse is characterized by consumption of large amounts over a short time, often to the point of intoxication. Even though an

adolescent may drink "only" with friends at weekend parties, he or she can still be the victim of a fatal motor-vehicle accident while driving home intoxicated after a party.

Few physical findings are associated with most chronic adolescent substance use, except in cases of intoxication or overdose (Tables 7–24 and 7–25). However, this does not mean that the commonly used substances are harmless. Hallucinogens such as phencyclidine ("angel dust") or LSD can trigger psychosis; methamphetamine and its derivatives can result in death from direct toxicity; the "club drugs" have both direct (e.g., coma and seizures) and indirect (e.g., sexual assault and dehydration) adverse effects; anabolic steroids also have both direct (e.g., gynecomastia and testicular atrophy) and indirect (e.g., mood swings and violence) adverse effects.

Acute Overdose. Many drugs (most commonly alcohol, amphetamines, opiates, and cocaine) can result in a toxicologic emergency. This most often occurs the first time an adolescent uses a substance, sometimes being unaware of its nature. Such an initial reaction makes identification of the offending agent difficult. Initial management should be directed at appropriate supportive medical treatment, with follow-up counseling after the toxic effects have diminished (Table 7–25).

Acute Illness. Heavy alcohol use can cause both acute gastritis and acute pancreatitis. Intravenous

Text continued on p. 292

TABLE 7–24
Effect, Duration of Action, Toxicity, Withdrawal Symptoms, and Treatment of Substance Abuse in Adolescents

Substance	Immediate Effects	Duration of Action	Toxicity	Signs and Symptoms of Withdrawal	Treatment of Overdose
Alcohol	Respiratory depressioin, CNS depression, ataxia, slurred speech	Depends on amount ingested and adolescent's tolerance	Cirrhosis, gastrointestinal hemorrhage, thiamine and folate deficiency, impaired motor performance and mental function, stupor, deep anesthesia, death	Insomnia, restlessness, anxiety, tremulousness, hypertension, tachycardia, diaphoresis; auditory or visual hallucinations or both, seizures, delirium tremens are rare in adolescents	Supportive ventilation if needed
Amphetamine, other stimulants (e.g., "club drugs" such as ecstasy)	↑ Blood pressure, activity, and alertness; tachycardia; insomnia, anorexia; ↓ fatigue; euphoria; excitation; aggression; hostility	2–8 hr	Agitation; ↑ heart rate, blood pressure, and temperature; hallucinations; paranoia, psychosis; convulsions; arrhythmias; vasculitis; death	Apathy, hallucinations, irritability, excessive sleep, depression, psychosis, suicidal, sudden death	Paranoia with haloperidol; seizures with diazepam
Tobacco	↑ Blood pressure and heart rate; ↓ temperature, CNS stimulation, skeletal muscle relaxation	Minutes	CNS stimulation	Restlessness, anxiety, insomnia, agitation, nausea, headache, ↑ appetite, inability to concentrate	None
Cocaine, crack	↑ Alertness, exultation, euphoria, insomnia; ↓ appetite; ↑ blood pressure and heart rate, aphrodisiac, local anesthesia	15–30 min	Agitation; ↑ temperature, pulse, and BP; tremors; convulsions, tachyarrhythmias; paranoia, psychosis; myocardial infarction; cerebral hemorrhage; death	Apathy, long periods of sleep, irritability, depression, suicidal, disorientation	Paranoia with haloperidol; seizures with diazepam; cooling for hyperthermia; nitroprusside, labetalol for hypertension

Drug	Effects	Duration	Complications	Withdrawal syndrome	Treatment
Inhalants (solvents, gasoline)	Respiratory depression, CNS depression, ataxia, slurred speech, bradycardia	5–30 min	Arrhythmias, ataxia, hallucinations, seizures, encephalopathy, renal tubular acidosis, peripheral neuropathy, lead poisoning, death	Rare: chills, hallucinations, headache, abdominal pain, muscle cramps, delirium tremens	See Chapter 3
LSD, other hallucinogens	Dysphoria; hallucination; anxiety; paranoia; psychosis; ↑ blood pressure, heart rate, and temperature; dilated pupils; incoordination; ↑ creativity	2–12 hr; can produce exhaustion lasting for days	Long, intense "trips"; psychotic reactions not always reversible; flashbacks; suicide attempts; deaths with some drugs	None	Reassurance; haloperidol
Marijuana, hashish	Euphoria, ↓ reaction time, ↓ inhibitions, ↑ appetite	2–4 hr	Dysphoria, acute anxiety attacks, acute psychosis, fatigue, paranoia, lack of motivation	Insomnia, hyperactivity, ↓ appetite	None
PCP and PCP analogs	Ataxia, nystagmus, ↑ blood pressure, slurred speech, dysphoria, hallucinations, paranoia, confusion	Hours to days	Psychosis; convulsions; paranoia; flashbacks; rhabdomyolysis; deaths have resulted from suicide, accidents	None	Haloperidol, diazepam
Opioids	Euphoria, ataxia, slurred speech, miosis, stupor	Hours	Respiratory depression, hypothermia, hypotension, pulmonary edema, apnea, coma, death	Increased sympathetic nervous system activity, hunger, antisocial behavior, gooseflesh, diaphoresis, rhinorrhea (flu), yawning; treatment with clonidine	Naloxone 2 mg IV, repeated up to 10 mg; ventilation

Data from Jones RL: Substance abuse. In Shearin RB, editor: *Handbook of adolescent medicine*, Kalamazoo, Mich, 1983, Upjohn; Abramowicz M, editor: *Med Lett* 38:43, 1996. *CNS*, Central nervous system; *LSD*, lysergic acid diethylamide; *PCP*, phencyclidine.

TABLE 7-25
Effects, Tolerance, Dependence, Adulteration, and Methods of Administration of Substances Abused by Adolescents

Substance	Long-Term Effects	Tolerance	Dependence Psychologic	Dependence Physical	Adulteration or Substitution	Method of Administration
Alcohol	Blackouts; behavioral changes; ↑ accidents; homicide; suicide; gastritis; peptic ulcer; alcoholic hepatitis; fatty liver; pancreatitis	Yes	Yes	Yes	Methanol	Ingested
Amphetamine, other stimulants	Weight loss, insomnia, anxiety, paranoia, hallucinations; skin abscesses and amphetamine psychosis following injections	Yes	High	Yes	More than 90% of speed is adulterated with caffeine, asthma medications, PCP, LSD, strychnine, sugars	Ingested, injected
Tobacco	↑ Risk of chronic bronchitis, heart disease, and cancer (oral cancer with smokeless tobacco)	Yes	Yes	Yes	No	Smoke inhaled, snuff dipping, chewed
Cocaine, crack	Nasal perforation with snorting; weight loss, insomnia, anxiety, paranoia, hallucinations, soft tissue abscesses with injections	Yes	High	Yes, especially following smoking or injection	Local anesthetics, sugars, PCP	Snorted, smoked, ingested, injected
Inhalants (e.g., solvents, gasoline, "white out")	Liver damage with toluene, trichloroethylene, gasoline; anemia with tetraethyl lead; leukemia with benzene; kidney damage with trichloroethylene	Yes, especially with toluene	Yes	Yes	None	Sniffing rags soaked with the compound, inhaling fumes through the mouth

Drug	Effects	Tolerance			Comments	Route of administration
LSD, other hallucinogens	Flashbacks, pronounced personality changes, ↑ risk of chronic psychosis	Yes, cross-tolerance with mescaline, DMT, and psilocybin	Degree unknown	No	Sold as tablets, in liquids, in micro-dots in many colors; often adulterated with or substituted for other drugs	Ingested, injected, sniffed
Marijuana, hashish	Great variety involving several body systems; ↓ motivation	Yes	Degree unknown	No	With PCP	Smoke inhaled, ingested
PCP and PCP analogs	Personality disorders, flashbacks, catatonia, neuropsychologic disturbances, increased risk of schizophrenia	Yes	High	Degree unknown	Often added to other drugs or advertised as other drugs	Ingested, injected, smoked
Opioids	↓ Motivation, antisocial behavior, crime to support habit, skin abscess, endocarditis, osteomyelitis, nephritis, hepatitis, HIV, amenorrhea	Yes	Yes	Yes	Quinine, sugar	Ingested, injected, subcutaneous (skin-popping), intravenous

Modified from Jones RLK: Substance abuse. In Shearin RB, editor: *Handbook of adolescent medicine*, Kalamazoo, Mich, 1983, Upjohn. *DMT*, Dimethyltryptamine; *HIV*, human immunodeficiency virus; *LSD*, lysergic acid diethylamide; *PCP*, phencyclidine.

drug use can result in right-sided bacterial endocarditis, vertebral or sternoclavicular osteomyelitis, septic pulmonary embolism, hepatitis B infection, or acquired immunodeficiency syndrome (AIDS). Chronic marijuana or tobacco use is associated with bronchoconstriction and bronchitis.

Chronic Use. Compulsive drug or alcohol use results in the adolescent's being unable to help himself or herself out of drug dependency and the psychosocial sequelae that attend such habituation (stealing, prostitution, drug dealing, unemployment, school failure, and social isolation).

Treatment. Specific management of substance use by adolescents depends on many individual patient factors. However, because of the highly addictive (physical or psychologic) nature of most substances, residential drug treatment facilities are increasingly being used, especially for younger adolescents.

REFERENCES

Behrman RE, Kliegman RM, Jenson HB, editors: *Nelson textbook of pediatrics,* ed 16, Philadelphia, 2000, WB Saunders, Chapter 113.
Johnston LD, O'Malley PM, Bachman JG: Monitoring the future: national survey results on drug use, 1975-1999. I. Secondary school students, NIH Publication No. 00-4802, Rockville, MD, 2000, National Institute on Drug Abuse. Available on-line at "http://monitoringthefuture.org/."
National Institute on Drug Abuse (NIDA). Information on-line at "http://www.drugabuse.gov/."
Partnership for a Drug-Free America. Information on-line at "http://www.drugfreeamerica.org/."
Substance Abuse and Mental Health Services Administration (SAMHSA). Information on-line at "http://www.samhsa.gov/."

FUNCTIONAL (PSYCHOSOMATIC) DISORDERS

Symptoms of pain or loss of function for which no physical cause is found are common during adolescence. Although the evidence for biologic disorders should be sought simultaneously with evidence for psychologic disorders, it must be realized that our knowledge regarding the relationship between these two domains remains primitive. For example, before research studies in the late 1970s clarifying the role of prostaglandins in causing most of the symptoms of dysmenorrhea, the condition was often labeled as "psychogenic." As knowledge about the molecular and physiologic underpinnings of symptoms emerges in the future, similar discoveries undoubtedly will be made about other poorly understood syndromes, transforming them from "nonorganic" to "organic" disorders.

The adolescent must not be led to believe that the physician, in finding no evidence of disease, judges the symptoms to be feigned or imaginary ("all in your head"). Psychologic factors may indeed play a role in such a situation, but rarely does the physician have the adolescent's trust and confidence required for the treatment to be effective. Even if the physician and adolescent can agree that psychologic factors are operating, this does not guarantee that there is no organic pathologic cause underlying the symptoms. Rather than labeling as "psychosomatic" those symptoms for which no organic cause can be determined, it is preferable to categorize the symptoms as "functional" (Table 7–26), which avoids the connotation that the symptoms are psychologic (they are somatic) and allows the difficulty to be recast in terms of disordered bodily functioning (rather than in terms of the imagination) triggered by previously unappreciated stressors.

The *chronic fatigue syndrome* is another problem in adolescents. It is often a postviral phenomenon, but its etiology is undetermined. It is often associated with a depression that can be incapacitating, in addition to the numerous physical complaints of fatigue.

REFERENCES

Behrman RE, Kliegman RM, Jenson HB, editors: *Nelson textbook of pediatrics,* ed 16, Philadelphia, 2000, WB Saunders, Chapter 19.
Buchwald D, Smith MS: Chronic fatigue. In McAnarney ER, Kreipe RE, Orr DP, et al, editors: *Textbook of adolescent medicine,* Philadelphia, 1992, WB Saunders.
Fritz GK, Fritsch S, Hagino O: Somatoform disorders in children and adolescents: a review of the past 10 years, *J Am Acad Child Adolesc Psychiatry* 36(10):1329–1338, 1997.

School Problems

School problems often indicate underlying psychologic or environmental difficulties. Common school problems are school phobia, truancy, and underachievement.

School Phobia

Adolescents who avoid or refuse to go to school may have histories of separation anxiety and multiple vague somatic complaints, such as headaches, abdominal pain, and fatigue. They often have been seen by numerous specialists and undergo elaborate medical evaluations. Their absence from school often is mistakenly seen as a consequence of their symptoms. In reality, the expression of their symptoms is a means of avoiding school and gaining the attention of a parent. These adolescents may have either a valid or an irrational concern about a parent and thus refuse to leave home, or they may have had an unpleasant experience in school. Rarely do they have a true phobia related to schoolwork. When challenged with the prospect of returning to school,

TABLE 7–26
Features of Functional (Psychosomatic) Disorders of Adolescents

Psychophysiologic Disorder
Presenting complaint is a physical symptom
Physical symptom caused by a known physiologic mechanism
Physical symptom is stress induced
Patient may recognize association between symptom and stress
Symptom responds to medication, biofeedback, and stress reduction

Conversion Reaction
(see also Chapter 1)
Presenting complaint is physical (loss of function, pain, or both)
Physical symptom not caused by a known physiologic mechanism
Physical symptom related to unconscious idea, fantasy, or conflict
Patient does not recognize association between symptom and the unconscious
Symptom responds slowly to resolution of unconscious factors

Somatization Disorder
Presenting complaint is >13 physical symptoms in females, >11 in males
Physical symptoms not caused by known physiologic or pathologic mechanism
Physical symptoms related to need to maintain the sick role
Patient convinced that symptoms unrelated to psychologic factors
Symptoms tend to either persist or change character despite treatment

Hypochondriasis
Presenting complaint is a physical sign or symptom
Physical sign or symptom is normal
Physical symptom is interpreted by patient to indicate disease
Conviction regarding illness may be related to depression or anxiety
Symptom does not respond to reassurance; medication directed at underlying psychologic problems often helpful

Malingering
Presenting complaint is a physical symptom
Physical symptom is under voluntary control
Physical symptom is used to gain reward (e.g., money, avoidance of military service)
Patient consciously recognizes symptom as factitious
Symptom may not lessen once reward is attained (need to retain reward)

Factitious Disorder (e.g., Munchausen syndrome)
Presenting complaint is symptom complex mimicking known syndrome
Symptom complex is under voluntary control
Symptom complex is used to attain medical treatment (including surgery)
Patient consciously recognizes symptom complex as factitious, but is often very psychologically disturbed, so that unconscious factors also are operating
Symptom complex often results in multiple diagnoses and multiple operations

these young people often become extremely anxious and incapacitated with escalating symptoms. School phobia that first becomes manifest during adolescence may be an expression of a severe underlying psychopathologic condition. If there is no medical contraindication for the young person to return to school and if he or she refuses to return, psychiatric consultation is indicated.

Truancy

Truancy is absenteeism from school without permission. It is often peer initiated. Truancy is more common in adolescents from lower socioeconomic status and low educational backgrounds. The truant adolescent leaves home, ostensibly to attend school, but either does not go to school or, once having arrived at school, leaves early. A review of the young person's curriculum for appropriateness and formal education testing is indicated because truancy is often a sign of borderline intellectual abilities or a learning disability. Young people who are truant often drop out of school when they reach 16 years of age.

Academic Failure

Academic difficulty is common during adolescence and often is a reflection of increasing demands of high school work and inability of adolescents to keep up with these demands for any number of reasons. Causes of academic failure should be sought. An initial history, physical examination, and laboratory evaluation by the pediatrician may define a physical cause, such as visual or hearing impairment or neurologic dysfunction, or previously undiagnosed chronic illness, such as anemia. A careful behavioral assessment may reveal undiagnosed depression. School records should be sought to compare academic capability measured by intelligence quotient (IQ) tests, teacher observations of the student's ability, and the student's actual performance reflected in school grades. Formal educational and psychologic evaluation may be indicated if information in the school records is insufficient to identify the cause of academic failure. Intervention involves development of a concerted plan to remedy the situation. The adolescent, the parents, the pediatrician, and the school authorities should participate in this planning.

REFERENCES

Behrman RE, Kliegman RM, Jenson HB, editors: *Nelson textbook of pediatrics,* ed 16, Philadelphia, 2000, WB Saunders, Chapters 22, 25, 29.
Koplewicz HS, Gallagher R: School-related anxiety and related conditions. In McAnarney ER, Kreipe RE, Orr DP, et al, editors: *Textbook of adolescent medicine,* Philadelphia, 1992, WB Saunders.
Sahler OJZ: The teenager with failing grades, *Pediatr Rev* 4:293–300, 1983.

SERIOUS PSYCHIATRIC ILLNESS

Psychoses related to drug ingestion, schizophrenia, or manic-depressive illness or psychoses as isolated episodes of decompensation during emotional stress often first occur during adolescence. It is unusual for an adult with psychosis to have had an uneventful adolescence. If there is any question about the possibility of psychosis, or impending psychosis, early psychiatric evaluation is indicated.

Schizophrenia generally presents before adulthood. It is characterized by loosening of associative thought patterns, inappropriate affect, ambivalent emotional state, and gradual but marked withdrawal from family, school, and peers. Perceptual disturbances are frequent. Health care providers frequently see adolescents in the early stage of their schizophrenic decompensation because of behavioral or somatic symptoms.

Manic-depressive (bipolar) disorder often is mislabeled as schizophrenia during adolescence. The distinct periods of elevated, expansive, or irritable moods associated with hyperactivity and distractibility may alternate rapidly with periods of severe depression lasting for several days or weeks. The family history usually is positive for mental illness.

Acute confusional states can be related to numerous panic inducers, including drugs. The hallucinogens (most notably lysergic acid diethylamide [LSD] and phencyclidine [PCP]), amphetamines, and marijuana all have been associated with an acute, toxic psychosis marked by confusion, disorientation, anxiety, agitation, and disturbances of perception, judgment, or reason. Major tranquilizers and a quiet, safe, nonthreatening environment are helpful in such cases (Table 7–24).

REFERENCES

American Academy of Child and Adolescent Psychiatry. On-line information available at "http://www.aacap.org."
Behrman RE, Kliegman RM, Jenson HB, editors: *Nelson textbook of pediatrics,* ed 16, Philadelphia, 2000, WB Saunders, Chapters 23, 27.
McAnarney ER, Kreipe RE, Orr DP, et al, editors: *Textbook of adolescent medicine,* Philadelphia, 1992, WB Saunders.

MISCELLANEOUS CONDITIONS
Runaway Behavior

Nearly 1 million young people run away from their families of origin during adolescence. Running away from home may indicate environmental stress, including abuse (more than two thirds of female runaways report sexual abuse), or it may indicate intrapsychic problems of the adolescent. Psychologic evaluation of the adolescent includes seeking evidence of depression, characterologic personality disturbance, or a combination of these conditions. Runaway youths are at particularly high risk of being used by adults for illicit activities such as drug-related crimes or prostitution. Hotlines are available for runaway youths to seek help.

Abuse

Abuse of adolescents may be physical, verbal, or sexual. Adults often believe that adolescents are unlikely to be abused because they have developed the capacity to ask for outside help or to leave the family to seek care. However, adolescents may be reluctant to report the abusive situation because they may want to protect the abusing parent or may be too embarrassed to seek help. Evidence of physical trauma, including unexplained bruises and cuts, should be considered as evidence of abuse, as it would be in younger children. Sexual abuse or exploitation, either in incestuous relationships or for prostitution, may become evident when adolescents, particularly early adolescents, become pregnant. If a pregnant adolescent is unable to identify the father of the baby openly to the clinician, either incest or prostitution should be suspected.

Adolescents who are the victims of abuse as children are more likely to abuse others as they get older. It is estimated that up to three fourths of adolescent boys who sexually abuse younger boys were themselves abused as children. In addition, in the United States adolescents are the perpetrators of up to one third of all rapes and one half of all child sexual abuse.

REFERENCES

Behrman RE, Kliegman RM, Jenson HB, editors: *Nelson textbook of pediatrics*, ed 16, Philadelphia, 2000, WB Saunders, Chapters 35, 39.

CHAPTER 8

Immunology and Allergy

Elizabeth C. TePas ▼ Dale T. Umetsu

THE IMMUNE SYSTEM

The body resists infection by means of a number of integrated systems, including anatomic barriers, a complex set of interacting serum proteins, and bone marrow–derived cells collectively known as the immune system. When functioning effectively, host defenses rapidly eliminate pathogens and toxins. The hallmarks of immunodeficiency (frequent or unusually severe infections) appear when the immune system is ineffective or deficient. When the immune system develops inappropriate and deleterious responses, autoimmune or allergic disease results.

Children with *primary immunodeficiencies,* which are relatively rare diseases, exhibit infection. The pediatrician must be able to distinguish the rare child with true immunodeficiency from the immunologically normal child who has recurrent infections. The evaluation of children with recurrent infections, therefore, must be based on a comprehensive understanding of the immune system and the patient's age, the site, and the pathogens involved in those opportunistic infections (Table 8–1).

Major Components of the Host Defense

The major components of host defense are as follows:
- Anatomic-mucociliary barrier mechanisms
- Innate immunity
- Cellular components (phagocytes, dendritic cells, and natural killer [NK] cells)
- Soluble factors (complement, acute-phase proteins, and cytokines)
- Adaptive immunity
- B-cell compartment (the major component of humoral immunity)
- T-cell compartment (the major component of cell-mediated immunity)

Innate immunity, which includes both cellular components and soluble factors, initiates antigen-nonspecific mechanisms as a first line of defense against pathogens, before the development of more versatile *adaptive immune* responses, which involve antigen-specific T cells and B cells. Defects may occur in one or more of these compartments and lead to recurrent, opportunistic, or life-threatening infections. In addition, anatomic integrity at the interface (skin and mucous membranes) between the body and its environment is essential for protection against infection (Table 8–2). Such defects must not be overlooked as a potential source in children with recurrent infection.

Innate Immunity

Cellular Components

Phagocytic cells engulf and digest foreign antigens and microorganisms. The predominant phagocytic cell in blood is the *polymorphonuclear neutrophil* (PMN), which has a circulating half-life of 6–10 hours, is antigen nonspecific, and does not divide. Its major function is to ingest pyogenic bacteria and some fungi, in particular *Aspergillus.* Recruitment and chemotaxis of PMNs to sites of inflammation are greatly aided by *adhesion molecules (selectins, integrins, and chemokines),* which regulate specific interactions between PMNs and endothelial cells. Phagocytosis is initiated by the recognition of a foreign antigen; this is greatly facilitated by cell surface receptors for the Fc portion of immunoglobulin and three receptors for complement (CR1, CR2, CR3). These receptors allow antigen-specific immunoglobulin (with complement) to enhance recognition and phagocytosis of foreign material. Phagocytosis also triggers the cell's NADPH oxidase system that generates superoxide and hydrogen peroxide, which greatly aid in the killing of ingested organisms. Hydrolytic enzymes in granules, such as lysozyme and myeloperoxidase, also aid in the killing of microorganisms.

TABLE 8–1
Clinical Characteristics of Primary Immunodeficiencies

B-Cell Defects

Recurrent pyogenic infections with extracellular encapsulated organisms, such as pneumococci, *Haemophilus influenzae*, and streptococci

Otitis, sinusitis, recurrent pneumonia, bronchiectasis, and conjunctivitis

Few problems with fungal or viral infections (except enterovirus encephalitis and poliomyelitis)

Decreased levels of immunoglobulins in serum and secretions

Diarrhea common, especially secondary to infection with *Giardia lamblia*

Growth retardation not striking

Compatible with survival to adulthood or for several years after onset unless complications occur

T-Cell Defects

Recurrent infections with less virulent or opportunistic organisms such as fungi, mycobacteria, viruses, and protozoa

Growth retardation, malabsorption, diarrhea, and failure to thrive common

Anergy

Susceptible to graft-versus-host reactions if given unirradiated blood

T-Cell Defects—cont'd

Fatal reactions may occur from live virus or BCG vaccination

High incidence of malignancy

Poor survival beyond infancy or childhood

Phagocytic Defects

Recurrent dermatologic infections with bacteria and fungi, such as *Staphylococcus, Pseudomonas, Escherichia coli*, and *Aspergillus*

Subcutaneous, lymph node, lung, and liver abscesses

Pulmonary infections common, including abscess and pneumatocele formation, contributing to chronic disease

Bone and joint infection common

Complement Defects

Recurrent bacterial infections with extracellular pyogenic organisms, such as pneumococcus and *H. influenzae*

Unusual susceptibility to recurrent *gonococcal* and *meningococcal* infections

Increased incidence of autoimmune disease (SLE)

Severe or recurrent skin and respiratory tract infection

BCG, Bacille Calmette-Guérin; *SLE,* systemic lupus erythematosus.

TABLE 8–2
Anatomic and Mucociliary Defects That Result in Recurrent or Opportunistic Infections

Anatomic Defects in Upper Airways

Aspiration syndromes (gastroesophageal reflux, ineffective cough, foreign body)

Cleft palate, eustachian tube dysfunction

Adenoidal hypertrophy

Nasal polyps

Obstruction of paranasal sinus drainage (osteomeatal complex disease), encephaloceles

Posttraumatic or congenital sinus tracts (CSF rhinorrhea)

Anatomic Defects in the Tracheobronchial Tree

Tracheal esophageal fistula, bronchobiliary fistula

Pulmonary sequestration, bronchogenic cysts, vascular ring

Tumor, foreign body, or enlarged nodes

Physiologic Defects in Upper and Lower Airways

Primary ciliary dyskinesia syndromes, Young syndrome

Cystic fibrosis, bronchopulmonary dysplasia, bronchiectasis

Allergic disease (allergic rhinitis, asthma)

Chronic cigarette smoke exposure

Other Defects

Burns

Chronic atopic dermatitis

Ureteral obstruction/vesicoureteral reflux

Intravenous drug use

Central venous lines, artificial heart valves, CSF shunts, peritoneal dialysis catheter, urinary catheter

CSF, Cerebrospinal fluid.

Short peptides called *defensins* (29–42 amino acids), which constitute about 5% of the total cellular protein of neutrophils, have important antimicrobial and cytotoxic functions against pathogens. Defensins aggregate and produce holes in the membranes of bacteria, mycobacteria, and fungi. Defensins are also secreted by tracheal cells and are important in resisting infection in the lungs.

The *macrophage,* another cell type in the phagocytic compartment, is a long-lived phagocytic cell that develops from circulating monocytes. Macrophages populate the lung, liver, kidneys, spleen, brain, and lymph nodes and are effective in killing facultative intracellular organisms such as *Mycobacterium, Toxoplasma,* and *Legionella.* Macrophages are most effective when activated by IFN-γ. T cells cross-link CD40 molecules on macrophages, resulting in the expression of nitric oxide synthase, B7-1 (CD80) and B7-2 (CD86) costimulatory molecules and in the production of interleukin-12 (IL-12). The expression of B7 molecules and the production of IL-12 enhance the capacity of macrophages to present antigens to T cells and to induce cell-mediated immunity (the development of Th1 cells and cytotoxic T cells).

Natural killer (NK) cells, which express CD16 and CD56 antigens but not T-cell receptors, play a major role in innate immunity by mediating cytotoxic activity against virally infected cells and cancer cells. NK cells recognize target cells that do not express major histocompatibility complex (MHC) molecules, allowing NK cells to kill rapidly cells to which they have not been previously sensitized. NK cells thus kill virus-infected cells or tumor cells, in which MHC expression is suppressed. The recognition of target cells by NK cells is mediated by killer-inhibitory receptors, which recognize MHC class I molecules and inhibit lytic activity. IL-12 and IL-2 enhance the development of NK cells, which secrete large quantities of IFN-γ and tumor necrosis factor-α (TNF-α). As part of the immune system, NK cells respond rapidly to pathogens early during immune responses and before immunologic memory (characteristics of adaptive immunity with T cells and B cells) becomes effective.

Recognition of pathogens by the innate immune system is facilitated by other receptors on macrophages, NK cells and neutrophils, which recognize conserved pathogen motifs called pathogen-associated molecular patterns (PAMPs). PAMPs include lipopolysaccharide (LPS) in gram-negative bacteria, lipoteichoic acid in gram-positive bacteria, mannans in yeast, and specific nucleotide sequences (cytosine adjacent to guanine) in bacterial and viral DNA. One type of pattern-recognition receptor binds to microbial cell wall components and leads to the phagocytosis and processing of microbial antigens. Peptide-MHC molecule complexes are then generated and are presented to T cells. Another of the PAMP receptors, which include toll-like receptors, activates signaling pathways, causing up-regulation of B7 costimulatory molecule expression in antigen-presenting cells and production of chemokines and cytokines, including IL-1, IL-6, and IL-12. These chemokines and cytokines have significant effects on the adaptive immune system by enhancing antigen presentation and providing costimulatory signals for T-cell activation.

Soluble Factors of the Innate Immune System

The complement system consists of 20 well-defined plasma complement components, five cell membrane regulatory proteins, and seven cell membrane receptors. The complement system can be activated through three pathways—classic, alternative, and lectin—that lead to the cascade-like, sequential activation of multiple factors. Activated factors have various biologic activities that enhance phagocytosis and antibody-dependent and -independent cell lysis (Fig. 8–1). The classical pathway is activated by antigen-antibody complexes and, nonimmunologically, by C-reactive protein and trypsin-like enzymes. The alternative pathway may be activated by C3b generated through classic complement activation and, nonimmunologically, by endotoxin or fungal antigens (zymogen). The lectin pathway is initiated by the interaction of mannose-binding lectin with microbial carbohydrate, with subsequent activation of associated proteases that cleave C2 and C4. The complement components amplify immunologic stimuli in an antigen-nonspecific manner, although complement can be activated in the classical pathway by aggregated antigen-specific antibody. Because the three pathways converge at C3 (after which the activation sequences are identical), C3 is a pivotal factor and is the most abundant, with a plasma concentration of 1 mg/mL. When activated, complement components have potent opsonizing (C3b, iC3b), chemotactic (C5a), mast cell–activating (C3a, C5a), and lytic (membrane attack complex, C5bBC9) activity. They can also activate neutrophil respiratory burst activity (C3a, C5a).

Other important soluble factors in innate immunity are acute-phase proteins, cytokines, and chemokines (Table 8–3). Proinflammatory acute-phase proteins include C-reactive protein and mannose-binding lectin. They are involved in recognition of damaged cells and pathogens. In addition, they can activate complement and induce production of inflammatory cytokines. Other acute-phase proteins have antiinflammatory activity and are involved in wound healing.

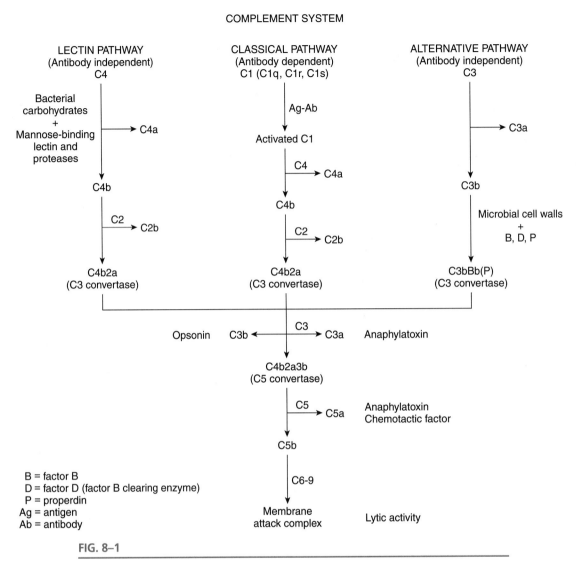

COMPLEMENT SYSTEM

FIG. 8–1

Complement component cascade involving the classical, alternate, and lectin pathways. The initiating events for the pathways differ but result in production of C3 cleaving enzyme activity, which is the pivotal step as the three pathways converge to the terminal activation sequences. *Ag-Ab,* Antigen-antibody complex.

Chemokines have a broad range of activities, including the recruitment and activation of inflammatory cells. The pattern of chemokines produced determines the type and location of inflammatory infiltrate. Cytokines are the immune system's messengers. They are involved in the regulation of the immune response and may also have a direct role in defense.

Adaptive Immunity

The innate immune system functions to rapidly recognize and deal with pathogens and tissue injury and to activate the more deliberate adaptive immune system. The key feature of the adaptive immune system is the development of immunologic memory, produced by the expansion and maturation of antigen-specific T cells and B cells.

B-Cell Compartment

Humoral immunity involves the capacity of serum components to combat infection. The major components of humoral immunity are the immunoglobulins, but the term also signifies other circulating components (complement proteins) that are involved in humoral defenses. Immunoglobulins, produced by B cells, attach specifically to antigens (glycoproteins,

TABLE 8–3
Cytokines and Chemokines and Their Functions

Factor	Source	Function
IL-1	Macrophages	Costimulatory effect on T cells enhances antigen presentation
IL-2	T cells	Primary T-cell growth factor; B- and NK-cell growth factor
IL-3	T cells	Mast cell growth factor; multicolony-stimulating factor
IL-4	T cells	T-cell growth factor; enhances IgE synthesis; enhances B-cell differentiation; mast cell growth
IL-5	T cells	Enhances immunoglobulin synthesis; enhances IgA synthesis; enhances eosinophil differentiation
IL-6	T cells, macrophages, fibroblasts, endothelium	Enhances immunoglobulin synthesis, antiviral activity, and hepatocyte-stimulating factor
IL-7	Stromal cells	Enhances growth of pre-B cells and pre-T cells
IL-8	T cells, macrophages, epithelium	Neutrophil-activating protein; T lymphocyte, neutrophil chemotactic factor
IL-9	T cells	Acts in synergy with IL-4 to induce IgE production, mast cell growth
IL-10	T cells, macrophages	Cytokine synthesis inhibitory factor; suppresses macrophage function; enhances B-cell growth; inhibits IL-12 production
IL-12	Macrophages, neutrophils	Natural killer cell stimulatory factor; cytotoxic lymphocyte maturation factor; enhances IFN-γ synthesis; inhibits IL-4 synthesis
IL-13	T cells	Enhances IgE synthesis; enhances B-cell growth; inhibits macrophage activation; causes airway hyperreactivity
IL-18	Macrophages	Enhances IFN-γ synthesis
IFN-γ	T cells	Macrophage activation; inhibits IgE synthesis; antiviral activity
TGF-β	T cells, many cells	Inhibits T-cell and B-cell proliferation and activation
RANTES	T cells, endothelium	Chemoattractant (chemokine) for monocytes, T cells, eosinophils
MIP-1α	Mononuclear cells, endothelium	Chemoattractant for T cells; enhances differentiation of CD4+ T cells
Eotaxin 1, 2, and 3	Epithelium, endothelium, eosinophils, fibroblasts, macrophages	Chemoattractant for eosinophils, basophils, and Th2 cells
IP-10	Monocytes, macrophages, endothelium	Chemoattractant for activated T cells, monocytes, and NK cells; T cells activate NK cells

IFN, Interferon; *Ig,* immunoglobulin; *RANTES,* regulated upon *a*ctivation, *n*ormal *T* *e*xpressed and secreted; *Th2,* T helper 2.

carbohydrates, and toxins) and inactivate or agglutinate the antigen, opsonize the antigen for phagocytosis, or allow the activation of complement, causing pathogen cytolysis. Five major immunoglobulin (Ig) isotypes, IgG, IgM, IgA, IgD, and IgE, are distinguished by antigenic and functional differences in their heavy chains.

IgG is the major serum immunoglobulin (representing 70–75% of all immunoglobulin) and is the ma-

jor immunoglobulin produced in secondary responses. IgG diffuses well into tissues, crosses the placenta, and has one of the longest half-lives of serum proteins (~21 days). IgG can be further subdivided into four subclasses—IgG1, IgG2, IgG3, and IgG4C—based on heavy-chain differences. In general, antibody responses to polysaccharide antigens reside in the IgG2 subclass, whereas responses to protein antigens reside in the IgG1 and IgG3 subclasses.

IgM represents 10% of all immunoglobulins and is confined to the intravascular pool. IgM circulates in the blood as a pentamer, joined by a J chain. IgM is rapidly secreted following primary antigenic stimulation. It binds complement efficiently and assists the reticuloendothelial system in clearing circulating bacteria by opsonization and agglutination.

IgA constitutes 15–20% of the serum immunoglobulin pool but is also the major protective antibody *(secretory IgA)* in saliva, lacrimal fluid, and colostrum. IgA is present in nasal, bronchial, and intestinal secretions, but because it does not activate complement, IgA is thought to function by clearing antigens from mucosal sites without evoking inflammatory responses. Secretory IgA (sIgA) is distinguished from serum IgA by the presence of a component called secretory piece and by a short polypeptide J chain.

IgD accounts for less than 1% of total immunoglobulin and serves as an antigen receptor or receptor site on circulating B cells.

IgE is present in serum in very small amounts but is the principal mediator of immediate hypersensitivity reactions. IgE may play a role in immunity to metazoan parasites (helminths).

Immunoglobulin is produced by B lymphocytes after they become activated and differentiate into plasma cells (Fig. 8–2). B cells express cell surface receptors for the Fc region of IgG and for complement and express major histocompatibility (MHC) class I and II molecules. They can be identified by staining for the CD19 and CD20 molecules.

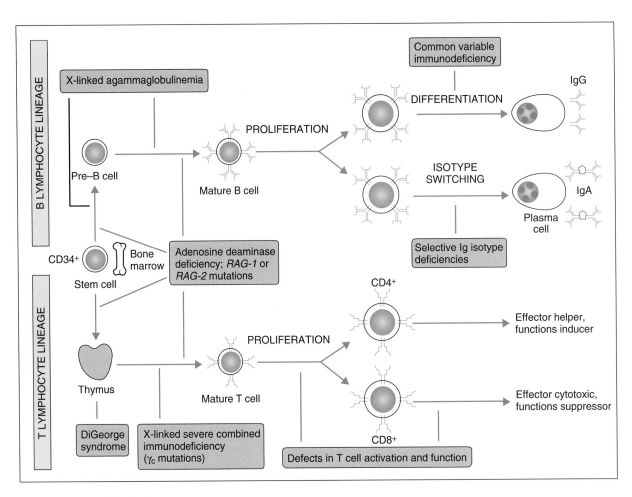

FIG. 8–2

Sites of cellular abnormalities in congenital immunodeficiencies. In different congenital (primary) immunodeficiencies, the maturation or activation of B or T lymphocytes may be blocked at different stages. (From Abbas AK, Lichtman AH, Pober JS: *Cellular and molecular immunology,* ed 3, Philadelphia, 1997, WB Saunders.)

T-Cell Compartment

T lymphocytes are responsible for the cytolysis of virus-infected cells, the induction of B-cell activation and differentiation, and the recruitment, by means of their soluble products, of macrophages, neutrophils, eosinophils, basophils, and mast cells. T cells are greatly involved in immunity to intracellular organisms (e.g., viruses, *Mycobacterium, Toxoplasma, Legionella,* and *Brucella*), fungal organisms (e.g., *Histoplasma* and *Candida*), and protozoa; in immune surveillance for cancer cells; and in causing graft-versus-host disease and transplant graft rejection. T cells can be divided into two major subsets: CD4+ and CD8+ T cells (Fig. 8–2).

CD4+ T cells, the helper-inducer subset, induce B-cell production of antibody and help regulate immune responses by producing a wide variety of cytokines, such as IL-2, IL-3, IL-4, IL-5, IL-10, and IFN-γ (Table 8–3). CD4+ T helper cells can be further subdivided into Th1 cells, which secrete cytokines such as IFN-γ and IL-2, and Th2 cells, which secrete cytokines such as IL-4, IL-5, IL-10, and IL-13. CD4+ Th1 cells are important in activating macrophages and in cell-mediated immunity. Th2 cells are critical for the activation and differentiation of B cells (humoral immunity) and in down-regulating immune responses. Development of Th cells expressing inappropriate cytokine profiles can exacerbate infection and cause allergy (Th2), autoimmunity (Th1), and graft-versus-host disease.

CD8+ T cells (cytotoxic suppressor cells) kill virus-infected cells or tumor cells and suppress or limit immune responses. They kill target cells through several mechanisms, such as pore formation by enzymes (porphyrin and granzyme B) stored in the lytic granules of CD8+ cells and induction of programmed cell death by the triggering of *Fas* antigen (CD95) on target cells and the *Fas* ligand on cytotoxic effector cells.

Tumor-infiltrating lymphocytes (TILs) are *CD3+ T cells* found in solid tumors that can be expanded in vitro when stimulated with IL-2. These cells are thought to be cytotoxic and tumor specific. When they are reinfused in the donor, they cause regression of the target tumor.

Ontogeny of the Immune System

T cells, B cells, neutrophils, and monocytes all derive from CD34+ stem cells in the bone marrow (Fig. 8–2). T cells mature in the thymus through a complex process involving both positive and negative selection that determines the T-cell receptor repertoire. More than 90% of the developing T cells are eliminated by *negative selection,* eliminating autoreactive T cells, and by *positive selection,* eliminating T cells with receptors that do not recognize self-MHC antigens. T cells that leave the thymus circulate and repopulate the lymphoid organs, including the lymph nodes, the spleen, and Peyer's patches.

B-cell development begins in the bone marrow and depends on the function of a gene called *Bruton tyrosine kinase (Btk),* which is dysfunctional in patients with Bruton X-linked agammaglobulinemia. In the bone marrow, B-cell differentiation involves deletional recombination of immunoglobulin genes and VDJ gene rearrangement. This process allows B cells to express cell surface IgM molecules and to circulate and populate lymphoid follicles in the spleen, lymph nodes, tonsils, and Peyer's patches.

Random recombination of the genes in the variable region, splicing inaccuracies, and insertion of additional nucleotides by the enzyme terminal deoxyribonucleotidyltransferase (TdT) generate the diversity of B- and T-cell receptors. Unlike T-cell receptors, B-cell receptors can be further altered in the germinal centers of secondary lymphoid organs by receptor editing and somatic hypermutation.

Phagocytes also differentiate from stem cells. Phagocytes include circulating monocytes, from which tissue macrophages and dendritic cells differentiate. Granulocytes, such as neutrophils, eosinophils, and basophils, develop in the bone marrow before circulating in the blood. Mast cells develop from stem cells as a separate lineage, leave the bone marrow in an immature state, and complete their differentiation in the tissues.

Initiation of Immune Responses (Fig. 8–3)

Immune responses are initiated by the presence of foreign materials or pathogens, which are taken up by antigen-presenting cells (APCs), such as dendritic cells, antigen-specific B cells, and macrophages. The initiation requires that the foreign material be accompanied by a "danger" signal provided by endotoxin, other bacterial products, and viral DNA or by tissue necrosis. These signals activate the APC, allowing more efficient antigen presentation. In the absence of this "danger" signal, T-cell tolerance or anergy occurs. Dendritic cells are APCs in the skin, lung, and tissues. These cells sample antigen and then migrate to regional lymph nodes, where they mature and activate naïve T cells and B cells, permitting the development of immunologic memory. After uptake by dendritic cells or macrophages, the antigen is processed and antigen peptides associate with MHC class I or class II molecules. The antigen peptide–MHC complex is then expressed on the surface of the APC for recognition by T cells. T-cell activation occurs if the T-cell receptor binds to the MHC-peptide complex and aggregates

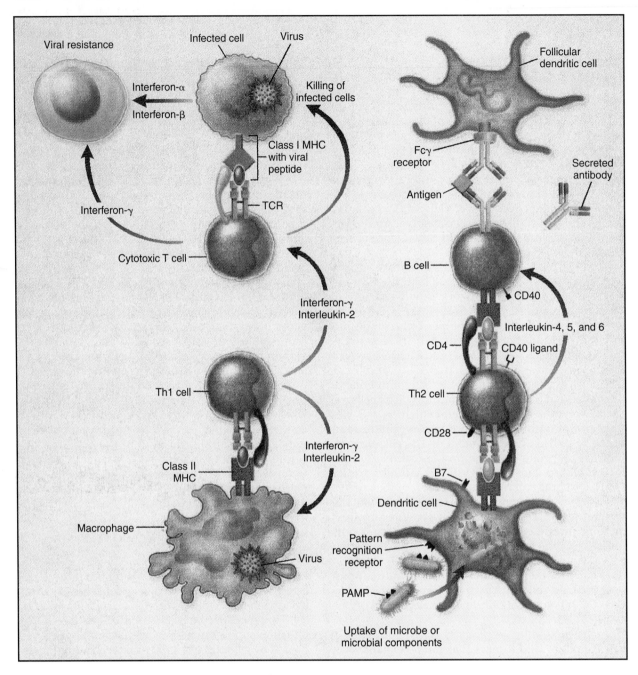

FIG. 8–3

An overview of lymphocyte responses. T cells characteristically possess T-cell receptors (TCRs) that recognize processed antigen presented by major histocompatibility complex (MHC) molecules, as shown on the left-hand side of the figure. Most cytotoxic T cells are positive for CD8, recognize processed antigen presented by MHC class I molecules, and kill infected cells, thereby preventing viral replication. Activated cytotoxic T cells secrete interferon-γ that, together with interferon-α and interferon-β produced by the infected cells themselves, sets up a state of cellular resistance to viral infection. As shown on the right-hand side of the figure, helper T cells are generally positive for CD4, recognize processed antigen presented by MHC class II molecules, and can be divided into two major populations. Type 1 (Th1) helper T cells secrete interferon-γ and interleukin-2, which activate macrophages and cytotoxic T cells to kill intracellular organisms; type 2 (Th2) helper T cells secrete interleukin-4, 5, and 6, which help B cells secrete protective antibodies. B cells recognize antigen either directly or in the form of immune complexes on follicular dendritic cells in germinal centers. (Modified from Delves PJ, Roitt IM: *N Engl J Med* 343[2]:108–117, 2000.)

and if the APC also delivers costimulatory signals to the T cell through the expression of cell surface molecules, such as B7-1 (CD80), B7-2 (CD86), and intercellular adhesion molecule-1 (ICAM-1). T-cell activation results in the phosphorylation of multiple membrane and cytoplasmic proteins, hydrolyzation of membrane phosphatidylinositol bisphosphate, and an increase in intracellular free calcium. Activation is manifested by T-cell proliferation and production of cytokines such as IL-2.

The activation of T cells sets off a number of events in the immune system, triggered by cell-cell interaction and by secreted cytokines. Activation of T cells induces the T cell to differentiate and produce other cytokines, such as IFN-γ and, in some instances, IL-4, IL-5, and IL-10. Activation of the T cell also induces T-cell expression of other cell surface molecules, such as CD40 ligand, which is critical in activating dendritic cells and macrophages. Cross-linking of CD40 on the surface of dendritic cells and macrophages by CD40 ligand (CD154), in the presence of IFN-γ, activates dendritic cells and macrophages to produce IL-12, which greatly enhances the production of IFN-γ from T cells and NK cells and the development of cytotoxic T cells. Activated macrophages can also produce nitric oxide, which effectively kills intracellular organisms such as *Mycobacterium, Listeria, Leishmania, Toxoplasma,* and other intracellular parasites. Cross-linking of CD40 on the surface of B cells, in the presence of IL-2, IL-4, and IL-5, induces B-cell differentiation, isotype switch, and immunoglobulin production.

Physiologic Immunodeficiency in the Neonate

Because immunity in young children (particularly neonates) is deficient compared with that in adults, children are more susceptible to infections than adults. The immune system in children is still developing and requires several years before reaching maturity. Infants produce only small amounts of immunoglobulin before 4–6 months of age. At birth they have received all of their immunoglobulins (IgG) transplacentally from the mother during the third trimester of gestation. Premature infants are frequently hypogammaglobulinemic because they receive only a fraction of the usual maternal antibody. The fetus can produce antibody, but mostly of the IgM isotype. Neonates do respond to immunization, generally to potent proteins, but the ability to respond to bacterial antigens (carbohydrates) is not consistently acquired until after 2 years of age. Normal levels of serum immunoglobulins reach a nadir at around 4–6 months of age and increase slowly over several years. Acquisition of adult levels of IgM

occurs by 1 year of age, whereas adult levels of IgG are noted at 5–7 years and adult levels of IgA are achieved at 10–14 years of age.

T-cell function in young children is reduced, mainly because neonatal T cells are immature and produce reduced quantities of IFN-γ, IL-4, IL-5, and other cytokines. T-cell help for B cells in young children is thus limited. In addition, neonatal T cells express CD40L poorly; this expression is required for cognate interaction with B cells in the induction of antibody synthesis. Cytotoxic responses are also reduced in the neonate, as is neutrophil function, which is dependent on exposure to IFN-γ. In neonates the production of neutrophils is reduced and neutrophil chemotaxis is poor. Complement levels (particularly C8 and C9) are decreased; the neonate has less than 20% of the normal adult activity. Thus multiple factors in the neonate contribute to the increased susceptibility to infection.

IMMUNODEFICIENCY DISORDERS

The hallmark of immunodeficiency is increased susceptibility to infection. Affected patients also have infections with increased severity or infections with opportunistic organisms, and they may be predisposed to the development of autoimmune disease and malignancy. Infections primarily occur in the respiratory tract, the gastrointestinal tract (resulting in diarrhea or malabsorption), or the skin. Primary immunodeficiencies can be classified according to the immunologic compartment that is defective (e.g., B-cell, T-cell, phagocytic, NK cells, or complement compartment). Deficiencies can exist in one or more of these compartments. The deficiency may be congenital (X-linked [Bruton] agammaglobulinemia) or secondary (Table 8–4). There are more than 95 different primary (inherited) immunodeficiencies. Although primary immunodeficiencies are rare, the overall frequency of these disorders is about 1 in 10,000. Patients with B-cell defects constitute about 50% of primary immunodeficiencies, whereas about 30% of primary immunodeficiencies are the result of T-cell defects. Phagocytic defects are even less common (~18% of all cases of primary immunodeficiency). Primary complement defects are the least common (~2% of all cases). Primary immunodeficiencies are genetic diseases, and consequently consanguinity is often present.

B-Cell Defects: Antibody Deficiency States

B-cell deficiencies are caused by the absence of B cells, abnormal B-cell differentiation, or secondary to abnormal T-cell function (Table 8–5). Defects of

---

TABLE 8–4
Causes of Secondary Immunodeficiency

Viral Infections
Measles (inhibits interleukin-12 production in
macrophages)
Roseola (human herpesvirus-6)
Epstein-Barr virus (X-linked lymphoproliferative
disease—Duncan syndrome)
Cytomegalovirus
Human immunodeficiency virus (destroys CD4+
T cells)

Metabolic Disorders
Diabetes mellitus
Malnutrition
Uremia
Sickle cell disease
Zinc deficiency
Multiple carboxylase deficiency
Burns

Protein-Losing States
Nephrotic syndrome
Protein-losing enteropathy

Other Causes
Prematurity
Immunosuppressive agents (e.g., corticosteroids,
radiation, and antimetabolites)
Malignancy (leukemia, Hodgkin disease,
nonlymphoid cancer)
Acquired asplenia
Periodontias
Chronic (acute) blood transfusions
Acquired neutropenia (autoimmune, viral, or drug
induced)
Bone marrow transplantation/graft-versus-host
disease
Systemic lupus erythematosus
Sarcoidosis

---

antibody production may involve all antibody classes, selective antibody classes, selective deficiency of IgG subclasses, or an inability to respond to a specific antigen.

The *clinical manifestations* of abnormal B-cell function include recurrent sinopulmonary infections (e.g., otitis media, sinusitis, and pneumonia) and bacteremia with encapsulated bacteria, such as *Streptococcus pneumoniae, Haemophilus influenzae,* and *Staphylococcus aureus* (Table 8–1). Antibody defi-

ciency states do not become manifest until after 6 months of age, when transplacentally acquired maternal IgG has been depleted. Patients with deficiency of IgG synthesis can exhibit the condition in the first year of life (through X-linked agammaglobulinemia) or later in childhood or early adulthood (through common variable agammaglobulinemia) (Table 8–5). Isolated deficiency of IgA is associated with recurrent infection, but because many individuals with low IgA levels are asymptomatic, the precise mechanism that causes recurrent infection when IgA levels are low is unclear. Similarly, isolated IgG2 subclass deficiency is associated with a propensity for development of recurrent sinopulmonary infection, although asymptomatic individuals with low IgG2 levels have been observed.

X-Linked Agammaglobulinemia

X-linked agammaglobulinemia is a congenital immunodeficiency in males characterized by a profound deficiency of B cells, resulting in severe hypogammaglobulinemia and absence of lymphoid tissue (Fig. 8–2 and Table 8–5). The defect is limited to the B-cell lineage and is caused by mutations of the B-cell–specific, Tec family tyrosine kinase *Btk* on chromosome Xq22. The major consequence is the arrest of B-cell development at the pre–B-cell state. Non–X-linked gene defects that lead to agammaglobulinemia include mutations in the μ heavy-chain gene on chromosome 14, the λ surrogate light chain, Igα (B-cell antigen receptor), and B-cell linker (BLNK). Patients with X-linked agammaglobulinemia usually exhibit the condition after the first few months of life; 20% of patients experience initial symptoms after 12 months or as late as 3–5 years. These patients develop infections with *S. pneumoniae, H. influenzae, Staphylococcus aureus,* and *Pseudomonas* species, organisms for which antibody is an important opsonin. Gastrointestinal problems, except for enteroviral infection and giardiasis, are relatively rare, in contrast to the frequency of gastrointestinal symptoms seen in **common variable immunodeficiency** (described further in this chapter). Immunization with live poliomyelitis vaccine has resulted in poliomyelitis.

Hyper-IgM Syndrome

Hyper-IgM syndrome is characterized by elevated serum levels of IgM but normal levels of IgG and IgA and by absent B-cell function (an inability to produce antigen-specific antibody). Recurrent sinopulmonary infections, infection with *Pneumocystis carinii,* thrombocytopenia, hemolytic anemia, hypothyroidism, and neutropenia are common. The X-linked form of the disease is caused by mutations in the gene coding for the CD40 ligand, an antigen

TABLE 8–5
Disorders of Lymphocyte Function

Disorder	Genetics	Onset	Manifestations	Pathogenesis	Associated Features
Bruton agammaglobulinemia	X-linked (Xq22)	Infancy (6–9 mo)	Recurrent high-grade infections, sinusitis, pneumonia, meningitis	Arrest in B-cell differentiation (pre-B level); mutation in the *Btk* gene	Lymphoid hypoplasia
Common variable immunodeficiency	AR; AD	Second to third decade	Sinusitis, bronchitis, pneumonia, chronic diarrhea	Arrest in B-cell to plasma cell differentiation	Autoimmune disease, RA, SLE, Graves disease, ITP, malignancy
Transient hypogammaglobulinemia of infancy		Infancy (3–7 mo)	Recurrent viral and pyogenic infections	Delayed development of plasma cell maturation	Frequently in families with immunodeficiencies
IgA deficiency	X-linked, AR, ? 6p21.3	Variable	Sinopulmonary infections	Failure of IgA expressing B-cell differentiation	IgG subclass deficiency, common variable immunodeficiency, autoimmune diseases
IgG subclass deficiency	AR 2p11; 14q32.3	Variable	Gastrointestinal infections; may be normal	Defect in isotype IgG production	IgA deficiency, ataxia-telangiectasia
IgM deficiency	AR	First year	Variable (normal to recurrent sinopulmonary infections and gastrointestinal infections)	Defective helper T-cell–B-cell interaction	Whipple disease, regional enteritis, lymphoid hyperplasia
Immunodeficiency with increased IgM	X-linked, AR, ? (Xq26)	2–3 yr	Recurrent septicemia, pneumococcus, *Haemophilus influenzae*	Defect in IgG and IgA synthesis and of CD40 ligand	Hematologic autoimmune disease
DiGeorge anomaly	? (22q11.2)	Early infancy	Recurrent pyogenic infections (e.g., otitis media, sinusitis, tonsillitis, pneumonia)	Hypoplasia of third and fourth pharyngeal pouch	Hypoparathyroidism, aortic arch anomalies, micrognathia, hypertelorism
Wiskott-Aldrich syndrome	X-linked (Xp11.22)	Early infancy	Variable	53-kD protein (WASP) defect	Recurrent infections, atopic dermatitis, platelet dysfunction, thrombocytopenia

Continued

Modified from Boxer L, Blackwood K: Recurrent infection. In Kliegman RM, Nieder ML, Super DM, editors: *Practical strategies in pediatric diagnostics and therapy*, Philadelphia, 1996, WB Saunders.
ADA, Adenosine deaminase; *AR*, autosomal recessive; *dATP*, deoxyadenosine triphosphate; *dGTP*, deoxyguanosine triphosphate; *Ig*, immunoglobulin; *IL*, interleukin; *IL-2R γ*, interleukin-2 receptor gamma chain; *ITP*, idiopathic thrombocytopenic purpura; *PNP*, purine nucleoside phosphorylase; *RA*, rheumatoid arthritis.

TABLE 8-5
Disorders of Lymphocyte Function—cont'd

Disorder	Genetics	Onset	Manifestations	Pathogenesis	Associated Features
Ataxia-telangiectasia	AR (11q22.3)	2–5 yr	Recurrent otitis media, pneumonia, meningitis with encapsulated organisms	AT gene mutation (PI3 kinase)	Neurologic and endocrine dysfunction, malignancy, telangiectasis; sensitive to radiation
Nijmegen breakage syndrome	AR (8q21)	Infancy	Sinopulmonary infections, bronchiectasis, urinary tract infections	Defect in chromosomal repair mechanisms	Sensitivity to ionizing radiation; microcephaly with mild neurologic impairment; malignancy
Cartilage-hair hypoplasia (short-limbed dwarf)	AR (9p13–21)	Birth	Variable	Unknown	Metaphyseal dysplasia, short extremities
Severe combined immunodeficiency (common γ chain)	X-linked (Xq13.1), AR	1–3 mo	Candidiasis, all types of infections (bacterial, viral, fungal, protozoal)	IL-2R common γ-chain mutation (severe T-cell depletion) ZAP-70 (2q12), Jak-3 kinase (19p13.1), or IL-7R α-chain deficiency (15p13 deficiency)	Severe graft-versus-host disease from maternal fetal transfusions
Severe combined immunodeficiency (ADA deficiency)	AR (20q13.11)	1–3 mo	Candidiasis, all types of infections (bacterial, viral, fungal, protozoal)	Adenosine deaminase deficiency resulting in dATP-induced lymphocyte toxicity	Multiple skeletal abnormalities, chondroosseous dysplasia
Severe combined immunodeficiency (PNP deficiency)	AR 14q13.1	1–3 mo	Candidiasis, all types of infections (bacterial, viral, fungal, protozoal)	Purine nucleosidase deficiency resulting in dGTP-induced T-cell toxicity	Neurologic disorders, severe graft-versus-host disease from transfusions
Severe combined immunodeficiency (reticular dysgenesis)	AR	1–3 mo	Candidiasis, all types of infections (bacterial, viral, fungal, protozoal)	Defective maturation of common stem cell affecting myeloid and lymphoid cells	Agammaglobulinemia, alymphocytosis, agranulocytosis

Condition	Inheritance	Age of Onset	Infections	Molecular Defect	Associated Features
…enn syndrome	AR (11p13)	1–3 mo	Candidiasis, all types of infections (bacterial, viral, fungal, protozoal)	Mutations of recombinase-activating genes (RAG-1 and RAG-2)	Exfoliative erythroderma, eosinophilia, elevated IgE, lymphadenopathy, hepatosplenomegaly
Bare lymphocyte syndrome (MHC class I)	AR (6p21.3)	First decade	Sinopulmonary infections	TAP1 (transporter associated with antigen processing) and TAP2 mutations	Chronic lung inflammation
Bare lymphocyte syndrome (MHC class II)	AR	Early infancy	Respiratory tract infections, chronic diarrhea, CNS viral infections	Mutations in RFX5, RFXAP, CIITA, and RFX-B (DNA binding factors)	Autoimmune disease
Chronic mucocutaneous candidiasis	AR	3–5 yr	Candidal infections of mucous membranes, skin, and nails	Unknown	Autoimmune endocrinopathies
Lymphoproliferative syndrome	X-linked (Xq25)	Variable	Variable decrease in T-, B-, and NK-cell function and hypogammaglobulinemia following EBV infection	SAP (SLA-associated protein) defect	Life-threatening EBV infection, lymphoma or Hodgkin's disease, aplastic anemia, lymphohistiocytic disorder
Lymphoproliferative syndrome	AR (10p14–15)	Variable	IL-2 receptor α-chain gene defect	CD25 deficiency, with autoimmunity	

Modified from Boxer L, Blackwood K: Recurrent infection. In Kliegman RM, Nieder ML, Super DM, editors: *Practical strategies in pediatric diagnostics and therapy*, Philadelphia, 1996, WB Saunders.

ADA, Adenosine deaminase; *AR,* autosomal recessive; *dATP,* deoxyadenosine triphosphate; *dGTP,* deoxyguanosine triphosphate; *Ig,* immunoglobulin; *IL,* interleukin; *IL-2R* γ, interleukin-2 receptor gamma chain; *ITP,* idiopathic thrombocytopenic purpura; *PNP,* purine nucleoside phosphorylase; *RA,* rheumatoid arthritis.

expressed on the surface of T cells, making the T cells unable to interact with CD40 molecules on the surface of B cells and macrophages. B cells in such individuals, therefore, cannot undergo isotype switch, and macrophages cannot be activated to produce cytokines such as IL-12. The result is an inability to generate normal antibody responses and a predisposition to infection with intracellular pathogens. The defect in B-cell activation also affects deletion of autoreactive B cells by apoptosis, resulting in the production of autoantibodies.

Common Variable Immunodeficiency

Common variable immunodeficiency (CVID) is a heterogeneous disorder characterized by initial normal immune function that is followed by a severe reduction in serum IgG (generally <250 mg/dL), IgA, and IgM and by recurrent sinopulmonary infections. Antibody titers to protein antigens such as tetanus and diphtheria are absent, but T-cell function (proliferation to mitogens) is normal. B cells may be present. Patients exhibit normal-sized or enlarged tonsils and lymph nodes and may have splenomegaly. Patients also have frequent respiratory tract infections. As many as 50% of patients have gastrointestinal disease (e.g., malabsorption or chronic diarrhea) of unclear etiology, as well as autoimmune diseases such as hemolytic anemia, thrombocytopenia, and neutropenia. Malignancy is observed in 6–16%. These observations suggest that T-cell helper function may also be quantitatively abnormal. CVID is frequently observed in families with IgA deficiency. It may also occur as an idiosyncratic reaction to some drugs (e.g., phenytoin).

Selective IgA Deficiency

Selective IgA deficiency is defined as serum IgA levels below 5–10 mg/dL accompanied by normal or increased levels of other immunoglobulins. It occurs in approximately 1 in 600 individuals. Some patients with selective IgA deficiency are asymptomatic. However, in others it is associated with recurrent sinopulmonary infections, IgG2 subclass deficiency, food allergy, autoimmune or rheumatologic disease, and celiac disease. IgA deficiency occurs in families, suggesting an autosomal inheritance. It also is seen in families with CVID. The genes for IgA deficiency (and for some forms of CVID) may reside in the MHC class III (complement) region on chromosome 6.

Immunoglobulin G Subclass Deficiency

IgG subclass deficiency occurs when the level of antibodies in one or more of the four IgG subclasses is decreased. IgG2 subclass deficiency is the most common of these deficiencies and is often associated with IgA deficiency, ataxia-telangiectasias, and a reduced capacity to produce antibody against carbohydrate antigens. In some patients, IgG2 subclass deficiency resolves spontaneously; in others it progresses to CVID.

Transient Hypogammaglobulinemia of Infancy

Transient hypogammaglobulinemia of infancy is a temporary condition characterized by delayed immunoglobulin production. It is thought to be caused by delayed development of CD4+ T cell helper activity. The normal low point at 3–5 months of age is accentuated, with immunoglobulin levels of less than 200 mg/dL. B and T cells are present, and antibodies can be synthesized to protein antigens such as diphtheria and tetanus toxoid. Immunoglobulin levels remain diminished throughout the first year of life but increase to normal, age-appropriate levels, usually between 18 and 36 months of age. The incidence of sinopulmonary infection is increased.

Specific Therapies for B-Cell Diseases

The *treatment* of X-linked agammaglobulinemia, CVID, and hyper-IgM syndrome is replacement of IgG with intravenous human pooled immunoglobulin (IVIG), 400–500 mg/kg/dose, given every 4 weeks. In spite of IVIG therapy, patients may continue to have sinusitis and bronchitis, requiring aggressive antibiotic therapy and prophylactic antibiotics. Chronic bronchitis and bronchiectasis may develop, in which case chest physiotherapy and serial pulmonary function studies may be useful. Patients with other antibody deficiency states benefit from prophylactic antibiotics, but IVIG should be used in such patients only if prophylactic antibiotic therapy fails and when B-cell responsiveness on antigen challenge is impaired. In all patients appropriate antibiotic therapy is indicated for specific infections as determined by culture and epidemiology (Table 8–1).

Complement Deficiencies

Complement deficiencies are rare diseases that occur when an individual is born without one of the 30 proteins that compose the complement system. The deficiencies may also occur secondary to either increased consumption or decreased synthesis of any of the complement components. Deficiency may result in recurrent pyogenic infection, infection with *Neisseria* species, lupus-like disease, or vasculitis (Table 8–6). Acquired deficiency usually results from consumption of complement components caused by immune complex deposition (e.g., systemic lupus erythematosus, bacterial endocarditis, or hepatitis) or protein loss. Sickle cell disease is associated with a defect in alternative pathway function that is required for opsonization of pneumococci.

TABLE 8–6
Deficiency of Complement and Associated Disease

Deficient Protein	Associated Disease
C1q, C1r	SLE, glomerulonephritis; occasional pneumococcal infection
C2	SLE, arthritis, JRA, recurrent infections in some patients, rare glomerulonephritis
C3	Recurrent infections, rare glomerulonephritis, or SLE
C4	SLE-like disease, pyogenic infection
C5	Recurrent meningococcal or gonococcal infections, rare glomerulonephritis, or SLE
C6	Recurrent meningococcal or gonococcal infections, rare glomerulonephritis, or SLE
C7	Recurrent meningococcal or gonococcal infections, Raynaud phenomenon
C8	Recurrent meningococcal or gonococcal infections
C9	Occasional meningococcal infection, autoimmune disease in some patients
Properdin	Recurrent infections, meningococcemia (often fatal)
Factor H	Glomerulonephritis, meningococcal infection
Factor I	Recurrent infections
C4-binding protein	Collagen-vascular disease
C5a inhibitor	Familial Mediterranean fever
C3b receptor	SLE
C1 inhibitor	Hereditary angioedema

JRA, Juvenile rheumatoid arthritis; *SLE,* systemic lupus erythematosus.

C1 esterase inhibitor deficiency, or hereditary angioedema (HAE), results in recurrent episodes of angioedema lasting 24–72 hours; angioedema is nonpruritic and occurs after trauma, stress, or anxiety. Angioedema can occur in any tissue. Abdominal edema can cause acute abdominal pain, and edema of the upper airway can be life threatening and may necessitate emergency tracheostomy. The *diagnosis* is suggested by family history (the disorder is transmitted as an autosomal dominant trait) and by chronically decreased C4 levels and decreased C2 levels during acute attacks. C1 inhibitor protein is markedly reduced or, if present, is not functional.

Specific *treatment of complement deficiencies* with component replacement is not available; frequent and long courses of antibiotics constitute the therapy. Immunization of patients and close contacts with pneumococcal and meningococcal vaccines may be useful. Patients with C1 esterase inhibitor deficiency and frequent episodes of angioedema respond to prophylactic use of an oral attenuated androgen (stanozolol or danazol), which increases serum concentrations of C1 esterase inhibitor. The use of androgens should be limited, however, because of side effects that include masculinization in females, growth arrest, and hepatitis. For example, prophylactic administration of fresh frozen plasma before surgery can prevent angioedema, but administration during an acute episode may exacerbate the episode. Angioedema of the airway can present as an acute emergency, necessitating tracheostomy, since administration of epinephrine, antihistamines, or corticosteroids is ineffective in reversing this type of angioedema. Purified C1 esterase inhibitor can be used prophylactically (e.g., before surgery) and during acute episodes of angioedema. Angiotensin-converting enzyme (ACE) inhibitors such as captopril should be avoided in patients with C1 esterase inhibitor deficiency because they can precipitate episodes of angioedema by inhibiting degradation of kinins that mediate edema formation.

Mannose-Binding Protein

An antigen-nonspecific humoral factor of major importance in host defense is the *mannose-binding protein.* It binds and opsonizes high mannose–containing glycoproteins on the membranes of bacteria, mycobacteria, and yeast and activates the classical complement pathway. Patients with mannose–binding protein defects exhibit skin infections, sepsis, chronic diarrhea, and failure to thrive.

Disorders of T-Cell Immunity

Because T cells have a wide range of functions, T-cell disorders have a broad range of *clinical manifestations*

(Fig. 8–1 and Table 8–5). Classically, patients with T-cell disorders have infections with fungi or pathogens that proliferate intracellularly in somatic cells and in macrophages (viruses, mycobacteria, toxoplasmosis, and *Leishmania*). CD8+ cytotoxic cells and CD4+ helper T cells that activate macrophages may be absent. In severe T-cell deficiency, B-cell function, which requires T-cell help, may also be impaired, leading to susceptibility to opportunistic infections (e.g., *Candida albicans* or *Pneumocystis carinii*) and severe infections with common pathogens (e.g., varicella, adenovirus, respiratory syncytial virus, parainfluenza virus, cytomegalovirus, and Epstein-Barr virus).

DiGeorge Syndrome

DiGeorge syndrome is the classic example of T-cell deficiency that is the result of dysmorphogenesis of the third and fourth pharyngeal pouches, resulting in hypoplasia of the thymus through which T cells must mature (Fig. 8–1 and Table 8–5). Genetically, the syndrome represents a subset of patients with a field defect on chromosome 22q11.2, the **velocardiofacial syndrome,** or **CATCH 22 syndrome** (*c*ardiac anomalies, *a*bnormal facies, *t*hymic hypoplasia, *c*left palate, and *h*ypocalcemia) (see Chapter 4). DiGeorge syndrome is classically characterized by hypocalcemic tetany, conotruncal and aortic arch anomalies (such as interrupted aortic arch type B, tetralogy of Fallot, and truncus arteriosus), and increased infections.

The *diagnosis* of CATCH 22 is made by fluorescent in situ hybridization (FISH) with a DNA probe to detect microdeletions in chromosome 22q11.2. Immunodeficiency in this syndrome varies markedly; indeed, immunologically significant defects are relatively rare. In severe cases complete absence of T-cell function can occur, resulting in severe combined immunodeficiency (SCID) (lack of both T-cell and B-cell function). In patients with partial thymic function, improvement in T-cell function is observed with time.

Severe Combined Immunodeficiency

SCID is characterized by a profound lack of T-cell and B-cell function (Fig. 8–2 and Table 8–5). Many specific genetic mutations cause this syndrome, and consequently the clinical severity and manifestations of this disease are heterogeneous. In patients with the most common form of SCID, which is caused by mutations in the gene on chromosome Xq13.1 coding for the common γ-chain of the IL-2 receptor (this chain is also used by the receptors for IL-4, IL-7, IL-13, IL-9, and IL-15), no T cells or NK cells are found in the peripheral blood (but normal B-cell numbers are present). Immunoglobulin levels are low or undetectable, and lymph nodes and tonsils are absent.

Clinical manifestations include failure to thrive, severe bacterial infection within the first month of life, chronic candidiasis, infection with *P. carinii* and other opportunistic organisms, and intractable diarrhea. Patients often have skin disease similar to eczema, possibly related to graft-versus-host disease from maternal lymphocytes.

Autosomal recessive forms of SCID can be caused by defects of various tyrosine kinases (e.g., Janus tyrosine kinase 3 [Jak3] or ZAP-70 kinase) that are important in T-cell activation. In **Jak3 deficiency,** B cells can be present in normal numbers but are not functional. In **ZAP-70 deficiency,** normal numbers of nonfunctional CD4+ T cells are present. Mutations in the gene for the α chain of the IL-7 receptor result in SCID, associated with the presence of B cells and NK cells. **Omenn syndrome** is another variant form of SCID that is characterized by exfoliative erythroderma, lymphadenopathy, hepatosplenomegaly, marked eosinophilia, elevated serum IgE, and impaired T-cell function. This syndrome is caused by mutations in the recombination-activating genes RAG1 and RAG2 that are required for immunoglobulin and T-cell receptor gene rearrangement. In **bare lymphocyte syndrome** either MHC class II or MHC class I is deficient because of mutations in genes that regulate expression of class II molecules or genes that affect transport of antigen peptides. Lymphoid tissue and B cells may be present in normal amounts, but CD4+ T cells are absent in class II deficiency, whereas CD8+ cells are absent in class I deficiency.

Adenosine deaminase (ADA) deficiency accounts for about 20% of all SCID patients. It is caused by mutations in the ADA gene on chromosome 20q13, which affects purine metabolic pathways. T cells are particularly sensitive to the accumulation of toxic purine metabolites, especially deoxyadenosine triphosphate and deoxyadenosine. This results in absent or markedly reduced T-cell function, often with absent or reduced B-cell function. Although most patients exhibit severe infection early in life, diagnosis in a number of patients with partial immune function has been made after the age of 5 years. Patients with late onset are generally lymphopenic; they have B cells and normal total immunoglobulin levels but little functional antibody **(Nezelof syndrome).** Immune function in these patients appears to wane with time.

Treatment of Severe T-Cell Disorders. The therapy for severe T-cell disorders is bone marrow or stem cell transplantation, preferably from an HLA-matched sibling. In patients with an accompanying humoral immunodeficiency, IVIG is also useful. Patients with the ADA deficiency form of SCID who lack histocompatible sibling donors can receive repeated intramuscular replacement doses of ADA, stabilized by coupling to polyethylene glycol (PEG-ADA). Gene therapy has been performed in several patients with the γ-chain deficiency form and ADA deficiency form of SCID by transfer of a normal gene into bone marrow stem cells, which were then infused into the patient.

Prenatal *diagnosis* is possible for ADA deficiencies in families with T-cell disorders. Prenatal diagnosis of other immunodeficiency disorders (e.g., Wiskott-Aldrich syndrome, ZAP-70 deficiency, or CD40L deficiency) can be made in specialized laboratories by gene sequencing when DNA or complementary DNA (cDNA) from the index case is available.

Partial Combined Defects

Several disorders feature a combination of T-cell and B-cell defects that are less severe than those of SCID. The **Wiskott-Aldrich syndrome** is an X-linked disorder characterized by thrombocytopenia, eczema, disorders in cell-mediated and humoral immunity, and a predisposition to lymphoproliferative disease. It is caused by mutations of the gene on chromosome Xp11.22 coding for the 53-kD Wiskott-Aldrich syndrome protein (WASP), which is expressed in lymphocytes, platelets, and monocytes. WASP deficiency results in elevated levels of IgE and IgA, decreased IgM, poor responses to polysaccharide antigens, waning T-cell function, and profound thrombocytopenia. Opportunistic infections and autoimmune cytopenias become problematic in older children. **Isolated X-linked thrombocytopenia** also results from mutations of the identical gene. One third of patients with Wiskott-Aldrich syndrome die from hemorrhage, and two thirds die from recurrent infection caused by bacteria, cytomegalovirus, *P. carinii,* or herpes simplex virus. Bone marrow or stem cell transplantation has corrected the immunologic and hematologic problems in some patients.

Ataxia-Telangiectasia

Ataxia-telangiectasia (AT) is a syndrome caused by the ATM (AT, mutated) gene on chromosome 11q22.3, which codes for a phosphatidylinositol-3 kinase. Patients have cutaneous and conjunctival telangiectasias and progressive cerebellar ataxia with degeneration of Purkinje cells. IgA deficiency, IgG2 subclass deficiency of variable severity, low IgE levels, and variably depressed T-cell function may also be seen. The normal function of the ATM gene is not clear, but it appears to be involved in detecting DNA damage, blocking cell growth division until the damage is repaired, or both. AT cells are exquisitely sensitive to irradiation. Leukemias, lymphomas, and diabetes may also be present, and sexual maturation is delayed. There is no uniformly effective therapy for this disease, but antimicrobial therapy and IVIG replacement therapy (with IgA-deficient preparations) may be helpful.

Chronic Mucocutaneous Candidiasis

Patients with CMCC have chronic or recurrent candidal infections of the mucous membranes, skin, and nails. They have normal antibody production but have significantly decreased or absent lymphocyte proliferation and delayed skin reactivity to *Candida*. Patients usually do not respond to topical antifungal therapy and must be treated with oral agents. In most patients, an autoimmune endocrinopathic condition such as hypoparathyroidism and Addison's disease develops by early adulthood. Other autoimmune disorders, such as autoimmune hemolytic anemia, have also been reported. Because the onset of these endocrine disorders can be insidious, patients must be evaluated frequently.

X-Linked Lymphoproliferative Disease

Patients with X-linked lymphoproliferative (XLP) disease have a defect in immune responsiveness to EBV. Boys with this disease are essentially normal until they become infected with EBV (infectious mononucleosis), which is fatal in 80% of patients. A mutation in the SAP gene (also called SH2D1A gene) at chromosome Xq25 codes for an adapter protein that normally inhibits signal transduction in proliferating T cells; in EBV infection the mutation results in extensive expansion of CD8 T cells, hepatic necrosis, and death. Boys who survive the EBV infection have significant hypogammaglobulinemia associated with aplastic anemia and lymphoma. Treatment of the acute EBV infection with prednisone and acyclovir may be helpful, as may VP-16 and anti-CD20 mAb. IVIG for hypogammaglobulinemia is also indicated. Bone marrow transplantation has been attempted in some patients and has prevented disease progression.

Hyper-IgE Syndrome

Patients with hyper-IgE syndrome have markedly elevated serum IgE levels, a rash that resembles atopic dermatitis, and eosinophilia, associated with staphylococcal abscesses of the skin, lungs, joints, and viscera. Infections with *H. influenzae, Candida,* and *Aspergillus* may also occur. These patients have coarse facial features, develop osteopenia, and may have giant pneumatoceles in the lungs following staphylococcal pneumonias. Although serum IgG, IgA, and IgM concentrations are near normal, humoral immune responses to specific antigens are reduced, as is cell-mediated immunity. Chronic treatment with antistaphylococcal medications is indicated, and IVIG therapy may be helpful.

Disorders of the Phagocytic Compartment

Disorders of the phagocytic compartment can be divided into those of deficient cell numbers (see Chapter 14) and those with insufficient function (Table 8–7). They are characterized by mucous membrane infections (e.g., gingivitis and abscesses in the skin and viscera), lymphadenitis, poor wound healing, delayed umbilical cord separation, and absence of pus (in disorders of cell numbers or of leukocyte migration). Microorganisms include *S. aureus*, certain fungi, and gram-negative bacteria.

Chronic Granulomatous Disease

Chronic granulomatous disease (CGD) is a rare disorder of white blood cells that results from defective intracellular killing of bacteria and intracellular pathogens by neutrophils and macrophages. The X-linked form of CGD (the more severe form) is caused by mutations in the gp91-*phox* gene on chromosome Xp21.1. CGD can also be inherited in an autosomal recessive fashion as the result of mutations in several genes (e.g., p22-*phox*, 16q24; p47-*phox*, 7q11.23; or p67-*phox*, 1q25) that result in the failure of the cytochrome b_{558} NADPH system to produce superoxide. Patients characteristically have lymphadenopathy, hypergammaglobulinemia, hepatosplenomegaly, dermatitis, failure to thrive, anemia, chronic diarrhea, and abscesses. Infections occur in the lungs, resulting in chronic bronchitis, as well as in the middle ear, gastrointestinal tract, skin, urinary tract, lymph nodes, liver, and bones. Granulomas may obstruct the pylorus or ureters. Common organisms include catalase-positive bacteria, such as *S. aureus*; enteric gram-negative bacteria (e.g., *Salmonella, Proteus, Klebsiella, E. coli, Serratia marcescens,* and *Burkholderia cepacia*); and fungi (e.g., *Aspergillus fumigatus, C. albicans,* and *Torulopsis glabrata*).

Treatment of Neutrophil Disorders

Frequent courses of antibiotics (trimethoprim/ sulfamethoxazole prophylaxis in the case of CGD)

TABLE 8–7
Phagocytic Disorders

Name	Defect	Comment
Chronic granulomatous disease	Bactericidal	X-linked recessive (66%), autosomal recessive (33%); eczema, osteomyelitis, granulomas, abscesses caused by *Staphylococcus aureus, Burkholderia cepacia, Aspergillus fumigatus;* X-linked defect in cytochrome b produces negative result on nitroblue tetrazolium test
Chédiak-Higashi syndrome (1q42I–44)	Bactericidal plus chemotaxis; poor natural killer function	Autosomal recessive; oculocutaneous albinism, neuropathy, giant neutrophilic cytoplasmic inclusions; malignancy, neutropenia
Hyperimmunoglobulin E (Job syndrome)	Chemotaxis, opsonization	Eczema, staphylococcal abscesses, red hair; granulocyte and monocyte chemotaxis affected; antistaphylococcal IgE
Myeloperoxidase deficiency	Bactericidal, fungicidal	Reduced chemiluminescence; autosomal recessive (1:4000); persistent candidiasis in diabetics
Glucose-6-phosphate dehydrogenase deficiency	Bactericidal	Phenotypically similar to chronic granulomatous disease
Burns, malnutrition	Bactericidal plus chemotaxis	Reversible defects
Lazy leukocyte syndrome	Chemotaxis	Normal bone marrow cells but poor migration; granulocytopenia
Leukocyte adhesion deficiency; CD18 deficiency (21q22.3)	Adherence, chemotaxis, phagocytosis; reduced lymphocyte cytotoxicity	Delayed separation or infection of umbilical cord; lethal bacterial infections without pus; autosomal recessive; neutrophilia; deficiency of LFA-1, Mac-1, CR3
Schwachman syndrome	Chemotaxis, neutropenia	Pancreatic insufficiency, metaphyseal chondrodysplasia; autosomal recessive

and surgical débridement of infections are required. Because *A. fumigatus* can cause serious infection in patients with CGD, moldy hay, decomposing compost, and other nests of fungi must be avoided. The frequency of infection in CGD is also lessened by treatment with recombinant IFN-γ administered subcutaneously 3 times/wk. Recombinant granulocyte-colony-stimulating factor (G-CSF) and granulocyte monocyte-colony-stimulating factor (GM-CSF) also appear to be effective against some forms of neutropenia. Bone marrow transplantation may be needed in other cases.

Clinical Evaluation of Suspected Immunodeficiency Syndromes (Fig. 8–4)

The frequency, type, location, and severity of infections must be assessed. Separate episodes must be differentiated from a relapse or recurrence of a single episode, which often occurs when episodes of otitis media or sinusitis are inadequately treated. Recurrent episodes of severe infection such as meningitis or sepsis are much more worrisome than recurrent otitis media, but antibody deficiency states initially manifest with common infections, such as otitis media and sinusitis. In patients with antibody deficiency states, ciliary dyskinesia, T-cell deficiencies, or neutrophil disorders, infections develop at multiple sites (e.g., ears, sinuses, lungs, and skin), whereas in individuals with anatomic problems (e.g., sequestered pulmonary lobe or ureteral reflux), infections are confined to a single anatomic site, such as a single pulmonary lobe or the urinary tract. Identification of the specific pathogens causing infections is helpful in the evaluation (Tables 8–1, 8–5, and 8–7). Patients with primary immunodeficiency acquire infection with opportunistic organisms that do not ordinarily cause disease.

Recurrent infection in immunologically deficient children is associated with incomplete recovery at sites of infection; this leads to scarring of the tympanic membrane (TM) or of the skin, abnormal hearing, persistent perforation of the tympanic membrane, persistent ear drainage, chronic lung disease, persistent cough and sputum production, failure to thrive, digital clubbing, or anemia of chronic disease. The accrual of substantial morbidity from repeated infections (including minor infections) suggests the presence of significant immunologic disease. In addition, a history of persistent, atypical rashes may suggest immunodeficiency. Atypical, generalized rashes suggest graft-versus-host disease. Persistent eczema or petechiae suggest Wiskott-Aldrich syndrome, and telangiectasia suggests ataxia-telangiectasia. A history of neonatal tetany (DiGeorge), cardiac disease (DiGeorge), micrognathia (DiGeorge), delay in umbilical cord detachment (LFA-1 deficiency), or chronic atypical diarrhea and malabsorption (graft-versus-host disease, CVID, or chronic viral infection) is an important fact that may suggest an immunologic diagnosis. The family history is also critical, because primary immunodeficiencies are genetic diseases. The family history of infants dying from infection or human immunodeficiency virus (HIV) risk factors (see Chapter 10) is important. Because primary immunodeficiency is rare, symptoms consistent with **anatomic disease** or **secondary immunodeficiency** should always be sought.

The height and weight percentiles, nutritional status, and presence of subcutaneous fat should be assessed. Evidence of persistent infection should be sought (e.g., thrush in the mouth, purulent nasal or otic discharge, chronic rales, and scarring of the tympanic membranes or of the skin). Lymphoid tissue, such as the tonsils, and lymph nodes should be examined. Absence of tonsils suggests SCID or X-linked agammaglobulinemia, whereas increased size of lymphoid tissue suggests common variable agammaglobulinemia or HIV infection.

Laboratory Evaluation of Suspected Immunodeficiency

Screening tests can be used initially for many patients (Table 8–8). More specific tests should be reserved for severe disease or for when the history, physical examination, or screening tests suggest a specific immunologic diagnosis (Fig. 8–4).

B-Cell Disease

Patients with B-cell disorders have decreased serum immunoglobulin levels. Normal values vary with age, with a physiologic nadir occurring at 6–8 months of age. Low albumin levels with low immunoglobulin levels suggest low synthetic rates for all proteins or increased loss of proteins (as in nephrotic syndrome or protein-losing enteropathy). High immunoglobulin levels suggest intact B-cell immunity (CGD, immotile cilia syndrome, or cystic fibrosis). Very high levels suggest HIV infection.

In some patients with normal total immunoglobulin levels, it may be important to determine whether antibody function is present (Table 8–8). If titers are low, the patient can be immunized with tetanus, diphtheria, or *H. influenzae* vaccines and with pneumococcal vaccine. Titers are reexamined 2–4 weeks later to check for response to the immunization(s). Inadequate responses to bacterial polysaccharide antigens normally occur before the age of 2 years, but they are also associated with IgG subclass deficiency in older children. Immunoglobulins and antibody

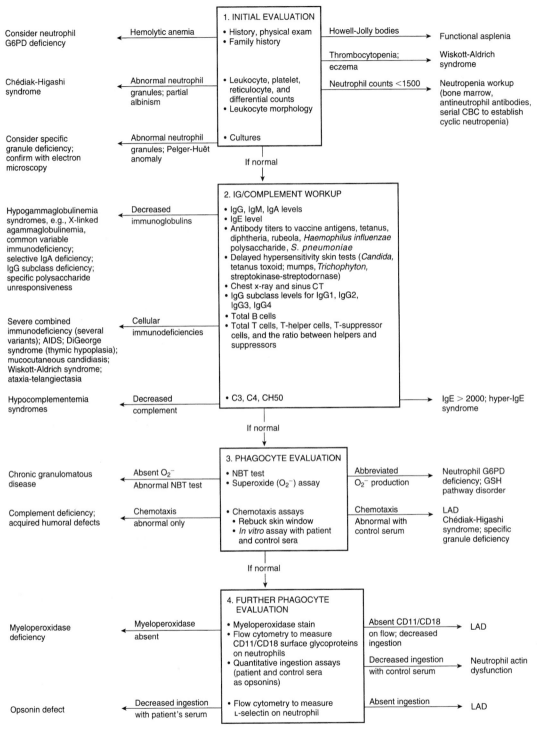

FIG. 8–4

Algorithm for the workup of a patient with recurrent infections. *AIDS,* Acquired immunodeficiency syndrome; *CBC,* complete blood count; *Ig,* immunoglobulin; *G6PD,* glucose-6-phosphate dehydrogenase; *GSH,* reduced glutathione; *NBT,* nitroblue tetrazolium; *LAD,* leukocyte adhesion deficiency syndrome. (From Boxer L, Blackwood R. In Kliegman RM, Nieder ML, Super DM, editors: *Practical strategies in pediatric diagnosis and therapy,* Philadelphia, 1996, WB Saunders.)

TABLE 8–8
Tests for Suspected Immune Deficiency*

General

Complete blood count, including hemoglobin, differential white blood cell count and morphology, and platelet count

Roentgenograms to document infection in chest, sinus, mastoids, and long bones, if indicated by clinical history

Cultures, if appropriate

Erythrocyte sedimentation rate

Antibody-Mediated Immunity

Quantitative immunoglobulin levels: IgG, IgA, IgM, IgE

Isohemagglutinin titers (anti-A, anti-B): measures IgM function

Preexisting antibody levels: diphtheria, tetanus, polio, rubella, *Haemophilus influenzae, Streptococcus pneumoniae*

Cell-Mediated Immunity

Lymphocyte count and morphology

Delayed hypersensitivity skin tests (*Candida,* tetanus toxoid, tuberculin, mumps): measures T-cell and macrophage function

T- and B-cell subset enumeration by FACS analysis

T-lymphocyte function analyses

Phagocytosis

Neutrophil cell count and morphology

Nitroblue tetrazolium dye test

Staphylococcal killing, chemotaxis assay

Myeloperoxidase stain

Complement

Total hemolytic complement (CH50): measures complement activity

C3, C4 levels: measure important pathway components

*Initial screening tests for less severe disease are in bold italics.

---

titers are absent in patients with X-linked agammaglobulinemia. These patients also do not have circulating B cells, as assessed by flow cytometry.

T-Cell Disease

T-cell disorders demonstrate lymphopenia and the absence of delayed type hypersensitivity (DTH) skin test reactions (tetanus, diphtheria, or *Candida*). Because negative DTH reactions are observed in 10–20% of normal individuals, individuals with negative results on DTH tests should receive boosters with tetanus or diphtheria toxoids and should be retested 2–4 weeks later. T-cell (and B-cell) subsets can be assessed by flow cytometry to enumerate total numbers of CD4+ and CD8+ cells, NK cells, and monocytes and to evaluate expression of HLA antigens. In addition, functional T-cell studies—in vitro proliferation of T cells in response to mitogens (phytohemagglutinin, concanavalin A, or pokeweed mitogen) or antigens (tetanus toxoid or *Candida*)—can also be performed. Tests for IL-2, IL-4, or IFN-γ production; expression of IL-2 receptor; and the presence of specific tyrosine kinases may be performed in specialized research laboratories. In patients thought to have DiGeorge syndrome, FISH studies for microdeletions of chromosome 22 can be helpful. In patients suspected of having ataxia telangiectasia, chromosomal studies for multiple breakage of chromosomes 7 and 14 are useful.

Complement Deficiency Diseases

The total hemolytic activity of serum (CH50) is a widely available test dependent on the presence of normal levels of the major components of complement. If the CH50 level is abnormal, individual components must be analyzed in specialized laboratories.

Phagocytic Disease

Evaluation of neutrophil disorders begins with the complete blood count (CBC) and examination of neutrophil number and morphology. Further studies include the nitroblue tetrazolium test (NBT) for chronic granulomatous disease and in vitro tests for evaluation of neutrophil phagocytosis, chemotaxis, and bacterial killing. In addition, tests for expression of CD18 (LFA-1, Mac-1) cell antigens and for myeloperoxidase activity can be performed.

General Management of Patients With Recurrent Infections

Table 8–9 lists guidelines for the management of immunocompromised children. Immediate culture and aggressive antibiotic therapy should be instituted for fever or other manifestations of infection because infection may rapidly disseminate and become life threatening. Continuous prophylaxis with antibacterial, antiviral, or antifungal agents may also be warranted if infection is difficult to control and likely to disseminate rapidly. Infections with uncommonly encountered organisms develop in children with immunodeficiency; poor response to commonly used antibiotics suggests the presence of a resistant or atypical pathogen, which must be specifically identified by culture or biopsy.

TABLE 8–9
General Management of Patients with Immunodeficiency

Avoid transfusions with blood products unless they are irradiated and cytomegalovirus negative.

Avoid live virus vaccines, especially in patients with severe T-cell deficiencies or severe agammaglobulinemia, and in household members.

Follow pulmonary function in patients with recurrent pneumonia.

Use chest physiotherapy, postural drainage in patients with recurrent pneumonia.

Use prophylactic antibiotics, since minor infections can quickly disseminate.

Examine diarrheal stools for *Giardia* and *Clostridium difficile.*

Avoid unnecessary exposure to individuals with infection.

Use intravenous immune globulin for severe antibody deficiency states at a dose of 400–500 mg/kg q3–4 wk IV

REFERENCES

Behrman RE, Kliegman RM, Jenson HB, editors: *Nelson textbook of pediatrics,* ed 16, Philadelphia, 2000, WB Saunders, Chapters 122–134.

Buckley RH: Primary immunodeficiency diseases due to defect in lymphocytes, *N Engl J Med* 343(18):1313–1324, 2000.

Buckley RH: Primary immunodeficiency diseases. In Middleton E Jr, Reed CE, Ellis EF, et al, editors: *Allergy principles and practice,* ed 5, vol 2, St Louis, 1998, Mosby.

Delves PJ, Roitt IM: The immune system, *N Engl J Med* 343(1):37–49 and 343(2):108–117, 2000.

Flake A, Roncarolo M, Puck J, et al: Treatment of X-linked severe combined immunodeficiency by in utero transplantation of paternal bone marrow, *N Engl J Med* 335(24):1806–1810, 1996.

Medzhitov R, Janeway C: Innate immunity, *N Engl J Med* 343(5):338–344, 2000.

Ozsahin H, Le Deist F, Benkerrou M, et al: Bone marrow transplantation in 26 patients with Wiskott-Aldrich syndrome from a single center, *J Pediatr* 129(2):238–244, 1996.

Stiehm ER: *Immunologic disorders in infants and children,* ed 4, Philadelphia, 1996, WB Saunders.

HYPERSENSITIVITY REACTIONS

Hypersensitivity reactions are caused by an untoward, inappropriate immunologic response to a "foreign" substance involving antigen-specific antibody or antigen-specific memory lymphocytes. There are four major types of hypersensitivity reactions.

Type I reactions (IgE-mediated immediate hypersensitivity) are triggered by the binding of antigen to IgE molecules attached to IgE receptors (FcεRI) on the surface of mast cells (or basophils). This results in mast cell degranulation and the release of preformed mediators such as histamine and eosinophil chemotactic factors, causing urticaria, pruritus, mucus production, sneezing, wheezing, and hypotension within 20 minutes. The most severe, life-threatening form of this reaction is *anaphylaxis.* The most common causes of anaphylaxis are penicillin (and other drugs), foods such as peanuts, pollen extracts, latex, and insect venom. Type I reactions against allergens encountered in the respiratory mucosa also cause symptoms of allergic rhinitis and allergic asthma. Four to 12 hours after the initial response, a *late-phase reaction* may develop, characterized by local influx of basophils, eosinophils, monocytes, lymphocytes, and neutrophils and causing persistent, more profound, and difficult-to-manage symptoms. Late-phase allergic inflammatory responses in the respiratory tract are associated with nasal or bronchial *hyperreactivity.* The infiltrating cells in the inflammatory response produce leukotrienes C4, D4, and E4; prostaglandins; and Th2 cytokines IL-4, IL-5, and IL-13, which amplify and prolong allergic inflammation by enhancing the growth and differentiation of eosinophils, basophils, mast cells, and B cells producing IgE.

Type II reactions (antibody cytotoxicity) involve IgG (or IgM) antibodies binding to cell surface or tissue antigens with complement and a variety of Fc receptor-bearing effector cells that damage cells and surrounding tissues. The target antigens can be cell surface membrane antigens such as red blood cell or platelet cell surface molecules, leading to hemolysis or thrombocytopenia, respectively; basement membrane molecules in the kidney, leading to Goodpasture syndrome; the α-chain of the acetylcholine receptor at the neuromuscular junction, resulting in myasthenia gravis; and the thyroid-stimulating hormone (TSH) receptor on thyroid cells, causing Graves disease. Other target antigens include drugs such as quinidine, which when bound to red cell membranes act as haptens, resulting in drug-induced hemolysis via complement activation.

Type III reactions involve the formation of soluble immune complexes of antigen and antibody (often IgG). Large immune complexes are removed by the reticuloendothelial system in the liver, spleen, and lungs; smaller complexes persist in the circulation and localize at the glomerular basement membrane or in the endothelium of other target organs (e.g, synovium or skin). Tissue deposition may be facilitated by the generation of C3a and C5a, which have anaphylactic and chemotactic properties, and occasionally by release of vasoactive amines from mast cells and basophils when antigen-specific IgE is present. Immune-complex activation of complement attracts polymorphonuclear leukocytes, resulting in increased capillary permeability, release of proteases, and tissue damage. Local reactions caused by the injection of antigen into tissue are called **Arthus reactions.** Systemic administration of large amounts of foreign protein, some of which enters the circulation, leads to antigen-antibody complex deposition and **serum sickness,** with a clinical picture of fever, arthralgia, urticaria-like rash, lymphadenopathy, and proteinuria. Other type III–mediated diseases are farmer's lung, caused by inhalation of large quantities of mold spores, and some vasculitic syndromes (e.g., Kawasaki disease and Henoch-Schönlein purpura).

Type IV reactions (delayed hypersensitivity) are mediated by antigen-specific T cells and macrophages and reach their peak 24–48 hours after antigen exposure. Memory T cells recognize antigen peptide/MHC class II complexes on APCs and release inflammatory cytokines (IFN-γ, TNF-α, and GM-CSF) that activate macrophages. Type IV hypersensitivity includes contact hypersensitivity—for example, to pentadecacatechol (poison ivy) or nickel. Classically, tuberculin skin test results manifest the characteristics of type IV reactions. In addition, organ transplant rejection and graft-versus-host disease are type IV reactions.

Atopic Disorders

Atopy is a condition in certain individuals that predisposes toward the development of disorders (e.g., allergic rhinitis, asthma, and atopic dermatitis [eczema]) characterized by elevated IgE production and eosinophilia and thought to be caused by the overproduction of IL-4, IL-5, and IL-13 by CD4+ Th2 cells. Both genetic and environmental factors contribute to the development of the atopy. Children of an atopic parent have a 30% risk for development of an atopic disorder and are more likely to become sensitized when exposed to allergens. Multiple genes predispose toward the development of atopy, although none have been conclusively identified. Candidate genes include the FcεR1β chain of the high-affinity receptor for IgE on chromosome 11q13; genes in a cluster at chromosome 5q31 (IL-4, IL-5, IL-9, IL-13, and the β$_2$-adrenergic receptor); glutathione S-transferase; the IL-4 receptor α; nitric oxide synthase 1; IL-10; and TGF-β.

Despite the existence of several potential genetic causes, genetic factors cannot explain the doubling in the prevalence of allergic disease and asthma that has occurred over the past two decades. The increase in prevalence of atopy may be a result of changes in the environment, such as the reduction in exposure to bacterial infections, which protects against the de-

TABLE 8–10
Disorders Associated with Elevated Serum Immunoglobulin E
Allergic disease
Atopic dermatitis (eczema)
Helminthic infections
Hyperimmunoglobulin-E syndrome
Allergic bronchopulmonary aspergillosis
Wiskott-Aldrich syndrome
Bone marrow transplantation
Hodgkin disease
Bullous pemphigoid
Idiopathic nephrotic syndrome
Mononucleosis

velopment of atopy. For example, the risk of developing asthma is reduced in individuals who have strong tuberculin skin test reactivity, in children living in farming environments (direct exposure to livestock), in children from large families (especially in the youngest siblings), and in children who have been placed in day care before 6 months of age. Passive tobacco smoke exposure has been associated with the development of childhood asthma but not with allergic sensitization. Environmental exposure to pollution such as diesel exhaust can worsen pre-existing conditions such as allergic rhinitis and asthma but does not increase the risk of developing allergic disease. Feeding hydrolyzed formulas or breast milk delays, but does not prevent, the development of allergic disease.

Atopic individuals frequently have elevated levels of serum IgE (other diseases are also associated with elevated IgE) (Table 8–10) and eosinophilia (3–10% or >250 eosinophils/mm^3). Extreme eosinophilia suggests a nonallergic disorder, such as infection with helminth parasites, drug reaction, immunodeficiency, or infiltrative lung disease (eosinophilic pneumonia).

Asthma

Asthma is defined as reversible obstruction of large and small airways as the result of hyperresponsiveness to various immunologic and nonimmunologic stimuli. The disease is intermittent and characterized by recurrent episodes of cough, chest tightness, dyspnea, and wheezing. Among children with asthma, 80–90% have the first episode by 4–5 years of age. In the United States 5 million children have asthma, and the prevalence of asthma is expected to double by 2020. It is the most common chronic disease of childhood and is a leading cause of emergency room visits, hospital admissions, and school absenteeism. The economic cost in the United States is estimated at $14 billion in the year 2000.

Pathophysiology. An allergic-type inflammatory response occurs in the airway mucosa of patients with asthma, resulting in bronchial hyperreactivity, the hallmark of asthma. Bronchial hyperreactivity has been linked to a chromosomal locus (5q31) containing genes for a number of cytokines, including IL-3, IL-4, and GM-CSF. This is consistent with the idea that the airways inflammation in asthma is an allergic type, associated with the production of Th2-type cytokines (IL-4 and IL-5). It is also consistent with the observation that the risk for development of asthma is associated with elevated serum IgE levels and hypersensitivity to perennial allergens. Viral respiratory infection (e.g., respiratory syncytial virus, parainfluenza virus, adenovirus, and rhinovirus), bacterial infection in the large airways and sinuses, or mycoplasmal respiratory infection can also increase airway inflammation and bronchial hyperreactivity.

Three major pathologic events contribute to airway obstruction: mucosal edema, smooth muscle contraction, and production of mucus. Obstruction occurs during expiration as the airway approaches the closing volume, and results in distal airway gas trapping; more severe asthma may have diminished air flow during inspiration. A number of anatomic and physiologic characteristics predispose infants and young children to an increased risk of airway obstruction: smaller airway size, lower elastic recoil of the lung, decreased smooth muscle support of the small airways, relative mucous gland hyperplasia, and decreased collateral channels of ventilation (pores of Cohn) between alveoli.

In the setting of airway hyperreactivity a number of triggers can initiate asthmatic symptoms. These include type 1 hypersensitivity (IgE-mediated) responses to allergens such as dust mites and pollens in sensitized individuals; irritants such as cold air, pollutants, or cigarette smoke; viral infections; and exercise, which acts by increasing the exposure of the airways to cool, dry air. In some individuals, particularly those with nasal polyps, aspirin and other nonsteroidal antiinflammatory drugs (NSAIDs) can trigger severe asthma symptoms, presumably by inhibiting prostaglandin and increasing leukotriene production via blockade of the cyclooxygenase pathway (Table 8–11). **Gastroesophageal reflux** (GER) has been associated with difficult-to-manage asthma, possibly by cholinergic mechanisms or as a direct result of aspiration. **Sinusitis,** a common problem in children, frequently aggravates asthma; **allergic bronchopulmonary aspergillosis** (ABPA) occurs in a small number of difficult-to-treat asthmatic individuals.

Clinical Manifestations and Diagnosis. Wheeze, cough, dyspnea, tachypnea, and chest pain are common during acute exacerbations but are late signs of asthma and may not always be present. A history of persistent cough (cough-variant asthma), night cough, exercise-induced cough, posttussive emesis, and cough following cold air exposure or with laughter is suggestive of asthma.

During acute episodes, the physical examination reveals a hyperinflated chest that is hyperresonant to percussion. Tachypnea, tachycardia, cough, inspiratory and (more usually) expiratory wheezing, a prolonged expiratory phase, and squeaky, musical inspiratory rales are often present. As the attack progresses, the following signs develop: cyanosis, use of accessory muscles of respiration, decreased breath sounds (tight chest) and diminished wheezing, agitation, inability to speak, tripod sitting position, diaphoresis, and increased pulsus paradoxus.

Differential Diagnosis. Causes of wheezing are listed in Table 8–12. Wheezing before 3 months of age suggests another condition, such as infection, pulmonary malformations, cardiac and gastrointestinal abnormalities, or cystic fibrosis (especially in the presence of malabsorption or clubbing, which is not seen in asthma). In infants and toddlers, bronchiolitis caused by respiratory syncytial virus is a common cause of wheezing. A foreign body in the airway or esophagus should be considered in patients above 1–2 years of age who have sudden onset of wheezing or coughing and diminished breath sounds localized to one region.

ABPA results from a hypersensitivity-like reaction in the lung to antigens of the mold *Aspergillus fumigatus.* It is not a result of fungal invasiveness. ABPA has been identified in patients with corticosteroid-dependent asthma, cystic fibrosis, and bronchiectasis.

ABPA often is diagnosed initially as asthma with peripheral eosinophilia; irreversible lung damage may occur before the correct diagnosis is made. In addition, patients often demonstrate marked immediate skin reactivity to *A. fumigatus.* Acute exacerbations are characterized by anorexia, headache, fever, fatigue, and increased sputum production. Rales, wheezing, and bronchial breathing may be present, resembling an acute exacerbation of asthma.

Peripheral blood eosinophils generally are greater than $1000/mm^3$ in cases of ABPA. Large numbers of eosinophils and fungal mycelia may be present in the sputum. Specific IgE or IgG levels (aspergillus precipitans) may be elevated. Administration of high doses of prednisone is the treatment of choice for ABPA because it reduces the clinical symptoms and sputum production, decreases the incidence of

TABLE 8–11
Classification and Treatment of Asthma Severity

Asthma Severity	Symptom Severity	Nighttime Symptoms	Lung Function in Patients Who Can Use a Spirometer or Peak Flow Meter	Short-Acting Beta₂-Agonist Use
Severe persistent	Continual symptoms Limited physical activity Frequent exacerbations interfere with normal activities	Frequent	FEV_1 or PEF ≤60% predicted PEF variability >30%	Daily qid use does NOT completely relieve symptoms
Moderate persistent	Daily symptoms Exacerbations ≥2 times/week; may last days; may affect activities	>1 time/week	FEV_1 of PEF >60% to <80% predicted PEF variability >30%	Daily
Mild persistent	Symptoms >2 times/week but <1 time/day Exacerbations may affect activities	>2 times/month	FEV_1 or PEF >80% predicted PEF variability 20–30%	>2 times/week but <1 time/day
Mild intermittent	Symptoms ≤2 times/week Asymptomatic and normal PEF between exacerbations Exacerbations brief (from a few hours to a few days); intensity may vary	≤2 times/month	FEV_1 or PEF ≥80% predicted PEF variability <20%	≤2 times/week

From American Academy of Allergy Asthma and Immunology: *The allergy report*, Milwaukee, 2000, The Academy.

TABLE 8–12
Differential Diagnosis of Wheezing

Respiratory
Common
Bronchial asthma
Respiratory infection
Foreign body
Cystic fibrosis
Vocal cord dysfunction
Laryngotracheomalacia
Uncommon
Bronchopulmonary dysplasia
Alpha$_1$-antitrypsin deficiency
Allergic bronchopulmonary aspergillosis
Ciliary dyskinesia syndrome
Hypersensitivity pneumonitis
Bronchiectasis
Pulmonary hemosiderosis

Cardiovascular (Uncommon)
Congenital heart disease
Vascular rings and slings
Cardiac failure

Gastrointestinal
Gastroesophageal reflux
H-type tracheoesophageal fistula
Foreign body

Miscellaneous
Immunodeficiency disorders
Vasculitis, collagen-vascular disease
Psychogenic cough
Mediastinal mass (tumor, lymphadenopathy)

(FEV_1), forced vital capacity (FVC), and average flow between 25% and 75% FVC ($FEV_{25-75\%}$) is useful in assessing and monitoring large and small airways obstruction in less symptomatic children. Spirometry with bronchial provocation (exercise or methacholine) is particularly useful in evaluating airway hyperreactivity and in diagnosing asthma when the history is unclear. Such studies can be performed only in cooperative children, usually older than 5–6 years. In the management of chronic asthma, skin testing and radioallergosorbent testing (RAST) are particularly useful in identification of environmental triggers. Skin testing is more sensitive and provides results within 30 minutes, but it cannot be performed in acutely ill children, patients with diffuse skin disease, or those who are receiving antihistamines. It is also unreliable in patients with significant dermatographism.

In status asthmaticus, routine use of arterial blood gases is not needed if pulse oximetry is available. However, during severe episodes of wheezing, arterial blood gases are essential to evaluation of respiratory ventilation. Because of V/Q mismatch (see Chapter 12), hypoxia develops in many patients with severe acute asthma. As airway obstruction worsens and chest compliance diminishes, CO_2 retention develops. In the face of tachypnea, a "normal" Pco_2 (40 mm Hg) suggests moderate to severe disease, whereas hypercapnia, respiratory acidosis, and hypoxia-associated metabolic acidosis indicate severe disease and impending respiratory arrest.

Treatment. The overall goals of therapy are, first, to reverse asthmatic symptoms and, second, to prevent or diminish the frequency of recurrent symptoms, maintain normal or close to normal pulmonary function, and maintain normal activity levels, including exercise. Although treatment of asthma in inpatient and emergency department settings is common, the ultimate goal is prevention of serious exacerbations requiring hospital-based therapy. In the management of chronic asthma, there are four components to therapy:
1. Patient education
2. Assessment and monitoring of asthma severity with objective measures of lung function
3. Avoidance or control of asthma triggers
4. Establishment of comprehensive plans of pharmacologic therapy, including plans for managing exacerbations (Table 8–13)

Patient education provides information and training to enhance the effectiveness of and improve compliance with recommended therapy. Successful education involves improving patient skills in the use of spacer devices for metered-dose inhalers (MDIs), in the use of peak flow monitoring, and in the use of self-management and environmental con-

positive sputum cultures, and clears roentgenographic lesions. The total serum IgE level typically declines within 2 months of initiation of prednisone therapy in patients with ABPA. Adjunctive therapy with itraconazole may be beneficial.

Laboratory Findings. The evaluation of patients with suspected moderate to severe asthma includes radiographic examination of the chest with both posteroanterior and lateral views to identify anatomic abnormalities, atelectasis, pneumomediastinum, pneumothorax, foreign bodies, or neoplasms. Such x-ray studies are particularly important in patients who respond poorly to bronchodilators. Peak expiratory flow rate (PEFR) monitoring is helpful in assessing the severity of disease and response to therapy in the acute phases of asthma. Spirometry, with measurement of forced expired volume in 1 second trol measures. Education also includes information about medications and their side effects and about when and how to respond to changes in symptoms.

The severity of asthma exacerbation is often underestimated by patients and physicians; therefore, objective assessment and monitoring of asthma severity and lung function are essential to prevent undertreatment and potentially fatal asthma (Table 8–11). Measurement of respiratory function with home peak-flow monitoring, which can be performed in children older than 5 years, improves compliance by providing patients the capacity to self-manage their disease and allowing more appropriate use of asthma medications. Peak flow determinations between 50% and 80% of a patient's personal best efforts necessitate changes in medical therapy, and repeated determinations below 50% of a patient's personal best efforts may necessitate acute intervention.

Specific triggers for asthma (e.g., allergens and cigarette or wood-burning stove smoke exposure) should be identified, and steps to avoid or reduce exposure should be instituted; avoidance of such triggers can decrease airway inflammation and hyperresponsiveness. With individuals allergic to dust mites, house dust mite control measures should be followed, including encasement of mattresses and pillows in nonpermeable covers, removal of carpets, and elimination of mites from stuffed toys. With patients allergic to animal dander, exposure to animals should be minimized, preferably by removal of the household pet. Aspirin and other NSAIDs and beta-blocker drugs should be avoided.

Pharmacologic treatment complements environmental avoidance measures and is based on disease severity and the frequency of symptoms. In patients with chronic asthma, pharmacologic intervention focuses on preventive, *antiinflammatory therapies* (Tables 8–11 and 8–13). Such agents include inhaled cromolyn sodium (Intal) and nedocromil sodium (Tilade), which inhibit mast cell degranulation. Both drugs inhibit early- and late-phase allergen-induced bronchospasm and acute bronchospasm after exercise or cold air; neither is a bronchodilator. Both are useful as prophylactic agents in children with mild asthma, particularly since they have virtually no known side effects. However, these agents are not particularly helpful in children with moderate to severe disease.

Inhaled corticosteroids (ICSs) represent another type of antiinflammatory agent. These include fluticasone (Flovent), budesonide (Pulmicort) (available as a nebulized solution and as a metered dose inhaler), beclomethasone (Vanceril or Beclovent), triamcinolone (Azmacort), and flunisolide (AeroBid), and *oral corticosteroids*. ICSs are generally safe and provide extremely effective therapy for chronic asthma. Regular use decreases airway hyperreactivity, reduces the need for rescue bronchodilator therapy, and decreases the risk of hospitalization and of death from asthma. Side effects caused by local drug-carrier deposition include dysphonia and oral candidiasis; these can be decreased by using a spacer device and rinsing the mouth after inhalation (or by using a dry-powder inhaler). Although effective in severe asthma, long-term, high-dose regimens of ICS in doses above 1 mg/day may be associated with systemic effects such as slowing of linear growth, suppression of the hypothalamic-pituitary-adrenal axis, cataracts, glaucoma, dermal thinning, and decreased bone density. Although the newer ICSs such as fluticasone have greater topical potency with reduced systemic availability compared with older ICSs, use of these potent corticosteroids in high doses can be associated with side effects. However, these adverse effects are significantly less than those associated with chronic use of *oral* corticosteroids. Long-term use of oral corticosteroids should be reserved for chronic asthma only if other therapies fail. If possible, an alternate-day oral dosage schedule is preferable to daily oral use because alternate-day therapy reduces (but does not eliminate) the incidence of side effects such as decreased linear growth, weight gain, hypertension, diabetes, cataracts, immunosuppression, and osteoporosis. The side effects associated with short courses (<7 days) of oral corticosteroids are significantly less than those associated with long-term use. Short courses of oral corticosteroids are beneficial in minimizing acute exacerbations in moderate to severe asthma.

Selective *beta$_2$-adrenergic agonists* are useful for the treatment of both acute and chronic asthma but alone do not give long-term control because they do not affect airway inflammation. Beta$_2$-adrenergic agonists relax airway smooth muscle, enhance mucociliary clearance, and may decrease mediator release from mast cells and basophils. They are available as metered-dose inhalers that are more effective when used with spacer devices and as nebulized aerosol, which is particularly useful in young children. Although beta$_2$-adrenergic agents are also available for oral administration, these cause more numerous and severe side effects (e.g., cardiovascular stimulation, tremor, and hypokalemia) than do inhaled agents. *Short-acting* inhaled beta$_2$-adrenergic agents are beneficial for *acute* exacerbations of asthma, for the pretreatment of exercise-induced asthma, and for rescue (quick-relief) therapy in the treatment of chronic asthma. Some of these agents are albuterol sulfate (Proventil, Ventolin), pirbuterol (Maxair), bitolterol mesylate (Tornalate), and levalbuterol (Xopenex). Levalbuterol, the R-isomer of racemic albuterol, may have fewer side effects than albuterol, but the difference between the two forms

TABLE 8-13
Stepwise Approach for Managing Asthma in Infants and Children With Chronic Asthma Symptoms—cont'd

	Infants and Young Children (≤5 Years of Age)		Children > 5 Years of Age	
	Long-Term Control	Quick Relief	Long-Term Control	Quick Relief
Step 4: Severe Persistent	Daily antiinflammatory medications: High-dose inhaled corticosteroid with spacer/holding chamber and facemask If needed, add systemic corticosteroids 2 mg/kg/day and reduce to lowest daily or alternate-day dose that stabilizes symptoms	Short-acting bronchodilator as needed for symptoms. Intensity of treatment depends on severity of exacerbation Either: inhaled short-acting beta$_2$-agonist by nebulizer or MDI with spacer/holding chamber and facemask OR oral beta$_2$-agonist **Daily or increasing use of short-acting inhaled beta$_2$-agonists indicates need for additional long-term control therapy**	Daily medications: High dose inhaled corticosteroids, AND Long-acting bronchodilator (e.g., long-acting inhaled beta2-agonist or sustained-release theophylline) Leukotrienes modifiers may be considered, although their position in therapy is not fully established If required, oral corticosteroid	Short-acting bronchodilator: inhaled beta$_2$-agonist as needed for symptoms; intensity of treatment depends on severity of exacerbation **Daily or increasing use of short-acting inhaled beta$_2$-agonist indicates need for additional long-term control therapy**
Step 3: Moderate Persistent	Daily antiinflammatory medications: Either: medium-dose inhaled corticosteroid with spacer/holding chamber and facemask OR once control is established, low to medium-dose inhaled corticosteroid and nedocromil OR low to medium-dose inhaled corticosteroid and long-acting bronchodilator (theophylline)	Short-acting bronchodilator as needed for symptoms; intensity of treatment depends on severity of exacerbation Either: inhaled short-acting beta$_2$-agonist by nebulizer or MDI with spacer-holding chamber and facemask OR oral beta$_2$-agonist **Daily or increasing use of short-acting inhaled beta$_2$-agonists indicates need for additional long-term control therapy**	Daily medication: Either: medium-dose inhaled corticosteroid OR low-to-medium dose inhaled corticosteroid Plus: long-acting bronchodilator: (e.g., long-acting inhaled beta2-agonist or sustained-release theophylline) Leukotriene modifiers may be considered, although their position in therapy is not fully established In needed, medium-to-high dose inhaled corticosteroids and long-acting broncho-dilator, especially for nighttime symptoms	Short-acting bronchodilator: inhaled beta$_2$-agonist as needed for symptoms; intensity of treatment depends on severity of exacerbation **Daily or increasing use of short-acting inhaled beta$_2$-agonist indicates need for additional long-term control therapy**

Step 2: Mild Persistent	Daily antiinflammatory medications: Either: Cromolyn (nebulizer preferred, or MDI) or nedocromil (MDI) tid-qid Infants and young children usually begin with a trial of cromolyn or nedocromil OR low-dose inhaled corticosteroid with spacer/holding chamber and facemask	Short-acting bronchodilator as needed for symptoms; intensity of treatment depends on severity of exacerbation Either: inhaled short-acting beta$_2$-agonist by nebulizer or MDI with spacer/holding chamber and facemask OR oral beta$_2$-agonist **Daily or increasing use of short-acting inhaled beta$_2$-agonists indicates need for additional long-term control therapy**	One daily medication: Either: low-dose inhaled corticosteroid, OR Cromolyn or nedocromil Sustained-release theophylline (to serum concentration of 5–15 μg/mL) is an alternative, but not preferred, therapy Leukotriene modifiers may be considered although their position in therapy is not fully established
			Short-acting bronchodilator: inhaled beta$_2$-agonist as needed for symptoms; intensity of treatment depends on severity of exacerbation **Daily or increasing use of short-acting inhaled beta$_2$-agonist indicates need for additional long-term control therapy**
Step 1: Intermittent	No daily medication	Short-acting bronchodilator as needed for symptoms occurring more than two times a week; intensity of treatment depends on severity of exacerbation Either: inhaled short-acting beta$_2$-agonist by nebulizer or MDI with spacer/holding chamber and facemask OR oral beta$_2$-agonist **2 times weekly or increasing use of short-acting inhaled beta$_2$-agonists indicates need for additional long-term control therapy**	No daily medication
			Short-acting bronchodilator: inhaled beta$_2$-agonist as needed for symptoms; intensity of treatment depends on severity of exacerbation **Use of short-acting inhaled beta$_2$-agonist >2 times per week indicates need for additional long-term control therapy**

Step Down
Review treatment every 1 to 6 months; a gradual stepwise reduction in treatment may be possible

Step Up
If control is not maintained, consider step up. First, review patient medication technique, adherence, and environmental control (avoidance of allergens and/or other factors that contribute to asthma severity)

From American Academy of Allergy, Asthma, and Immunology: *The allergy report*, Milwaukee, 2000, The Academy.

does not appear to be clinically significant. If frequent or regularly scheduled use of short-acting inhaled beta$_2$-adrenergic agents is required for symptomatic control, inhaled antiinflammatory agents should be added to control symptoms, because chronic use of inhaled beta$_2$-adrenergic agents alone has been associated with diminished control of asthma. *Long-acting* inhaled beta$_2$-adrenergic agents such as salmeterol xinafoate (Serevent) have a duration of action of more than 12 hours and are particularly useful for treating *chronic asthma* that is unresponsive to inhaled antiinflammatory agents alone. These long-acting agents are also useful for treating nighttime cough. Adding salmeterol to ICS therapy has been shown to be more effective than increasing the dose of ICS in terms of rescue albuterol use, symptom scores, and measures of pulmonary function. A new single inhaler containing both salmeterol and fluticasone (Advir Diskus) may also improve compliance. Long-acting agents must not be used for acute exacerbations.

Among other antiinflammatory agents are *leukotriene antagonists* and *lipoxygenase inhibitors.* Montelukast (Singulair) and zafirlukast (Accolate), both oral leukotriene D4 receptor antagonists, and zileuton (Zyflo), a 5-lipoxygenase inhibitor, have been shown to be modestly effective in the treatment of mild intermittent or mild persistent asthma. These medications are not bronchodilators, but the first dose of leukotriene receptor antagonists may rapidly and significantly improve pulmonary function. Although they are less effective as monotherapy than are inhaled corticosteroids, leukotriene antagonists may be used as adjunctive measures for the treatment of chronic asthma, particularly in patients with aspirin sensitivity. Zafirlukast and zileuton are both metabolized by cytochrome P450. Patients taking zileuton must be monitored for hepatic toxicity. Zafirlukast cannot be taken with food, because food significantly decreases the drug's bioavailability.

Sustained-release preparations of *theophylline,* a bronchodilator with mild antiinflammatory effects, are occasionally used for the treatment of asthma. However, theophylline use can be associated with significant adverse effects, including gastrointestinal symptoms, behavior problems, cardiovascular effects, and seizures. These effects can be reduced substantially by using low doses, aiming for serum levels of 5–10 µg/mL rather than the "therapeutic levels" of 10–20 µg/mL. Serum levels must be monitored when high doses are administered, to prevent the development of adverse side effects, because liver metabolism is altered with febrile illness, pregnancy, liver disease, congestive heart failure, or concomitant use of ciprofloxacin, cimetidine, or macrolide antibiotics, except azithromycin (Zithromax). Theophylline

can be recommended when inhaled corticosteroids and inhaled beta$_2$-adrenergic agents fail to control symptoms, particularly nocturnal asthma, and if patient compliance is improved by once-daily or twice-daily oral (rather than inhaled) medication.

Anticholinergic agents, such as ipratropium bromide (Atrovent), are available in metered-dose inhalers and as nebulized solutions. These drugs are potent bronchodilators that may also block reflex bronchoconstriction caused by inhaled irritants. They are less effective as bronchodilators than beta$_2$-adrenergic agents for the treatment of asthma but may be useful when nebulized together with a beta$_2$-adrenergic agent, especially for acute exacerbations.

Subcutaneous or intravenous therapy with a *humanized anti-IgE monoclonal antibody* (rhuMAb-E25) has recently been shown to improve peak flow and quality-of-life scores significantly, reduce the frequency of asthma exacerbations, and reduce β-agonist and oral corticosteroid use in patients with asthma. However, the cost of the drug is not yet clear, nor is which subgroups of patients would benefit most from use of anti-IgE monoclonal antibody.

Treatment with *allergen immunotherapy* should also be considered in patients with stable allergic asthma. Multiple studies have demonstrated its effectiveness in patients with asthma who are sensitized to allergens such as cat dander, dust mites, mold, and grass, ragweed, and tree pollens. In addition, allergen immunotherapy can prevent the progression from allergen sensitization to the development of asthma in patients with allergic rhinitis, thus altering the course of asthma and eventually curing patients. Patients with asthma have an increased risk of systemic reactions from immunotherapy. Therefore, patients with brittle asthma or frequent exacerbations are not candidates for immunotherapy. However, concomitant therapy with anti-IgE monoclonal antibody (rhuMAb-E25) may decrease the adverse allergic reactions associated with allergen immunotherapy.

Selection of specific medications or combinations depends on the severity of the asthma. Consideration is given to patient preference for oral versus inhaled medications and to the side effect profile in individual patients. Table 8–13 illustrates a stepwise approach to therapy, in which the number and frequency of medications are increased with increasing asthma severity. The goal is to achieve optimal symptom control with the least possible medication. If symptoms develop while a specific regimen is being prescribed, the next higher step in therapy is recommended. Plans for medical treatment of symptomatic exacerbation and for responding to changes in peak expiratory flow should be written out for every patient as part of the educational program for asthma self-management. Treatment of associated sinusitis or gastroesophageal reflux is essential.

Emergency Treatment. In patients with significant airway hyperreactivity, asthma exacerbation can readily occur secondary to viral respiratory infection, acute sinusitis, bronchitis, or exposure to a major trigger (allergen). Exacerbation is characterized by significant respiratory distress, dyspnea, wheezing, cough, and major reduction in peak expiratory flow rates. Deterioration may progress over several days or occur precipitously, and it may range in severity from mild to life threatening. Evaluation should include assessment of the degree of cyanosis, breathlessness, mental status, respiratory rate, accessory muscle use, wheezing, pulsus paradoxus, PEFR, and oxygen saturation (in room air). In the emergency department, treatment should include repetitive administration of inhaled beta$_2$-agonists, oxygen, and early use of systemic corticosteroids. Epinephrine by subcutaneous or intramuscular injection is rarely indicated and is reserved for acute anaphylaxis or severe asthma unresponsive to continuous administration of inhaled beta$_2$-agonists. Arterial blood gases should be obtained if the PEFR is 30–50% of predicted value, if severe distress persists after initial treatment, or when oxygen saturation remains below 90% in room air. If the patient responds well to therapy (PEFR >70% of predicted, oxygen saturation >95% in room air, and marked reduction or elimination of symptoms), discharge is indicated, with a step-up in maintenance medication and plans for outpatient follow-up.

Hospital admission is indicated if:
1. Patient response is inadequate and symptoms persist.
2. PEFR is below 70% of predicted value, particularly in patients at high risk for death (e.g., recent withdrawal from systemic corticosteroids, hospitalization or emergency care for asthma in the past year, previous intubation for asthma, psychiatric disease or psychosocial problems, or noncompliance with asthma medication plan).
3. Respiratory arrest is impending (e.g., signs of deterioration, confusion, Po_2 <60 mm Hg, and/or Pco_2 >40–45 mm Hg).

Inpatient therapy for asthma includes the use of inhaled beta-agonists up to every 1–2 hours or the use of beta-agonists by continuous nebulized aerosols and systemic corticosteroids (methylprednisolone, 2–4 mg/kg/24 hr, divided every 6 hours). Intravenous aminophylline (5 mg/kg loading dose, followed by 0.7–1.2 mg/kg/hr infusion) or intravenous terbutaline may be beneficial in patients who do not respond to aerosols and intravenous steroids; endotracheal intubation with mechanical ventilation may be required in the event of severe hypoxia and respiratory failure. Sedation is contraindicated unless the patient is intubated.

Discharge from the hospital is appropriate when:
1. Inhaled beta-agonists are being used no more than every 4 hours.
2. Clinical findings are normal or near normal.
3. PEFR is above 70–80% of predicted value after the use of a short-acting inhaled beta$_2$-agonist.
4. PEF variability is below 20%.
5. Asthma education has been initiated (correct use of inhaler devices, development of an action plan, and plans for discharge medication and outpatient follow-up understood, as appropriate, by patient and parent).

Prognosis. Although asthma can be a fatal disease, the long-term prognosis of childhood asthma is good. Most children with an onset of asthma before the age of 5 years are symptom free by adolescence. Risk factors for persistence of asthma include severe asthma, concurrent allergic rhinitis, dust mite and cat allergies, a family history of asthma, lower respiratory tract infection in infancy, and maternal smoking. In patients who are dependent on corticosteroids, Cushing habitus, growth failure, acne, osteoporosis, cataracts, and opportunistic infections may develop.

REFERENCES

Adkinson NF, Eggleston PA, Eney D, et al: A controlled trial of immunotherapy for asthma in allergic children, *N Engl J Med* 336(5):324–331, 1997.

American Academy of Allergy Asthma and Immunology: *The allergy report,* Milwaukee, Wis, 2000, The Academy.

Behrman RE, Kliegman RM, Jenson HB, editors: *Nelson textbook of pediatrics,* ed 16, Philadelphia, 2000, WB Saunders, Chapters 141, 145.

Drugs for asthma, *Med Lett* 42:19–24, 2000.

Harding SM, Richter JE, Guzzo MR, et al: Asthma and gastroesophageal reflux: acid suppressive therapy improves asthma outcome, *Am J Med* 100(4):395–405, 1996.

Keeley D, Rees J: New guidelines on asthma management, *BMJ* 314(7077):315–316, 1997.

McFadden ER, Hejal R: Asthma, *Lancet* 345(8959):1215–1220, 1995.

Postma DS, Bleecker ER, Amelung PJ, et al: Genetic susceptibility to asthma-bronchial hyperresponsiveness coinherited with a major gene for atopy, *N Engl J Med* 333(14):894–900, 1995.

Strachan D, Carey IM: Home environment and severe asthma in adolescence: a population based case-control study, *BMJ* 311(7012):1053–1056, 1995.

Suissa S, Dennis R, Ernest P, et al: Effectiveness of the leukotriene receptor antagonist zafirlukast for mild-to-moderate asthma, *Ann Intern Med* 126(3):177–183, 1997.

von Mutius E: The environmental predictors of allergic disease, *J Allergy Clin Immunol* 105(1 pt 1):9–19, 2000.

Allergic Rhinitis

Allergic rhinitis is the most prevalent chronic condition in the pediatric population. Estimates of the prevalence of allergic rhinitis in children range from 5–40%. Although not a life-threatening disorder, allergic rhinitis is a significant problem in terms of morbidity and health care costs, impeding education within the classroom, limiting outdoor or indoor activity, and predisposing to the development of sinusitis, otitis media, and asthma.

Pathogenesis. Allergic rhinitis is caused by a type I allergic response, either to wind-borne pollens of grasses, trees, and weeds (classified as *seasonal allergic rhinitis*) or to house dust mite allergen, pet dander, or mold spores (classified as *perennial allergic rhinitis*). Both types of rhinitis may occur concomitantly.

Clinical Manifestations. Symptoms of allergic rhinitis include chronic, recurrent sneezing; nasal congestion; clear rhinorrhea; and pruritus of the nose, eyes, soft palate, and ears. Patients frequently rub the nose with the palm of the hand *(allergic salute)* or rub the soft palate with the tongue, producing clucking sounds. Allergic symptoms, such as sneezing, classically occur immediately (within 20 minutes) following exposure to an offending allergen. Often, a more severe and persistent reaction, with nasal congestion, sneezing, and rhinorrhea, occurs 6–12 hours later. Seasonal symptoms caused by tree pollen occur in late winter and early spring (in temperate climates), whereas symptoms caused by grasses occur in the spring to early summer. Symptoms caused by weeds occur in the late summer. In perennial allergic rhinitis, chronic rather than intermittent exposure to allergen results in less acute symptoms than in seasonal rhinitis, which often obfuscates associations between exposure and onset of symptoms. Prominent symptoms in such patients include significant nasal congestion and snoring. Although seasonal allergic rhinitis rarely begins before the second year of life, perennial allergic rhinitis may occur occasionally before 2 years of age if exposure to indoor allergens is great. Patients with allergic rhinitis often have a personal or family history of asthma or atopic dermatitis.

The *physical examination* demonstrates a clear nasal discharge and enlarged, often pale, turbinates. A transverse nasal crease may be present, secondary to the chronic practice of the allergic salute. The sclera may be injected, pruritic, and rarely edematous (chemosis); the lower eyelids may be darkened with **allergic shiners** from venous stasis and creased with **Dennie's lines** from intermittent edema. In severe perennial rhinitis, an "allergic facies" with mouth breathing, high arched palate, and dental malocclusion or overbite is observed. **Cobblestoning** of the posterior pharynx from lymphoid hyperplasia is also seen. Nasal polyps (gray, glistening membranous tissue, often with fine blood vessels) are uncommon and are seen mainly in older allergic children and adults. When **vernal conjunctivitis** is present, the palpebral conjunctiva is cobblestoned. A **geographic tongue** is common in atopic patients. The middle ear may contain fluid or may be infected. Examination of the chest may reveal wheezing, rales, or rhonchi. Signs of asthma and atopic dermatitis may be present.

Laboratory Findings. The specific allergens to which the patient is allergic can be identified by (immediate) skin tests or by in vitro serum testing (RAST). For inhalant allergens, skin testing is sensitive and less costly and gives results in minutes rather than days, as is the case with RAST. Skin testing can provoke significant anxiety in young children. Identification of allergens is critical if specific environmental control measures are to be prescribed or if allergen immunotherapy is contemplated. Another relevant laboratory study is nasal cytology, which may show eosinophils (instead of neutrophils, as in sinusitis). An elevated serum IgE level suggests the presence of allergic disease. Because considerable overlap exists between the values of normal and allergic individuals, the total IgE test has low sensitivity and low specificity. IgE is also elevated in other conditions (Table 8–10).

Differential Diagnosis. Problems that may be confused with allergic rhinitis are noted in Tables 8–14 and 8–15.

Treatment. The treatment of allergic rhinitis is based on disease severity, impact of the disease on the patient, and expected capacity of the patient to comply with recommendations. Treatment modalities include:

1. Environmental control and avoidance of allergens
2. Pharmacologic therapy (systemic and topical)
3. Allergen immunotherapy

Less severe disease can be treated solely with the first modality.

Environmental Control. Indoor allergens include many agents. Specific control measures should be guided by symptom history and by results of skin testing that identify specific allergens. The house dust mite is a major indoor allergen, particularly in humid and warm conditions. Dust mite control measures are focused on reducing mite content in reservoirs, primarily mattresses, pillows, carpets, stuffed toys, blankets, and upholstered furniture. Environmental control measures (e.g., covering, cleaning, or eliminating mite reservoirs) are very effective and should especially be applied within the bedroom. Exposure to pet dander and wind-borne pollens is somewhat more difficult to manage, but avoidance measures can be effective in reducing symptoms. Measures include avoidance of outdoor activity during high pollen count days, use of air conditioning and HEPA filters, washing hands and face and

TABLE 8–14
Differential Diagnosis of Nasal Symptoms in Childhood

Congenital
Choanal atresia
Posterior choanal stenosis
Encephalocele
Dermoid cyst
Glioma
Syphilis

Anatomic
Septal anatomic deviation
Adenoidal hypertrophy
Foreign body

Inflammatory
Eosinophilic
Allergic
Nonallergic (NARES)
Neutrophilic (infection)
Nasopharyngitis
Sinusitis
Nasal polyps

Inflammatory—cont'd
Mastocytosis
Granulomatous (Wegener)

Noninflammatory
Rhinitis medicamentosa
Vasomotor rhinitis
Hypothyroidism, pregnancy, oral contraceptive agents
Cerebrospinal fluid rhinorrhea
Encephalocele

Neoplastic
Benign
Angiofibroma
Papilloma
Hemangioma
Malignant
Lymphoma
Rhabdomyosarcoma
Neuroblastoma

NARES, Nonallergic rhinitis with eosinophilia syndrome.

TABLE 8–15
Differential Diagnosis of Rhinitis

Diagnosis	Character of Nasal Discharge	Comments
Allergic rhinitis		
Seasonal rhinitis	Clear	Acute symptoms
Perennial rhinitis	Clear	Chronic nasal congestion and allergic shiners
Viral upper respiratory infection	Clear	Symptoms last 7–10 days; associated with sore throat, fever, poor appetite, exposure to others with upper respiratory infection
Sinusitis	Purulent or clear	Symptoms last >10 days, associated with cough, headache, and halitosis; abnormal sinus CT
NARES (nonallergic rhinitis with eosinophilia syndrome)	Clear	Negative skin tests; eosinophils on nasal smear
Vasomotor rhinitis	Clear	Profuse nasal discharge triggered by exercise, strong odors, cold air or heat
Rhinitis medicamentosa	Clear	Caused by overuse of topical decongestants
Nasal polyps	Purulent or clear	Associated with cystic fibrosis, the aspirin triad (aspirin sensitivity, asthma, nasal polyps with chronic/recurrent sinusitis), and chronic rhinitis

changing clothing after outdoor activity to remove pollen, and removing pets from the home (or at least keeping them out of the bedroom).

Symptom Therapy. *Topical nasal corticosteroids* (Flonase, Rhinocort, Nasonex, Vancenase, and Beconase) are the most effective agents for treatment of allergic rhinitis. They provide the greatest benefit for the broadest range of symptoms. They are the first-line therapy for patients who have prominent symptoms of nasal congestion and blockage. Systemic effects rarely occur in children. Systemic corticosteroids are generally not indicated for the treatment of allergic rhinitis.

Antihistamines (H_1 antagonists) are safe and effective medications for the treatment and prevention of allergic reactions. They are particularly useful in controlling the symptoms of sneezing, nasal pruritus, and rhinorrhea but generally are not effective for the treatment of nasal congestion. Although diphenhydramine (Benadryl) and hydroxyzine (Atarax) are effective in relieving acute allergic reactions, these should be avoided because they are especially sedating. Loratadine (Claritin), cetirizine (Zyrtec), and fexofenadine (Allegra) are nonsedating (but costly) antihistamines; the first two are available as both pills and liquids. A topical form of antihistamine, azelastine (Astelin), is also available, but systemic absorption of this can cause sedation and some patients dislike the bitter taste.

Topical decongestants, such as oxymetazoline hydrochloride (Afrin) and phenylephrine hydrochloride (Neo-Synephrine) should not be used for the treatment of allergic rhinitis because prolonged use causes severe rebound edema *(rhinitis medicamentosa).* *Oral decongestants,* such as pseudoephedrine (Sudafed), are effective in relieving symptoms of nasal obstruction but have significant potential side effects. Combination oral antihistamine-decongestant products are available (Claritin D and Allegra D).

Cromolyn sodium 4% nasal solution (Nasalcrom), a *topical mast cell stabilizer,* is effective in preventing the symptoms of allergic rhinitis and is quite safe. However, it is not as effective as nasal steroids or antihistamines and must be used 4–6 times per day to achieve maximum benefit. *Leukotriene modifiers* (montelukast [Singulair], zarfirlukast [Accolate], and zileuton [Zileuton]) may be effective therapy in allergic rhinitis. Ipratropium bromide (Atrovent nasal spray 0.03%, 0.06%) is used primarily for vasomotor rhinitis and rhinitis associated with viral upper respiratory infection, but it can also be used as adjunctive therapy for allergic rhinitis associated with profuse nonpurulent rhinorrhea.

Immunotherapy. Allergen immunotherapy, which involves the subcutaneous administration of increasing doses of allergen, is highly effective in the patient with allergic rhinitis in whom specific allergens are identified. It decreases clinical symptoms by reversing established allergen sensitivities through a process called *immune deviation,* in which the activity of allergen-specific Th2 cells is reduced. Immunotherapy is the only treatment currently available that alters the natural course of and potentially cures allergic disease. This effect is maintained for years after cessation of immunotherapy in patients who have been treated for at least 3 years. Because of the costs involved (of time, pain, and money), allergen immunotherapy is generally reserved for older children with relatively severe allergic rhinitis. However, given that immunotherapy has now been shown to prevent polysensitization and also prevent the progression toward asthma, more liberal use should be considered. As a result of a small but real risk of anaphylaxis, allergen immunotherapy must be administered in a physician's office, where treatment for systemic reactions is readily available.

REFERENCES

Behrman RE, Kliegman RM, Jenson HB, editors: *Nelson textbook of pediatrics,* ed 16, Philadelphia, 2000, WB Saunders, Chapter 144.

Beltrani VS, editor: Atopic dermatitis, *J Allergy Clin Immunol* 104(3 Pt 2):S85–S98, 1999.

Berhisel-Broadbent J, Sampson HA: Food hypersensitivity and atopic dermatitis, *Pediatr Clin North Am* 35(5):1115–1130, 1988.

Tan B, Weald D, Strickland I, et al: Double-blind controlled trial of effect of house dust mites allergen avoidance on atopic dermatitis, *Lancet* 347(8993):15–18, 1996.

Atopic Dermatitis

Atopic dermatitis (AD), or eczema, is a common skin disorder of infancy and childhood, affecting 3–5% of children before 5 years of age. In approximately 50% of affected children, atopic dermatitis develops within the first year of life; in 80%, it occurs within the first 5 years. Eczema has a genetic component, such that 70% of affected children have first-degree relatives exhibiting some form of allergic disease; in 50–80% of children with eczema, allergic rhinitis or asthma develops later.

Pathogenesis. Abnormalities within the skin and in lymphocytes may contribute to the pathogenesis of AD. Patients have a reduced threshold for pruritus and irritant responsiveness. The skin reacts abnormally to light strokes (white dermographism) and demonstrates abnormal rates of cooling and warming, which suggests the existence of an abnormal balance between beta-adrenergic and cholinergic activity. Pruritus leads to skin trauma inflicted by scratching, which plays an important role in exacerbating the skin lesions and can lead to skin infections. Abnormal cutaneous cellular immune responses also predispose to skin infections with viruses (e.g., herpes simplex, vaccinia, molluscum contagiosum, and papillomavirus), fungi (e.g., *Trichophyton rubrum* and *Pityrosporum ovale*), and bacteria *(S. aureus)*.

Because AD is seen in immunodeficiency (with Wiskott-Aldrich and Omenn syndromes) but is eliminated after bone marrow transplantation, bone marrow–derived cells also appear to be involved. Serum IgE levels are elevated in 80–85% of patients with AD. Elevated levels of Th2 cytokines (IL-4, IL-5, and IL-10) are observed in the skin lesions of patients.

Food allergies can be demonstrated in 35–40% of infants and young children with moderate to severe AD. The most common food allergies seen in patients with AD are the usual offenders—milk, soy, egg, wheat, and peanut. Improvement in AD can be seen after the causal food(s) is removed from the diet. Because most food allergies resolve by 3–4 years of age (with several exceptions, including peanut), the food(s) usually can be reintroduced later. Aeroallergen exposure (e.g., to dust mites), either by inhalation or by direct contact, can also exacerbate AD.

Diagnosis and Clinical Manifestations. Because AD has no specific feature or laboratory marker, the diagnosis is based on the history and physical findings (Table 8–16).

The most useful clue is the distribution of the lesions, which is very typical but varies with age. In the infantile form (2 months to 5 years) the face, extensor surface of the arms, and chest are affected with erythematous papules and vesicles. The diaper area is spared. In older children (4–12 years), the lesions appear in the antecubital and popliteal fossa and on the wrists and hands. Typically the lesions are erythematous, dry, papular, excoriated or lichenified, and hyperpigmented. In the adult form the dorsal surface of the hands and feet, the eyelids, the neck, the flexor folds, and the upper arms are affected. Associated findings include pityriasis alba (scaly, hypopigmented patches of skin, worse with sun exposure) and keratosis pilaris (keratinized papules at the mouths of hair follicles, usually on the extensor surfaces of arms and thighs).

The *prognosis* in most patients with atopic dermatitis is extremely good, with a tendency for remission at 3–5 years of age. Approximately 75% of patients outgrow the problem by adolescence. Any "eczematoid" lesion can have the appearance of, and must be distinguished from, atopic dermatitis (Table 8–17).

Laboratory Findings. In rare circumstances, laboratory studies and skin biopsy are performed to rule out other diseases that may mimic AD. Skin tests or RAST may be useful if food allergy is suspected but should be performed mainly when aggressive skin care fails.

Treatment. The goals of therapy are to assess disease severity, which will vary with time, and to provide appropriate measures to control the symptoms. General measures include reduction or avoidance of triggers such as chemicals, frequent handwashing, overuse of soap, allergens, wool or acrylic clothing that can dry or irritate the skin, and overheating and stress that can increase pruritus. Because pruritus is a significant feature of AD and because injury to the skin from scratching aggravates the disease, fingernails should be trimmed often.

TABLE 8–16
Criteria for the Diagnosis of Atopic Dermatitis in Children

Major Features (Must Have Three)	Minor or Less Specific Features—cont'd
1. Pruritus	3. Ichthyosis, hyperlinear palms, or keratosis pilaris
2. Typical morphology and distribution	4. IgE reactivity (increased serum IgE, RAST, or prick test positivity)
a. Facial and extensor involvement during infancy and early childhood	5. Hand or foot dermatitis
b. Flexural lichenification by adolescence	6. Cheilitis
3. Chronic or chronically relapsing dermatitis	7. Scalp dermatitis (cradle cap)
4. Personal or family history of atopy	8. Susceptibility to cutaneous infections (especially *Staphylococcus aureus* and herpes simplex)
Minor or Less Specific Features	9. Perifollicular accentuation (especially in pigmented races)
1. Xerosis	
2. Periauricular fissures	

Modified from Hanifin JM: *Pediatr Clin North Am* 38(4):763–789, 1991.
IgE, Immunoglobulin E; *RAST,* radioallergosorbent test.

TABLE 8–17
Differential Diagnosis of Atopic Dermatitis

Disease	Comment
Seborrheic dermatitis	Usually on scalp (cradle cap), sides of nose, with greasy, scaly lesions
Diaper dermatitis	Diaper area spared by atopic dermatitis
Contact dermatitis	Generally not chronic and recurring; distribution on exposed sites
Tinea dermatitis	Found in skin folds (neck, diaper area) rather than with distribution of atopic dermatitis
Langerhans cell histiocytosis (histiocytosis X)	Lesions generally hemorrhagic
Psoriasis	Lesions of raised plaques with sharply demarcated, irregular borders and silvery scales, occurring mainly on scalp, knees, elbows, and genitalia
Pyoderma	Lesions generally pustular
Other	

Immunodeficiency disorders (Wiskott-Aldrich syndrome, severe combined immunodeficiency disease, Omenn syndrome, hyper-IgE syndrome, Leiner disease [C5 deficiency], ataxia-telangiectasia, agammaglobulinemia)
Metabolic disorders (Hartnup syndrome, phenylketonuria, histidinemia, pellagra, acrodermatitis enteropathica [zinc deficiency], biotinidase deficiency)
Ectodermal dysplasia, ichthyosis
Scabies

Skin hydration can significantly reduce pruritus and therefore is a major component of therapy. Although frequent baths with water can result in drying of the skin, which has led some physicians to recommend limitations on bathing, improved skin hydration can be achieved by baths and showers one to four times per day, followed *immediately* by the application of lubricants to trap moisture in the skin. Depending on the severity of the problem, fragrance-free creams, mineral oil, or petroleum jelly (e.g., Vaseline) can be used, but never lotions. More severe disease requires greater occlusion, but greater occlusion can occasionally result in folliculitis, particularly in hot weather. Conversely, increased occlusion (as well as humidification of the air) is required in winter months, when drying of the skin is worse because of the use of indoor heat.

Another major component of treatment is the use of *topical steroids,* which are applied to affected skin, usually only on erythematous areas. These agents decrease pruritus, reduce inflammation, and cause vasoconstriction. Topical steroids are available in different strengths and in different vehicles. Compared with creams, ointments provide better penetration and therefore increased potency, whereas gels and lotions often dry the skin. Only low-potency steroids (e.g., 1% hydrocortisone) should be used on the face, to avoid skin atopy. High-potency steroids (e.g., 0.05% fluocinonide and 0.1% halcinonide) should be avoided except for limited periods of time and in limited areas, because systemic side effects can occur if large areas of the body are treated.

Systemic steroids are not necessary for the treatment of AD.

A third component in the treatment of AD consists of *antihistamines,* which are very effective in decreasing pruritus. Frequently used agents include hydroxyzine (Atarax, Vistaril); diphenhydramine (Benadryl); cetirizine (Zyrtec), a metabolite of hydroxyzine without the sedative effects of hydroxyzine; and doxepin (Sinequan), a tricyclic compound with potent H_1 and H_2 receptor blocking action. Topical doxepin (Zonalon cream) may be used for short periods. Because pruritus and scratching are usually worse at night, nighttime doses of oral antihistamines are important.

Because of the potential local and systemic side effects of topical corticosteroids, especially with long-term use of high-potency formulations in patients with severe AD, alternative treatments have been sought. The most promising of these new therapies is topical tacrolimus (FK506) ointment. The ointment has a broad range of antiinflammatory activities and has been shown to be highly effective in treating AD. It has good percutaneous penetration but does not appear to have any systemic side effects. Tacrolimus does not cause skin atrophy because it does not affect collagen synthesis.

TABLE 8–18
Mechanisms for Development of Adverse Reactions to Food

Mechanism	Example
IgE-mediated allergy	Anaphylaxis, urticaria, angioedema (peanuts, eggs)
Delayed allergic responses	Atopic dermatitis
Immune (non-IgE) mediated	Celiac disease, cow's milk protein enteropathy, eosinophilic gastroenteropathy
Food poisoning (toxins)	Botulism, *Staphylococcus aureus*, *Bacillus cereus*, *Escherichia coli*
Infection	Viral, *Salmonella*, *Shigella*
Pharmacologic effect	Caffeine, alcohol, tyramine, histamine
Gastrointestinal disorders	Peptic ulcer disease, lactase deficiency, cholelithiasis, inflammatory bowel disease
Reaction to additives	Sodium nitrate headaches, monosodium glutamate (headache, flushing), sorbitol (diarrhea)
Metabolic	Organic acidemias, hyperammonemias
Psychogenic	School phobia

Most patients respond to treatment with good skin care, topical steroids, and antihistamines. In children who are resistant to such care, food allergies should be sought. In addition, patients with AD are more likely to develop fungal skin infections. Therefore, it is critical that scaly, erythematous lesions without the usual distribution of AD and that are unresponsive to the usual therapy for eczema be examined for hyphae and treated with antifungal medications instead of topical steroids.

Disease severity in a particular patient waxes and wanes. Acute exacerbations, caused by increased scratching, stress, heat, or infection, are characterized by increased pruritus and the development of new skin lesions. These episodes should be treated with more aggressive skin care, including more frequent baths or cool soaks, one to four times per day. When lesions become crusted, weepy, or vesicular, infection with *S. aureus* or herpes simplex (eczema herpeticum) should be suspected. Steroid medications and emollients should be discontinued at the involved sites. Staphylococcal infections should be treated with topical povidone, soaks with Burow's solution, and topical or systemic antibiotics if necessary, whereas herpes simplex infections can be treated with topical or systemic acyclovir.

REFERENCES

Behrman RE, Kliegman RM, Jenson HB, editors: *Nelson textbook of pediatrics*, ed 16, Philadelphia, 2000, WB Saunders, Chapter 146.
Beltrani VS, editor: Atopic dermatitis, *J Allergy Clin Immunol* 104(3 Pt 2):S85–S86, 1999.
Berhisel-Broadbent J, Sampson HA: Food hypersensitivity and atopic dermatitis, *Pediatr Clin North Am* 35(5):1115–1130, 1988.
Tan BB, Weald D, Strickland I, et al: Double-blind controlled trial of effect of housedust-mites allergen avoidance on atopic dermatitis, *Lancet* 347(8993):15–18, 1996.

Food Allergy

Adverse reactions to foods are common. When severe reactions such as anaphylaxis occur immediately after ingestion, identifying the offending food may be easy. However, if symptoms are more vague (as in headache, fatigue, increased irritability, behavior disorders, colic, diarrhea, and vomiting) and do not occur immediately after ingestion of the food, identification of an offending food can be extremely difficult. Much of this difficulty is a result of the fact that reactions to foods can occur via multiple mechanisms (Table 8–18), most of which are poorly understood. Food reactions are difficult to identify because reliable tests for *non*–IgE-mediated reactions are not available. To minimize the confusion regarding adverse reactions to food, the term "food allergy" is defined here as an abnormal response to a food that is triggered by an IgE-mediated immunologic reaction. IgE-mediated food reactions occur with higher frequency in families in which atopic diseases occur.

Clinical Manifestations

Symptoms of food allergy include urticaria, exacerbation of atopic dermatitis, angioedema, nausea, vomiting, abdominal pain and diarrhea, wheezing, nasal congestion, sneezing, laryngeal edema, and anaphylaxis. In infants, food allergies may cause colic, vomiting, feeding problems, or growth failure. In young children, other reactions such as colitis, intestinal blood loss, and malabsorption may occur, in which case the mechanism may include T cells or immune complexes rather than IgE. Most food allergies in young children resolve with time, although IgE-mediated allergies to specific allergens (e.g., peanuts), which can be particularly severe, remain for life.

Diagnosis and Laboratory Findings

The diagnosis of food allergy is based on a careful history, with regard to the reproducibility of the reaction, timing of the reaction (reactions occurring soon after ingestion are more likely to be confirmed), and response to elimination of the food from the diet. The most common foods causing IgE-mediated reactions are cow's milk, eggs, legumes (peanuts and soy), shellfish, and wheat. Adverse reactions resulting from food poisoning, pharmacologic effects, and gastrointestinal disorders must be ruled out. A positive family history of food allergy or atopic dermatitis is common. IgA deficiency may be present. The specific problematic food must be identified so that specific dietary recommendations can be made.

Skin tests (or RAST) for foods can be performed to confirm IgE-mediated food allergies. The sensitivity of these tests is good, such that a negative result can eliminate the likelihood of IgE-mediated food allergy and can provide a guide for elimination diets and food challenge. However, food skin testing has a relatively low specificity; results may be positive in patients not experiencing allergic reactions to the particular food. Positive results with skin tests or RAST need to be confirmed by response to diet elimination and reintroduction (except in the case of severe reactions with a clear-cut history). Open oral challenges can also be performed.

The gold standard for diagnosis of food allergies is the double-blind, placebo-controlled food challenge (DBPCFC). It is a more definitive but more time-consuming test than RAST or skin testing. With this method, the patient is given increasing oral doses of the suspected food, placed in gelatin capsules in a blinded fashion. Only about 40% of suspected food allergies by history are confirmed by this test.

Treatment

Treatment for food allergy is dietary avoidance of the offending food or foods, with a diet that continues to meet the child's nutritional requirements. In infants, non–IgE-mediated allergy to cow's milk or soy (frequency, ~2–7% of all infants) can be treated with hypoallergenic formulas, such as Pregestimil, Nutramigen, or Alimentum. With older children, the patient or parent must read food product labels carefully and communicate effectively with restaurants and schools to avoid the offending foods. Some foods, such as celery, are easily eliminated from the diet. Careful dietary planning is needed to avoid other foods, such as milk, eggs, and wheat, which are added to many different products. Overzealous dietary restriction may cause malnutrition and failure to thrive; therefore, substituted foods must be recommended. Because accidental ingestion of offending foods can occur despite precautions, antihistamines and bronchodilators for mild reactions and epinephrine for more severe reactions (e.g., anaphylaxis) should be available for administration. Patients with a history of food-induced anaphylaxis should be taught how to self-administer epinephrine using an EpiPen or Ana-Kit and should wear a Medic-Alert bracelet.

Prevention

In children with a strong family history of atopic disease, delayed exposure to food antigens may inhibit or postpone the development of food allergy. Breast-feeding as the only source of nutrients for 6 months is nutritionally sound and may prevent or delay the development of allergy. Because antigens from foods ingested by the mother are excreted into breast milk, breast-feeding decreases but does not eliminate exposure of the infant to food allergens. If breast-feeding is not possible, the infant at risk may be fed hydrolyzed milk-based formulas. Some recommend that eggs, fish, and nuts be avoided by such infants until 12 months of age.

REFERENCES

Behrman RE, Kliegman RM, Jenson HB, editors: *Nelson textbook of pediatrics*, ed 16, Philadelphia, 2000, WB Saunders, Chapter 153.
Bock SA: Prospective appraisal of complaints of adverse reactions to foods in children during the first 3 years of life, *Pediatrics* 79(5):683–688, 1987.
Sampson HA, Mendelson L, Rosen JP: Fatal and near-fatal anaphylactic reactions to food in children and adolescents, *N Engl J Med* 327(6):380–384, 1992.
Sampson HA: Food allergy, *J Allergy Clin Immunol* 103(5):717–728 and 103(6):981–989, 1999.
Yunginger JW: Lethal food allergy in children, *N Engl J Med* 327(6):421–422, 1992.

Anaphylaxis

Anaphylaxis is an acute, generalized allergic reaction that is immune mediated. IgE cross-linking by allergen results in mediator release from tissue mast cells and peripheral blood cells, leading to systemic symptoms. An *anaphylactoid reaction* is clinically similar or identical to anaphylaxis, but it is not immunologically mediated. It occurs in the absence of an antigen-antibody interaction (e.g., with radiocontrast material or opioids).

Etiology. Antigen can be introduced by inhaled, oral, topical, and parenteral routes. Most cases of anaphylaxis are caused by the following:

1. Hypersensitivity to drugs (e.g., antibiotics, blood products)
2. Food (e.g., peanuts, egg, seafood, milk)
3. Latex (particularly in patients with myelodysplasia or multiple surgeries)
4. Insect stings

Penicillin causes anaphylaxis more frequently than any other drug. Latex allergy has increased in prevalence, in part as a result of universal precautions that have led to more frequent glove use in the healthcare setting. Exposure to latex can occur through several routes: mucous membranes (catheters), skin, intravascular, and inhalation (from glove powder). Occasionally, in recurrent idiopathic anaphylaxis or exercise-induced anaphylaxis, no etiologic agent is found.

Pathophysiology. Anaphylaxis is a type I hypersensitivity reaction mediated by IgE bound to mast cells, leading to release of granules containing histamine, tryptase, tumor necrosis factor (TNF), prostaglandin D2, leukotriene C4, and platelet-activating factor (PAF) and to the release of IL-1, IL-4, IL-5, and IL-6. Histamine, TNF, and PAF all cause the production of nitric oxide, which results in vascular dilation and leakage. Agents that directly cause mast cell degranulation (opiates and complement components) do induce interleukin production but do not cause late-phase reactions.

Clinical Manifestations and Diagnosis. The symptoms of anaphylaxis are generalized urticaria, inspiratory stridor, laryngeal edema, difficulty swallowing, wheezing, nasal congestion, abdominal cramps, diarrhea, hypotension (decreased systemic vascular resistance and increased vascular permeability), and vascular collapse. Sneezing, pruritus (especially of the hands and soles), a feeling of impending doom, or hoarseness in the throat and dysphonia may initiate the episode. Life-threatening manifestations usually involve respiratory symptoms (e.g., upper airway obstruction or bronchospasm) or cardiovascular involvement. The severity of the reaction is often proportional to the rapidity of onset and in general parallels the magnitude of the stimulus.

Anaphylaxis can be *protracted* or *biphasic*, presumably as a result of the development of late-phase responses. Concurrent illness, underlying asthma, or use of beta-blockers (Inderal) can also predispose to a more severe episode of anaphylaxis. Vasovagal reactions (bradycardia, nausea, weakness, sweating, and hypotension), hypoglycemic reactions to insulin, sepsis, and cardiac arrests can mimic and must be distinguished from anaphylaxis. These episodes are not associated with skin manifestations (except for diaphoresis). Elevated histamine or tryptase levels can retrospectively help in diagnosis of the problem, as can cautious skin testing or RAST to specific antigens.

Treatment. Successful treatment of anaphylaxis requires prompt recognition and the immediate institution of appropriate therapy. The causative agent should be identified and exposure discontinued. Epinephrine 0.01 mL/kg (up to 0.3–0.5 mL) subcutaneously or intramuscularly is indicated. If anaphylaxis is caused by an insect sting or allergy shot, another dose of epinephrine is indicated at the site of the sting or shot and a tourniquet should be placed around the involved extremity. Supplemental oxygen should be administered and the patient's airway assessed and maintained. Intubation or tracheotomy may be required. If the blood pressure is reduced, IV fluids (normal saline, 10–20 mL/kg or more if needed) should be administered. An epinephrine drip may be started if necessary. Diphenhydramine, 1–2 mg/kg IM, IV, or PO, can be administered first in less severe cases or concurrently with epinephrine in more severe cases. Cimetidine, an H_2 receptor antagonist, may also be helpful in a dose of 4 mg/kg. Corticosteroids, such as methylprednisolone (Solu-Medrol) IV, or prednisone, 1–2 mg/kg PO, when given early, may be helpful in limiting late-phase or prolonged responses. Inhaled bronchodilator therapy (albuterol sulfate) or aminophylline may also help patients with wheezing.

Patients having anaphylaxis who improve rapidly with treatment should be observed closely for late-phase reactions, which may occur 8–12 hours after the initial episode.

Prevention. The management of known causes of anaphylaxis focuses on avoidance. Patients with latex allergy need to be aware of the many products that may contain latex, such as balloons, pacifiers, and bath toys. Schools and healthcare providers should be notified so that latex precautions may be taken. Some patients may also need to avoid avocado, banana, kiwi, and chestnut because these can cross-react with latex.

Patients with a history of severe bee-sting anaphylaxis benefit from immunotherapy with bee venom and from appropriate measures to avoid insects (including avoidance of perfumes, bright-colored clothes, and walking barefoot outdoors). Patients with a history of food, bee-sting, or latex allergy and anaphylaxis should also be taught how to self-administer epinephrine using an EpiPen or Ana-Kit. They also should wear a Medic-Alert bracelet and should have antihistamines available.

Patients taking beta-blockers who are at risk for another anaphylaxis episode should be given a substitute for the beta-blocker if possible. Patients with radiocontrast allergy who require repeated imaging should be pretreated with oral steroids and antihistamines and given only low-ionic-strength contrast agents.

In rare instances, patients with a history of egg anaphylaxis may be at risk for anaphylaxis when given vaccines that contain egg protein (influenza and yellow fever vaccines). Skin testing with these vaccines before vaccine administration is prudent, and rapid desensitization can be performed in the event of a positive skin test result. Measles, mumps, rubella (MMR) vaccine (produced in chicken fibro-blasts) does not contain sufficient egg antigens to cause anaphylaxis in allergic patients, although caution is advised when MMR vaccine is given to such patients.

REFERENCES

American Academy of Allergy Asthma and Immunology: *The allergy report 2000*, Milwaukee, Wis, 2000, The Academy.

Behrman RE, Kliegman RM, Jenson HB, editors: *Nelson textbook of pediatrics*, ed 16, Philadelphia, 2000, WB Saunders, Chapter 148.

Bochner B, Lichtenstein L: Anaphylaxis, *N Engl J Med* 324(25): 1785–1790, 1991.

Yunginger JW: Anaphylaxis, *Curr Prob Pediatr* 22(3):130–146, 1992.

Penicillin Hypersensitivity

Penicillin is the most common cause of serious allergic drug reactions in children. Anaphylaxis has been reported to occur after parenteral, oral, topical, and inhalational administration, although parenteral treatment is the most likely route to produce anaphylaxis (in approximately 0.02% of treatments). Conversely, because of inappropriate diagnosis, as many as 85% of patients reported to have had some reaction to penicillin may be able to tolerate the drug on readministration.

Pathophysiology. Penicillin is a low-molecular-weight compound that is unable to elicit an immune response unless it combines with a carrier, such as a protein, polysaccharide, or cell membrane. When penicillin G (benzylpenicillin) is degraded, the beta-lactam ring opens and reacts with tissue proteins to form the benzylpenicilloyl (BPO) group, which is referred to as the "major determinant" because approximately 95% of benzylpenicillin reacts in this manner. The remaining available haptens, or "minor determinants," account for 5% of products, but these determinants are more important in inducing IgE production and in causing immediate reactions.

Penicillin can elicit antibody responses of all major classes and can also produce delayed-type hypersensitivity. Immediate reactions occurring within 1 hour after administration are mediated by IgE that is directed against the minor determinants and on rare occasions against the major determinants. Accelerated reactions, occurring between 1 and 72 hours, and delayed reactions, occurring later than 72 hours after administration, are mediated by BPO-specific IgE, which may be modified by the presence of BPO-specific IgG acting as a "blocking antibody." BPO-specific IgG and IgM have been associated with hemolytic anemia, maculopapular eruptions, and urticaria. Delayed-type hypersensitivity reactions have been associated with contact dermatitis.

Clinical Manifestations. Penicillin may produce a wide variety of hypersensitivity reactions. Reactions may be systemic (e.g., anaphylaxis or vasculitis), cutaneous (e.g, urticaria, angioedema, or maculopapular eruptions), hematologic (e.g., Coombs-positive hemolytic anemia), and renal (e.g., interstitial nephritis). Occasionally, penicillin may be responsible for more severe cutaneous eruptions, such as Stevens-Johnson syndrome, exfoliative dermatitis, and toxic epidermal necrolysis.

A maculopapular, nonurticarial rash occurs during *ampicillin* administration in 5–10% of patients. This rash is non–IgE-mediated and does not correlate with a history of penicillin therapy. The incidence of the rash is higher in certain viral infections, such as mononucleosis and cytomegalovirus. The maculopapular eruption is not necessarily an indication to discontinue the drug, and the rash may resolve despite continued therapy. To avoid falsely labeling patients as allergic to penicillin, the physician should distinguish between penicillin hypersensitivity and the ampicillin rash.

Diagnosis. The diagnosis of penicillin hypersensitivity can be made by skin testing. Skin testing with both the major and minor determinants must be performed to detect the full spectrum of IgE activity. The major determinant is commercially available as a benzylpenicilloyl polylysine (Pre-Pen). The minor determinants are not commercially produced but are available at certain medical centers. Some persons sensitized to minor determinants can be identified by skin tests with diluted penicillin G. Skin testing is performed with a combination of prick testing and, if results are negative, intradermal testing with appropriate dilutions of the above antigens. Testing with both Pre-Pen and penicillin G identifies 95% of potential reactors. Skin tests are not predictive in non–IgE-mediated reactions.

Treatment. The treatment of a penicillin reaction is discontinuation of the drug. If penicillin administration is mandatory in a penicillin-allergic patient, penicillin desensitization may be necessary. The desensitization procedure varies with the level of sensitivity and the route of drug administration. Desensitization has been successfully accomplished using the oral, subcutaneous, and intravenous routes. The desensitization process involves the administration of gradually increasing amounts of drug over a short time by personnel experienced in the procedure and capable of treating anaphylaxis. Once penicillin has been stopped for more than 48 hours following a desensitization procedure, the patient is no longer considered "desensitized" and future administration would require similar precautions.

REFERENCES

Behrman RE, Kliegman RM, Jenson HB, editors: *Nelson textbook of pediatrics*, ed 16, Philadelphia, 2000, WB Saunders, Chapter 150.
Boguniewicz M, Leung D: Hypersensitivity reactions to antibiotics commonly used in children, *Pediatr Infect Dis J* 14(3): 221–231, 1995.

Insect Hypersensitivity

Stinging Insects

Allergic reactions to insect stings result in significant morbidity in children. Stinging female insects of the order Hymenoptera include honeybees, wasps, yellow jackets, hornets, and fire ants. Although most allergic reactions occur in individuals younger than 20 years of age, children are at lower risk than adults for subsequent serious systemic reactions.

Clinical Manifestations. Reactions are classified as *immediate*, occurring within minutes to several hours after the sting, or *delayed*, occurring from several hours to weeks after the sting (Table 8–19). The prevalence of sensitization (positive result on the skin test or RAST) in the general population is 10–30%, whereas anaphylaxis, the most serious reaction, occurs in only 1–2% of the population. Symptoms of anaphylaxis may involve the skin (e.g., generalized urticaria, flushing, or angioedema), the cardiovascular system (e.g., circulatory collapse and hypotension), the respiratory tract (e.g., upper airway edema of the pharynx, epiglottis, and trachea, or bronchospasm), and gastrointestinal tract (e.g., diarrhea or cramps).

Pathophysiology. Venom-specific IgE antibodies are produced following an initial exposure to insect venom and become bound to tissue mast cells and circulating basophils. Local reactions are the result of venom-associated histamine, formic acid, hyaluronidase, and kinins. After a sting, degranulation and release of mediators may result in local signs and symptoms or in anaphylaxis.

Diagnosis. A positive history of immediate systemic reaction is necessary before venom testing and immunotherapy should be considered. Identifying the offending insect is helpful but usually difficult. Information that may help in diagnosis includes a description of the insect and its nest (including location). The honeybee has a barbed stinger that remains embedded after a sting. Even unprovoked, the more aggressive yellow jacket and hornet may sting repeatedly.

Laboratory Findings. Venom skin testing is the most sensitive means of detecting venom-specific IgE. Five purified venoms are available: honeybee, yellow jacket, wasp, white hornet, and yellow hornet. Whole-body extract is available for fire ants. No good correlation exists between severity of the systemic reaction and degree of skin test positivity. Venom-specific IgE antibodies may also be measured by in vitro tests, although 15–20% of patients with positive skin tests do not have positive immunoassays.

TABLE 8–19
Classification of Sting Reactions

Immediate	
Normal	Localized swelling (<2 inches), transient pain, erythema, all lasting less than 24 hr
Toxic	Follows multiple stings, produced by exogenous vasoactive amines in venom
Large local	Swelling contiguous to sting lasting more than 24 hr
Systemic	Generalized symptoms involving signs or symptoms remote from sting site; may be non-life-threatening (distal urticaria, angioedema), or life-threatening (laryngeal edema, bronchospasm, hypotension)
Delayed	
Systemic	May take several clinical forms, including serum sickness–like reactions, myocarditis, transverse myelitis, nephrosis

Treatment. Avoiding brightly colored clothing and exterminating infested areas decrease the risk of accidental stings. Local reactions should be treated initially by removing the stinger if present, cleaning the site, applying cold compresses, and administering oral antihistamines and analgesics. In cases of severe, large local reactions, a short course of prednisone may be recommended.

Treatment of systemic reactions should be very aggressive. Epinephrine, 0.01 mL/kg of a 1:1000 solution (with a maximum of 0.3 mL), is the drug of choice instead of an antihistamine, although both drugs may be administered concurrently. Theophylline, pressor agents, and intravenous colloid solutions may be necessary for more severe reactions. Glucocorticoids are not first-line drugs for the systemic reactions because of their delayed onset of action, but they should be administered to prevent recurrent or prolonged symptoms.

Patients who are at risk for systemic reactions should be instructed in the use of injectable epinephrine. Automatic injections, such as EpiPen (delivering 0.3 mg) and EpiPen Jr. (delivering 0.15 mg), are especially useful.

Venom *immunotherapy* is recommended for pediatric patients exhibiting a systemic reaction that involves the cardiovascular or respiratory tracts, but not for patients having only cutaneous reactions. Children who have had anaphylaxis to insect stings carry a 10% risk that a systemic reaction will occur again on re-sting. Immunotherapy is quite effective in this population, with an almost 99% nonreaction rate on subsequent stings. In patients younger than 16 years old who have had only a mild systemic reaction (e.g., generalized urticaria), the risk of a subsequent severe systemic reaction is the same as that in the general population. Therefore, skin testing and immunotherapy are not recommended for this group of patients. Patients with a history of normal, large local, toxic, or delayed systemic reactions are also not candidates for immunotherapy.

Biting Insects

In certain susceptible patients, unusually large local reactions to the salivary secretions of biting insects (e.g., mosquitos, flies, and fleas) may develop. The reaction appears urticarial (papular urticaria) and probably results from vasoactive or irritant substances present in the insect secretions. The immune mechanism is unknown. *Treatment* consists of avoidance, antihistamines for pruritus, topical corticosteroids, and therapy for secondary infection, if present. Anaphylactic reactions have been reported after insect bites from the kissing bug (*Triatoma*). Immunotherapy with *T. protracta* salivary gland extract may be effective.

REFERENCES

Behrman RE, Kliegman RM, Jenson HB, editors: *Nelson textbook of pediatrics,* ed 16, Philadelphia, 2000, WB Saunders, Chapter 151.

Valentine M, Schuberth K, Kagey-Sobotka A, et al: The value of immunotherapy with venom in children with allergy to insect stings, *N Engl J Med* 323(23):1601–1603, 1990.

Yunginger JW: Insect allergy. In Middleton E Jr, Reed CE, Ellis EF, et al, editors: *Allergy principles and practice,* ed 5, St Louis, 1998, Mosby.

Serum Sickness

Serum sickness is a type III hypersensitivity reaction that results from an immunologic response to foreign proteins, mediated by the deposition of immune complexes. The reaction is frequently seen in response to heterologous (animal-derived) antisera (e.g., antilymphocyte, anti–snake venom, and antibotulism), in response to drugs (e.g., penicillin and cephalosporins), and, occasionally, with chronic viral infection.

Pathogenesis. Serum sickness follows the administration of large doses of antigen. Antigen must enter the circulation, where it forms soluble antigen-antibody complexes (in moderate antigen excess). These immune complexes deposit in small blood vessels; fix complement, producing C3a, C5a, and C5,6,7; and recruit polymorphonuclear leukocytes (PMNs). Capillary leak is triggered by vasoactive amines released either by antigen activation of IgE-coated mast cells or basophils or by complement activation with IgG and IgM; this results in anaphylatoxin production. Proteolytic enzymes released from the lysosomal granules of the neutrophils mediate tissue damage and produce the vasculitis.

Clinical Manifestations. Serum sickness is characterized by pruritus, fever, polyarticular arthritis and arthralgia (particularly in the small joints of the hand and feet), lymphadenopathy, and urticaria and angioedema. It usually begins 7–14 days after antigen administration as antibody forms and begins to circulate. An accelerated reaction may develop within 2–4 days if prior sensitization has occurred. Symptoms generally improve in 1–2 weeks as antigen is cleared. Skin eruptions occur in 90% of cases and may include urticaria, erythema multiforme, angioedema, and maculopapular and purpuric lesions (as a result of vasculitis). A characteristic serpiginous erythematous eruption on the sides of the hands and feet has been described. Generalized lymphadenopathy associated with splenomegaly may occur, as may gastrointestinal complaints (e.g., cramping, diarrhea, and nausea). Cardiovascular (e.g., myocarditis and pericarditis), pulmonary (e.g., pleuritis and wheezing), and renal involvement is uncommon, although proteinuria is frequently seen. Involvement of the nervous system, including cranial nerve palsies, optic neuritis, transient hemiplegia, and Guillain-Barré syndrome, may occur rarely.

Laboratory Findings. Findings include an elevated erythrocyte sedimentation rate (ESR); proteinuria; microscopic hematuria; hyaline casts; and thrombocytopenia, leukopenia, or leukocytosis, with or without associated eosinophilia. Serum C3 and C4 levels are variably depressed, and circulating immune complexes are occasionally observed. Circulating plasma cells are uncommon but are thought to be specific for serum sickness.

Treatment. Treatment involves discontinuation of antigen administration, after which symptoms begin to improve slowly. Antihistamines may relieve the urticaria and, if given prophylactically at the time of antigen exposure, may potentially decrease immune complex deposition. Aspirin and other nonsteroidal agents are effective for fever and joint pain. If organs are involved, prednisone (1–2 mg/kg/24 hr) should be administered. Immediate skin testing with antigen does not predict the likelihood of serum sickness development.

REFERENCES

Behrman RE, Kliegman RM, Jenson HB, editors: *Nelson textbook of pediatrics*, ed 16, Philadelphia, 2000, WB Saunders, Chapter 149.

Bielory L, Gascon P, Lawley TJ, et al: Human serum sickness: a prospective analysis of 35 patients treated with equine antithymocyte globulin for bone marrow failure, *Medicine (Baltimore)* 67(1):40–57, 1988.

Heckbert S, Stryker W, Coltin K, et al: Serum sickness in children after antibiotic exposure: estimates of occurrence and morbidity in a health maintenance organization population, *Am J Epidemiol* 132(2):336–342, 1990.

Lawley TJ, Frank MM: Immune complexes and allergic disease. In Middleton E Jr, Reed CE, Ellis EF, et al, editors: *Allergy principles and practice*, ed 4, St Louis, 1993, Mosby.

URTICARIA AND ANGIOEDEMA

Urticaria (hives) is characterized by raised, pruritic, erythematous lesions that are evanescent and vary in size and pattern. Angioedema affects subcutaneous tissues and may accompany urticaria. When angioedema occurs alone, it is not pruritic. Urticaria can be "acute," present for less than 6 weeks, or "chronic," occurring episodically for more than 6 weeks.

Etiology and Diagnosis. Both acute and chronic urticaria may be produced by a number of factors (Table 8-20). A careful history regarding the specific appearance of the lesions, including how and when they are provoked, often provides useful clues about the etiology of the urticaria. Factors that produce cutaneous vasodilation (e.g., exertion, heat, fever, and hyperthyroidism) can exacerbate urticaria. Acute urticaria is more likely to be IgE mediated, whereas allergy does not generally play a significant role in the pathogenesis of chronic urticaria. In younger patients, acute urticaria is usually a benign condition. The cause of acute urticaria is often found, in contrast to chronic urticaria, which is usually categorized as idiopathic because of a lack of identifiable etiology. Of adult patients with chronic idiopathic urticaria, 25–50% have been found to have functional anti-IgE and anti-FcεR1 (high-affinity IgE receptor α-chain) autoantibodies.

Skin testing or RAST may help identify the cause of acute urticaria. Laboratory tests are not beneficial in evaluating chronic urticaria except to rule out collagen-vascular diseases. Therefore, a CBC with differential, ESR, and urinalysis are more helpful for evaluation of chronic urticaria than skin testing or RAST.

Treatment. The mainstay of treatment in acute and chronic urticaria is administration of antihistamines

---

TABLE 8–20
Etiology of Urticaria

Agent	Example
Drugs	Antibiotics (penicillin), aspirin, codeine, blood products
Foods and food additives	Eggs, peanuts, fish
Infectious diseases	Streptococcal pharyngitis, sinusitis, hepatitis, mononucleosis, viral infection, *Mycoplasma*, parasites
Insect stings	Bee stings, flea bites, mite bites
Collagen-vascular diseases	Lupus erythematosus, vasculitis, polymyositis
Inhalant allergens	Cat, horse
Idiopathic	Unknown
Physical agents	Dermatographism, cold, heat, solar, cholinergic, pressure, water, vibration
Contact allergens	Cat scratches, moth scales, caterpillars, nettle plants
Neoplasms	Hodgkin disease, leukemia
Mastocytosis	Urticaria pigmentosa
Endocrine disease	Hyperthyroidism, pregnancy, hypothyroidism

(H$_1$ receptor antagonists). Hydroxyzine (Atarax) and diphenhydramine (Benadryl) are very effective but can be sedating. Nonsedating antihistamines such as cetirizine (Zyrtec), fexofenadine (Allegra), and loratadine (Claritin) are also effective but more expensive. The tricyclic antihistamine doxepin may also be useful. H$_2$ receptor antagonists can be tried in refractory cases. If the offending agent can be identified, its avoidance will bring about rapid and dramatic improvement.

ANGIOEDEMA

When angioedema occurs in the absence of urticaria, the diagnosis of C1 esterase inhibitor deficiency must be ruled out. Two forms exist: inherited and acquired. The inherited form, or hereditary angioedema (HAE), is discussed earlier in this chapter under Complement Deficiencies. Acquired C1-esterase inhibitor deficiency is associated with lymphoma, other syndromes with expanded B-cell populations, and autoimmune deficiency with an autoantibody directed against the C1-esterase inhibitor. Patients with acquired C1-esterase inhibitor deficiency, in contrast to patients with HAE, have reduced levels of C1q.

Treatment is that of the underlying lymphoproliferative disease.

REFERENCES

Behrman RE, Kliegman RM, Jenson HB, editors: *Nelson textbook of pediatrics*, ed 16, Philadelphia, 2000, WB Saunders, Chapter 147.

Greaves M: Chronic urticaria, *J Allergy Clin Immunol* 105:664, 2000.

Huston DP, Bressler RB: Urticaria and angioedema, *Med Clin North Am* 76:804, 1992.

Kaplan AP: Urticaria and angioedema. In Middleton E Jr, Reed CE, Ellis EF, et al, editors: *Allergy, principles and practice*, ed 4, St Louis, 1993, Mosby.

CHAPTER 9

Rheumatic Diseases of Childhood

Judyann C. Olson

The rheumatic diseases of childhood (autoimmune, collagen-vascular, or connective tissue diseases) are conditions characterized by inflammation and autoimmunity. Common manifestations of rheumatic diseases include **synovitis** (arthritis), or inflammation of the joint synovium (Table 9–1); **enthesopathy,** or inflammation at the insertion of a ligament to a bone (sacroiliac joint arthritis, Achilles tendinitis, and plantar fasciitis); **serositis,** or inflammation of a serosal lining (Table 9–2); **myositis,** or muscle inflammation; **autoantibody** production (Table 9–3); and **vasculitis** (Table 9–4). Inflammation may be localized in one joint or tendon group, or it may be generalized. Local inflammation is characterized by pain, swelling, erythema, limited range of motion, and warmth. Systemic inflammation is manifested as fever, malaise, anorexia, weight loss, and myalgias.

Currently, rheumatology is a descriptive subspecialty, with most conditions diagnosed by clinical findings or the fulfillment of classification criteria. Inflammation and tissue injury in rheumatic diseases are mediated by the immune response from the activation of monocytes, lymphocytes, polymorphonuclear leukocytes, complement, and antibodies. Specific autoantibodies may be produced, such as antiplatelet antibodies in **systemic lupus erythematosus** (SLE), or the injury may be mediated by deposition of non–tissue-specific antigen–antibody complexes in organs with large capillary beds, such as the glomerulus of the kidney. Furthermore, tissue damage may be mediated by local activation of macrophages and lymphocytes, as occurs in the synovium of patients with adult-type rheumatoid arthritis (RA). In RA, local inflammatory cells accumulate as a result of immune complexes and activate complement, which attracts more inflammatory cells. Cytokines, phospholipids, kinins, and other mediators of inflammation are released into the tissue, and hydrolytic enzymes (e.g., proteases and col-

| TABLE 9–1 |
| **Causes of Childhood Arthritis (Synovitis)** |

Common
Juvenile rheumatoid arthritis
Rheumatic fever
Systemic lupus erythematosus
Henoch-Schönlein purpura
Pyogenic infection (septic or immune complex)
Viral infection (e.g., parvovirus, rubella, or mumps; possibly toxic synovitis)
Lyme disease (*Borrelia burgdorferi*)
Serum sickness
Kawasaki disease

Less Common
Hemophilia
Endocarditis
Leukemia
Reiter syndrome (enteric, genital)
Inflammatory bowel disease
Dermatomyositis
Psoriatic

Rare
Acneiform arthritis
Wegener granulomatosis
Sarcoidosis
Scleroderma

lagenases) are released, producing local damage. Synovitis produces synovial hypertrophy (pannus) that migrates into the articular cartilage. This hypertrophy, together with hydrolytic enzymes, further destroys and demineralizes the tissue, as well as enhancing mechanical injury of the tissue. Although

TABLE 9–2
Serositis

Manifestations	Differential Diagnosis—cont'd
Pericarditis	Tuberculosis
Peritonitis	Viral (coxsackievirus)
Pleuritis	Bacterial (pneumococcus, *Staphylococcus aureus*, group A streptococcus)
	Immune complex (meningococcus, gonococcus)
Differential Diagnosis	Malignancy
Juvenile rheumatoid arthritis	Spontaneous peritonitis (pneumococcus, *Escherichia coli*)
Systemic lupus erythematosus	

TABLE 9–3
Manifestations of Autoantibodies

Coombs-positive hemolytic anemia	Double-stranded DNA* (SLE, renal disease)
Immune neutropenia	DNA-histone (drug-induced SLE)
Immune thrombocytopenia	Sm (Smith) (SLE, renal, central nervous system)
Thrombosis (anticardiolipin, antiphospholipid, lupus anticoagulant)	RNP (ribonucleoprotein) (SLE, Sjögren syndrome, scleroderma, polymyositis, MCTD)
Immune lymphopenia	Ro (Robert: SSA) (SLE, neonatal lupus–congenital heart block, Sjögren syndrome)
Antimitochondrial (primary biliary cirrhosis, SLE)	La (Lane: SSB) (SLE, Sjögren syndrome)
Antimicrosomal (chronic active hepatitis, SLE)	Jo-1 (polymyositis, dermatomyositis)
Antithyroid (thyroiditis, SLE)	Sc1-70 (scleroderma)
Antineutrophil cytoplasmic antibody (ANCA-cytoplasmic) (Wegener granulomatosis)	Centromere (CREST syndrome, variant scleroderma)
ANCA-perinuclear (microscopic polyangiitis)	PM-Sc1 (scleroderma, UCTD)
Antinuclear Antibodies to Specific Nuclear Antigens and Associated Manifestations	
Single-stranded DNA* (nonspecific, indicates inflammation)	

Adapted from Condemi J: The autoimmune diseases, *JAMA* 268(20):2882–2892, 1992.
*Because antibodies to single-stranded DNA (ssDNA) are a nonspecific response to inflammatory diseases and because ssDNA may contaminate double-stranded DNA (dsDNA) preparations, the purer, circular dsDNA of *Crithidia luciliae* (crithidia test) is preferred.
CREST syndrome, Calcinosis, Raynaud phenomenon, *e*sophageal dysfunction, *s*clerodactyly, *t*elangiectasia; *DNA,* deoxyribonucleic acid; *MCTD,* mixed connective tissue disease; *SLE,* systemic lupus erythematosus; *SSA,* Sjögren syndrome antigen A; *SSB,* Sjögren syndrome antigen B; *UCTD,* undifferentiated connective tissue disease.

TABLE 9–4
Vasculitis Syndrome

Type	Comment
Polyarteritis Nodosa Group	
Polyarteritis nodosa	Multisystem—kidney, nerve, liver, skin; necrotizing vasculitis of small and medium muscular arteries
Churg-Strauss syndrome (allergic angiitis and granulomatosis)	Skin and pulmonary involvement; eosinophilia and asthma; granulomatous vasculitis of small and medium arteries
Polyangiitis overlap	Overlap of more than one of any type vasculitis with skin, lung, kidney, nerve involvement
Hypersensitivity Syndromes	
Henoch-Schönlein purpura	Palpable purpura, kidney, joint, intestine; inflammation of arteriole, capillary, and venule; leukocytoclastic vasculitis, IgA immune complexes
Serum sickness (e.g., drug-related)	Antigen-antibody hypocomplementemic, skin, joint, kidney
Vasculitis with infections	Meningococcemia, Rocky Mountain spotted fever, endocarditis, HIV, EBV, parvovirus B19, syphilis, hepatitis B and C
Connective tissue vasculitis	SLE, JRA
Wegener granulomatosis	Necrotizing granulomas; small and medium arteries; upper and lower respiratory tract, glomerulonephritis; positive antineutrophil cytoplasm antibodies
Giant Cell Arteritis	
Temporal/cranial	Medium-large arteries; retinal arteritis may cause blindness
Takayasu	Young women, inflammation of aortic arch
Others	
Behçet disease	Recurrent oral, gastrointestinal, and genital ulcers; uveitis; skin
Kawasaki disease	Arteritis, coronary artery aneurysm; immune complexes
Hypocomplementemic disease	Chronic urticaria

EBV, Epstein-Barr virus; *HIV*, human immunodeficiency virus; *Ig*, immunoglobulin; *JRA*, juvenile rheumatoid arthritis; *SLE*, systemic lupus erythematosus.

the clinical features of each of the rheumatic diseases are distinct, an individual patient may have overlapping signs and symptoms that make a precise diagnosis difficult.

LABORATORY TESTS USED TO ASSESS RHEUMATIC DISEASES
Acute-Phase Reactants

The Westergren sedimentation rate (WSR), or erythrocyte sedimentation rate (ESR), is the most commonly used test for assessing the activity of a rheumatic disease. It is nonspecifically increased in response to systemic inflammation (rheumatic disease, infection, or malignancy). The sedimentation rate requires erythrocyte rouleaux formation and an interaction with fibrinogen or macroglobulins; afibrinogenemia, anemia, and sickle cell anemia may reduce the sedimentation rate. Other acute-phase reactants whose levels are elevated in response to inflammation are the C-reactive protein, which is rapidly synthesized by the liver; platelet count; ferritin; and total hemolytic complement (CH50). Any of the acute-phase reactants may be helpful in following the disease course in a particular patient, but some patients have active inflammatory disease with normal values for one or more acute-phase reactants.

Rheumatoid Factors

Rheumatoid factors are antibodies directed against the Fc portion of immunoglobulin G (IgG). Most of the conventional tests for rheumatoid factor, such as the latex agglutination titer, detect rheumatoid factors that are IgM; IgG, IgA, and IgE rheumatoid factors can be measured by other techniques.

A positive result from a rheumatoid factor test is not diagnostic. Eighty-five to ninety-five percent of children with **juvenile rheumatoid arthritis** (JRA) have a negative test result for conventional rheumatoid factors, whereas children with SLE and Henoch-Schönlein purpura may have rheumatoid factors. Rheumatoid factors also are present in viral infections such as hepatitis B and in other conditions, including bacterial endocarditis, sarcoidosis, tuberculosis, and congenital TORCH infections (*t*oxoplasmosis, *o*ther conditions, *r*ubella, *c*ytomegalovirus, and *h*erpes simplex).

Antinuclear and Anticytoplasmic Antibodies

Autoantibodies against nuclear, as well as cytoplasmic, constituents often are found in the serum of patients with connective tissue diseases, but antibodies are also found in individuals with nonrheumatic conditions (e.g., mononucleosis, endocarditis, chronic active hepatitis, malaria, and drug therapy such as hydralazine) (Table 9–3). The presence of antinuclear antibodies (ANAs) is determined by indirect immunofluorescent antibody (IFA) tests in which the patient's serum is incubated with a source of nuclei and a fluorescent-labeled immunoglobulin; the greatest dilution of serum at which a positive immunofluorescent pattern is observed is recorded. Normal ranges differ in various laboratories, but frequently a 1:40 titer is the lowest dilution considered a positive test result. Other methods (ELISA kits) have become available for the detection of ANA. A recent study found IFA tests outperformed ELISA kits for clinical utility in JRA.

Between 60% and 70% of children with a positive test result for ANAs have autoimmune disease, which is often evident at the time of the positive ANA test result. JRA is the most common of these, followed by SLE, dermatomyositis, undifferentiated connective tissue disease, and uveitis. Patients may have a positive ANA test result but no evidence of autoimmune disease.

Complement

The levels of the various complement components (see Chapter 8, Fig. 8–2) and the level of the total hemolytic complement may be elevated, as the acute-phase reactants are in rheumatic diseases. Decreased complement levels are noted in active SLE, particularly in SLE with nephritis. Determining the level of total hemolytic complement is an important screening test; the complement level is depressed in SLE and in various vasculitides. In addition, hereditary complement component deficiencies have been associated with familial cases of SLE and vasculitis.

Histocompatibility Antigens

Children with the human leukocyte antigen (HLA) B27 locus are at increased risk for ankylosing spondylitis, Reiter syndrome, psoriatic arthritis, and arthritis associated with inflammatory bowel disease. Seropositive polyarticular JRA is associated with the HLA-DR4 locus.

REFERENCES

Behrman RE, Kliegman RM, Jenson HB, editors: *Nelson textbook of pediatrics*, ed 16, Philadelphia, 2000, WB Saunders, Chapter 154.

Deane P, Liard G, Siegel D, et al: The outcome of children referred to a pediatric rheumatology clinic with a positive antinuclear antibody test but without an autoimmune disease, *Pediatrics* 95(6):892–895, 1995.

Eichenfield AH, Athreya BH, Doughty RA, et al: Utility of rheumatoid factor in the diagnosis of juvenile rheumatoid arthritis, *Pediatrics* 78(3):480–484, 1986.

Fawcett PT, Rose CD, Gibney KM, et al: Use of ELISA to measure antinuclear antibodies in children with juvenile rheumatoid arthritis, *J Rheumatol* 26(8):1822–1826, 1999.

JUVENILE RHEUMATOID ARTHRITIS

JRA has an incidence of 5–18 per 100,000 children in Europe and America. Prevalence is between 30–150 per 100,000 children. The peak age of onset is between 1–3 years, and a second peak occurs in the early teenage years.

Classification

Traditionally, chronic arthritis persisting for at least 6 weeks in an individual 16 years of age or younger suggests JRA when there is no other reason for the arthritis. JRA is divided into three broad onset types based on the clinical manifestations in the first 6 months of illness. The most common type is **pauciarticular disease,** which involves four or fewer joints. The next most common is **polyarticular disease,** with involvement of five or more joints. The least common is **systemic-onset disease,** which begins with high, spiking fevers to greater than 39.4°C (103°F). The fever is frequently accompanied by a rheumatoid rash that comes and goes with temperature elevations. Joint involvement may occur either at onset or later in the course of the disease.

It has recently been proposed that the nomenclature and classification criteria for diagnosis of childhood arthritis be changed so that terminology would be more consistent internationally. Juvenile idiopathic arthritis is diagnosed when arthritis occurs before the sixteenth birthday and has been present for at least 6 weeks with no other apparent diagnosis. The arthritis may be unclassified between 6 weeks and 6 months, after which time it is assigned to one of seven subtypes: systemic arthritis; polyarthritis—rheumatoid factor positive; polyarthritis—rheumatoid factor negative; oligoarthritis (pauci); extended oligoarthritis (one to four joints in the first 6 months with cumulative total of five or more joints after 6 months); enthesis-related arthritis; and psoriatic arthritis. Because a recent study of the new criteria recommended changes before the criteria are incorporated into clinical practice, this section is written using the traditional nomenclature.

Pauciarticular Juvenile Rheumatoid Arthritis

JRA has a pauciarticular onset in about half of all children affected by the disease. Two prominent subgroups of pauciarticular JRA are recognized: a younger group of patients, primarily female, who often have chronic uveitis; and older children with later onset of disease, more frequently male, who may demonstrate features of a spondyloarthropathy syndrome.

Clinical Manifestations. Pauciarticular arthritis in the *younger* child has a peak age of onset of about 2 years. These children appear healthy, with few systemic signs of illness. The large joints are most commonly involved. The knee is the most frequently involved joint, followed by ankles and elbows. Hip involvement is very rare. The child occasionally may have swelling in the small joints of the hands or feet. Pain is uncommon in these children, and the diagnosis may be made after months of asymptomatic swelling, leading to the slow development of contractures. The joint disease rarely is destructive. Localized growth disturbance may occur as a result of asymmetric joint disease. This growth disturbance is particularly noticeable in the knees because it may lead to an overgrowth in the length of the affected leg. Signs and symptoms of uveitis are few (e.g., occasionally poor vision or red eye), and the diagnosis usually is made at the time of a regularly scheduled slit-lamp examination. Therefore, a risk of blindness exists. The differential diagnosis includes Lyme disease (Table 9–5) because of the pattern of few joints being involved.

Results of most *laboratory tests* are normal; these tests include the hemoglobin level, sedimentation rate, and white blood cell count. Rheumatoid factor rarely is present, but many of the children have positive results with tests for ANAs (>50%). The presence of ANAs in the very young female patient with pauciarticular arthritis is closely associated with the development of chronic iridocyclitis.

Treatment of uveitis with local steroid eyedrops and dilating agents usually is successful. A minority of patients may require systemic steroids for severe eye disease. Severe arthritis occurs in 10% of patients. Some patients progress to a polyarticular course (extended oligoarthritis). If there is a *significant leg length discrepancy* from overgrowth of a leg, the child may have a severe pelvic tilt, compensatory scoliosis, and a gait abnormality that is easily corrected by placing a lift on the shoe of the normal (shorter) leg. The lift equalizes leg length and normalizes gait.

Pauciarticular arthritis in *older* children usually occurs after 8 years of age and has a propensity to involve the joints of the lower extremity in an asymmetric fashion; enthesopathy of the Achilles tendon, patellar tendon, or plantar fascia often occurs. Hips commonly are involved. The knee is the most commonly involved joint, and the ankle and the first metatarsophalangeal joint are the next. Some children have asymmetric upper extremity joint involvement. Many children have a positive family history of significant low back pain, psoriasis, inflammatory bowel disease, ankylosing spondylitis, or reactive (e.g., Reiter) arthritis.

Frequently there is slowly diminishing motor performance that may manifest with difficulties in sports or physical education. Commonly, the patient has a history of slowly decreasing exercise capacity, malaise, and nagging aches and pains. Occasionally the child may have significant systemic signs accompanied by weight loss, fever, anorexia, and diffuse arthralgia or myalgia. In the first years of their illness, most children complain of painful inflammation at points of insertion of tendons and ligaments **(entheses).** Joint swelling and back pain may develop later in the course. Uveitis, when it occurs, tends to be acute in nature (decreased visual acuity and erythema). This is in contrast with the younger children, who may have asymptomatic chronic uveitis. The differential diagnosis of seronegative spondyloarthropathy (inflammatory low back pain, enthesitis, and asymmetric lower joint involvement) includes juvenile ankylosing spondylitis, Reiter disease, psoriatic arthritis, and arthropathies of inflammatory bowel disease.

Laboratory Tests. Older children with pauciarticular arthritis inevitably have normal findings on laboratory tests, except perhaps children with constitutional symptoms, who may have markedly elevated sedimentation rates or depressed hemoglobin levels; these children frequently have positive test results for HLA-B27. Rheumatoid factor and ANA test results are negative.

TABLE 9–5
Differential Diagnosis of Pediatric Arthritis Syndromes

Characteristic	Systemic Lupus Erythematosus	Juvenile Rheumatoid Arthritis	Rheumatic Fever
Sex	F > M	Type-dependent	M = F
Age	10–20 yr	2–16 yr	5–15 yr
Arthralgia	Yes	Yes	Yes
Morning stiffness	Yes	Yes	No
Rash	Butterfly; discoid	Salmon-pink macules (systemic onset)	Erythema marginatum
Monoarticular, pauciarticular	Yes	50%	No
Polyarticular	Yes	Yes	Yes
Small joints	Yes	Yes	No
Temporomandibular joint	No	Rare	No
Eye disease	Uveitis/retinitis	Iridocyclitis (rare in systemic)	No
Total WBC count	Decreased	Increased (decreased in macrophage activation syndrome)	Normal to increased
ANA	Positive	Positive (50%)	Negative
Rheumatoid factor	Positive	Positive (10%) (poly-onset)	Negative
Other laboratory results	↓Complement ↑Antibodies to double-stranded DNA	—	↑ASO anti-DNAase B
Erosive arthritis	No, rare	Yes	No, rare
Other clinical manifestations	Proteinuria, serositis	Fever, serositis (systemic onset)	Carditis, nodules, chorea
Pathogenesis	Autoimmune	Autoimmune	Group A streptococcus
Treatment	NSAIDs, steroids, hydroxy-chloroquine, immunosuppressive agents	NSAIDs, etanercept, methotrexate for resistant disease	Penicillin prophylaxis, aspirin, steroids

ANA, Antinuclear antibody; *ASO*, antistreptolysin-O titer; *GC*, gonococcus; *NSAID*, nonsteroidal antiinflammatory drug; *WBC*, white blood cell.

Polyarticular Juvenile Rheumatoid Arthritis

Children with the polyarticular onset of JRA (five or more joints involved in the first 6 months) are further subcategorized into those who are seronegative (more common) and those who are seropositive for rheumatoid factor. Girls outnumber boys in both categories.

Polyarticular disease characteristically involves the small joints of the hands and feet. Large joint involvement also is common. The cervical spine, temporomandibular joint, sternoclavicular joint, and distal interphalangeal joints also may be affected. Systemic manifestations of disease are more frequently seen than in children with pauciarticular disease. Mild anemia of chronic disease, leukocytosis, fever, lymphadenopathy, and hepatosplenomegaly may be seen. Fatigue is common, and anorexia may occur.

Approximately one fourth of the *seronegative polyarticular JRA* patients have positive test results for ANAs; a few of these patients have associated chronic uveitis. The onset of illness usually occurs when the child is 10 years old or younger. The course of the disease in this type of illness generally is favorable, with few extraarticular manifestations and 10–15% of cases finally being categorized in functional class III or IV (Table 9–6). In general, seronegative JRA patients respond better to treatment

Lyme Disease	Leukemia	Gonococcemia	Kawasaki Disease
M = F	M = F	F > M	M = F
2–20 yr	2–10 yr	>12 yr	<4 yr
Yes	Yes	Yes	Yes
No	No	No	No
Erythema chronicum migrans	No	Palms/soles papulo-pustules	Diffuse maculopapular (nonspecific)
Yes	Yes	Yes	—
Rare	Yes	No	Yes
No	Yes	No	Yes
Rare	No	No	No
Keratitis	No	No	Conjunctivitis, uveitis
Normal	Increased or neutropenia ± blasts	Increased	Increased
Negative	Negative	Negative	Negative
Negative	Negative	Negative	Negative
↑Cryoglobulin, ↑immune complexes	+ Bone marrow	+ Culture for GC	Thrombocytosis, ↑immune complexes
Rare	No	Yes	No
Carditis, neuropathy	Thrombocytopenia	Sexual activity, menses	Fever, lymphadenopathy, swollen hands/feet, mouth lesions
Borrelia burgdorferi	Acute lymphoblastic leukemia	*Neisseria gonorrhoeae*	Unknown
Penicillin, tetracycline, ceftriaxone	Steroids, chemotherapy	Ceftriaxone, cefoxitin	Aspirin, intravenous immunoglobulins

with nonsteroidal antiinflammatory drugs (NSAIDs) than do seropositive patients. The *differential diagnosis* includes Lyme disease, rheumatic fever, and SLE (Table 9–5).

Only about 5–8% of all children with chronic arthritis are *seropositive for rheumatoid factor*. The onset of illness usually occurs when the child is 9–16 years of age. Most of these children demonstrate evidence of erosive, destructive arthritis on roentgenograms at the end of 1 year of illness. Nodules over the tendons (of the elbows, knees, and scalp) are seen more frequently in seropositive than in seronegative polyarticular disease and are thought to indicate severe disease. Vasculitis (of the lungs or skin) occurs uncommonly. Approximately half of these adolescents have severe, unremitting disease with a functional outcome that puts them in class III or IV. Disease persists into adulthood, and the natural history is similar to that of adult-onset RA. About 50% of patients have positive results on ANA tests. The disease is associated with HLA antigens DW4 and DR4 (similar to adult RA).

Systemic-Onset Juvenile Rheumatoid Arthritis

Systemic-onset JRA is the most dramatic and least common form of the illness. It is the only type of JRA that affects males as frequently as it affects females.

TABLE 9-6
American College of Rheumatology Revised Criteria for Classification of Functional Status in Rheumatoid Arthritis*

Class I	Completely able to perform usual activities of daily living (self-care, vocational, and avocational)
Class II	Able to perform usual self-care and vocational activities, but limited in avocational activities
Class III	Able to perform usual self-care activities, but limited in vocational and avocational activities
Class IV	Limited in ability to perform usual self-care, vocational, and avocational activities

From *Arthritis Rheum* 35:498, 1992.
*Usual self-care activities include dressing, feeding, bathing, grooming, and toileting. Avocational (recreational and/or leisure) and vocational (work, school, homemaking) activities are patient desired and age and sex specific.

Clinical Manifestations. The age of onset in children is usually 16 years or younger, and the sexes are equally affected. These patients usually appear ill and often have high, spiking fevers of at least 39.4° C (103° F) for many weeks. They usually have associated erythematous macular rash, splenomegaly, hepatomegaly, and lymphadenopathy. Irritability and arthralgia and myalgia are prominent features, particularly during fever spikes. The characteristic rash consists of small, salmon-colored macules located on the trunk and extremities that come and go with the fever spikes; rarely, the rash is pruritic. Arthritis often is absent during the first weeks or even 6–8 months of illness. Later in the course, chronic polyarticular arthritis may occur; it may be severe. Therefore, JRA becomes a suspected diagnosis, and one of exclusion. The *differential diagnosis* includes occult infection (Epstein-Barr virus), systemic vasculitis, inflammatory bowel disease, malignancy (leukemia or neuroblastoma), and acute rheumatic fever (Table 9–5).

Other systemic features of JRA include pericarditis, pleuritis, and, uncommonly, abdominal serositis. Myocarditis occasionally is seen. Growth retardation is a prominent feature of this type of illness, particularly if long-term corticosteroid therapy has been required. Though uncommon, life-threatening abnormalities of coagulation have been seen. Bony fusion of the cervical spine can occur. Chronic uveitis is a rare manifestation of systemic JRA.

Laboratory Findings. There are no diagnostic laboratory features of systemic-onset JRA. The affected child typically has anemia that may be profound and is generally the normocytic-normochromic anemia of chronic disease. The white blood cell count frequently is markedly elevated and may show a shift to the left; often platelet counts are elevated, as are acute-phase reactants. Ferritin levels may be markedly elevated. The sedimentation rate usually is extremely high. The serum is uniformly negative for rheumatoid factors and ANA.

Prognosis. Some children have intermittent episodes of febrile illness for years after onset; others (25%) progress to severe chronic, destructive polyarticular joint disease without recurrent fevers. Death is uncommon in the course of JRA, but it is most likely to occur in the child with systemic-onset disease. Death usually is a result of myocarditis or infection, especially if the child has been immunosuppressed. The coagulopathy syndrome (macrophage activation syndrome) associated with JRA may also be life threatening.

GENERAL CHARACTERISTICS OF ARTHRITIS IN CHILDHOOD

Morning stiffness is characteristic of JRA. Children rarely complain of stiffness but often respond to questions asking them if they need time to "loosen up" in the morning. This morning stiffness may be ameliorated by the setting of an earlier time for arising, provision of a warm morning bath, and use of heating pads or electric blankets at night. Stretching exercises may also be beneficial. Stiffness also occurs after periods of immobility, and teachers need to be reminded that children with arthritis need extra freedom to move about the classroom throughout the day.

Pain is variable in JRA. Many children feel little or no pain. Later in life this lack of pain often may conceal the presence of a long-standing arthritis, possibly accompanied by significant flexion contractures, before the joint disease finally is appreciated. Contractures may occur as the child avoids the extremes of motion—the points at which pain may occur. Some children have significant pain or discomfort.

Generalized **growth retardation** may occur in the systemic form of the disease and in severe polyarticular disease and is accentuated if corticosteroids have been used. If the systemic illness remits, some catch-up growth occurs, but many children have such prolonged disease that their final height will be reduced.

Localized overgrowth and undergrowth occur in areas of asymmetric arthritis. In this case, generally marked overgrowth occurs and epiphyseal maturation accelerates in the affected joints; the result, for example, is that the leg with the arthritic knee becomes much longer than the normal leg. If the cervical spine is involved, neck instability, stiffness, and torticollis may develop. Undergrowth of the mandible may result in a marked micrognathia and severe cosmetic and orthodontic deformity.

Although **roentgenographic changes** may be minimal, one study found that after 13 years, 28% of pauciarticular, 54% of polyarticular, and 45% of systemic-onset JRA patients developed joint space narrowing or erosions characteristic of significant damage to the joints. MRI is more sensitive for revealing cartilage loss and erosions earlier in the disease than radiographs. A child who has severe JRA for many years may have only osteopenia. Joint space narrowing may occur. Older children who are seropositive for rheumatoid factor may have evidence of erosive disease.

Prognosis of Juvenile Rheumatoid Arthritis

Most parents are interested in knowing what to expect for their child's outcome. Although information is available about outcome for aggregate groups of patients, predicting with certainty how an individual child will do is impossible. New instruments to measure health status, function, and disability have been developed so that outcome studies are more standardized (Table 9–6). Generally, children with pauciarticular disease do well. Some with an extended course of disease have a more guarded outcome. Rheumatoid factor positivity and the clinical finding of subcutaneous nodules are associated with risk of severe disease. Some children with systemic-onset JRA have very aggressive disease. Outcome studies that evaluate status after longer follow-up intervals find more patients with disability. The course of JRA is often characterized by periods of active disease and periods of remission.

Treatment. Most children respond to NSAIDs with improvement in joint swelling and diminished symptoms of inflammation. Aspirin historically has been the initial treatment for JRA; because of the association with Reye syndrome, more frequent dosage schedules, gastritis, and hepatotoxicity, NSAIDs now are often preferred. For severe disease, methotrexate 10 mg/m² is often used as the initial disease-modifying agent. Recently, etanercept (0.4 mg/kg subcutaneously, twice a week, up to adult dose) has been approved for polyarticular-course disease that is nonresponsive to methotrexate or in cases involving methotrexate intolerance. Systemic corticosterioids are indicated for serious complications such as pericarditis or cases in which cricoarytenoid joint involvement obstructs the airway. Intraarticular corticosterioids may be used to control local joint involvement and may help minimize leg length discrepancy. Influenza vaccine should be considered for children receiving immunosuppressive therapy. Varicella vaccine should be considered before initiation of immunosuppressive treatment if clinically possible.

Osteopenia may develop in some children with JRA. This is aggravated in children who have required systemic corticosteroid therapy. Adequate calcium intake and weight-bearing activity are important to minimize the osteopenia.

Occupational and physical therapy for range of motion exercises, strengthening, conditioning, and adaptions for activity of daily living are important aspects of the treatment plan. Joint splinting is used for refractory contractures. Joint replacement surgery may be needed for pain control and to improve function in severely affected joints.

Many children need supportive care to deal with the chronic aspects of their disease. Social workers and psychologists are often part of the treatment team for children with JRA.

REFERENCES

Behrman RE, Kliegman RM, Jenson HB, editors: *Nelson textbook of pediatrics,* ed 16, Philadelphia, 2000, WB Saunders, Chapters 155–156.

Foeldvari I, Bidde M: Validation of the proposed ILAR classification criteria for juvenile idiopathic arthritis, *J Rheumatol* 27(4): 1069–1072, 2000.

Gare BA: Epidemiology, *Baillieres Clin Rheumatol* 12(2):191–208, 1998.

Henderson CJ, Specker BL, Sierra RI, et al: Total-body bone mineral content in non-corticosteroid-treated postpubertal females with juvenile rheumatoid arthritis, *Arthritis Rheum* 43(3):531–540, 2000.

Lovell DJ, Giannini EN, Reiff A, et al: Etanercept in children with polyarticular juvenile rheumatoid arthritis, *N Engl J Med* 342(11):763–769, 2000.

Prahalad S, Passo MH: Long-term outcome among patients with juvenile rheumatoid arthritis, *Front Biosci* 3:e13–e22, 1998.

Schneider R, Lang B, Reilly B, et al: Prognostic indicators of joint destruction in systemic-onset juvenile rheumatoid arthritis, *J Pediatr* 120(2 Pt 1):200–205, 1992.

Wallace CA, Levinson JE: Juvenile rheumatoid arthritis, *Rheum Dis Clin North Am* 17(4):891–905, 1991.

SYSTEMIC LUPUS ERYTHEMATOSUS

SLE is an autoimmune disease that may involve nearly every organ system in an inflammatory process. SLE occurs more frequently in females and has a higher incidence in the black population than in Caucasians. Peak ages of onset correlate roughly with menarche and menopause; the preponderance of females demonstrating onset of the disease

---

TABLE 9–7
Clinical Diagnostic Criteria for Systemic Lupus Erythematosus*

Physical Signs Butterfly rash (malar) Discoid lupus Photosensitivity Oral and nasopharyngeal ulcers Nonerosive arthritis (two or more joints with effusion and tenderness) Pleuritis *or* pericarditis (serositis) Seizures *or* psychosis in absence of metabolic toxins or drugs	*Hematologic Disease* Hemolytic anemia with reticulocytosis *or* Leukopenia (<4000 on two occasions) *or* Lymphopenia (<1500 on two occasions) *or* Thrombocytopenia (<100,000)
	Serologic Data Positive anti-dsDNA *or* Positive anti-Sm *or* Positive LE prep *or* False-positive VDRL for >6 months Positive ANA in absence of drugs known to induce lupus
Laboratory Data *Renal Disease (Nephritis)* Proteinuria (greater than 500 mg/24 hr) *or* Cellular casts (RBC, granular, or tubular)	

LE, Lupus erythematosus; *RBC,* red blood cell.
*Table shows the 1982 revised criteria for diagnosing SLE. A patient must have four of the 11 criteria in order to establish the diagnosis of SLE. These criteria may be present at the same or at different times during the patient's illness. Additional, less diagnostic manifestations are noted in Table 9–8.

---

during these ages and in the postpartum period is even more striking than the number of individuals with SLE onset before puberty.

Clinical Manifestations. Arthritis or arthralgia, weight loss, fever, malaise, and rash are frequent symptoms at the onset of illness. The arthritis affects small more than large joints and is disproportionately painful relative to the physical findings. Many patients have a typical "butterfly" rash over the malar area of the face, sparing the nasolabial folds. Many other rashes are common with SLE and may vary from papular to bullous in character; some of these rashes exhibit photosensitivity. Any serosal surface also may be inflamed, resulting in pericarditis, pleuritis, or acute abdominal pain secondary to abdominal serositis. Vasculitis, myositis, pancreatitis, and the antiphospholipid antibody syndrome (with propensity for thrombosis) may be seen.

Renal disease is frequent in SLE, although in some patients it may be clinically inapparent. Renal biopsy demonstrates various lesions accompanied by deposition of complement and immunoglobulins within the glomerulus. Renal biopsy also helps differentiate acute inflammatory changes from chronic changes and scarring. At the onset of disease, some patients have a diffuse proliferative nephritis with compromised renal function; others may have a mild mesangial involvement that may not be progressive.

Hematologic disorders are common and again reflect autoantibody formation. Disorders include Coombs-positive hemolytic anemia, leukopenia secondary to antineutrophil antibodies, and thrombocytopenia associated with antiplatelet antibodies.

A broad spectrum of neurologic disorders may result from SLE, the most common being seizures or psychotic states. The level of cerebrospinal fluid (CSF) protein may be elevated mildly, and an MRI study may yield abnormal results. Neuropsychologic testing may be helpful. Other causes of central nervous system (CNS) symptoms, such as steroid psychosis, hypertension, uremia, infection (with toxoplasmosis, cryptococcosis, *Nocardia,* or *Listeria*), or stroke (from the antiphospholipid antibody syndrome), must be considered in the differential diagnosis. *Diagnostic criteria* for SLE and additional clinical manifestations are presented in Tables 9–7 and 9–8, respectively.

Laboratory Findings. Nearly all patients have positive results on tests for ANAs, although this is a screening test and is not diagnostic (Table 9–3). Most patients with SLE have antibodies to double-stranded DNA and decreased levels of total hemolytic complement. With effective therapy, complement levels may return to normal, except in rare patients with familial complement deficiencies. Other less specific test results may be seen, such as a

TABLE 9–8
Additional Manifestations of Systemic Lupus Erythematosus

Systemic	Neuropsychiatric—cont'd	Gastrointestinal—cont'd	Hematologic—cont'd
Fever	Chorea	Hepatitis (chronic-lupoid)	Antiphospholipid
Malaise	Transverse myelitis	Splenomegaly	antibodies (lupus
Weight loss	Migraine headaches		anticoagulant
Fatigue	Depression	**Renal**	causing
		Nephritis	thrombosis)
Musculoskeletal	**Cardiopulmonary**	Nephrosis	
Myositis, myalgia	Endocarditis	Uremia	**Endocrine**
Arthralgia	Myocarditis	Hypertension	Hypothyroidism
	Pneumonitis		Hyperthyroidism
Cutaneous		**Reproduction**	
Raynaud phenomenon	**Ocular**	Infertility	**Treatment-Induced**
Alopecia	Episcleritis	Repeat spontaneous	Steroid toxicity
Urticaria-angioedema	Sicca syndrome	abortions	Immunosuppression
Panniculitis	Retinal cytoid bodies	Neonatal lupus	Opportunistic
Livedo reticularis		Congenital heart block	infections
	Gastrointestinal		
Neuropsychiatric	Pancreatitis	**Hematologic**	
Personality disorders	Mesenteric arteritis	Anticoagulants (factors	
Stroke	Serositis	VIII, IX, XII, others	
Peripheral neuropathy	Hepatomegaly	causing hemorrhage)	

false-positive test for syphilis (VDRL) or the presence of a rheumatoid factor. A usually reversible form of SLE also may be induced by various drugs (e.g., hydralazine, procainamide, isoniazid, chlorpromazine, phenytoin, carbamazepine, quinidine, minocycline, and propylthiouracil); in 95% of patients, this condition is associated with antihistone antibodies. When the drug is withdrawn, the lupus-like syndrome resolves.

Treatment. Treatment varies with the disease manifestation. Arthritis and less serious manifestations usually are managed with NSAIDs. The skin manifestations of lupus respond to sunscreens and sun avoidance. Hydroxychloroquine may be used for skin and joint involvement and may have a steroid-sparing effect. Many patients have widespread organ system involvement that requires use of oral corticosteroids or, with very serious disease, intravenous pulses of steroids. Severe recalcitrant disease sometimes necessitates the use of cytotoxic agents (e.g., cyclophosphamide or azathioprine). Patients who have had a thrombotic event and evidence of the antiphospholipid antibody syndrome may require anticoagulation. Serologic parameters and complement levels may reflect disease activity. The goal of treatment is to allow the physician to use the lowest possible doses of medication for the shortest possible period.

Hypertension is a frequent complication of renal disease and steroid therapy and may necessitate aggressive use of antihypertensive agents. End-stage renal disease may be managed with dialysis or transplantation. Children with CNS lupus and seizures require antiseizure medications in addition to the therapy for the lupus itself.

Prognosis. The outlook for long-term survival has improved in childhood lupus; most centers, using a variety of treatment regimens, report a better-than-85% 5-year survival rate. With earlier diagnosis and treatment, renal failure is less commonly a cause of death, but secondary infection with opportunistic organisms has become a leading cause of mortality. Cerebritis, vasculitis, and acute nephritis are less common causes of mortality.

As with any child with chronic disease, psychologic support is crucial to the long-term well-being of the patient with lupus.

REFERENCES

Akin E, Miller LC, Tucker LB: Minocycline-induced lupus in adolescents, *Pediatrics* 101(5):926, 1998.

Behrman RE, Kliegman RM, Jenson HB, editors: *Nelson textbook of pediatrics*, ed 16, Philadelphia, 2000, WB Saunders, Chapter 159.

Lehman T: A practical guide to systemic lupus erythematosus, *Pediatr Clin North Am* 42(5):1223–1238, 1995.

McCurdy D, Lehman T, Bernstein B, et al: Lupus nephritis: prognostic factors in children, *Pediatrics* 89(2):240–246, 1992.

NEONATAL LUPUS SYNDROME

See Chapter 6.

DERMATOMYOSITIS

Dermatomyositis is an inflammatory disease with characteristic skin changes and striated muscle involvement manifesting as proximal muscle weakness. Gastrointestinal involvement occurs in some patients, and an underlying vasculopathy may be present. The illness is more common in females and tends to peak between 8 and 12 years of age, although disease is seen from infancy to adulthood.

Clinical Manifestations. The clinical syndrome is associated with a characteristic rash, symmetric proximal muscle weakness, elevated muscle enzyme levels, an abnormal electromyogram, and a muscle biopsy that shows loss of muscle fibrils commensurate with damage to the blood supply of the affected muscle. MRI can provide additional information about muscle edema and disease activity. The typical pattern of onset is insidious, and when the patient finally comes to medical attention, the history is one of very slowly diminishing capabilities, unnoticed by parents and teachers alike until some major motor dysfunction is apparent (e.g., the child may no longer be able to climb stairs, step onto the school bus, comb his or her own hair, or get up out of a chair). In retrospect, the child may have had malaise or worsening endurance, but usually there have been no specific complaints. The fatigue and nonspecific complaints may have caused the parents to seek medical attention.

The rash is said to be pathognomonic, but similar rashes occur in other disease entities. However, the rash is exceedingly characteristic and often overlooked. A "heliotrope" rash of purplish discoloration is present over the upper eyelids and is associated with periorbital edema and redness in the malar region. *Gottron papules* are areas of erythema, atrophy, or hyperkeratosis over the metacarpophalangeal and proximal interphalangeal joints, without associated arthritis. Commonly an associated nonspecific papular eruption covers the elbows and knees and, on occasion, also occurs in the sun-exposed "V"-area of the neck. Telangiectasias of the nail fold capillaries may occur. A magnification aid, such as use of the ophthalmoscope, helps in visualization. Calcifications over pressure points (e.g., knee and elbow) or in soft tissue may occur later in the course of the illness. If the characteristic rash is present, only three of the other four criteria are necessary for diagnosis (Table 9–9).

Rarely, children may exhibit fulminant dermatomyositis and polymyositis with an acute course of proximal muscle weakness, often with dysphagia or respiratory muscle compromise. The rash may not be appreciated at onset, and its course may be rapid enough to necessitate intensive care support. Cardiac involvement (e.g., conduction abnormalities or myopericarditis) may be present but is uncommon. A history of regurgitating liquids through the nose and laboratory evidence of markedly diminished vital capacity indicate that such a child must be placed immediately in an intensive care facility. The status of palatal function and voluntary respiratory muscle function (spirometry) must be followed. Proximal muscle weakness also should be monitored and scored according to loss of function (Table 9–10). Hip, shoulder, neck flexor, and abdominal muscle weakness are common.

Involvement of the gastrointestinal tract with vasculopathy may result in massive gastrointestinal bleeding or intestinal perforation. Pulmonary involvement may be secondary to muscle weakness,

---

TABLE 9–9
Dermatomyositis: Criteria for Diagnosis

Rash typical of dermatomyositis
Symmetric proximal muscle weakness
Elevated muscle enzymes (SGOT, SGPT, LDH, CPK, and aldolase)
EMG abnormalities typical of dermatomyositis (fasciculations, needle insertion irritability, and high-frequency discharges)
Positive muscle biopsy with chronic inflammation

CPK, Creatine phosphokinase; *EMG,* electromyographic; *LDH,* lactic dehydrogenase; *SGOT,* serum glutamic oxaloacetic transaminase; *SGPT,* serum glutamic pyruvic transaminase.

TABLE 9–10
Scoring System for Muscle Weakness

Score	Function
0	No movement or contraction
1	Contraction without extremity movement
2	No movement against gravity
3	Movement only against gravity
4	Movement against examiner resistance
5	Normal movement and strength

interstitial pneumonitis, or the development of fibrosing alveolitis.

Muscle-specific antibodies have been recognized in adults with dermatomyositis, and some have been correlated with different clinical courses. Muscle-specific antibodies have been identified in a small number of children, although their clinical utility needs further evaluation.

The *differential diagnosis* includes relatively uncommon disorders, such as trichinosis, tropical pyomyositis, hypereosinophilic syndromes, steroid myopathy, metabolic myopathies, SLE, overlap syndrome, emetine abuse, azidothymidine, and hyperthyroidism or hypothyroidism. Chronic myositis also may be caused by persistent coxsackievirus infection. Acute viral (e.g., enterovirus or influenza) myositis is common and associated with rhabdomyolysis, myoglobinuria, elevated creatine phosphokinase, and tender muscles.

Treatment. Most pediatric rheumatologists recommend 2 mg/kg of prednisone equivalent per day as initial therapy unless the child is so severely affected that intravenous pulse steroids are indicated. Usually a child responds within weeks with improved muscle function and markedly decreased muscle enzymes; the steroid dose then can be tapered slowly over the course of months. Most children do not tolerate alternate-day steroids until they are well into their recovery. The natural history of the active disease spans approximately 2–3 years, so most physicians plan a treatment regimen that involves at least alternate-day, low-dose steroids for a total duration of 2 years.

For children with steroid-dependent or steroid-nonresponsive disease, a variety of other treatment measures have been used, including methotrexate, intravenous immunoglobulin, cyclosporin, and cyclophosphamide. Optimal treatment regimens are yet to be determined.

Prognosis. Before the advent of steroids, one third of children died in the acute phase of illness, one third were severely compromised by disease, and one third recovered. Currently the mortality rate from dermatomyositis is significantly less than 10%. Most children totally recover after their disease has run its course. Some children have a remitting and exacerbating course, and a few unfortunate children have severe and unremitting disease, which may require them to receive immunosuppression with drugs such as methotrexate.

A complication of dermatomyositis is **calcinosis,** which occurs in patients with a prolonged disease course (at least 1 year in duration) and therefore is not seen in patients during the acute onset of disease. The calcium deposition may be minimal, sporadic, and unimportant or may be severe enough to significantly retard movement in all joints, resulting in a major disability. No effective treatment exists for the calcinosis of dermatomyositis; it may remit spontaneously or progress unremittingly and produce severe debilitation.

REFERENCES

Behrman RE, Kliegman RM, Jenson HB, editors: *Nelson textbook of pediatrics,* ed 16, Philadelphia, 2000, WB Saunders, Chapter 160.

Pachman LM: Juvenile dermatomyositis, *Pediatr Clin North Am* 42(5):1071–1098, 1995.

Rider LG, Miller FW, Targoff IN, et al: A broadened spectrum of juvenile myositis, *Arthritis Rheum* 37(10):1534–1538, 1994.

SCLERODERMA

In childhood, scleroderma (hardening of the skin) is a very rare condition that can be subdivided into localized and general disease entities. Girls are affected more than boys.

Clinical Manifestations. *Localized* scleroderma is the most frequent type of scleroderma in childhood and may appear as morphea or patch-like scleroderma on the trunk or as linear scleroderma that involves an extremity. The initial lesion may be inflammatory, exhibiting purplish discoloration and raised borders, some heat, and mild pain. Rapidly progressing scleroderma lesions evolve into areas with hypopigmentation and atrophy. Even localized scleroderma can be a "full-thickness" entity in which not only skin and subcutaneous tissue but also muscle, supporting structures, and even bone are involved; in linear scleroderma this extensive involvement can lead to marked contractures and undergrowth of limbs, resulting in disability. When linear scleroderma involves the scalp, extension to underlying structures can produce seizures, hypoplasia of the face, and severe cosmetic problems. Skin softening may occur. The lesions of morphea are particularly likely to regress.

Localized scleroderma is differentiated from **progressive systemic sclerosis** (PSS), which involves organ systems that include the kidneys, resulting in severe hypertension and renal failure; the gastrointestinal tract, leading to esophageal and intestinal motility problems; the lungs, causing restrictive disease and pulmonary hypertension; and the joints, resulting in arthritis.

Progressive systemic sclerosis is extremely uncommon in childhood. **Raynaud phenomenon** is frequent and may be one of the first manifestations of the disease. The skin may initially be edematous and then becomes sclerotic. The hard, tightened skin is bound to subcutaneous structures. Digital involvement is common and may result in flexion contractures. Bone in the distal phalangeal tuft often disintegrates, resulting in tapering of the ends of the fingers, termed "sclerodactyly." Calcinosis is relatively common in patients with PSS. Skin involvement proximal to the metacarpophalangeal or metatarsophalangeal joints is an important feature of PSS. Antibodies to Sc1-70 may be seen.

The **CREST syndrome** represents a more benign pattern of illness that involves *c*alcinosis, *R*aynaud phenomenon, *e*sophageal hypomotility, *s*clerodactyly, and *t*elangiectasia. *Raynaud phenomenon,* which may precede scleroderma for as many as 10 years, is characterized by intense pallor (vasoconstriction), followed by cyanosis (partial recirculation) and then by marked erythema (recirculation of blood) of the fingers in response to cold or stress. Anticentromere antibodies may be seen.

Scleroderma-like conditions may occur secondary to drugs (bleomycin), toxins (polyvinyl chloride), and chronic graft-versus-host disease following bone marrow transplantation.

Differential Diagnosis. The differential diagnosis includes idiopathic Raynaud disease (rather than phenomenon), eosinophilic fasciitis, toxin exposure (e.g., toxic oil or vinyl chloride), carcinoid syndrome, hereditary telangiectasia, porphyria, lichen sclerosus et atrophicus, idiopathic pulmonary hypertension, and mixed connective tissue disease (MCTD). MCTD is an overlap syndrome with manifestations of arthritis, SLE, scleroderma, and myositis. Levels of antibodies to extractable nuclear antigen and ribonucleoprotein are elevated in MCTD.

Laboratory Findings. There is no pathognomonic test for scleroderma, although the presence of ANAs, anticentromere antibodies, and anti-Sc1-70 antibodies are common. Capillaroscopy may reveal nail fold capillary changes, such as enlarged capillary loops, disruption or loss of capillaries, tortuosity, and pseudoglomerular (bushy) capillaries. Vital capacity and carbon monoxide diffusion capacity are useful tests for evaluation of pulmonary interstitial fibrosis and pulmonary endothelial damage, respectively.

Treatment. The treatment of localized scleroderma is not firmly established. Corticosteroids, methotrexate, calcitriol, D-penicillamine, and hydroxychloroquine have been used. Physical therapy is important if joint contractures have occurred.

The treatment of progressive systemic sclerosis or CREST syndrome is directed to the particular problems the patient has. Proton-pump inhibitors have been useful for gastroesophageal reflux occurring in adults. Hypertension is treated with angiotensin-converting enzyme inhibitors. Intravenous epoprostenol therapy for pulmonary hypertension in scleroderma has recently been used in adults.

Raynaud phenomenon is best treated by preventive measures, such as cold avoidance. Calcium channel blockers, such as nifedipine, may be of benefit. Biofeedback also may be of benefit.

REFERENCES

Badesch DB, Tapson UF, McGoon M, et al: Continuous intravenous epoprostenol for pulmonary hypertension due to the scleroderma spectrum of disease: a randomized controlled trial, *Ann Intern Med* 132(6):425–434, 2000.

Behrman RE, Kliegman RM, Jenson HB, editors: *Nelson textbook of pediatrics,* ed 16, Philadelphia, 2000, WB Saunders, Chapter 161.

Uziel Y, Miller M, Laxer R: Scleroderma in childhood, *Pediatr Clin North Am* 42(5):1171–1203, 1995.

VASCULITIS

Henoch-Schönlein Purpura

Henoch-Schönlein purpura (HSP) is the most common vasculitis of childhood and is characterized by palpable, nonthrombocytopenic purpura; periarticular, scrotal, and scalp swelling, edema, and inflammation; gastrointestinal bleeding (with or without intussusception); and nephritis (Table 9–4). The cutaneous manifestations are striking, with circular purpuric lesions 2–3 cm in size typically occurring over the buttocks and the posterior surfaces of the arms and legs. Skin lesions and the renal glomeruli may contain IgA immune complexes.

Clinical Manifestations. The onset of the illness often follows a nonspecific upper respiratory tract infection in a 4–10-year-old child. The skin lesions are the hallmark of the disease, but cramping, intermittent abdominal pain; hematochezia; periarticular swelling; and tense scalp or scrotal edema may be present. Glomerulonephritis may occur within 1–2 months of onset and becomes manifest as asymptomatic hematuria, with or without proteinuria. Fewer than 5% of patients have acute renal insufficiency, and another 5% have a slow progression, with renal failure developing months to years later. Initial manifestations of nephritis, nephrotic syndrome, or nephritic nephrosis increase the long-term risks of hypertension, renal impairment, or preeclampsia. Encephalopathy and pulmonary hemorrhage are rare manifestations of HSP. Most patients recover without therapy, but a small percentage relapse, and another small group has a much slower rate of recovery accompanied by the persistence of hematuria for 1–2 years.

Treatment. Therapy is symptomatic because 90% of patients have a self-limited illness. Corticosteroids may relieve abdominal pain and joint, scalp, or scrotal edema, but this has not been proven in controlled studies. Steroids do not have a beneficial effect on established renal disease. Although the optimal treatment regimen for HSP severe nephritis is not known, immunosuppressive therapy may be of benefit. Renal transplantation may be needed for the few patients with irreversible renal insufficiency; in some patients who have received a transplant, HSP has recurred in the transplanted kidney.

REFERENCES

Behrman RE, Kliegman RM, Jenson HB, editors: *Nelson textbook of pediatrics*, ed 16, Philadelphia, 2000, WB Saunders, Chapter 167.

Foster BJ, Chantal B, Drummond KA, et al: Effective therapy for severe Henoch-Schönlein purpura nephritis with prednisone and azathioprine: a clinical and histopathologic study, *J Pediatr* 136(3):370–375, 2000.

Goldstein A, White R, Akuse R, et al: Long-term follow-up of childhood Henoch-Schönlein nephritis, *Lancet* 339(8788):280–282, 1992.

Mills J, Michel B, Bloch D, et al: The American College of Rheumatology 1990 criteria for the classification of Henoch-Schönlein purpura, *Arthritis Rheum* 33(8):1114–11221, 1990.

Kawasaki Disease

Kawasaki disease, first described in Japan, now has been found throughout the world. The disease has a marked predilection in children of Japanese ancestry. It occurs in childhood, mostly in very young children, particularly under the age of 5 years. The etiology is unknown, although many believe it is viral or toxin mediated in origin.

Clinical Manifestations. Kawasaki disease is primarily a multisystem vasculitis; a significant number of untreated children (20–25%) have coronary artery aneurysms as sequelae to the disease. Criteria for diagnosing Kawasaki disease are listed in Table 9–11; five of the six criteria are required to make a diagnosis, although incomplete forms of the disease are recognized. Other disease manifestations are noted in Table 9–12. In addition, other disease processes must be excluded (Table 9–13).

The disease can be divided into three stages. The *acute phase* lasts about 10 days, during which most of the diagnostic criteria are likely to be present. In the acute phase, children have high fever, conjunctivitis, changes in oral mucous membranes, extremity changes (e.g., puffiness of the hands and feet and redness of the palms and soles), and rash. A desquamating perineal rash may be present. Cervical lymphadenopathy is less frequent. Irritability is profound in children with Kawasaki disease, and aseptic meningitis frequently is found. Myocarditis and pericarditis may occur.

The *subacute phase* (from days 11 through 21) usually is associated with a decrease in fever. Arthritis occurs in many children at this time, although in a few children arthritis has already appeared in the acute phase of the disease. A dramatic skin desquamation occurs in virtually all children beginning on about day 14; usually this desquamation begins at the junction of the nail and the fingertip, is very thick in nature, and is not painful. It is most common on the hands and feet but may occur in other regions.

The third phase, the *convalescent phase*, begins about day 21. During this phase, coronary artery aneurysms are often detected by echocardiogram. Arthritis and thrombocytosis may persist, but generally the acute-phase reactants subside. Myocardial infarctions and rupture of aneurysms may occur in either the subacute or convalescent phases.

TABLE 9–11
Kawasaki Disease: Criteria for Diagnosis

Fever persisting for 5 days or more
Changes of peripheral extremities
  Initial stage: reddening of palms and soles, indurative edema
  Convalescent stage: membranous desquamation from fingertips
Polymorphous exanthem
Bilateral conjunctival congestion
Changes of lips and oral cavity: reddening of lips, strawberry tongue, diffuse injection of oral and pharyngeal mucosa
Acute, nonpurulent cervical lymphadenopathy (>1.5 cm in diameter)

TABLE 9–12
Complications of Kawasaki Disease

Coronary artery thrombosis
Peripheral artery aneurysm
Coronary artery aneurysms
Myocardial infarction
Myopericarditis
Congestive heart failure
Hydrops of gallbladder
Aseptic meningitis
Irritability
Arthritis
Sterile pyuria (urethritis)
Thombocytosis (late)
Diarrhea
Pancreatitis
Peripheral gangrene

TABLE 9–13
Differential Diagnosis of Kawasaki Disease

Scarlet fever
Staphylococcal toxic shock syndrome
Stevens-Johnson syndrome (erythema multiforme)
Leptospirosis
Epstein-Barr virus
Juvenile rheumatoid arthritis (systemic-onset)
Measles
Acrodynia
Polyarteritis nodosa
Rocky Mountain spotted fever
Drug reaction
Scalded skin syndrome
Adenovirus

Treatment. High doses of aspirin (100 mg/kg/24 hr) generally are used in the acute phase and shorten the duration of fever; as the child improves, low doses of aspirin generally are used for their effect in preventing platelet aggregation. Low-dose aspirin therapy (3–5 mg/kg/24 hr) generally is continued until both the thrombocytosis and the other acute-phase reactants have returned to normal (i.e., the end of the convalescent phase), provided coronary artery changes have not occurred, in which case therapy is continued. Intravenous immunoglobulin therapy (2 g/kg for 1 dose) during the acute phase reduces coronary aneurysm formation.

When Kawasaki disease was first described, the death rate was about 3%; this rate has dramatically decreased over the last 20 years.

REFERENCES

Barron KS, Shulman ST, Rowley A, et al: Report of the National Institutes of Health workshop on Kawasaki disease, *J Rheumatol* 26(1):170–190, 1999.
Behrman RE, Kliegman RM, Jenson HB, editors: *Nelson textbook of pediatrics,* ed 16, Philadelphia, 2000, WB Saunders, Chapter 166.
Shulman ST, De Inocencio J, Hirsh R: Kawasaki disease, *Pediatr Clin North Am* 42(5):1205–1222, 1995.

Polyarteritis Nodosa

Polyarteritis nodosa (PAN) is an uncommon form of vasculitis characterized by inflammation of small and medium-sized arteries. Systemic features are weight loss, malaise, and anorexia. Multisystem organ involvement can occur and most commonly involves joints, muscles, the kidneys, peripheral nerves, and the skin. Cutaneous nodules may be seen; a biopsy or angiography may help establish the *diagnosis.* Livedo reticularis and peripheral gangrene may occur. Other major organs may also be involved.

The etiology is not known; it may be associated with hepatitis B infection in adults and streptococcal infections in childhood. The outlook in the systemic form of the disease is guarded.

Treatment includes corticosteroids and cytotoxic agents. Patients with a more limited form, known as cutaneous PAN, may have a better outlook and require less aggressive treatment.

REFERENCES

Behrman RE, Kliegman RM, Jenson HB, editors: *Nelson textbook of pediatrics,* ed 16, Philadelphia, 2000, WB Saunders, Chapter 167.
Sheth AP, Olson JC, Esterly NB: Cutaneous polyarteritis nodosa of childhood, *J Am Acad Dermatol* 31(4):561–566, 1994.

Wegener Granulomatosis

Wegener granulomatosis is an uncommon vasculitis in childhood (Table 9–4). The disease may resemble HSP, exhibiting renal, skin, joint, and gastrointestinal involvement, or it may resemble an adult-type vasculitis, with lung, renal, sinus or nasopharynx, eye, and joint disease. Necrotizing midline upper respiratory tract granulomas (in the sinus, subglottic stenosis, nose, or otitis) accompanied by renal vasculitis and pulmonary lesions (cavitary or nodular infiltrates or pulmonary hemorrhage) are typical in both age groups. Sinus disease is an early manifestation, demonstrating inflammation of the paranasal sinuses and, rarely, nasal septum perforation. Secondary infection may produce pyogenic sinusitis. Renal involvement may occur late and becomes manifest as hematuria, proteinuria, renal failure, and hypertension. Other manifestations include rash, arthralgia, peripheral neuropathy, and dacryocystitis.

Wegener granulomatosis can be differentiated from HSP by the presence of lung involvement, the absence of IgA immune complexes in dermal capillaries, and the presence of antineutrophil cytoplasmic antibodies and granulomas.

Without treatment the prognosis is poor. Treatment with both cyclophosphamide and corticosteroids has resulted in improved prognosis.

REFERENCES

Behrman RE, Kliegman RM, Jenson HB, editors: *Nelson textbook of pediatrics,* ed 16, Philadelphia, 2000, WB Saunders, Chapter 167.
Rottem M, Fauci A, Hallahan C, et al: Wegener granulomatosis in children and adolescents: clinical presentation and outcome, *J Pediatr* 122(1):26–31, 1993.

ACUTE RHEUMATIC FEVER

See Chapter 13.

PAIN SYNDROMES IN CHILDHOOD
Recurrent Limb Pain

Many children, most frequently between the ages of 5 and 12 years, complain of recurrent evening or nighttime limb pains. These pains usually are intermittent and occur around and behind the knee, in the calves and thigh areas, and sometimes in the shins; occasionally upper extremity pain occurs. The pain typically occurs at the end of a day of strenuous activity and is resolved totally by the following morning. There is no associated limp, but the pain may interfere with normal sleep. Historically, these are likely to represent what people have called growing pains.

Growth and development are normal, as is the physical examination. No associated effusions, limitations of joint motion, features of hypermobility syndrome, or "trigger points" are present. Systemic signs are absent and roentgenograms and laboratory studies are normal. In one study, children with growing pains were rated by their parents as having different temperamental and behavioral profiles than a control group of children.

Treatment consists of reassurance and comfort measures, such as local heat and rubbing the limb. Stretching exercise for the Achilles tendons and hamstrings may be beneficial. Pain medication, such as acetaminophen, may be helpful. Recurrent limb pains may be episodic and may reappear over the course of months or years. Ultimately, the child outgrows the propensity for having these pains.

Fibromyalgia

Fibromyalgia is a benign, intermittent, noninflammatory musculoskeletal pain syndrome seen in children and in adults; it is more common in females (5:1) and tends to occur much more often in adolescents than in younger children. Arthralgia is present, but not synovitis. A number of characteristically tender trigger points exist: those on the anterior chest (costochondral); on the inner aspect of the scapula medially (supraspinatus muscle); around the knee but beyond the joint margin; over the greater trochanters; and near the gluteus medius, low cervical spine (C5–C7), and low lumbar ligaments (L4–S1). Many patients relate their symptoms to changes in the weather, and some often have an associated depression, morning stiffness, and a disturbance in sleep pattern. Many of these children miss an extraordinary amount of school. Some children may improve over time. Associated nonrheumatic illnesses are headache, irritable bowel syndrome, major depression, and panic disorder.

The *treatment* of fibromyalgia includes educating the patient that fibromyalgia is not a crippling, deforming disease. NSAIDs may have an analgesic effect, but most controlled studies have not found them to be more effective than placebo. Amitriptyline and cyclobenzaprine have been more effective than placebo in adults. Controlled studies in adults have shown benefit from cardiovascular fitness training, electromyography-biofeedback, electroacupuncture, and hypnotherapy. Cognitive-behavioral interventions have been successful in some children.

Reflex Sympathetic Dystrophy

Chronic, unilateral extremity pain may be the result of reflex sympathetic dystrophy, which is characterized by local, burning pain; hyperalgesia; allodynia (pain from usually nonpainful stimuli, such as light touch); cyanosis; sweating; mottling; coldness; excessive hair growth; swelling; and, if not treated, contractures, demineralization, and atrophy. The patient may have a history of mild-moderate trauma.

Benign Hypermobility Syndrome

Benign hypermobility syndrome is diagnosed in children with excessive joint mobility in the absence of a congenital disease of connective tissue, such as **Ehlers-Danlos syndrome** or **Marfan syndrome.** Some authors question whether this is a distinct entity or might represent a mild variant of Ehlers-Danos syndrome. It likely represents a variation in normal joint range of motion. Children who meet three or more criteria (Fig. 9–1) are said to be hypermobile. Some children with joint hypermobility have episodic arthralgia. It is generally thought that symptoms improve with maturation.

REFERENCES

Behrman RE, Kliegman RM, Jenson HB, editors: *Nelson textbook of pediatrics,* ed 16, Philadelphia, 2000, WB Saunders, Chapters 168–169.

Buskila D, Neumann L, Hershman E, et al: Fibromyalgia syndrome in children: an outcome study, *J Rheumatol* 22(3):525–528, 1995.

Gedalia A, Brewer EJ: Joint hypermobility in pediatric practice: a review, *J Rheumatol* 20(2):371–374, 1993.

Oberklaid F, Amos D, Liu C, et al: Growing pains: clinical and behavioral correlates in a community sample, *J Dev Behav Pediatr* 18(2):102–106, 1997.

Wilder R, Berde C, Wolohan M, et al: Reflex sympathetic dystrophy in children, *J Bone Joint Surg Am* 74(6):910–919, 1992.

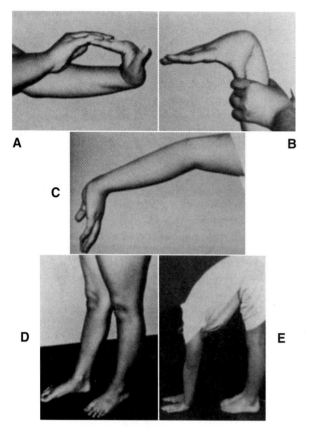

FIG. 9–1

Features of hypermobility in children. **A,** Hyperextension of fingers. **B,** Apposition of thumbs. **C,** Hyperextension of elbows. **D,** Hyperextension of knees. **E,** Flexion of trunk. (From Gedalia A, Brewer EJ: *J Rheumatol* 20[2]:371–374, 1993.)

tion varies by age, with children 4 years old or younger demonstrating skin lesions, arthritis, and uveitis. This presentation may mimic JRA. Older children have a disease presentation similar to that in adults, with lung, lymph node, and eye involvement. Sarcoidosis is more common in African-Americans.

The *clinical manifestations* of sarcoidosis include weight loss, cough, fatigue, bone or joint pain, lymphadenopathy, dyspnea, parotid enlargement, fever, uveitis, nodules, maculopapular rash, neurologic involvement, erythema nodosum, and hepatosplenomegaly. Hilar adenopathy with pulmonary nodules or interstitial infiltrates also is common.

Laboratory findings are not specific, but hypercalcemia, polyclonal gammopathy, and elevated angiotensin-converting enzyme levels are common. Slit-lamp examination reveals granulomatous anterior uveitis, and tissue biopsy demonstrates noncaseating granulomas. Pulmonary function tests may show a restrictive pattern, and gallium scanning demonstrates increased pulmonary uptake. Computed tomography may help define pulmonary involvement. Renal disease becomes manifest as hematuria and proteinuria. Cutaneous anergy is common.

Treatment includes corticosteroids. The *prognosis* is fair to good; only 40–50% of patients remain symptomatic for 5 years after therapy.

REFERENCES

Behrman RE, Kliegman RM, Jenson HB, editors: *Nelson textbook of pediatrics,* ed 16, Philadelphia, 2000, WB Saunders, Chapter 715.

Hafner R, Vogel P: Sarcoidosis of early onset: a challenge for the pediatric rheumatologist, *Clin Exp Rheumatol* 11(6):685–691, 1993.

SARCOIDOSIS

Sarcoidosis is a chronic disease of unknown cause. Multisystem involvement (more than five systems) is common. In pediatric patients the peak age for this disease is during adolescence, but it has occurred in children as young as 2 months of age. The presenta-

CHAPTER 10

Infectious Diseases

Alice Prince

BASIC PRINCIPLES OF PEDIATRIC INFECTIOUS DISEASES

Epidemiology

The ability to diagnose and appropriately treat specific childhood infections depends on an understanding of the epidemiology and risk factors associated with each infectious agent, as well as the population at risk for certain pathogens. Susceptibility to specific infectious agents is a direct consequence of the maturity of the immune system, exposure to potential infectious agents, and the presence of underlying diseases. The host response varies with age. Thus before the development of their own immunologic repertoire, neonates are at risk for different types of infections than school-aged children or adolescents. Clinical consequences of an excessive inflammatory response may be more deleterious than the injury directly attributed to the pathogen. To approach the diverse types of infections seen in pediatrics, the clinician must consider the following questions:

1. Who gets a specific disease?
2. Does this occur in a normal host, a globally immunocompromised patient, or a child with a specific immunologic defect, or is the child at risk because of medical devices (e.g., central lines or shunts)?
3. What organisms are involved?
4. Is the presentation one of a benign viral illness or more suggestive of bacterial infection?
5. How can the etiologic agent be identified?
6. What antimicrobial agents are available for treatment?
7. What can be done to prevent this disease?
8. What is the nature of the host immune response?

The likelihood of many infections can be estimated by historical factors and host evaluation. Sociologic factors are important; for infants the ade-quacy of prenatal care, gestational age, maternal risk-taking behavior, and appropriate screening tests for congenital infection are helpful clues. The immunization history and living conditions, including exposure to infected adults or to other infants in a closed setting such as day care or an informal baby-sitting arrangement, may be factors in the transmission of common infections. Other environmental factors such as travel, exposure to air conditioners, the season, construction sites, insects, and animals or exotic pets may help the clinician assess the possibility of specific etiologic agents. Adopted infants from countries with disorganized health care delivery systems and children who have lived in refugee camps may be at risk for infections not typically seen in developed countries.

A careful and complete physical examination is critical to the diagnosis of many infectious diseases. Although initial complaints, particularly in infants, may be nonspecific (e.g., irritability, poor feeding, or lethargy), certain physical findings, such as specific rashes, may be diagnostic. Particular care should be given to identifying the sites of infection (Table 10–1). Knowledge of these common sites permits identification of the infecting organism and guides appropriate treatment. Rashes are a common manifestation of infections; appropriate classification of the rash morphology can be diagnostic for many infections (Table 10–2).

Prevention

The prevention of many previously fatal childhood diseases has been a triumph of pediatrics and has been accomplished through the use of routine vaccination (Fig. 10–1 and Table 10–3). Vaccines may be live attenuated viruses (e.g., measles, mumps, rubella, varicella, and polio) or may consist of

Text continued on p. 365

TABLE 10–1
Localizing Manifestations of Infection

Site	Symptoms	Signs
Upper respiratory	Rhinorrhea, sneezing, cough, sore throat, drooling, stridor, trismus, sinus pain, fever, ear pain or drainage, tooth pain	Nasal congestion; pharyngeal erythema; enlarged tonsils with exudate; swollen, red epiglottis; red, bulging tympanic membrane; regional lymphadenopathy
Lower respiratory	Cough, fever, chest pain, dyspnea; sputum production	Rales, wheezing, localized diminished breath sounds, intercostal retractions, tachypnea
Gastrointestinal	Vomiting, diarrhea, abdominal pain, anorexia, fever	Hyperactive bowel sounds, abdominal tenderness, hematochezia
Hepatic	Anorexia, vomiting; dark urine, light stools	Jaundice, hepatomegaly, hepatic tenderness, hemorrhage, coma
Genitourinary	Dysuria, frequency, urgency, fever, flank or suprapubic pain, vaginal discharge	Costovertebral angle or suprapubic tenderness, cervical motion and adnexal tenderness
Skeletal	Limp, bone pain, fever, pseudoparalysis	Local swelling, erythema, warmth, limited range of motion, tenderness
Central nervous system	Fever, lethargy, irritability, headache, neck stiffness, seizures	Kernig or Brudzinski sign, bulging fontanel, focal neurologic deficits, coma
Cardiovascular	Dyspnea, palpitations, exercise intolerance, chest pain, fever, shock	Tachycardia, hypotension, cardiomegaly, hepatomegaly, splenomegaly, rales, petechiae, Osler nodes, Janeway lesions, new murmur, distended neck veins, pericardial friction rub, muffled heart tones

TABLE 10–2
Differential Diagnosis of Fever and Rash

Lesion	Pathogen or Associated Factor
Maculopapular or macular rash	**Viruses** Measles, rubella, roseola (human herpesvirus-6 or -7), fifth disease (parvovirus), Epstein-Barr virus, enteroviruses, hepatitis B virus (papular acrodermatitis or Gianotti-Crosti syndrome), human immunodeficiency virus **Bacteria** Rheumatic fever (group A streptococcus), scarlet fever, erysipelas, *Arcanobacterium haemolyticum*, secondary syphilis, leptospirosis, *Pseudomonas*, meningococcal infection (early), *Salmonella*, Lyme disease **Rickettsiae** Early Rocky Mountain spotted fever, typhus (scrub, endemic), ehrlichiosis **Other** Kawasaki disease, rheumatoid arthritis, drug reaction
Diffuse erythroderma	**Bacteria** Scarlet fever (group A streptococcus), toxic shock syndrome (*Staphylococcus aureus*) **Fungi** *Candida albicans*

TABLE 10–2
Differential Diagnosis of Fever and Rash—cont'd

Lesion	Pathogen or Associated Factor
Urticarial rash	**Viruses** Epstein-Barr virus, hepatitis B, human immunodeficiency virus **Bacteria** *Mycoplasma pneumoniae,* group A streptococci **Other** Drug reaction
Vesicular, bullous, pustular	**Viruses** Herpes simplex, varicella-zoster, coxsackievirus **Bacteria** Staphylococcal scalded skin syndrome, staphylococcal bullous impetigo, group A streptococcal crusted impetigo **Other** Toxic epidermal necrolysis, erythema multiforme (Stevens-Johnson syndrome), rickettsialpox
Petechial-purpuric	**Viruses** Atypical measles, congenital rubella, cytomegalovirus, enterovirus, human immunodeficiency virus, hemorrhagic fever viruses **Bacteria** Sepsis (meningococcal, gonococcal, pneumococcal, *Haemophilus influenzae*), endocarditis **Rickettsiae** Rocky Mountain spotted fever, epidemic typhus, ehrlichiosis **Other** Vasculitis, thrombocytopenia, Henoch-Schönlein purpura, malaria
Erythema nodosum	**Viruses** Epstein-Barr, hepatitis B **Bacteria** Group A streptococcus, tuberculosis, *Yersinia,* cat-scratch disease **Fungi** Coccidioidomycosis, histoplasmosis **Other** Sarcoidosis, inflammatory bowel disease, estrogen-containing oral contraceptives, systemic lupus erythematosus, Behçet disease
Distinctive Rashes	
Ecthyma gangrenosum	*Pseudomonas aeruginosa*
Erythema chronicum migrans	Lyme disease
Necrotic eschar	Aspergillosis, mucormycosis
Erysipelas	Group A streptococcus
Koplik spots	Measles
Erythema marginatum	Rheumatic fever

Recommended Childhood Immunization Schedule
United States, January–December 2001

Vaccines[1] are listed under routinely recommended ages. Bars indicate range of recommended ages for immunization. Any dose not given at the recommended age should be given as a "catch-up" immunization at any subsequent visit when indicated and feasible. Ovals indicate vaccines to be given if previously recommended doses were missed or given earlier than the recommended minimum age.

Age ▲ / Vaccine ▼	Birth	1 mo	2 mo	4 mo	6 mo	12 mo	15 mo	18 mo	24 mo	4-6 yr	11-12 yr	14-18 yr
Hepatitis B[2]	Hep B #1	Hep B #2			Hep B #3						Hep B[2]	
Diphtheria, Tetanus, Pertussis[3]			DTaP	DTaP	DTaP		DTaP[3]			DTaP	Td	Td
H. influenzae type b[4]			Hib	Hib	Hib	Hib						
Inactivated Polio[5]			IPV	IPV	IPV[5]					IPV[5]		
Pneumococcal Conjugate[6]			PCV	PCV	PCV	PCV						
Measles, Mumps, Rubella[7]						MMR				MMR[7]	MMR[7]	
Varicella[8]						Var					Var[8]	
Hepatitis A[9]									Hep A — in selected areas[9]			

Approved by the Advisory Committee on Immunization Practices (ACIP), the American Academy of Pediatrics (AAP), and the American Academy of Family Physicians (AAFP).

* This schedule indicates the recommended ages for routine administration of currently licensed childhood vaccines as of November 1, 2000, for children through age 18 years. Additional vaccines may be licensed and recommended during the year. Licensed combination vaccines may be used whenever any components of the combination are indicated and the vaccine's other components are not contraindicated. Providers should consult the manufacturer's package inserts for detailed recommendations.

† **Infants born to hepatitis B surface antigen (HBsAg)-negative mothers** should receive the first dose of hepatitis B vaccine (Hep B) by age 2 months. The second dose should be administered at least 1 month after the first dose. The third dose should be administered at least 4 months after the first dose and at least 2 months after the second dose, but not before age 6 months. **Infants born to HBsAg-positive mothers** should receive Hep B and 0.5 mL hepatitis B immune globulin (HBIG) within 12 hours of birth at separate sites. The second dose is recommended at age 1–2 months and the third dose at age 6 months. **Infants born to mothers whose HBsAg status is unkown** should receive Hep B within 12 hours of birth. Maternal blood should be drawn at delivery to determine the mother's HBsAg status; if the HBsAg test is positive, the infant should receive HBIG as soon as possible (no later than age 1 week). **All children and adolescents (through age 18 years)** who have not been immunized against hepatitis B should begin the series during any visit. Providers should make special efforts to immunize children who were born in or whose parents were born in areas of the world where hepatitis B virus infection is moderately or highly endemic.

§ The fourth dose of diphtheria and tetanus toxoids and acellular pertussis vaccine (DTaP) may be administered as early as age 12 months, provided 6 months have elapsed since the third dose and the child is unlikely to return to age 15–18 months. Tetanus and diphtheria toxoids (Td) is recommended at age 11–12 years if at least 5 years have elapsed since the last dose of diphtheria and tetanus toxoids and pertussis vaccine (DTP), DTaP, or diphtheria and tetanus toxoids (DT). Subsequent routine Td boosters are recommended every 10 years.

¶ Three *Haemophilus influenzae* type b (Hib) conjugate vaccines are licensed for infant use. If Hib conjugate vaccine (PRP-OMP) (PedvaxHIB or ComVax [Merck]) is administered at ages 2 and 4 months, a dose at age 6 months is not required. Because clinical studies in infants have demonstrated that using some combination products may, induce a lower immune response to the Hib vaccine component, DTaP/Hib combination products should not be used for primary immunization in infants at ages 2, 4, or 6 months unless approved by the Food and Drug Administration for these ages.

** An all-inactivated poliovirus vaccine (IPV) schedule is recommended for routine childhood polio vaccination in the United States. All children should receive four doses of IPV at age 2 months, age 4 months, between ages 6 and 18 months, and between ages 4 and 6 years. Oral poliovirus vaccine should be used only in selected circumstances (1).

†† The heptavalent pneumococcal conjugate vaccine (PVC) is recommended for all children age 2–23 months. It is also recommended for certain children age 24–59 months (2).

§§ The second dose of measles, mumps, and rubella vaccine (MMR) is recommended routinely at age 4–6 years but may be administered during any visit, provided at least 4 weeks have elapsed since receipt of the first dose and that both doses are administered beginning at or after age 12 months. Those who previously have not received the second dose should complete the schedule no later than the routine visit to a health-care provider at age 11–12 years.

¶¶ Varicella vaccine (Var) is recommended at any visit on or after the first birthday for susceptible children (i.e., those who lack a reliable history of chickenpox [as judged by a health-care provider] and who have not been immunized]). Susceptible persons aged ≥13 years should receive two doses given at least 4 weeks apart.

*** Hepatitis A vaccine (Hep A) is recommended for use in selected states and/or regions, and for certain high-risk groups. Information is available from local public health authorities (3).

Additional information about the immunization schedule is available on the National Immunization Program World-Wide Web site, http://www.cdc.gov/nip, or by telephone, (800)232-2522 (English) or (800)232-0233 (Spanish).

FIG. 10–1

Recommended childhood immunization schedule, United States, January–December 2001. (Modified from Centers for Disease Control and Prevention, *MMWR* 50:7, 2001.)

TABLE 10–3
Recommended Immunization Schedules for Children Not Immunized in the First Year of Life*

Recommended Time/Age	Immunization(s)	Comments
Younger Than 7 Years		
First visit	DTaP, Hib, HBV, MMR	If indicated, tuberculin testing may be done at same visit
		If child is 5 yr of age or older, Hib is not indicated in most circumstances
Interval after first visit		
1 mo (4 wk)	DTaP, IPV, HBV, Var	The second dose of IPV may be given if accelerated poliomyelitis immunization is necessary, such as for travelers to areas where polio is endemic
2 mo	DTaP, Hib, IPV	Second dose of Hib is indicated only if the first dose was received when younger than 15 mo
≥8 mo	DTaP, HBV, IPV	IPV and HBV are not given if the third doses were given earlier
Age 4–6 yr (at or before school entry)	DTaP, IPV, MMR	DTaP is not necessary if the fourth dose was given after the fourth birthday; IPV is not necessary if the third dose was given after the fourth birthday
Age 11–12 yr	See Fig. 10–1	
7–12 Years		
First visit	HBV, MMR, dT, IPV	
Interval after first visit		
2 mo (8 wk)	HBV, MMR, Var, dT, IPV	IPV also may be given 1 mo after the first visit if accelerated poliomyelitis immunization is necessary
8–14 mo	HBV, dT, IPV	IPV is not given if the third dose was given earlier

From American Academy of Pediatrics: *Red book 2000*, ed 25, Chicago, Ill, 2000, The Academy.
DTaP, Diphtheria and tetanus toxoids and acellular pertussis; *dT*, adult tetanus toxoid (full dose) and diphtheria toxoid (reduced dose); *HBV*, hepatitis B virus; *Hib, Haemophilus influenzae* type b conjugate; *IPV*, inactivated poliovirus; *MMR*, live measles-mumps-rubella; *Var*, varicella.
*Table is not completely consistent with all package inserts. For products used, also consult manufacturer's package insert for instructions on storage, handling, dosage, and administration. Biologics prepared by different manufacturers may vary, and package inserts of the same manufacturer may change. Therefore, the physician should be aware of the contents of the current package insert.

TABLE 10–4
Additional Special Vaccines

Vaccine	Indication
Meningococcal (polysaccharide A/C/Y/W135)	Functional or anatomic asplenia, travel to an endemic area, patients with terminal complement deficiency; college freshmen; type B meningococcus not covered
Influenza (inactivated virus)	Patients with asthma, cystic fibosis, bronchopulmonary dysplasia, sickle cell anemia, diabetes, chronic heart disease
Bacille Calmette-Guérin (BCG) (live attenuated *M. bovis* vaccine)	Infants in high tuberculosis incidence areas
Typhoid (live attenuated bacteria)	Oral vaccine for travel to or living in endemic areas. Exposure to *S. typhi* chronic carrier; recommended for children >6 yr of age
Rabies (human diploid cell vaccine)	
Preexposure	High-risk groups (e.g., veterinarians, animal handlers, and laboratory workers)
Postexposure	Must include human rabies immune globulin passive immunization, plus vaccine on days 1, 3, 7, 14, and 28, following high-risk animal bites: dog, raccoon, skunk, fox, cat, coyote, and bat

TOPV, Trivalent oral polio vaccine.

inactivated immunogenic components of either viruses or bacteria (e.g., polio, hepatitis B, pertussis, influenza, diphtheria, tetanus, *Haemophilus influenzae* type b, and pneumococcus). Vaccine efficacy depends on the age of the child, the immune status, appropriate administration, and booster immunizations.

In addition to those vaccines recommended for all children, various high-risk situations (e.g., repeated exposure to a pathogen, altered cardiopulmonary status, or increased susceptibility to various bacteria) warrant additional vaccinations (Table 10–4). When there are no specific effective vaccines and the patient is at increased risk for the infectious disease because of repeated exposure or increased host susceptibility, antimicrobial prophylaxis is administered for as long as the patient remains at risk (Table 10–5).

Clinical Use of the Microbiology Laboratory

Laboratory diagnosis of infection involves a variety of techniques, ranging from the simple microscopic examination of bacterial morphology using the Gram stain to the more technical molecular microbiologic methods, such as the polymerase chain reaction (PCR). Current practices include the following:

- Routine culture methods for isolation of specific pathogens from infected sites

TABLE 10–5
Antimicrobial Prophylaxis

	Pathogen	Preventive Therapy
Pertussis	*Bordetella pertussis*	Erythromycin, azithromycin
Diphtheria	*Corynebacterium diphtheriae*	Penicillin, erythromycin
Meningitis	*Haemophilus influenzae* type b	Rifampin
	Neisseria meningitidis	Rifampin, ceftriaxone
Tuberculosis	*Mycobacterium tuberculosis*	Isoniazid
Sepsis/asplenia*	*Streptococcus pneumoniae*	Penicillin
	Haemophilus influenzae type b	Amoxicillin
Rheumatic fever	Group A streptococci	Penicillin
Interstitial pneumonia	*Pneumocystis carinii*	Trimethoprim/sulfamethoxazole, pentamidine
Influenza	Influenza virus	Amantadine (influenza A): oseltamivir
Hepatitis A	HAV	Immune serum globulin†
Hepatitis B	HBV	Hepatitis B immune globulin (HBIG)†
Chickenpox	Varicella-zoster virus	Varicella-zoster immune globulin (VZIG)†
RSV	RSV	RSV-immune globulin
AIDS	HIV	Maternal prepartum and intrapartum plus neonatal postpartum therapy with AZT‡
Neonatal sepsis	Group B streptococcus	Intrapartum ampicillin for at-risk mothers
Neonatal conjunctivitis	*Chlamydia trachomatis*	0.5% erythromycin topically
	Neisseria gonorrhoeae	1% silver nitrate or 0.5% erythromycin topically
Bacterial endocarditis		
Dental procedure	Streptococci	Amoxicillin (PO), ampicillin and gentamicin (IV)
Genitourinary/ gastrointestinal procedure	Enterococcus	Amoxicillin (PO), ampicillin and gentamicin (IV) (see Chapter 13)

AIDS, Acquired immunodeficiency syndrome; *AZT*, zidovudine (azidothymidine); *HAV*, hepatitis A virus; *HBV*, hepatitis B virus; *HIV*, human immunodeficiency virus; *RSV*, respiratory syncytial virus.
*Including sickle cell disease.
†Early administration of vaccine may also be effective after exposure with immune globulin.
‡Accidental occupational exposure (e.g., needle stick) managed with AZT plus additional antiretroviral agents (e.g., lamivudine with indinavir or nelfinavir).

- Antigen detection using either latex agglutination or fluorescent antibody
- Detection of genomic deoxyribonucleic acid (DNA) or ribonucleic acid (RNA) sequences of pathogens using complementary probes and PCR
- Demonstration of an antibody response to an infection by serologic testing or Western hybridization technique
- Tissue culture to identify viruses and intracellular pathogens

The laboratory also can provide critical information to optimize therapy and prevent toxicity, such as antimicrobial susceptibility testing, mean inhibitory (MIC) or bactericidal (MBC) concentrations of antimicrobial agents, or peak and trough drug levels.

FEVER

Healthy individuals maintain their core body temperatures within 1°–1.5° C (37°–38° C). Normal body temperature is considered to be 98.6° F (37° C, range from 97°–99.6° F). Most individuals have a diurnal variation, with maximal levels achieved in the late afternoon. The normal body temperature is maintained by the anterior hypothalamus using a complex regulatory system. Rectal temperatures greater than 38° C (100.4° F) generally are considered abnormal.

Pathogenesis of Fever

All infections can produce fever, which begins with the release of endogenous pyrogens into the circulation after an infectious or immunologically mediated event. Endogenous pyrogens are cytokines (interleukin [IL]-1, IL-6, tumor necrosis factor [TNF], and the interferons), which are released by monocytes, macrophages, mesangial cells, glial cells, epithelial cells, and B lymphocytes. The endogenous pyrogens reach the anterior hypothalamus via the arterial blood supply, liberating arachidonic acid, which is metabolized to prostaglandin E_2 (PGE_2), resulting in an elevation of the hypothalamic thermostat. Antipyretics work by altering the synthesis of prostaglandins, reducing production of PGE_2.

Intense muscle contraction (as in cocaine overdose) or muscle metabolism altered by drugs (e.g., neuroleptic agents) or anesthetics produces **malignant hyperthermia** (see Chapter 18). Heat stroke, a potentially fatal febrile illness, is caused by excessively high environmental temperatures and failure of physiologic body heat–losing mechanisms.

The *pattern* of fever in children may vary, depending on the age of the child and the nature of the illness. Neonates may not have a febrile response or may be hypothermic despite a significant infection, whereas older infants and children younger than 5 years may have an exaggerated febrile response, with temperatures as high as 105° F in response to either a serious bacterial infection or a benign viral process. Fevers to this latter degree are unusual in older children and adolescents and suggest a significant pathologic process. Except in unusual circumstances, the fever pattern does not distinguish fever caused by bacterial, viral, fungal, or parasitic organisms from that resulting from malignancy, autoimmune diseases, or drugs.

Most febrile illness in children may be categorized according to the following list:

- Fever of short duration accompanied by localizing signs and symptoms, in which a diagnosis can be established by clinical history and physical examination
- Fever without localizing signs, usually occurring in a child younger than 3 years of age, in which a history and physical examination fail to establish a cause but a diagnosis may be suggested by laboratory studies
- Fever of unknown origin (FUO), fever present for more than 14 days *(in a child)* that does not have an etiology despite history, physical examination, and routine laboratory tests. (In older children and adolescents, an FUO usually is defined as a fever over 38° C for more than 2 weeks that remains undiagnosed despite detailed comprehensive evaluation for 7 days.)

Fever Without a Source: Occult Bacteremia

A common clinical pediatric problem is the evaluation of the febrile but well-appearing child with no localizing signs of infection. Although most of these children have self-limited viral infections, some (usually younger than 3 years of age) have bacteremia, and a few have severe and potentially life-threatening illnesses such as bacterial meningitis. Particularly in the early stages of such illness, it is difficult even for experienced clinicians to differentiate patients with bacteremia from those with benign illness (Table 10–6).

Fever in Children Between 3 Months and 2 Years of Age

Etiology. Children between 3 months and 2 years of age are at risk for infection resulting from organisms with polysaccharide capsules, such as *Streptococcus pneumoniae*, *H. influenzae* type b, meningococci, and *Salmonella*. Effective phagocytosis of these organisms requires opsonic antibody. Although neonates receive maternal immunoglobulin G (IgG)

TABLE 10–6
Differentiating Viral from Bacterial Infections

Variable	Viral	Bacterial
Petechiae	Present	Present
Purpura	Rare	If severe
Leukocytosis	Uncommon*	Common
Shift to left (↑ bands)	Uncommon	Common
Neutropenia	Possible	Suggests overwhelming infection
↑ESR	Unusual*	Common
↑CRP	Unusual	Common
↑TNF, IL-1, PAF	Uncommon	Common
Meningitis (pleocytosis)	Lymphocytic†	Neutrophilic
Meningeal signs positive‡	Present	Present

CRP, C-reactive protein; *ESR,* erythrocyte sedimentation rate; *IL,* interleukin; *PAF,* platelet-activating factor; *TNF,* tumor necrosis factor.
*Adenovirus and herpes simplex may cause leukocytosis and increased ESR; Epstein-Barr virus may cause petechiae and increased ESR.
†Early viral (enterovirus, arbovirus) meningitis may initially have a neutrophilic pleocytosis.
‡Nuchal rigidity, bulging fontanel, Kernig or Brudzinski sign.

transplacentally, this protection is gradually lost (over 3–6 months), leaving the infant at risk for infection caused by encapsulated organisms until their own IgM and IgG are produced. In the United States, widespread use of the conjugate vaccine against *H. influenzae* type b has dramatically reduced the incidence of infections caused by this organism. It is anticipated that use of the conjugate pneumococcal vaccine will reduce but not eliminate occult bacteremia caused by *S. pneumoniae.*

Clinical Manifestations and Diagnosis. In children between 3 months and 2 years of age, many febrile episodes demonstrate an obvious source of infection as elicited by history or physical examination (e.g., pharyngitis, otitis media, pneumonia, or upper respiratory tract infection). The evaluation of infants who are febrile and well appearing but without a focus of infection depends on the clinical assessment, which may include a complete blood count (CBC) with white blood cell (WBC) differential, erythrocyte sedimentation rate (ESR), blood culture, urinalysis with urine culture, and a chest radiograph (if respiratory symptoms are present) to attempt to find an infectious focus. Bacteremia is more likely in patients with fever higher than 39° C.

The WBC count does not always predict accurately whether a child has bacteremia. Nonetheless, it can be helpful in dividing the population into high-risk and low-risk (>5000 to <15,000/L) groups. This division may help select patients for further investigation or therapy. The ESR is no more useful than the WBC count in predicting bacteremia in ambulatory febrile patients. Elevated C-reactive protein (CRP) and TNF levels have been correlated with bacterial disease. With or without thrombocytopenia, the finding of petechiae in a febrile child is suggestive of bacteremia and warrants close attention. All patients should have a urinalysis to measure urine nitrites and leukocyte esterase, the presence of which suggests a urinary tract infection (see Chapter 16). Patients with diarrhea should have a stool checked for leukocytes. Variables that may help in differentiating viral from bacterial disease are noted in Table 10–6.

Occult bacteremia caused by pneumococcus in otherwise healthy children between 3 and 24 months of age may be transient, with serious infections developing in a small but important percentage of infants. In contrast, bacteremias caused by *H. influenzae* type b and *Neisseria meningitidis* are often less benign, and serious localizing infections such as meningitis, septic arthritis, and pericarditis are possible sequelae.

Children with **sickle cell anemia** have deficiencies of splenic function and properdin-dependent opsonization, placing them at high risk for bacteremia, especially during the first 5 years of life (see Chapter 14). Pneumococcal sepsis accompanied by meningitis, and (less commonly) bacteremia and meningitis caused by *H. influenzae* type b, are potentially serious and fulminant infections in patients with sickle cell disease. *Salmonella* bacteremia may lead to osteomyelitis.

Treatment. Because of the low incidence of occult bacteremia (4–5% of children) and because most episodes of occult bacteremia are caused by pneumococci and may be transient in healthy immunocompetent children, most physicians do not routinely administer antibiotics to all febrile infants whose infection has no focus or to those patients who do not appear to be septic. After obtaining blood and urine specimens for culture, some physicians administer ceftriaxone IM and discharge the well-appearing infant with follow-up within 24 hours.

Any ill-appearing infant should be considered seriously infected, admitted to the hospital, and treated with antibiotics. A well-appearing febrile infant between 3 and 24 months of age should be carefully evaluated. A blood specimen from the infant should be obtained and the child sent home with follow-up in 24 hours. If the blood culture becomes positive for pneumococci and the child is afebrile, appears well, and has no localizing signs, the child does not need to be treated; a subsequent blood specimen should be obtained. If the initial blood culture tests positive for pneumococcus or the child remains febrile or has localizing signs suggestive of pneumonia or meningitis, the child should be treated with appropriate antibiotics in the hospital.

If the bacteremia is caused by *H. influenzae* type b or *N. meningitidis*, the child should be immediately reevaluated, a lumbar puncture performed, and parenteral antibiotics administered. Before the administration of antibiotics, another blood specimen should be obtained in all children to determine the persistence of the bacteremia. Antibiotic dosages are noted in Appendix I.

Fever in Infants Younger Than 3 Months of Age

Fever in infants younger than 3 months of age may be associated with a higher risk of serious bacterial infections than fever in older infants. These younger infants may not demonstrate localizing signs, and bacteremia, meningitis, urinary tract infection, and pneumonia may be present in the infant exhibiting nonspecific signs such as poor feeding. Often fever is the only manifestation of serious bacterial infection in very young infants. Urinary tract infection (with *E. coli*), bacteremia (caused by *Salmonella*, group B streptococci, pneumococcus, *H. influenzae*, or meningococcus), pneumonia (*Staphylococcus aureus* or pneumococcus), meningitis (viral or group B streptococci, meningococcus, pneumococcus, or *H. influenzae* type b), and osteomyelitis (*S. aureus* or group B streptococci) are common types of infection. Nonetheless, most febrile diseases in this age group are caused by common viral pathogens.

Differentiation between viral and bacterial infections often is difficult (Table 10–6). Therefore, infants younger than 3 months of age who appear sick and all infants younger than 1 month of age (especially with uncertain follow-up) usually are admitted to the hospital.

After blood, urine, and cerebrospinal fluid (CSF) specimens are obtained for culture, broad-spectrum antibiotics are administered to many of these infants. The choice of antibiotics depends on the possible pathogens involved and any localizing findings, such as pneumonia, septic arthritis and osteomyelitis, or meningitis. Well-appearing febrile infants without an infectious focus (e.g., otitis media, skin, soft tissue, bone, or joint); who are older than 1 month of age; with good follow-up; no history of prematurity or prior antimicrobial therapy; and a WBC count between 5000 and 15,000, fewer than 10 WBCs/high-power field (hpf) on examination of urine (or negative leukocyte esterase); and fewer than 5 WBCs/hpf on examination of stool (in infants with diarrhea) may be discharged home without therapy. Some physicians administer ceftriaxone IM to these infants after obtaining a blood specimen for culture. In either case, careful outpatient management requires close phone contact for 48 hours and a return visit within 24 hours.

REFERENCES

Baker MD, Bell LM, Avner JR: The efficacy of routine outpatient management without antibiotics of fever in selected infants, *Pediatrics* 103(3):627–631, 1999.

Behrman RE, Kliegman RM, Jenson HB, editors: *Nelson textbook of pediatrics*, ed 15, Philadelphia, 2000, WB Saunders, Chapters 170–172.

Chiu C, Lin T, Bullard M: Identification of febrile neonates unlikely to have bacterial infections, *Pediatr Infect Dis J* 16(1):59–63, 1997.

Finkelstein JA, Christiansen CL, Platt R: Fever in pediatric primary care: occurrence, management, and outcomes, *Pediatrics* 105(1 Pt 3):260–266, 2000.

Netea MG, Kullberg BJ, Van der Meer JWM: Circulating cytokines as mediators of fever, *Clin Infect Dis* 31(Suppl 5):S178–S184, 2000.

Rothrock S, Harper M, Green S, et al: Do oral antibiotics prevent meningitis and serious bacterial infections in children with *Streptococcus pneumoniae* occult bacteremia? A meta-analysis, *Pediatrics* 99(3):438–444, 1997.

Fever of Unknown Origin

FUO (fever >100.4° F lasting for more than 14 days with no obvious cause despite a complete history, physical examination, and routine laboratory evaluation) historically was a difficult problem because most patients remained undiagnosed despite in-hospital evaluation for 1 week. The differential diagnosis between occult infections and neoplasms may require invasive procedures. With the improved capability of diagnostic imaging techniques (combined with imaging-guided needle biopsy), including ultrasound, computed tomography (CT), magnetic resonance imaging (MRI), and radionuclide scanning with gallium or technetium, the number of undiagnosed patients in this category has decreased substantially.

Etiology. The evaluation must take into consideration whether the patient is a normal or immunocompromised host. In addition to a careful documentation of several instances of an elevated temperature, a thorough *history* should be undertaken, including the impact the fever has had on the child's health;

weight loss; the presence of an associated disease, such as diabetes mellitus, malignancy, or rheumatologic conditions; involvement of vital organs such as the liver, heart, or brain; the use of drugs, medications, or immunosuppressive therapy; exposure to industrial or hobby-related chemicals; blood transfusions; domestic or foreign travel to endemic areas (e.g., with malaria, dengue fever, tick- or mosquito-borne diseases [Lyme, ehrlichiosis, encephalitis, hanta virus] or endemic fungal diseases [histoplasmosis, coccidioidomycosis, or *Cryptococcus neoformans*]); genetic background; recent surgical procedure or dental work; and sexual activity. Specific attention should be given to the social history and exposure to pathogens (e.g., malaria, tuberculosis, or day care) or animals (e.g., birds, livestock, bats, reptiles, or pets) and insects (e.g., tick or mosquito).

Because the etiology of most occult infections in the normal host involves an unusual presentation of a common disease, an evaluation for diseases typical to a geographic locale should be pursued. Thus an adolescent from an urban area with an FUO requires a careful evaluation for bacterial diseases, including tuberculosis, salmonellae, and spirochetes, as well as viral entities such as Epstein-Barr virus (EBV), cytomegalovirus (CMV), human immunodeficiency virus (HIV), and hepatitis A, B, and C viruses. Inhabitants of or travelers to rural areas should be evaluated for zoonosis and insect- or water-borne pathogens.

In the absence of localizing signs (e.g., heart murmur, abdominal pain, or abnormal liver function), it may be difficult to focus the evaluation. Furthermore, entities such as sinusitis, endocarditis, intraabdominal abscesses (perinephric, intrahepatic, or subdiaphragmatic), and central nervous system (CNS) lesions (e.g., tuberculoma, cysticercosis, abscess, or toxoplasmosis) may be relatively asymptomatic. An FUO also may be the presentation of an immunodeficiency disease.

Differential Diagnosis (Table 10–7). The three most common categories of FUO in children are infectious

---

TABLE 10–7
Causes of Fever of Unknown Origin in Children

Infections	***Spirochetal Diseases***
Bacterial Diseases	*Borrelia* (borreliosis: *B. recurrentis, B. burgdorferi;* Lyme disease)
Specific organism causing systemic disease	Leptospirosis
Bartonellosis (e.g., cat scratch disease)	*Spirillum minus*
Brucellosis	Syphilis
Campylobacter	***Viral Diseases***
Gonococcemia (chronic)	Cytomegalovirus
Meningococcemia (chronic)	Hepatitis
Salmonellosis	Human immunodeficiency virus (and its opportunistic-associated infections)
Streptobacillus moniliformis	Infectious mononucleosis (Epstein-Barr virus)
Tuberculosis	Unidentified presumed virus
Tularemia	***Chlamydial Diseases***
Localized infections	Lymphogranuloma venereum
Abscesses: abdominal, dental, hepatic, pelvic, perinephric, rectal, subphrenic, splenic, periappendiceal, psoas	Psittacosis
	Rickettsial Diseases
Cholangitis	*Ehrlichia canis*
Endocarditis	Q fever
Mastoiditis	Rocky Mountain spotted fever
Osteomyelitis	***Fungal Diseases***
Pneumonia	Blastomycosis (nonpulmonary)
Pyelonephritis	Coccidioidomycosis (disseminated)
Sinusitis	Histoplasmosis (disseminated)

Modified from Behrman RE, Kliegman RM, Jenson HB, editors: *Nelson textbook of pediatrics,* ed 16, Philadelphia, 2000, WB Saunders.

Continued

TABLE 10–7
Causes of Fever of Unknown Origin in Children—cont'd

Parasitic Diseases
Extraintestinal amebiasis
Babesiosis
Giardiasis
Malaria
Toxoplasmosis
Trypanosomiasis
Visceral larva migrans

Autoimmune Hypersensitivity Diseases
Drug fever
Hypersensitivity pneumonitis
Juvenile rheumatoid arthritis (systemic onset, Still
   disease)
Polyarteritis nodosa
Rheumatic fever
Serum sickness
Systemic lupus erythematosus
Undefined vasculitis

Neoplasms
Atrial myxoma
Ewing sarcoma
Hepatoma
Hodgkin disease
Leukemia
Lymphoma
Neuroblastoma

Granulomatous Diseases
Granulomatous hepatitis
Sarcoidosis
Crohn disease

Familial-Hereditary Diseases
Anhidrotic ectodermal dysplasia
Cyclic neutropenia
Deafness, urticaria, amyloidosis syndrome
Fabry disease
Familial dysautonomia
Familial Mediterranean fever
Hypertriglyceridemia
Ichthyosis

Miscellaneous
Behçet syndrome
Chronic active hepatitis
Diabetes insipidus (central and nephrogenic)
Factitious fever
Hemophagocytic syndromes
Histiocytosis syndromes
Hypothalamic-central fever
Infantile cortical hyperostosis
Inflammatory bowel disease
Kawasaki disease
Pancreatitis
Periodic fever
Postoperative (pericardiotomy, craniectomy)
Pulmonary embolism
Spinal cord injury–crisis
Thyrotoxicosis
Central fever

Undiagnosed Fever
Persistent
Recurrent
Resolved

Modified from Behrman RE, Kliegman RM, Jenson HB, editors: *Nelson textbook of pediatrics*, ed 16, Philadelphia, 2000, WB Saunders.

diseases, inflammatory or rheumatologic diseases, and neoplasms. A diagnosis is not established in 10–20% of children with FUO.

The diseases most commonly identifiable in children can be grouped into two categories: *generalized* infections caused by specific organisms, and *localized* infections caused by a variety of organisms. In the United States organisms and conditions most frequently associated with FUO in children that produce a generalized infection are *Bartonella* (cat-scratch disease), ehrlichiosis, *Salmonella*, mycobacteria, brucellosis, tularemia, spirochetes (leptospirosis, Lyme disease, rat-bite fever, and syphilis), HIV, CMV, hepatitis viruses, and EBV. Localized infections are endocarditis, intraabdominal or liver abscess, sinusitis, mastoiditis, osteomyelitis, pneumonia, and pyelonephritis or perinephric abscess.

The inflammatory diseases that most commonly manifest as FUO are juvenile rheumatoid arthritis (JRA), systemic lupus erythematosus (SLE), polyarteritis nodosa, rheumatic fever, inflammatory bowel disease, and undefined vasculitis (see Chapter 9).

Malignancies are a less common cause of FUO in children than in adults, accounting for about 10% of all episodes. Malignancies that may be associated with FUO are Hodgkin and non-Hodgkin lymphoma, leukemia, Ewing sarcoma, and neuroblastoma.

Factitious fever is another important consideration, particularly if family members are health care providers. Fever should be recorded in the hospital by a reliable individual who remains with the patient when the temperature is taken. Psychiatric disorders frequently are masked by the family's denial and desire to find an organic cause for their child's problems. Continuously observing the patient over a long period of time and repetitive evaluation are indicated.

For children with underlying disorders (e.g., immunosuppression, HIV, or malignancy), an aggressive evaluation to find an occult infection is justified. Infections in these patients can involve viral infections such as hepatitis A, B, or C or EBV, CMV and other herpesviruses, including HHV 6 or 7, or systemic bacterial infections caused by organisms such as *Bartonella,* ehrlichiae, *Salmonella,* or mycobacteria. With transplanted organs, the graft itself may be infected (e.g., in CMV or Chagas disease). Localized infections (e.g., sinusitis; endocarditis; intraabdominal, splenic, or endovascular abscesses; osteomyelitis; pneumonia; or pyelonephritis or perinephric abscesses) may be relatively asymptomatic. These entities are also important causes of fever in the normal host and can be diagnosed during an exhaustive workup. Following cardiovascular and other major surgical procedures, infection caused by relatively indolent bacteria such as the coagulase-negative staphylococci must be considered. Endocarditis is a leading diagnosis in patients who have had cardiac surgery.

Clinical Manifestations. Two major patterns of presentation are seen: prolonged, daily fevers that are true FUOs, and repeated, discrete febrile episodes over a prolonged period of time, which may indicate a different pathogenesis such as hyperimmunoglobulin-D syndrome, cyclic neutropenia, familial Mediterranean fever, periodic fevers with aphthous ulcers, or other rheumatologic diseases. Systemic illness may be manifested by anorexia, malaise, night sweats, and fatigue. These will also affect the patient's nutritional status.

Noninfectious causes may be suggested by specific physical findings. Fever in the absence of sweating may be associated with anhidrotic ectodermal dysplasia, exposure to atropine, nephrogenic or central diabetes insipidus, and familial dysautonomia. Patients with **dysautonomia** lack tears, have smooth tongues that lack fungiform papillae, are insensitive to pain, and have failure to thrive and gastroesophageal reflux. Fever caused by hypothalamic dysfunction may also be accompanied by the failure of the pupils to constrict, since the sphincter-constrictor muscle develops embryologically at the same time that the hypothalamus undergoes differentiation.

A meticulous physical examination may provide clues to focus the diagnostic evaluation. A careful HEENT examination to elicit tenderness to tapping over the sinuses or teeth, which may be followed with more sophisticated imaging techniques, often leads to the diagnosis of sinusitis or dental abscess. Oral candidiasis or mucosal ulcers may suggest a number of immunologic disorders, especially HIV infection. Mucosal ulcers are indicative of several different viral, bacterial, and immunologic disorders ranging from Behçet syndrome to the common coxsackievirus infection (hand-foot-mouth syndrome) and herpes simplex infections. The **syndrome of periodic fevers, aphthous stomatitis, pharyngitis, and adenitis** may be considered in children younger than 5 years of age. More commonly, herpesvirus infections, EBV, CMV, Behçet syndrome, streptococcal infections, or pharyngitis caused by *C. hemolyticum* present with injection of the pharynx without an exudate. The acute presentation of primary HIV infection includes fever and malaise, pharyngitis, lymphadenitis, and a maculopapular rash and should be considered because this is treated with antiretroviral agents.

Ocular findings may suggest a specific etiology, particularly in conjunction with other systemic manifestations of infection. Conjunctivitis and red, weepy eyes may be indicative of superantigen-mediated disease such as toxic shock syndrome or Kawasaki disease; viral infection; or symptoms of rheumatologic disease indicative of systemic diseases, particularly vasculitis, such as that associated with polyarteritis nodosa, sarcoidosis, inflammatory bowel disease, or JRA. These systemic disorders are more frequently associated with bulbar conjunctivitis, whereas palpebral conjunctivitis is more typical of viral infection such as measles, coxsackievirus, or adenovirus. Careful ophthalmologic evaluation and a slit-lamp examination may be useful to diagnose intraocular manifestations of rheumatologic disease or embolic phenomena suggestive of endocarditis or endovascular infection, or manifestations of fungal *(Candida),* parasitic (toxoplasmosis), or granulomatous (TB and sarcoidosis) diseases.

Repetitive chills and fevers, suggestive of septicemia, indicate the release of immunostimulatory components of the infecting organism and the host response. This can be elicited by cell wall fragments from gram-positive bacteria, lipopolysaccharide-endotoxin from gram-negative bacteria, mycobacterial lipoproteins, protozoal lipoproteins, fungal arabinogalactan, or viral antigens and may continue during appropriate antimicrobial chemotherapy.

The muscles and bones should be palpated carefully. Point tenderness over a bone suggests osteomyelitis or neoplastic bone marrow invasion. Tenderness over the trapezius muscle may be a clue to a subdiaphragmatic abscess. Generalized muscle tenderness suggests dermatomyositis, trichinosis, polyarteritis, or *Mycoplasma,* influenza, or arboviral infection.

Rectal or pelvic examination may reveal tenderness and suggest a deep pelvic abscess, iliac or mesenteric adenitis, or pelvic osteomyelitis. A guaiac test on stool should be performed because occult blood loss suggests inflammatory bowel disease. Hyperactive deep tendon reflexes suggest thyrotoxicosis.

Diagnosis. Children with unexplained fever should be evaluated in a logical sequence beginning with a meticulous history, comprehensive physical examination, and compilation of screening laboratory data. An organ-system approach is helpful. The urgency of further testing depends on the clinical status of the patient and the tempo of the disease processes. Not all patients with unexplained fever need to be evaluated for all of the conditions associated with FUO. Young infants with unexplained fever frequently have undefined viral illnesses such as EBV infections.

Other causes of FUO in infants are pyogenic bacterial infections, JRA, and Kawasaki disease. A more aggressive approach is required to evaluate an infant with daily fever spikes to 105° F and significant toxicity.

The immune function of the host often must be evaluated. The WBC and differential cell counts provide an indication of granulocyte and lymphocyte numbers, the presence of immature forms, leukocytosis, or lymphocytosis. Leukocyte markers can be readily determined to establish the proportions of T and B cells and to further identify T-cell subsets and helper and cytotoxic cells. The function of these cells can be assessed by measuring immunoglobulins and isohemagglutinins; skin testing with anergy panels to monitor T-cell function; and measurement of complement. Additional tests for the evaluation of an FUO are listed in Fig. 10–2. These additional tests should be used judiciously and should focus on areas suggested by the screening tests, physical findings, or historical data.

Central Nervous System Disease. The child with headache, possible sinusitis, or other signs suggestive of CNS involvement should first have a computed tomography (CT) scan. Analysis of the CSF may be useful to determine CNS involvement as a manifestation of an FUO, looking for cells, protein, and immunoglobulins. This is particularly important in the evaluation for CNS Lyme disease, syphilis, or immunologic diseases such as SLE. Increased protein may suggest a parameningeal infection that could be better delineated by CT with contrast or MRI. Small CNS lesions, tuberculomas, toxoplasmosis, cysticercosis, and small abscesses would also require neuroimaging techniques.

Cardiovascular Disease. Bacterial endocarditis is an important cause of FUO but may be difficult to diagnose because patients frequently are given oral antibiotics that sterilize blood cultures but are inadequate to sterilize intracardiac vegetations (see Chapter 13). While endocarditis may be considered in the patient with rheumatic heart disease or following cardiac surgery, patients with abnormal natural valves (mitral valve prolapse, bicuspid aortic valves) or intracardiac defects that lead to turbulent blood flow, damaged endothelium, and platelet and fibrin deposition are also at risk for endocarditis with organisms that are "adhesive" and routinely cause transient bacteremias (e.g., oral streptococci, enterococci, and HACEK bacteria). Patients with indwelling intravascular catheters are at risk for endocarditis because of staphylococcal species and occasionally fungi. The evaluation of myocarditis, endocarditis, or pericarditis involves echocardiography and both transthoracic and transesophageal echocardiography.

Pulmonary Disease. Even in the absence of respiratory manifestations, pulmonary disease may be a cause of FUO. Patients with significant parenchymal disease, pleural disease, mediastinal widening, or hilar adenopathy may be asymptomatic. The determination of arterial blood gases may be helpful to define alveolar disease. CT scan or MRI may assist in the assessment of the extent of disease and suggest a diagnosis. Hilar adenopathy may suggest lymphoma, sarcoidosis, histoplasmosis, or tuberculosis. The diagnosis of sarcoidosis may require bronchioalveolar lavage, a tissue biopsy via fiberoptic or rigid bronchoscopy, or thoracoscopy. Interstitial infiltrates may be associated with histiocytosis, CMV, or *Pneumocystis carinii* with or without HIV infection. Bronchoalveolar lavage to recover an organism is indicated in such patients.

Gastrointestinal Disease. Many causes of FUO originate in the gastrointestinal tract, either as walled-off occult abscesses from clinically inapparent appendiceal perforations or hepatic, pelvic, and splenic abscesses or as inflammatory bowel disease. CT with

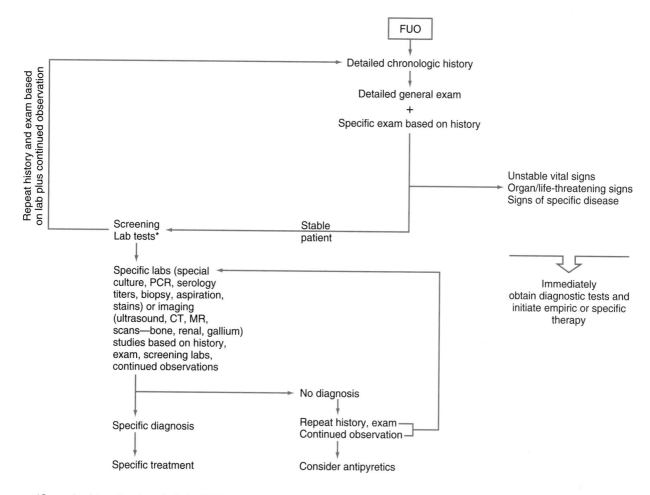

*Screening laboratory tests include CBC with differential; ESR; CRP; urinalysis; liver enzymes; direct and indirect bilirubin; CPK; blood, urine, and stool culture (including ova and parasites); serology, VDRL, ANA, Monospot-EBV titers; and radiologic studies such as chest x-ray.

FIG. 10–2

Approach to the evaluation of fever of unknown origin (FUO) in children. *ANA*, Antinuclear antibody; *CBC*, complete blood count; *CPK*, creatine phosphokinase; *CRP*, C-reactive protein; *CT*, computed tomography; *EBV*, Epstein-Barr virus; *ESR*, erythrocyte sedimentation rate; *MR*, magnetic resonance (imaging); *PCR*, polymerase chain reaction; *VDRL*, Venereal Disease Research Laboratory (test for syphilis). (Modified from Corder WT, Aranoff SC: Fever of unknown origin. In Kliegman RM, editor: *Practical strategies in pediatric diagnosis and therapy,* Philadelphia, 1996, WB Saunders.)

contrast or MRI may be helpful after screening ultrasonography. These tests are useful in ruling out mass lesions and evaluating the integrity of the gastrointestional tract and bowel wall. When inflammatory bowel disease is suspected in children, contrast studies and endoscopy with mucosal biopsy are required.

Weight loss and diarrhea may indicate parasitic infection, which may occur in a normal or immunodeficient child. In addition to the screening tests discussed in the preceding paragraph, careful evaluation for parasites may involve a total eosinophil count and a stool examination for *Giardia* and other organisms. In HIV-infected patients, usually innocuous organisms such as *Blastocystis hominis, Cryptosporidium,* or *Cyclospora* may be associated with significant symptoms.

Genitourinary Disease. The genitourinary tract may be the source of several causes of FUO, including bacterial urinary tract infection, tuberculosis (heralded by sterile pyuria), perinephric abscess, and neuroblastoma. Ultrasound followed by CT or renal scan is used in the evaluation of possible renal pathology, pelvic abscess, pelvic inflammatory disease (PID), or other occult genitourinary infections.

Musculoskeletal Disease. The usual presentation of osteomyelitis or septic arthritis is that of an acute localized infection. However, vertebral or pelvic osteomyelitis that is not apparent may cause FUO. Similarly, a psoas abscess may present as vague back pain and limp without localizing signs. Technetium pyrophosphate radionuclide imaging, which is highly sensitive for osteoclast and osteoblast activity, is extremely useful in detecting bony involvement. Similarly, a gallium scan, which indicates collections of polymorphonuclear leukocytes, may be useful to screen for abscesses. CT scan or MRI is helpful in demonstrating the presence of Ewing sarcoma, which often presents as bone pain with FUO.

The presence or history of arthritis in the patient or family, even if evanescent or migratory, may be quite important in establishing the diagnosis of Lyme disease, autoimmune processes (see Chapter 9), or one of the postinfectious arthritides such as Reiter syndrome. Appropriate screening serologic tests may be helpful (Fig. 10–2). Myositis frequently is suggested by myalgias, muscle tenderness, and a high serum creatine phosphokinase (CPK) level.

Hematologic Disease. Children with FUO, chronic infection, or both are frequently anemic. Examination of a peripheral blood smear may indicate findings suggestive of the "anemia of chronic disease" or the toxic granulations suggestive of bacterial infection. An examination of the bone marrow may be indicated to exclude hematologic malignancy or storage cells. Bone marrow aspirates should be examined and cultured for fungi (histoplasmosis) and mycobacteria (*Mycobacterium tuberculosis* and *M. avium-intracellulare*), as well as for other bacteria (*Brucella*).

Treatment. By definition, an FUO is a chronic process. Every effort should be made to arrive at a specific diagnosis before initiating therapy, particularly with modalities that may mask significant underlying diseases.

REFERENCES

Behrman RE, Kliegman RM, Jenson HB, editors: *Nelson textbook of pediatrics*, ed 16, Philadelphia, 2000, WB Saunders, Chapter 172.
Knockaert DC, Vanneste LJ, Vanneste SB, et al: Fever of unknown origin in the 1980s: an update of the diagnostic spectrum, *Arch Intern Med* 152(1):51–55, 1992.
Miller L, Sisson B, Tucker L, et al: Prolonged fevers of unknown origin in children: patterns of presentation and outcome, *J Pediatr* 129(3):419–423, 1996.
Steele RW, Jones SM, Lowe BA, et al: Usefulness of scanning procedures for diagnosis of fever of unknown origin in children, *J Pediatr* 119(4):526–530, 1991.

Fever in the Immunocompromised Host

The evaluation of fever in immunologically impaired patients is quite different from that in normal hosts. Although an FUO may be the initial presentation of an immune deficiency, it is more commonly seen in a febrile patient with a known immunodeficiency. The types of infections and their management can be predicted by which parts of the immune system are abnormal.

An increasing number of children are being successfully treated for malignancies and genetic disorders with stem cell transplantation, as well as the many children who are receiving organ transplants for cardiac, renal, hepatic, pulmonary, and gastrointestinal disease. Febrile episodes in immunocompromised postsurgical patients occur both at the time of transplantation and later while these patients remain on immunosuppressive therapy. The use of corticosteroids and immunosuppressants that impair the activation of T cells (cyclosporine, tacrolimus, sirolimus) increases the risk for pathogens that normally are controlled by T cell–mediated responses. At the time of solid organ transplantation, these patients are at significant risk of infection, but since they retain normal neutrophil function, they are usually managed with relatively brief courses of prophylactic antimicrobial agents (antibacterial and antifungal agents), often followed by chronic prophylaxis to prevent CMV, herpesvirus, and *P. carinii* infection, with regimens including trimethoprim/sulfamethoxazole, acyclovir, or ganciclovir. Children receiving stem cell transplants are exposed to significantly greater immunosuppression as a consequence of the myeloablative conditioning regimens; children receiving allogeneic transplants are at greater risk for infection than those receiving autologous transplants. The time to hematologic engraftment is a significant factor in the development of infection in these patients. Episodes of fever and neutropenia are common; these patients are at significant risk of hematogenous infection from their own bacterial or fungal flora until their marrow function and circulating PMNs return. Most clinicians feel that these patients are at significant risk for invasive infection and warrant prophylactic antimicrobial agents, often fluoroquinolones and azole antifungals. The use of corticosteroids puts these patients at risk for infections because of intracellular pathogens such as *P. carinii*, salmonellae, *Listeria*, mycobacteria, and many fungi. They have a high incidence of viral infection caused by CMV, EBV, and the herpes simplex viruses, including varicella-zoster.

Fever and Neutropenia

Infection is a major cause of death in patients with hematologic malignancy and following stem cell or solid organ transplantation. The use of chemotherapeutic agents that target rapidly dividing cells causes myelosuppression and mucositis. These patients require antimicrobial therapy until the source of their fever is identified. However, whether "clinically well" patients with fever and neutropenia, in the setting of treatment for a hematologic or other malignancy, can be treated with oral agents, or even with parenteral regimens in an outpatient setting, has received great discussion. Avoidance of hospitalization and exposure to the many nosocomial pathogens transmitted in the hospital setting has advantages in this group of patients.

Most positive blood cultures in these patients are the result of gram-positive bacteria and fungi; gram-negative rods had been most common previously. The use of central indwelling catheters provides a source of infection. Coagulase-negative staphylococci are frequently associated with catheter infections; *Streptococcus viridans* and enterococci, which can be resistant to β-lactam antibiotics and vancomycin, are isolated with increasing frequency. As the peripheral WBC count decreases below 500, patients are at risk for bacterial sepsis caused by their own endogenous flora. Techniques to decrease the incidence of infection, such as the prophylactic use of fluoroquinolone antibiotics, fluconazole, or acyclovir/ganciclovir to prevent infection caused by gram-negative bacteria, *Candida* species, or herpesviruses (including CMV), respectively, may also predispose these patients to infection from highly drug-resistant organisms. Although the use of prophylactic antimicrobial agents does increase the risk of drug resistance, the net effect in decreasing episodes of fever and bacteriologically confirmed infection may outweigh the potential increase in the incidence of infection caused by drug-resistant organisms.

Febrile episodes in neutropenic patients routinely are treated with combinations of broad-spectrum antimicrobial agents (e.g., vancomycin or nafcillin-ceftazidime or antipseudomonal penicillins–aminoglycosides) until the WBC count improves; some patients are prescribed prophylactic antimicrobial agents to prevent sepsis. The use of recombinant granulocyte colony–stimulating factor or granulocyte-macrophage colony–stimulating factor stimulates neutrophil production by the bone marrow, reduces the duration and severity of neutropenia, and decreases the risk of infection.

Fungal infection (e.g., *Candida* or aspergillosis) also becomes a problem in persistently neutropenic patients. A febrile neutropenic patient treated with prophylactic antifungal drugs may have infection as a result of resistant organisms and often is treated with intravenous amphotericin B. Fungal infections may produce fungemia, sinusitis, pneumonia, endophthalmitis, and soft tissue, hepatic, splenic, or renal abscesses.

In the absence of neutrophils to localize an infection, it often is difficult to determine the source of infection by physical examination. For example, chest examination findings may be negative despite significant infection, but abnormalities may be revealed by chest radiographic examination and arterial blood gases. Bronchoalveolar lavage may help identify pulmonary pathogens. Many patients have indwelling central venous catheters to facilitate chemotherapy and the drawing of blood. Coagulase-negative staphylococci frequently colonize these catheters and are a source of infection in the absence of signs. Sinus infection (e.g., with bacteria, *Aspergillus*, or Zygomycetes) is common in neutropenic hosts and may be appreciated only on CT scan. Perirectal abscess is another focus of infection in neutropenic hosts; tenderness and erythema may be the only clues to a significant local infection.

REFERENCES

Arceci RJ: Fever and neutropenia: changing patterns of medical practice, *Pediatr Hematol Oncol* 22(5):397, 2000.

Behrman RE, Kliegman RM, Jenson HB, editors: *Nelson textbook of pediatrics*, ed 16, Philadelphia, 2000, WB Saunders, Chapter 179.

Centers for Disease Control and Prevention: Guidelines for preventing opportunistic infections among hematopoietic stem cell transplant recipients: Recommendations of CDC, Infectious Disease Society of America, and American Society of Blood and Marrow Transplantion, *MMWR* 49(RR-10):1–125, 2000.

BACTEREMIA AND SEPTICEMIA

Bacteremia is a bloodstream infection and is documented by positive blood cultures. This is distinguished from *sepsis*, which is the systemic response to infection and includes tachypnea, tachycardia, hyperthermia or hypothermia, and neutropenia or leukocytosis. The **sepsis syndrome,** also called the systemic inflammatory response syndrome (SIRS), involves the clinical diagnosis of sepsis with evidence of altered organ perfusion, including hypoxemia, oliguria, or elevated blood lactate levels. In approximately 10% of patients with a sepsis syndrome the blood culture is negative. **Septic shock** includes the clinical diagnosis of the sepsis syndrome plus hypotension despite fluid resuscitation. See Chapter 3 and Table 3–18 for discussion of shock.

Etiology and Epidemiology. The age and immunization status of the child are important factors in determining which organisms must be considered (Table 10–8). In neonatal sepsis the important

---

TABLE 10–8
Risk Factors for Bacterial Sepsis

Age	**Associated Disease States—cont'd**
Premature greater risk than full term	Galactosemia
Full term greater than infant less than 2 years of age	Intravenous drug abuse
	Paraplegia
Immunodeficiency	Gonococcal genitourinary infection
Severe combined immunodeficiency syndrome	Contact with *Neisseria meningitidis* or *Haemophilus in-*
B-cell defects (agammaglobulinemia)	*fluenzae* (e.g., day care)
Neutropenia and immunosuppression (malignancy)	
Complement deficiency	**Medical Instrumentation/Procedures**
Sickle cell anemia *plus* other asplenic conditions	Indwelling intravascular catheters
Acquired immunodeficiency syndrome	Indwelling urinary catheter
Neutrophil chemotactic defects	Endotracheal intubation
Malnutrition	Ventriculoatrial shunts
	Continuous peritoneal dialysis
Associated Disease States	Surgery
Malignancy	Prosthetic heart valves
Nephrotic syndrome	

---

microorganisms are group B streptococci, *E. coli,* other streptococci, *S. aureus, Staphylococcus epidermidis* (coagulase-negative staphylococci), and *Listeria monocytogenes.* In preterm infants infection caused by coagulase-negative staphylococci is common; *Candida* species must also be considered. In the immunocompetent older febrile child with no localizing findings, the most common pathogens are *S. pneumoniae, N. meningitidis, Salmonella, S. aureus,* and group A streptococci. *H. influenzae* is now rarely seen, except in infants who have not been immunized. Infants with galactosemia and children with pyelonephritis often have gram-negative bacteremia (e.g., *E. coli*).

Immunocompromised children (those with asplenia, sickle cell disease, neutropenia, malignancy, AIDS, or indwelling foreign bodies) are infected by a broader spectrum of organisms and are more susceptible to the development of septicemia. Illness may be caused by common organisms or may be associated with a wide variety of bacteria or fungi in immunocompromised children.

In some patients bacteremia or septicemia may precede or occur during focal infections (e.g., pyelonephritis, pneumonia, cellulitis, osteomyelitis, endocarditis, or meningitis). In such cases, when bacteremia or septicemia is strongly suspected, specimens should be obtained for culture and intravenous broad-spectrum antibiotics administered.

Pathophysiology of Septic Shock. The pathophysiology of septic shock is based in large part on the body's response to microbial products: peptidoglycan fragments from gram-positive bacteria and lipopolysaccharide (LPS) from gram-negative organisms. LPS, peptidoglycan, and lipoproteins interact with host cells through recognition of a family of "toll-like receptors" (TLRs) present on macrophages, endothelial cells, and epithelial cells. Activation of the TLRs in addition to ligation of LPS-binding protein and CD14 on immune cells stimulates the transcription of proinflammatory cytokines, initiating the cascade of physiologic responses that produce the clinical manifestations of "sepsis" or the systemic inflammatory response syndrome. These include the production of IL-1, TNF-α, IL-6, IL-8, and platelet-activating factor, activation of the coagulation cascade, stimulation of arachidonate metabolism, and production of prostaglandins and nitric oxide. Neutrophils are released from both the marginating pool and the bone marrow and are recruited to specific sites of infection by local accumulation of chemokines. Systemic manifestations include fever, profound vasodilation, increased vascular permeability, and resultant hypotension. In the lung this response is manifested as acute respiratory distress syndrome and failure of gas exchange, and elsewhere as multi–organ-system failure (see Chapter 3).

Certain bacteria, particularly *S. aureus* and *S. pyogenes,* may be associated with an unusually severe systemic inflammatory response syndrome, such as staphylococcal toxic shock syndrome. TSST-1 is a *superantigen,* a bacterial antigen that can interact with a superficial component of the T-cell receptor, without the usual requirement for presentation of a bacterial antigen within the context of the major histocompatibility complex (MHC) and the antigen-binding groove. Superantigens can activate entire classes of T cells, which trigger cytokine production and initiate a cascade of biologic responses leading to shock. The clinical picture is that of shock accompanied by multisystem dysfunction such as a sunburn-type rash, renal failure, disseminated intravascular coagulation (DIC), hepatic abnormalities, hypoxia, and hypotension.

Clinical Manifestations. A clinical diagnosis of presumptive septicemia should be made when the child's fever and toxic appearance (e.g., tachycardia, hyperventilation, agitation, lethargy, or poor perfusion) suggest serious illness. The history and physical examination may indicate the site of origin. The early features of septicemia are similar to those of many infections. The child usually is febrile; however, hypothermia may be an important sign of sepsis in the neonate, the neutropenic immunosuppressed patient, or the burn patient. Chills, hyperventilation, tachycardia, hypotension, and peripheral vasodilation are early signs. Petechiae and purpura may be present. Apprehension, confusion, and agitation also are often early signs of septic shock, which often progresses to lethargy and coma. Profound hypotension with cold, clammy, mottled skin, cyanosis, poor capillary refill, a weak pulse, lethargy, and coma is observed later in the progression of shock.

Cutaneous lesions such as purpura and petechiae classically are seen in meningococcemia but may occur in infection with other organisms. *Pseudomonas aeruginosa* causes a characteristic skin lesion called **ecthyma gangrenosum.** These lesions are single round or oval lesions that look like a bull's eye, with a necrotic ulcer in the center surrounded by a rim of redness and induration. DIC is common and becomes manifest as purpura and bleeding from puncture sites. Hypotension may lead to peripheral gangrene, anuric renal failure, and lactic acidosis.

Diagnosis and Differential Diagnosis. In all patients, especially those immunocompromised by an underlying disease or by cancer therapy, the outcome of sepsis depends on early diagnosis and treatment. A careful physical examination to identify potential sources of infection is important. Establishment of venous access and fluid resuscitation to maintain intravascular volume is critical. Following cultures of blood and identification of other possible sites of infection (e.g., indwelling urinary catheters, intravenous or arterial lines, surgical or other wounds, packing material), broad-spectrum bactericidal antimicrobial agents should be administered immediately.

Neutropenia is an important early laboratory finding caused by infection-mediated neutrophil storage pool depletion and margination of cells. Thrombocytopenia and reduced factor VIII concentration reflect DIC, whereas fibrin split products are the result of fibrinolysis. Activation of the clotting cascade results in a consumption coagulopathy with platelet aggregation and intravascular coagulation. Lactic acidosis is caused by circulatory insufficiency, pulmonary insufficiency, or both.

Several specific infectious and noninfectious diseases can present with clinical signs and symptoms similar to the findings of sepsis. Toxic shock syndrome caused by either staphylococcal or streptococcal superantigens, the viral hemorrhagic fevers such as Hanta virus or hemorrhagic dengue fever, rickettsial disease (Rocky Mountain spotted fever), *Yersinia pestis* (plague), and leptospirosis all can have similar toxic presentations. Anaphylaxis, hemorrhagic shock in which vasoconstriction is prominent, a midgut volvulus, a perforated viscus, or toxic ingestion can present with similar cardiovascular collapse.

Treatment. The initial treatment of shock involves supportive therapy to maintain blood pressure, perfusion, and oxygenation, as well as antimicrobial therapy. Broad-spectrum antibiotics that are bactericidal against both gram-negative and gram-positive bacteria should be initiated before the causative bacteria are identified. Therapy for suspected gram-negative sepsis involves an aminoglycoside plus an anti-*Pseudomonas* penicillin combined with a beta-lactamase inhibitor or a broad-spectrum third-generation cephalosporin (such as ceftazidime) (see Appendix I for dosages). Treatment of nosocomial infections may be aided by knowledge of the susceptibility patterns of bacteria prevalent in the hospital setting. When methicillin-resistant *S. aureus* or coagulase-negative staphylococci are suspected, vancomycin should be added. The possibility of vancomycin-resistant organisms (e.g., vancomycin-resistant enterococcus) necessitates the use of linezolid. Anaerobic bacteremia frequently complicates infections of the mouth, abdomen, rectum, or pelvis and necessitates therapy with either clindamycin or metronidazole, in addition to antibiotics active against gram-negative enteric pathogens. Identifying the specific bacteria and performing antimicrobial susceptibility tests form the basis for subsequently administering antibiotics having a narrow spectrum, which prevents superinfection by yeast or resistant bacteria and reduces antibiotic toxicity.

Supportive care for shock is best performed in a pediatric intensive care unit, where continuous monitoring of vital signs is possible (see Chapter 3). Venodilation, transcapillary fluid losses, and hemorrhage necessitate the expansion of the circulating blood volume (with crystalloid solutions) to maintain the perfusion of vital organs. In addition to volume replacement, septic shock must be treated with sympathomimetic drugs such as dopamine, dobutamine, and epinephrine. These drugs improve cardiac output and renal and systemic perfusion and may increase vascular tone. The mortality rate for patients with septic shock is 40–70%. When multiple organ systems fail (e.g., in ARDS or renal or hepatic failure), the mortality rate approaches 90–100%.

REFERENCES

Behrman RE, Kliegman RM, Jenson HB, editors: *Nelson textbook of pediatrics,* ed 15, Philadelphia, 2000, WB Saunders, Chapter 173.

Bone RC, Balk RA, Cerra FB, et al: Definitions for sepsis and organ failure and guidelines for the use of innovative therapies in sepsis, *Chest* 101(6):644–655, 1992.

Wenzel RP, Pinsky MR, Ulevitch RJ, et al: Current understanding of sepsis, *Clin Infect Dis* 22(3):407–412, 1996.

OSTEOMYELITIS AND SEPTIC ARTHRITIS

Infections of bones (osteomyelitis) and joints (septic arthritis) usually are caused by bacterial pathogens and must be differentiated from cellulitis, trauma, inflammatory reactions, and malignancy.

Osteomyelitis

Osteomyelitis may occur at any age but is most common in children between the ages of 3 and 12 years. It affects boys twice as frequently as girls.

Pathogenesis. Infections of the bone may result from hematogenous dissemination or by direct spread from a contiguous focus of infection. Osteomyelitis in children is most often the consequence of bacteremia and involves rapidly growing bone, particularly the metaphyses of long bones (e.g., distal femur, proximal tibia, distal humerus, and distal radius). Bacteria lodge in sharp loops of nutrient arteries supplying the growth plates of these bones. Blood in the large sinusoidal veins flows slowly, and no phagocytic cells are present in this area. Obstruction of flow by bacterial microemboli produces small areas of avascular necrosis with a resultant metaphyseal abscess. Trauma often is noted before the onset of osteomyelitis and may lead to local areas of bone injury that predispose to infection. This may mislead the clinician to think the bone symptoms are the result of trauma. In infants younger than 1 year of age, the capillaries perforate the epiphyseal growth plate, permitting spread across the epiphysis, which causes a septic arthritis (Fig. 10–3). In older children the infection is contained in the metaphyseal sinusoidal veins because the vessels no longer cross the epiphyseal plate (Fig. 10–4). Osteoarthritis also may be seen

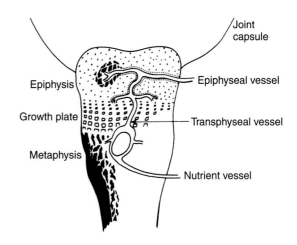

FIG. 10–3

Major structures of the bone of an infant prior to maturation of the epiphyseal growth plate. Note the transphyseal vessel, which connects the vascular supply of the epiphysis and metaphysis, facilitating spread of infection between these two areas. (From Gutman LT: *Curr Probl Pediatr* 15:6, 1985.)

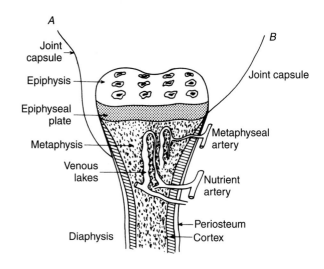

FIG. 10–4

Major structures of the bone of a child. Joint capsule *A* inserts below the epiphyseal growth plate, as in the hip, elbow, ankle, and shoulder. Rupture of a metaphyseal abscess in these bones is likely to produce pyarthrosis. Joint capsule *B* inserts at the epiphyseal growth plate, as in other tubular bones. Rupture of a metaphyseal abscess in these bones is likely to lead to a subperiosteal abscess but seldom to an associated pyarthrosis. (From Gutman LT: *Curr Probl Pediatr* 15:7, 1985.)

in joints where the capsule inserts on the metaphysis proximal to the epiphyseal plate. Pyarthritis complicating osteomyelitis is common in these joints (e.g., the hip, elbow, shoulder, and knee) (Fig. 10–4). Infection spreads through the haversian system and Volk-

TABLE 10–9
Clinical Manifestations of Acute Hematogenous Osteomyelitis by Age Groups

Age	Usual Site of Involvement	Symptoms and Signs	Expected Organism
Neonate	Varied; 40% may have multiple sites	Usually few systemic signs; local edema; reduced limb motion; joint effusion (60–70%)	Group B streptococci, *Escherichia coli*, *Staphylococcus aureus*, or *Candida*
1–24 mo	Long bones; may involve joints	Pseudoparalysis, fever, limp	*S. aureus*, group B streptococci
2–20 yr	Metaphysis of long bones; rarely, vertebral bodies or pelvis	Focal pain with fever (90%) for days to weeks; focal tenderness (70%); focal swelling (70%) or joint effusion (20%)	*S. aureus* (60–90%), streptococci (10%), *Salmonella* (especially with sickle cell anemia); rarely, gram-negative bacilli, anaerobes, or fungi

mann canals; as infection spreads laterally, the periosteum is lifted. In chronic osteomyelitis the infected periosteum may calcify into a shell of new bone around the infected portion of the shaft; this is called an *involucrum*. The host defense mechanisms may wall off a metaphyseal abscess, producing a chronic infection with a sclerotic rim called a *Brodie abscess*. Dead bone within this space is called *sequestrum*.

Contiguous osteomyelitis is less common in children and usually occurs after the spread of cellulitis as a result of an infected wound, such as a decubitus or sinus or periodontal disease, or after a surgical procedure. Osteomyelitis also may result from direct inoculation from a penetrating wound and from heel punctures, paronychia, open fracture, orthopedic surgery, and human or animal bites.

Etiology. *S. aureus* is responsible for most infections. Group B (in neonates) or other streptococci, anaerobic microorganisms, gram-negative enteric bacteria, and *M. tuberculosis* also cause osteomyelitis. Other factors that predispose the patient to osteomyelitis are furunculosis, infected lesions of varicella, infected burns, prolonged intravenous or central parenteral alimentation, intravenous drug abuse, and trauma. Sickle cell anemia and other hemoglobinopathies predispose the patient to osteomyelitis caused by *Salmonella* or *Staphylococcus* species or, less commonly, *S. pneumoniae*. Osteomyelitis secondary to dog or cat bites may be caused by *Pasteurella multocida*. *Pseudomonas* osteomyelitis commonly follows puncture wounds of the foot (in sneaker wearers) or intravenous drug abuse (see Chapter 19). Infection as a result of *H. influenzae* type b is rarely seen in an immunized population.

Clinical Manifestations. Hematogenous osteomyelitis in children usually involves a single bone (after infancy) and occurs either as an acute illness with fever, focal bone pain, and sepsis or as a subacute illness with mild systemic signs but with local complaints at the site of involved bone. Complaints include severe localized pain, exquisite tenderness, warmth, erythema, and swelling. Weight bearing and spontaneous or requested motion are refused, which mimics paralysis (pseudoparalysis). Muscle spasm may make the extremity difficult to examine. Hematogenous osteomyelitis involving the vertebrae is notable for an insidious onset, vague symptomatology, backache, occasional spinal cord compression, and usually little associated fever or systemic toxicity. This must be differentiated from a more common entity—discitis—usually seen in younger children and presenting more acutely (see Chapter 19). With osteomyelitis of the pelvis, presenting signs may include limp; abdominal, hip, groin, or thigh pain; and fever. Table 10–9 presents features of acute hematogenous osteomyelitis.

Diagnosis. Marked tenderness over the involved site identifies the infected bone. Leukocytosis may be present. The ESR and CRP usually are elevated and are of great help in monitoring the response to treatment. Blood specimens (positive in 60%), cultures of an aspirate of cellulitis, and a diagnostic aspirate of the periosteal space (or, if negative, of the bone itself) should be obtained before antibiotic therapy is begun. The evaluation of patients with chronic disease includes a tuberculin test and a chest roentgenogram. The tuberculin test and chest x-ray examination may be especially helpful in establishing a diagnosis in vertebral osteomyelitis.

Radiographs or CT scans of the affected areas should be obtained to allow observation of soft tissue swelling, periosteal elevation and calcification, and bone destruction and to allow consideration of a possible alternative diagnosis such as bone tumors, bone cysts, leukemia, or histiocytosis. Plain films of the bone generally are normal during the early phase (at 10–14 days); the radionuclide technetium-99m bone scan may be valuable if plain films are normal. MRI is particularly useful for delineating the extent of infection in complex cases or when infection is a complication of trauma, surgery, or sickle cell anemia. MRI helps distinguish vertebral osteomyelitis from discitis. Ultrasonography of the hip may help identify toxic synovitis, a nonbacterial condition (see Chapter 19).

Treatment. Initial intravenous antibiotic therapy should be based on results of Gram stain of bone aspirate, blood culture reports, age, and associated diseases. Initial therapy should cover the staphylococci, all of which must be assumed to be penicillinase producing (oxacillin, nafcillin, methicillin, and clindamycin) (see Appendix I for dosages); the possibility of methicillin-resistant staphylococci should be considered. In patients with sickle cell anemia, *Salmonella* and *S. aureus* must both be covered (with cefotaxime and ceftriaxone). Gram-negative organisms may be present if wound contamination or a history of intravenous drug abuse is discovered. *Candida, Aspergillus,* and *Rhizopus* are potential pathogens in immunocompromised patients or patients receiving long-term parenteral hyperalimentation; these patients require appropriate antifungal therapy (amphotericin B).

The response to appropriate intravenous antibiotics usually occurs within 48 hours; lack of improvement in fever and pain after this time indicates that surgical drainage may be necessary or that an unusual pathogen (e.g., *M. tuberculosis*) may be present. Surgical drainage may be appropriate at an earlier time if a sequestrum is present, if the disease is chronic or atypical, if the hip joint is involved, or if the disease occurs in the presence of spinal cord compression.

Standard therapy usually consists of administering antibiotics for 4–6 weeks or longer. Oral antibiotics are effective after a good response to intravenous therapy (discussed in the next section, Septic Arthritis). Ensuring that patients are compliant with oral regimens is essential; this may entail the assistance of social services.

Inadequate or delayed antibiotic therapy for osteomyelitis often leads to chronic abscess formation, draining sinus tracts, pathologic fractures, orthopedic deformity, and the late onset of amyloidosis.

Septic Arthritis

Septic or suppurative arthritis is a serious infection of the joint space. It occurs most commonly during the first 2 years of life and during adolescence.

Pathogenesis. Septic arthritis results from hematogenous dissemination of bacteria, contiguous spread from surrounding soft tissues, and spread of osteomyelitis through the epiphysis into the joint space in young children (Figs. 10–3 and 10–4). Septic arthritis must be differentiated from postinfectious joint effusions, which are sterile and often caused by antigen-antibody complex deposition. Joint effusions developing after 7 days of a bacterial illness (e.g., bacteremia, meningitis, diarrhea, or urethritis) more often are immunologically mediated, whereas those presenting in the first 3 days more often represent the hematogenous spread of bacteria.

Etiology. *S. aureus* is the most common agent, followed by streptococci, pneumococci, and meningococci. Joint effusions may develop in patients with meningococcal sepsis and meningitis (discussed in the preceding section, Pathogenesis). Meningococcal arthritis may occur in the absence of sepsis or meningitis. Gonococcal arthritis associated with disseminated gonococcal infection is the most common cause of polyarthritis and monoarticular arthritis in adolescents. In endemic areas Lyme arthritis also must be considered. *H. influenzae* type b was the most common etiologic factor in children ages 3 months to 4 years but is now rarely seen in an immunized population.

Clinical Manifestations. The presentation has the typical features of infection: erythema, warmth, swelling, and tenderness over the affected joint, with a palpable effusion and decreased range of movement. The onset may be sudden, resulting in an ill-appearing child with fever and chills; or insidious, with symptoms noted only when the joint is moved, such as during a diaper change, or if parents become aware of decreased voluntary movement (pseudoparalysis) of a joint or limb. Toddlers may demonstrate a limp. It is often difficult to assess septic arthritis of the hip, which may cause referred pain to the knee. The limb may be positioned in external rotation and flexion to minimize pain from pressure on the hip's joint capsule. Similarly, the knee and elbow joints usually are held in flexion. An acute septic arthritis most often involves a single joint (e.g., the knee, hip, ankle, shoulder, elbow, or wrist), with multiple joints affected in fewer than 10% of cases.

Diagnosis and Differential Diagnosis. Leukocytosis and an elevated ESR or CRP are common. Arthrocentesis is the test of choice for rapid diagnosis of suppurative arthritis (Table 10–10). During arthrocentesis, it is important to avoid crossing an overlying area of cellulitis to prevent the inoculation of bacteria and the conversion of a deep cellulitis into septic arthritis. Blood or joint cultures are positive in up to 85% of patients infected with *H. influenzae*. Joint fluid that exhibits the characteristics of pyogenic infection may not reveal bacterial pathogens in up to 30% of patients who have never received antibiotic therapy, because synovial fluid exerts a bacteriostatic effect. Gram stain, potassium hydroxide (KOH) preparation for fungi (in neonates and

TABLE 10–10
Synovial Fluid Findings in Various Joint Diseases

Condition	Appearance	White Blood Cell Count (µg/L)	Polymorphonuclear Cells (%)	Mucin Clot	Synovial Fluid–to–Blood Glucose Difference (mg/dL)	Comment
Normal	Clear, yellow	0–200 (200)*	<10	Good	No difference	—
Trauma	Clear, turbid, or hemorrhagic	50–4000 (600)	<30	Good	No difference	Common in hemophilia
Systemic lupus erythematosus	Clear or slightly turbid	0–9000 (3000)	<20	Good to fair	No difference	LE cell positive, complement decreased
Rheumatoid arthritis reactive arthritis (Reiter syndrome, inflammatory bowel disease)	Turbid	250–80,000 (19,000)	>70	Poor	30	Decreased complement
Infectious						
Pyogenic infection	Turbid	10,000–250,000 (80,000)	>90	Poor	50–90	Positive culture, positive Gram stain
Tuberculosis	Turbid	2500–100,000 (20,000)	>60	Poor	40–70	Positive culture, PPD, and acid-fast stain
Lyme arthritis	Turbid	500–100,000 (20,000)	>60	Poor	70	History of tick bite or erythema chronicum migrans

LE, Lupus erythematosus; *PPD*, purified protein derivative of tuberculin.
*Average in parentheses.

immunosuppressed patients), and acid-fast stain are helpful if no bacteria are recovered. In chronic arthritis, synovial biopsy may distinguish between an infectious and a noninfectious process. Because septic arthritis may be present with osteomyelitis, roentgenograms or bone scans of the adjacent bone usually are indicated. Adolescents with acute septic arthritis should have urethral, cervical, rectal, and pharyngeal culture examination for *N. gonorrhoeae*.

The *differential diagnosis* of suppurative arthritis involves infectious (septic bursitis), postinfectious (Reiter syndrome, rheumatic fever), and noninfectious (rheumatoid arthritis, SLE, other collagen-vascular diseases, serum sickness, and inflammatory bowel disease) diseases. Other entities that should be considered include Henoch-Schönlein purpura, leukemia, metabolic diseases involving joints, foreign bodies, and traumatic arthritis. Viral infections (e.g., rubella, rubella vaccine, parvovirus, hepatitis B) may cause arthritis.

Toxic tenosynovitis of the hip is presumed to be viral in etiology and is a common condition of children ages 3–6 years (see Chapter 19). This self-limited disorder is far more common than septic arthritis. Other bacterial infections causing arthritis are tuberculosis, syphilis, and Lyme disease. These infections must be considered in the child or adolescent with the signs of an acutely inflamed joint or joints but without typical findings of pyogenic infection.

Treatment. Therapy for septic arthritis is based on knowledge of the likely organism, the Gram stain of joint fluid, and the host's immunologic status. Parenteral antimicrobial agents are the mainstay of therapy, with surgical intervention reserved for specific situations. Pyogenic arthritis of the hip or shoulder caused by *S. aureus* usually necessitates prompt surgical drainage to prevent joint destruction and long-term sequelae. However, staphylococcal infection of the knee may be treated with repeated arthrocenteses to remove infected fluid and with continuation of appropriate parenteral antibiotics. Irrigation of the joints with antimicrobial agents is rarely, if ever, indicated. Infections caused by gonococci or meningococci rarely require surgical intervention in a normal host.

A number of antimicrobial agents are available that provide adequate antibiotic levels in joint spaces to eradicate the typical bacterial infections. For empiric therapy in the neonate, an antibiotic with activity against staphylococci, group B streptococci, and aerobic gram-negative rods (cefotaxime or ticarcillin/clavulanate) may be used, depending on the results of the joint fluid Gram stain. Infants aged 3 months to 4 years should receive antibiotics active against *S. aureus* and *H. influenzae* type b until culture results are known. These antibiotics include cefotaxime or ampicillin/sulbactam. Intravenous methicillin (or nafcillin or oxacillin) is the treatment of choice for *S. aureus;* methicillin-resistant organisms are treated with vancomycin. The length of therapy depends on clinical resolution (e.g., patient is afebrile and has less pain) and reduction of the ESR. Infection with organisms such as *S. aureus* usually necessitates more lengthy treatment (14–21 days or more), whereas gonococcal or meningococcal arthritis responds to 7 days of penicillin. Ceftriaxone is preferred for gonococcal arthritis because of the large number of penicillin-resistant isolates. Treatment may be changed to oral antibiotics (discussed earlier in this chapter under Osteomyelitis) for staphylococcal and other infections if compliance can be ensured. Oral agents with excellent activity against *S. aureus* are augmentin, cloxacillin, dicloxacillin, cephalexin, clindamycin, and ciprofloxacin (in older children); these are often used to complete therapy.

REFERENCES

Behrman RE, Kliegman RM, Jenson HB, editors: *Nelson textbook of pediatrics*, ed 16, Philadelphia, 2000, WB Saunders, Chapter 178.

Lew D, Waldvogel F: Osteomyelitis, *N Engl J Med* 336(14): 999–1007, 1997.

Rodriguez AF, Kaplan SL: Outpatient management of skeletal infections in children, *Semin Pediatr Infect Dis* 1:365, 1990.

CENTRAL NERVOUS SYSTEM INFECTIONS

Acute Bacterial Meningitis Beyond the Neonatal Period

Meningitis is an inflammation of the leptomeninges. Although this may be caused by bacteria, viruses, or rarely fungi, bacterial meningitis is a common complication of septicemia in children and must be treated as an emergency. A limited number of bacteria are associated with meningitis in normal hosts; thus the principles of supportive management and the initial choice of antibiotics can be generalized. Meningitis during the neonatal period is discussed in Chapter 6.

Etiology. Bacterial meningitis in children 2 months to 12 years of age usually is the result of *S. pneumoniae* or *N. meningitidis*. *H. influenzae* type b was the most common cause of meningitis in children younger than 4 years of age; the incidence of *H. influenzae* disease has decreased dramatically after the introduction of conjugated vaccine against the organism. Meningitis associated with ventricular-peritoneal shunts generally is the result of coagulase-negative staphylococci or corynebacteria; meningitis in patients with an open neural tube defect may be the result of *S. aureus* or enteric bacteria. Immuno-suppressed patients with T-cell defects are suscepti-ble to cryptococcal and *L. monocytogenes* meningitis. Pneumococcal meningitis is common in patients with CSF leaks caused by sinus fractures, whereas in patients with penetrating head trauma or neuro-surgical procedures, staphylococcal disease often develops.

Epidemiology. Bacterial meningitis occurs more frequently in the winter and spring, more in males than in females, and most often between 2 months and 2 years of age. Close contact with a nasopha-ryngeal carrier (as in a day care setting) or with a pa-tient ill with meningococcal infection has been asso-ciated with an increased risk of meningitis. Meningococcal disease often follows viral upper res-piratory tract infections such as influenza.

Pathogenesis. Bacterial meningitis is usually the result of hematogenous dissemination of microor-ganisms from a distant site of infection; bacteremia precedes the condition or occurs at the same time. The microorganisms are acquired by aerosol or droplet; this leads to nasopharyngeal colonization, replication, invasion, and bacteremia. The hosts at risk for meningitis resulting from encapsulated or-ganisms (e.g., *S. pneumoniae*, *N. meningitidis*, and *H. influenzae* type b) lack preformed anticapsular anti-body. High-grade bacteremia is followed by menin-geal seeding; binding of organisms to specific recep-tors and production of local cytokines initiates inflammation. Meningitis rarely may be the result of bacterial spread from a contiguous focus of infection, such as sinusitis, otitis media, or mastoiditis. More often, brain abscesses or epidural or subdural empyema follows contiguous infections. Bacterial meningitis in children with otitis media generally follows bacteremia. Hematogenous spread to the meninges may occur with infective endocarditis, pneumonia, or thrombophlebitis. When there is a di-rect communication between the skin and meninges, the meninges may be invaded from a dermoid sinus tract or meningomyelocele. Fracture of the cribri-form plate and CSF rhinorrhea predispose to pneu-mococcal meningitis. Osteomyelitis of the skull or vertebral column also may produce meningitis.

Children with sickle cell anemia or asplenia have an increased incidence of meningitis caused by *S. pneumoniae*. Without antimicrobial prophylaxis, pneumococcal meningitis develops before 4 years of age in approximately 1 in 24 patients with sickle cell anemia. Terminal complement deficiency pre-disposes some children to *Neisseria* sepsis and meningitis.

The clinical manifestations of bacterial meningi-tis are caused by the local immune response to un-opposed bacterial replication, specifically to the im-munogenic fragments of bacterial peptidoglycan. Endothelial cells and macrophages are activated, and local production of cytokines (IL-1β, TNF-β) is stimulated.

Neutrophil migration from capillaries is trig-gered, and the release of toxic neutrophil products further increases local damage. The ensuing inflam-matory response increases the blood-brain barrier permeability, producing cerebral edema and in-creased intracranial pressure and activation of the coagulation system, which produces local thrombo-sis and infarction. Increased CSF protein is the result of this inflammatory response, whereas the reduced CSF glucose is the result of alterations of the blood-brain barrier and increased CNS glucose utilization.

Clinical Manifestations. Manifestations of bacterial meningitis may be preceded by several days of up-per respiratory tract symptoms. Rapid onset (<1 day) is common with *S. pneumoniae* or *N. meningi-tidis*, whereas the course may be subacute (2–3 days) with *H. influenzae*. In young infants signs of men-ingeal inflammation may be minimal; only irritabil-ity, restlessness, and poor feeding may be noted. Fever usually is present. Inflammation of the me-ninges is associated with headache, irritability, nau-sea, vomiting, anorexia, nuchal rigidity, lethargy, and occasionally photophobia. The older child may be confused and may complain of back pain and usu-ally demonstrates the Kernig and Brudzinski signs. Seizures and coma may occur.

Increased intracranial pressure may be reflected in complaints of headache and diplopia. A bulging fontanel may be present. Ptosis, sixth nerve palsy, anisocoria, bradycardia with hypertension, and ap-nea are common signs of increased intracranial pressure and brain herniation, whereas a bulging fontanel is not always associated with herniation. Papilledema is uncommon unless there are occlu-sions of the venous sinuses, subdural empyema, or a brain abscess. Focal neurologic signs, arthralgia, myalgia, transient arthritis, anemia, petechial or purpuric lesions, and signs of DIC are additional manifestations.

Diagnosis and Differential Diagnosis. Lumbar punc-ture should be performed in every child when bacte-rial meningitis is suspected, except when signs (other than a bulging fontanel) of increased intracranial pressure are present. Infection at the lumbar punc-ture site, suspicion of a mass lesion, and extreme pa-tient instability are other reasons to defer a spinal tap. CSF examination should include a WBC count, dif-ferential, measurement of protein and glucose levels, and Gram stain (Table 10–11). Specimens for culture should be obtained to look for bacteria and, when ap-propriate, for fungi, viruses, and mycobacteria. The

TABLE 10–11
Cerebrospinal Fluid (CSF) Findings in Various Central Nervous System Disorders

Condition	Pressure	Leukocytes (/μL)	Protein (mg/dL)	Glucose (mg/dL)	Comments
Normal	50–180 mm H$_2$O	<4; 60–70% lymphocytes, 30–40% monocytes, 1–3% neutrophils	20–45	>50 or 75% blood glucose	
Acute bacterial meningitis	Usually elevated	100–60,000+; usually a few thousand; PMNs predominate	100–500	Depressed compared with blood glucose; usually <40	Organism may be seen on Gram stain and recovered by culture
Partially treated bacterial meningitis	Normal or elevated	1–10,000; PMNs usual but mononuclear cells may predominate if pretreated for extended period	100+	Depressed or normal	Organisms may be seen; pretreatment may render CSF sterile in pneumococcal and meningococcal disease, but antigen may be detected
Tuberculous meningitis	Usually elevated; may be low because of block in advanced stages	10–500; PMNs early but lymphocytes and monocytes predominate later	100–500; may be higher in presence of block	<50 usual; decreases with time if treatment not provided	Acid-fast organisms may be seen on smear; organism can be recovered in culture or by PCR; PPD, chest x-ray positive
Fungal	Usually elevated	25–500; PMNs early; mononuclear cells predominate later	20–500	<50; decreases with time if treatment not provided	Budding yeast may be seen; organism may be recovered in culture; India ink preparation or antigen may be positive in cryptococcal disease
Viral meningitis or meningoencephalitis	Normal or slightly elevated	PMNs early; mononuclear cells predominate later; rarely more than 1000 cells except in eastern equine	20–100	Generally normal; may be depressed to 40 in some viral diseases (15–20% of mumps)	Enteroviruses may be recovered from CSF by appropriate viral cultures or PCR; HSV by PCR
Abscess (parameningeal infection)	Normal or elevated	0–100 PMNs unless rupture into CSF	20–200	Normal	Profile may be completely normal

DNA, Deoxyribonucleic acid; *HSV,* herpes simplex virus; *PCR,* polymerase chain reaction; *PMN,* polymorphonuclear leukocyte; *PPD,* purified protein derivative of tuberculin.

Gram stain is helpful in 90% of patients with bacterial meningitis. Additional diagnostic tests include blood cultures (positive in 50–90% of patients), a complete blood count, and a sickle cell screening test.

Tuberculous meningitis, fungal meningitis, aseptic meningitis, spirochete infection (e.g., in syphilis or Lyme disease), brain abscess, encephalitis, Rocky Mountain spotted fever, intracranial or spinal epidural abscesses, bacterial endocarditis with embolism, subdural empyema (with or without thrombophlebitis), subarachnoid hemorrhage, and brain tumors may mimic bacterial meningitis. The differentiation of these disorders depends on careful examination of CSF and additional laboratory tests and roentgenographic studies (Table 10–11). The CSF in aseptic meningitis may also have a PMN predominance.

Treatment. Treatment of bacterial meningitis focuses on decreasing the CNS damage caused by the inflammatory response, sterilization of the CSF by the use of appropriate antimicrobial agents that achieve cidal levels, and the maintenance of adequate CNS and systemic perfusion. The selection of empiric antimicrobial agents is problematic. To cover *S. pneumoniae,* many of which are relatively resistant to penicillin (MIC 0.1–1.0 μg/ml), cefotaxime (200–300 mg/kg/24 hr) or ceftriaxone (100 mg/kg/ 24 hr) should be used, *plus* vancomycin (60 mg/ kg/24 hr), until antibiotic susceptibility testing is available. A third-generation cephalosporin (cefotaxime or ceftriaxone) is also adequate to cover *N. meningitidis* or *H. influenzae* type b. For sensitive meningococci or pneumococci, penicillin G (300,000 units/kg/24 hr) is recommended. For infants younger than 2 months of age, ampicillin (200 mg/ kg every 6 hours) is added to cover the possibility of *L. monocytogenes.* Treatment for 7 days (for meningococcus) or 10 days (for *S. pneumoniae* or *H. influenzae*) is adequate because less antibiotic will cross the blood-brain barrier as the inflammation decreases.

Supportive therapy involves the treatment of shock, DIC, inappropriate antidiuretic hormone secretion, seizures, increased intracranial pressure, apnea, arrhythmias, and coma. Supportive therapy also involves the maintenance of adequate CNS perfusion in the presence of cerebral edema. Hypotension and hypoperfusion are much more common clinically than inappropriate antidiuretic hormone secretion, which may occur in severely ill patients. Subdural effusions (detected by CT scan) are common in infection with *H. influenzae* type b. Most subdural effusions are asymptomatic and do not necessitate drainage unless associated with increased intracranial pressure or focal neurologic signs. Persistent fever is common with *H. influenzae* type b infection but also may suggest a subdural effusion, pericardial or joint effusions, drug fever, thrombophlebitis,

or nosocomial infection. Another lumbar puncture is not indicated for fever in the absence of other signs of persistent CNS infection.

Prevention. Chemoprophylaxis with rifampin for family contacts of individuals with *H. influenzae* type b and *N. meningitidis* infections is recommended. Vaccines or prophylactic antibiotics against *N. meningitidis* are recommended for at-risk individuals and should be considered in adolescents starting college; routine immunization against *H. influenzae* is recommended for all infants (Tables 10–3 and 10–5). Use of the conjugate pneumococcal vaccine should also have an effect in reducing the incidence of pneumococcal meningitis.

Prognosis. Even with appropriate antibiotic therapy, the mortality rate for bacterial meningitis in children is significant (8% for *H. influenzae;* 15% for meningococcal; 25% for pneumococcal). As many as 35% of the survivors (particularly following pneumococcal infection) have some sequelae resulting from their disease, including, in order of frequency, the following: deafness, seizures, learning disabilities, blindness, paresis, ataxia, or hydrocephalus. All patients with meningitis should have a hearing evaluation before discharge.

Poor prognosis is associated with young age, long duration of illness before effective antibiotic therapy, late-onset seizures, coma at presentation, shock, low or absent CSF WBC count in the presence of visible bacteria on Gram stain of the CSF, and immunocompromised status.

Relapse may occur 3–14 days after treatment and is caused by the same pathogen, possibly from parameningeal foci; *recrudescence* occurs during inappropriate therapy; and *recurrence* takes place later and is caused by the same pathogen. This may indicate an underlying immunologic or anatomic defect that predisposes the patient to infection of the CNS, or, as in the case of group B streptococci, may indicate a reservoir of intracellular bacteria.

REFERENCES

Behrman RE, Kliegman RM, Jenson HB, editors: *Nelson textbook of pediatrics,* ed 16, Philadelphia, 2000, WB Saunders, Chapter 174.

Negrini B, Kelleher KJ, Wald ER: Cerebrospinal fluid findings in aseptic versus bacterial meningitis, *Pediatrics* 105(2):316–319, 2000.

Pomeroy SL, Holmes SJ, Dodge PR, et al: Seizures and other neurologic sequelae of bacterial meningitis in children, *N Engl J Med* 323(24):1651–1657, 1990.

Quagliarello V, Scheld W: Treatment of bacterial meningitis, *N Engl J Med* 336(10):708–716, 1997.

Spanos A, Harrell FE, Durack DT: Differential diagnosis of acute meningitis: an analysis of the predictive value of initial observations, *JAMA* 262(19):2700–2707, 1989.

Tunkel AR, Scheld WM: Pathogenesis and pathophysiology of bacterial meningitis, *Annu Rev Med* 44:103–120, 1993.

Tuomanen EI, Austrian R, Masure HR: Pathogenesis of pneumococcal infection, *N Engl J Med* 332(19):1280–1284, 1995.

Acute Aseptic Meningitis

Aseptic meningitis, an acute inflammation of the meninges, is a common illness with many causes. CSF usually is characterized by lymphocytic pleocytosis (although many have PMN predominance), normal glucose levels, normal or slightly elevated protein levels, and the absence of bacterial microorganisms on Gram stain or culture.

Etiology. Although an etiologic agent is not always identified, viruses are usually the responsible agents. Enteroviruses cause approximately 85% of all cases of aseptic meningitis; coxsackievirus B5 and echoviruses 4, 6, 9, and 11 are the most common types. St. Louis and California encephalitis viruses are the most commonly implicated arboviruses in the United States, accounting for 5–7% of all cases of aseptic meningitis. Other etiologic viral agents are human herpes virus 6 and 7; HIV; varicella; EBV; lymphocytic choriomeningitis; measles, mumps, rubella, or polio; rabies; influenza; and parainfluenza. A primary genital herpes simplex virus infection (type 2) in the adolescent can also be associated with a self-limited aseptic meningitis. Acute aseptic meningitis also may be caused by *Mycoplasma, Chlamydia,* various fungi and protozoa, and other parasites, as well as by postinfectious reactions to various viruses.

The most common cause of nonviral aseptic meningitis is partially or inappropriately treated bacterial disease; tuberculosis, parameningeal infections, toxoplasmosis, and Kawasaki disease should be considered. Less common causes include leptospirosis, syphilis, cryptococcosis, Lyme disease, Rocky Mountain spotted fever, malignancy, intracranial hemorrhage, and reactions to nonsteroidal antiinflammatory drugs (NSAIDs), intravenous immunoglobulins, or trimethoprim/sulfamethoxazole.

Epidemiology. Because 85% of cases are a result of enteroviral infections, the epidemiologic pattern is typical of these agents. In temperate climates most cases occur in the summer and fall. The epidemiology of aseptic meningitis caused by other agents also depends on season, geography, climatic conditions, exposures to animals or insects, and other factors related to the specific pathogens.

Clinical Manifestations. The onset usually is acute, although it may be insidious or preceded by a nonspecific febrile illness. In older children, the initial manifestation is severe headache; in infants, it is irritability. Fever, nausea, and other neurologic complaints, such as vomiting, a stiff neck, photophobia, and retrobulbar pain, are frequent, but convulsions are uncommon. Examination often reveals nuchal rigidity without significant localizing neurologic signs. Exanthems that precede or accompany the infection may occur, especially in infections with echoviruses and coxsackieviruses. Parotitis or orchi-

tis is noted with mumps, lymphadenopathy, and hepatosplenomegaly with CMV, HIV, or EBV infections, and petechiae with Rocky Mountain spotted fever. The child with aseptic viral meningitis usually appears less ill than the child with bacterial meningitis; however, the two may be indistinguishable (Table 10–6).

Acute aseptic meningitis may become manifest in a meningeal or an encephalitic pattern. The children exhibiting the encephalitic pattern have a great incidence of headache, confusion, altered consciousness, and seizures.

Diagnosis. The CSF contains a few to several thousand cells per microliter, which are often polymorphonuclear leukocytes (Table 10–11). No organisms are seen on laboratory stain, and the protein level is normal to slightly elevated. The CSF glucose concentration is normal in most viral infections; glucose may be decreased with medulloblastoma, leukemia infiltration, *Mycoplasma pneumoniae* infection, inadequately treated bacterial meningitis, tuberculosis, and, rarely, certain viral infections. CSF, throat swabs, and stool specimens should be taken for viral culture. Antigenic or genomic (PCR) methods also help determine the etiology. A serum specimen should be obtained early in the illness and again in 2–3 weeks for serologic identification of the virus.

Treatment. Aseptic viral meningitis is usually a benign, self-limited disease. Hospitalization usually is necessary in young infants or more acutely ill children because of the possibility of bacterial disease. Treatment is supportive for viral meningitis, except for aseptic meningitis caused by herpes simplex. Meningoencephalitis resulting from herpes simplex or complicated herpes zoster should be treated with acyclovir. Lyme disease should be treated with high-dose parenteral ceftriaxone. Headache, which may be severe in all cases of aseptic meningitis, should be treated with NSAIDs or mild narcotics such as codeine.

REFERENCES

Behrman RE, Kliegman RM, Jenson HB, editors: *Nelson textbook of pediatrics,* ed 16, Philadelphia, 2000, WB Saunders, Chapter 174.
Lyall E, Hons B, Hons C: Human herpes virus 6: primary infection and the central nervous system, *Pediatr Infect Dis J* 15(8):693–696, 1996.
Nigrovic L: What's new with enteroviral infections? *Curr Opin Pediatr* 13(1):89–94, 2001.

Encephalitis

Encephalitis is an inflammatory process of the brain parenchyma that is usually an acute process but may be a postinfectious encephalomyelitis, a chronic degenerative disease, or a slow virus infection. The diagnosis is established with absolute certainty by brain biopsy, but it usually is made in the presence of neurologic signs, epidemiologic data, and laboratory (e.g., CSF, electroencephalography [EEG], and brain imaging techniques) evidence of infection. Encephalitis may be diffuse or localized (e.g., cerebellar ataxia, brainstem encephalitis, a meningoencephalitis, and meningoencephalomyeloradiculitis). Considerable overlap exists between viral aseptic meningitis and meningoencephalitis. Neurologic manifestations suggestive of encephalitis but occurring in the absence of inflammation (e.g., intoxication, Reye syndrome, anoxia, and inborn errors of metabolism) indicate **encephalopathy.**

Etiology. Encephalitis usually is caused by direct viral infection of the brain via a hematogenous or neuronal (peripheral or cranial) route. During epidemic seasons (summer or fall), arboviruses and enteroviruses are common pathogens. Other causes of encephalitis are varicella, mumps, measles, EBV, rubella, lymphocytic choriomeningitis, influenza, parainfluenza, adenovirus, and respiratory syncytial virus. Herpes simplex, the most common cause of sporadic encephalitis (herpes simplex virus [HSV] type I), is also a common encephalitis seen in neonates (HSV type II is seen more than type I). Cerebellar ataxia commonly is caused by the varicella virus. Postinfectious, allergic demyelinating encephalitis may follow either vaccination or a viral infection and is an autoimmune process. HIV is an increasingly common cause of encephalitis in children and may present as an acute febrile illness, but more commonly it is insidious in onset (discussed later in the chapter under Human Immunodeficiency Virus Infection). Opportunistic CNS infections or lymphoma may also complicate HIV infection.

Epidemiology. The St. Louis encephalitis virus, which is spread from the bird reservoir, is the most common arboviral (arthropod-borne) agent and is present throughout the United States. The California encephalitis virus, common in the Midwest, is carried by rodents and spread by mosquitoes. The eastern equine encephalitis virus is limited to the East Coast, in mosquitoes and birds, whereas the western equine encephalitis virus is present throughout the Midwest and West in mosquitoes and birds. The spread of disease depends on the geographic area, season, arthropod vector, and animal reservoir. Epizootics in horses often precede human cases of eastern equine encephalitis, but the horse is not a direct source of disease to humans. Outbreaks of mosquito-borne West Nile encephalitis in the northeast United States produce a broad spectrum of illness from asymptomatic to death. Children with encephalitis may also have a maculopapular rash and severe complications such as fulminant coma, transverse myelitis, or peripheral neuropathy.

HSV infections account for approximately 10% of nonneonatal cases. Sporadic encephalitis caused by HSV occurs in newborn infants born to mothers with an active primary infection, or in adults as a primary infection or reactivation of latent virus (discussed later in the chapter under Herpes Simplex Virus Infection). HHV-6 and HHV-7, associated with roseola in infants, may cause encephalitis in immunocompromised patients. Diagnosis can be made by PCR; treatment is with anti-HSV agents.

Rabies is a rare but important cause of encephalitis in developing countries and is endemic in parts of the United States. In the Northeast, raccoons and bats may be infected; in the Southeast, foxes and bats are potential sources. Management after exposure to potentially infected animals involves the aggressive postexposure use of vaccine plus hyperimmune globulin to prevent infection.

Slow viral diseases present months to years after infection with dementia, poor cognition, and personality changes. Agents include HIV, natural or vaccine-related measles (in subacute sclerosing panencephalitis), rubella, HSV (in Mollaret meningitis), and papovavirus (in progressive multifocal leukoencephalopathy). Slow CNS infection may be the result of small proteinaceous particles *(prions);* illness includes kuru or Creutzfeldt-Jakob disease. The incidence of these infections has increased significantly in Europe; this is believed to be caused by transmission of prions associated with bovine spongiform encephalitis after consumption of infected beef. Slow viral or prion diseases are progressive and fatal; treatment is available only for HIV encephalopathy.

Clinical Manifestations. Signs and symptoms are similar to those in aseptic meningitis; in encephalitis, however, more abnormalities of mental function are noted. Headache and fever are associated with confusion, delirium, irritability, hallucinations, memory loss, combativeness, coma, seizures (sometimes focal), ataxia, and signs of increased intracranial pressure.

Diagnosis and Differential Diagnosis. A patient's history should take into account possible exposures to persons and animals with illnesses, to mosquitoes, and to ticks; the history also should note any extent of travel. Encephalopathy caused by toxins, hypoglycemia, hypervitaminosis A, Reye syndrome, inborn errors of metabolism, or trauma should be considered. A patient with concurrent or recent mumps, measles, or varicella is at risk for infectious or postinfectious encephalitis; neurologic involvement may precede the development of other manifestations of these diseases.

Bacterial diseases to be considered are mycoplasmal infection, tuberculosis, syphilis, leptospirosis, rickettsia, Lyme disease, cat-scratch disease, and borreliosis. Parasites associated with encephalitis are *Toxoplasma gondii,* trypanosomiasis, cysticercosis, and malaria. Cryptococcal disease presents as an encephalitis and is common in older children with

HIV infection. Noninfectious causes of an encephalitic disease are malignancy, sarcoidosis, Kawasaki disease, and primary CNS or systemic vasculitis.

Examination of the CSF in viral encephalitis usually reveals abnormalities. The findings may resemble those in aseptic meningitis, with elevated protein and lymphocytosis. Increased erythrocytes may be seen with HSV, whereas extreme elevations of protein and reductions of glucose suggest tuberculosis or cryptococcal infection. The diagnosis of cryptococcal disease can be made by India ink smear and determination of CSF cryptococcal antigen. The EEG, CT scan, and MRI may be nonspecific, but in HSV infection they often reveal a temporal lobe focus. Many causes of temporal lobe disease exist, and when HSV is suspected on clinical grounds, biopsy confirms the diagnosis in only 40%–50% of cases. Viral cultures of the nasopharynx, rectum, and CSF for HSV occasionally are helpful. PCR has been most valuable in rapid diagnosis of HSV, enteroviral, and HHV-6 and HHV-7 encephalitis. In many cases of viral encephalitis, paired serology of plasma is needed to determine a rise of specific antibodies. Brain biopsy may be necessary for definitive diagnosis, especially in patients with focal neurologic findings or at risk for CNS lymphoma or toxoplasmosis (both treatable).

Treatment. For HSV infections, acyclovir is the treatment of choice (see Appendix I). HIV infections may be treated with a combination of antiretroviral agents. *M. pneumoniae* infections may be treated with doxycycline, erythromycin, azithromycin, or clarithromycin. Enteroviral disease is treated with pleconaril. Supportive care is extremely important to decrease elevated intracranial pressure and maintain cardiopulmonary function.

Prognosis. Most children with encephalitis recover without major sequelae. Disease caused by HSV, rabies, or *M. pneumoniae* is associated with a poorer prognosis. Encephalitis may be severe in young children (younger than 1 year of age) and those with coma. Although most patients with epidemic forms of encephalitis (St. Louis, California, and enteroviral infections) do well, eastern equine encephalitis has a poorer outcome.

REFERENCES

Behrman RE, Kliegman RM, Jenson HB, editors: *Nelson textbook of pediatrics,* ed 16, Philadelphia, 2000, WB Saunders, Chapter 174.

Cinque P, Cleator G, Weber T, et al: The role of laboratory investigation in the diagnosis and management of patients with suspected herpes simplex encephalitis: a consensus report, *J Neurol Neurosurg Psychiatry* 61(4):339–345, 1996.

Craven R, Roehrig J: West Nile virus, *JAMA* 286(6):651–653, 2001.

Jeffery K, Read S, Peto T, et al: Diagnosis of viral infections of the central nervous system: clinical interpretation of PCR results, *Lancet* 349(9048):313–317, 1997.

Rautonen J, Koskiniemi M, Vaheri A: Prognostic factors in childhood acute encephalitis, *Pediatr Infect Dis J* 10(6):441–446, 1991.

RESPIRATORY TRACT INFECTIONS
Upper Respiratory Tract Infections
Ear Infections

Otitis Externa ("Swimmer's Ear"). Otitis externa is an acute infection of the external auditory canal. Trauma or prolonged exposure to moisture predisposes to infection. *P. aeruginosa* is the leading cause, followed by *S. aureus* and other skin flora. The infected child has severe unilateral pain localized to the ear. Exquisite tenderness is noted on manipulation of the pinna or tragus, a finding not observed in patients with otitis media. In otitis externa the tympanic membrane is normal, whereas the canal is erythematous. **Malignant otitis externa** is noted in patients with diabetes and presents as a severe cellulitis caused by *P. aeruginosa.* Rarely, herpes zoster may produce otitis externa.

The *differential diagnosis* involves the presence of a foreign body, such as small toys or insects; trauma; and referred pain. *Treatment* of uncomplicated otitis externa involves irrigation and topical antibiotics. For abscess formation, incision and drainage are necessary; for severe cellulitis, parenteral antistaphylococcal and anti-*Pseudomonas* antibiotics are necessary.

Otitis Media. Otitis media is a suppurative infection of the middle ear cavity and is most common in healthy children between 6 months and 2 years of age; in certain high-risk populations, such as children with HIV, cleft palate, and Down syndrome; and in Inuits and Native Americans. Otitis media is also more common in boys, in patients of lower socioeconomic status, in formula-fed infants, and in the winter months.

Pathogenesis. Bacteria gain access to the middle ear when the normal patency of the eustachian tube is blocked by local infection, pharyngitis, or hypertrophied adenoids. Air trapped in the middle ear is reabsorbed, creating negative pressure in this cavity; this permits reflux of bacteria. This bacterial reflux, plus obstruction of the flow of secretions from the middle ear to the pharynx, leads to a middle ear effusion that becomes infected by nasopharyngeal bacteria. The common bacterial pathogens are the pneumococci, nontypable *H. influenzae, Moraxella catarrhalis,* and, less frequently, group A streptococci. Relatively resistant (to penicillin, MIC 0.1–1.0 μg/mL) and highly resistant *S. pneumoniae* (to penicillin, MIC >2 μg/mL) are being isolated with increasing frequency from young children, particularly from those who attend day care and those who have recently received antibiotics. Bacteria recovered from the nasopharynx do not correlate with those isolated by tympanocentesis. Viruses (e.g., respiratory syncytial virus [RSV], CMV, and rhinovirus) have been recovered as copathogens or alone in 20–25% of patients.

Clinical Manifestations. Patients with otitis media are often febrile and irritable and may inconsistently pull at their ears. The disease usually occurs 1–7 days after a nasopharyngitis. Vomiting, diarrhea, a bulging fontanel, vertigo, tinnitus, and a draining ear (with tympanic membrane perforation) also may be seen. The normal eardrum moves freely when negative or positive pressure is generated by the otoscope; it appears pink and translucent, and a cone of reflected light usually is noted radiating from the center to the anteroinferior margin. The otoscopic examination in otitis media reveals a bulging, immobile, erythematous tympanic membrane, with loss of identifiable landmarks such as the short process and handle of the malleus. Perforation of the tympanic membrane also may occur and usually is associated with acute relief of pain. Otitis media may be associated with an ipsilateral conjunctivitis; both usually are caused by nontypable *H. influenzae.*

Treatment. Use of the conjugate vaccine for *S. pneumoniae* has been associated with only a small decrease in incidence of otitis media. Oral antibiotics frequently used to treat otitis media are amoxicillin, amoxicillin/clavulanate, trimethoprim/sulfamethoxazole, and erythromycin/sulfisoxazole. Oral cephalosporins (cefaclor, cefuroxime, cefixime, cefpodoxime, cefprozil, cefdinir, and loracarbef) have also been approved for the treatment of otitis media caused by β-lactamase–producing organisms and have convenient once-a-day or twice-a-day dose schedules. These regimens are expensive. *S. pneumoniae* remains the most common significant pathogen causing acute otitis media; relatively and highly resistant pneumococci that are not susceptible to the discussed agents are increasingly frequent causes of infection. Higher doses of amoxicillin/clavulanate or clindamycin or a single dose of parenteral ceftriaxone may be efficacious, but no generally agreed-on regimens exist for therapy of otitis media caused by highly resistant pneumococci. Tympanocentesis may be needed in patients who are difficult to treat or those who do not respond to therapy (see Appendix I).

Decongestants or antihistamines are not effective alone or when combined with antibiotics. The *complications* of otitis media are hearing loss, chronic effusion, cholesteatoma formation (mass-like keratinized epithelial growth), petrositis, intracranial extension (brain abscess, subdural empyema, or venous thrombosis), and mastoiditis.

Acute mastoiditis is a suppurative complication of otitis media, with inflammation and potential destruction of the mastoid air spaces. The disease progresses from a periostitis to an osteitis with mastoid abscess formation and draining tracts (e.g., through the tympanic membrane or into the neck). Posterior auricular tenderness and swelling and erythema, in addition to the signs of otitis media, are present. The pinna is displaced downward and outward. Roentgenograms or CT of the mastoid reveals clouding of the air cells, demineralization, or bone destruction. Bacteria that cause acute otitis media are also those responsible for acute mastoiditis. *S. aureus, P. aeruginosa,* and anaerobic bacteria may be recovered in chronic cases. Culturing swabs of the external ear is not as specific as obtaining fluid by tympanocentesis, aspiration of posterior auricular cellulitis or the mastoid at surgery, or, rarely, a blood culture.

Treatment involves systemic antibiotics and incision and drainage if the disease has progressed to abscess formation.

Nasopharyngitis

Rhinorrhea (Nasal Discharge). Rhinorrhea is a common manifestation of infectious, allergic, or mechanical conditions. Infectious rhinitis is associated with a mucopurulent discharge that contains polymorphonuclear leukocytes and is the result of rhinovirus and other respiratory viruses, such as RSV. Low-grade fever, nasal stuffiness, and sneezing may be present. Hypersensitivity to allergens is another common cause of rhinitis and is characterized by a lack of fever, eosinophils in the discharge, and other allergic manifestations, such as allergic shiners; nasal polyps; a pale, edematous, nasal turbinate mucosa; and a transverse crease on the nasal bridge (see Chapter 8). Other, less common causes of rhinorrhea are foreign body, choanal atresia,vasomotor rhinitis, CSF fistula, diphtheria, tumor, congenital syphilis, and Wegener granulomatosis. Persistent rhinorrhea following a cold suggests sinusitis.

The *treatment* of viral rhinorrhea is usually supportive, with normal saline nose drops, steam, and, occasionally, decongestants.

Sinusitis. Sinusitis is a suppurative infection of the paranasal sinuses and often complicates the common cold and allergic rhinitis. Indeed, patients with rhinitis often have thickened sinus mucosa. Patients with cyanotic heart disease, cystic fibrosis, immunoglobulin deficiency (total or subclass), HIV infection, nasotracheal intubation, immotile cilia syndrome, or dental infection have an increased incidence of sinusitis. It is also a frequent problem in immunocompromised children following organ transplantation. The maxillary, ethmoid, and sphenoid sinuses are present at birth, whereas the frontal sinus develops at 1 year of life. Pneumatization of the sinuses is delayed relative to sinus formation; the frontal sinuses may not appear as air-filled spaces until 10 years of age.

Etiology. Obstruction to mucociliary flow (preceding viral rhinitis) predisposes to bacterial proliferation. The bacteria producing acute sinusitis are pneumococci, nontypable *H. influenzae, M. catarrhalis,* anaerobic bacteria, and, rarely, streptococci and staphylococci. Nosocomial sinusitis occurs in children with indwelling nasogastric tubes and may be caused by gram-negative bacteria (*Klebsiella, Pseudomonas,* or *Enterobacter*); antibiotic-resistant organisms are often selected out by prior systemic antibiotic therapy. Sinusitis may develop in neutropenic immunosuppressed patients as a result of infection by *Aspergillus* species or Zygomycetes. Culture of the nasal mucosa is not helpful in identifying the responsible bacteria. If necessary, antral puncture (for maxillary sinusitis) is the diagnostic procedure of choice.

Clinical Manifestations. Clinical manifestations include persistent mucopurulent rhinorrhea; cough (especially at night); nasal stuffiness; a nasal quality to the voice; facial swelling, tenderness, and pain; and headache. CT reveals clouding, thickened mucosa, or an air-fluid level. Sinus aspiration usually is not needed in patients with uncomplicated sinusitis.

Treatment. Amoxicillin or amoxicillin/clavulanate is usually effective in the treatment of uncomplicated sinusitis (see Appendix I). *Complications* should be treated with drainage and, if indicated, broad-spectrum parenteral antibiotics; complications are orbital cellulitis, epidural or subdural empyema, brain abscess, dural sinus thrombosis, osteomyelitis of the outer or inner table of the frontal sinus (Pott's puffy tumor), and meningitis. Sinusitis also may exacerbate bronchoconstriction in asthmatic patients.

Orbital Cellulitis. Orbital cellulitis is a complication of sinusitis following spread of bacteria into the orbit through the wall of the infected sinus. Typically, ethmoid sinusitis spreads through the lamina papyracea, a thin, bony plate that separates the orbit and the ethmoid sinus. Infection of the extraocular structures of the orbit progresses through the following stages:

1. An inflammatory edema
2. Orbital cellulitis (edema plus chemosis; mild proptosis; limited extraocular muscle motion, with or without reduced visual acuity)
3. A subperiosteal abscess (down-and-out position of the globe in proptosis, resulting from abscess formation in the periosteum)
4. An orbital abscess (involvement of the orbital fat, muscle, and posterior cone of the orbit; severe ophthalmoplegia; vision loss; and proptosis)
5. Cavernous sinus thrombosis (headache; nuchal rigidity; involvement of cranial nerves III, IV, V, and VI)

The patient often has a high fever, orbital pain, limited extraocular motion (ophthalmoplegia), decreased vision, and proptosis. Infection of the orbit must be differentiated from that of the preseptal space (the anterior to palpebral fascia, separating the eyelids and the orbit) or periorbital space. **Periorbital cellulitis** (preseptal) usually occurs in young children (younger than 3 years of age); these children may, like those with orbital cellulitis, have fever and lid swelling and appear toxic but do not have ophthalmoplegia or proptosis. These infections may be caused by hematogenous infection (e.g., *S. pneumoniae; H. influenzae* type b is rarely seen in immunized children). Periorbital (preseptal) cellulitis may be a complication of sinusitis caused by the bacteria typically associated with sinusitis (*S. pneumoniae,* nontypable *H. influenzae,* and *M. catarrhalis*) and the anaerobic organisms found in the upper respiratory tract. Periorbital cellulitis associated with trauma is more often caused by *S. aureus* or *S. pyogenes.*

Diagnosis. Orbital cellulitis is confirmed by a CT scan of the orbit. This essential examination determines the extent of orbital infection and the need for surgical drainage. Blood culture, ESR, and CBC are additional laboratory studies to be performed. Disorders to be considered in the differential diagnosis are zygomycosis (mucormycosis), aspergillosis, rhabdomyosarcoma, neuroblastoma, Wegener granulomatosis, inflammatory pseudotumor of the orbit, and trichinosis.

Treatment. Therapy for orbital cellulitis involves broad-spectrum parenteral antibiotics, such as oxacillin and ceftriaxone (see Appendix I). Draining the infected sinus or orbital abscess also is indicated in *complicated cases.*

Pharyngitis (Pharyngotonsillitis). Patients with pharyngitis demonstrate cough, sore throat, dysphagia, and fever. Pharyngitis is one of the most common pediatric infections. Inflammation confined to the pharynx is unusual, but if involvement of the tonsils is prominent, the term *tonsillitis* is used.

Etiology. Pharyngitis in children younger than 2 years of age is often viral; group A streptococci are more common in children older than 5 years of age, and *Mycoplasma,* gonococcus, and *Arcanobacterium haemolyticum* are more common among adolescents. Viral pathogens are rhinovirus, coronavirus, adenovirus, enteroviruses, EBV, CMV, and HSV; the bacterial agent is predominantly group A streptococcus, which may be recovered from only 10–20% of patients. Pharyngitis is one component of primary HIV infection (along with fever, adenopathy, and a maculopapular rash) and should be considered in patients potentially at risk because therapy with antiretroviral agents is indicated. Less common causes are group C or G streptococcus, *Corynebacterium diphtheriae,* tularemia, toxoplasmosis, and gonorrhea.

Clinical Manifestations. Examination of the throat reveals erythema, exudate, palatine petechiae, enlarged tonsils, and, occasionally, anterior cervical lymphadenopathy. This appearance does not differentiate bacterial pathogens from viral pathogens. Nonetheless, vesiculation and ulceration suggest HSV and coxsackieviruses (herpangina); concomitant conjunctivitis suggests adenovirus; a gray-white fibrinous pseudomembrane with marked cervical swelling (bull neck), with or without carditis or neuropathy, suggests diphtheria; and a macular rash suggests group A beta-hemolytic streptococci (scarlet fever) or, less frequently, *A. haemolyticum*.

Rare *complications* of pharyngitis are extension to oropharyngeal or retropharyngeal spaces, peritonsillar abscess, and septic thrombophlebitis of the internal jugular vein **(Lemierre syndrome)**. Patients with Lemierre syndrome have painful adenopathy in the neck and often have evidence of metastatic foci of infection, such as pneumonia.

Diagnosis. The diagnosis of streptococcal pharyngitis is made by throat culture or by rapid streptococcal antigen detection kits. Identification of streptococcal pharyngitis in children is important because treatment reduces symptoms; prevents the poststreptococcal sequela of acute rheumatic fever; prevents local suppurative complications; and identifies the possibility of, but does not prevent the development of, the poststreptococcal sequela of acute glomerulonephritis. A CBC and heterophil testing may be used in the diagnosis of infectious mononucleosis. Cold agglutinins may be useful for mycoplasmal infection. Streptococcal pharyngitis may be present in 25% of patients with mononucleosis.

The *differential diagnosis* of infectious pharyngitis involves other local infections of the oral cavity, retropharyngeal abscesses (caused by *S. aureus*, streptococci, or anaerobes), peritonsillar abscesses (with quinsy sore throat; unilateral tonsil swelling; and infections caused by streptococci, anaerobes, or, rarely, *S. aureus*), Ludwig angina (mixed anaerobic bacterial cellulitis of the floor of the mouth, which may be the result of an odontogenic source), and epiglottitis (see Chapter 12). In addition, neutropenic mucositis (in leukemia or aplastic anemia), thrush (candidiasis secondary to T-cell immune deficiency), autoimmune ulceration (SLE or Behçet disease), and Kawasaki disease may cause pharyngitis. Signs suggesting that the disease is not a simple pharyngitis are persistent clinical manifestations for more than 1 week, stridor, trismus, poor clearance of oral secretions, difficulty swallowing, pain in the absence of erythema, presence of a mass, and blood in the pharynx.

Treatment. The treatment of choice for group A streptococcal pharyngitis is penicillin. Organisms associated with this condition have remained highly susceptible to penicillin. Erythromycin (or clarithromycin or azithromycin) is an acceptable alternative and is also active against *Mycoplasma* and *A. haemolyticum*. Failure to eradicate pharyngeal carriage of group A streptococci may be the result of colonization with β-lactamase–producing anaerobes, which destroy penicillin locally. Administration of clindamycin or amoxicillin/clavulanate usually eradicates the group A streptococci in these instances. Peritonsillar abscesses may be treated initially with high-dose penicillin and aspiration; following resolution of these abscesses, tonsillectomy may be indicated. Retropharyngeal abscesses frequently warrant drainage and the addition of antistaphylococcal antibiotics. Ludwig angina and other odontogenic infections may be treated with high-dose penicillin or ampicillin with sulbactam.

Epiglottitis. See Chapter 12.

REFERENCES

Alvarez A, Schreiber JR: Lemierre's syndrome in adolescent children: anaerobic sepsis with internal jugular vein thrombophlebitis following pharyngitis, *Pediatrics* 96(2 Pt 1):354–359, 1995.

Ambati BK, Ambati J, Azar N, et al: Periorbital and orbital cellulitis before and after the advent of *Haemophilus influenzae* type b vaccination, *Ophthalmology* 107(8):1450–1453, 2000.

Behrman RE, Kliegman RM, Jenson HB, editors: *Nelson textbook of pediatrics*, ed 16, Philadelphia, 2000, WB Saunders, Chapters 381, 382, 646.

Bluestone CD: Clinical course, complications, and sequelae of acute otitis media, *Pediatr Infect Dis J* 19(5 Suppl):S37–S46, 2000.

de Marie S, Tjon A, Tham RTO, et al: Clinical infections and nonsurgical treatment of parapharyngeal space infections complicating throat infection, *Rev Infect Dis* 11(6):975–982, 1989.

Ogle J, Laver B: Acute mastoiditis, *Am J Dis Child* 140(11): 1178–1182, 1986.

Shinefield HR, Black S: Efficacy of pneumococcal conjugate vaccines in large-scale field trials, *Pediatr Infect Dis J* 19(4):394–397, 2000.

Shoemaker M, Lampe R, Weir M: Peritonsillitis: abscess or cellulitis? *Pediatr Infect Dis* 5(4):435–439, 1986.

Shulman ST, Gerber MA, Tanz RR, et al: Streptococcal pharyngitis: the case for penicillin therapy, *Pediatr Infect Dis J* 13(1):1–7, 1994.

Wald ER: Sinusitis in children, *N Engl J Med* 326(5):319–323, 1992.

Lower Respiratory Tract Infections

Bronchiolitis

See Chapter 12.

Pneumonia

See Chapter 12.

URINARY TRACT INFECTIONS

See Chapter 16.

BACTERIAL INFECTIONS

Antibiotic Therapy

Dosages

See Appendix I.

Principles

The therapy for bacterial infections depends on the isolation of the offending agent, characterization of the agent's antibiotic susceptibility, and delivery of the appropriate antibiotic to the site of infection in sufficient quantities to either kill the bacteria (bactericidal) or alter it to permit the body's immune response to eventually kill it. The two major strategies are as follows:

1. Use broad-spectrum, empiric antibiotics in high-risk situations, such as neonatal sepsis or bacteremia in an immunocompromised host.
2. Tailor antibiotic treatment to the specific pathogen in lower risk, immunocompetent patients.

This second principle minimizes drug toxicity, the development of resistant microorganisms, superinfection by fungi and previously resistant bacteria, and cost to the family.

Antibiotic efficacy may be affected by several host factors. Antimicrobial agents are an adjunct to the host immune response. Infections of a foreign body, such as an intravascular catheter or a prosthetic device, are difficult to eradicate because polymorphonuclear leukocytes and macrophages do not readily engulf organisms on plastic surfaces. Similarly, in endocarditis it is difficult for phagocytic cells to eradicate bacteria amid vegetations of fibrin and platelets on infected heart valves. For these types of infections to be sterilized, prolonged therapy with bactericidal antibiotics is required and does not always result in a satisfactory outcome. Chronic osteomyelitis, with organisms sequestered from the circulation in abscesses or poorly perfused bone, is similarly difficult to cure without surgical débridement of the infected tissue and reestablishment of a good vascular supply. Antimicrobial therapy alone may not cure infections in closed spaces with limited perfusion.

Optimal antimicrobial therapy requires an understanding of the pharmacokinetic properties of the drugs being administered to specific patient populations. Dose schedules in the premature neonate account for the immaturity of renal function by increasing dose intervals. In patients with cystic fibrosis, who often have larger volume of distribution of the hydrophilic antibiotics and increased renal clearance, larger doses are required to achieve therapeutic levels. Obese children may receive significant antibiotic overdoses if they are given dosage regimens on a per-kilogram basis that exceed the maximal adult doses recommended. These patients may have a significantly smaller volume of distribution for hydrophilic drugs and do not necessarily require large doses as are required by a leaner child of equivalent weight.

Another variable affecting antimicrobial therapy is the oral absorption of drugs. The bioavailability of orally administered antibiotics is highly variable, depending on the acid stability of the antimicrobial agent, the amount of gastric acidity, and whether the drug is taken with food, antacids, H_2 blockers, or other medications.

The site of infection is another important consideration. Aminoglycosides, which are active only against aerobic organisms, have significantly reduced activity in abscesses and milieus with low pH and oxygen tension. Infections of the CNS or the eye necessitate treatment with antimicrobial agents that are able to penetrate and achieve levels in these sites.

Drug interactions must be considered when multiple antimicrobial agents are used to treat infection. For the empiric treatment of life-threatening infection, the use of two or more antimicrobial agents may be justified when broad-spectrum activity is needed prior to the identification of the organism. A few indications remain for the continuation of two drugs to treat infection, such as the use of a cell wall–active agent (β-lactam or vancomycin) plus an aminoglycoside to effectively treat infections caused by the highly resistant enterococci. Similarly, two drugs with different mechanisms of action are used against serious *P. aeruginosa* infections. Several drugs are dispensed together (trimethoprim/sulfamethoxazole, amoxicillin/clavulanate, ampicillin/sulbactam, and ticarcillin/clavulanate) because the activity of the antibiotics in combination is significantly greater than when they are used alone. The addition of clavulanic acid (a β-lactamase inhibitor with modest antibacterial activity) to amoxicillin broadens the spectrum of the penicillin, allowing it to be used against gram-negative β-lactamase producers such as *H. influenzae*, gram-positive organisms such as *S. aureus*, and anaerobes. The use of a bacteriostatic drug, such as a tetracycline, along with a β-lactam agent (which is effective only against growing organisms), may result in antibiotic *antagonism*—that is, less bacterial killing in the presence of both drugs than if either were used alone.

Selection of Antibiotics

The choice of antibiotics depends on the epidemiology of the condition, site of infection, localizing manifestations (Table 10–1), host factors, the need for antibiotic prophylaxis (Table 10–5), and the spectrum of bacterial pathogens susceptible to the antibiotic (Table 10–12). The treatment of specific bacterial infections is covered in the following text.

TABLE 10–12
Commonly Used Antibiotics for Bacterial Infection

Antibiotic	Mechanism of Action/Activity	Sensitive Bacteria/Indications	Comments
Penicillins	Bind to penicillin-binding proteins; inhibit transpeptidation reaction of cell wall, causing eventual cell lysis		No activity for *Staphylococcus epidermidis, Mycoplasma, Chlamydia*
Penicillin		Pneumococcus, meningococcus, gonococcus, streptococci, anaerobic bacteria (*Bacteroides melaninogenicus*), *Pasteurella multocida, Actinomyces* sp.	Penicillinase-producing gonococcus, some pneumococci, and many anaerobes are resistant
Ampicillin/amoxicillin	Extended spectrum; beta-lactamase susceptible	*Haemophilus influenzae, Listeria monocytogenes, Escherichia coli, Salmonella, Shigella, Proteus mirabilis, Enterococcus*	Many of these organisms produce beta-lactamases and are resistant
Ticarcillin	Anti-*Pseudomonas*	*E. coli, Pseudomonas aeruginosa, Proteus* sp.	Ureidopenicillins not beta-lactamase stable
Piperacillin/tazobactam	Anti-*Pseudomonas*	*P. aeruginosa, Klebsiella, Citrobacter, Acinetobacter, S. aureus,* anaerobes	Ureidopenicillins, tazobactam stable to penicillinases
Oxacillin/methicillin or nafcillin	Anti-*Staphylococcus*	*Staphylococcus aureus,* pneumococcus, *Streptococcus*	Penicillinase-resistant penicillins; *S. epidermidis* is usually resistant
Amoxicillin/clavulanic acid	Extended spectrum	As for ampicillin, plus *S. aureus, Enterococcus, Bacteroides fragilis, Moraxella catarrhalis*	Clavulanic acid inhibits beta-lactamases; PO prep
Ampicillin/sulbactam	Extended spectrum	As for amoxicillin/clavulanic acid, plus anaerobes	Sulbactam inhibits β-lactamase; IV prep
Ticarcillin/clavulanic acid	Extended spectrum	As above, plus broader gram-negative coverage	IV prep
Cephalosporins	Bind to penicillin-binding proteins; inhibit cell wall cross-linking; produce cell lysis		No activity against *Listeria* or *Enterococcus*
1st generation Cefazolin or cephalothin		*S. aureus, E. coli, Klebsiella*	Good for *S. aureus,* other gram-positive organisms; *H. influenzae* type b is resistant

Data from *Med Clin North Am* 71:1051–1216, 1987; *Med Lett* 34:49, 1992.
CNS, Central nervous system; *CSF,* cerebrospinal fluid; *DNA,* deoxyribonucleic acid; *RNA,* ribonucleic acid.

Continued

TABLE 10–12
Commonly Used Antibiotics for Bacterial Infection—cont'd

Antibiotic	Mechanism of Action/Activity	Sensitive Bacteria/Indications	Comments
2nd generation			
Cefuroxime	Beta-lactamase stable	*H. influenzae* type b, *S. aureus, Klebsiella, E. coli*	Poor blood drug levels
Cephamycins			
Cefoxitin, cefotetan	Anaerobic coverage	*B. melaninogenicus, Bacteroides fragilis, E. coli,* gonococcus	Abdominal and genital tract infections
3rd generation			
Cefotaxime or ceftriaxone	Extended spectrum	*E. coli, Klebsiella,* gonococcus, *H. influenzae,* pneumococcus, meningococcus, *S. aureus*	Better gram-negative enteric coverage, good CSF penetration
Ceftazidime, cefoperazone	Broad spectrum	Same as above, gram-negative plus *Pseudomonas;* not uniformly active against *Burkholderia cepacia*	Resistance may be induced during therapy
Aminoglycosides	Inhibition of bacterial protein synthesis at ribosomes		Ototoxicity and nephrotoxicity, must monitor peak and trough serum concentrations
Gentamicin, tobramycin, netilmicin		Gram-negative Enterobacteriaceae, including *Pseudomonas*	Broad spectrum, synergy with beta-lactams; enterococci are resistant
Amikacin		Same as above	Less susceptible to aminoglycoside-inactivating enzymes
Streptomycin		Plague, tularemia, brucellosis (plus tetracycline)	
Other Antibiotics			
Imipenem with cilastatin	Thienamycin drug: binds to penicillin-binding proteins; very broad spectrum	Most gram-positive and gram-negative bacteria, *Listeria, Bacillus* sp., *Pseudomonas, Acinetobacter*	*Stenotrophomonas maltophilia,* methicillin-resistant *S. aureus,* enterococci are resistant; requires cilastatin to inhibit renal degradation
Meropenem	Same as imipenem	Same as imipenem	Does not require cilastatin
Aztreonam	Monobactam drug: binds to penicillin-binding proteins of Enterobacteriaceae only; narrow spectrum	Most gram-negative bacteria	No action against anaerobic or gram-positive bacteria; *B. cepacia* is resistant; does not induce beta-lactamase production
Tetracyclines	Inhibition of protein synthesis	*Chlamydia, Mycoplasma,* gonococcus, *Actinomyces,* Lyme disease; pelvic inflammatory disease, Rocky Mountain spotted fever, urethritis, *Brucella* sp., tularemia, plague	Stains teeth, contraindicated before 10 yr of age

Data from *Med Clin North Am* 71:1051–1216, 1987; *Med Lett* 34:49, 1992.
CNS, Central nervous system; *CSF,* cerebrospinal fluid; *DNA,* deoxyribonucleic acid; *RNA,* ribonucleic acid.

TABLE 10–12
Commonly Used Antibiotics for Bacterial Infection—cont'd

Antibiotic	Mechanism of Action/Activity	Sensitive Bacteria/Indications	Comments
Chloramphenicol	Inhibition of protein synthesis	*Salmonella, H. influenzae,* meningococcus, pneumococcus, *Shigella, B. fragilis,* Rocky Mountain spotted fever, typhoid fever	Reversible bone marrow suppression, aplastic anemia, gray baby syndrome (rarely used in United States)
Rifampin	Inhibition of DNA-dependent RNA polymerase	*S. aureus, Mycobacterium tuberculosis, H. influenzae, Meningococcus*	Red discoloration of secretions; increases metabolism of drugs (e.g., oral contraceptives); resistance develops if used alone
Metronidazole	Damage of DNA by free radicals	*Bacteroides* sp., *Clostridium difficile,* anaerobic bacteria, *Gardnerella vaginalis, Capnocytophaga, Giardia, Entamoeba histolytica*	Seizures, encephalopathy, disulfiram reaction, metallic taste
Erythromycin	Macrolide: inhibits protein synthesis	*Corynebacterium diphtheriae, Mycoplasma, Chlamydia, Bordetella pertussis, Haemophilus ducreyi, Legionella* sp., *Campylobacter*	Often used as an alternative to penicillin G; nausea, hepatoxicity (estolate ester); increases theophylline and carbamazepine blood levels
Azithromycin	Macrolide	Less active than erythromycin against *S. aureus,* pneumococcus, streptococci, more active against *H. influenzae, Mycoplasma, Chlamydia,* gram-negative bacilli; active against *M. catarrhalis, C. pneumoniae, Legionella pneumophila, Borrelia burgdorferi, Neisseria gonorrhoeae*	Possible efficacy for *Mycobacterium avium, Toxoplasma* encephalitis, cryptosporidiosis; long half-life: single-dose treatment for uncomplicated *Chlamydia* urethritis or cervicitis Prolonged use may cause hearing loss
Clarithromycin	Macrolide	More active than erythromycin for *S. aureus,* pneumococcus, *Streptococcus*	Similar to azithromycin
Clindamycin	Similar to erythromycin	*S. aureus, Streptococcus,* most anaerobic bacteria, *Actinomyces* (penicillin-allergic patients)	Pseudomembranous colitis toxicity

Data from *Med Clin North Am* 71:1051–1216, 1987; *Med Lett* 34:49, 1992.
CNS, Central nervous system; *CSF,* cerebrospinal fluid; *DNA,* deoxyribonucleic acid; *RNA,* ribonucleic acid.

Continued

TABLE 10–12
Commonly Used Antibiotics for Bacterial Infection—cont'd

Antibiotic	Mechanism of Action/Activity	Sensitive Bacteria/Indications	Comments
Vancomycin	Inhibits cell wall synthesis	Methicillin-resistant *S. aureus, S. epidermidis,* JK diphtheroids, *C. difficile, Enterococcus,* anaerobic bacteria	Red man syndrome if injected too fast, nephrotoxic; resistance in enterococci a major problem
Trimethoprim/ sulfamethoxazole	Inhibition of bacterial folate synthesis at two separate sites of the folate pathway	*E. coli, Proteus mirabilis, Salmonella, Shigella, H. influenzae, Yersinia,* Pneumococcus, *S. aureus, Pneumocystis carinii, M. catarrhalis, Nocardia*	Group A streptococci may be resistant; *P. aeruginosa* and enterococci resistant, Stevens-Johnson syndrome—anemia, neutropenia, glucose-6-phosphate dehydrogenase hemolysis
Ciprofloxacin	Similar to nalidixic acid; inhibition of bacterial DNA gyrase; broad spectrum	*P. aeruginosa, Shigella, Salmonella, E. coli, Klebsiella, Proteus* sp., *S. aureus, H. influenzae,* gonococcus, *Chlamydia, Listeria monocytogenes*	May be given by mouth; arthritis; CNS toxicity; not approved for children <17 yr of age but widely used
Linezolid	Inhibits protein synthesis	Gram-positive bacteria, including vancomyin-resistant *Enterococcus faecium* and *E. faecalis, S. aureus,* coagulase-negative *Staphylococcus*	Reserve for antibiotic-resistant isolates; kinetics not fully known in children

Data from *Med Clin North Am* 71:1051–1216, 1987; *Med Lett* 34:49, 1992.
CNS, Central nervous system; *CSF,* cerebrospinal fluid; *DNA,* deoxyribonucleic acid; *RNA,* ribonucleic acid.

Anaerobic Infections

Etiology. Anaerobic bacteria are ubiquitous and are usually harmless commensal members of the normal human flora of the oropharynx, gastrointestinal tract, vagina, and skin. The fecal flora contains as many as 500 different species of anaerobes. Obligate anaerobes require special culture media to grow. Gram-negative nonsporulating rods include *Bacteroides* and *Fusobacterium* species; gram-positive nonsporulating rods include *Eubacterium* and *Propionibacterium;* cocci include *Peptostreptococcus, Peptococcus,* and *Veillonella.*

Epidemiology. Blood, peritoneum, oropharynx, lungs, and soft tissues are the main sites of anaerobic infection. Infection follows disruption of mucous membrane barriers. Several anaerobes, or both anaerobes and aerobes, may be recovered concomitantly from infected tissue.

The major clinical settings for anaerobic infection are as follows:
- In the neonate after prolonged rupture of the membranes, amnionitis, or obstetric difficulty
- Peritonitis or septicemia associated with intestinal obstruction or perforation (appendicitis)
- Aspiration pneumonia with lung abscess
- Salpingitis and tuboovarian abscess
- Orofacial infections
- Brain abscess

Clinical Manifestations. Anaerobic infections of the *upper respiratory tract* have many different clinical manifestations. Periodontal infection ("trench mouth") often is the result of poor dental hygiene. Periapical abscesses or anaerobic osteomyelitis of the mandible or maxilla may also be present. Anaerobic microorganisms may be present in chronic sinusitis, chronic otitis media, mastoiditis, peritonsillar and retropharyngeal abscesses, and cervical lymphadenitis. Fusobacteria are important in the development of **Vincent stomatitis,** an infection characterized by ulcers covered by a brown or gray, foul- smelling exudate. Extensive tissue destruction can lead to perforation of the carotid artery. **Ludwig angina** is an acute cellulitis of the sublingual and submandibular spaces that tends to spread rapidly, without lymph node involvement or abscess formation. Edema of the tongue and airway may cause respiratory obstruction and necessitate tracheotomy.

Anaerobic infection of the *lower respiratory tract* produces necrotizing pneumonia, putrid empyema, or lung abscess. A history of aspiration may be elicited. Aspiration pneumonia is a common problem in neurologically impaired children, who may have repeated episodes of inapparent aspiration and less well-defined areas of pneumonia.

Anaerobic infection of the *CNS* produces brain abscess, subdural empyema, or septic thrombophlebitis of cortical veins and venous sinuses. These lesions originate by direct spread from a contiguous infection or by hematogenous spread. Purulent meningitis rarely is caused by anaerobes; identification of anaerobes from the CSF indicates another focus, such as a brain abscess or subdural empyema.

Peritoneal spillage of gastrointestinal contents, especially that of the colon, is associated with a high incidence of anaerobic *intraabdominal infection*. Peritonitis and abscess formation (either subdiaphragmatic or pelvic) are common after intestinal perforation. In sexually active adolescents anaerobes are an important component of pelvic inflammatory disease, in addition to the typical sexually transmitted pathogens *N. gonorrhoeae* and *C. trachomatis*, and contribute to the formation of tuboovarian abscesses.

Anaerobic *bacteremia* is clinically indistinguishable from aerobic bacteremia. Anaerobic bacteremia frequently is associated with disease of the gastrointestinal and genitourinary systems.

Diagnosis. The diagnosis of anaerobic infection requires an awareness of anaerobe-associated infections and appropriate collection of specimens for cultures, with the use of special media and techniques. Factors that should increase the suspicion of an anaerobic infection include the following:

- Presence of a foul-smelling exudate or discharge
- Evidence of necrotic tissue, gangrene, or fasciitis
- Infection located in proximity to a mucosal surface

- Gas in tissue
- Gram stain of material that reveals multiple types of organisms
- Infection associated with tissue destruction (trauma or malignancy)
- Failure to respond to antibiotics, especially aminoglycosides
- Septic thrombophlebitis
- Abscess formation

Added clues that suggest anaerobes are the absence of growth on routine cultures (sterile pus); failure to grow, but the presence of bacteria on Gram stain; growth in thioglycollate broth or on media containing kanamycin, neomycin, or paromomycin; production of gas and a foul odor in culture; and development of characteristic colonies on agar plates incubated anaerobically.

Treatment. The pathogen usually can be predicted from the site of infection (above or below the diaphragm), and most anaerobes have predictable susceptibilities to antibiotic agents. Many anaerobic bacteria produce β-lactamases, and often therapy is presumptive so the antimicrobial susceptibility of the anaerobic pathogens may not be known. Cefoxitin, amoxicillin/clavulanate, clindamycin, or metronidazole may be used to treat anaerobic infections at other sites. Anaerobes also usually are susceptible to cefotetan, imipenem, merapenem, or piperacillin/tazobactam. Metronidazole is quite effective in treating anaerobic brain abscesses, whereas clindamycin is excellent for lung abscesses (see Appendix I).

REFERENCES

Behrman RE, Kliegman RM, Jenson HB, editors: *Nelson textbook of pediatrics,* ed 16, Philadelphia, 2000, WB Saunders, Chapter 211.
Styrt B, Gorbach SL: Recent developments in the understanding of the pathogenesis and treatment of anaerobic infections (first of two parts), *N Engl J Med* 321(4):240–246, 1989.
Styrt B, Gorbach SL: Recent developments in the understanding of the pathogenesis and treatment of anaerobic infections (second of two parts), *N Engl J Med* 321(5):298–302, 1989.

Clostridial Infections

Clostridial organisms have been associated with tetanus, gas gangrene (clostridial myonecrosis), food poisoning, necrotizing enteritis, antimicrobial-associated colitis, and botulism. Most of these disorders are the result of toxin elaboration by vegetative organisms.

Tetanus (Lockjaw)

Etiology. *Clostridium tetani* is an anaerobic, spore-forming, gram-positive bacillus. The spores are resistant to many injurious agents and processes, including boiling. The vegetative forms of *C. tetani* are susceptible to heat and many disinfectants. *C. tetani* survive in soil for years and may be found in house dust, salt and fresh water, the oral cavities of mammals, and feces of many animal species.

C. tetani causes disease through the production of exotoxins, tetanus toxin or tetanospasmin, and tetatanolysin, which is thought to potentiate the effect of tetanus toxin. This is a neurotoxin that migrates transsynaptically and inhibits acetylcholine release, particularly from inhibitory synapses, resulting in muscle contraction, characteristic localized spasms, and rigidity. The toxin can also block transmission at neuromuscular junctions and cause paralysis. These toxins are produced by the vegetative forms of the bacteria when they propagate under favorable growth conditions (i.e., low oxygen tension as created by poorly perfused tissue after crush injuries).

Epidemiology. Tetanus occurs throughout the world and is a major cause of mortality in developing countries, particularly in unvaccinated individuals. Neonatal tetanus follows contamination of the umbilical cord with these organisms. Only 2 cases have been reported in the United States since 1989.

In the United States tetanus is rare. Only 33 cases were reported in 1999. Almost all of these were in elderly individuals or intravenous drug users who either were unvaccinated or had not received booster immunizations in the preceding 10 years.

Clinical Manifestations. Tetanus has several clinical forms: localized, generalized, cephalic, and tetanus neonatorum. In each, an examination of the actual wound does not reveal an appearance that is different from that of an uninfected wound.

Localized Tetanus. Localized tetanus is uncommon in children but produces pain and continuous rigidity and spasm of muscles in proximity to the injury; symptoms may persist for weeks and resolve without sequelae.

Generalized Tetanus. Generalized tetanus has an insidious onset, with gradually increasing muscle stiffness; trismus is the presenting symptom in over 50% of cases. Spasm of the masseter muscles may be associated with stiffness of neck muscles and difficulty in swallowing. Tetanic seizures are characterized by sudden bursts of tonic contractions of various muscle groups. Spasm of the airway or respiratory muscles causes airway obstruction and respiratory insufficiency. Spasm may cause fractures and local hemorrhages. The patient is completely conscious during the clinical course and has intense pain. Signs and symptoms increase over 3–7 days, reach a plateau during the second week, and gradually abate. Recovery is complete in 2–6 weeks.

Cephalic Tetanus. Cephalic tetanus is rare and may precede generalized tetanus. The incubation period is 1–2 days after otitis media, trauma to the head and face, and the presence of nasal foreign bodies.

Tetanus Neonatorum. Tetanus neonatorum begins 3–10 days after birth and is generalized. Difficulty in sucking, excessive crying, difficulty in swallowing, rigidity, tonic contractions, and opisthotonos are common.

Diagnosis and Differential Diagnosis. The diagnosis of tetanus is made on clinical grounds. A history of a wound or bite, the characteristic facial appearance, and spasms aid in establishing the diagnosis. Most cases occur in unimmunized individuals or in their infants. Wound cultures are positive for *C. tetani* in one third of instances. Gram stains of the wound may show gram-positive rods with terminal, drumstick-like spores. Trismus may be associated with tooth, peritonsillar, or retropharyngeal abscesses. Spasms also may be seen in rabies, hypocalcemia, and strychnine or phenothiazine intoxication. Rabies and (rarely) tetanus may follow animal bites. Rabies causes pain and numbness at the bite, fever (not noted in tetanus), painful esophageal spasm on drinking, CSF pleocytosis, and, eventually, coma and paralysis.

Treatment. The objectives of therapy are to remove the source of tetanospasmin, to neutralize remaining circulating toxin before it reaches the CNS, and to provide supportive care until tetanospasmin, which is fixed to neural tissue, can be metabolized. Supportive care includes meperidine for pain, benzodiazepines, endotracheal intubation and paralysis (if needed), and ventilatory support. Human tetanus immune globulin (antitoxin) (3000–6000 U, one dose) should be given, part of the dose injected directly into the wound. Wounds should be irrigated and debrided. Penicillin therapy is indicated to eradicate vegetative *C. tetani* organisms. There is no transmission to humans, but body substance isolation should be used until rabies is excluded.

Prevention. Immediate and thorough surgical treatment of wounds is mandatory. The indications for active and passive immunoprophylaxis depend on the prior immunization status and the severity of the wound (Table 10–13). *Tetanus toxoid* should also be given following suspected tetanus infection because the disease does not induce natural immunity.

REFERENCES

Behrman RE, Kliegman RM, Jenson HB, editors: *Nelson textbook of pediatrics*, ed 16, Philadelphia, 2000, WB Saunders, Chapter 209.
Gergen JP, McQuillan GM, Kiely M, et al: A population-based serologic survey of immunity to tetanus in the United States, *N Engl J Med* 332:761–766, 1995.

TABLE 10–13
Tetanus Prevention Following Wounds

Tetanus Immunization History	Clean Td*	Minor TIG†	All Others‡ Td	All Others‡ TIG
Uncertain or incomplete (<3 doses)	Yes	No	Yes	Yes
Complete (>3 doses plus booster)	No§	No	No‖	No

Modified from Report of Committee on Infectious Diseases: *Red Book 2000*, Elk Grove Village, Ill, 2000, American Academy of Pediatrics.
DT, Diphtheria-tetanus vaccine; *Td*, tetanus-diphtheria toxoid (adult type); *TIG*, tetanus immune globulin.
*If younger than 7 years old, DT may be given.
†Tetanus immune globulin (human).
‡Other wounds include those contaminated with soil, dirt, feces, and saliva and punctures, avulsions, crush injuries, burns, frostbite, and wounds resulting from missiles. All wounds require appropriate irrigation and débridement.
§Yes, if longer than 10 years since last immunization.
‖Yes, if longer than 5 years since last immunization.

Botulism

Etiology. *Clostridium botulinum* is an anaerobic, gram-positive bacillus that produces heat-resistant spores. When spores survive food processing, they germinate in the container and elaborate neurotoxins. Seven antigenically distinct toxins have been identified (A–G). All except D have been associated with human disease. *C. botulinum* toxins bind irreversibly to the presynaptic nerve terminals, are internalized by endocytosis, and block acetylcholine release. Neural transmission at ganglionic, postganglionic, and neuromuscular junctions is inhibited.

Epidemiology. Botulism has three forms, responsible for an average of 110 cases reported to the CDC each year:

1. *Infant botulism,* the most common cause of botulism in the United States, caused by germination of spores of *C. botulinum* in the gastrointestinal tract accompanied by toxin produced in vivo rather than by the ingestion of preformed toxin.
2. *Food-borne botulism,* an intoxication from preformed botulinum toxin present in improperly preserved food. Home-preserved foods are the most frequent cause of this type of botulism in the United States.
3. *Wound botulism,* a rare botulism resulting from local wound infection and toxin production by *C. botulinum.*

Infant botulism usually occurs in children younger than 6 months of age, has a peak onset from 1–3 months, and is caused by type A and B strains. Adults also have had this type of botulism. Sources for spores include soil, house and vacuum cleaner dust, honey, and possibly corn syrup. The majority of patients have been reported from California, Pennsylvania, Hawaii, and Utah, clusters correlating with areas of high soil spore concentration of *C. botulinum.* Alterations in the normal host intestinal flora, perhaps pH changes, and altered gut motility may predispose the infant to this disease.

Clinical Manifestations

Infant Botulism. The course of infant botulism varies from mild constipation and poor feeding to severe neurologic deterioration and sudden, at times unexplained, death. Typically, a previously healthy, afebrile infant has constipation and poor sucking and swallowing. A weak cry and smile develop, and bilateral ptosis, hypotonia, and poor head control are present. Symmetric, descending paralysis progresses over hours to days, involving facial muscles, trunk, and limbs. Ileus, bladder atony, nonreactive dilated pupils, and decreased tearing and salivation may be present. Infants require ventilatory support for apnea or hypoventilation. Because the CNS is not affected, the child is awake and may even appear alert.

Food-borne botulism. Incubation usually takes 12–36 hours but can range from several hours to a week. Nausea, vomiting, diplopia, dysphagia, dysarthria, and dry mouth are common during the course of disease. Weakness, postural hypotension, absent or diminished deep tendon reflexes, urinary retention, and constipation (not diarrhea) also may develop.

Wound botulism. The course may be similar to that exhibited after ingestion of *C. botulinum* toxin but is usually milder and more prolonged. The incubation period is 4–14 days.

Diagnosis and Differential Diagnosis. The diagnosis of botulism is established by identifying *C. botulinum* organisms or toxin in feces, blood, or food products.

Infant botulism should be differentiated from septicemia, myasthenia gravis, poliomyelitis, Werdnig-Hoffmann disease, spinal cord injury, an acute life-threatening event (SIDS), hypothyroidism, and inborn errors of metabolism.

Food-borne botulism must be differentiated from myasthenia gravis, poliomyelitis, Guillain-Barré syndrome, drug intoxication, trichinosis, diphtheria, and various forms of electrolyte or mineral imbalances.

The diagnosis of *wound botulism* is made by demonstrating the organisms in the wound or the toxin in blood. An electromyogram with brief, small, abundant potentials suggests botulism.

Treatment. Antitoxin is of uncertain value in *infant botulism*. Intensive care alone usually is sufficient. Antibiotics do not shorten the clinical course or decrease intestinal colonization. Aminoglycosides exacerbate or accelerate paralysis and produce respiratory failure as a result of synergistic inhibition of neurotransmission at the neuromuscular junction. A cleansing enema may eliminate the site of toxin production.

All children with *food-borne botulism* must be hospitalized. Vomiting should be induced and gastric lavage initiated. Cathartics may be placed in the stomach at the conclusion of lavage and an enema given to facilitate elimination of unabsorbed toxin. Equine antitoxin has been efficacious in treating food-borne disease. The polyvalent preparation is preferred until the toxin type has been identified. Skin sensitivity testing is mandatory before administration. Penicillin G is given to kill *C. botulinum*, which may continue to produce toxin.

Wound botulism requires débriding and draining the wound. Performing supportive intensive care measures and administering antitoxin and antibiotics also are indicated.

Supportive care involves monitoring cardiorespiratory functions in anticipation of apnea, hypotension, or aspiration.

Prevention. Boiling food for 10 minutes destroys the toxin. A pressure cooker is required to kill spores of *C. botulinum*; pressure requirements vary with the food being processed. Because 10% of retail honey in the United States may contain *C. botulinum* spores, it should not be fed to infants younger than 6 months of age. Breast-feeding may lessen the severity of the illness.

Prognosis. Most infants recover without sequelae if adequate intensive care and supportive therapy prevent hypoxia. Severity of illness in food-borne botulism is directly related to the titer of toxin ingested and inversely related to the duration of the incubation period. Complete recovery is delayed for many months and requires regeneration of the previously destroyed presynaptic terminals. Because the toxin does not cross the blood-brain barrier, intelligence is normal in the absence of prior hypoxic episodes.

REFERENCES

Behrman RE, Kliegman RM, Jenson HB, editors: *Nelson textbook of pediatrics*, ed 16, Philadelphia, 2000, WB Saunders, Chapter 192.

Schreiner MS, Field E, Ruddy R: Infant botulism: a review of 12 years' experience at the Children's Hospital of Philadelphia, *Pediatrics* 87:159–165, 1991.

Shapiro RL, Hatheway C, Swerdlow DL: Botulism in the United States: a clinical and epidemiologic review, *Ann Intern Med* 129:221–228, 1998.

Infection Caused by Corynebacterium Diphtheriae

Etiology and Pathophysiology. *C. diphtheriae* is a gram-positive, nonsporulating bacillus. Infection of *C. diphtheriae* by a lysogenic bacteriophage containing the gene for the toxin is required to produce disease. Only strains that produce toxin are responsible for myocarditis and neuritis.

Diphtheria is characterized by local inflammation and the production of a pseudomembrane composed of necrotic epithelium and coagulated inflammatory cells in the upper respiratory tract (nasal or oral pharynx), which may cause airway obstruction. In addition, toxin production causes injury to distant visceral tissues (e.g., nerve, heart, and kidney). Diphtheria toxin is an extremely potent inhibitor of protein synthesis that acts by adenosine diphosphate (ADP)–ribosylating elongation factor-2 (EF-2).

Epidemiology. Humans are the only known reservoir of *C. diphtheriae*. From 1980–1999, only 49 cases were reported in the United States, mostly in unimmunized or inadequately immunized adults. Outbreaks in the countries of the former Soviet Union have affected more than 50,000 individuals, with 1500 deaths in 1995. These outbreaks have been largely attributed to failure to immunize children and waning immunity in adults, but not to lack of efficacy of the available vaccine.

Diphtheria is acquired by close contact with respiratory droplets from either an asymptomatic carrier or a person with the disease. Fomites and dust occasionally are vehicles of transmission. The incubation period is 2–4 days.

Tonsillar or pharyngeal diphtheria is the most common type, beginning insidiously with malaise, low-grade fever, and a mild sore throat. Within 1–2 days, a membrane forms; its size and extent vary according to the host's immune status. The membrane initially is thin, white, and localized; as the disease progresses, it coalesces and extends from the tonsil to the contiguous soft or hard palate, pharyngeal wall, larynx, and trachea. This pattern distinguishes diphtheria from other diseases producing membranous tonsillitis. The membrane becomes gray, and the breath may have a foul, garlic odor. Removal of the exudate is followed by bleeding. Bilateral cervical lymphadenitis is variable. Ten percent of patients have high fever, toxicity, rapid progression of the pseudomembrane, and edema of the soft tissues of the neck (bull neck).

Laryngeal diphtheria usually results when the

membrane extends downward from the pharynx. In 10% of cases, only the larynx is involved. Hoarseness and stridor produce acute and potentially fatal obstruction if the membrane occludes the airway. In severe cases the membrane may extend downward, forming a cast over the entire tracheobronchial tree.

Cardiac toxicity occurs in 10% of patients, appears between the 7th and 14th day of illness, and is characterized by heart failure, atrioventricular nodal block, and arrhythmias. Isolated peripheral neuropathies involving the palate, pharynx, larynx, extraocular muscles, or diaphragm appear in 2–6 weeks. Paralysis of the extremities and elevated CSF protein resembling Guillain-Barré syndrome may occur. Hepatitis, nephritis, and gastritis also may occur.

Diagnosis and Differential Diagnosis. Determining the diagnosis requires isolating *C. diphtheriae* from the membrane or the exudate beneath the membrane. The bacillus is readily recovered on selective media (tellurite) using inhibitors that retard the growth of other microorganisms. Microscopic examination of diphtheritic lesions is unreliable. *C. diphtheriae* should be tested for toxigenicity.

Tonsillar and pharyngeal diphtheria must be differentiated from streptococcal pharyngitis, EBV infection, viral tonsillitis, primary herpetic tonsillitis, thrush, blood dyscrasias (such as agranulocytosis and leukemia), toxoplasmosis, cytomegalovirus, *Francisella tularensis,* and Vincent angina. Laryngeal diphtheria must be differentiated from viral croup, the presence of foreign bodies, retropharyngeal abscesses, and laryngeal tumors (e.g., papillomas, hemangiomas, lymphangiomas).

Treatment. Treatment of diphtheria requires neutralizing the circulating toxin and eradicating *C. diphtheriae* with antibiotics. Equine antitoxin must be given as soon as possible because once toxin is bound to tissue, antitoxin has no effect. Antibiotics help stop the production of additional toxin. Penicillin and erythromycin are effective against most strains of *C. diphtheriae* but do not alter the evolution of the disease. The diphtheria carrier state can be treated with penicillin G benzathine, penicillin G, or oral erythromycin. The endpoint of antibiotic therapy and infectivity is indicated by three consecutive negative cultures. Supportive care may include endotracheal intubation for respiratory insufficiency resulting from airway obstruction or paralysis.

Prevention. Prevention requires isolation of the patient and treatment of close contacts who are likely to become ill (if nonimmune) or become carriers. Previously immunized carriers should be given a booster injection of diphtheria toxoid and should be treated with penicillin or erythromycin. Nonimmunized asymptomatic carriers should have samples taken for culture, should receive diphtheria toxoid and penicillin or erythromycin, and should be examined carefully for 7 days. Because diphtheria does not always produce persistent immunity, patients should receive toxoid after the illness.

Prognosis. Before the use of antitoxin and antibiotics, the mortality rate from diphtheria was 30–50%. Death was most common in younger children (younger than 4 years old) and often resulted from airway obstruction by the diphtheritic pseudomembrane. Today the mortality rate is less than 5%, and death is the result of severe myocarditis. Nasopharyngeal persistence of *C. diphtheriae* may be noted in 5–10% of convalescing patients.

REFERENCES

Behrman RE, Kliegman RM, Jenson HB, editors: *Nelson textbook of pediatrics,* ed 16, Philadelphia, 2000, WB Saunders, Chapter 187.

Centers for Disease Control and Prevention: Diphtheria epidemic: new independent states of the former Soviet Union, 1990–1994, *MMWR* 44:177, 1995.

Rappuoli R, Perugini M, Falsen E: Molecular epidemiology of the 1984–1986 outbreak of diphtheria in Sweden, *N Engl J Med* 318:12–14, 1988.

Infection Caused by *Haemophilus Influenzae*

General Considerations

Etiology. *H. influenzae* are nonmotile, small, fastidious, pleomorphic gram-negative coccobacilli. Encapsulated strains are classified according to their soluble capsular polysaccharides (polyribosyl ribitol phosphate [PRP]) and are designated as types a through f. Type b produces serious invasive infections (e.g., meningitis, septic arthritis, epiglottitis, pericarditis, facial cellulitis, and pneumonia) in children. Infants lacking anti-PRP immunoglobulin G (IgG) have deficient opsonization of these encapsulated organisms. Nontypable unencapsulated strains are associated with sinusitis, conjunctivitis, otitis media, and bronchitis. Some strains produce beta-lactamase and thus are resistant to ampicillin.

Epidemiology. *H. influenzae* is a part of the normal commensal flora of the upper respiratory tract; most children have unencapsulated strains in their pharynx, and 2–5% carry type b organisms. The mode of transmission is by breathing respiratory droplets or by directly contacting secretions. Children with asplenia (from congenital and surgical causes and sickle cell anemia), those with antibody deficiencies (e.g., IgG2), and patients receiving chemotherapy for malignancies are at an increased risk for infection.

Invasive disease caused by *H. influenzae* type b is more common in children younger than 4 years of age and in specific ethnic groups, including the Inuit in Alaska and Native Americans (Navajo and

Apaches). Before effective vaccines were available, *H. influenzae* type b caused approximately 10,000 cases of meningitis per year in the United States. The peak incidence of meningitis caused by this organism was in infants younger than 12 months of age. Children in day care settings were also at risk for outbreaks of disease caused by *H. influenzae* type b.

Infections Caused by Haemophilus Influenzae Type B

Clinical Manifestations

Meningitis. *H. influenzae* type b was a common cause of bacterial meningitis in children between ages 1 months and 4 years before the widespread use of Hib vaccine. Meningitis caused by *H. influenzae* cannot be distinguished from that caused by *N. meningitidis* or *S. pneumoniae* on the basis of clinical presentation. The illness may be complicated at the time of presentation or later by other sites of infection with *H. influenzae,* including pneumonia, arthritis, osteomyelitis, pericarditis, cellulitis, and endophthalmitis.

Acute Epiglottitis. Acute epiglottitis is potentially a lethal condition that may result in airway obstruction from an acutely inflamed epiglottis. It usually occurs in children between 2 and 7 years old (see Chapter 12).

Pneumonia. The incidence of *H. influenzae* pneumonia in children is unknown, but it is most common in children under 6 years of age. The signs and symptoms of pneumonia caused by *H. influenzae* cannot be distinguished from those caused by other microorganisms. Pleural effusions and lobar and patchy infiltrates may be noted. Associated infections include otitis media, meningitis, and epiglottitis.

Septic Arthritis. *H. influenzae* type b was the most common agent producing septic arthritis in children younger than 3 years of age. Large joints, such as knees, hips, ankles, and elbows, commonly are affected, often in association with infections such as meningitis. Arthritis that appears late in the course of *H. influenzae* meningitis infection may be an antigen-antibody reaction and not a true joint space infection. Septic arthritis caused by *H. influenzae* type b is indistinguishable from that caused by other bacterial pathogens.

Cellulitis. More than 85% of children with *H. influenzae* type b cellulitis were 3 years of age or younger. Frequently, an upper respiratory tract infection precedes the acute onset of cellulitis. High fever, marked toxicity, bacteremia, and leukocytosis without a prior history of local trauma are present. The face and neck, particularly the cheek (buccal) and the periorbital area, are the most common sites. The lesion has indistinct margins, is tender and indurated, and may have a violaceous or bluish purple color. Meningitis with facial cellulitis may occur.

Pericarditis. *H. influenzae* type b caused up to 15% of bacterial pericarditis cases in children. Children are usually 2–4 years of age and often have had an antecedent upper respiratory tract infection or adjacent pneumonia.

Bacteremia Without an Associated Focus. Bacteremia caused by *H. influenzae* type b may occur without any apparent focus of infection other than signs of an upper respiratory tract infection or pharyngitis. Although affected children may appear only mildly ill at the initial visit, they are at substantial risk for development of pneumonia or meningitis, a finding that is in marked contrast to occult pneumococcal bacteremia, which has a much lower risk of metastatic foci or infection following bacteremia without a source.

Neonatal Disease. In the neonate, nontypable *H. influenzae* is more common than type b. Septicemia, pneumonia, meningitis, and respiratory distress syndrome produced by nontypable *H. influenzae* are indistinguishable from those caused by other neonatal bacterial pathogens. Nontypable *H. influenzae* is acquired by the infant from the mother's genitourinary tract.

Diagnosis. Specimens of CSF, blood, synovial fluid, cellulitis aspirate, or other material should be obtained for culture on a selective medium, such as chocolate agar. Antibiotic susceptibility tests should be performed on all isolates to determine resistance to ampicillin and cephalosporins.

Treatment. (Also discussed in this chapter under Central Nervous System Infections.) Invasive infections presumed to be caused by *H. influenzae* initially should be treated with intravenous ceftriaxone or cefotaxime. Since much of the pathology associated with *H. influenzae* type b meningitis is the result of the host inflammatory response, administration of dexamethasone *prior* to the first dose of antibiotic is recommended and appears to be associated with a decrease in neurologic sequelae, *if* given prior to the antibiotic (see Appendix I).

Prevention. Conjugate vaccines with PRP covalently linked to diphtheria toxoid or OMP (outer membrane protein of *N. meningitidis*) should be administered to infants at 2, 4, 6, and 15 months and to unimmunized children 24–60 months old (Fig. 10–1). Because the risk for secondary infection caused by *H. influenzae* type b in close contacts is high, rifampin is recommended for all family contacts (adults, index case, plus young children) of individuals with *H. influenzae* disease when there are other susceptible (not fully immunized) children in the household who are younger than 4 years of age. Close contacts in day care centers also may be candidates for rifampin therapy.

REFERENCES

Behrman RE, Kliegman RM, Jenson HB, editors: *Nelson textbook of pediatrics,* ed 16, Philadelphia, 2000, WB Saunders, Chapter 193.

Dawson KG, Emerson JC, Burns JL: Fifteen years of experience with bacterial meningitis, *Infect Dis J* 18:816–822, 1999.

Korones DN, Marshall GS, Shapiro ED: Outcome of children with occult bacteremia caused by *Haemophilus influenzae* type b, *Pediatr Infect Dis J* 11:516–520, 1992.

Rosenstein NE, Perkins BA: Update on *Haemophilus influenzae* serotype b and meningococcal vaccines, *Pediatr Clin North Am* 47:337–352, 2000.

Mycobacterial Infections

Tuberculosis

Etiology. Tuberculosis is caused by *Mycobacterium tuberculosis,* an aerobic, slow-growing organism with a complex cell wall structure containing mycolic acid, a 70–80 carbon fatty acid, and arabinogalactan, linked to muramic acid. The high lipid content gives the organism its "acid-fast" staining properties (resistance to decolorization with acid–alcohol), as used in the Ziehl-Neelsen or Kinyoun staining methods used to identify these organisms. *M. tuberculosis* can be differentiated from other mycobacteria by its lack of pigmentation, by its slow growth rate, with a doubling time of 24–36 hours, and by the use of specific DNA probes.

Epidemiology. Worldwide, TB is a major cause of morbidity and is estimated by the World Health Organization to cause approximately 3 million deaths per year, primarily in developing countries and in populations in which HIV infection is common. TB has decreased in people born in the United States but has increased among the foreign born. Reservoirs of tuberculosis are the elderly, immigrants (Asian, African, and Latin American), the homeless, and patients with AIDS. Tuberculosis is more common in crowded semiindustrialized societies and among the poor. Infection in children occurs after inhalation of contaminated respiratory droplets (from coughing or sneezing) from heavily infected respiratory tract secretions. Infection in children typically is the result of prolonged close contact with an individual having untreated, active, cavitary, sputum-positive disease. The incubation period from infection to development of a positive tuberculin skin test is 2–6 weeks.

Pathogenesis. Tubercle bacilli, which are resistant to drying, are inhaled in small droplet nuclei and deposited in the distal airways. The organisms are ingested by alveolar macrophages, where they replicated intracellularly, resisting the lytic effects of phagolysosomal fusion. These infected macrophages migrate to the hilar lymph nodes; bacterial antigens are presented to T cells, primarily CD4+ cells, and activate them to cause "delayed-type hypersensitivity."

The pathology is caused by the host immune response to the organisms. From these lymph nodes the bacilli can disseminate through the lymphatics or hematogenously throughout the body. The induced immune response, chiefly activated macrophages, may contain replication of the organism, as evidence by the formation of granulomas consisting of epithelioid cells, Langerhans giant cells, and lymphocytes. The presence of a delayed hypersensitivity response to *M. tuberculosis* is evaluated by skin testing, using a purified protein antigen extract of heat-killed mycobacteria. These foci of infection may calcify, forming a Ghon complex (lung and node calcification), which may be inactive for years. However, under the appropriate conditions, and most often within the first 2 years following infection, the organisms evade macrophage killing, begin to replicate locally, and cause reactivation disease, typically in the apical parts of the lung or elsewhere in the body. Factors that increase the likelihood of reactivation are underlying conditions that diminish CD4+ T-cell (helper) function, such as HIV infection; age (less than 3 years); immunosuppressive therapy, particularly with corticosteroids and antibody to tumor necrosis factor; malnutrition; genetic factors; puberty; and pregnancy.

Primary pulmonary tuberculosis in older infants and children is usually an asymptomatic infection. The diagnosis is confirmed only by a positive skin test, often with minimal abnormalities (infiltrate with hilar adenopathy) on the chest roentgenogram. Malaise, low-grade fever, erythema nodosum, or symptoms resulting from lymph node enlargement may occur after the development of delayed hypersensitivity.

In **progressive primary disease,** as may be seen in infants and young children, a primary pneumonia may develop shortly after the initial infection. Progression of the primary complex to pulmonary disease, or disseminated miliary disease, or progression of CNS granulomas to meningitis occurs most commonly in the first year of life. Hilar adenopathy may compress the bronchi or trachea, producing airway obstruction and wheezing; compression of the recurrent laryngeal nerve may result in hoarseness. When the phrenic nerve is impinged, diaphragmatic paralysis may result; more extensive inflammatory responses can result in a superior vena cava syndrome.

Tuberculous pleural effusion, which may accompany primary infection, generally represents the immune response to the organisms. Pleurocentesis reveals lymphocytes and an increased protein level, but usually does not contain bacilli. A pleural biopsy may be necessary to find tissue with the expected granuloma formation and acid-fast organisms.

Reactivation pulmonary tuberculosis, common in

adolescents, usually is confined to apical segments of upper lobes or superior segments of lower lobes. There is usually little lymphadenopathy and no extrathoracic infection as a result of established hypersensitivity. This is a manifestation of a secondary expansion of infection at a site seeded years previously during primary infection. Cavitation and endobronchial spread of bacilli occur and are associated with fever, night sweats, malaise, and weight loss. A productive cough and hemoptysis often herald cavitation and bronchial erosion.

Tuberculosis in HIV-infected patients has a more variable presentation. In adolescents who would be expected to develop reactivation disease with cavity formation, more diffuse infiltrates may be present. In younger infants hilar adenopathy and nonspecific pulmonary infiltrates may indicate tuberculosis; upper lobe cavitary disease may also be seen.

Tuberculous pericarditis usually occurs when organisms from the lung or pleura spread to the contiguous surfaces of the pericardium. Activation of an immune response results in the accumulation of fluid with lymphocytic infiltration. Persistent inflammations may result in a more cellular response, with rupture of granulomas into the pericardial space and the development of constrictive pericarditis. In addition to antimycobacterial therapy, TB pericarditis is managed with corticosteroids to decrease inflammation.

Lymphadenopathy is common in primary pulmonary disease. The most common extrathoracic sites of adenitis are the cervical, supraclavicular, and submandibular areas (e.g., scrofula). The illness usually is insidious, unilateral more often than bilateral, and associated with a history of exposure to an infected family member. The nodes are nontender and firm. Chest radiographic examination may also reveal pulmonary tuberculosis. Suppuration of the nodes may lead to fluctuance and draining sinus tracts. Enlargement may cause compression of adjacent structures. Differential diagnosis includes infections caused by atypical mycobacteria, cat-scratch disease, fungal infection, viral or bacterial disease, toxoplasmosis, sarcoidosis, drug reactions, and malignancy. Diagnosis may be confirmed by fine-needle aspiration but may necessitate excisional biopsy accompanied by appropriate histologic and microbiologic studies.

Miliary tuberculosis refers to widespread hematogenous dissemination with infection of multiple organs. The lesions are of roughly the same size as that of a millet seed, from which the name miliary is derived. Miliary tuberculosis is characterized by fever, weakness, malaise, anorexia, weight loss, lymphadenopathy, night sweats, and hepatosplenomegaly. Diffuse bilateral pneumonitis is present, and meningitis may be noted. Anemia, monocytosis, thrombocytopenia, hyponatremia, hypokalemia, and abnormal liver function tests are common. The chest radiographic examination reveals bilateral miliary infiltrates, demonstrating overwhelming infection. The tuberculin skin test may be nonreactive as a result of anergy. Liver or bone marrow biopsy may be needed for the diagnosis.

Tuberculous meningitis most commonly occurs in children younger than 5 years of age and often within 6 months of the primary infection. Most patients have a family member with active tuberculosis. Tubercle bacilli that seeded the meninges during the primary infection replicate, triggering an inflammatory response. This may have an insidious onset, initially characterized by low-grade fever, headache, and subtle personality change. Progression of the infection results in a basilar meningitis with impingement of the cranial nerves and is manifested by meningeal irritation, positive Kernig and Brudzinski signs, cranial nerve palsies, seizures, and eventually increased intracranial pressure, deterioration of mental status, and coma.

The majority of patients have abnormal findings on chest x-ray films: hilar adenopathy, parenchymal disease, and miliary disease are common. CT scans demonstrate hydrocephalus, edema, periventricular lucencies, and infarctions. CSF analysis reveals increased cell number (50–500 leukocytes/μL), which may be either lymphocytes or polymorphonuclear leukocytes early in the course of disease. Glucose is low and protein significantly elevated. Most patients do not have acid-fast bacilli detected in the CSF by either routine or fluorescent staining procedures. Although culture is the gold standard for diagnosis, PCR for *M. tuberculosis* is widely available and may be useful to make this diagnosis. Many patients with CNS tuberculosis have negative tuberculin tests, often because of anergy. Prompt diagnosis and treatment are essential to decrease morbidity. Treatment regimens for TB meningitis generally include four antituberculosis drugs and corticosteroids.

In some children an expanding mass presenting as a CNS infection with focal neurologic signs and low-grade fever may be caused by a **tuberculoma of the CNS.** The CT scan may reveal a hypodense area surrounded by edema. As in tuberculous meningitis, children often come from endemic areas or have a history of contact with an infected adult, a positive skin test, and concurrent pulmonary disease.

In **skeletal tuberculosis,** mycobacterial infection of the bone results from either hematogenous seeding or direct extension from a caseous lymph node. This is usually a chronic disease with an insidious onset that may be mistaken for chronic osteomyelitis caused by *S. aureus.* Radiographs reveal cortical destruction; biopsy and culture are essential for proper diagnosis. Patients, particularly those from endemic areas, who fail to respond appropriately to anti-staphylococcal antimicrobial agents should be carefully evaluated for the possibility of tuberculosis. The spine **(Pott disease)** is the most common site, followed by the hip and the fingers and toes **(dactylitis).**

Abdominal tuberculosis occurs secondary to swallowing infected material, including contaminated milk or sputum. This is a relatively uncommon complication in developed nations, where dairy herds are inspected for bovine tuberculosis. Manifestations include dysphagia, pain, or signs of obstruction, perforation, hemorrhage, fistula formation, or colitis. Tuberculous peritonitis presents as fever, anorexia, and abdominal pain. The diagnosis depends on skin test results and on histology and culture of involved tissue and peritoneal fluid.

Urogenital tuberculosis is a late reactivation complication and is rare in children. Symptomatic illness presents as dysuria, frequency, urgency, hematuria, and "sterile" pyuria.

Diagnosis. The *skin test* response to tuberculin antigen is a manifestation of a T cell–mediated delayed hypersensitivity. It is usually positive 2–6 weeks after onset of infection (occasionally 3 months) and at the time of symptomatic illness. The *Mantoux test,* an intradermal injection, usually on the volar surface of the forearm, of 5 TU (tuberculin units) (intermediate test strength) of Tween-stabilized purified tuberculous antigen (purified protein derivative, standard [PPD-S]) is the standard for screening high-risk populations and for diagnosis in all ill patients or contacts. The likelihood that a positive skin test represents a true infection is dependent on the prevalence of *M. tuberculosis* in the population. In the United States the prevalence of tuberculosis is low. Thus the criteria (Table 10–14) for a positive skin test reflect the increased likelihood that small reactions to PPD may represent cross reactivity to atypical mycobacteria and are less likely to indicate true infection. This is not necessarily true in other populations. False-negative responses may occur early in the illness, with use of inactivated antigen (as a result of poor storage practice or inadequate administration), or as a result of immunosuppression (secondary to underlying illness, AIDS, malnutrition, or overwhelming tuberculosis). Tests with questionable results should be repeated after several weeks of therapy and adequate nutrition. An antigen panel should be included with the PPD-S to determine a more global state of anergy.

The ultimate diagnostic confirmation relies on *culture* of the organism, a process that usually is more successful when tissue is utilized (e.g., pleural biopsy, pericardial membrane), rather than only the pleural or pericardial fluid. In young infants, gastric

---

TABLE 10–14
Definitions of Positive Tuberculin Skin Test Results in Infants, Children, and Adolescents*

Induration ≥5 mm
Children in Close Contact With Known or Suspected Contagious Cases of Tuberculosis Disease:
Households with active or previously active cases if treatment cannot be verified as adequate before exposure, treatment was initiated after the child's contact, or reactivation of latent tuberculosis infection is suspected
Children Suspected To Have Tuberculosis Disease:
Chest radiograph consistent with active or previously active tuberculosis
Clinical evidence of tuberculosis disease†
Children Receiving Immunosuppressive Therapy or With Immunosuppressive Conditions, Including HIV Infection‡

Induration ≥10 mm
Children at Increased Risk of Disseminated Disease:
Young age; younger than 4 years of age
Other medical conditions, including Hodgkin disease, lymphoma, diabetes mellitus, chronic renal failure, or malnutrition
Children With Increased Exposure to Tuberculosis Disease:
Born or whose parents were born in high-prevalence regions of the world
Frequently exposed to adults who are HIV infected, homeless, users of illicit drugs, residents of nursing homes, incarcerated or institutionalized persons, and migrant farm workers
Travel and exposure to high-prevalence regions of the world

Induration ≥15 mm
Children 4 years of age or older without any risk factors

From American Academy of Pediatrics: *Red book 2000,* ed 25, Elk Grove, Ill, 2000, The Academy.
The test should be read at 48–72 hours after placement.
HIV, Human immunodeficiency virus.
*These definitions apply, regardless of previous bacille Calmette-Guérin (BCG) immunization; erythema at tuberculin skin test site does not indicate a positive test result.
†Evidence by physical examination or laboratory assessment that would include tuberculosis in the working differential diagnosis (e.g., meningitis).
‡Including immunosuppressive doses of corticosteroids.

material (often mixed with swallowed sputum) may yield positive results when sputum is unobtainable. Large volumes of fluid (CSF, pericardial fluid) yield a higher rate of recovery of organisms, but slow growth of the mycobacteria makes culture less helpful in very ill children. Once the organism is grown, the drug susceptibilities should be determined because of the increasing incidence of resistant organisms. Antigen detection and DNA probes have expedited diagnosis, especially in CNS disease.

Treatment. Effective treatment of cavitary disease must take into account the large numbers of bacilli found in cavitary lesions and the potential for selecting out mutant antibiotic resistant clones from this population. The slow growth rate of *M. tuberculosis* necessitates prolonged antimicrobial therapy to effectively inhibit the metabolism of the organisms. In contrast, therapy for latent infection (i.e., tuberculin skin test reactivity in the absence of signs of active disease) is aimed at eradicating the presumably small inoculum of organisms sequestered within macrophages and suppressed by normal T-cell activity. To prevent reactivation of these latent bacilli, therapy with a single agent (usually isoniazid for 9 months) is suggested, or with a rifamycin derivative plus pyrazinamide for 2 months. Rifampin administered as a single agent for 4 months could also be used. These alternative regimens would be preferred if the patient is known to have been in close contact with a person harboring INH-resistant bacilli (approximately 8% of U.S. isolates). For active infection, four drugs are initiated and continued until susceptibility testing is performed and clinical and bacteriologic improvement is established (Table 10–15).

The "first-line" agents for tuberculosis are isoniazid, rifampin (rifabutin), pyrazinamide, ethambutol, and streptomycin. Combinations of these drugs are selected to initiate therapy in patients with active disease until susceptibility testing is performed to guide therapy. Although *M. tuberculosis* isolates in the United States are generally susceptible, this is not necessarily the case worldwide. Attention must be paid to drug-drug interactions. This is especially important in patients who are also taking or should be taking antiretroviral agents that are metabolized by the CP3/P450 cytochrome enzymes. The use of rifampin, a potent inducer of the p450 cytochrome system, is generally avoided in this patient group, and rifabutin, a less potent inducer, is preferred.

Although hospitalization is not required to either evaluate or treat patients with latent infection, it is important to involve public health personnel to try to establish the source of the infection. Targeted screening is preferred to identify individuals at high risk of contracting tuberculosis from an index case, as opposed to screening populations that generally are at low risk for the disease.

Infants and young children with active tuberculosis are usually hospitalized to facilitate workup and establish effective therapy. It is also important to provide the appropriate social support network for family members to receive appropriate evaluation and therapy if necessary. For children or adolescents with cavitary disease, hospitalization and respiratory isolation are generally recommended for the first 2 weeks of therapy with four drugs, at which time the sputum are generally sterile, even if acid-fast organisms (hopefully nonviable) may still be detected with highly sensitive methods. Since the incidence of tuberculosis is quite high in HIV-infected individuals, these patients should be screened for HIV disease.

Corticosteroids are useful in the initial therapy of tuberculous meningitis to lower increased intracranial pressure, and in endobronchial tuberculosis and tuberculous pleuritis or pericarditis to speed the resolution of fluid and obstruction. Steroids should never be used in a patient with tuberculosis without concomitant antituberculosis therapy.

Pregnancy During Tuberculosis. Pregnant women should be screened for tuberculosis; the relative immunosuppression that accompanies pregnancy does not cause false-negative tuberculin skin tests in the absence of other factors. Although pregnant women are often asymptomatic during pregnancy, the disease may be activated postpartum, putting both the mother and infant at risk. Pregnant women with positive skin tests for TB should be evaluated with chest radiographs as soon as the abdomen can be appropriately shielded. If there is no evidence of active disease, treatment for latent tuberculosis should be deferred until 3 months postpartum to avoid the increased hepatotoxicity of INH seen during pregnancy. Pregnant women with active TB should receive multidrug treatment, usually INH, rifampin, ethambutol, and pyridoxine.

Infants Born to Mothers with Tuberculosis. Because of decreased T-cell function, the tuberculin skin test is relatively unreliable in young infants, and even in congenital disease may not be positive for 6 months. Infants born to mothers with newly diagnosed latent infection (positive skin tests but no pulmonary disease) can be followed with skin testing at 4–6 weeks of age and again at 3–4 months. Infants exposed to family members with active disease should be evaluated with skin testing, chest radiographs, and if negative, treated as if for latent infection with INH. If repeat skin testing remains negative, the INH can be discontinued at 3–4 months. Infants exposed to patients with known INH-resistant organisms

TABLE 10–15
Recommended Treatment Regimens for Drug-Susceptible Tuberculosis in Infants, Children, and Adolescents*

Infection of Disease Category	Regimen	Remarks
Latent Tuberculosis Infection (positive TST, no disease)		
Isoniazid susceptible	9 mo of isoniazid once a day	If daily therapy is not possible, therapy twice a week DOT may be used for 9 mo; HIV-infected children should be treated for 9–12 mo
Isoniazid resistant	6 mo of rifampin once a day	
Isoniazid-rifampin resistant*	Consult a tuberculosis specialist	
Pulmonary	**6-Month Regimens**	
	2 mo of isoniazid, rifampin, and pyrazinamide once a day, followed by 4 mo of isoniazid and rifampin daily	If possible drug resistance is a concern, another drug (ethambutol or streptomycin) is added to the initial three-drug therapy until drug susceptibilities are determined
	OR	
	2 mo of isoniazid, rifampin, and pyrazinamide daily, followed by 4 mo of isoniazid and rifampin twice a week	Drugs can be given 2 or 3 times per week under DOT in the initial phase if nonadherence is likely
	9-Month Regimens	
	9-mo alternative regimens (for hilar adenopathy only): 9 mo of isoniazid and rifampin once a day	Regimens consisting of 6 mo of isoniazid and rifampin once a day, and 1 mo of isoniazid and rifampin once a day, followed by 5 mo of isoniazid and rifampin DOT twice a week have been successful in areas where drug resistance is rare
	OR	
	1 mo of isoniazid and rifampin once a day, followed by 8 mo of isoniazid and rifampin twice a week	
Extrapulmonary: meningitis, disseminated (miliary), bone or joint disease	2 mo of isoniazid, rifampin, pyrazinamide, and streptomycin once a day, followed by 7–10 mo of isoniazid and rifampin once a day	Streptomycin is given with initial therapy until drug susceptibility is known
	OR	
	2 mo of isoniazid, rifampin, pyazinamide, and streptomycin once a day, followed by 7–10 mo of isoniazid and rifampin twice a week (9–12 mo total)	For patients who may have acquired tuberculosis in geographic areas where resistance to streptomycin is common, capreomycin (15–30 mg/kg/day) or kanamycin (15–30 mg/kg/day) may be used instead of streptomycin
Other (e.g., cervical lymphadenopathy)	Same as for pulmonary disease	See **Pulmonary**

From American Academy of Pediatrics: *Red book 2000*, ed 25, Elk Grove, Ill, 2000, The Academy.
DOT, Directly observed therapy; *TST*, tuberculin skin test.
*Duration of therapy is longer for human immunodeficiency virus (HIV)-infected persons, and additional drugs may be indicated.

should be treated "prophylactically" with a regimen expected to have activity against the index patient's isolate, such as rifampin and pyrazinamide. The transmission rate from an adult with cavitary disease, or a high inoculum of organisms as occurs in HIV-infected individuals, to an infant in the household approaches 50%. If congenital TB (hepatic, pulmonary, miliary pattern) is suspected, prompt four-drug therapy must be initiated. If the mother has active untreated TB, the infant must be separated from her until the mother is no longer contagious.

REFERENCES

American Thoracic Society, Centers for Disease Control and Prevention: Targeted tuberculin testing and treatment of latent tuberculosis infection, *Am J Resp Crit Care* Med 161:S221, 2000.

Behrman RE, Kliegman RM, Jenson HB, editors: *Nelson textbook of pediatrics*, ed 16, Philadelphia, 2000, WB Saunders, Chapter 212.

Centers for Disease Control and Prevention: Initial therapy for tuberculosis in the era of multidrug resistance, *MMWR* 42:(RR1)1, 1993.

Cohn DL: Treatment of latent tuberculosis infection: renewed opportunity for tuberculosis control, *Clin Infect Dis* 31:120–124, 2000.

Hussey G, Chisholm T, Kibel M: Miliary tuberculosis in children: a review of 94 cases, *Pediatr Infect Dis J* 10:832–836, 1991.

Starke JR, Jacobs RF, Jereb J: Resurgence of tuberculosis in children, *J Pediatr* 120:839–855, 1992.

Waecker NJ Jr, Connor JD: Central nervous system tuberculosis in children: a review of 30 cases, *Pediatr Infect Dis J* 9:539–543, 1990.

Yaramis A, Gurkan F, Elevli M, et al: Central nervous system tuberculosis in children: a review of 214 cases, *Pediatrics* 102:E49, 1998.

Atypical Mycobacterial Infection

Etiology. The atypical mycobacteria are common in the environment but are uncommonly associated with disease in normal hosts. These "nontuberculous" mycobacteria are acid-fast bacilli that have structural and morphologic characteristics similar to *M. tuberculosis* but differ in a number of other distinguishing features, such as growth pattern and pigment production. They are classified in Runyon groups as follows:

- *Group I*—Photochromogens, which form pigment when exposed to light (*M. kansasii, M. marinum*)
- *Group II*—Scotochromogens, which form pigment in the dark (*M. scrofulaceum*)
- *Group III*—Nonchromogens—*M. avium-intracellulare* complex (MAC)
- *Group IV*—rapid growers (*M. fortuitum-chelonei*)

Epidemiology. Mycobacterial agents are distributed worldwide and exist in soil, vegetation, dust, and water. Infection occurs by inoculation of the skin or by inhalation. Atypical mycobacterial infections in immunocompetent patients are more common in warm, humid, rural environments, such as the southern states. No evidence exists for person-to-person spread. Nosocomial infection with *M. chelonei* and *M. fortuitum* have occurred, and opportunistic infection with *M. avium-intracellulare* organisms affects patients with advanced AIDS.

Clinical Manifestations. The most frequent manifestation of infection in children is lymphadenitis. This is usually a unilateral cervical, submandibular, or preauricular (less commonly axillary and inguinal) swelling in a 1–5-year-old child with a normal chest x-ray and no history of exposure to tuberculosis. The node may suppurate and drain but usually is hard and painless. In the United States, lymphadenitis is associated with several atypical mycobacterial species, depending on the epidemiology of the infection. *M. tuberculosis* is a less common cause of isolated lymphadenopathy. In the southeastern United States, *M. avium-intracellulare* is often a causative organism, as is *M. scrofulaceum* and less commonly *M. kansasii*.

HIV-infected children and adolescents usually receive prophylaxis against disseminated MAC disease with clarithromycin or azithromycin if they have low CD4+ T-lymphocyte counts, depending on their age (<50 cells/µL for children >6 years, with higher thresholds for younger children). Few HIV-infected children who are receiving highly active antiretroviral therapy have disseminated atypical mycobacterial infection. Differential diagnosis should rule out infection caused by *M. tuberculosis*, fungi, or bacteria, as well as cat-scratch disease, toxoplasmosis, sarcoidosis, lymphoma, and drug reaction. Diagnosis and therapy both are made by excisional biopsy. These organisms are usually highly drug resistant, and therapy must be guided by antimicrobial susceptibility tests.

Cutaneous disease is usually the result of inoculation with *M. marinum* (swimming pool granuloma or fish tank granuloma) or with *M. fortuitum-chelonei*. The initial papule or nodule may enlarge and ulcerate. Infection in healthy children often is self-limited. *M. marinum* is treated for 3–4 months with doxycycline, rifampin, and ethambutol, or trimethoprim/sulfamethoxazole. *M. fortuitum-chelonei* infection usually develops secondary to abrasions, puncture wounds, or foreign body placement during surgery and requires débridement, drainage, and often antibiotic therapy (with amikacin, cefoxitin, or clarithromycin for *M. chelonei*).

Pulmonary infection with these bacterial agents is uncommon in children and resembles tuberculosis. It may occur rarely with *M. kansasii* in adolescent patients.

Disseminated disease with bacteremia, pneumonia, diarrhea, and fever usually occurs in immunocompromised individuals and often is caused by the *M. avium-intracellulare* complex, especially in patients with AIDS. Disseminated MAC infection in these patients often presents with unremitting fevers in the absence of specific symptoms along with weight loss, night sweats, and evidence of bone marrow suppression; most commonly, it occurs in patients with long-standing HIV infection and severe depletion of CD4 T cells and high viral loads. Multiple blood cultures should be examined to isolate the organisms. Therapy usually consists of a multidrug regimen. Prophylaxis for MAC in AIDS patients with low CD4 cell counts is often recommended.

Diagnosis. The diagnosis of atypical mycobacterial infection requires the culture or PCR of either secretions or biopsy material. Skin test reactivity to purified protein derivative (PPD) is variable and may be officially negative (5–10 mm induration) in the presence of atypical mycobacterial infection.

REFERENCES

1999 USPHS/IDDSA guidelines for the prevention of opportunistic infections in persons infected with human immunodeficiency virus, *MMWR* 48(RR-10), 1999.

Behrman RE, Kliegman RM, Jenson HB, editors: *Nelson textbook of pediatrics,* ed 16, Philadelphia, 2000, WB Saunders, Chapter 214.

Wolinsky E: Mycobacterial diseases other than tuberculosis, *Clin Infect Dis* 15:1–10, 1992.

Infections Caused by Neisseriae

Neisseriae are gram-negative, spherical or oval diplococci. The bacteria are observed within polymorphonuclear leukocytes obtained from diseased areas of the body. Neisseriae are aerobic and can be cultured on blood agar, but recovery is enhanced by use of appropriate media. Neisseriae normally are found in the nasal mucosa, pharynx, vagina, and lower intestinal tract. Human disease most commonly is caused by infection with *N. meningitidis* and *N. gonorrhoeae* (see Chapter 7).

Neisseria Meningitidis

N. meningitidis is exclusively a human pathogen often associated with fulminant sepsis with or without meningitis. Organisms colonize the nasopharynx and elude the mucosal barrier through the expression of IgA proteases. They are ingested by receptor-mediated endocytosis and transported across the epithelium. In the absence of preformed IgG, bacteremia and sepsis can then ensue. These organisms express a number of virulence factors, including siderophores to scavenge iron, pili that facilitate mucosal attachment, and capsular polysaccharides that require either specific IgG or complement for opsonization. Most important, the lipopolysaccharide moieties of *N. meningitidis* are highly immunogenic, activating a florid immune response, activating macrophages and T cells, and causing cytokine expression and the recruitment of neutrophils. Once in the bloodstream, in the absence of preformed anticapsular antibody or complement, they cause bacteremia and sepsis. These organisms are frequently associated with the "sepsis syndrome" as described earlier with profound immunologic, cardiovascular, and hematologic sequelae.

Thirteen serogroups of *N. meningitidis* have been identified on the basis of specific capsular polysaccharides. Serogroup prevalence varies across the United States: in a 1992–1996 survey, serogroup C was associated with 35% of cases, serogroup B with 32% of cases, and serogroup Y with 26%. Children less than 2 years of age more frequently were infected with serogroup B, whereas older children and adolescents had infections caused by serogroup C, which was associated with several outbreaks in colleges and other institutions.

Epidemiology. The rates of asymptomatic carriers of *N. meningitidis* vary from 2–5% in healthy children to as high as 90% in military personnel during epidemics. Meningococcal meningitis is a disease of young children who acquire *N. meningitidis* from an adult carrier, usually in the same family. Person-to-person transmission is through infected respiratory droplets. Age-specific attack rates are greatest for infants under 1 year of age; 80% of cases of meningococcal disease occur in children under 10 years of age. A second peak appears during adolescence. The estimated likelihood of meningococcal disease in close contacts, usually occurring within 1 week of the first case (incubation period is 3–4 days), is 1%. This is 1000-fold greater than the risk in the community. Persons with deficiency of terminal complement component (C5–9) and IgG2 subclass are at high risk for recurrent disease. Meningococcal disease often follows viral upper respiratory tract infections. Epidemic *N. meningitidis* is a common problem in sub-Saharan Africa, the "meningitis belt," as well as in other developing countries. These outbreaks may last several years and are usually caused by type A organisms; the annual incidence may be up to 400 cases per 100,000.

Clinical Manifestations. Meningococcal infections can lead to sepsis or meningitis. Acute meningococcemia initially manifests as a nonspecific illness accompanied by fever and malaise, but rapidly progresses within hours to days. In its most fulminant form septic shock occurs, a syndrome caused by the host response to the large amounts of circulating meningococcal LPS (endotoxin) that activates macrophages, T cells, and endothelial cells, causing an outpouring of proinflammatory cytokines, stimulation of prostaglandins and mediators of arachidonic acid metabolism, activation of the coagulation cascade, and the physiologic response to these mediators. Fever, hypotension, and coagulopathy are frequent, manifested initially as petechiae, then purpuric lesions, and finally by frank ecchymoses accompanied by the failure to perfuse distal extremities with subsequent necrosis and gangrene. This fulminant clinical syndrome has been associated with a 40% fatality rate. Septic shock is accompanied by many systemic abnormalities: oliguria, renal failure, hepatic failure, altered mental status, and ARDS. Disseminated organisms can cause local infections throughout the body, including enophthalmitis, peritonitis, arthritis, and pneumonia. Adrenal hemorrhage (Waterhouse-Friderichsen syndrome) and associated adrenal insufficiency are common. Less commonly, acute endocarditis, myocarditis, and pericarditis can occur.

Meningococcal meningitis occurs with or without the concomitant sepsis syndrome and represents meningeal seeding of organisms during high-grade meningococcemia. As compared with other causes of bacterial meningitis, meningococcal meningitis does not elicit as profound a suppurative response, and patients generally do better with reported mortality in the 1–2% range.

Some patients do not have a fulminant reponse to *N. meningitidis;* instead, a low-grade bacteremia and a syndrome of chronic meningococcemia develop. This is characterized by intermittent fever, malaise, a maculopapular rash, arthralgias, and arthritis, perhaps caused by immune complexes.

Diagnosis and Differential Diagnosis. The diagnosis of meningococcal disease is established by stains and culture of blood, CSF, skin lesions, or other usually sterile sites. When meningitis is present, the laboratory characteristics of CSF reflect an acute bacterial meningitis. A poor prognostic sign is a normal CSF profile with no leukocytes but with sheets of gram-negative diplococci. Alternatively, the Gram stain and culture may be negative if the patient was pretreated with antibiotics.

The petechial or purpuric rash of meningococcemia is similar to that of diseases characterized by generalized vasculitis, including septicemia caused by gram-negative and gram-positive organisms; bacterial endocarditis; gonococcemia; Henoch-Schönlein purpura; Rocky Mountain spotted fever; endemic typhus; atypical measles; and infection with echoviruses and coxsackieviruses. The morbilliform rash occasionally observed may be confused with any macular or maculopapular viral exanthem (Table 10–2).

Treatment. Intravenous penicillin is the drug of choice for patients with invasive disease. Ceftriaxone and cefotaxime are alternative antibiotics (see Appendix I). Penicillin-resistant strains have been re-

ported from all over the world, including Europe, Africa, and the United States (less frequently). These strains have mutations in PBP2 (penicillin-binding protein), a transpeptidase normally inhibited by penicillin. Cefotaxime is active against these organisms. Supportive measures include careful monitoring and treatment of shock, myocarditis, pericarditis, septic arthritis, ARDS, DIC, and necrotic cutaneous or extremity lesions. Recombinant protein therapy that increases bactericidal permeability may improve the outcome. Activated protein C (an anticoagulant) infusions may improve the outcome of severe sepsis complicated by purpura fulminans.

Prevention. Meningococcal vaccine against serogroups A, C, Y, and W135 is available but is not routinely recommended for children. Outbreaks in college-age adolescents have stimulated interest in vaccinating this population; data suggest that 60% of cases could be prevented. Vaccine should be administered to children over 2 years of age who have functional or anatomic asplenia and to those with terminal complement component or properdin deficiencies. A serogroup C meningococcal-conjugate vaccine for use in infants, who do not respond to polysaccharaide vaccines, has been developed and licensed in the United Kingdom. The incidence of invasive meningococcal disease in household contacts of primary cases is 500–1000 times that of the general population; 50% of secondary cases occur within the first week; therefore, this group should receive prophylaxis with rifampin 5 mg/kg (<1 month) or 10 mg/kg (600 mg maximum) q24h for 2 days, ceftriaxone 125 (<12 years) or 250 mg IM as a single dose, or ciprofloxacin (500 mg for adults as a single dose). The patient should be placed in respiratory isolation for 24 hours after admission and should receive rifampin before discharge.

Prognosis. The mortality rate of acute meningococcemia with septic shock may be as high as 20–50%. The mortality rate for patients with isolated meningococcal meningitis is less than 3%, if treated early. Poor prognostic signs include the development of hypotension, coma, rapidly progressive purpura (within 12 hours), DIC, absence of meningitis, absence of leukocytosis, thrombocytopenia, high antigen concentrations in serum and CSF, and a low sedimentation rate. Survival for 48 hours following initiation of therapy is a good prognostic sign. Sloughing of necrotic skin over purpuric areas usually heals uneventfully.

REFERENCES

Behrman RE, Kliegman RM, Jenson HB, editors: *Nelson textbook of pediatrics,* ed 16, Philadelphia, 2000, WB Saunders, Chapter 191.
Centers for Disease Control and Prevention: Prevention and control of meningococcal disease and college students: recommendations of the Advisory Committee on Immunization Practices, *MMWR* 49:13, 2000.

DeWals P, De Serres G, Niyonsenga T: Effectiveness of a mass immunization campaign against serogroup C meningococcal disease in Quebec, *JAMA* 285:177–181, 2001.

Levin M, Quint PA, Goldstein B, et al: Recombinant bactericidal/permeability-increasing protein (rBPI$_{21}$) as adjunctive treatment for children with severe meningococcal sepsis: a randomized trial, *Lancet* 356:961–967, 2000.

Richmond P, Borrow R, Goldblatt D, et al: Ability of 3 different meningococcal C conjugate vaccines to induce immunologic memory after a single dose in UK toddlers, *J Infect Dis* 183:160–163, 2001.

Pertussis

(Whooping Cough)

Etiology. Pertussis, which means "intense cough," is predominantly caused by *Bordetella pertussis*. *B. pertussis* organisms are gram-negative, pleomorphic bacilli with fastidious requirements for growth provided by Bordet-Gengou media.

Epidemiology. Pertussis is highly contagious, producing attack rates of more than 90% in susceptible populations. Humans are the only known host of *B. pertussis*; transmission is by droplets released during intense coughing. The incubation period has a mean of 6 days and a range of 6–14 days. Patients are most contagious during the preparoxysmal stage. Risk of disease is highest in children under 5 years of age; 30% of cases in the United States occur in infants under 6 months of age. Mortality is greatest in infants under 1 year of age.

Immunization reduces the incidence and mortality rate of pertussis, but immunity is neither complete nor permanent. Outbreaks of pertussis have been common in urban areas, even in children who were fully immunized. Many adolescents and adults, despite previous vaccination or disease, are susceptible to infection and are the major reservoir for infection of infants. In adults, the syndrome often is atypical, becoming manifest as a severe, protracted cough without a whoop. Intrafamily spread is common. The younger the child, the more atypical the signs and symptoms of the disease; infants less than 6 months of age may have apnea, cyanotic spells, and cough but no whoop. Pertussis is increasing in frequency in areas where immunization has declined.

Clinical Manifestations. Symptomatic illness lasts from 6–8 weeks, although many patients have cough for 3 weeks or less. The illness generally is divided into three states: (1) *catarrhal* (prodromal, preparoxysmal), (2) *paroxysmal* (spasmodic cough), and (3) *convalescent.* The clinical manifestations depend on the specific pathogen, the patient's age, and the host's immunization status. The organism adheres to airway epithelial cells, activating cytokines and stimulating apoptosis. This results in inflammation and cell necrosis, causing bronchitis, atelectasis, and bronchopneumonia. The perihilar infiltrates produce the "shaggy" heart border on chest roentgenograms characteristic of pertussis.

Catarrhal Stage (1–2 weeks). Rhinorrhea (clear to mucoid), conjunctival injection, lacrimation, mild cough, wheezing, and low-grade fever are noted. Unfortunately, a diagnosis of pertussis usually is not considered during this stage, even though at this time the organisms are present in the greatest concentration, because the manifestations are similar to those of most nonspecific viral upper respiratory tract infections.

Paroxysmal Stage (2–4 weeks or longer). Episodes of coughing increase in severity and frequency. Multiple coughs during an expiration are followed by a sudden massive inspiration, producing the whoop, as air is forcefully inhaled against a narrowed glottis. The whoop may be absent in children younger than 6 months of age or in adults. Facial petechiae and redness, venous engorgement, and cyanosis may be prominent during the attack. Posttussive vomiting should raise the suspicion of pertussis. Recurrent episodes are exhausting; patients appear apathetic and lose weight. Paroxysms may produce anoxic brain damage; alternately, pertussis may produce encephalopathy.

Convalescent Stage (1–2 weeks). Paroxysmal coughing and vomiting decrease in frequency and severity. During this phase, chronic cough may persist for several months. Rarely, paroxysmal cough recurs accompanied by subsequent upper respiratory tract infections in the ensuing months.

Diagnosis and Differential Diagnosis. Pertussis is clinically suspected during the typical paroxysmal stage. Outbreaks of pertussis in older children and adolescents are difficult to diagnose. In this population and in adults, pertussis may be associated with coryza or a paroxsymal cough and vomiting lasting more than 4 weeks. A history of incomplete immunization and of contact with a known case is helpful. Leukocytosis (counts of 20,000–100,000 cells/L) with an absolute lymphocytosis is characteristic at the end of the catarrhal stage and during the paroxysmal stage of the disease. Lymphocytosis may not be evident in partially immunized or very young infants. Chest x-ray examination may show perihilar infiltrates, atelectasis, or emphysema.

The diagnosis depends on isolation of *B. pertussis,* usually accomplished during the early phases of illness by culture of nasopharyngeal swabs on glycerin-potato-blood agar medium (Bordet-Gengou) to which penicillin has been added to inhibit growth of other organisms. *B. parapertussis* and *B. bronchiseptica,* both morphologically similar to *B. pertussis,* may require identification by a reference laboratory. Fluorescent antibody staining is technically difficult and has low specificity. PCR may be useful.

Differential diagnosis includes infection caused by other organisms that provoke an intense cough response, such as *B. parapertussis, C. pneumoniae, C. trachomatis, B. bronchoseptica,* and adenoviruses. A foreign body produces similar coughing and can be distinguished by sudden onset of symptoms and by roentgenography and endoscopy.

Complications. The most frequent complication is pneumonia caused by *B. pertussis* itself or resulting from secondary bacterial infection (pneumococcus, *H. influenzae, S. aureus*). Atelectasis may be secondary to mucous plugs. Otitis media and sinusitis may occur. The force of the paroxysm may rupture alveoli and produce pneumomediastinum, pneumothorax, or interstitial or subcutaneous emphysema. Bronchiectasis may develop. Increased intrathoracic pressure and venous engorgement may cause epistaxis, retinal and subconjunctival hemorrhages, intraventricular and subarachnoid hemorrhage, rupture of the diaphragm, and inguinal hernia. Tetanic seizures may be associated with alkalosis related to persistent vomiting. Convulsions and encephalopathy occur in 2.5% and 0.5% of infants, respectively.

Treatment. Erythromycin, given early in the course of illness, can eradicate nasopharyngeal carriage of organisms within 3–4 days but is not effective in the paroxysmal stage. When given to infants under 4 weeks of age, erythromycin has been rarely associated with pyloric stenosis. Azithromycin or clarithromycin can be given for shorter duration. Trimethoprim/sulfamethoxazole is an unproven alternative. Codeine may be needed for coughing.

Prevention. As a result of limited immunity in adults and lack of transplacental immunity, infants are highly susceptible to infection. Active immunity can be induced with an "acellular" pertussis vaccine (DTaP). Pertussis vaccine has an efficacy of 70–90%; efficacy declines with fewer vaccinations. In the United States an acellular pertussis vaccine combined with diphtheria and tetanus toxoids, combined with *Haemophilus influenzae* type b, is given to all infants. The acellular vaccines contain one or more antigens isolated from *B. pertussis,* such as pertussis toxin, pertactin, or the filamentous hemagglutinin, and each preparation currently licensed appears to provide equivalent protection. These acellular vaccines have a significantly lower rate of side effects (e.g., drowsiness, irritability, or anorexia), as well as lower rates of local reactions. Serious side effects, including prolonged crying, hypotonic-hyporesponsive episodes, and high fever (>104.8° F) have been reported with the acellular vaccines, but at a substantially lower frequency than the 1:1750 incidence of serious side effects reported with the older whole-cell vaccines. Infants who receive subsequent pertussis vaccine after a significant side effect have no further adverse affects. Erythromycin is effective in preventing disease in newborn infants and adults exposed to pertussis. Close contacts younger than 7 years of age who have received four doses of vaccine should receive a booster dose of DTaP unless a booster dose has been given within the preceding 3 years. They also should be given erythromycin. Close contacts older than 7 years of age should receive prophylactic erythromycin for 10–14 days but not the vaccine. For the primary immunization schedule and contraindications for DPT or DTaP, see Fig. 10–1. If pertussis exposure is probable, because of endemic or epidemic disease, the vaccine may be given at 2 weeks of age. Patients who have pertussis do not require further pertussis vaccinations because the disease produces lifelong immunity.

REFERENCES

Aoyama T, Sunakawa K, Iwata S, et al: Efficacy of short term treatment of pertussis with clarithromycin and azithromycin, *J Pediatr* 129:761–764, 1996.

Bace A, Zrnic, Begovac J, et al: Short-term treatment of pertussis with azithromycin infants and young children, *Eur J Clin Microbiol Infect Dis* 18:296–298, 1999.

Behrman RE, Kliegman RM, Jenson HB, editors: *Nelson textbook of pediatrics,* ed 16, Philadelphia, 2000, WB Saunders, Chapter 195.

Braun MM, Mootrey GT, Salive ME, et al: Infant immunization with acellular pertussis vaccines in the United States: assessment of the first two years data from the vaccine adverse event reporting system, *Pediatrics* 106:E51, 2000.

DuVernoy TS, Braun MM: Hypotonic-hyporesponsive episodes reported to the vaccine adverse event reporting team, *Pediatrics* 106:E52, 2000.

Yih WK, Lett SM, Vignes FN, et al: The increasing incidence of pertussis in Massachusetts adolescents and adults, 1989-1998, *J Infect Dis* 182:1409–1416, 2000.

Infections Caused by *Streptococcus Pneumoniae* (Pneumococcal Infections)

Streptococcus pneumoniae (pneumococcus) may colonize the upper respiratory tract or cause invasive disease: otitis media, pneumonia, bacteremia, and meningitis.

Etiology. *S. pneumoniae* are gram-positive, lancet-shaped diplococci. Ninety serogroups have been identified; of these, serotypes 4, 6B, 9V, 14, 18C, 19F, and 23F are responsible for most of the invasive disease in children in the United States. Serotypes 6B, 9V, 14, 19A, 19F, and 23F are often resistant to penicillin.

S. pneumoniae bind to the polymeric IgG receptor and are transported across the airway epithelial cell. In the absence of preformed anticapsular antibody, these encapsulated organisms can cause focal infections, especially otitis media and pneumonia, or invade the bloodstream to cause bacteremia and can seed the meninges to cause meningitis. Their main virulence factor is the capsule, which thwarts effective phagocytosis in the absence of type-specific anticapsular antibody. They cause disease chiefly by activating the host PMN response. In addition, pneumococci are naturally transformable and take up DNA fragments from related organisms. DNA fragments from antibiotic-resistant streptococci in the oral flora, and especially from penicillin-resistant pneumococci, are incorporated into the genome of virulent encapsulated organisms by genetic recombination, giving rise to penicillin-resistant pneumococci as either colonizers or causes of invasive infection.

Epidemiology. Pneumococci commonly colonize the upper respiratory tract and are readily transmitted from person to person by contaminated secretions and droplets. Person-to-person transmission in a day care setting is common; prior viral infection increases susceptibility to pneumococcal infection. Several patient populations appear to be at increased risk for pneumococcal infections, such as African American and Native American populations, males more than females (3:2), and immunocompromised patients with poorly controlled HIV infection, low CD4+ counts, and high viral loads and patients with decreased or absent splenic function, sickle cell anemia or other hemoglobinopathies that affect reticuloendothelial function, nephrotic syndrome or hypogammaglobulinemia, decreased T-cell function after organ transplantation, chronic pulmonary or renal disease, and heart failure. Patients with anatomic deformities that affect the blood-brain barrier, such as cribriform plate fractures, or CSF leaks after trauma, are at increased risk for pneumococcal meningitis. Infections caused by *S. pneumoniae* are most common in the winter, presumably because of increased person-to-person transmission and concomitant viral infections. The rate of pneumococcal disease is greatest in children 1 year of age or younger (~150 cases/100,000 in 1999).

Clinical Manifestations. *S. pneumoniae* is the most frequent cause of bacterial otitis media, bacterial pneumonia, bacteremia, and bacterial meningitis in infants and children. The classic presentation of pneumococcal pneumonia in an older child or an adult is the relatively abrupt onset of fever and a shaking chill, following a brief period of nonspecific upper respiratory symptoms, accompanied by cough and the production of rusty sputum. Findings of lobar consolidation on physical examination and confirmation of a lobar infiltrate on chest film would be typical, along with an elevated WBC count with a PMN predominance. Pleural effusions are common, and empyemas, with extension of the inflammatory response into the pleural space, necessitate chest tube drainage. In younger children the signs and symptoms are less well localized; bilateral disease

may be present. However, relatively high fever and elevated WBCs are typical. Bacteremic infection may produce signs of the sepsis syndrome, or *S. pneumoniae* may seed the meninges, causing a brisk inflammatory response characterized by PMN infiltration and breakdown of the blood-brain barrier, with loss of tight junctions in the capillary endothelial cells. In the absence of type-specific antibody, the organisms are not efficiently phagocytosed, although the recruited PMNs release elastase and reactive oxygen intermediates that further stimulate local inflammation. TNF-α production and IL-1 release by both the local dendritic cells, as well as by macrophages and endothelial cells, further amplify the local inflammation. Although the organisms do not invade the brain directly, the local inflammation causes edema, poor perfusion, and local infarction. *S. pneumoniae* cell wall components mimic platelet-activating factor, triggering small vessel thromboses and further disrupting oxygenation and perfusion.

Pneumococcal bacteremia facilitates distant infections, septic arthritis, endocarditis in children with damaged endovascular tissues, or peritonitis in children with nephrotic syndrome. In addition to these clinically evident infections, *S. pneumoniae* is a common cause of "occult bacteremia," a cause of fever without localizing signs in children 3 months to 2 years of age, which often resolves without antibiotic therapy. Despite the increasing rates of penicillin resistance, studies do not indicate a poorer outcome with pneumonia or meningitis caused by penicillin-nonsusceptible isolates treated with cefotaxime or ceftriaxone.

Diagnosis. The diagnosis is confirmed in older patients by Gram stain and a culture of sputum and in all patients by recovering pneumococci from blood or CSF culture. Isolation of pneumococci from the nose or throat of patients with otitis media, sinusitis, pneumonia, septicemia, or meningitis is not proof of causation because the frequency of the carrier state is high. The total white blood cell count is elevated (20,000–30,000/L), as is the ESR in serious pneumococcal disease. Paracentesis, Gram stain, and culture are required to differentiate pneumococcal from other pathogens (e.g., *Escherichia coli*) in patients with peritonitis.

Treatment. *S. pneumoniae*, once uniformly susceptible to penicillin (MIC ≤0.06 μg/ml), is now more often "relatively resistant" (MIC 0.1–1.0 μg/ml). The most common source of resistant organisms is young children (younger than 5 years of age) in day care; most uncomplicated infections in this setting, such as otitis media, can be readily treated using higher doses of conventional antimicrobial agents such as amoxicillin or amoxicillin/clavulate combinations for a 5-day course of treatment or a single dose of intramuscular ceftriaxone. Clindamycin or macrolides (azithromycin or clarithromycin) are alternatives. Unfortunately, many of the penicillin-resistant isolates are often multidrug resistant, and surveys report 15% resistance to erythromycin and 29% to trimethoprim/sulfamethoxazole in penicillin-resistant pneumococci.

Tympanocentesis and cultures of middle ear fluid should be considered if the child does not respond to the usual empiric therapy to cover antibiotic-resistant pneumococci, as well as β-lactamase–producing *H. influenzae* or *Moraxella catarrhalis*.

For more serious infections, high doses of cefotaxime or ceftriaxone may be used; however, these may not achieve adequate levels in the CSF to treat meningitis caused by resistant organisms. For life-threatening infections, vancomycin is added to a third-generation cephalosporin. Vancomycin at 60 mg/kg should be used. Susceptibility testing of blood and CSF isolates must be performed, and penicillin susceptibility is determined using a 1-μg oxacillin disc. There is a 7.7% fatality rate in children with pneumococcal meningitis; no deaths are the result of documented failure of treatment caused by penicillin resistance.

Prevention. A pneumococcal-conjugate vaccine (PCV7) is recommended for use in all infants, to be given concurrently with the other vaccines at 2, 4, 6, and 12 to 15 months of age, as well as to chronically ill at-risk children ages 24–59 months or others at increased risk for invasive pneumococcal disease (Blacks and Native Americans, in group day care, frequent or complicated otitis media, children who are socially or economically disadvantaged [Fig. 10–1]). This vaccine includes the capsular antigens for types 4, 6B, 9V, 14, 19F, 23F, and 18C conjugated to CRM_{197}. It elicits protective antibody against these serotypes with a 97.4% efficacy in fully immunized children against disease caused by pneumococcal types included in the vaccine and an 89% efficacy against all pneumococci. Use of the vaccine was associated with a decrease of otitis media and pneumonia.

A 23-valent pneumococcal polysaccharide vaccine for *S. pneumoniae,* has been available, but its lack of immunogenicity in children less than 2 years of age, who have the highest prevalence of pneumococcal disease, has limited its efficacy. It has been used in older children with sickle cell disease or asplenia along with penicillin prophylaxis. Two doses of PCV7 are recommended for children 24–59 months of age, with a high or moderate risk of invasive pneumococcal disease, followed by a dose of the 23-valent polysaccharide vaccine to expand the serotypes covered. The serotypes covered by the PCV7 vaccine and the 23-valent polysaccharide vaccine are responsible for 78% and 88% of the penicillin-resistant strains.

Administration of gamma globulin to children with hypogammaglobulinemia (IgG <200 mg/dL) reduces the risk of pneumococcal bacteremia and meningitis, but not necessarily pneumococcal respiratory infections. Oral penicillin (amoxicillin) should be given continuously to all infants with sickle cell anemia and to other patients who are anatomically or functionally asplenic, to prevent sepsis.

REFERENCES

Bachur R, Harper MB: Reevaluation of outpatients with *Streptococcus pneumoniae* bacteremia, *Pediatrics* 105:502–509, 2000.

Behrman RE, Kliegman RM, Jenson HB, editors: *Nelson textbook of pediatrics,* ed 16, Philadelphia, 2000, WB Saunders, Chapter 183.

Black S, Shinefield H, Fireman B, et al: Efficacy, safety, and immunogenicity of heptavalent pneumococcal conjugate vaccine in children, *Pediatr Infect Dis J* 19:187–195, 2000.

Committee on Infectious Diseases Policy Statement: Recommendations for the preventions of pneumococcal polysacharide vaccine and antibiotic prophylaxis, *Pediatrics* 106:362, 2000.

Fiore AE, Moroney JF, Farley MM, et al: Clinical outcomes of meningitis caused by *Streptococcus pneumoniae* in the era of antibiotic resistance, *Clin Infect Dis* 30:71–77, 2000.

Overturf G: Technical report: prevention of pneumococcal infections, including the use of pneumococcal conjugate vaccine, pneumococcal polysaccharide vaccine and antibiotic prophylaxis, *Pediatrics* 106:367–376, 2000.

Infections Caused by Salmonellae

Salmonellae are important pathogens of animals and humans. Humans become infected by ingesting contaminated water or food, typically beef, poultry, milk, and eggs. Systemic infection with *Salmonella typhi* (typhoid fever) is uncommon in the United States but is endemic and epidemic in other parts of the world. Infections caused by other types of salmonellae are common throughout the United States.

Etiology. Salmonellae are gram-negative, facultative anaerobic bacilli and unable to ferment lactose. The principal antigens are the flagellum (H) antigens, the cell wall (O) antigens, and the envelope (Vi) heat-labile antigens. A typing scheme using O and H antigens permits the differentiation of more than 2200 *Salmonella* serotypes. Salmonellae are divided into serogroups designated A, B, C1, C2, D, and E on the basis of the O antigen. Although *S. typhi* and *S. paratyphi* are human pathogens, most other serotypes are widely distributed in animals.

Organisms are usually ingested from a contaminated source, and a large inoculum is required because salmonellae are killed by gastric acidity. Salmonellae express a number of specific virulence factors that enable them to elude the normal mucosal defenses. These bacteria attach and invade via specific receptors in the intestinal epithelium found on "M" cells, which are in direct contact with intestinal reticuloendothelial cells of the Peyer patches.

The organisms are phagocytosed by macrophages and reside in "spacious phagosomes." Replication occurs within the macrophages in the mesenteric lymph nodes. Salmonellae can be released into the bloodstream, causing bacteremia or sepsis. Disseminated infection can occur, particularly with *S. cholerasuis* and in immunocompromised patients, including patients with sickle cell disease and HIV infection, and produces bacteremia and metastatic complications.

Salmonella Gastroenteritis

(Nontyphoidal)

Epidemiology. *Salmonella* gastroenteritis is most common in children younger than 4 years of age; infants younger than 1 year of age have the highest rates of infection, although it can occur at any age. Patients with decreased gastric acidity, especially young infants and older people, are particularly at risk. Infected animals are the major reservoir for the nontyphoid salmonellae. Infected poultry, eggs, and egg products, as well as contaminated meats and pet reptiles, such as turtles and iguanas, are frequent sources of infection. Concern is growing that the widespread use of antibiotics in animal feeds has contributed to the increasing incidence of antibiotic-resistant salmonellae.

Humans are important carriers of *Salmonella* species and can cause localized epidemics of food poisoning by fecal-oral contamination of food at large gatherings such as picnics. Intrafamilial transmission of salmonellosis is frequent.

The incubation period for gastroenteritis is from 6–72 hours but usually is less than 24 hours.

Clinical Manifestations. *Salmonella* gastroenteritis is typically a self-limited disease lasting from 3-7 days. It has a peak incidence in the late summer and early fall, correlating with food-borne outbreaks. Epidemics and disease found in small family clusters occur throughout the year. Onset is abrupt and is characterized by nausea, vomiting, and crampy abdominal pain followed by loose, watery stools that may contain mucus, leukocytes, and blood. Systemic signs of malaise, headache, and chills occasionally are noted. Fever of 38.3°–38.9° C (101°–102° F) is noted in 70% of patients and lasts for 48 hours. Symptoms subside within 2–5 days in healthy individuals. Patients with impaired immune function are at risk for complications from *Salmonella*; intact T-cell function is critical. HIV infection, organ transplantation, and lymphoproliferative diseases are risk factors. In addition, patients with impaired reticuloendothelial clearance, such as sickle cell disease and other hemoglobinopathies, chronic granulomatous disease, and malaria, are at higher risk, along with patients who are either very old or very young.

Interleukin-12 is critical for the ability to handle this organism, and patients lacking the IL-12 receptor are highly susceptible to *Salmonella* and mycobacterial infections. Septicemia accompanied by toxic appearance and high fever is much more common in the first 3 months of life. Bacteremia in young infants and older children may clear spontaneously. Nonetheless, salmonellae can localize and cause pneumonia, empyema, abscesses, osteomyelitis, septic arthritis, pyelonephritis, and meningitis. Neonates may become infected at birth, and sepsis and meningitis develop. Most individuals will have a positive stool culture for several weeks, and neonates may be positive for months.

Complications. Enteritis may produce significant dehydration, electrolyte disturbances, and hypovolemic shock. Other complications of nontyphoidal salmonellosis are unusual and are limited to the extraintestinal lesions noted above. A postinfectious arthritis is associated with *Salmonella* infection, occuring more frequently in patients who have a positive test result for HLA-B27. This is an immunologically mediated arthritis, not associated with active infection of the joints.

Diagnosis. Culture of stool is indicated when fever is present and in the presence of blood, mucus, or leukocytes in the stool. Blood specimens should be obtained for culture in young infants and immunocompromised patients. Cultures of stool, blood, urine, bone marrow aspirate, CSF, and foci of infection should be obtained in more complicated cases. Although three consecutive negative stool cultures suggest that infection has ceased, excretion may be intermittent. *Salmonella* gastroenteritis must be distinguished from other viral and bacterial causes of diarrhea (see Chapter 11). Rarely, the clinical course and roentgenographic findings suggest ulcerative colitis.

Treatment. Correction of shock, dehydration, and electrolyte imbalances is the most important aspect of the therapy for *Salmonella* gastroenteritis. Uncomplicated enteritis in healthy children usually is improving when stool culture results are known; these children require no antibiotics. Antibiotics are indicated for high-risk individuals because of the possibility of dissemination of disease (infants under 3 months of age or children with immunologic deficiency, malnutrition, malignancy, or intravascular catheters or other foreign material).

Children with septicemia, enteric fever, or metastatic sites of infection initially should be treated with ceftriaxone or cefotaxime. Alternative antibiotics are determined on antimicrobial resistance patterns; useful agents for susceptible *Salmonella* are amoxicillin, trimethoprim/sulfamethoxazole, or quinolones. Fluoroquinolones are particularly effective for *Salmonella* infections and are considerably safer than alternatives such as chloramphenicol (see Appendix I).

Typhoid Fever

(Enteric Fever)

Epidemiology. In the United States, approximately 400 cases of typhoid fever occur each year. The majority of reported cases occur in persons under 20 years of age and are imported from other countries. Worldwide there are an estimated 16 million cases of typhoid fever annually, resulting in 600,000 deaths. The typhoid bacillus infects only humans, and chronic carriers therefore are responsible for new cases.

Pathogenesis. The upper small bowel is the predominant site of invasion. Monocytes phagocytose but do not kill the bacilli early in the disease, and they carry the organisms from the blood to the mesenteric lymph nodes and other reticuloendothelial sites in which bacteria proliferate to produce inflammation in the lymph nodes, liver, and spleen. Secondary septicemia is disseminated from these sites and usually is prolonged, seeding other organs. The gallbladder is particularly susceptible and is infected from the liver via the biliary system or from the blood. Microorganisms that multiply in the gallbladder eventually are discharged into the intestine.

Clinical Manifestations. The pattern of typhoid fever in infants ranges from mild gastroenteritis to severe septicemia without diarrhea. Fever, hepatomegaly, jaundice, anorexia, lethargy, and weight loss can be marked.

In older children, the course is characterized by high fever, malaise, lethargy, myalgia, headache, rash, hepatosplenomegaly, and abdominal pain and tenderness. Diarrhea occurs in fewer than half of older children in the early stage, but constipation is noted in the later stages. The patient may become severely obtunded and exhibit delirium and confusion. At this stage of the disease, the spleen generally is enlarged and abdominal tenderness is present. A macular (rose spots) or maculopapular rash is observable on the skin in approximately 30% of patients. The paradoxic relationship of a high temperature and low pulse rate may be observed. Typically, for each degree rise above 38.3° C (101° F), the pulse should rise 10 beats/min. Leukopenia is common.

Complications. Intestinal perforation at the site of inoculation, usually in the ileum, occurs in 0.5–3%, and severe gastrointestinal hemorrhage occurs in 1–10%, of children with typhoid fever. Most complications occur during the second (dissemination) stage of disease and are preceded by a fall in temperature and blood pressure and a rise in pulse rate. Toxic encephalopathy, cerebral thrombosis, acute cerebellar ataxia, optic neuritis, aphasia, deafness,

transverse myelitis, and acute cholecystitis may occur. Pneumonia is common during the second stage of illness but is caused by a superinfection. Pyelonephritis, endocarditis, meningitis, osteomyelitis, and septic arthritis are rare in the normal host. Septic arthritis and osteomyelitis are seen in individuals with hemoglobinopathies.

Diagnosis and Differential Diagnosis. Blood cultures are positive early in the disease, whereas urine and stool cultures become positive following the secondary septicemia. Because of the relatively small number of organisms, blood cultures may be negative. Bone marrow, lymph nodes, and reticuloendothelial tissues often contain organisms after the blood has been sterilized. In suspected cases with negative cultures, a culture of aspirated bone marrow or duodenal fluid (to evaluate possible biliary infection) may be helpful.

During the initial stage of typhoid fever, the clinical diagnosis may be bronchitis, bronchopneumonia, gastroenteritis, or influenza. Subsequently, other infectious conditions caused by intracellular microorganisms may need to be considered. Concern about an acute abdomen may lead to unnecessary surgical intervention.

Treatment. Antibiotic resistance is common. Based on susceptibility, ceftriaxone, ampicillin, chloramphenicol, trimethoprim/sulfamethoxazole, and ciprofloxacin are useful drugs Azithromycin may be effective for multiply resistant isolates from endemic areas (see Appendix I).

Third-generation cephalosporins, particularly drugs that are metabolized in the liver, may cure carriers. Cholecystectomy may be indicated to eliminate the carrier state.

Prognosis. Antimicrobial therapy has reduced the mortality rate to less than 1% in most areas, but the presence of underlying debilitating disease, perforation of the gastrointestinal tract, severe hemorrhage, or coma increases the mortality rate. Meningitis or endocarditis may be associated with high morbidity and mortality rates. Relapse occurs in up to 10% of those who are not treated with antibiotics.

Individuals who excrete *S. typhi* for 3 or more months are usually excreters at 1 year and often for life. The risk of becoming a chronic carrier is low in children; fluoroquinolones usually eradicate the carrier state.

Prevention. Two typhoid vaccines are available for use in the United States and are recommended to travelers to endemic areas and household contacts with known carriers. The efficacy is 55–77%. An oral live-attenuated vaccine from Ty21a strain of *S. typhi* is approved for use in children older than 6 years of age (but should not be given with mefloquine, often used for malaria prophylaxis). Four doses of the capsules are required. The longevity of the immune response is not well documented; a booster series is suggested every 5 years. An injectable polysaccharide vaccine, ViCPS, is also available for children younger than 2 years of age; it requires booster doses every 2 years.

REFERENCES

Behrman RE, Kliegman RM, Jenson HB, editors: *Nelson textbook of pediatrics*, ed 16, Philadelphia, 2000, WB Saunders, Chapter 196.

Dunne EF, Fey PD, Ludt P, et al: Emergence of domestically acquired ceftriaxone-resistant *Salmonella* infections associated with AmpC β-lactamase, *JAMA* 284:3151–3156, 2000.

Frenck RW Jr, Nakhla I, Sultan Y, et al: Azithromycin versus ceftriaxone for the treatment of uncomplicated typhoid fever in children, *Infect Dis* 31:1134–1138, 2000.

Shigellosis

(Bacillary Dysentery)
See also Chapter 11.

Etiology. Shigellae are non–lactose-fermenting gram-negative rods. The genus *Shigella* includes *S. dysenteriae* (group A) and is important worldwide but rarely isolated in the United States; *S. flexneri* (group B); *S. boydii* (group C); and the most common isolate, *S. sonnei* (group D). Unlike the case with salmonellae, only a very small inoculum of ingested shigellae is needed to cause disease. The organisms bind to receptors on M cells, specialized intestinal epithelial cells overlying the Peyer patches. They are propelled within the epithelial cells by their ability to polymerize host cell actin filaments and can invade and spread laterally from one epithelial cell to the next. This invasion triggers host cell cytokine release and apoptosis, resulting in the recruitment of polymorphonuclear leukocytes and other inflammatory cells. In addition, some strains of *Shigella* produce Shiga toxin, a potent cytotoxin that acts by inhibiting mammalian protein synthesis and is associated with hemolytic-uremic syndrome.

Epidemiology. Shigellosis is a common disease occurring primarily in young children between the ages of 1–10 years, when fecal-oral transmission may be more likely to occur. Humans are the major reservoir of infection. The organisms survive readily on inanimate objects, facilitating transmission in child care settings, in nursery schools, and within families. In developing countries, water supplies are commonly contaminated. The incubation period varies from 1–7 days, and infected adults may shed organisms for a month.

Clinical Manifestations. Shigellae are prototypic invasive pathogens that destroy the superficial epithelial cells, producing inflammation, edema, microabscess formation, and ulceration with bleeding.

Mild *Shigella* infections result in watery diarrhea with minimal systemic symptoms. In severe cases, crampy abdominal pain, temperature greater than 40° C (104° F) lasting 1–3 days, and diarrhea containing blood and mucus can occur. The child may have nonlocalized lower abdominal tenderness. Shigellosis may mimic CNS diseases such as meningitis, particularly when high fever is associated with seizures. Seizures occur in 30% of children with *Shigella* gastroenteritis and are more common if the temperature exceeds 40° C (104° F).

Shigella infrequently may cause conjunctivitis and vaginitis from autoinoculation. Nonsuppurative arthritis and Reiter syndrome have been associated with *Shigella* infection. Hemolytic-uremic syndrome, possibly associated with toxin production, may coincide with or follow enteritis.

Diagnosis. Stool should reveal leukocytes and red blood cells. The complete blood count displays leukocytosis composed of immature forms. The diagnosis is established by isolating the organism from stool or rectal cultures. Shigellosis must be differentiated from other causes of dysentery, such as infection with invasive or enterohemorrhagic *E. coli,* amebae, *Campylobacter jejuni, Yersinia enterocolitica,* and *Salmonella,* as well as from intussusception and acute appendicitis.

Treatment. Particularly in young infants, fluid and electrolyte replacement, using oral rehydration solutions when possible, is critical. Antimicrobial therapy is complicated by widespread antimicrobial resistance. Appropriate treatment decreases further intestinal shedding of the organisms and further transmission of infection to others. Although oral ampicillin (but not amoxicillin, which does not achieve sufficient luminal concentrations) was recommended, few isolates remain susceptible. Trimethoprim/sulfamethoxazole can be used if isolates are susceptible. Parenteral ceftriaxone is efficacious, as are the fluoroquinolones, which are often the only therapeutic option and have been safely used for this indication (see Appendix I).

REFERENCES

Behrman RE, Kliegman RM, Jenson HB, editors: *Nelson textbook of pediatrics*, ed 16, Philadelphia, 2000, WB Saunders, Chapter 197.

Leibovitz E, Janco J, Piglansky L, et al: Oral ciprofloxacin versus intramuscular ceftriaxone as empiric treatment of acute invasive diarrhea in children, *Pediatr Infect Dis J* 19:1060–1067, 2000.

Mohle-Boetani JC, Stapletone M, Finger R, et al: Community-wide shigellosis: control of an outbreak and risk factors in child day-care centers, *Am J Public Health* 85:812–816, 1995.

Staphylococcal Infections

Staphylococci are a common cause of pyogenic infections in infants and children. These organisms are gram-positive cocci that grow aerobically or as facultative anaerobes and appear in grape-like clusters. Strains are classified as *S. aureus* (coagulase protein A and mannitol positive), *S. epidermidis* species (coagulase protein A and mannitol negative and novobiocin sensitive), and *S. saprophyticus* (coagulase negative, mannitol positive, novobiocin resistant). They are extremely hardy organisms, able to persist on toys and hard surfaces and to withstand drying.

Infections Caused by Staphylococcus Aureus

Etiology. Staphylococci cause disease by a number of mechanisms:

1. Local destruction by exoenzymes (e.g., catalase, hyaluronidase, coagulase, or phospholipases), which also interfere with host defense mechanisms
2. The secretion of toxins, which can act locally or at a distant site (enterotoxins and TSST-1, the toxic shock toxin)
3. Superantigens, which activate T-cell receptor Vβ chains without requiring processing α- or β-chain specificity (TSST-1)
4. The organism's ability to elude normal host polymorphonuclear killing by binding the Fc portion of IgG and interfering with efficient opsonophagocytosis

Strains of *S. aureus* can be classified by bacteriophage group typing. Exfoliative toxin, associated with phage group 2 and some non–group 2 staphylococci, is the cause of "scalded skin syndrome" **(Ritter disease)** and bullous impetigo. Staphylococcal enterotoxin is elaborated by most strains of *S. aureus*. Ingestion of preformed enterotoxin is associated with vomiting and diarrhea and, in some cases, with the development of profound hypotension.

Epidemiology. *S. aureus* is part of normal human flora and is present in the anterior nares and moist areas of the body in about 30% of asymptomatic people. Transmission of *S. aureus* generally occurs via hands, nasal discharge, person-to-person contact, and, rarely, through air. Newborn infants are extremely susceptible to staphylococci; the nasopharynx, skin, and umbilical stump are the most common sites of colonization.

S. aureus colonizes skin and mucous membranes through its affinity for host glycoconjugates and intracellular matrix components, such as fibronectin, laminin, and collagen. Any break in the epidermis provides a niche for the organism. Infants with a very thin epidermis and impaired host defenses are particularly at risk, as are hospitalized patients with intravascular access devices or decreased polymorphonuclear leukocyte function caused by corticosteroids or cancer chemotherapy. Person-to-person transmission of virulent organisms is common because nasal carriage is frequent in hospital personnel and is a potential source of infection.

Clinical Manifestations. *S. aureus* causes a wide variety of suppurative lesions, as well as septicemia and toxin-related diseases, including scalded skin syndrome, toxic shock syndrome, and food poisoning.

Skin. Pyogenic skin infections may be primary or secondary to wounds or to a superinfection of other noninfectious skin disease (e.g., eczema) and include impetigo contagiosa, bullous impetigo, pustules, cellulitis, folliculitis, furuncles, and carbuncles. Toxins produce staphylococcal scalded skin syndrome (Ritter disease), toxic shock syndrome, and a rash resembling that in scarlet fever. In these conditions, staphylococci are not present in the lesions.

Respiratory Tract. Infections of the upper respiratory tract caused by *S. aureus* are rare, considering the rate of colonization of this area. Sinusitis caused by *S. aureus* may occur. Suppurative parotitis is a rare infection, but *S. aureus* is a common cause. *S. aureus* is a common cause of suppurative cervical adenitis. Tracheitis resembling viral croup but with high fever and toxicity may be caused by *S. aureus*. Pneumonia caused by *S. aureus* is noted in children under 1 year of age and is associated with pneumatoceles, empyema, and sepsis.

Sepsis. Staphylococcal bacteremia and sepsis may be primary infections without an initiating focus or localized lesion. Later, organisms may localize in the lungs, heart valves, joints, bones, kidneys, and brain. Disseminated staphylococcal disease has been associated with deep vein thrombophlebitis and septic pulmonary emboli.

Muscle. Localized staphylococcal abscesses in muscle associated with elevation of muscle enzymes have been called **pyomyositis.** Multiple abscesses occur in 30–40% of cases. Surgical drainage and appropriate antibiotic therapy are essential.

Bones and Joints. *S. aureus* is the most common cause of osteomyelitis and septic arthritis in children. These diseases are derived from hematogenous dissemination rather than direct extension of infection from an adjacent skin or soft tissue lesion.

Central Nervous System. Meningitis caused by *S. aureus* is rare but may follow bacteremia or may originate from direct extension of otitis media or osteomyelitis of the skull or vertebrae. Trauma or infection of meningomyelocele also may predispose the patient to *S. aureus* meningitis. Staphylococcal infection following neurosurgical procedures generally is the result of *S. epidermidis*. *S. aureus* can be recovered from brain abscesses after CNS trauma and spinal epidural abscess.

Heart. Acute bacterial endocarditis in children may follow staphylococcal bacteremia and occur in the absence of valvular heart disease, as well as in patients with minimal valvular abnormalities, such as bicuspid mitral valves. Perforation of heart valves, myocardial abscesses, heart block, acute hemopericardium, purulent pericarditis, and sudden death may ensue.

Kidney. S. aureus is a common cause of renal and perinephric abscess. Uncomplicated urinary tract infection caused by *S. aureus* is unusual. Coagulase-negative staphylococci, particularly *S. saprophyticus*, are an important cause of urinary tract infection in adolescent girls.

Intestinal Tract. Food poisoning may be caused by ingestion of preformed staphylococcal enterotoxins that contaminate foods. The short (1–7 hour) incubation period, lack of fever, short illness, and profuse emesis help differentiate it from other causes of food poisoning. Enterotoxins A and D are the most common causes in the United States.

Diagnosis. The diagnosis of staphylococcal infection follows the isolation of the organisms from skin lesions, abscess cavities, blood, CSF, or other usually sterile sites. Gram stains reveal gram-positive cocci in clusters. After isolation, identification is made on the basis of Gram stain and coagulase and mannitol reactivity. Patterns of susceptibility to antibiotics should be assessed to guide therapy. Diagnosis of staphylococcal food poisoning is made on the basis of epidemiologic (e.g., unrefrigerated meats, mayonnaise, or creamed foods) and clinical findings. Food suspected of contamination should be examined by Gram stain culture and tested for enterotoxin.

Treatment. Loculated collections of purulent material must be incised and drained. Foreign bodies associated with infection may need to be removed. Virtually all staphylococci are resistant to penicillin; therefore, therapy for *S. aureus* should include a penicillinase-resistant antibiotic, such as methicillin, oxacillin, and nafcillin, or first-generation cephalosporins (cephalothin and cefazolin), or clindamycin. Vancomycin may be used to treat methicillin-resistant *S. aureus* or *S. epidermidis*. Methicillin resistance is the result of the expression of mec-A, an altered penicillin-binding protein with diminished affinity for penicillins and cephalosporins (see Appendix I). Strains that hyperproduce beta-lactamase may often be treated with amoxicillin/clavulanate, ticarcillin/clavulanate, ampicillin/sulbactam, imipenem, first-generation cephalosporins, fluoroquinolones, or vancomycin. Some mecA$^+$ strains also produce large amounts of beta-lactamase.

Although there have been isolated reports of low-level vancomycin resistance in staphylococci, this has not yet become a problem for therapy.

Prevention. Staphylococcal infection is transmitted by hand-to-hand contact. Observance of strict hand-washing techniques is the most effective measure for preventing the spread of staphylococci. Local antibiotic ointment (mupirocin), antiseptic dyes, rifampin, or ciprofloxacin may be useful in reducing the carrier state.

REFERENCES

Archer GL, Climo MW: *Staphylococcus aureus* bacteremia—consider the source, *N Engl J Med* 344:55–56, 2001.

Behrman RE, Kliegman RM, Jenson HB, editors: *Nelson textbook of pediatrics*, ed 16, Philadelphia, 2000, WB Saunders, Chapter 182.

Dinges MM, Orwin PM, Schlievert PM: Exotoxins of *Staphylococcus aureus, Clin Microbiol Rev* 13:16–34, 2000.

Hodes DS, Barzilai A: Invasive and toxin-mediated *Staphylococcus aureus* diseases in children, *Adv Pediatr Infect Dis* 5:35–68, 1990.

Shopsin B, Mathema B, Martinez J, et al: Prevalence of methicillin-resistant and methicillin-susceptible *Staphylococcus aureus* in the community, *J Infect Dis* 182:359–362, 2000.

Toxic Shock Syndrome

Toxic shock syndrome is an acute, multisystem disease characterized by high fever, hypotension, an erythematous rash, and other less specific manifestations.

Etiology and Epidemiology. Toxic shock syndrome is caused by staphylococcal toxins, which function as superantigens, activating entire subsets of T cells by binding to specific Vβ chains of the T-cell receptor without Vα specificity. The activation of a large number of immune cells results in an outpouring of cytokines with profound physiologic consequences, including fever, vasodilation, hypotension, and multisystem organ involvement. The expression of TSST is upregulated by certain environmental conditions. The initial cases of toxic shock syndrome were associated with use of tampons, described in women who were using hyperabsorbent tampons that chelated local Mg, providing an environment that triggered TSST-1 expression. Recognition that other staphylococcal (and streptococcal) infections could result in this clinical syndrome has led to increased awareness of this disease and more prompt and effective therapy.

Clinical Manifestations. The onset is abrupt, with high fever, vomiting, diarrhea, and myalgias, with or without sore throat, headache, and malaise. A diffuse erythematous sunburn-like macular rash appears within 24 hours and is associated with hyperemia of pharyngeal, conjunctival, and vaginal mucous membranes. Symptoms often include alterations in the level of consciousness, oliguria, and hypotension, which may progress to shock or may be postural in mild cases. Coagulopathy, hypocalcemia, hypoalbuminemia, leukocytosis, and elevated levels of blood urea nitrogen, creatinine, serum glutamic oxaloacetic transaminase, or CPK may be present.

Recovery occurs within 7–10 days and is accompanied by desquamation of the palms and soles; hair and nail loss may be observed.

Differential Diagnosis. Kawasaki disease resembles toxic shock syndrome, but many features of toxic shock syndrome are absent or rare in Kawasaki disease, including diffuse myalgia, vomiting, abdominal pain, diarrhea, azotemia, hypotension, ARDS, and shock. In addition, Kawasaki disease occurs in children under 5 years of age; these children often have aneurysms of the coronary artery or other arteries. Scarlet fever, Rocky Mountain spotted fever, leptospirosis, toxic epidermal necrolysis, drug rash, and measles should be considered.

Treatment and Prevention. Fluid replacement should be aggressive to prevent or treat hypotension. Eradication of the source of toxin-producing *S. aureus* (e.g., tampon, nasal packing, or abscess) is necessary. Parenteral administration of a beta-lactamase–resistant antistaphylococcal antibiotic, such as nafcillin, oxacillin, or methicillin, is indicated in all cases for treatment and prevention of recurrences.

REFERENCES

Behrman RE, Kliegman RM, Jenson HB, editors: *Nelson textbook of pediatrics*, ed 16, Philadelphia, 2000, WB Saunders, Chapter 182.

Resnick SD: Toxic shock syndrome: recent developments in pathogenesis, *J Pediatr* 116:321, 1990.

Schafer R, Sheil JM: Superantigens and their role in infectious disease, *Adv Pediatr Infect Dis* 10:369, 1995.

Infections Caused by Coagulase-Negative Staphylococci

Etiology. Coagulase-negative staphylococci are common, usually nonpathogenic skin flora that are important causes of nosocomial infection as a result of their ability to colonize intravascular venous access devices.

Epidemiology. Coagulase-negative staphylococci are ubiquitous organisms that have affinity for plastic as a result of surface hydrophobicity, as well as the elaboration of an extracellular "slime." Although most, if not all, intravascular catheters become colonized by these organisms, large numbers of coagulase-negative staphylococci and the production of this slime are associated with bacteremia and clinical signs of local or systemic infection. These infections assume major clinical importance if they involve small neonates or CNS shunts. Bacteremias caused by coagulase-negative staphylococci are common in children with indwelling intravascular catheters for chemotherapy or nutrition.

Clinical Manifestations. In premature neonates, infection caused by coagulase-negative staphylococci presents as noscomial sepsis with or without an indwelling line (see Chapter 6).

In older children bacteremia may be accompanied by intermittent fever; patients generally have few other signs of systemic infection. Persistent bacteremia may represent an infected thrombus or endocarditis in patients with prosthetic valves or Dacron grafts. Such infections often are more indolent than those caused by *S. aureus* and may be difficult to diagnose. Often, single positive blood cultures with *S. epidermidis* are considered contaminants, when they may, in fact, represent a significant infection. Coagulase-negative staphylococci are common causes of infection in CNS ventriculoperitoneal shunts.

Staphylococcus saprophyticus is a cause of urinary tract infection, particularly in adolescent girls. Urine cultures that grow gram-positive cocci in symptomatic girls should not be dismissed as contaminants.

Treatment. These bacteria synthesize β-lactamases and have altered penicillin-binding proteins, producing resistance to all of the β-lactam antibiotics. Treatment therefore requires vancomycin. Rifampin also may be added to treat CNS infections. Infected intravenous catheters may be treated without removal in many instances, but CNS shunts must be replaced. *S. saprophyticus* may be treated with amoxicillin or one of the quinolones.

REFERENCES

Behrman RE, Kliegman RM, Jenson HB, editors: *Nelson textbook of pediatrics*, ed 16, Philadelphia, 2000, WB Saunders, Chapter 182.

Lyytikainen O, Saxen H, Ryhanen R, et al: Persistence of a multiresistant clone of *Staphylococcus epidermidis* in a neonatal intensive care unit for a four-year period, *Clin Infect Dis* 20:24–29, 1995.

Villari P, Sarnataro C, Iacuzio L: Molecular epidemiology of *Staphylococcus epidermidis* in a neonatal intensive care unit over a three-year period, *J Clin Microbiol* 38:1740–1746, 2000.

Group A Streptococcal Infections

Etiology. Streptococci are gram-positive cocci that grow in chains and that are classified by their ability to produce a zone of hemolysis on blood agar: those producing the enzyme hemolysin that causes partial hemolysis (alpha-hemolytic), those causing complete hemolysis (beta-hemolytic), and those with no hemolysis (gamma-hemolytic). Streptococci are further subdivided on the basis of differences in carbohydrate cell wall components; streptococcal Lancefield groups (A–H and K–V) have been identified.

The Lancefield group A streptococci (*S. pyogenes*) are beta-hemolytic and express several important virulence factors. The *M protein* is a surface structure that inhibits complement-mediated opsonophagocytosis. It has homology with certain mammalian proteins (tropomyosin) that may be the basis for some of the nonsuppurative complications of group A streptococcal infection.

More than 100 different types of M proteins have been identified and are linked to outbreaks. Immunity to one type does not necessarily protect against infection caused by strains with immunologically distinct M proteins; thus repeated group A streptococcal infections are possible.

Streptococci express numerous exotoxins associated with tissue damage, such as streptolysins, hyaluronidase, DNAse, and a lipoproteinase; they also express an erythrogenic toxin (pyrogenic toxin), the product of the *speA* or *speC* genes, which are phage-encoded superantigens functioning by activating entire classes of T cells by binding to specific V chains without antigen processing. This toxin accounts for the rash of scarlet fever, the streptococcal toxic shock syndrome, and many of the manifestations of severe, invasive group A streptococcal disease. This array of virulence factors enables the organism to produce human disease by three distinct mechanisms:

- Locally invasive disease (skin and soft tissue infection)
- Severe multisystem failure associated with toxin expression (streptococcal toxic shock)
- Nonsuppurative sequelae, including rheumatic fever and glomerulonephritis

Epidemiology. Group A streptococci are normal inhabitants of the nasopharynx; colonization is present in 15–20% of the population throughout the year. The incidence of pharyngeal disease is highest in school-aged children (5–15 years of age), in the winter, in northern climates, and in settings of crowding and close contact. Person-to-person spread is by droplets from sneezing and coughing. Occasionally, a pet dog or contaminated food may be the source of infection. Streptococcal infection of the skin is most common in children under 6 years of age and during summer or in warmer climates, in which skin abrasions or insect bites become infected.

Clinical Manifestations. The incubation period of streptococcal pharyngitis is 2–5 days.

Respiratory Tract Infection. Streptococcal pharyngitis is associated with an acute sore throat with fever, headache, and tender anterior cervical lymph nodes. Occasionally, vomiting, abdominal pain, and rash may be present. The tonsils are hyperemic, edematous, and covered with exudate. The pharynx is inflamed and covered by a membrane in severe cases. The tongue may be edematous and reddened.

Scarlet Fever. Scarlet fever is caused by infection with group A streptococci, which elaborate an erythrogenic toxin associated with a characteristic rash appearing 24–48 hours after the onset of pharyngitis. The epidemiology, symptoms, sequelae, and treatment of scarlet fever are the same as those of streptococcal pharyngitis.

The exanthem is red, punctate, or finely papular. In some patients, it may be palpated more readily than it is seen, having the texture of coarse sandpaper (goose flesh). The rash first appears in the axillae, groin, and neck but within 24 hours becomes generalized. Areas of more intense erythema are noted in the creases of the fingers and groin and the antecubital fossae (Pastia lines). The face appears flushed, and there is circumoral pallor. The rash begins to fade 3–4 days after the onset; desquamation of fine flakes from the face and peeling of the palms and fingers may occur after 1 week. The tongue has a white coat through which the red and edematous papillae project (white strawberry tongue). After several days, the white coat desquamates; the red tongue with prominent papillae persists (red strawberry tongue).

Scarlet fever rarely may follow infection of wounds (surgical scarlet fever), burns, or streptococcal skin infection. Scarlet fever must be distinguished from measles, rubella, erythema infectiosum, infectious mononucleosis, enteroviral infections, roseola, severe sunburn, toxic shock syndrome, drug reactions, and Kawasaki disease.

Skin infections. The most common skin infection caused by group A beta-hemolytic streptococci is superficial pyoderma **(impetigo)**, which begins as a single papulovesicular lesion surrounded by erythema that later becomes one or many golden yellow–crusted, weeping lesions. Fever and systemic signs other than regional lymphadenopathy are uncommon. Acute poststreptococcal glomerulonephritis may follow impetigo despite adequate treatment (see Chapter 16).

Erysipelas. Erysipelas is an acute cellulitis and lymphangitis of the skin with rapid progression to contiguous skin. The lesion is very erythematous and indurated; the margins have a raised, firm border. Lymphyangitis and regional lymphadenitis are common. Erysipelas is associated with fever, vomiting, toxicity, and irritability; progression to bacteremia or abscesses is common. Cellulitis caused by *S. aureus* is characterized by diffuse, brawny edema without discrete margins, whereas that caused by *H. influenzae* appears purple and is usually located on the face.

Bacteremia. Streptococcal bacteremia may follow streptococcal disease of the skin, respiratory tract, rectum, or vagina and has been noted without an obvious focus. DIC, shock, and peripheral gangrene can occur. Hematogenous dissemination may result in meningitis, osteomyelitis, arthritis, soft tissue abscesses, pneumonia, or endocarditis.

Necrotizing Fasciitis. Group A streptococcal infection of deep subcutaneous tissues can spread rapidly along tissue planes, causing necrosis. This may be a complication of infected varicella lesions or of a surgical wound. Fever, severe pain, marked leukocytosis, and elevated creatine phosphokinase levels help make the diagnosis. A compartment syndrome may develop. Mortality and morbidity are high, with a 10% fatality rate. Extensive débridement and excision of necrotic and gangrenous tissue are essential. Varicella vaccination should prevent many of these cases.

Streptococcal toxic shock syndrome manifests as hypotension, multisystem organ dysfunction, and musculoskeletal complaints, with or without an erythematous macular rash. It may occur after streptococcal superinfection of varicella lesions. Bacteremia resulting from a virulent pyrogenic exotoxin A–producing group A streptococcus is present in many cases. This syndrome is associated with a high mortality.

Vaginitis. Group A streptococci are a common cause of vaginitis in prepubertal girls. There usually are a serous discharge, marked erythema, and irritation of the vulvar area, accompanied by discomfort on walking and on urination. Proctitis is rare but may be seen in either sex.

Diagnosis. The diagnosis of streptococcal infection should be established by isolating organisms from throat, skin, or blood or by rapid diagnostic tests that are specific for the group A antigen. If results of such tests are positive, a throat culture is not necessary; if they are negative, a throat culture is warranted. The immunologic response to streptococcal antigen can be assessed by measuring titers to antistreptolysin O (ASO), antideoxyribonuclease B (the best serologic test for pyoderma), and antihyaluronidase (elevated with less regularity than ASO titers). Unfortunately they are of no value in the immediate diagnosis and management of acute streptococcal infection. Throat swabs incubated on blood agar demonstrate a zone of hemolysis, with growth inhibited by bacitracin, which typically inhibits only group A streptococci.

The *differential diagnosis* of acute pharyngitis includes infectious mononucleosis, acute HIV infection, HSV, adenovirus, diphtheria, *Arcanobacterium haemolyticum,* tularemia, toxoplasmosis, and, rarely, aplastic anemia. Pharyngitis and scarlatiniform rash in adolescents may be caused by *A. haemolyticum.* Streptococcal pyoderma and cellulitis must be differentiated from staphylococcal skin disease. Bullous impetigo is usually staphylococcal, whereas the golden crusted lesions are caused by streptococci.

Complications. Complications are the result of extension of local infection from the nasopharynx, which results in sinusitis, otitis media, mastoiditis, cervical adenitis, retropharyngeal and peritonsillar abscess, or bronchopneumonia. Hematogenous dissemination of streptococci may cause meningitis, osteomyelitis, or septic arthritis. Nonsuppurative complications include rheumatic fever (see Chapter 13) and acute glomerulonephritis (see Chapter 16).

Treatment and Prevention. Penicillin is the treatment of choice for most streptococcal infections, although many prefer clindamycin for infections associated with toxin production or necrotizing fasciitis. Clindamycin inhibits protein (toxin) synthesis. If the patient is allergic to penicillin, erythromycin or clindamycin is used. Penicillin failures in the treatment of pharyngitis are often attributed to local destruction of the drug by β-lactamase–producing commensal flora. Affected patients often respond to another course of therapy, including a β-lactamase inhibitor (amoxicillin/clavulanate) or clindamycin. Impetigo is treated locally with mupirocin or with oral erythromycin.

Treatment of group A streptococcal pharyngitis is effective in preventing rheumatic heart disease. Administration of daily oral or monthly intramuscular, long-acting penicillin in patients with an episode of rheumatic fever prevents most cases of streptococcal disease and recurrent illness. Treatment with antibiotics does not prevent poststreptococcal glomerulonephritis, but recurrent episodes are rare. Patients treated with penicillin for pharyngitis may be considered noncontagious within 48 hours of therapy.

REFERENCES

Ayoub E, Ahmed S: Update on complications of group A streptococcal infections, *Curr Probl Pediatr* 27:90, 1997.

Behrman RE, Kliegman RM, Jenson HB, editors: *Nelson textbook of pediatrics*, ed 15, Philadelphia, 2000, WB Saunders, Chapter 184.

Laupland KB, Davies HD, Low De, et al: Ontario Group A Streptococcal Study Group: invasive group A streptococcal disease in children and association with varicella-zoster virus infection, *Pediatrics* 105:E60, 2000.

Zimbelman J, Palmer A, Todd J: Improved outcome of clindamycin compared with beta-lactam antibiotic treatment for invasive *Streptococcus pyogenes* infection, *Pediatr Infect Dis J* 18:1096–1100, 1999.

Infections Caused by Pseudomonas Aeruginosa

Etiology. *P. aeruginosa* are ubiquitous organisms that thrive in any moist environment (e.g., sinks, water fountains, plants, puddles, and hospitals). They are motile, gram-negative rods that do not ferment sugars but are oxidase positive. Although generally considered aerobes, they can use nitrite as a terminal electron acceptor and grow in anaerobic environments.

Epidemiology. *P. aeruginosa* rarely infects normal hosts but is a common cause of serious infection in immunocompromised patients, as a nosocomial pathogen, and as the major cause of pulmonary infection in patients with cystic fibrosis. In normal hosts it can be associated with superficial infections such as otitis externa (swimmer's ear), folliculitis associated with hot tubs, keratitis associated with contact lenses, and osteomyelitis caused by a puncture wound acquired through *Pseudomonas*-contaminated sneakers. It has been associated with primary pneumonias in HIV-infected infants.

P. aeruginosa can develop resistance to most antimicrobial agents. Thus it is often selected out following therapy for more susceptible bacterial infections. It expresses a number of virulence factors, including enzymes to destroy host tissues such as phospholipases, proteases, and ADP ribosylating enzymes that stop host protein synthesis (exotoxin A and exoenzymes S and T), pili to facilitate mucosal attachment, and an extracellular polysaccharide that inhibits phagocytosis (pathognomic for strains isolated from cystic fibrosis patients).

Clinical Manifestations

Superficial Infections. *P. aeruginosa* is a common cause of otitis externa, which develops when there is moisture and trauma to the external auditory canal that enables the organisms to attach and stimulate inflammation. Similarly, *P. aeruginosa* folliculitis develops after immersion in improperly disinfected hot tubs, where the organisms proliferate and are able to establish infection through microabrasions or small defects in the normal epidermis. Although highly resistant to many antimicrobial agents, in the normal host these infections often respond to topical therapy. *P. aeruginosa* can also cause superificial infections in burns; these infections can progress rapidly and necessitate débridement, as well as parenteral and topical therapy.

Pulmonary Infection. Patients with cystic fibrosis are at high risk for the development of airway infection, first with environmental strains of *P. aeruginosa*, followed by the selection of mucoid strains that express mucoexopolysaccharide. Several factors have been implicated in the pathogenesis, including a diminished clearance of the organisms from the airway because of defective killing by innate mechanisms, poor physical clearance resulting from mucous plugs and dehydrated mucins, and increased adherence of *P. aeruginosa* to CF cells, which stimulates an excessive inflammatory response. Infection is intermittent at first, followed by chronic colonization that leads to deterioration of pulmonary infection.

Infection in the Compromised Host. *P. aeruginosa* is not usually a part of the commensal flora, but in hospitalized patients it is often selected out by antibiotic therapy to which other organisms are more suscep-

tible. In neutropenic patients, often with chemotherapy-induced disruption of their mucosal integrity or colonization of intravascular catheters, bacteremia and sepsis develop. Ecthyma gangrenosum associated with *P. aeruginosa* sepsis represents peripheral cutaneous infections characterized by tissue necrosis. Patients with endotracheal tubes may become colonized with *P. aeruginosa* and aspirate the organisms causing pneumonia. *P. aeruginosa* is a cause of urinary tract infection, usually in a hospital setting in a patient who has had a urinary catheter and often has had previous antibiotic therapy.

Treatment. The selection of drugs is based on the specific susceptibility pattern of the infecting organism and the pharmokinetic properties of the possible drugs. For sepsis, usually two agents such as a beta-lactam and an aminoglycoside (an anti-*Pseudomonas* penicillin such as piperacillin/tazobactam or ceftazidime and tobramycin) are given either to achieve a potentially synergistic combination or in anticipation of the development of resistance. Carbapenems and ciprofloxacin also have anti–*P. aeruginosa* activity. Although these organisms express an inducible chromosomal beta-lactamase, they also have potent efflux systems that pump many antimicrobial agents out of the cell. In cystic fibrosis, usually two anti-*Pseudomonas* agents are used for acute exacerbations of pulmonary infection. In affected patients with cystic fibrosis, tobramycin is often given by aerosolization, with good results.

REFERENCES

Berhman RE, Kliegman RM, Jenson HB: *Nelson textbook of pediatrics*, ed 16, Philadelphia, 2000, WB Saunders, Chapter 203.

Chatzinikolaou I, Abi-Said D, Bodey GP, et al: Recent experience with *Pseudomonas aeruginosa* bacteremia in patients with cancer: retrospective analysis of 245 episodes, *Arch Intern Med* 160:501–509, 2000.

Foca M, Jakob K, Whittier S, et al: Endemic *Pseudomonas aeruginosa* infection in a neonatal intensive care unit, *N Engl J Med* 343:695–700, 2000.

Infections Caused by Escherichia Coli

Etiology. *E. coli* are the predominant aerobic intestinal gram-negative bacteria in the gut and are versatile both as commensal flora and as pathogens. *E. coli* are facultative anaerobes that are motile, lactose fermenters. The expression of a K1 capsule is associated with virulence.

Epidemiology. *E. coli* cause disease when they either acquire or activate the expression of specific virulence factors that enable them to become invasive, or interact with host structures to activate inflammation. *E. coli* associated with diarrheal disease express specific pili or fimbriae that facilitate bacterial attachment to epithelial surfaces, and express specific toxins that activate cAMP or cGMP to cause diarrhea or stimulate cytokine responses associated with urinary tract infection. Alternatively, commensal E. coli cause disease when normal mucosal defenses are broached and the organisms contaminate normally sterile sites, such as the blood or central nervous system. This occurs during the mucositis that accompanies chemotherapy for malignancies providing a route for E. coli translocations from the gut to cause sepsis, or occurs in neonates who are contaminated with E. coli at the time of delivery and in whom sepsis and meningitis develop because of specific encapsulated types of bacteria that are inefficiently phagocytosed.

Clinical Manifestations

Bacteremia and Sepsis. E. coli are frequently associated with neonatal sepsis and meningitis, in infants born to mothers with prolonged rupture of membranes or presumably contaminated at delivery. The E. coli that cause sepsis in neonates frequently express the K1 polysaccharide on their surfaces, which thwarts effective phagocytosis. The polysaccharaide mimics normal host glycoconjugates that are heavily sialylated, thus evading the activations of normal immune surveillance mechanisms. In addition, many E. coli associated with neonatal meningitis express fimbriae that adhere to the vascular endothelium and to brain cells. As a gram-negative organism, E. coli LPS activates T cells and macrophages to cause the many physiologic consequences of gram-negative sepsis and the sepsis syndrome, causing hypotension, generalized vasodilatation, DIC, and pulmonary edema. The use of ampicillin prophylaxis to prevent group B streptococcal disease in neonates may increase the prevalence of E. coli as a major cause of sepsis, pneumonia, and meningitis in the newborn. Treatment of E. coli sepsis includes ampicillin or cefotaxime and an aminoglycoside. The treatment of E. coli meningitis includes cefotaxime and ampicillin. There is an incidence of ampicillin resistance; therefore, sensitivities must be determined.

Diarrheal Disease. E. coli can acquire specific genes to cause diarrhea. These include the genes for pili to allow attachment. Several proteins that direct the injection of toxins directly into the host epithelial cells through the type III secretion apparatus are also expressed. These enteropathogenic E. coli (EPEC) bind closely to mucosal cells and stimulate the reassembly of host cytoskeletal components, producing an "attaching-effacing" lesion. Disruption of normal cellular absorption and secretory processes leads to diarrhea. This is a self-limited process in well-nourished patients; it is a major cause of diarrhea and a significant cause of infant mortality in developing nations.

Acquisition of the Shiga or Shiga-like toxin by E. coli leads to the toxigenic organisms that cause hemolytic-uremic syndrome. The prototype are the E. coli O157:H7 (although Shiga-like toxin produc-

tion is not limited to this serotype), which has been associated with contaminated food, including unpasteurized apple juice, water, and especially improperly cooked beef distributed to fast-food restaurants. These organisms are associated with a self-limited form of gastroenteritis, usually with bloody diarrhea. However, the production of this toxin, which blocks host cell protein synthesis, affects vascular endothelial cells and the glomeruli and leads to a microangiopathic hemolytic anemia, thrombocytopenia, and renal failure typical of HUS. Although HUS develops in only a few (less than 15%) of children with EHEC, mortality is approximately 5%; a fraction of affected children have chronic renal failure. It is important to note that the incidence of HUS is higher in children who received antimicrobial agents.

Traveler's Diarrhea. E. coli (ETEC) can also produce a heat-labile toxin that has properties similar to that of cholera toxin. After pili-mediated attachment, the organisms secrete toxins that activate epithelial cAMP. Enteroinvasive E. coli produces disease similar to the shigellae.

Urinary Tract Infection. E. coli is the major cause of urinary tract infections both in young infants with possible urogenital structural abnormalities and in sexually active adolescent females. The organisms express pili or fimbriae that bind to specific carbohydrate receptors on either the bladder epithelium or the cells lining the upper tracts. Bacterial attachment activates host cell cytokine production and initiates a PMN reponse. In addition, some of these organisms may be internalized into bladder epithelial cells, forming a nidus for recurrent infection. The intracellular bacteria are generally protected from many of the antimicrobial agents used to treat urinary tract infections and from antibody and other types of mucosal surface defenses.

REFERENCES

Behrman RE, Kliegman RM, Jenson HB, editors: *Nelson textbook of pediatrics*, ed 16, Philadelphia, 2000, WB Saunders, Chapter 198.

Mulvey MA, Schilling JD, Martinez JJ, et al: From the cover: bad bugs and beleaguered bladders: interplay between uropathogenic *Escherichia coli* and innate host defenses, *Proc Natl Acad Sci* 97:8829–8835, 2000.

Vallance BA, Finlay BB: Exploitation of host cells by enteropathogenic *Escherichia coli*, *Proc Natl Acad Sci* 97(16):8799–8806, 2000.

Wong CS, Jelacic S, Habeeb RL, et al: The risk of the hemolytic-uremic syndrome after antibiotic treatment of *Escherichia coli* O157:H7 infections, *N Engl J Med* 342(26):1930–1936, 2000.

Campylobacter Infections

Etiology and Epidemiology. Campylobacter are motile, gram-negative rods that commonly infect humans and animals, causing diarrheal disease and sepsis in immunocompromised patients. *Campy-*

lobacter jejuni are considered microaerophilic and grow best at 42° C. They are commonly isolated from wild and domestic animals, including sheep, cattle, goats, dogs, and fowl. *C. fetus* is more commonly associated with sepsis in immunocompromised hosts. In the United States, Campylobacter has been isolated as frequently as either salmonellae or shigellae.

Clinical Manifestations. *C. jejuni* produces gastroenteritis indistinguishable from that of other enteric bacterial pathogens. There is often a prodrome of fever, headache, and malaise, followed by abdominal pain and diarrhea. Disease is typically a colitis, associated with local inflammation and bleeding. The illness is often self-limited, lasting approximately 1 week, but occasionally longer. Diarrhea may be watery or frankly bloody.

Campylobacter fetus is more typically associated with sepsis. This organism has a superficial S-protein layer that acts like a capsule to impede the attachment of complement and evade phagocytosis.

Treatment. Erythromycin and azithromycin and the fluoroquinolones shorten the duration of illness when given early. Parenteral therapy for patients with bacteremia should be based on the susceptibilities of the specific isolate, which is usually susceptible to carbapenems (imipenem and meropenem) and aminoglycosides.

Yersinia Enterocolitica and *Yersinia Pseudotuberculosis* Infections

Etiology. *Y. enterocolitica* and *Y. pseudotuberculosis* are oxidase-negative, gram-negative bacilli. *Y. enterocolitica* has 35 serotypes, and *Y. pseudotuberculosis* has five.

Epidemiology. The sources of the organisms include wild and domestic animals, milk, chitterlings, oysters, and water supplies. Common source infections after ingestion of contaminated foods have been reported. Infection from dogs and human-to-human spread occur. Infants and children appear most susceptible. The incubation period varies from 1–3 weeks.

Clinical Manifestations. *Y. enterocolitica* commonly is associated with enteritis and enterocolitis, which mimic inflammatory bowel disease and become manifest as fever and bloody diarrhea with mucus and abdominal pain. Young infants may have a nonspecific gastroenteritis or dysentery-like disease. Other manifestations are acute mesenteric adenitis, pharyngitis, hepatosplenic abscesses, arthritis, osteomyelitis, hepatitis, carditis, meningitis, Reiter syndrome, septicemia, and erythema nodosum. Septicemia has been associated with iron intoxication and has occurred after accidental overdose of oral iron in previously healthy children. Treatment with desferoxamine, an iron siderophore that chelates iron in hypertransfused patients with chronic anemia or iron intoxication, is associated with an increased risk of infection. Mesenteric adenitis typically affects older children and adolescents; the severe abdominal pain may simulate appendicitis. The duration of the illness generally is 2–3 weeks without treatment, but occasionally diarrhea may persist for several months and simulate inflammatory bowel disease.

Y. pseudotuberculosis has been associated with mesenteric adenitis and terminal ileitis. Abdominal pain may be severe and may suggest acute appendicitis. Septicemia is unusual; other findings are diarrhea and erythema nodosum.

Diagnosis. The diagnosis may be established by identifying the organism in stool, mesenteric lymph nodes, bowel mucosa at endoscopy, peritoneal fluid, or blood. Because identification requires special techniques, laboratory personnel should be notified.

Treatment. Most strains of *Y. enterocolitica* and *Y. pseudotuberculosis* are susceptible to trimethoprim/ sulfamethoxazole, aminoglycosides, cefotaxime, and ceftazidime. Patients with septicemia or sites of infection outside the gastrointestinal tract should receive therapy. Parenteral ceftriaxone or cefotaxime has been used successfully as a single agent or with an aminoglycoside. The benefits of treating patients with enterocolitis or mesenteric adenitis are unknown (see Appendix I).

REFERENCES

Abdel-Haq NM, Asmar BL, Abuhammour WM, et al: *Yersinia enterocolitica* infection in children, *Pediatr Infect Dis J* 19:954–958, 2000.
Ackers ML, Schoenfeld S, Markman J, et al: An outbreak of *Yersinia enterocolitica* O:8 infections associated with pasteurized milk, *J Infect Dis* 181:1834–1837, 2000.
Behrman RE, Kliegman RM, Jenson HB, editors: *Nelson textbook of pediatrics*, ed 16, Philadelphia, 2000, WB Saunders, Chapter 201.

Spirochetal Infections
Syphilis

Etiology. Syphilis is caused by *Treponema pallidum*, a long, slender, coiled spirochete. It cannot routinely be cultivated in vitro but can be seen by darkfield microscopy.

Epidemiology. Syphilis is acquired through sexual contact, transplacentally from an infected mother to her fetus and, less commonly, at birth, in the postpartum period, or by infected blood. Infants with congenital syphilis often are born to women who are HIV positive or are drug abusers. Isolated outbreaks have been reported. Infection in males is 3 times more common than in females. Sexual abuse should be considered in young children who have acquired syphilis. The incubation period for primary syphilis is 10–90 days after exposure.

Clinical Manifestations

Congenital Syphilis. Early manifestations occurring between birth and the first year of life are fever, anemia, failure to thrive, irritability, local mucocutaneous lesions (e.g., maculopapular rash on trunk, palms, and soles; condylomata lata; bullous eruptions), persistent rhinitis (snuffles), hepatosplenomegaly, lymphadenopathy, dactylitis, and pseudoparalysis resulting from osteochondritis. *Laboratory evaluation* may show direct hyperbilirubinemia, elevated liver function tests, multiple sites of osteochondritis, CSF pleocytosis, thrombocytopenia, Coombs-negative hemolytic anemia, and leukocytosis.

The moist secretions of early congenital syphilis are highly contagious. In an untreated pregnant woman, syphilis may be transmitted to the fetus at any time; however, transmission to the fetus is more common during the first year after syphilis has been acquired by the mother. Although some newborns demonstrate symptoms of the disease within the first 4–8 weeks after birth, many infants are symptomatic at birth and exhibit nonimmune hydrops with anemia; thrombocytopenia; leukopenia; pneumonia; hepatitis, with or without nephrosis; and osteochondritis.

Late congenital syphilis appears many years after birth and becomes manifest as multiple bone signs (frontal bossing or saber shins), Hutchinson teeth (peg or screw-like), mulberry molars, a saddle-nose deformity, rhagades (perioral linear scars), juvenile paresis, juvenile tabes, interstitial keratitis, eighth nerve deafness, and Clutton joints (painless joint effusions). These manifestations are all rare in the modern era, in which penicillin therapy is used to control congenital syphilis.

Acquired Primary Syphilis. Three to 6 weeks after inoculation, a single painless papule appears, becomes indurated, and progresses to a painless ulcer (chancre). This ulcer usually is found on the genitalia but may appear at any other site of inoculation.

Secondary Syphilis. An influenza-like illness occurs 6–8 weeks after the primary chancre, with generalized adenopathy and a generalized erythematous, maculopapular rash, which is present on the palms and soles. Plaque-like skin lesions (condylomata lata) and mucous membrane lesions also occur and are all infectious. Other manifestations of secondary syphilis that may be present are meningitis, hepatitis, glomerulonephritis, bursitis, and periostitis.

Other Types of Syphilis. *Latent* syphilis has no clinical manifestations, but a history of untreated syphilis and serologic evidence of infection may be discovered. *Late* syphilis, a slowly progressive disease typically involving the CNS and heart, is not seen in children.

Diagnosis. Serologic tests for syphilis include the nontreponemal reagin antibody tests, which are directed against a poorly characterized lipoidal antigen. These tests include (1) the Venereal Disease Research Laboratory (VDRL) test, (2) a rapid plasma reagin (RPR) test, and (3) an automated reagin test (ART). The specific test is the fluorescent treponemal antibody–absorption (FTA-ABS) test. The specific test is less likely to be falsely reactive in collagen-vascular disease, pregnancy, drug addiction, malaria, Lyme disease, infectious mononucleosis, and other infectious diseases ("biologic false-positive tests") than the nontreponemal tests. The serologic tests are uniformly positive in secondary and later stages of syphilis. The VDRL test becomes positive within 4–6 weeks after infection. Treatment results in declining titers of the VDRL test, RPR test, and ART, but not the FTA-ABS test.

In the process of identifying congenital syphilis, maternal transplacentally passed antibody often confuses the diagnosis. It is frequently difficult to determine whether the infant has only passive acquisition of antibody. This is particularly true in HIV-infected patients, who may have absent or exaggerated antibody responses. Positive CSF VDRL or RPR tests warrant therapy for CNS syphilis in congenital or acquired disease. Darkfield examination of chancres, mucous membranes, or cutaneous lesions may reveal motile organisms.

Treatment. *T. pallidum* is extremely sensitive to penicillin, which remains the drug of choice for therapy of all forms of syphilis. Primary, secondary, and early latent syphilis are treated with a single dose of benzathine penicillin; all other types necessitate multiple doses (e.g., neurosyphilis, tertiary, or late latent). Alternative therapy includes tetracycline or erythromycin; however, neither is recommended during pregnancy, and if the patient is allergic, penicillin desensitization is preferred. Dosage regimens vary according to stage of disease and the presence of neurologic involvement and congenital infection. Neonates must be treated with regimens to provide effective concentrations of penicillin in the CNS. Current regimens for therapy of gonorrhea also effectively treat incubating syphilis. Exposure to a documented case of syphilis warrants "prophylactic" therapy and serologic follow-up. A pregnant woman with documented or possible syphilis should be treated with penicillin to prevent illness in the mother and her offspring. HIV-infected patients with evidence of syphilis should have a lumbar puncture to determine whether CNS infection is present, which necessitates more prolonged therapy. A systemic, febrile reaction (*Jarisch-Herxheimer reaction*) occurs in 15–20% of syphilitic patients treated with penicillin. Patients with syphilis who also have AIDS may require prolonged therapy. Health care providers should be aware that patients are often infected with multiple sexually transmitted pathogens. Patients being evaluated for syphilis should also be screened for HIV, gonorrhea, chlamydia, and if appropriate, human papilloma virus.

REFERENCES

Azimi PH, Janner D, Berne P, et al: Concentrations of procaine and aqueous penicillin in the cerebrospinal fluid of infants treated for congenital syphilis, *J Pediatr* 124:64, 1994.

Behrman RE, Kliegman RM, Jenson HB, editors: *Nelson textbook of pediatrics*, ed 16, Philadelphia, 2000, WB Saunders, Chapter 215.

Dorfman DH, Glaser JH: Congenital syphilis presenting in infants after the newborn period, *N Engl J Med* 323:1299, 1990.

Hook EW III, Marra CM: Acquired syphilis in adults, *N Engl J Med* 326:1060, 1992.

Mobley JA, McKeown RE, Jackson KL, et al: Risk factors for congenital syphilis in infants of women with syphilis in South Carolina, *Am J Public Health* 88:597–602, 1998.

Borrelia Burgdorferi Infection

(Lyme Disease)

Etiology. Lyme disease is a tick-borne illness caused by a fastidious spirochete, *B. burgdorferi.* Ticks of the *Ixodes* genus and possibly other blood-sucking insects feed off animal reservoirs, such as the white-footed mouse, the deer, and the dog.

Epidemiology. Lyme disease has been reported in 49 states; 92% of reported cases were from northeastern and mid-Atlantic states, as well as Minnesota and Wisconsin. The predominant vector is *I. dammini* in the East and Midwest and *I. pacificus* in the West. In Europe, Lyme disease may be atypical relative to the clinical presentation in the United States and may be associated with other ticks. Because exposure to ticks is more common in warm months, Lyme disease is noted predominantly in summer.

Clinical Manifestations

Stage 1: Early Infection (Local Disease). Although not all patients recall a tick bite, the typical pattern of disease evolves from this bite. Seven to 14 days after a tick bite, the site forms an erythematous papule that expands to form a red, raised border and a clear center. Multiple rings may form, and new areas of this annular lesion may appear distal to the original site. The lesion, *erythema chronicum migrans,* may be 15 cm wide, may be pruritic or painful, and may contain *B. burgdorferi* organisms. This skin lesion is not present in all patients. The lesions fade within 1 month. During this early stage, systemic manifestations include malaise, lethargy, fever, headache, arthralgias, stiff neck, myalgias, and lymphadenopathy. All of these early manifestations resolve without treatment in 1 month.

Stage 2: Early Infection (Disseminated Disease). Cardiac manifestations occur within 5 weeks and include myocarditis, atrioventricular node block (occasionally requiring external pacemakers), ST depression, and T wave inversion. Cardiac disease is serious, present in approximately 10% of patients, and reversible.

Neurologic manifestations occur within 4 weeks and include lymphocytic "aseptic" meningitis, encephalitis, papilledema, cranial neuritis (Bell palsy of nerve VII), pseudotumor, polyradiculitis, peripheral neuropathy, mononeuritis multiplex, or transverse myelitis. Neurologic manifestations usually resolve by 3 months but may recur or become chronic.

Stage 3: Persistent Infection. Arthritis may develop in 50–60% of patients within weeks to years of the tick bite. Intermittent arthritis also is noted in stage 2 and may be monoarticular, pauciarticular, or polyarticular, resembling JRA. The knee, shoulder, elbow, and, rarely, the small joints of the hands are involved. Chronic erosive arthritis may persist in 10% of patients, with involvement of the knee more than other joints. The male-to-female ratio is 7:1. Popliteal cysts may develop, and joint fluid is typically inflammatory, with leukocytic predominance and a total WBC count between 500 and 100,000 cells/L (Table 10–10). These patients are negative for rheumatoid factor and antinuclear antibody (ANA).

Diagnosis. A history of a tick bite and the classic rash are helpful but not present in all cases. The ESR is elevated, and complement may be reduced in patients with arthritis. The VDRL test may be falsely positive. Cryoglobulins and circulating immune complexes may precede or coincide with arthritis. CSF reveals a lymphocytic pleocytosis with normal glucose levels and slightly raised protein levels. Demonstration of intrathecal production of antibodies is confirmatory.

The diagnosis is confirmed by serologic tests specific for *B. burgdorferi.* Because of high false-positive rates, the ELISA must be confirmed by a Western blot. The *differential diagnoses* are many and relate to the organ involved, as discussed under aseptic meningitis, arthritis, and myocarditis. In children, JRA must be considered (see Chapter 9).

Treatment. Stage 1 disease, especially erythema chronicum migrans, may be treated with oral amoxicillin or, in older children, doxycycline for 2–3 weeks. Jarisch-Herxheimer reaction has been seen during the first 24 hours of therapy. Early treatment may prevent carditis and meningitis. Stages 2 and 3 usually are treated with high-dose parenteral ceftriaxone (75–100 mg/kg/24 hr; max. 2 g) or penicillin G (300,000 U/kg/24 hr, max. 20 million U/24 hr) for 2–3 weeks, if severe complications are present. The great majority of cases resolve without sequelae, particularly those treated early.

Prevention. An OspA Lyme vaccine has been licensed by the FDA for individuals 15–70 years of age. This vaccine is based on antibody-mediated killing of the spirochete in the tick (OspA is not expressed in humans). As transmission of *B. burgdoferi* from infected ticks is thought to involve prolonged (more than 36 hours) attachment, human antibody interacts with the spirochetes within the tick. Reported antibody titers in children ages 2–5 appear excellent; however, the efficacy of the vaccine is variable, and the longevity of the antibody response is not known. Most clinicians prefer to rely upon general methods to prevent tick-borne infections in endemic areas. Recent studies suggest that a single dose of doxycycline given within 72 hours of a documented *Ixodes scapularis* tick bite can prevent the development of Lyme disease.

REFERENCES

Behrman RE, Kliegman RM, Jenson HB, editors: *Nelson textbook of pediatrics,* ed 16, Philadelphia, 2000, WB Saunders, Chapter 219.

Gerber MA, Shapiro E, Burke G, et al: Lyme disease in children in southeastern Connecticut, *N Engl J Med* 335:1270–1274, 1996.

Nadelman RB et al: Prophylaxis with single-dose doxycycline for prevention of Lyme disease after an *Ixodes scapularis* tick bite, *N Engl J Med* 345:79–84, 2001.

Orloski KA, Hayes EB, Campbell GL, et al: Surveillance for Lyme disease: Unites States, 1992-1998, MMWR 49(3):1–11, 2000.

Seltzer EG, Gerber MA, Carter ML, et al: Long-term outcomes of persons with Lyme disease, *JAMA* 283:609–616, 2000.

Szer IS, Taylor E, Steere AC: The long-term course of Lyme arthritis in children, *N Engl J Med* 325:159–163, 1991.

Wormser GP, Nadelman RB, Dattwyler RJ, et al: Practice guidelines for the treatment of Lyme disease, *Clin Infect Dis* 31:S1–S14, 2000.

Chlamydial Infection

Etiology. Chlamydiae are obligate intracellular bacteria that contain DNA and RNA. Infected cells contain cytoplasmic Giemsa stain–positive inclusions.

Chlamydia Trachomatis Infection

Chlamydia trachomatis is one of three species associated with human disease. There are many serologically distinct serovars of *C. trachomatis* associated with specific infections: the common oculogenital infections, trachoma, and lymphogranuloma venereum.

The organisms have a biphasic life cycle, existing as relatively inert elementary bodies in their extracellular form, and as reticulate bodies when phagocytosed and replicating within a phagosome. Reticulate bodies divide by binary fission and after 48–72 hours of intracellular infection have reorganized into elementary bodies that can be released from the cell. These organisms can infect nonciliated squamocolumnar cells or the transitional epithelial cells that line the mucosa of the conjunctivae, urethra, cervix, and rectum.

Epidemiology. *C. trachomatis* causes infection in neonates (conjunctivitis and pneumonia); oculogenital infection, lymphogranuloma venereum, and ocular trachoma. Conjunctivitis is seen in the neonate of an infected mother and appears from 3 days to 6 weeks after delivery; it must be distinguished from gonococcal and chemical conjunctivitis. Residual eye damage is rare. Trachoma is a chronic follicular keratoconjunctivitis resulting from repeated infections and eventually leads to blindness resulting from extensive local scarring and inflammation.

Pneumonia caused by *C. trachomatis* typically occurs in infants 4–12 weeks of age and presents with tachypnea, cough, and rales in an afebrile infant, often with a history of conjunctivitis. Confirmatory laboratory data would be a chest film demonstrating hyperinflation and symmetric interstitial infiltrates, eosinophilia, and elevated immunoglobulins. This syndrome must be differentiated from RSV infection, in which wheezing is predominant, *Ureaplasma*, and other viral infections.

Genital infection associated with *C. trachomatis* is common, found in up to 50% of males and females, with symptoms of pelvic cervicitis, pelvic inflammatory disease, urethritis, or epididymitis. It may produce tubal infertility. *Chlamydia* infection may be associated with premature birth. Infants born to infected mothers are culture positive in at least one site in 50% of cases; asymptomatic colonization may persist for months. Lymphogranuloma venereum is endemic in tropical areas but rare in the United States. It is manifested primarily as lymphadenitis at the site of the original infection.

Clinical Manifestations. *Conjunctivitis* caused by *Chlamydia* in the neonate may appear from 3 days to 6 weeks after delivery, but it usually occurs in the second week of life. The eyes are inflamed, with purulent discharge issuing from one or both eyes. Recurrences can occur even with appropriate therapy, but residual eye damage is rare. **Trachoma** is a chronic follicular keratoconjunctivitis resulting from repeated infection and may result in blindness in older children or adults because of extensive local scarring and inflammation.

Pneumonitis develops at 3–10 weeks of age. The child generally appears well and is afebrile, but has tachypnea and a cough. Apnea also may occur. One half of affected patients have concomitant conjunctivitis. Examination reveals rales and wheezing. Roentgenograms of the chest reveal hyperinflation and diffuse interstitial or patchy infiltrates. Mild eosinophilia (about 400/L), hypergammaglobulinemia, and mild hypoxemia are common. The illness is self-limiting but may last for weeks.

As a cause of genital infection, males often have dysuria and a mucopurulent discharge, although many (approximately 25%) may be asymptomatic. Women are more often asymptomatic (approximately 70%) or may have minimal symptoms, including dysuria, mild abdominal pain, or a vaginal discharge. Prepubertal girls may have vaginitis; conjunctival infection occurs in both sexes.

Diagnosis. *Chlamydia* can be grown in tissue culture; this remains the standard procedure. Many non-culture assay systems are under development, and several molecular techniques appear to be more sensitive than culture, such as a ligase chain reaction performed on urine. Fluorescent antibody testing is available, as are DNA probes and PCR techniques.

Conjunctivitis must be differentiated from inflammation (red eye) caused by silver nitrate (chemical), gonococcal infection, or viral infection (Table 10–16).

The adenopathy of LGV must be differentiated from that caused by cat-scratch disease, pyogenic bacteria, chancroid, granuloma inguinale, syphilis, HSV, and neoplasms. Examination of the node may reveal inclusions using Giemsa stain. Chlamydial cultures may be positive. Serology usually is diagnostic.

Treatment. Although topical therapy of conjunctivitis using sulfonamides is effective, oral erythromycin or sulfisoxazole also should be administered to treat either conjunctivitis (to eradicate the nasopharyngeal colonization and risk of subsequent pneumonitis) or pneumonitis. Prophylactic therapy of the infected mother and her sexual partner can decrease the rate of infection in the newborn. For uncomplicated genital tract infection caused by *C. trachomatis* in adolescents and adults, doxycycline,

TABLE 10–16
The Red Eye

Condition	Etiology	Signs and Symptoms	Treatment
Bacterial conjunctivitis	*Haemophilus influenzae, Haemophilus aegyptius, Streptococcus pneumoniae Neisseria gonorrhoeae*	Mucopurulent unilateral or bilateral discharge, normal vision, photophobia Conjunctival injection and edema (chemosis); gritty sensation	Topical antibiotics, parenteral ceftriaxone for gonococcus, *H. influenzae*
Viral conjunctivitis	Adenovirus, ECHO virus, coxsackievirus	As above; may be hemorrhagic, unilateral	Self-limited
Neonatal conjunctivitis	*Chlamydia trachomatis,* gonococcus, chemical (silver nitrate), *Staphylococcus aureus*	Palpebral conjunctival follicle or papillae; as above	Ceftriaxone for gonococcus and oral erythromycin for *C. trachomatis*
Allergic conjunctivitis	Seasonal pollens or allergen exposure	Itching, incidence of bilateral chemosis (edema) greater than that of erythema, tarsal papillae	Antihistamines, steroids, cromolyn
Keratitis	Herpes simplex, adenovirus, *S. pneumoniae, S. aureus, Pseudomonas, Acanthamoeba,* chemicals	Severe pain, corneal swelling, clouding, limbus erythema, hypopyon, cataracts; contact lens history with amebic infection	Specific antibiotics for bacterial/fungal infections; keratoplasty, acyclovir for herpes
Endophthalmitis	*S. aureus, S. pneumoniae, Candida albicans,* associated surgery or trauma	Acute onset, pain, loss of vision, swelling, chemosis, redness; hypopyon and vitreous haze	Antibiotics
Anterior uveitis (iridocyclitis)	JRA, Reiter syndrome, sarcoidosis, Behçet disease, inflammatory bowel disease	Unilateral/bilateral; erythema, ciliary flush, irregular pupil, iris adhesions; pain, photophobia, small pupil, poor vision	Topical steroids, plus therapy for primary disease

Data from *Am J Med* 79:545, 1985; *BMJ* 296:1720, 1988; *Lancet* 338:1498, 1991; *Pediatr Ann* 22:353, 1993.
CMV, Cytomegalovirus; *EBV,* Epstein-Barr virus; *JRA,* juvenile rheumatoid arthritis; *SLE,* systemic lupus erythematosus.

Continued

TABLE 10–16
The Red Eye—cont'd

Condition	Etiology	Signs and Symptoms	Treatment
Posterior uveitis (choroiditis)	Toxplasmosis, histoplasmosis, *Toxocara canis*	No signs of erythema, decreased vision	Specific therapy for pathogen
Episcleritis/scleritis	Idiopathic autoimmune disease (e.g., SLE, Henoch-Schönlein purpura)	Localized pain, intense erythema, unilateral; blood vessels bigger than in conjunctivitis; scleritis may cause globe perforation	Episcleritis is self-limiting; topical steroids for fast relief
Foreign body	Occupational or other exposure	Unilateral, red, gritty feeling; visible or microscopic size	Irrigation, removal; check for ulceration
Blepharitis	*S. aureus, Staphylococcus epidermidis*, seborrheic, blocked lacrimal duct; rarely molluscum contagiosum, *Phthirus pubis, Pediculus capitis*	Bilateral, irritation, itching, hyperemia, crusting, affecting lid margins	Topical antibiotics, warm compresses
Dacryocystitis	Obstructed lacrimal sac: *S. aureus, H. influenzae*, pneumococcus	Pain, tenderness, erythema and exudate in areas of lacrimal sac (inferomedial to inner canthus); tearing (epiphora); possible orbital cellulitis	Systemic, topical antibiotics; surgical drainage
Dacryoadenitis	*S. aureus, Streptococcus*, CMV, measles, EBV, enteroviruses; trauma, sarcoidosis, leukemia	Pain, tenderness, edema, erythema over gland area (upper temporal lid); fever, leukocytosis	Systemic antibiotics; drainage of orbital abscesses
Orbital cellulitis (postseptal cellulitis)	Paranasal sinusitis: *H. influenzae, S. aureus, S. pneumoniae*, streptococci Trauma: *S. aureus* Fungi: *Aspergillus, Mucor* spp. if immunodeficient	Rhinorrhea, chemosis, vision loss, painful extraocular motion, proptosis, ophthalmoplegia, fever, lid edema, leukocytosis	Systemic antibiotics, drainage of orbital abscesses
Periorbital cellulitis (preseptal cellulitis)	Trauma: *S. aureus*, streptococci Bacteremia: pneumococcus, streptococci, *H. influenzae*	Cutaneous erythema, warmth, normal vision, minimal involvement of orbit; fever, leukocytosis, toxic appearance	Systemic antibiotics

Data from *Am J Med* 79:545, 1985; *BMJ* 296:1720, 1988; *Lancet* 338:1498, 1991; *Pediatr Ann* 22:353, 1993.
CMV, Cytomegalovirus; *EBV*, Epstein-Barr virus; *JRA*, juvenile rheumatoid arthritis; *SLE*, systemic lupus erythematosus.

azithromycin, or ofloxacin is recommended. LGV is treated with tetracycline or sulfonamides (see Appendix I).

REFERENCES

Behrman RE, Kliegman RM, Jenson HB, editors: *Nelson textbook of pediatrics,* ed 16, Philadelphia, 2000, WB Saunders, Chapter 223.

Bell TA, Stamm WE, Pin Wang S, et al: Chronic *Chlamydia trachomatis* infections in infants, *JAMA* 267:400–402, 1992.

Brasfield DM, Stagno S, Whitley RJ, et al: Infant pneumonitis associated with cytomegalovirus, *Chlamydia, Pneumocystis,* and *Ureaplasma:* follow up, *Pediatrics* 79:76–83, 1987.

Martin DH, Mroczkowski TF, Dalu ZA, et al: A controlled trial of a single dose of azithromycin for the treatment of chlamydial urethritis and cervicitis, *N Engl J Med* 327:921–925, 1992.

Rettig PJ: Infection due to *Chlamydia trachomatis* from infancy to adolescence, *Pediatr Infect Dis* 5:449–457, 1986.

Chlamydia Pneumoniae Infection

C. pneumoniae is an important cause of respiratory disease in children and adults. Serologic studies demonstrate that primary infection usually occurs in school-aged children; reinfections during adulthood are common. Symptoms are indistinguishable from those of infection caused by *Mycoplasma;* pharyngitis, hoarseness, bronchitis, and pneumonia are commonly seen. Symptoms are generally mild but prolonged. *C. pneumoniae* has been associated with 6–10% of cases of pneumonia in adults. *C. pneumoniae* causes significant pulmonary disease in immunocompromised patients, particularly those receiving stem cell transplants.

There are data linking *C. pneumoniae* to the pathogenesis of atherosclerosis. In addition to serologic and epidemiologic studies, *C. pneumoniae* have been demonstrated in atherosclerotic plaques.

Treatment with erythromycins or with tetracyclines in older patients is recommended.

REFERENCES

Heinemann M, Kern WV, Bunjes D, et al: Severe *Chlamydia pneumoniae* infection in patients with neutropenia: case reports and literature review, *Clin Infect Dis* 31:181–184, 2000.

Kauppinen M, Saikku P: Pneumonia due to *Chlamydia pneumoniae:* prevalence, clinical features, diagnosis and treatment, *Clin Infect Dis* 21:S44–S52, 1995.

Mycoplasmal Infection

Etiology. Mycoplasmas are the smallest free-living organisms. They lack a cell wall and are distinct from bacteria but grow on artificial media and are not viruses. Pathogenic species of mycoplasmas include *M. pneumoniae* (pneumonia, systemic infection), *M. hominis* (genitourinary tract infection), and *Ureaplasma urealyticum* (genitourinary tract, neonatal pneumonia).

Epidemiology. M. pneumoniae is a major cause of illness in school-aged children and young adults. The organism is highly transmissible through person-to-person spread. Although pneumonia is uncommon before 4–5 years of age, serologic studies suggest it is associated with mild infections in young children. It is the main cause of pneumonia in school-age children. *M. pneumoniae* is estimated to cause one-half million cases of pneumonia and more than 11 million cases of tracheobronchitis in the United States annually. Illness occurs at irregular intervals, tending to begin in the fall with smoldering epidemics. Transmission is presumed to be by droplet spread from symptomatic patients. The incubation period is 2–3 weeks.

Clinical Manifestations. Onset of illness (atypical pneumonia) is gradual, with headache, malaise, fever, sore throat, and cough. Sputum production, rales, and pleural effusions are frequent. Severe pulmonary disease has been reported in children with sickle cell anemia. Other manifestations include skin eruptions (maculopapular rashes, urticaria, erythema nodosum, Stevens-Johnson syndrome), hemolytic anemia, thrombocytopenia, myocarditis, and pericarditis. Less commonly, there are neurologic manifestations, including meningoencephalitis, Guillain-Barré syndrome, and transverse myelitis. Confirmation of the diagnosis is demonstrated by an increase of specific IgM antibodies, using complement fixation or immuofluorescence techniques. Mycoplasma PCR is also useful.

Treatment. Erythromycin or doxycycline (in children over 10 years of age) is the drug of choice (see Appendix I).

REFERENCES

Behrman RE, Kliegman RM, Jenson HB, editors: *Nelson textbook of pediatrics,* ed 15, Philadelphia, 2000, WB Saunders, Chapter 220.

McCracken GH Jr: Etiology and treatment of pneumonia, *Pediatr Infect Dis J* 19:373–377, 2000.

Smith R, Eviatar L: Neurologic manifestations of *Mycoplasma pneumoniae* infections: diverse spectrum of diseases: a report of six cases and review of the literature, *Clin Pediatr* 39:195–201, 2000.

Cat-Scratch Disease

Etiology. The cat-scratch disease agent *Bartonella henselae* is a small, pleomorphic, gram-negative bacillus that stains with Warthin-Starry silver impregnation of material from aspirated lymph nodes. It also causes bacillary angiomatosis and peliosis hepatis in immunosuppressed (HIV) and, occasionally, in immunocompetent patients.

Epidemiology. Cat-scratch disease has a worldwide distribution, is more common in males, and occurs in temperate climates in the fall and winter months. In more than 90% of cases, the disease follows the scratch (rarely, a lick) of a kitten (less often, of an older cat). The cats are not sick but may be bacteremic. Rare cases have occurred in association with dogs, thorns, or wood splinters.

Clinical Manifestations. A primary cutaneous papule or conjunctival granuloma develops 3–10 days after the initial contact. Lymphadenopathy localized to the draining regional nodes develops 2 weeks (range, 1–7 weeks) later, usually on the head, neck, and axilla. The nodes enlarge to 1–8 cm, may suppurate, and are painful in the early stage of the illness. There is no lymphangitis and usually few systemic signs, although fever and malaise may be noted in 30% of patients. Lymphadenopathy lasts 1–4 months. Additional but rare features are erythema nodosum, osteolytic lesions, encephalitis, sepsis-like appearance, oculoglandular (Parinaud) syndrome, polyneuritis, transverse myelitis, hepatic or splenic granulomas, endocarditis, thrombocytopenia, and pneumonia.

Diagnosis. Usually, cat-scratch disease is suspected by a history of exposure to cats, the primary lesion localized at the site of the scratch or bite, and a single, enlarged node. Aspiration of the node with subsequent microscopic evidence of the bacillus by Warthin-Starry silver stain is diagnostic and may be curative. Antibody titers to *B. henselae* are also useful.

Treatment. Usually, no treatment is required because the lymphadenopathy resolves in 2–4 months without sequelae. Aspiration is indicated for large, painful, and uncomfortable lesions. Azithromycin, rifampin, ciprofloxacin, gentamicin, or trimethoprim/sulfamethoxazole may enhance resolution of more severe disease. Bacillary angiomatosis, bacillary peliosis, or relapsing bacteremia may respond to erythromycin (clarithromycin, azithromycin) plus rifampin or doxycycline for 4–6 weeks. After an illness, immunity is lifelong. The disease is not contagious; therefore, the patient does not need to be isolated.

REFERENCES

Bass J, Vincent J, Person D: The expanding spectrum of *Bartonella* infections II: cat-scratch disease, *Pediatr Infect Dis J* 16:163, 1997.
Behrman RE, Kliegman RM, Jenson HB, editors: *Nelson textbook of pediatrics*, ed 15, Philadelphia, 2000, WB Saunders, Chapter 207.
Margileth AM: Recent advances in diagnosis and treatment of cat-scratch disease, *Curr Infect Dis Rep* 2(2):141–146, 2000.

VIRAL DISEASES
Antiviral Chemotherapy

Therapy against viral disease must take into consideration the intracellular nature of viral replication and, to avoid toxicity to the host's cells, must be directed at viral specific proteins. Viral enzymes (e.g., HIV neu-raminidase and reverse transcriptase) or enzymes with different substrate specificity compared with the host's enzyme (thymidine kinase, DNA polymerase of herpes viruses) are targets for antiviral chemotherapy. In addition, recombinant human factors that naturally reduce virus replication and kill viruses, such as interferon and high-dose intravenous immunoglobulin, have been used. To date, the most successful antiviral agents are those nucleoside analogs that interfere with viral DNA or RNA synthesis (Table 10–17).

Adenoviral Infection

Etiology. Adenoviruses are double-stranded DNA viruses. More than 51 distinct types have been associated with human illness.

Epidemiology. Adenoviruses produce respiratory tract disease year round, with a higher incidence in the spring, early summer, and midwinter. Infection occurs early in childhood by respiratory, fecal, oral, and, possibly, conjunctival inoculation. Transmission occurs from person to person, usually by respiratory spread. Asymptomatic infections are common. Enteric strains of adenovirus may be transmitted by the fecal-oral route. The period of communicability is highest during the first several days of illness. The incubation period ranges from 2–14 days for respiratory disease and 3–10 days for gastrointestinal disease.

Clinical Manifestations. Many adenoviral infections are asymptomatic or are manifested as self-limited upper respiratory illnesses. Infection is more common in children in day care and includes fever, pharyngeal exudate, and cervical lymphadenopathy. This is distinct from adenoviral pharyngeal-conjunctival fever, a rare syndrome that includes high fever and a follicular conjunctivitis.

Lower respiratory tract infection, especially with adenovirus types 3 and 7, is severe, causing bronchiolitis and pneumonia. Adenovirus infections may be a risk factor for the later development of chronic obstructive lung disease or airway reactivity. Disseminated adenoviral disease is seen in immunocompromised patients, particularly bone marrow transplant recipients. This can present as pneumonia, hepatitis, and gastroenteritis.

Epidemic keratoconjunctivitis, also caused by adenoviruses (types 8, 19, and 37), is a severe disease lasting from 4–6 weeks and is seen more commonly in adults.

Gastrointestinal illness is usually caused by types 40 and 4, typically producing gastroenteritis in young children. These infections are similar to those attributed to rotavirus but persist longer (1–2 weeks). Adenoviruses have also been associated with intussusception. Hepatitis associated with adenoviruses is seen in transplant patients, particularly recipients of

TABLE 10–17
Antiviral Chemotherapy

Drugs	Mechanism of Action	Indication	Comments
Acyclovir (valacyclovir, famciclovir—increases absorption of prodrug)	Requires viral thymidine kinase to produce acyclovir monophosphate, which inhibits DNA polymerase	Herpes simplex 1 and 2, varicella-zoster (systemic, mucocutaneous)	Oral, intravenous, topical; varicella requires higher drug levels; toxic encephalopathy, renal dysfunction
Amantadine/rimantadine	Inhibits viral replication	Influenza A	Prophylaxis and therapy; CNS toxicity with poor concentration, confusion
Oseltamivir	Neuraminidase inhibitor	Influenza A & B	Oral; as therapy or prevention after exposure
Zanamavir	Neuraminidase inhibitor	Influenza A & B	Inhalation; as therapy or prevention
Ganciclovir	As acyclovir	CMV, herpes viruses	Neutropenia, recurrence when discontinued
Foscarnet	Inhibits viral DNA polymerase	CMV retinitis, ganciclovir-resistant CMV; acyclovir-resistant HSV and varicella-zoster virus	Nonmyelosuppressive; nephrotoxic, $\uparrow\downarrow Ca^2$, Mg^2
Pleconaril	Inhibits viral attachment and uncoating	Enteroviruses	Oral
Ribavirin	Inhibits RNA synthesis and reverse transcriptase	Parenteral for influenza, Lassa virus, use for RSV controversial	Aerosol has few side effects, avoid exposure in pregnancy
Zidovudine (azidothymidine [AZT])	Inhibits viral reverse transcriptase	HIV-AIDS	Bone marrow depression
Didanosine (DDI)	Inhibits reverse transcriptase	Advanced AIDS if intolerant of or deteriorating on AZT	Painful peripheral neuropathy, pancreatitis
Stavudine (d4T)	Nucleoside analog; inhibits reverse transcriptase	HIV-AIDS	Peripheral neuropathy
Lamivudine (3TC)	Nucleoside analog	HIV-AIDS	Increases bone marrow suppression with AZT
Abacavir	Nucleoside reverse transcriptase inhibitor	HIV-AIDS	Hypersensitivity reaction: rash, fever, hypotension
Efavirenz	Nonnucleoside inhibitor	HIV-AIDS	Dizziness, headache, insomnia, rash
Viramune	Non-nucleoside inhibitor of reverse transcriptase	HIV-AIDS	Rash; must be used in combination (AZT, DDI)
Saquinavir	Viral protease inhibitor	HIV-AIDS	GI distress, diarrhea, drug interaction with rifampin
Ritonavir	Protease inhibitor	HIV-AIDS	Bad taste, circumoral paresthesias, diarrhea, drug interactions
Indinavir	Protease inhibitor	HIV-AIDS	Nephrolithiasis, drug interactions
Nelfinavir	Protease inhibitor	HIV-AIDS	Diarrhea
Ampsenavir	Protease inhibitor	HIV-AIDS	Nausea, diarrhea, rash, vomiting, perioral paresthesias

AIDS, Acquired immunodeficiency virus; *CMV*, cytomegalovirus; *CNS*, central nervous system; *DNA*, deoxyribonucleic acid; *GI*, gastrointestinal; *HIV*, human immunodeficiency virus; *HSV*, herpes simplex virus.

liver transplants. Adenoviruses cause hemorrhagic cystitis, which occurs in transplant recipients, but may also be seen in normal hosts.

Diagnosis. Adenoviruses can be isolated by tissue culture using a variety of cell lines. DNA amplification techniques are available. The ESR and WBC count may be elevated.

Treatment. For most adenoviral infections, treatment is supportive. The successful use of cidofovir, ribavirin, and ganciclovir has been reported in individual cases of severe adenoviral infection in immunocompromised patients (neonates and transplant patients).

REFERENCES

Behrman RE, Kliegman RM, Jenson HB, editors: *Nelson textbook of pediatrics*, ed 16, Philadelphia, 2000, WB Saunders, Chapter 254.

Howard DS, Phillips II GL, Reece DE, et al: Adenovirus infections in hematopoietic stem cell transplant recipients, *Clin Infect Dis* 29:1494–1501, 1999.

Ruuskanen O, Meurman O, Sarkkinen H: Adenoviral diseases in children: a study of 105 hospital cases, *Pediatrics* 76:79–83, 1985.

Enteroviruses

Enteroviruses, a group of RNA viruses, include 23 group A coxsackieviruses (types A1–A24, except type A23), six group B coxsackieviruses (B1–B6), three polioviruses, and 31 echoviruses (types 1–33, except types 10 and 28). More recent isolates are designated enteroviruses (types 68–71). They are common causes of infection in children, ranging from aseptic meningitis to nonspecific febrile illnesses. Clinical manifestations include conjunctivitis, colds, pharyngitis, herpangina, hepatitis, hand-foot-mouth syndrome, exanthems, encephalitis, paralytic polio, vomiting, diarrhea, pericarditis, and myocarditis.

Epidemiology. These hardy viruses maintain activity for days at room temperature. They are spread from person to person, primarily by the fecal-oral route and, possibly, by the respiratory route, especially among susceptible children in lower socioeconomic status groups and in developing countries. There is a peak incidence in summer and fall in temperate climates that is less evident in the tropics. Males and females are equally affected by the disease, although males are more likely to become symptomatically ill. Young children frequently are infected; the disease in neonates may be fulminant, whereas older children have more benign illness unless paralysis or significant myocarditis is present. The incubation period is 3–6 days.

Pathogenesis. After initial upper respiratory tract infection, viral replication occurs in regional lymph nodes, followed several days later by a low-grade (minor) viremia. This viremia may involve many secondary sites (e.g., heart, skin, pericardium, pleura, lung, liver, brain, and spinal cord). Viral replication in these sites coincides with clinical illness and the second (major) viremia. Viral replication is halted by the appearance of antibody on approximately the seventh day of infection. Gastrointestinal tract viral replication and shedding are generally of longer duration but do not necessarily produce gastrointestinal symptoms.

Pathology and Pathophysiology. Each of the groups of enteroviruses has a predilection for specific organ systems. The pathognomonic finding in **poliomyelitis** is viral multiplication in motor neurons, a process that occurs predominantly in the spinal cord (especially anterior horn cells), but the medulla, midbrain, thalamus, hypothalamus, pallidum, and motor cortex also may be involved. Typical organ involvement by *coxsackieviruses* includes pharyngitis (**herpangina**); skin (**hand-foot-mouth disease**); myocarditis; meningoencephalitis; and involvement of adrenal glands, pancreas, liver, pleura, pericardium, and, at times, the lung. Hepatic necrosis has been observed in some severe *echovirus* infections. Myositis, pneumonia, and adrenal involvement may also occur.

Clinical Manifestations

Polioviruses. As a result of the success of immunization programs the western hemisphere has been free of wild-type paralytic poliomyelitis since 1994. The only cases of poliomyelitis are the rare vaccine-associated paralytic polio in immunosuppressed patients or caused by reversion of the vaccine-attenuated strains. Vaccine-associated polio is most common in young infants after they receive the first dose of live attenuated vaccine, but has also been reported in unimmunized children. The features of infection are similar to those of wild-type polio, with viral infection of motor and autonomic neurons causing inflammation and destruction. In symptomatic infections there is a prodrome consisting of headache, malaise, and meningeal signs, accompanied by CSF pleocytosis. Severe myalgias and meningismus are then followed by weakness and flaccid paralysis. The distribution is typically asymmetric, with proximal muscles more involved than distal muscles. Involvement of the cranial nerves (bulbar polio) results in dysphagia and the inability to handle secretions. Progression of paralysis may continue for up to 1 week; the prognosis can be determined 1 month after infection. Sensory function remains intact, unlike other causes of paralysis such as Guillain-Barré syndrome. Some degree of permanent damage is seen in the majority of patients, although those with bulbar paralysis generally recover completely. Nonpolio enteroviruses rarely produce a paralytic illness.

As paralytic polio in the western hemisphere is now entirely the result of the vaccine-associated strains, current recommendations for immunization in the United States suggest the use of the inactivated polio vaccine (Fig. 10–1).

The major forms and clinical manifestations of poliomyelitis are outlined in Table 10–18. The clinician must be vigilant regarding respiratory insufficiency resulting from respiratory muscle or central respiratory center involvement. Such involvement may result in anxiety; jerky, breathless speaking; tachypnea; signs of respiratory distress (nasal flaring, use of accessory muscles of respiration); decreased cough; paradoxic abdominal movement; and immobility of intercostal spaces. Arm and deltoid weakness is a clue to impending respiratory paralysis.

In **bulbar poliomyelitis,** a nasal twang in the voice indicates palatal and pharyngeal weakness, as do pooling of saliva; poor cough; nasal regurgitation of saliva and other fluids; deviation of palate, uvula, or tongue; hoarseness; and aphonia. Changes in respiratory and cardiac function or vasomotor function (blood pressure changes, flushing and mottling of the skin) point toward central involvement of the key regulatory nuclei of the brainstem. The differential diagnosis includes Guillain-Barré syndrome, other types of viral encephalitis, botulism, tetanus, demyelinating encephalomyelitis, tick paralysis, CNS tumor, and trauma. In the United States, most cases of paralytic poliomyelitis are caused by the vaccine virus in normal or immunoincompetent hosts.

NONPOLIO ENTEROVIRAL INFECTION. Unlike the rare or declining occurrence of polio in most developed countries resulting from successful vaccination, the nonpolio enteroviruses remain common. Their manifestations may be biphasic, in which the patient experiences several days of well-being that occur between periods of 1–4 days of illness. Less than 50% of patients with enteroviral infection are *asymptomatic.*

The most common manifestation of all types of enteroviral infection is *nonspecific febrile illness.* It generally lasts 3 days and is associated with fever, malaise, headache, pharyngitis, and myalgia. In neonates, gastrointestinal tract symptoms may occur.

The enteroviruses have been associated with a variety of *respiratory tract illnesses,* including conjunctivitis, pharyngitis, herpangina, stomatitis, parotitis, croup, bronchitis, pneumonia, and pleurodynia. Pharyngitis is associated with pharyngeal erythema and, at times, with exudate. **Herpangina** (coxsackievirus A) is associated with fever, oral ulcers, and vesicles surrounded by erythema, usually in the posterior pharynx but also the anterior tonsillar pillars, palate, uvula, and posterior buccal surfaces. The duration is 3–6 days. **Pleurodynia** (Bornholm disease, devil's grip), an acute febrile illness, typically is associated with intense pleuritic chest and upper abdominal muscular pain that occurs in spasms and is intensified by breathing or coughing. The pain may mimic acute pulmonary or abdominal surgical processes and is the result of intercostal muscle infection. This illness, often caused by a member of the coxsackie B group, generally occurs in outbreaks and may be associated with the other manifestations of enteroviral infection. Chest roentgenograms usually are normal, and the WBC count may be normal or elevated, with an increased percentage of myeloid cells.

Gastrointestinal manifestations commonly are associated with outbreaks of enteroviral infection. They include vomiting (in about 50% of cases), diarrhea (without blood), abdominal pain, mesenteric adenitis, and pseudoappendicitis.

Acute hemorrhagic conjunctivitis, particularly that

TABLE 10–18
Clinical Manifestations of Poliovirus Infection (Poliomyelitis)

Asymptomatic infection	95% of infected persons are asymptomatic
Abortive form (nonspecific febrile illness)	Fever, malaise, anorexia, nausea, vomiting, headache, pharyngitis, abdominal pain
Nonparalytic form (aseptic meningitis)	Similar to the abortive form plus stiff neck and signs of meningeal inflammation, soreness of back muscles, tripod sign, positive Kernig and Brudzinski signs, and bulging fontanel; decrease in both superficial (cremasteric, abdominal) and deep tendon reflexes heralds paralysis
Paralytic form	Similar to the nonparalytic form, plus weakness of skeletal or cranial muscle groups; with deeper brain involvement the signs and symptoms may be pain, spasticity, hypertonia, respiratory and cardiac arrhythmias, blood pressure and vasomotor changes, and bladder and bowel dysfunction; hallmark is asymmetric, flaccid paralysis in spinal, bulbar, and encephalitic forms
Spinal form	Axial and extremity muscle weakness that may involve intercostal muscles and diaphragm
Bulbar form	Cranial nerve weakness and respiratory and circulatory disturbances
Encephalitic form	Irritability, disorientation, drowsiness, and tremors

associated with coxsackievirus A24 and enterovirus 70, may become manifest as eye pain, photophobia, blurred vision, lacrimation, erythema, congestion of the eye as a result of edema, chemotic eyelids, and eye discharge. Subconjunctival hemorrhages, conjunctivitis, keratitis, and preauricular adenopathy are present. Outbreaks have occurred in tropical and temperate climates.

Pericarditis and *myocarditis* commonly are caused by enteroviruses, especially coxsackieviruses B1–B5, and must be distinguished from acute rheumatic fever and acute bacterial endocarditis. Myocarditis carries a significant mortality rate from acute disease, especially in neonates and young infants. Older patients may experience chronic congestive heart failure and dilated cardiomyopathy after coxsackievirus myocarditis.

Genitourinary tract manifestations of the group B coxsackieviruses include orchitis and epididymitis. Rare manifestations include glomerulonephritis, pyuria, hematuria, cystitis, and vaginal ulcerative lesions.

Myositis, arthritis, and a dermatomyositis-like syndrome occurring in immunodeficient patients (usually with B-cell defects) have been linked to chronic enteroviral infection.

Hand-foot-mouth syndrome, often associated with coxsackievirus A16 or enterovirus 7, is characterized by small intraoral ulcers on the tongue and buccal mucosa associated with vesicular or erythematous macular lesions on the hands, feet, and, occasionally, the buttocks. Nonspecific maculopapular and even petechial rashes also are common during enteroviral infection.

The enteroviruses are the most common cause of seasonal *aseptic meningitis syndrome,* which occurs in summer and fall in temperate climates. This syndrome may be associated with other manifestations of enteroviral infection or may be the sole manifestation of the condition. Rash (erythematous, maculopapular, or petechial), sore throat, muscle pain, and signs of meningeal irritation are common, except in infants under 12 months of age, who commonly are infected. CSF usually reveals an early polymorphonuclear cell predominance, which may or may not shift to a lymphocytic predominance in 12–24 hours. The median number of cells is 100–150/L, but occasionally thousands of cells per microliter are seen. The CSF protein level is mildly elevated, and the glucose level is normal. The duration of illness is generally 4–6 days of fever and 7–14 days of neurologic signs or symptoms. The enteroviruses also are probably the most common cause of seasonal *encephalitis* in locales with low arthropod-mediated arboviral activity.

As with poliovirus, the other enteroviruses uncommonly can cause an acute anterior horn cell infection resulting in *paralysis.* Peripheral neuritis and acute hemiplegia also have been associated with enteroviral infection.

Neonatal nonspecific febrile illness may be acquired transplacentally from a mildly ill mother or, more usually, at birth from the sick mother, another sick family member, or a nursery contact. The illness is characterized by fever, irritability, anorexia, mild vomiting, or diarrhea and often is indistinguishable from bacterial sepsis. The duration of the illness is 3–4 days. The peripheral WBC count often is elevated, accompanied by a predominance of polymorphonuclear leukocytes. This illness must be differentiated from neonatal bacterial sepsis, and hospitalization is usually required for diagnostic evaluation and empiric antimicrobial therapy. Echovirus 11 has been associated with fulminating neonatal hepatic necrosis.

Myocarditis in the neonate often is the result of coxsackieviruses B1–B5. Illness begins abruptly with fever, tachycardia, cardiomegaly, electrocardiographic changes, transient systolic murmurs, shock, and respiratory distress. In the newborn, fulminant *encephalomyocarditis* can occur.

Diagnosis. Although the season, location, age of the patient, exposure, and clinical manifestations may suggest enteroviral infection, it often is difficult to differentiate this infection from bacterial infection or other viral infections. The definitive diagnosis may be made by PCR or by culturing enterovirus from a normally sterile site or from biopsy material. Recovering virus from stool or pharyngeal secretions suggests, but does not prove, that infection exists because a significant number of infants may be asymptomatically shedding enterovirus during an epidemic or continue to shed vaccine strains after polio immunization. Viral growth requires 3–7 days in tissue culture. If polio virus is isolated, it should be sent to the Centers for Disease Control and Prevention (CDC) in Atlanta to distinguish wild polio from vaccine strains. Serum collected at the initial presentation of the patient with the illness and 2–4 weeks later may confirm or refute infection, especially in the infant with fecal shedding of virus or in one who has an unusual illness. RNA hybridization with complementary DNA (cDNA) probes may identify the viral genome in infected tissues or fluids (CSF).

Treatment. There are no available approved specific antiviral therapies for enteroviral infections. Pleconaril has been highly effective in immunocompromised patients. In immunocompetent patients, therapy is aimed at anticipating and preventing complications and preparing for the more prolonged phases of rehabilitation, when necessary. Corticosteroid therapy is of no value in any form of the enteroviral infection and has worsened experimental murine coxsackievirus myocarditis. Supportive therapy for myocarditis and meningitis is essential and includes providing cardiorespiratory care and controlling increased intracranial pressure, respectively.

Prevention. Poliovirus infection can be prevented almost entirely by vaccination (live oral or inactivated injected preparations) (Fig. 10–1). Because of the concern of vaccine-associated paralytic polio (VAPP), in the absence of wild-type disease in the United States, the American Academy of Pediatrics suggests that inactivated polio vaccine (IPV) be used solely. OPV is recommended in areas of the world where poliomyelitis has *not* been eradicated, to control outbreaks of paralytic polio where the ease of administration, lower cost, and advantages to excretion of a live virus in the development of herd immunity are obvious advantages.

REFERENCES

Behrman RE, Kliegman RM, Jenson HB, editors: *Nelson textbook of pediatrics,* ed 16, Philadelphia, 2000, WB Saunders, Chapter 209.

Hennessey KA, Marx A, Ashgar R, et al: Widespread paralytic poliomyelitis in Pakistan: a case-controlled study to determine risk factors and implications for poliomyelitis eradication, *J Infect Dis* 182:6–11, 2000.

Rotbart HA: Antiviral therapy for enteroviral infections, *Pediatr Infect Dis J* 18:632–633, 1999.

Sutter RW, Prevots DR, Cochi SL: Poliovirus vaccines: progress toward global poliomyelitis eradication and changing routine immunization recommendations in the United States, *Pediatr Clin North Am* 47:287–308, 2000.

Human Parvovirus Infection

(Erythema Infectiosum, or Fifth Disease)

Etiology. Erythema infectiosum is the clinical designation given to infection caused by the human parvovirus B19. Although this is a benign viral exanthem in normal children, the affinity of this virus to red blood cell progenitor cells makes it an important cause of aplastic crisis in patients with hemolytic anemias, including sickle cell disease, spherocytosis, and thalassemia (see Chapter 14). It also causes fetal anemia and hydrops fetalis when primary infection occurs during pregnancy. The erythrocyte P antigen is the cellular receptor for parvovirus B19; the virus replicates in actively dividing erythroid stem cells. The virus is acquired via the respiratory tract and causes transient viremia.

Epidemiology. This is a common disease; community epidemics usually occur in the spring. The virus is transmitted by respiratory secretions or by blood product transfusions. Virus can be detected by PCR techniques. Patients may shed the virus prior to the onset of the rash. Seroprevalence studies suggest that 40–60% of adults have antibody to parvovirus B19.

Clinical Manifestations. Parvovirus B19 infections usually begin with a mild, nonspecific illness characterized by fever, malaise, myalgias, and headache. In some cases this is followed by the characteristic rash 7–10 days later. Erythema infectiosum becomes manifest by rash, low-grade or no fever, and, occasionally, by pharyngitis and mild conjunctivitis. The rash appears in three stages. The initial stage typically is demonstrated by erythematous cheeks, which gives a "slapped cheek" appearance with circumoral pallor. One to 4 days later, an erythematous symmetric, maculopapular, truncal rash appears but later fades as central clearing takes place, giving a distinctive lacy-reticulated rash that lasts 2–40 days (mean, 11 days). This rash often is pruritic; does not desquamate; and may recur with exercise, bathing, rubbing, or stress. Adolescents and adults may experience myalgia, significant arthralgia or arthritis, headache, pharyngitis, coryza, and gastrointestinal upset. Parvovirus may produce pancytopenia in immunosuppressed patients. Patients with hemolytic anemias (sickle cell disease) may have a transient aplastic crisis. Case reports link parvovirus infection with myocarditis, meningitis, and a significant association with rheumatologic disease (vasculitis).

Diagnosis and Differential Diagnosis. Serologic tests demonstrating antibody response to parvovirus and the presence of specific IgM antibody to parvovirus are diagnostic. In serum specimens taken during the acute stage, the virus has been detected by immune electron microscopy and DNA hybridization. A mild leukopenia, thrombocytopenia, and reticulocytopenia may be present. This illness is characteristic, although atypical cases may be confused with other viral exanthems (such as measles, rubella, and enterovirus), as well as with drug rashes or SLE.

Treatment. There is no specific therapy. Respiratory isolation is advisable for 7 days after the onset of illness. Patients with sickle cell anemia or fetuses with hydrops may require transfusion. Immunosuppressed patients may develop pancytopenia, which may be treated with IVIG. These patients, as well as those with aplastic crises, are highly contagious; droplet precautions should be used, and pregnant health care workers who may be at risk should be alerted.

REFERENCES

Behrman RE, Kliegman RM, Jenson HB, editors: *Nelson textbook of pediatrics,* ed 16, Philadelphia, 2000, WB Saunders, Chapter 244.

Brown KE, Hibbs JR, Gallinella G, et al: Resistance to parvovirus B19 infection due to lack of reception (erythrocyte P antigen), *N Engl J Med* 330:1192, 1994.

Hare L, Staussberg R, Rudich H, et al: Raynaud's phemomenon as a manifestation of parvovirus B19 infection: case reports and review of parvovirus B19 rheumatic and vasculitis syndromes, *Clin Infect Dis* 30:500–503, 2000.

Valeur-Jensen AK, Pedersen CB, Westergaard T, et al: Risk factors for parvovirus B19 infection in pregnancy, *JAMA* 281:1099–1105, 1999.

Hepatitis

See Chapter 11.

Herpesvirus Infections

The human herpesvirus family consists of cytomegalovirus, EBV, herpes simplex virus, varicella-zoster virus, human herpesvirus-6 (HHV6), human herpesvirus-7 (HHV7), and human herpesvirus-8 (Kaposi sarcoma–associated virus). The herpesviruses cause acute primary infection, maintain a state of latency in lymphoid and neuronal tissues, and reactivate and occasionally induce a clinical recurrence, especially in immunocompromised individuals.

Cytomegalovirus Infection

Etiology. CMV is a large, enveloped, double-stranded DNA virus with an icosahedral capsid. After fusion of the viral envelope with host cell membranes, viral replication occurs within the cell nucleus and new viral particles bud through the nuclear membrane and are released through the cell membrane. Infection of host mucosal surfaces occurs via the respiratory or genital tract. Following viremia, the virus disseminates to various tissues and is isolated from many sites.

Epidemiology. CMV is a ubiquitous virus. It is the most commonly known human virus that is transmitted *vertically* to the fetus (transplacentally, during birth, and by breast milk), but transmission also occurs *horizontally* from person to person. In addition, CMV persists in a latent form after a primary infection, and reactivation may occur, particularly during immunosuppression. Infection rates are inversely correlated with socioeconomic status. In the United States, 20–50% of childbearing-age women are infected; in developing countries, the infection rate approaches 100%. From 4–10% of pregnant women excrete virus in cervical secretions or in their urine, and 5–25% shed it in milk during lactation. From 1–3% of children are infected before birth, and 10–20% acquire infection in the neonatal period. Day care centers are important areas of CMV transmission in infants and young children. These infected infants act as a source of infection for their seronegative parents.

The transmission of CMV infection requires close contact. Epidemic outbreaks have not been reported, although transmission is common in families, in day care centers, and among sexual partners. CMV can be isolated from saliva, urine, nasopharyngeal secretions, milk, semen, blood, and donor organs (e.g., kidneys and bone marrow). The incidence of CMV excretion in day care centers may reach 50–70% in 1–2 year olds. Although infection of the fetus can result from either primary or recurrent disease in the mother, it is the primary form in the mother that results in symptomatic neonatal illness, which is estimated to occur in 5–10% of infants of mothers with primary infection. Horizontal transmission probably occurs most commonly via saliva, but urine also may be an important medium, especially in day care

centers. Blood transfusion with CMV-infected blood cells may induce a mononucleosis-like syndrome in susceptible individuals, which is prevented by the use of filters that exclude leukocytes. Immunocompromised patients often experience severe primary infection or may reactivate latent infection.

Clinical Manifestations. These vary according to age and immune status of the host.

Neonatal Infection. More than 90% of congenitally infected infants are asymptomatic. A significant number (15%) of infants born to women with asymptomatic or symptomatic primary infection occurring early in pregnancy will have a TORCH syndrome (*t*oxoplasmosis, *o*ther, *r*ubella, *C*MV, and *h*erpes simplex) (see Chapter 6). Infants infected during maternal reactivation have less severe disease. Premature neonates who are CMV seronegative and who receive blood from CMV-positive donors may develop a syndrome characterized by respiratory distress, pallor, sepsis-like signs, hepatosplenomegaly, neutropenia, thrombocytopenia, and lymphocytosis. In a small number of term infants with perinatally acquired disease, CMV pneumonitis, petechial rash, intracranial calcifications, and hepatosplenomegaly occur. Some congenitally infected infants who appear to be asymptomatic at birth will have hearing loss or learning disability in infancy or childhood.

Older Children. Asymptomatic infections are the most common type in older children. A characteristic syndrome caused by CMV in healthy children is a mononucleosis-like syndrome and hepatitis. The former often includes fever, malaise, myalgia, headache, anorexia, abdominal pain, and hepatosplenomegaly. The degree of pharyngitis and lymphadenopathy generally is less striking than that seen in the EBV-induced mononucleosis syndrome. As occurs in patients with infectious mononucleosis, an ampicillin-induced rash and abnormal serologic reactions, including the presence of cold agglutinins, ANAs, rheumatoid factor, and cryoglobulins, may occur in this CMV syndrome. A CMV hepatitis syndrome without other manifestations of the mononucleosis syndrome may occur.

Immunocompromised Hosts. CMV commonly causes serious infection in immunocompromised hosts: In HIV-infected patients, CMV causes retinitis, pneumonia, gastrointestinal ulcers, and encephalitis. The spectrum of disease is different in organ or bone marrow transplant recipients in whom CMV pneumonitis and neutropenia are major problems. Transplantation of CMV-negative tissue into CMV-negative patients is recommended. CMV-positive patients may reactivate endogenous infection or may acquire new strains from CMV-positive donors. Active CMV infection may be associated with organ rejection.

Diagnosis. The diagnosis may be difficult to establish because of the high rate of asymptomatic excretion, the frequency of reactivation infections, and the presence of IgM antibody in some episodes of reactivation.

Neonatal Infection. The diagnosis of congenital disease (TORCH) relies on demonstrating CMV in urine, pharyngeal secretions, or peripheral blood leukocytes during the first week of life or on demonstrating a positive CMV-IgM serologic test. The serologic diagnosis is complicated by maternal transplacental IgG antibody and the common occurrence of perinatally acquired disease, which makes studies after the first few weeks of life inconclusive in establishing the diagnosis. Negative serologic studies of the infant generally exclude the latter diagnosis, as do negative maternal serologic studies.

The *differential diagnosis* of congenital CMV includes infection with *Toxoplasma,* syphilis, rubella, HSV, HIV, *Listeria monocytogenes,* varicella, and enterovirus.

Acquired Infection. Diagnosis of CMV depends on viral isolation from a target organ, whereas the recovery of virus from secretions may be transient. Viremia may be detected. Diagnosis is especially complicated in immunosuppressed patients, who may not mount an immune response and in whom the finding of CMV in the urine is so common as to be nondiagnostic. Thus diagnosis of CMV hepatitis or pneumonitis may rest on isolation of CMV from the specific site by biopsy, bronchoscopy (bronchoalveolar lavage), or other invasive tests. The isolation of CMV from blood or buffy coat cells has been associated with the presence of invasive CMV disease. Appropriate serologic tests should exclude infection caused by hepatitis A, B, and C viruses and EBV. PCR-based tests are highly sensitive but may be difficult to interpret.

Treatment. Ganciclovir, foscarnet, and cidofovir act by inhibiting the CMV DNA polymerase and have been approved for use in the treatment of CMV infection. Ganciclovir has been used most widely, and resistance has been increasing, especially in patients who have been treated either chronically or repeatedly for CMV infection. Treatment for CMV pneumonia often includes the use of CMV-IVIG, and many transplant patients routinely receive prophylaxis with antiviral drugs to prevent CMV disease.

Prevention. Serologic testing may be done to identify persons at risk. Asymptomatic shedding of CMV is so common as to be unavoidable in many circumstances.

Blood transfusions were once a common source of CMV. This has been virtually eliminated by the use of filters, freezing red blood cells in glycerol, and the use of CMV-negative donors.

Prognosis. Symptomatic congenital infection carries a guarded outlook regarding neurologic sequelae, especially in the child with microcephaly or intracranial calcifications. Hearing loss is a common complication of asymptomatic or symptomatic congenital CMV infection. Acquired infection in the healthy host usually is self-limited, whereas it may be fatal in the immunocompromised host as a result of pneumonitis, encephalitis, or secondary opportunistic infections.

REFERENCES

American Society of Blood and Bone Marrow Transplantation: Guidelines for preventing opportunistic infections among hematopoetic stem cell transplant recipients, *MMWR* 49/RR-10, 2000.

Behrman RE, Kliegman RM, Jenson HB, editors: *Nelson textbook of pediatrics,* ed 16, Philadelphia, 2000, WB Saunders, Chapter 248.

Boppana SB, Fowler K, Vaid Y, et al: Neuroradiologic findings in the newborn period and long term outcome in children with symptomatic congenital cytomegalovirus infection, *Pediatrics* 99:409–414, 1997.

Lazzarotto T, Varani S, Guerra B, et al: Prenatal indicators of congenital cytomegalovirus infection, *J Pediatr* 137:90–95, 2000.

Ljungman P, Engelhard D, Link H, et al: Treatment of interstitial pneumonitis due to cytomegalovirus with ganciclovir and intravenous immune globulin: experience of European bone marrow transplant group, *Clin Infect Dis* 14:831–835, 1992.

Noyola DE, Demmler GJ, Williamson WD, et al: Congenital CMV Longitudinal Study Group: Cytomegalovirus urinary excretion and long-term outcome in children with congenital cytomegalovirus infection, *Pediatr Infect Dis J* 19:505–510, 2000.

Epstein-Barr Virus Infection

(Infectious Mononucleosis)

Etiology. EBV, a double-stranded DNA virus, contains a capsid, a protein tegument, and a lipid outer envelope. The virus infects permissive cells and is maintained as an episome. Pharyngeal epithelial cells are probably the initial target of viral infection and replication. Viral genes are transcribed in a sequential pattern, first the early antigens, which are viral enzymes necessary for DNA replication, followed by DNA replication and expression of the capsid antigen. These specific gene products provide the basis for the serologic diagnosis of primary or reactivation of EBV infection. EBV infects B cells and immortalizes them, maintaining itself within the nucleus. These B cells are widely disseminated until the immune system, particularly natural killer and T cells, is activated. The atypical lymphocytes present during acute EBV infections are cytotoxic T cells, activated in response to EBV-infected B cells. The ability of this virus to transform B cells is also associated with the X-linked lymphoproliferative syndrome and the posttransplant lymphoproliferative syndromes caused by EBV infection.

Epidemiology. EBV infection occurs at an early age in persons in developing countries; most children are seropositive by 3 years of age. In developed countries, age of infection is inversely related to socioeconomic level; 60–80% of adolescents from lower socioeconomic levels are seropositive. In higher socioeconomic levels, infection typically occurs during high school or college attendance. Susceptible Yale University students demonstrated a 15% seroconversion rate per year. Endemic disease in group settings of adolescents is common.

EBV is transmitted by salivary exchange, contact with contaminated objects, or, less commonly, blood transfusions. It is spread by intimate contact, and EBV is shed in the saliva before and during clinically apparent infection. In addition, 10–20% of healthy seropositive individuals and 60% of seropositive immunosuppressed individuals shed virus intermittently; therefore, the period of communicability is not known. The incubation period is 30–50 days.

Clinical Manifestations. The clinical manifestations of EBV are related to age and range from asymptomatic to fatal infections. Infants and young children infected with EBV usually are asymptomatic or experience mild disease that may include tonsillitis, fever, or upper respiratory tract disease. In older children and young adults, a typical infectious mononucleosis syndrome (pharyngitis, fever, lymphadenopathy, hepatosplenomegaly, lymphocytosis) may develop after EBV infection.

The prodromal period of infectious mononucleosis includes malaise, fatigue, headache, nausea, and abdominal pain lasting 1–2 weeks. The typical symptoms and signs of mononucleosis are pharyngitis (with enlarged tonsils and exudate), an enanthema (pharyngeal petechiae), fever, lymphadenopathy (posterior cervical; epitrochlear; less commonly, generalized), splenomegaly (up to 50% of patients), and hepatomegaly (10–20%). Eyelid edema and maculopapular or urticarial rash occur in 5–15% of cases. Group A streptococci may be recovered from the pharynx in 30% of children. A diffuse, erythematous rash develops in approximately 80% of patients treated with ampicillin. The symptoms last 2–4 weeks, then slowly abate.

Oncogenicity of EBV. EBV is probably the initiator of African Burkitt lymphoma in children and of adult nasopharyngeal carcinoma in Asia. Polyclonal B-cell lymphoma in immunocompromised patients and X-linked lymphoproliferative disease (discussed under Complications) have been shown to be associated with EBV.

Complications. As a result of rapid swelling, splenic rupture may occur. The pharyngeal tonsillar hypertrophy may cause airway obstruction. Neurologic complications may occur in the absence of classic features of mononucleosis and include seizures, ataxia, aseptic meningitis syndrome, Bell palsy, transverse myelitis, encephalitis, combative behavior, headache, and Guillain-Barré syndrome. Other complications are hepatitis (85% of cases); myocarditis; interstitial pneumonia; Coombs-positive hemolytic anemia; antibody-mediated thrombocytopenia; hemophagocytic syndrome; and, rarely, aplastic anemia, pancreatitis, parotitis, orchitis, and Reye syndrome.

In several kindreds, a rare syndrome of *X-linked lymphoproliferative disease* (Duncan syndrome) following EBV infection has occurred. The affected males may die of overwhelming infection; they may survive, and B-cell lymphoproliferative disease may develop; or hypoplastic syndromes may develop, such as aplastic anemia or hypogammaglobulinemia. Rarely, immunocompromised patients (e.g., from transplantation, AIDS, ataxia-telangiectasia, or severe combined immunodeficiency disorders) and apparently healthy patients may have the same fate.

Diagnosis. Nonspecific findings often include a leukocytosis of 10,000–20,000 cells/L, with at least 20–40% being atypical lymphocytes. These lymphocytes are T cells responding to EBV-infected B cells. Children under 5 years of age have less striking atypical lymphocytosis. Mild thrombocytopenia occurs in 50% of individuals, and elevated liver enzymes occur in approximately 85%.

Nonspecific tests for the heterophil antibody are based on the appearance of IgM antibody against sheep, horse, or oxen red blood cells not absorbable by guinea pig kidney cells. These are present in the serum for up to 6 months after EBV infection. This antibody response generally is absent in children under 5 years of age but identifies about 90% of cases in older children and adults. Specific diagnosis of EBV infection involves analysis for several types of antibodies against specific EBV antigens.

Serologic Response to EBV Infection. The most commonly performed test is that for detecting antibodies to viral capsid antigen (VCA). At the time of the onset of symptoms, most patients have high IgG anti-VCA and IgM anti-VCA antibodies, as well as antibodies to early antigen (EA). The absence or low level of antibody to Epstein-Barr nuclear antigen (EBNA) and the presence of the anti-VCA antibody indicates acute infection. High levels of IgG anti-VCA and anti-EBNA and absence of IgM anti-VCA and anti-EA indicate previous (not acute) infection. Absence of all anti-EBV antibodies indicates a susceptible, uninfected individual. These serologic tests are particularly useful for evaluating young patients who have heterophil-negative infectious mononucleosis or for those with isolated organ manifestations, such as myocarditis, FUO, and encephalitis.

EBV DNA also can be demonstrated in infected cells by DNA hybridization.

Differential Diagnosis. The differential diagnosis includes cytomegalovirus infection, toxoplasmosis, hepatitis A, lymphoma, and leukemia. Less commonly confused conditions are rubella, leptospirosis, Kawasaki syndrome, HIV infection, human herpesvirus-6, and streptococcal infection.

Treatment. The typical patient with mononucleosis requires no antiviral therapy. Bed rest is indicated by the patient's needs and does not improve the course. Acyclovir may have some beneficial effects in life-threatening EBV infection. Corticosteroids have been used for respiratory distress resulting from tonsillar hypertrophy, thrombocytopenia, hemolytic anemia, and neurologic complications. Although steroids have been shown to shorten the course of the acute illness, they should not be used in uncomplicated cases. EBV-induced lymphoproliferative syndromes are generally managed by reducing the immunosuppression. Interferon has been used, with some success.

Prevention. There are no measures to prevent EBV infection. Patients with recent EBV infection should not donate blood. Splenic trauma should be avoided by limiting athletics and repeated examinations.

REFERENCES

Behrman RE, Kliegman RM, Jenson HB, editors: *Nelson textbook of pediatrics*, ed 16, Philadelphia, 2000, WB Saunders, Chapter 247.

Cohen JI: Epstein-Barr virus infection, *N Engl J Med* 343:481–490, 2000.

Jenson HB: Acute complications of Epstein-Barr virus infectious mononucleosis, *Curr Opin Pediatr* 12:263, 2000.

Herpes Simplex Virus Infection

Etiology. Herpes simplex viruses (HSV-1 and HSV-2) are large double-stranded DNA viruses that consist of a linear genome contained within an icosahedral capsid. There is significant DNA homology between types 1 and 2. The virus initially infects mucosal surfaces or injured skin and enters cutaneous neurons, where it migrates along the axons to the sensory ganglia. Viral replication occurs in these ganglia, and infectious virus then moves down the axon to infect and destroy the epithelial cells. In immunocompromised patients and in the neonate, viral replication persists and disseminates to other organs.

Latency is established within neurons, where virus is maintained but undergoes active replication only at sporadic intervals triggered by undefined events. Although antibody production in response to infection is associated with recovery from primary HSV infection and maternal transmission of antibody to the neonate appears to be protective in neonatal infections, it does not prevent reactivation disease.

Although either virus can be found in any site, nongenital type 1 (HSV-1) usually occurs above the waist (CNS, eyes, mouth), and genital type 2 (HSV-2) generally involves the genitalia and skin below the waist; HSV type 2 generally occurs in the neonate at any site. *Primary infection* occurs in nonimmune individuals who have never been previously infected. This infection often is asymptomatic but may cause a typical clinical syndrome. In most infected individuals, the virus attains a state of *latency* in neural tissue. *Reactivation* of latent virus may result in a characteristic clinical syndrome of herpetic *recurrence.* In addition, another exposure to a second type or even a second strain of the same type can result in exogenous *reinfection.*

Epidemiology. The incubation period is 2–12 days, with a mean of 6–7 days. Approximately 85% of infections are asymptomatic. Institutional and family outbreaks have occurred. Close body contact (e.g., saliva, kissing, wrestling, or sexual) and inoculation of mucous membranes or disrupted skin are required for infection. After the loss of transplacental antibodies, infants and young children begin to be infected with HSV-1. At the onset of sexual activity, HSV-2 infection becomes more common. HSV infection occurs more frequently in individuals from lower socioeconomic status groups. Approximately 2–5% of healthy individuals shed HSV in oral secretions at any time.

Pathology. The classic findings are intranuclear inclusion bodies and multinucleated giant cells. Immunity requires T-cell–mediated activity and anti-HSV antibodies.

Clinical Manifestations

Skin and Mucous Membranes. Primary infection of the skin in neonates is common. Autoinoculation from another site may cause a localized vesicular eruption on an erythematous base. Healing is complete in 7–14 days. Recurrences occur at the same site. Infection of a digit causes a viral paronychia, referred to as a **herpetic whitlow,** which is painful, erythematous, and occasionally presents with a vesicular eruption. It is found in children who suck their thumbs and bite their nails. In older children it may be found concomitantly with genital herpes; in health care professionals, it usually is nosocomially acquired. Abraded or burned skin is quite susceptible to HSV infection. In this setting the lesions often are atypical, with ulcers predominating. Wrestlers and rugby players acquire cutaneous herpes from close body contact with the cutaneous infections of other players **(herpes gladiatorum and herpes rugbiaforum).** Erythema multiforme also is associated with HSV.

Acute Herpetic Gingivostomatitis. Acute herpetic gingivostomatitis is the most common clinical manifestation of primary HSV infection in infants and children beyond the neonatal period. It generally occurs in 1–3-year-olds, although it may occur at any age. The onset is abrupt, with mouth pain, salivation, fetor oris, dysphagia, anorexia, and fever. The vesicles usually rupture, and the typical lesion is ulcerative. The anterior and, less commonly, the posterior oropharynx are involved, with lesions in the gingiva, buccal mucosa, tongue, and lips and, following autoinoculation, on the skin of the neck and nose. Regional lymphadenopathy is common. The illness lasts 7–14 days. *Herpangina,* an enteroviral infection, may be differentiated by its vesicles and ulcers, which occur predominantly in the posterior pharynx. In adolescents, a severe exudative pharyngitis may be the manifestation of primary oral HSV infection.

Recurrent stomatitis is the typical fever blister that occurs on the mucocutaneous junction. These lesions are a recurrence of oral HSV infection and are not associated with systemic signs or symptoms.

Eczema Herpeticum (Kaposi Varicelliform Eruption). This is a serious, usually primary HSV infection that occurs in individuals with eczema. It may be generalized and involve many areas of skin, producing vesicles, ulcers, and hemorrhagic crusts. Fever (40.0°–40.5° C [104°–105° F]) occurs for 7–10 days, and recurrent attacks are common. In severe cases the widespread infection acts as a burn, causing fluid loss and hyponatremia. Dissemination to visceral organs or the brain may occur. In previous times this infection had to be differentiated from vaccinia, variola, and varicella.

Ocular Lesions. Conjunctivitis and keratoconjunctivitis may be manifestations of primary or recurrent infection at any age. The conjunctiva is erythematous and swollen, without purulence. Corneal lesions may occur as dendritic or ameboid ulcers or more commonly, in recurrent infection, as a deep keratitis. Vesicular lid lesions, if present, should suggest the diagnosis. HSV, along with bacteria and other viruses, always should be included in the differential diagnosis of conjunctivitis (Table 10–16). Steroids, which worsen HSV ocular infection, should not be used in patients with herpes conjunctivitis. Ocular manifestations of neonates infected with HSV may include cataracts, uveitis, and chorioretinitis (in utero), in addition to conjunctivitis and keratoconjunctivitis (perinatal).

Encephalitis. HSV is the most common cause of fatal, sporadic viral encephalitis. Beyond the neonatal period, it is predominantly caused by HSV-1. It may be a manifestation of primary or recurrent disease. Although HSV resembles other forms of encephalitis with alterations of mentation, fever, and seizures, the characteristic features of HSV encephalitis are clinical signs of *focal* CNS disease, as evidenced by EEG, CT, or MRI or neuroradiologic signs of focality, especially in the temporal lobe. The spinal fluid usually reveals lymphocytosis, an elevated protein level, a normal glucose level, and red blood cells. The CSF culture is negative for bacteria or HSV (HSV may be recovered in neonatal disease). Detection of HSV antigen or more often DNA, by PCR from the CSF, confirms the diagnosis.

Genital Herpes. This condition occurs most commonly in adolescents or young adults. It may be a sign of early sexual activity or child abuse in younger children. Many genital infections in young adults are caused by HSV-1 and HSV-2. Primary symptomatic infection becomes manifest by vesicular, ulcerative, and crusted lesions in the genital areas of males or females. In females, the cervix is involved as well. Systemic symptoms of fever, adenopathy, paresthesia, and dysuria are common. The course of illness lasts 10–20 days. In patients practicing rectal intercourse, a similar syndrome involving the perirectal area occurs.

Recurrent genital tract disease is characterized by localized vesicles, ulcers, and crusts that last for several days without systemic symptoms. Recurrences occur in 50–80% of patients with primary symptomatic genital tract disease.

Complications of primary genital tract herpes infection include a self-limited aseptic meningitis syndrome. HSV infection of the genital tract of pregnant women can result in the transmission of infection to their offspring.

Neonatal Infection. The majority of cases of neonatal HSV are caused by HSV-2 and are acquired when the infant passes through an infected birth canal. The risk of neonatal infection is 30–50% with a primary maternal infection; it is 1-3% after recurrent genital infection. Infants also can be infected by nongenital maternal or nosocomial sources. Most infected mothers are asymptomatic, and usually no history of maternal or paternal genital HSV infection is discovered. The incidence of premature birth is higher than expected. HSV infection in the neonate is classified as (1) localized skin, eye, and mouth disease, (2) CNS disease (encephalitis), or (3) disseminated disease. Skin, eye, or mouth disease is usually diagnosed in the first 2 weeks of life as vesicles often arising at a site of trauma, such as a fetal scalp monitor or after circumcision. If not treated promptly, the infection spreads and usually becomes disseminated. CNS disease more typically presents at 2 weeks of age with fever, lethargy, and seizures, often focal and difficult to manage. Only half of these infants will have any cutaneous manifestations of infection at the onset. CSF findings characteristically include elevated protein and mild pleocytosis with mononuculear cells. CT, MRI, or EEG typically shows diffuse abnormalities. Disseminated disease, seen in the first few days of life, is more severe and often initially diagnosed as bacterial sepsis with hypotension, thrombocytopenia, and disseminated intravascular coagulation. With current diagnostic techniques and aggressive antiviral treatment, survival associated with SEM disease is excellent, whereas CNS involvement is associated with 15% mortality, and disseminated disease with greater than 50% mortality. After the initial episode of infection, many affected infants have recurrent infection, which mandates retreatment and consideration of prophylactic antiviral therapy. Thus *any* manifestation of HSV infection in the neonate should be treated with antiviral chemotherapy. If the neonate is left untreated, the mortality of neonatal HSV infection is 50%, with 50% of survivors having significant sequelae. Even localized disease of the skin, eyes, and mouth is associated with sequelae in 10–15% of infants.

Immunocompromised Patients. Patients with T-cell disorders, severe combined immunodeficiency, AIDS, lymphoma, leukemia, or severe malnutrition and those undergoing chemotherapy or transplantation procedures have a significant increase in susceptibility to serious HSV infection. This becomes manifest rarely as disseminated disease but frequently as severe recurrences, which are typically focal, necrotic, painful lesions that heal slowly. Rarely, these lesions disseminate to other areas of skin or visceral organs. In immunosuppressed patients, HSV commonly causes mucositis and esophagitis as a result of local spread from oral infection. Less commonly, pneumonitis, hepatitis, and, rarely, chronic encephalitis occur.

Diagnosis. Cytologic examination (Tzanck stain) or direct fluorescent antibody stains may reveal cells with characteristic intranuclear inclusions or giant cells. These indicate either HSV or varicella-zoster virus infection. Antigen detection tests, such as fluorescent antibody and enzyme-linked immunoassays, are rapid and specific but are only 50–80% sensitive. The test of choice is PCR or (if it is not available) tissue culture for viral cytopathic effects, which is rapid (2–5 days), specific, and sensitive.

Acute and convalescent antibody testing may be diagnostic in primary infection but is not helpful for making clinically useful decisions. Most neonates have transplacental anti-HSV antibody, patients with recurrences have high and stable levels of antibody, and severely immunosuppressed children may fail to produce any antibody.

Treatment. Therapy for HSV infection depends on the type of the disease (primary or recurrent), the anatomic sites involved, and, most important, the immune status of the host. No treatment is needed for mild, self-limited infection in immunocompetent children (gingivostomatitis, "cold sores"). Acyclovir is used either orally for uncomplicated infections (primary genital lesions) or intravenously for more serious (encephalitis) or disseminated (immunocompromised host, neonate) infections. Topical therapy with trifluridine or iododeoxyuridine is indicated for ocular infection.

Prevention. Prepartum HSV cultures do not predict the presence of the virus at the time of delivery. Women at term with active genital lesions at the time of deliver and ruptured membrane should have a cesarean delivery; the risk of neonatal infection is decreased if performed within 4–6 hours of membrane rupture.

Many clinicians elect to treat neonates born to mothers with primary genital herpes simplex infection because their risk of infection is greater than 50%. Chronic acyclovir occasionally is used in patients with frequent or severe recurrences of herpes infections (particularly HIV-infected patients); acyclovir resistance has occurred in this setting. The use of condoms provides some protection against sexual transmission of herpes simplex.

REFERENCES

Behrman RE, Kliegman RM, Jenson HB, editors: *Nelson textbook of pediatrics,* ed 16, Philadelphia, 2000, WB Saunders, Chapter 245.

Jacobs RF: Neonatal herpes simplex virus infections, *Semin Perinatol* 22:64–71, 1998.

Kimberlin DW, Lakeman FD, Arvin AM, et al: Application of the polymerase chain reaction to the diagnosis and management of neonatal herpes simplex virus disease: National Institute of Allergy and Infectious Diseases collaborative antiviral study group, *J Infect Dis* 174:1162–1167, 1996.

Langenberg AG, Corey L, Ashley RL, et al: A prospective study of new infections with herpes simplex virus type 1 and type 2: Chiron HSV Vaccine Study Group, *N Engl J Med* 341: 1432–1438, 1999.

Varicella-Zoster Virus Infection

Etiology. Varicella-zoster virus (VZV) is a member of the Herpesviridae family. It is an enveloped, icosahedral, double-stranded DNA virus that causes varicella as a primary infection or an endogenously reactivated recurrent infection (herpes zoster or shingles). The virus infects susceptible individuals by the conjunctivae or respiratory tract and replicates in the nasopharynx and upper respiratory tract. It then disseminates by a primary viremia and infects regional lymph nodes, the liver, the spleen, and other organs. A secondary viremia follows, resulting in a cutaneous infection with the typical vesicular rash. There is one antigenic type of varicella, and humans are the only host. The organism has been found in dorsal root ganglia cells in individuals with herpes zoster infection.

Varicella (Chickenpox)

Epidemiology. Varicella is a highly contagious infection of childhood. The peak age of occurrence is 5–10 years; 90% of children in temperate climates are infected by age 10. The secondary household attack rate in susceptible individuals is 90%. The peak seasonal infection rate is late winter and spring. Transmission is by direct contact, droplet, and air. The incubation period is generally 14–16 days, with a range of 11–20 days after contact. The period of communicability ranges from 2 days before to 7 days after the onset of the rash, when all lesions are crusted. Patients with zoster may cause varicella in seronegative contacts.

Clinical Manifestations

Chickenpox. Primary infection with VZV results in chickenpox. Prodromal symptoms (fever, malaise, and anorexia) may precede the rash by 1 day. The characteristic rash appears initially as small red papules that rapidly progress to nonumbilicated, oval, "teardrop" vesicles on an erythematous base. The fluid progresses from clear to cloudy, and the vesicles ulcerate, crust, and heal. New crops appear for 3–4 days, usually beginning on the trunk and then the head, the face, and, less commonly, the extremities. In total, there may be 100–300 lesions, with all forms of lesions being present at the same time. Pruritus is almost universal. Lesions may be present on all mucous membranes. Lymphadenopathy may be generalized. The severity of the rash varies, as do systemic signs and fever, which generally abate after 3–4 days.

Congenital Varicella. Varicella in the pregnant woman may result in fetal varicella infection, characterized by low birth weight, cortical atrophy, seizures, mental retardation, chorioretinitis, cataracts, microcephaly, intracranial calcifications, and diagnostic cicatricial scarring of the body or extremities.

In mothers with varicella (not shingles) occurring 5 days before or 2 days after delivery, a severe neonatal varicella syndrome develops that is thought to be caused by the lack of transplacental antibody. These infants should be treated as soon as possible with zoster immune globulin (ZIG) to attempt to prevent or ameliorate their infection. In children who were exposed in utero to VZV, zoster may develop early in life without ever exhibiting varicella.

Complications. Although VZV infection is generally a mild disease, complications are common. Varicella is a more severe disease for neonates, adults, and immunosuppressed individuals. HIV-infected children frequently have a prolonged course and may have recurrent episodes of varicella. Secondary infection of skin lesions by streptococci or staphylococci is the most common complication. Such infections may be mild or life threatening (e.g., toxic shock or necrotizing fasciitis). Thrombocytopenia and hemorrhagic lesions or bleeding also may occur (purpura fulminans, varicella gangrenosa). Pneumonia is uncommon in healthy children but occurs in 15–20% of healthy adults and immunosuppressed patients. Myocarditis, pericarditis, orchitis, hepatitis, ulcerative gastritis, glomerulonephritis, and arthritis complicate VZV. Reye syndrome may be preceded by varicella; therefore, aspirin should be avoided during varicella infection.

Neurologic complications are postinfectious encephalitis, cerebellar ataxia, nystagmus, and tremor. Guillain-Barré syndrome, transverse myelitis, cranial nerve palsies, optic neuritis, and hypothalamic syndrome have been associated with varicella.

In immunodeficient or immunosuppressed children, primary varicella can be a fatal disease as a result of visceral dissemination, encephalitis, and pneumonitis. In children with leukemia who have not received prophylaxis or therapy for varicella, the mortality rate approaches 10%.

Diagnosis. Vesicles contain polymorphonuclear leukocytes. Cytology and electron microscopy of vesicular fluid or scrapings may reveal intranuclear inclusions, giant cells, and virus particles. VZV is fastidious and difficult to culture. If the cytology is consistent with either HSV or VZV but is culture negative, it may indicate VZV. Infection can be confirmed by detection of varicella-specific antigen in vesicular fluid with immunofluorescence of monoclonal antibodies or by testing acute and convalescent antibody for VZV antibody.

Treatment. Symptomatic therapy of varicella includes nonaspirin antipyretics, cool baths, and careful hygiene. Intravenous acyclovir is effective in treating varicella in immunocompromised patients. Early therapy prevents severe complications, including pneumonia, encephalitis, and death. Oral acyclovir shortens the duration of illness in normal children; however, it is uncertain whether acyclovir's cost justifies its use in otherwise healthy children. VZIG is not effective therapy once the disease has been contracted.

Oral acyclovir given within 24 hours of the appearance of the first cutaneous lesion is associated with clinical benefit in healthy patients. In adolescents and adults, early administration of acyclovir may decrease the incidence of varicella pneumonia. In patients receiving corticosteroids or a chronic regimen of salicylates, its use in uncomplicated varicella is recommended. The dose of acyclovir for varicella-zoster infections is higher than for herpes simplex.

Prevention. A live attenuated varicella vaccine was licensed for use in 1995 (Fig. 10–1). A single dose is recommended for use in healthy children ages 1–12 years. It is effective but not as protective as the measles vaccine; household exposure to varicella within 5 years of vaccination results in mild disease (>50 skin lesions) in about 20% of exposed children. The major adverse effects of the vaccine are local tenderness at the injection site and a sparse maculopapular rash occurring within 1 month of immunization in approximately 5% of vaccinees. Transmission of the vaccine virus from a healthy vaccinee is possible.

Passive immunity can be induced by use of VZIG, which is indicated within 96 hours of exposure for susceptible individuals at risk for severe illness. Candidates for VZIG are immunocompromised or immunosuppressed individuals, neonates of infected mothers who had onset of chickenpox within 5 days before delivery or 48 hours after delivery, premature infants younger than 28 weeks or those born to mothers without a history of chickenpox, and possibly children older than 15 years or adults with a close exposure to varicella. Administration of VZIG does not eliminate the possibility of disease in recipients and prolongs the incubation period to 28 days. Children should not return to school until all vesicles have crusted. The hospitalized child with varicella should be isolated in a room that will prevent the air-circulation system from transmitting the virus.

Herpes Zoster (Shingles)

Epidemiology. Shingles is a recurrence of VZV in individuals previously infected. After the episode of chickenpox, VZV remains latent in nerve ganglion cells, but for unknown reasons (other than immunosuppression) a local recurrence occurs. Herpes zoster is unusual in children under 10 years of age. Infants and young children with herpes zoster often have a history of early or presumed in utero varicella. Immunocompromised or immunosuppressed children have an increased incidence of herpes zoster.

Clinical Manifestations. The preeruption phase of shingles includes intense localized pain and tenderness along a dermatome, accompanied by malaise and fever. In several days, the eruption of papules, which quickly vesiculate, occurs in the dermatome or in two adjacent dermatomes. Groups of lesions occur for 1–7 days then progress to crusts and healing. The typical areas involved are dorsal and lumbar, although cephalic and sacral lesions may develop. Lesions generally are unilateral and are accompanied by regional lymphadenopathy. In one third of patients, a few vesicles occur outside the primary dermatome.

Any branch of cranial nerve V may be involved, which also may cause corneal and intraoral lesions. Involvement of cranial nerve VII may result in facial paralysis and ear canal vesicles **(Ramsay Hunt syndrome).** Ophthalmic zoster may be associated with ipsilateral cerebral angiitis and stroke. Immunocompromised patients may have unusually severe, painful herpes zoster that involves cutaneous and, rarely, visceral dissemination (to liver, lungs, and CNS). Skin lesions may be chronic and hemorrhagic. Postherpetic neuralgia and ocular complications are rare in normal children. Secondary bacterial infections may occur.

Diagnosis. The differentiation between VZV and HSV infections is difficult because HSV may cause infection in a dermatome distribution. The previously healthy patient with more than one recurrence probably has HSV infection, which can be confirmed by culture.

Treatment. VZV infection in immunocompromised patients is treated with acyclovir, either orally or parenterally, depending on the severity of the infection. Acyclovir therapy decreases pain, shortens the duration of viral shedding, and decreases visceral dissemination.

Prevention. There is no clinically useful way to prevent herpes zoster. Patients with herpes zoster are infectious to VZV-susceptible individuals.

REFERENCES

Behrman RE, Kliegman RM, Jenson HB, editors: *Nelson textbook of pediatrics,* ed 16, Philadelphia, 2000, WB Saunders, Chapter 246.

Brunell PA: Varicella in pregnancy, the fetus, and the newborn: problems in management, *J Infect Dis* 166(Suppl 1):S42, 1992.

Dunkle LM, Arvin AM, Whitley RJ, et al: A controlled trial of acyclovir for chickenpox in normal children, *N Engl J Med* 32:1539, 1991.

Kelley R, Mancao M, Lee F, et al: Varicella in children with perinatally acquired human immunodeficiency virus infection, *J Pediatr* 124:271, 1994.

Human Herpesvirus-6 and Human Herpesvirus-7

(Exanthem Subitum, Roseola Infantum)

Etiology. HHV-6, a member of the herpesvirus family, is a large, enveloped double-stranded DNA virus. It is the infectious agent of roseola, also called exanthem subitum or sixth disease. This virus is ubiquitous and is likely to be transmitted by respiratory secretions. It infects mature T cells, B cells, astrocytes, and macrophages and causes a relatively prolonged (3–5 days) viremia during primary infection. HHV-6 can be detected in the saliva of healthy adults, which suggests that, as with other herpesviruses, there are latent infection and intermittent shedding of virus.

Epidemiology. Most children become seropositive for HHV-6 by 2 years of age, and most primary infections occur in the first year of life after 6 months of age. HHV-6 is a major cause of acute febrile illnesses in infants and in one study was responsible for 20% of the visits to the emergency department for infants 6–18 months of age. There is a notable lack of history of exposure to other children with similar illnesses, which suggests that the virus is acquired from asymptomatic adults. HHV-7 has many similarities to HHV-6. HHV-7 infection occurs at an older age (2 years versus 9 months) and may have a higher incidence of seizures. Both viruses cause encephalitis in immunocompromised patients.

Clinical Manifestations. The most reliable characteristic of HHV-6 infection is high fever, often 40° C or more, with an abrupt onset and lasting 3–7 days. In roseola, a maculopapular rash erupts coincident with defervescence, although it may also be present earlier. Respiratory symptoms, nasal congestion, erythematous tympanic membranes, and cough may occur, and gastrointestinal symptoms are often described: most commonly, patients are irritable and appear toxic. CNS findings are common, with a bulging anterior fontanel often associated with roseola; seizures occur in some patients, suggesting that this virus may be responsible for many febrile seizures.

Laboratory findings include a relatively low WBC count, particularly reduced numbers of lymphocytes. Infection in immunocompromised hosts, transplant patients, or children infected with HIV can be disseminated and severe. Reactivation of HHV-6 may be a cause of bone marrow suppression following bone marrow transplantation.

Differential Diagnosis. The characteristic timing of the onset of rash immediately after defervescence of fever is not typical of other viral exanthems (e.g., rubella, rubeola, or enteroviral infection). The differential diagnosis of the infant with high fever must include local infections (otitis media, pneumonia, pyelonephritis, meningitis) and nonlocalized bacteremia (especially pneumococcal). Assays for the diagnosis of primary HHV-6 infection are being developed. Serologic tests, including indirect immunofluorescent and enzyme immunosorbent assays, are available.

Treatment. Management of HHV-6 infections is primarily supportive, providing control of fever and symptomatic relief. For immunocompromised patients, ganciclovir and foscarnet, which have in vitro activity against the virus, have been tried, but there are no controlled clinical trials available.

REFERENCES

Behrman RE, Kliegman RM, Jenson HB, editors: *Nelson textbook of pediatrics*, ed 16, Philadelphia, 2000, WB Saunders, Chapter 249.

Caserta MT, Hall CB, Schnabel K, et al: Primary human herpesvirus-7 infection: a comparison of human herpesvirus-7 and human herpesvirus-6 infections in children, *J Pediatr* 133:386–389, 1998.

Kimberlin DW: Human herpesviruses 6 and 7: identification of newly recognized viral pathogens and their association with human disease, *Pediatr Infect Dis J* 17:59–67, 1998.

Peiris M: Human herpesvirus-6 (HHV-6) and HHV-7 infections in bone marrow transplant recipients, *Crit Rev Oncol Hematol* 32:187–196, 1998.

Human Immunodeficiency Virus Infection

(Acquired Immunodeficiency Syndrome)

Etiology. The cause of AIDS in infants, children, and adults is HIV. Human immunodeficiency viruses are RNA retroviruses that produce a reverse transcriptase enabling the viral RNA to act as a template for DNA transcription and incorporation into the host genome. HIV-1 is most common in the United States. HIV-2 is a related virus rarely seen in the United States, but is more common in Africa.

Pathogenesis. HIV selectively infects human helper T cells via an interaction between the CD4 and a number of chemokine surface receptors on the T cell and the viral protein gp120. Because helper T cells are important for delayed hypersensitivity, for T cell–dependent B-cell antibody production, and for T cell–mediated lymphokine activation of macrophages, their destruction produces a profound combined (B and T cell) immunodeficiency. Lack of T-cell regulation and unrestrained antigenic stimulation result in a nonspecific and ineffective polyclonal hypergammaglobulinemia. Infection of macrophages disseminates the virus throughout the body and passes the virus to uninfected CD4+ T cells. Infection of brain tissue accounts for the encephalopathy and cerebral atrophy associated with the condition.

HIV is a chronic, progressive process with a variable period of clinical latency. Sensitive assays for HIV nucleic acids demonstrate that virtually all untreated patients have evidence of ongoing viral replication. As long as the host continues to replace the CD4 cells destroyed by infection, there are no overt manifestations of immunodeficiency. When CD4 cell numbers become progressively depleted, clinical immunodeficiency results. The ability to quantify the viral load has become important in management. Patients with more virus have a more rapid depletion of the CD4 cells accompanied by the development of the typical opportunistic infections (*P. carinii* and *M. avium-intracellulare* complex).

Epidemiology. Unprotected sexual contact (heterosexual or homosexual), intravenous drug use, and birth to or breast-feeding by an HIV-infected mother leads to a high risk of infection. Many routes of infection, such as contaminated blood and blood products, have been eliminated in developed countries, but are a risk in less developed areas.

Perinatal transmission of HIV infection may occur either transplacentally or more likely perinatally and is preventable with perinatal antiretroviral therapy. Other risk factors are prematurity, rupture of membranes more than 4 hours, and high circulating levels of virus at the time of delivery. Perinatal transmission can be decreased from approximately 25% to less than 8% with treatment of the mother with zidovudine before delivery and treatment of the infant postnatally. The minimum treatment needed to protect the infant in areas where antiretroviral drugs are limited is still under investigation. Breast-feeding by HIV-infected mothers increases the risk of neonatal HIV infection by 50–100%.

The epidemiology of HIV infection in the pediatric population has shifted in developed countries as fewer infants are infected. Many cases are now in young adults who engage in unprotected sexual activities. In areas of Africa and Asia, infection rates as high as 40% are largely the result of heterosexual transmission.

Clinical Manifestations. In the United States, most high-risk pregnant women are screened and treated for HIV infection. Their infants similarly receive prophylactic therapy and are prospectively tested for infection. The diagnosis of HIV infection in most infants born in the United States is made before there are clinical signs of infection. This is in contrast to previous eras, in which the diagnosis of the condition was made in infants when they demonstrated serious opportunistic infection and clear-cut evidence of immunodeficiency (Tables 10–19 and 10–20). In such untreated patients the mean incubation period after vertical transmission is 5 months, ranging from 1–24 months. In older patients the incubation period is generally 7–10 years. The major manifestations of HIV infections and the basis for the classification of the disease are the opportunistic infections related to the depletion of CD4+ T cells (Tables 10–19 and 10–20).

Pulmonary Disease. Pulmonary manifestations of HIV infection are common and include *Pneumocystis carinii* (PCP) infection, which can present early in infancy as a primary pneumonia characterized by profound hypoxia, accompanying tachypnea, retrac-

tions, elevated serum LDH, and fever. Neonates at risk for vertical transmission of HIV infection receive anti-PCP prophylaxis, usually with trimethoprim/sulfamethoxazole. In older patients, the risk of PCP is directly related to the CD4+ count and specific recommendations have been established. In untreated infants, lymphoid interstitial pneumonitis was commonly seen, probably representing HIV pulmonary infection, but is rarely seen in children receiving antiretroviral therapy.

AIDS-defining illnesses are similar to those described in adults but include lymphoid interstitial pneumonitis and lymphoid hyperplasia, as well as lymphadenitis. For children older than 13 years of age there is an expanded CDC case definition that can be applied.

An acute retroviral syndrome consists of fever, malaise, weight loss, pharyngitis, lymphadenopathy, and a maculopapular rash. This syndrome develops 2–6 weeks after an HIV infection and coincides with the appearance of anti-HIV antibodies. Prompt treatment of individuals with acute HIV infection with potent combinations of antiretroviral agents may be highly effective.

Diagnosis. To diagnose HIV infection in a neonate it is necessary to demonstrate active viral infection because maternal transplacental anti-HIV antibodies

---

TABLE 10–19

CDC Classification for Children (Below 13 Years of Age) with Human Immunodeficiency Virus (HIV) Infection

Clinical Categories	Diagnostic Criteria
N: Not Symptomatic: No signs or symptoms of HIV infection or only one of the conditions listed in Category A	If < 18 months of age has two positive results on separate determinations from one or more of the following: (a) HIV culture, (b) HIV PCR or (c) HIV p24 antigen If 18 months is HIV antibody positive by repeatedly reactive ELISA and confirmatory test (e.g., Western blot or IFA)
A: Mildly Symptomatic: Two or more of the conditions listed, but none of the conditions listed in Categories B or C	Lymphadenopathy (0.5 cm at more than two sites; bilateral one site) Hepatomegaly Splenomegaly Dermatitis Parotitis Recurrent or persistent upper respiratory infection, sinusitis, or OM

Modified from Centers for Disease Control and Prevention: *MMWR* 43(RR-12):1–19, 1994.
AIDS, Acquired immunodeficiency syndrome; *CMV,* cytomegalovirus; *CT,* computed tomography; *HSV,* herpes simplex virus; *LIP,* lymphoid interstitial pneumonia; *MRI,* magnetic resonance imaging; *OFC,* occipitofrontal circumference; *OM,* otitis media; *PCR,* polymerase chain reaction.

Continued

TABLE 10–19
CDC Classification for Children (Below 13 Years of Age) with Human Immunodeficiency Virus (HIV) Infection—cont'd

Clinical Categories	Diagnostic Criteria
B: Moderately Symptomatic: Symptoms of HIV infection other than those listed for Categories A or C Examples include but are not limited to those listed	Anemia (<8), neutropenia (<1,000), or thrombocytopenia (<100,000) persisting 30 days Bacterial meningitis, pneumonia or sepsis (single episode) Candidiasis, oropharyngeal thrush, persisting >2 mo in children >6 mo old Cardiomyopathy CMV infection, onset before 1 mo of age Diarrhea, recurrent or chronic Hepatitis HSV stomatitis, recurrent (more than 2 episodes within 1 year) HSV bronchitis, pneumonitis or esophagitis with onset before 1 mo of age Herpes zoster (shingles)—two episodes or more than one dermatome Leiomyosarcoma LIP or pulmonary lymphoid hyperplasia (AIDS defining, report to State) Nephropathy Nocardiosis Persistent fever (lasting >1 mo) Toxoplasmosis, onset before 1 mo of age Varicella, disseminated (complicated chickenpox)
C. Severely Symptomatic: Any condition listed in the 1987 surveillance case definition for AIDS, with the exception of LIP	Serious bacterial infection; 2 in 2 yr: sepsis, pneumonia, meningitis, bone or joint infection, abscess of organ or body cavity (excludes OM, skin or mucosal abscesses and indwelling catheter infections) Candidiasis (esophageal, tracheal, bronchial, pulmonary) Coccidioidomycosis, disseminated or extrapulmonary Cryptococcosis, extrapulmonary Cryptosporidiosis or isosporiasis >1 mo duration CMV disease (onset >1 mo), other than liver, spleen or lymph nodes Encephalopathy: more than one finding for >2 mo and no illness that explains: (a) failure to attain or loss of milestones or intellectual ability shown by neuropsychological tests; (b) impaired brain growth or acquired microcephaly shown by OFC measurements or brain atrophy on CT scan or MRI (serial imaging needed if <2 years old); (c) acquired symmetric motor deficit with 2 of: paresis, pathologic reflexes, ataxia or gait disturbances Herpes simplex (ulcer >1 mo duration or pneumonia or esophagitis >1 mo old) Histoplasmosis, disseminated or extrapulmonary Kaposi sarcoma Lymphoma, primary, in brain Lymphoma, B cell, non-Hodgkin lymphoma *Mycobacterium tuberculosis*, disseminated or extrapulmonary *Mycobacterium* infection, noncutaneous, extrapulmonary or disseminated (except leprosy)

Modified from Centers for Disease Control and Prevention: *MMWR* 43(RR-12):1–19, 1994.
AIDS, Acquired immunodeficiency syndrome; *CMV,* cytomegalovirus; *CT,* computed tomography; *HSV,* herpes simplex virus; *LIP,* lymphoid interstitial pneumonia; *MRI,* magnetic resonance imaging; *OFC,* occipitofrontal circumference; *OM,* otitis media; *PCR,* polymerase chain reaction.

TABLE 10–19
CDC Classification for Children (Below 13 Years of Age) with Human Immunodeficiency Virus (HIV) Infection—cont'd

Clinical Categories	Diagnostic Criteria
C. Severely Symptomatic—cont'd	*Pneumocystis carinii* pneumonia Progressive multifocal leukoencephalopathy *Salmonella* (nontyphoid) sepsis, recurrent Toxoplasmosis of the brain, onset >1 mo old Wasting syndrome—in absence of other illness that explains: (a) weight loss >10% of baseline *or* (b) downward crossing of two percentile lines on the weight chart in a child 1 yr *or* (c) <5th percentile on weight for height on two consecutive measures 30 days apart *plus* (1) chronic diarrhea (two loose stools/day for 30 days) *or* (2) documented fever for 30 days, intermittent or constant

Modified from Centers for Disease Control and Prevention: *MMWR* 43(RR-12):1–19, 1994.
AIDS, Acquired immunodeficiency syndrome; *CMV,* cytomegalovirus; *CT,* computed tomography; *HSV,* herpes simplex virus; *LIP,* lymphoid interstitial pneumonia; *MRI,* magnetic resonance imaging; *OFC,* occipitofrontal circumference; *OM,* otitis media; *PCR,* polymerase chain reaction.

TABLE 10–20
CDC Classification for Children (Below 13 Years of Age) with Human Immunodeficiency Virus (HIV) Infection

Immunologic Categories Based on Age-Specific CD4 +T-Lymphocyte Counts and Percent of Total Lymphocytes

	Age of Child					
	<12 mo		1–5 yr		6–12 yr	
Immunologic Category	µL	%	µL	%	µL	%
1. No suppression	31500	325	31000	325	3500	325
2. Moderate suppression	750–1499	15–24	500–999	15–24	200–499	15–24
3. Severe suppression	<750	<15	<500	<15	<200	<15

Pediatric HIV Classification Based on Degree of Immune Suppression and Clinical Category*

	Clinical Categories			
Immunologic Category	*N: No Signs/Symptoms*	*A: Mild Signs/Symptoms*	*B: Moderate Signs/Symptoms†*	*C: Severe Signs/Symptoms†*
1. No suppression	N1	A1	B1	C1
2. Moderate suppression	N2	A2	B2	C2
3. Severe suppression	N3	A3	B3	C3

From Centers for Disease Control and Prevention: *MMWR* 43(RR-12):1–19, 1994.
*Children whose HIV infection status is not confirmed are classified by placing the letter E (for perinatally exposed) before the classification code (e.g., EN1).
†Both Category C and lymphoid interstitial pneumonitis in Category B are reportable to state health departments as acquired immunodeficiency virus (AIDS).

will be detectable for up to 18 months. Virologic diagnostic tests include HIV culture, or detection of HIV DNA or RNA or HIV p24 antigen. An exposed infant is considered to be infected if virologic tests are positive on two separate occasions. If a child tests repeatedly negative by 6 months of age, the chance of infection is remote. All exposed infants should have an HIV antibody test done at 18 months of age to finalize the diagnosis, because all maternal IgG should be gone by this time. Older children may be screened for HIV antibody, confirmed by Western blot (specific for HIV) and assessed by viral load (virus culture or PCR).

The *differential diagnosis* includes primary immunodeficiency syndromes (usually found in HIV-negative children whose parents have no risk factors for HIV infection) and intrauterine infection caused by other agents.

Treatment. Three classes of drugs are available for the treatment of HIV infection. Zidovudine (AZT) has been shown to be effective in decreasing the transmission of HIV from the infected pregnant woman to the neonate when it is given in the perinatal period. Additional nucleoside analogs used in children are didanosine (dideoxyinosine), zalcitabine (dideoxycytidine), stavudine (D4T), and lamivudine (3TC). Nonnucleoside inhibitors of reverse transcriptase (Viramune [nevirapine]) are widely used, as are inhibitors of the HIV protease, an enzyme required to cleave the gag-pol precursor protein of HIV, which contains important structural and enzymatic elements required for viral maturation. The protease inhibitors are associated with significant drug-drug interactions because they can induce the cytochrome CYP3A4 P450 enzymes.

The ability of HIV to rapidly become resistant to antiretroviral agents and the development of cross-resistance to several classes of agents at once are also major problems. Therapeutic regimens involve drugs in combination, and consultation with an expert in this area is encouraged. Viral loads can be significantly reduced when such combination therapy is used with the amelioration of clinical symptoms and opportunistic infection.

The approach to the numerous opportunistic infections in HIV-infected patients involves both prophylaxis and treatment for infections likely to occur as CD4 cells are depleted. With potent antiretroviral therapy and immune reconstitution, routine prophylaxis for these common opportunistic infections depends on the child's age and CD4+ count. Infection caused by *P. carinii* can be prevented with trimethoprim/sulfamethoxazole, and *M. avium-intracellulare* infection can be prevented with prophylactic rifabutin in patients with CD4 cell counts less than 200. Pneumococcal sepsis is common, and

some patients may benefit from immunization or IVIG, since normal B-cell function is often impaired. Oral and gastrointestinal candidiasis is common and often responds to imidazole therapy. Varicella-zoster infection may be severe and should be treated with acyclovir. Recurrent herpes simplex infections may also require acyclovir prophylaxis. Other common infections in HIV-infected patients are toxoplasmosis, CMV, EBV, salmonellosis, and tuberculosis.

Opportunistic infections should be treated aggressively, as with any infection in an immunodeficient host. Treatment of PCP is possible with high-dose trimethoprim/sulfamethoxazole and steroids. Although routine immunizations may result in suboptimal antibody concentrations, they remain indicated except for the use of most live vaccines in symptomatically infected children. Because of the risk of fatal measles in children with AIDS, live measles vaccine is indicated in presymptomatic, HIV-seropositive patients. Children exposed to varicella or measles should receive ZIG or serum immune globulin, respectively. Household contacts of children with AIDS should receive inactivated, not live, poliovirus vaccine.

Prevention. Preventing AIDS or HIV infection in adults decreases the incidence of infection in children. Adult prevention may result from behavior changes ("safe sex," decrease in intravenous drug use, needle exchange), abortion, or avoidance of pregnancy and breast-feeding (in developed countries) in high-risk women. Screening of blood donors already has markedly reduced the risk of transmission from blood products, including those used to treat hemophilia. HIV infection almost never is transmitted in a casual or nonsexual household setting.

REFERENCES

Balotta C, Colombo C, Colucci G, et al: Plasma viremia and virus phenotype are correlates of disease progression in vertical human immunodeficiency virus type 1 infected children, *Pediatr Infect Dis J* 16:205, 1997.
Behrman RE, Kliegman RM, Jenson HB, editors: *Nelson textbook of pediatrics*, ed 16, Philadelphia, 2000, WB Saunders, Chapter 268.
Centers for Disease Control and Prevention: CDC 1999 US-PHA/IDSA guidelines for the prevention of opportunistic infections in persons infected with human immunodeficiency virus, *MMWR* 48(RR-10):1–59, 61–66, 1999.
Drugs for HIV infection, *Med Lett* 42:1, 2000.
Guidelines for the use of antiretroviral agents in pediatric HIV infection. Updated Jan 7, 2000. Available online at http://www.hivatis.org/trtgdlns.html#Pediatric.
Kourtis AP, Bulterys M, Nesheim SR, et al: Understanding the timing of HIV transmission from mother to infant, *JAMA* 285:709, 2001.
Kovacs JA, Masur H: Prophylaxis against opportunistic infections in patients with human immunodeficiency virus infection, *N Engl J Med* 342:1416, 2000.

Kuhn L, Abrams EJ, Weedon J, et al: Disease progression and early viral dynamics in human immunodeficiency virus–infected children exposed to zidovudine during prenatal and perinatal periods, *J Infect Dis* 182:104, 2000.

Lallemant M, Jourdain G, LeCoeur S, et al: A trial of shortened zidovudine regimens to prevent mother-to-child transmission of human immunodeficiency virus type 1, *N Engl J Med* 343:982, 2000.

Perlmutter BL, Glaser JB, Oyugi SO: How to recognize and treat acute HIV syndrome, *Am Fam Physician* 60:535, 1999.

Influenza Viral Infection

Etiology. Influenza viruses are RNA orthomyxoviruses with a segmented genome. The viruses infect animals, particularly birds and swine, as well as humans, facilitating genetic reassortments among the viruses infecting different species.

There are three major types: A, B, and C. A and B account for major epidemics and consist of (1) a negatively stranded RNA, which encodes 10 proteins including the hemagglutin (HA) that mediates viral binding to epithelial cells, and (2) neuraminidase (N), an enzyme that allows viral release from the cell surface. Major changes in HA account for *antigenic drift*, responsible for epidemics of disease occurring in a susceptible population. Minor variations in HA *(antigenic shift)* occur more frequently. These antigenic variants cause cycles of disease and allow for the classification of viruses as A/Hong Kong/68 (H3N2), for example, which is distinct from the H1N1 viruses. Specific antibodies to different viruses are important determinants of immunity.

Epidemiology. Influenza occurs seasonally in temperate climates, with annual epidemics of influenza A in the winter months. Influenza B causes outbreaks every 3–4 years; often both influenza A and B are found concurrently. Antigenic shift is responsible for major pandemics of influenza, which occur every 10–40 years, with antigenic drifts occurring more frequently (every 2–3 years). The virus is shed in infected respiratory secretions and is transmitted from person to person or by articles contaminated with nasopharyngeal secretions. The period of communicability begins 24 hours before symptoms develop and continues until resolution. The incubation period is from 1–3 days.

Pathogenesis. During the incubation period, virus is present in the respiratory tract but rarely in blood and other organs. Virus binds to respiratory epithelial cells, replicates, and causes cell death, desquamation, and decreased mucociliary clearance of bacteria. Immunity correlates better with secretory antibody than with serum antibody, although the latter is associated with protection.

Clinical Manifestations

Older Children and Adolescents. In this group the manifestations are similar to those seen in adults. There is an abrupt onset of high fever, flushed face, headache, myalgia, cough, and chills. Pharyngitis occurs in 50% of patients, and ocular symptoms (tearing, photophobia, burning, pain on eye motion) and nasal stuffiness are common. These symptoms last 2–5 days. As the systemic signs and symptoms resolve, the cough and nasal congestion become more prominent and last 4–10 days. Leukopenia occurs in 25% of patients, and 10% have clinical and roentgenographic evidence of bronchopneumonia.

Younger Children. The classic influenza illness is less common in younger children, who manifest laryngotracheitis, bronchiolitis, bronchitis, pneumonia, or a mild upper respiratory tract syndrome. Influenza B has been associated with myositis. Parotitis has been reported in influenza A infection. Fever tends to be higher in younger children than in older children. In neonates, the sudden fever and nonspecific signs simulate sepsis, although a nasal discharge may suggest the diagnosis of a viral respiratory tract infection. Influenza C infection has been associated with an upper respiratory tract syndrome.

Significant increases in hospitalizations for children of all ages occur during the influenza season. Morbidity for children with underlying diseases also increases.

Complications. The most important complication is secondary bacterial infection of the respiratory tract, including otitis media, sinusitis, and pneumonia. These complications should be treated with antibiotics effective against *Haemophilus*, pneumococci, and staphylococci. Virus-related complications are pneumonia, rarely neurologic syndromes, myocarditis, myositis with myoglobinuria, and Reye syndrome. Salicylates should be avoided in children and adolescents with influenza.

Diagnosis. In community-wide outbreaks of winter respiratory tract disease involving all age groups, influenza is the most likely agent. Virus may be isolated in 2–6 days from nasopharyngeal secretions in tissue culture. Rapid diagnosis may be made by PCR, immunofluorescent techniques, or ELISA. Serologic responses are helpful for retrospective diagnosis.

Treatment. Oral oseltamivir and inhaled zanamivir, two neuraminidase inhibitors, significantly improve the outcome of influenza A and B if started early in the infection. Side effects are minimal. Amantadine and rimantadine are useful for prophylaxis and, perhaps, very early in the treatment of only influenza A. Antibiotics should be avoided unless a bacterial superinfection is suspected. Non–aspirin-containing antipyretics increase the patient's comfort and do not carry the risk of the development of Reye syndrome.

Prevention. Inactivated vaccine, given on a yearly basis, is indicated for children at risk for complications and, probably, for other children and adults who live in a household with high-risk children. Examples of the latter are children with cardiovascular, pulmonary (cystic fibrosis, bronchopulmonary dysplasia), metabolic, renal, or neurologic disorders and those who are immunosuppressed or have a hemoglobinopathy, including sickle cell disease.

Oseltamivir and zanamivir are both effective in the prevention of influenza A and B if given after exposure in a family setting.

REFERENCES

Behrman RE, Kliegman RM, Jenson HB, editors: *Nelson textbook of pediatrics*, ed 16, Philadelphia, 2000, WB Saunders, Chapter 251.

Hayden FG, Gubareva LV, Monto AS, et al: Inhaled zanamivir for the prevention of influenza in families, *N Engl J Med* 343:1282, 2000.

Izurieta HS, Thompson WW, Kramarz P, et al: Influenza and the rates of hospitalization for respiratory disease among infants and young children, *N Engl J Med* 342:232, 2000.

Welliver R, Monto AS, Carewicz, et al: Effectiveness of oseltamivir in preventing influenza in household contacts, *JAMA* 285:748, 2001.

Whitley RJ, Hayden FG, Reisinger KS, et al: Oral oseltamivir treatment of influenza in children, *Pediatr Infect Dis J* 20:127, 2001.

Measles (Rubeola)

Etiology. Measles virus is an RNA paramyxovirus with one antigenic type. It is stable at room temperature for 1–2 days and can be cultivated in human or monkey cells, with cytopathic changes visible in 5–10 days.

Epidemiology. Measles is highly contagious, particularly by droplets during the prodromal (catarrhal) stage. The infected individual is contagious from 1–2 days before the development of the characteristic rash. There are few subclinical cases. Most neonates and young children are protected from measles by transplacental antibody but become susceptible toward the end of the first year of life. Passive immunity may interfere with effective vaccination until 12–15 months of age.

The incubation period is 8–12 days from exposure to the onset of symptoms and 14 days from exposure to the onset of rash. In areas where measles vaccination is not available, measles is endemic and responsible for about 1 million deaths per year. Since the widespread use of the measles vaccine, the number of cases has declined dramatically. Recent outbreaks have occurred as a result of decreased rates of immunization in susceptible infants and toddlers in crowded urban areas. Outbreaks of measles in adolescents, particularly on college campuses, have also been reported, and have been found to be caused by primary vaccine failure. This leads to the institution of a second dose of measles vaccine for American children at age 12 (middle school).

Pathogenesis. Viral particles infect the respiratory tract and spread to regional lymph nodes. A primary viremia disseminates the virus. After viral replication, a secondary viremia occurs 5–7 days after the initial infection as virally infected monocytes and other leukocytes spread the virus to the respiratory tract, skin, and other organs. These infected sites are manifested by rash and the classic symptoms of cough, conjunctivitis, and coryza. Histologic evidence includes the presence of multinucleated giant cells and syncytium formation. The virus is found in the respiratory secretions, blood, and urine of infected individuals.

Clinical Manifestations. The manifestations of the 3-day prodromal period are cough, coryza, conjunctivitis, and the pathognomonic Koplik spots (gray-white, sand grain–sized dots on the buccal mucosa opposite the lower molars) that last 12–24 hours. The conjunctiva may reveal a characteristic transverse line of inflammation along the eyelid margin (Stimson line). The rash phase often is accompanied by high fever (40.0°–40.5° C [104°–105° F]). The macular rash begins on the head (often above the hairline) and spreads over most of the body in 24 hours in a descending fashion. It fades in the same manner. The severity of the illness is related to the extent of the rash. It may be petechial or hemorrhagic (**black measles**). As the rash fades, it undergoes desquamation and brownish discoloration.

Cervical lymphadenitis, splenomegaly, and mesenteric lymphadenopathy (with abdominal pain) may be noted. Otitis media, pneumonia, and gastrointestinal tract symptoms are more common in infants. Liver involvement is more common in adults. Leukopenia is characteristic. In patients with acute encephalitis, the CSF reveals an increased protein, a lymphocytic pleocytosis, and normal glucose levels.

Complications. Measles often is complicated by otitis media. Interstitial pneumonia may be caused by measles or, more commonly, may be the result of a secondary bacterial infection. The anergy associated with measles may activate latent tuberculosis. Myocarditis and mesenteric adenitis are infrequent complications. Encephalomyelitis occurs in 1–2:1000 cases and usually occurs 2–5 days after the onset of the rash. Early encephalitis probably is caused by viral activity in the brain, whereas later onset encephalitis is a demyelinating and probably an immunopathologic phenomenon. **Subacute sclerosing panencephalitis** is a late neurologic complication of slow measles infection, occurring years (usually adolescence) after the acute illness.

Diagnosis. The clinical presentation is characteristic. Confirmation includes (1) multinucleated giant cells in nasal mucosal smears, (2) virus isolation in culture, and (3) diagnostic antibody rises in convalescent serum.

The rash must be differentiated from exanthem subitum, rubella, enteroviral or adenoviral infection, infectious mononucleosis, toxoplasmosis, meningococcemia, scarlet fever, rickettsial disease, Kawasaki syndrome, serum sickness, and drug rash. The constellation of fever, rash, cough, and conjunctivitis is fairly diagnostic for measles. Measles modified by transplacental or administered antibody may be less characteristic. Koplik spots usually are pathognomonic but are not always present at the time of the most pronounced rash.

Treatment. Therapy is supportive. Photophobia is intensified by strong light, which should be avoided. Immunoglobulin and steroids are of no proven value in established disease. Vitamin A improves outcome in infected malnourished infants (100,000 U, IV, ×1 for children 6 months to 1 year; 200,000 U, IV, ×1 for children older than 1 year). Vitamin A supplementation should be considered for populations at risk for severe complications, such as (1) infants aged 6 months to 2 years requiring hospitalization, (2) HIV-infected infants, or (3) infants from endemic areas. Intravenous ribavirin also may be of benefit in severe infections.

Prevention

Active Immunization. Live measles vaccine prevents infection and should be administered to children at 12–15 months and at 4–6 years of age (Fig. 10–1). The effects of vaccination are obstructed by transplacental antibody or passive immunization with immunoglobulin (~12 months in the former case, 3 months in the latter). The live vaccine is contraindicated in pregnant women, immunodeficient or immunosuppressed children (see Human Immunodeficiency Virus Infection) during a febrile illness, or if immunoglobulin has been administered within 3 months. If inadvertently vaccinated, immunocompromised patients should receive immunoglobulin. Vaccination shortly after exposure to measles may prevent illness.

Passive Immunization. Immune serum globulin may prevent or ameliorate measles if given within 5 days of exposure. Protection is indicated for chronically ill, immunosuppressed, or immunodeficient children. The usual dose is 0.25 mL/kg or 0.5 mL/kg for immunocompromised children (maximum, 15 mL).

REFERENCES

Behrman RE, Kliegman RM, editors: *Nelson textbook of pediatrics,* ed 16, Philadelphia, 2000, WB Saunders, Chapter 240.

Cutts FT, Henao-Restrepo A, Olive JM: Measles elimination: progress and challenges, *Vaccine* 17(Suppl 3):S47–S52, 1999.

Kaplan LJ, Daum RS, Smaron M, et al: Severe measles in immunocompromised patients, *JAMA* 267:1237–1241, 1992.

Villamor E, Fawzi WW: Vitamin A supplementation: implications for morbidity and mortality in children, *J Infect Dis* 182: S122–133, 2000.

Mumps

Etiology. Mumps is an enveloped, negative-stranded RNA virus of the paramyxovirus family. Humans are the only known host.

Epidemiology. Mumps occurs worldwide and spreads by direct contact, aerosolization of respiratory secretions, and fomites. Epidemics are most frequent in late winter and spring. The incidence of natural infection in developed countries has decreased as a result of immunization.

Although the virus may be isolated from saliva 6 days before and 9 days after the onset of parotid swelling, the illness can be transmitted 1 day before until 3 days after swelling. Transplacental antibody protects infants from infection in the first 6 months of life. Infection is associated with lifelong immunity. The incubation period is usually 16–18 days but may range from 12–25 days after exposure.

Pathogenesis. The mumps virus is acquired through infected respiratory secretions, replicates in the upper respiratory tract and regional lymphatics, and is spread systemically by a primary viremia. It has tropism for the salivary glands, where it causes lymphocytic infiltration and edema. CNS infection also occurs with spread along neuronal pathways.

Clinical Manifestations. Thirty to forty percent of the cases of infection are subclinical, but when symptoms occur, the onset is characterized by fever, muscle pain, headache, malaise, and pain and swelling in the parotid glands lasting 3–7 days. The swelling obscures the angle of the mandible and pushes the earlobe upward and outward. Pain is elicited by palpation of the gland and also by agents, such as citrus juice, that stimulate salivary flow. Swelling and erythema also surround the Stensen duct. Swelling also may be present in the pharynx and larynx and over the manubrium and upper chest (probably as a result of lymphatic obstruction). Swelling of the submandibular glands may accompany parotid swelling, and in 10–15% of cases they may be the only glands involved. The sublingual glands are involved less commonly.

Meningoencephalomyelitis. Sixty-five percent of patients with parotitis have CSF pleocytosis, and more than 10% have clinical manifestations of meningoencephalitis. In the preimmunization era, mumps was one of the most common causes of aseptic meningitis. Early-onset meningitis probably is the result of direct viral infection of the brain, whereas meningoencephalitis that occurs 10 days or more after the onset of illness is a postinfectious, demyelinating syndrome.

Orchitis, Epididymitis. Orchitis and epididymitis occur in 15–35% of adolescents and adults and rarely occur before puberty. They become manifest at the end of the first week of illness. Bilateral illness occurs in 3% of affected patients. The testes are red, swollen, and tender. Atrophy is common as a sequela, but infertility is rare.

Pancreatitis. Mild pancreatitis is common and may become manifest as epigastric pain, tenderness, and vomiting. An elevated serum amylase value usually is present in mumps, with or without clinical pancreatitis. It may indicate pancreatic or salivary gland involvement.

Rare Complications. Examples of rare complications are nephritis (viruria is common but nephritis is rare), thyroiditis, myocarditis, mastitis, deafness, ocular complications, arthritis, and thrombocytopenia. No firm evidence for a fetal mumps syndrome has been discovered.

Diagnosis. The diagnosis is made clinically. Elevated serum amylase is typical and its onset parallels parotid swelling. Specific diagnosis can be confirmed by isolation of the virus from saliva, urine, CSF, or blood by routine viral culture. A rise in serum antibody to mumps also is diagnostic.

Parotitis also may be caused by other viruses, such as enterovirus, lymphocytic choriomeningitis virus, and influenza A virus. CMV may cause parotitis in immunocompromised children, and infants with AIDS may exhibit parotitis. The diagnosis of suppurative parotitis, which usually is the result of *S. aureus,* can be confirmed by expression of purulent material containing bacteria through the Stensen duct. Other causes of swelling in the parotid area are salivary calculus, recurrent parotitis (etiology unknown), salivary gland tumors, lymphomas, and cervical adenitis, which may mimic parotitis.

Treatment. No therapy is available except for supportive care.

Prevention. Live attenuated mumps vaccine has markedly diminished the incidence of mumps and should be administered to children 12–15 months of age as part of their measles, mumps, and rubella (MMR) vaccine (Fig. 10–1). Parotitis and meningoencephalitis are rare complications of the highly protective mumps vaccination.

REFERENCES

Behrman RE, Kliegman RM, Jenson HB, editors: *Nelson textbook of pediatrics,* ed 16, Philadelphia, 2000, WB Saunders, Chapter 242.
Briss PA, Fehrs LJ, Parker RA, et al: Sustained transmission of mumps in a highly vaccinated population: assessment of primary vaccine failure and waning vaccine-induced immunity, *J Infect Dis* 169:77–82, 1994.
Findley SE, Irigoyen M, Schulman A: Children on the move and vaccination coverage in a low-income, urban Latino population, *Am J Public Health* 89:1728–1731, 1999.

Parainfluenza Viral Infection

Etiology. Parainfluenza viruses are RNA viruses of the paramyxovirus family. Four major serotypes (1–4) have been identified, although there is antigenic cross-reactivity among these. Types 1–3 occur in seasonal outbreak settings, whereas type 4 is usually endemic.

Epidemiology. By the age of 3 years, most children have been symptomatically infected with parainfluenza types 1–3. Type 4 infection also is common but usually asymptomatic. Symptomatic reinfection is common. Infection occurs worldwide, with epidemics occurring in the fall and endemic activity occurring throughout the year. Transmission is from person to person by direct contact, aerosolization of respiratory secretions, and articles contaminated by respiratory tract secretions. The period of contagiousness generally is 4–9 days but may last for up to 2–3 weeks. The incubation period is 2–4 days. Infection does not provide complete immunity, but reinfections are usually mild.

Clinical Manifestations. The major manifestations are laryngotracheitis (croup), bronchitis, bronchiolitis, and, less commonly, pneumonia, particularly in immunodeficient children. Illness lasts approximately 5 days. Less common manifestations are parotitis, Guillain-Barré syndrome, aseptic meningitis, and Reye syndrome. Secondary bacterial infections, including otitis media, tracheitis, and pneumonia, may occur. In the immunocompromised host, progressive pneumonia may occur.

Diagnosis. Tissue culture may be used to provide specific diagnosis within 1 week. Serologic diagnosis is possible, but results may be confused by cross-reactivity with other paramyxoviruses. Rapid identification of viral RNA by PCR or viral antigen in nasopharyngeal secretions through immunofluorescent techniques or ELISA may be used to establish the diagnosis. Differential diagnosis includes infection caused by other respiratory viruses (influenza virus, RSV, adenovirus, rhinovirus) and mycoplasma. In addition, bacterial infection (acute epiglottitis), aspirated foreign bodies, and angioneurotic edema must be differentiated from viral laryngotracheobronchitis.

Treatment. No specific antiviral therapy is available for parainfluenza infection. Secondary bacterial infections must be treated.

Prevention. No chemotherapeutic or vaccine modalities are available for prevention.

REFERENCES

Behrman RE, Kliegman RM, Jenson HB, editors: *Nelson textbook of pediatrics,* ed 15, Philadelphia, 2000, WB Saunders, Chapter 252.
Knott AM, Long CE, Hall CB: Parainfluenza viral infections in pediatric outpatients: seasonal patterns and clinical characteristics, *Pedatr Infect Dis J* 13:269–273, 1994.

Respiratory Syncytial Virus Infection

Etiology. RSV is a single-stranded RNA virus of the paramyxovirus family. Among its products are surface proteins F and G, the major antigenic determinants. The heavily glycosylated G protein binds to the cellular receptor. Antibody to the F (fusion) protein neutralizes infectivity. RSV can be divided into A and B subgroups that are antigenically distinct, and both can be present concurrently in a population. Humans are the only source of infection.

Epidemiology. Worldwide outbreaks of respiratory illness caused by RSV occur among infants each winter or early spring. These outbreaks lead to predictable, yearly increases in infant hospitalization for bronchiolitis and pneumonia. The partially protective effect of transplacental antibody probably accounts for the relative lack of severe infection before 4–6 weeks of life. Infection is universal by the age of 2 years. Reinfections are common and tend to be mild. RSV is responsible for 55–85% of cases of bronchiolitis, 15–25% of cases of childhood pneumonia, and 6–8% of cases of croup. Illness generally is introduced into families by an older sibling, parents with "colds," and infants exhibiting the more severe syndromes. Nosocomial infection is extremely common among infants during RSV epidemics. The virus is spread by large droplets delivered, either airborne or via the hands, to nose or eyes. The period of viral shedding is 3–8 days but may last for up to 4 weeks in young infants and longer in immunocompromised patients. The incubation period is 5–8 days.

Pathogenesis. RSV infects the respiratory epithelial cell and causes syncytium formation. The disease involves the small airways with obstruction from edema, mucus secretion, and inflammatory cells. This leads to distal atelectasis and hyperexpansion of the lung. The pathology can be attributed not only to viral destruction of the epithelium but also to the local immune response.

Clinical Manifestations. RSV causes acute respiratory tract disease in all ages, but in infants and young children it is the most important cause of bronchiolitis and pneumonia (see Chapter 12). The initial manifestations of RSV infection are rhinorrhea, pharyngitis, cough, tachypnea, and low-grade fever. If the illness progresses, the cough worsens, wheezing ensues, and signs of respiratory distress appear. Chest x-ray films usually reveal hyperexpansion and, at times, pneumonitis. In young infants, pneumonia may occur alone or concomitantly with bronchiolitis, a combination that often is associated with a paroxysmal cough resembling that of pertussis. In the very young infant, the premature infant, or the child with underlying respiratory or cardiac illness, only apnea and periodic breathing may occur. Long-term abnormalities in pulmonary function and subsequent wheezing that accompany respiratory infections have been reported in children with RSV bronchiolitis or pneumonia. RSV infection is very severe and life threatening in patients with pulmonary hypertension (congenital heart disease, bronchopulmonary dysplasia), immunosuppression, or immunodeficiency.

Diagnosis. The season of the year, the occurrence of community outbreaks, and the presence of a sibling with an upper respiratory tract infection should alert the physician to the likelihood of RSV infection in an infant with bronchiolitis or pneumonia. Routine laboratory tests are of little use in specific diagnosis. Tests of blood gases often reveal a higher level of hypoxemia than expected, and as the infant's condition worsens, hypercapnia ensues. Specific diagnosis can be made by virus isolation from nasopharyngeal secretions (2–5 days) or tests for rapid detection of RSV antigen or RSV RNA by PCR.

The differential diagnosis of RSV pneumonia in young infants must include infection caused by *Chlamydia,* which often is accompanied by conjunctivitis and eosinophilia; infection caused by pertussis, which usually occurs in an unimmunized child with lymphocytosis; or infection caused by other viral or bacterial agents.

Treatment. Symptomatic therapy is usually all that is necessary for most children with RSV infection. Oxygen is indicated for hypoxia. In the severely ill child or in high-risk patients, as noted earlier, the use of aerosolized ribavirin is controversial, and recent studies fail to discern a beneficial effect. Severely ill hospitalized infants are often treated with beta sympathomimetic aerosols. Immunocompromised patients, particularly those receiving bone marrow transplants, have a high mortality with RSV infection and have been treated with RSV-IgG in addition to ribavirin.

Prevention. No vaccines are available to prevent RSV infection. Breast-feeding has been linked to less severe illness in infants. The use of humanized mouse monoclonal RSV immune globulin (palivizumab) offers protection in young infants at high risk for complications of RSV infection (premature birth, chronic lung disease, and younger than 24 months old). It is of no value for therapy. In the hospital setting, meticulous handwashing and the use of gown, gloves, and eye and nose protection has been shown to decrease the occurrence of infection in staff and to decrease the nosocomial spread of RSV.

REFERENCES

Behrman RE, Kliegman RM, Jenson HB, editors: *Nelson textbook of pediatrics,* ed 16, Philadelphia, 2000, WB Saunders, Chapter 253.

Hall CB, Walsh EE, Schnabel KC, et al: Occurrence of groups A and B of respiratory syncytial virus over 15 years: associated epidemiologic and clinical characteristics in hospitalized and ambulatory children, *J Infect Dis* 162:1283–1290, 1990.

Synagis revisited, *Med Lett* 43:13–14, 2001.

Wheeler JG, Wofford J, Turner RB: Historical cohort evaluation of ribavirin efficacy in respiratory syncytial virus infection, *Pediatr Infect Dis J* 12:209–213, 1993.

Rubella (German or Three-Day Measles)

Etiology. Rubella, a single-stranded positive-sense RNA virus with a glycolipid envelope, is a member of the togavirus family. Although it is a pathogen of humans only, the virus is readily cultivated in a variety of tissue culture systems.

Pathogenesis. The virus is acquired from infected respiratory secretions; it invades the respiratory epithelium and is disseminated by a primary viremia. Following replication in the reticuloendothelial system, a secondary viremia ensues and virus can be isolated from peripheral blood monocytes. Virus is then found throughout the body (secretions, CSF, urine). Infection in utero results in significant morbidity. Maternal infection during the first trimester results in fetal infection in more than 90% of cases and in a generalized vasculitis; chronic infection affects virtually all organ systems (see Chapter 6).

Epidemiology. In unvaccinated populations, the illness occurs in 5–14 year olds. In vaccinated populations, it occurs more commonly in teenagers and young adults (especially in large institutions, such as colleges and hospitals). Health care personnel should be screened for rubella antibody and immunized if their status is seronegative. Maximum communicability of postnatal rubella appears to be 2 days before and 5–7 days after onset of the characteristic rash. The incubation period for postnatal rubella ranges from 14–21 days but most commonly is 16–18 days. Infants with congenital rubella may shed virus in nasopharyngeal secretions and urine for more than 1 year after birth and may transmit the virus to susceptible contacts.

Transplacental antibody is protective during the first 6 months of life. In closed populations the infection rate approaches 100%, whereas it is 50–60% among susceptible family members. Subclinical cases outnumber clinically apparent cases by a ratio of 2:1. Rubella generally occurs in the spring, with epidemics occurring in cycles of every 6–9 years in unvaccinated populations. Infection confers lifelong immunity. Surveys indicate that 10–20% of young adults are susceptible to rubella.

Clinical Manifestations. The prodromal phase of rubella (mild catarrhal symptoms) may go unnoticed. The characteristic signs of rubella are retroauricular, posterior cervical, and posterior occipital lymphadenopathy accompanied by an erythematous, maculopapular, discrete rash. The rash begins on the face and spreads to the body; it lasts for 3 days. An enanthem consisting of rose-colored spots on the soft palate may appear before the rash. Other signs are mild pharyngitis, conjunctivitis, anorexia, headache, malaise, and low-grade fever. Polyarthritis (usually of the hands) may occur, especially among older women, but it usually resolves without sequelae. Paresthesia and tendonitis may occur. The WBC count usually is normal or low, and thrombocytopenia rarely occurs.

Diagnosis. Rubella has a relatively nonspecific appearance. The clinical diagnosis can be made with confidence only during a rubella epidemic. The *differential diagnosis* includes scarlet fever, mild rubeola, roseola, enteroviral infection, infectious mononucleosis, and drug eruptions. Specific diagnosis can be established by viral isolation from nasopharyngeal secretions or by a fourfold antibody rise from acute to convalescent serum. Blood, urine, and CSF also may yield the virus, especially in infants with congenital infection.

Treatment. No antiviral therapy is available for rubella.

Prevention. Immunoglobulin should be used in pregnant, nonimmune women exposed to rubella who refuse to have an abortion even if documented infection has occurred. Serology determines the immune status of a pregnant, exposed woman.

Active immunization with a live attenuated vaccine prevents rubella (Fig. 10–1). Following vaccination, virus is shed from the nasopharynx for several weeks, but it is not readily communicable. In the United States, vaccination is indicated for all children (given at 12–15 months of age), for all nonimmune prepubescent children, and for all postpubescent females who are nonimmune and will not become pregnant within 3 months. This regimen has reduced the incidence of rubella and of the congenital rubella syndrome, primarily by preventing epidemics of rubella. In other countries, only pubescent girls are immunized. This policy does not prevent rubella outbreaks but may decrease the percentage of nonimmune pregnant women.

Although highly attenuated and not associated with fetal damage, the vaccine virus has been recovered from fetuses. Therefore, rubella vaccination is contraindicated in pregnant women. Inadvertent use of the vaccine in this setting is not an indication for abortion. Vaccination is contraindicated in patients with an immunodeficiency state, an immunosuppressed condition, vaccine hypersensitivity, or acute febrile illness in patients who have received immunoglobulin within the last 3 months. Fever, lymphadenopathy, rash, arthralgia, and arthritis (the latter two especially in older girls and women) may follow vaccination.

REFERENCES

Behrman RE, Kliegman RM, Jenson HB, editors: *Nelson textbook of pediatrics*, ed 16, Philadelphia, 2000, WB Saunders, Chapter 241.

Lee SH, Ewert DP, Frederick PD, et al: Resurgence of congenital rubella syndrome in the 1990s, *JAMA* 267:2616–2620, 1992.

McIntosh EDG, Menser MA: A fifty-year follow-up of congenital rubella, *Lancet* 340:414, 1992.

MYCOTIC INFECTIONS

Diseases caused by fungi frequently cause cutaneous (candidiasis, "ringworm," tinea) or mucocutaneous (candidal thrush, vulvovaginitis) infections in immunocompetent patients or systemic illnesses in immunoincompetent and immunosuppressed patients. Localized pulmonary diseases (histoplasmosis, blastomycosis, and cryptococcosis) are common among immunocompetent patients, whereas unusual or disseminated disease is more common among neutropenic, lymphopenic, or immunosuppressed patients. These latter infections include invasive mucormycosis or aspergillosis, disseminated candidiasis, and CNS cryptococcosis.

Treatment depends on the presence of underlying immunologic disease, the site of infection, and the specific fungus involved. Treatment of systemic fungal infections usually requires prolonged antifungal therapy using empiric antifungal agents because most laboratories do not routinely perform antifungal susceptibility testing (Table 10–21).

Coccidioidomycosis

Etiology. Coccidioidomycosis (San Joaquin fever, desert rheumatism) is caused by *Coccidioides immitis*, a dimorphic fungus.

Epidemiology. C. immitis is present in soil in the southwestern states, including western Texas, Arizona, New Mexico, and California. It also occurs in Mexico and certain areas of Central and South America. The infection is usually a childhood illness and, once contracted, confers permanent immunity. The spores are spread by inhalation or, less commonly, by

TABLE 10–21
Antifungal Agents

Drug	Mechanism of Action	Indications	Comments/Toxicity
Amphotericin B	Polyene component of drug combines with fungal membrane sterols	Blastomycosis, candidiasis, histoplasmosis, cryptococcosis, aspergillosis, mucormycosis, coccidioidomycosis, sporotrichosis (extracutaneous)	Fever, chills, azotemia, hypokalemia, toxicity; may be combined with flucytosine
Liposomal amphotericin B	Soluble (taken up by reticuloendothelial system)	Same as above	Less nephrotoxicity
Nystatin	As above	Candidiasis	Topical/oral use only
Caspofungin	Blocks cell wall synthesis	*Aspergillus, Candida*	Used if patients do not tolerate or respond to other antifungal agents
Flucytosine	Conversion to 5-fluorouracil, which interferes with DNA synthesis	Combined with amphotericin B; candidiasis, cryptococcosis, aspergillosis, mucormycosis	Not used as a single drug; neutropenia, thrombocytopenia, hepatitis
Ketoconazole	Interferes with membrane sterol formation	Candidiasis (mucosal), nonmeningeal blastomycosis, or histoplasmosis; ringworm, tinea versicolor	Oral drug; gastrointestinal toxicity; inhibits testosterone synthesis; multiple drug interaction (see Appendix I)
Fluconazole	As ketoconazole	Candidiasis (oral, esophagitis), cryptococcosis; some *Candida* species are resistant (*C. krusei*)	Intravenous or oral drug; gastrointestinal toxicity; drug interactions
Itraconazole	As ketoconazole	As ketoconazole; higher tissue levels, *Aspergillus*	Oral drug; headache, hypertension, edema; drug interactions
Griseofulvin	Disrupts mitotic spindle formation	Ringworm	Headache, gastrointestinal toxicity

Data from *Med Lett* 28:41, 1986; 30:30, 1988; 32:57, 1990.

implantation. Person-to-person spread does not occur. Hot summers, dry soil, and rodent burrows are an ideal environment for preservation of infectious spores. The incubation period is 10–16 days, with a range of 1 week to 1 month.

Clinical Manifestations. The primary pulmonary infection is asymptomatic in 60% of patients. Symptomatic disease may resemble an influenza syndrome. Skin manifestations may include a diffuse maculopapular rash; urticaria; and, frequently, erythema nodosum or, less often, erythema multiforme. Skin infection can occur following trauma or with dissemination of the fungus and often occurs with arthralgias. Pleural effusions as well as pneumonitis may be present. The chest x-ray examination often is more impressive than the findings on physical examination.

Infrequently, a cavity or chronic progressive fibrocavitary syndrome occurs. The fungus may occasionally disseminate to skin, bones, and meninges. Disseminated disease in HIV-infected patients has been seen in endemic areas.

Diagnosis. Histologic examination of pulmonary or other involved tissue reveals double-contoured spherules accompanied by endospores without budding. Obtaining specimens for culture on appropriate media should be performed cautiously because the fungus is highly contagious. In meningitis, the CSF almost always contains specific antibody. The level and persistence of complement fixation titers in serum and CSF are useful for determining the prognosis and for guiding therapy.

Treatment. Primary coccidioidal infection is self-limiting, and no specific therapy is required. Persistent cavitary disease may require surgical excision, usually combined with amphotericin B treatment. Amphotericin B is the agent of choice for treatment of disseminated coccidioidomycosis and may be followed by oral fluconazole or itraconazole therapy (see Appendix I). Fluconazole also has been used with success. For meningitis, intrathecal administration usually is utilized in addition to systemic therapy. Relapse, which is heralded by headache or by abnormal CSF chemistries, may occur years after therapy has ceased. Surgical débridement may be indicated for localized, symptomatic, or progressive lesions.

REFERENCES

Behrman RE, Kliegman RM, Jenson HB, editors: *Nelson textbook of pediatrics*, ed 16, Philadelphia, 2000, WB Saunders, Chapter 236.

Catanzaro A, Galgiani JN, Levine BE, et al: Fluconazole in the treatment of chronic pulmonary and nonmeningeal disseminated coccidioidomycoses, *Am J Med* 98:249–256, 1995.

Einstein HE, Johnson RH: Coccidioidomycosis: new aspects of epidemiology and therapy, *Clin Infect Dis* 16:349–354, 1993.

Histoplasmosis

Etiology. Histoplasmosis is caused by a dimorphic fungus, *Histoplasma capsulatum*.

Epidemiology. The organism grows particularly well in soil containing bird or bat droppings. In the United States, it is endemic in the Mississippi, Missouri, and Ohio river valleys. Infection is acquired by inhalation of airborne spores. Outbreaks have occurred following exploration and dust-raising activities in heavily contaminated areas. It is not transmitted from person to person. The incubation period is variable but is usually a few weeks from the time of exposure.

Pathogenesis. Histoplasmosis infection is much like tuberculosis. Inhalation of spores results in primary infection of the lung, with seeding of multiple organs. An effective immune response results in granulomatous containment of the organism, occasionally associated with calcification.

Clinical Manifestations. Pulmonary histoplasmosis is an influenza-like illness with hilar adenopathy. Splenomegaly and erythema nodosum or erythema multiforme may be present. Chest x-ray films reveal patchy infiltrates and hilar adenopathy in about 25% of patients. Involved areas eventually may calcify, resulting in the characteristic "buckshot" areas of healed histoplasmosis. This self-limiting illness persists for 3–4 weeks.

Disseminated histoplasmosis may occur as an acute illness in infants, young children, or immunocompromised patients. The disease progresses to involve the reticuloendothelial system, with diffuse adenopathy, hepatosplenomegaly, pneumonitis, and bone marrow involvement, resulting in anemia, leukopenia, and thrombocytopenia. Death is caused by respiratory failure, gastrointestinal tract bleeding, or bacterial sepsis.

Diagnosis. The diagnosis is made by culture from normally sterile sites or sputum using standard mycological media. For blood cultures, the lysis-centrifugation method yields best results. DNA probes are used to identify the organism, which grows slowly, often needing 2–6 weeks. Histoplasma polysaccharide antigens can be reliably detected by a radioimmunoassay system. Skin tests are not recommended for diagnosis.

Treatment. Acute histoplasmosis in older children and adults is a self-limited disease and does not necessitate therapy. Other forms of histoplasmosis, including symptomatic pulmonary disease in the infant and young child and disseminated disease, are treated with amphotericin B. In immunocompromised children (particularly those with AIDS), long-term suppressive therapy is required; itraconazole has been successfully used (see Appendix I).

TABLE 10–22
Superficial Fungal Infections

Name	Etiology	Manifestations	Diagnosis	Therapy
Tinea capitis (ringworm)	*Microsporum audouinii, Trichophyton tonsurans, M. canis*	Prepubertal infection of scalp, hairshafts; "black dot" alopecia; *T. tonsurans* common in blacks	*M. audouinii* fluorescence: blue-green with Wood lamp*; +KOH, culture	Griseofulvin; selenium sulfide shampoo
Kerion	Inflammatory reaction to tinea capitis	Swollen, boggy, crusted, purulent, tender mass with lymphadenopathy; secondary distal "id" reaction common	As above	As above, plus steroids for "id" reactions
Tinea corporis (ringworm)	*M. canis, T. rubrum,* others	Slightly pruritic ring-like, erythematous papules, plaques with scaling and slow outward expansion of the border; check cat or dog for *M. canis*	+KOH, culture; *M. canis* fluorescence: blue-green with Wood lamp; differential diagnosis: granuloma annulare, pityriasis rosea, nummular eczema, psoriasis	Local miconazole or clotrimazole
Tinea cruris (jock itch)	*Epidermophyton floccosum, T. mentagrophytes, T. rubrum*	Symmetric, pruritic, scrotal sparing, scaling plaques	+KOH, culture; differential diagnosis: erythrasma (*Corynebacterium minutissimum*)	Local miconazole, clotrimazole, undecylenic acid, or tolnaftate; wear loose cotton underwear
Tinea pedis (athlete's foot)	*T. rubrum, T. mentagrophytes*	Moccasin or interdigital distribution, dry scales, interdigital maceration with secondary bacterial infection	+KOH, culture; differential diagnosis: *C. minutissimum* erythrasma	Medications as above; wear cotton socks
Tinea unguium (onychomycosis)	*T. mentagrophytes, T. rubrum, Candida albicans*	Uncommon before puberty; peeling of distal nail plate; thickening, splitting of nails	+KOH, culture	Oral ketoconazole, itraconazole, or griseofulvin
Tinea versicolor	*Malassezia furfur*	Tropical climates, steroids or immunosuppressive drugs; uncommon before puberty; chest, back, arms; oval hypopigmented or hyperpigmented in blacks, red-brown in whites; scaling patches	+KOH; orange-gold fluorescence with Wood lamp; differential diagnosis: pityriasis alba	Selenium sulfide shampoo, topical sodium hyposulfite, oral ketoconazole
Candidiasis	*C. albicans*	Diaper area, intense erythematous plaques or pustules, isolated or confluent	+KOH, culture	Topical nystatin; oral nystatin treats concomitant oral thrush

*Wood lamp examination uses an ultraviolet source in a completely darkened room. *Trichophyton* usually has no fluorescence.
KOH, Potassium hydroxide.

REFERENCES

Behrman RE, Kliegman RM, Jenson HB: *Nelson textbook of pediatrics*, ed 15, Philadelphia, 2000, WB Saunders, Chapter 234.

Weinberg GA, Kleiman MB, Grosfeld JL, et al: Unusual manifestations of histoplasmosis in children, *Pediatrics* 72:99–105, 1983.

Wheat LJ, Connolly-Stringfield PA, Baker RL, et al: Disseminated histoplasmosis in the acquired immunodeficiency syndrome: clinical findings, diagnosis and review of the literature, *Medicine* 6:361–374, 1990.

Superficial Fungal Infections

Cutaneous manifestations of infection by relatively nonvirulent fungi are quite common (Table 10–22).

RICKETTSIAL DISEASE

Etiology. Rickettsiae are gram-negative coccobacillary organisms that resemble bacteria but have incomplete cell walls and have lost enzymes, and thus require an intracellular site for replication.

Epidemiology. Rickettsiae infect arthropod vectors and, with the exception of louse-borne epidemic typhus, are transmitted to humans only incidentally. Table 10–23 summarizes the agents, epidemiology, and serologic response to the more common rickettsial infections of humans. Rocky Mountain spotted fever is the most common human rickettsial illness in the United States. Rickettsiae have a limited geographic and seasonal occurrence related to arthropod life cycles, activity, and distribution.

Pathogenesis. The fundamental characteristic of the condition is infection of the blood vessels of skin, brain, and subcutaneous tissue resulting in vasculitis, increased vascular permeability, edema, and, eventually, decreased vascular volume, altered tissue perfusion, and widespread organ failure.

Clinical Manifestations. Local primary lesions are present in many rickettsial infections. Prominent features include fever, rash, headache, myalgias, and respiratory tract signs and symptoms. Patients with Q fever do not exhibit rash but may have pneumonia and hepatitis as part of their clinical presentation.

Diagnosis. Organisms can be detected in biopsy specimens (usually of skin) and by fluorescent antibodies. Serologic diagnosis may be accomplished by detection of specific antirickettsial antibodies (IgM and IgG). Culturing of rickettsiae is possible in animals or tissue culture. PCR-based diagnostic tests are under development.

Treatment. Therapy with tetracycline or fluoroquinolones is curative when begun early (see Appendix I).

Immunity. Prolonged immunity and some degree of cross-immunity to other rickettsial infections is conferred by infection. Recurrent or recrudescent activation of rickettsial infection years after the first attack (as in Brill disease or scrub typhus) is common. Humoral antibodies are produced during infections, but cell-mediated immunity is probably of greater importance.

Rocky Mountain Spotted Fever

Epidemiology. Rocky Mountain spotted fever is the most common rickettsial illness in the United States, occurring primarily in the Eastern coastal, the Southeast, and the Western states, especially among 5–9-year-old children. Although the illness is transmitted by various ticks, 15–20% of infected individuals are not able to describe tick bites or contacts. Most cases occur from April to September following outdoor activity in wooded areas.

Clinical Manifestations. The onset is nonspecific, with headache, malaise, and fever. In a few days, a pale, rose-red macular or maculopapular rash appears in 90% of cases. It begins peripherally and spreads to involve the entire body, including palms and soles. The early rash blanches on pressure and is accentuated by warmth. In several days, it progresses to a petechial and purpuric eruption. Fever, headache, myalgia, malaise, splenomegaly (33%), and facial edema become evident. In severe cases, symptoms of CNS inflammation, myocarditis, renal impairment, pneumonitis, and shock occur. Thrombocytopenia and hyponatremia are common findings and may be important clues to the etiology of this syndrome.

The illness is prolonged, lasting as long as 3 weeks with multisystem involvement (e.g., CNS, GI, renal, hematologic-DIC) and can be fatal. Permanent sequelae are common after severe disease.

Diagnosis. The epidemiologic data (locale, time of year, evidence of a tick bite) and clinical manifestations (especially the rash) should facilitate diagnosis. Absence of or failure to obtain appropriate information will greatly hinder diagnosis and increase the risk of a fatal outcome. Fever, headache, and myalgias lasting longer than 1 week are more indicative of Rocky Mountain spotted fever in endemic areas than of the typical influenza that usually has resolved or begins resolving after 1 week of duration. The *differential diagnosis* includes a broad spectrum of illnesses, such as measles, collagen-vascular diseases, viral infections, Henoch-Schönlein purpura, idiopathic thrombocytopenic purpura, infectious mononucleosis, ehrlichiosis (Table 10–20), and meningococcemia.

Treatment. Doxycycline is the drug of choice, despite possible staining of teeth in children younger than 8 years of age.

Prevention. Protection from tick bites and rapid removal of ticks can prevent Rocky Mountain spotted

TABLE 10–23
Rickettsial Diseases of Humans: Summary of Pertinent Features

Group Disease	Causative Agent	Arthropod Vector	Hosts	Incubation Period	Confirmatory Tests*	Geographic Distribution
Spotted Fever						
Rocky Mountain spotted fever	R. rickettsii	Tick	Dogs, rodents	1–8 days	IFA, DFA	Western hemisphere
Boutonneuse fever (Mediterranean spotted fever)	R. conorii	Tick	Dogs, rodents	3–15 days	IFA, DFA	Africa, Mediterranean region, India, Middle East
Rickettsialpox	R. akari	Mite	Mice	10–24 days	IFA	North America, Russia, Korea, South Africa
Ehrlichiosis	E. canis	Tick	Dogs	7–28 days	IFA	Southeast, north and south central United States
Typhus						
Epidemic typhus/ Brill-Zinsser disease	R. prowazekii	Body louse	Humans	—	IFA	Highlands of Africa, Asia, Central and South America
Flying squirrel–associated typhus fever	R. prowazekii	Lice, fleas	Flying squirrels	10–14 days	IFA	Eastern United States (including Texas)
Murine (endemic) typhus	R. typhi	Cat or rat flea, rat louse	Rats	8 days	IFA	Worldwide
Scrub Typhus						
Scrub typhus	R. tsutsugamushi	Mite	Rodents	8–10 days	IFA, IP	Pacific Islands, Australia, and central, eastern, and southeast Asia
Others						
Q fever	Coxiella burnetii	Ticks?	Cattle, sheep, goats, cats	18–20 days	IFA, CF	Worldwide

Adapted from Behrman RE, Kliegman RM, Jenson HB, editors: *Nelson textbook of pediatrics*, ed 16, Philadelphia, 2000, WB Saunders.
*Although not widely available or highly sensitive, a direct fluorescent antibody (DFA) test can be used to detect rickettsiae in skin biopsies or tissue samples. Preferred confirmatory serologic tests include indirect fluorescent antibody or microimmunofluorescent assay (IFA), complement fixation (CF), and immunoperoxidase (IP) assays. Cross-absorption of the patient's serum with specific rickettsial antigens can be done to distinguish the following infections: *R. rickettsii* versus *R. conorii* or *R. akari*; and *R. prowazekii* versus *R. typhi*.

fever. Ticks are best removed by gentle upward traction with forceps to avoid infecting the patient or oneself with material from the crushed tick.

REFERENCES

Abramson JS, Givner LB: Rocky Mountain spotted fever, *Pediatr Infect Dis J* 18(6):539–540, 1999.

Behrman RE, Kliegman RM, Jenson HB, editors: *Nelson textbook of pediatrics,* ed 16, Philadelphia, 2000, WB Saunders, Chapters 225–229.

Centers for Disease Control and Prevention: Consequences of delayed diagnosis of Rocky Mountain spotted fever in children—West Virginia, Michigan, Tennessee, and Oklahoma, May-July 2000, *MMWR* 49(39):885–888, 2000.

Kirk JL, Fine DP, Sexton DJ, et al: Rocky Mountain spotted fever: a clinical review based on 48 confirmed cases, 1943–1986, *Medicine* 69:35–45, 1990.

Kirkland KB, Marcom PK, Sexton DJ, et al: Rocky Mountain spotted fever complicated by gangrene: report of six cases and review, *Clin Infect Dis* 16:629–634, 1993.

Human Ehrlichiosis

Etiology. Human monocytic ehrlichiosis (caused by *Ehrlichia chaffeensis*) and granulocytic ehrlichiosis are common diseases in North America. Granulocytic ehrlichiosis, which is caused by several species of *Ehrlichia,* is the second-most prevalent tick-borne disease in the northeastern United States.

Epidemiology. The granulocytic disease is transmitted by the tick *Ixodes scapularis,* which is also the vector of Lyme disease *(Borrelia burgdorferi).* Although the distribution of these vectors is widespread, there are clusters of cases in the northeastern and upper midwestern United States, as well as in areas in the Southeast, where the tick *Amblyomma americanum,* which transmits *E. chaffeensis,* is common.

Clinical Manifestations. These zoonoses are acute febrile illnesses with systemic findings characterized by granulocytopenia, anemia, and hepatitis, but often without a rash. The typical presentation is what appears to be a "viral syndrome": fever, malaise, myalgias, headache, anorexia, and nausea, with rash developing in the second week. The symptoms persist and may progress to marrow hypoplasia, pulmonary infiltrates, and as occurs in Rocky Mountain spotted fever, disseminated intravascular coagulation, anemia, and CNS involvement. Most patients recover completely.

Diagnosis. An indirect immunofluorescence test is used to diagnose a fourfold or greater rise in antibody titer and is available in reference laboratories. Organisms may be seen in leukocytes.

Treatment. Doxycycline is the preferred drug and should be given early in the course of the disease. Because ehrlichiosis can be fatal, the potential of dental staining does not outweigh the benefits of effective therapy.

REFERENCES

Bakken JS, Krueth J, Wilson-Nordskog C, et al: Clinical and laboratory characteristics of human granulocytic erhlichiosis, *JAMA* 275:199–205, 1996.

Ido JW, Meek JI, Carter ML, et al: The emergence of another tick-borne infection in the 12-town area around Lyme, Connecticut: human granulocytic ehrlichiosis, *J Infect Dis* 181:1388–1393, 2000.

PARASITIC INFECTIONS

Although much attention is focused on bacterial and viral infections, protozoal and helminthic infections are a more significant health problem in most parts of the world. Malaria is estimated to kill more than 1 million individuals a year, mostly children.

Protozoal Disease

Protozoa are the simplest organisms of the animal kingdom. They are unicellular and most are free living, but some have a commensal or parasitic existence. Protozoal disease is considered under the groupings of intestinal and systemic protozoal infections.

Intestinal Protozoal Infections

Amebiasis

Etiology. Amebiasis is caused by *Entamoeba histolytica,* a protozoan that exists as a resistant infectious cyst (10–18 μm, with four nuclei) or as a motile, invasive trophozoite.

Epidemiology. Humans are the natural host and reservoir of *E. histolytica.* It is transmitted via contaminated food or water and by person-to-person contact.

Pathogenesis. Once ingested, a cyst becomes a trophozoite that can cause invasive disease and produce a characteristic flask-shaped ulcer in the intestinal mucosa. The amebas may disseminate to the liver or, less commonly, to other areas, such as the pleura, skin, brain, and lungs. The disease is distributed worldwide, although it is more prevalent in areas of poor sanitation. A patient is intermittently infectious if not treated.

Clinical Manifestations. Most infected individuals are asymptomatic, but some exhibit acute, cramping diarrhea. In 2–8% of infected persons, intestinal amebiasis may be associated with diarrhea that contains blood and mucus and that is associated with fever, abdominal pain, headache, and chills. Symptoms last for days to weeks and recur without therapy. *Ameboma* (a mass caused by amebas), extraintestinal lesions, or intestinal perforation and hemorrhage may occur. Twenty-five percent of patients have ulcerative lesions that can be visualized by sigmoidoscopy. These lesions may lead to perforation of the colon and subsequent peritonitis.

Hepatic amebiasis is the most common manifestation of disseminated infection. Amebic liver abscess with fever, abdominal pain, distention, and a tender liver occurs in 1% of infected individuals. These patients often do not have a history of intestinal amebiasis, and their stool is negative for amebas.

Diagnosis. The diagnosis of intestinal illness relies on demonstration of the organism in stool or biopsy of ulcers or liver abscess tissue. In invasive intestinal amebiasis and in cases of liver abscess, antibody to ameba is present in over 90% of cases. Ultrasound or CT will delineate the liver abscess, which is usually singular and located in the right lobe.

Treatment. Therapy of amebiasis depends on the type of illness. Metronidazole or tinidazole is recommended for forms that invade tissue, followed by iodoquinol for intraluminal organisms.

REFERENCES

Behrman RE, Kliegman RM, Jenson HB, editors: *Nelson textbook of pediatrics*, ed 16, Philadelphia, 2000, WB Saunders, Chapter 271.

Cryptosporidiosis

Etiology. *Cryptosporidium* is a coccidian protozoan that can produce an acute illness in immunocompetent and immunocompromised hosts (particularly those with AIDS).

Epidemiology. The oocysts of *Cryptosporidium* are hardy, withstand routine disinfectants, and survive in moist areas. Both person-to-person and zoonotic transmission is possible; infection from contaminated water sources causes large-scale outbreaks. *Cryptosporidium* frequently is a cause of diarrhea in young children in developing countries. The prevalence of infection may be as high as 4–7% in sporadic outbreaks of enteritis. The incubation period is 2–14 days.

Clinical Manifestations. Cryptosporidiosis can appear as an acute and self-limited enteritis in normal individuals who exhibit watery diarrhea, nausea, and cramps lasting 12–14 days. Although most immunocompetent hosts recover within 10–14 days, occasionally the disease is protracted and oocyst shedding persists for 2 weeks. In immunocompromised patients (particularly those with HIV), profuse, watery diarrhea with profound weight loss may occur. Biliary tract disease is also found.

Treatment. In normal hosts cryptosporidiosis is usually self-limited and supportive care is sufficient. In patients with more severe disease and in immunocompromised hosts, azithromycin and paromomycin along with appropriate fluid and electrolyte replacement have been efficacious.

REFERENCES

Behrman RE, Kliegman RM, Jenson HB, editors: *Nelson textbook of pediatrics*, ed 16, Philadelphia, 2000, WB Saunders, Chapter 273.
MacKenzie WR, Hoxie NJ, Proctor ME, et al: A massive outbreak in Milwaukee of *Cryptosporidium* infection transmitted through the public water supply, *N Engl J Med* 331:161, 1994.

Vargas SL, Shenep JL, Flynn PM, et al: Azithromycin for treatment of severe *Cryptosporidium* diarrhea in two children with cancer, *J Pediatr* 123:154–156, 1993.

Giardiasis

Etiology. Giardiasis is caused by *Giardia lamblia,* a flagellated protozoan. The hardy cysts are ingested (often in water) and are the infectious form. The trophozoites are liberated after ingestion and are responsible for symptoms. Giardiae live in the duodenum.

Epidemiology. *Giardia* has a worldwide distribution and infects humans, dogs, and wild animals (beavers). Transmission occurs from person to person by fecal-oral spread or by drinking or eating contaminated water or food. Outbreaks occur in day care centers, in institutions for the mentally retarded, and in travelers to the former Soviet Union and the Rocky Mountains.

Clinical Manifestations. Individuals vary in their response to infection and may have the following clinical manifestations: (1) asymptomatic; (2) an acute illness with a sudden onset of explosive, watery, foul-smelling stools, flatulence, abdominal distention, nausea, and anorexia; and (3) chronic diarrhea and malabsorption (including that of antibiotics and iron), with flatulence, abdominal distention, and abdominal pain, often lasting for months.

Diagnosis. Examination of several stool specimens is necessary for visualizing the organism, because intermittent excretion occurs. Examining duodenal contents obtained by direct aspiration or by use of a string test (Enterotest) is more sensitive. Rarely, duodenal intubation with fluid aspiration or biopsy may be required for diagnosis. ELISA can be used to detect *Giardia* antigen in stool specimens; PCR and DNA probes are also available to identify infected patients.

Treatment. Several drugs, including metronidazole, tinidazole, and furazolidine are effective in the treatment of giardiasis.

REFERENCES

Addiss DG, Juranek DD, Spencer HC: Treatment of children with asymptomatic and nondiarrheal *Giardia* infection, *Pediatr Infect Dis J* 10:843–846, 1991.
Behrman RE, Kliegman RM, Jenson HB, editors: *Nelson textbook of pediatrics*, ed 16, Philadelphia, 2000, WB Saunders, Chapter 272.
Gunasekaran TS, Hassall E: Giardiasis mimicking inflammatory bowel disease, *J Pediatr* 120:424–426, 1992.
Quick R, Paugh K, Addiss D, et al: Restaurant-associated outbreak of giardiasis, *J Infect Dis* 166:673–676, 1992.

Systemic Protozoal Infections

American Trypanosomiasis (Chagas Disease)

Etiology. American trypanosomiasis is a zoonosis caused by *Trypanosoma cruzi,* a protozoan hemoflagellate.

Epidemiology. *T. cruzi* is transmitted to humans by blood-sucking insects called reduviid bugs. The trypomastigotes are released as the insect defecates near its bite. The trypanosome gains entry, and amastigotes (intracellular forms) and trypomastigotes (vascular forms) are produced. The infected reduviid bugs have adapted to adobe, mud, and cane housing in most of South and Central America. It is estimated that 24 million South Americans are infected with *T. cruzi*. Several endogenous cases have occurred in Texas. Animal reservoirs, including rats, opossums, and raccoons, may be important. Although it is common to encounter infected reduviid bugs in the southwestern United States, infection in humans appears to be rare, possibly because of better housing, low adaptability of North American reduviids to domestic housing, or difference in *Trypanosoma* virulence. *T. cruzi* also may be transmitted congenitally or by infected blood. The incubation period is 1–2 weeks.

Clinical Manifestations

Acute Infection. Illness generally is asymptomatic or mild in young children in endemic areas. There may be local inflammation at the site of entry of the parasite. Half of infected children have unilateral eye swelling (Romaña sign), which is the first indication of disease. Some patients have a nodular skin lesion (chagoma) at the site of the original inoculation. Hematogenous dissemination results in malaise, fever, muscle pain, adenopathy, rash, hepatosplenomegaly, and, less often, meningoencephalitis. Myocardial involvement is noted in nearly one half of symptomatic patients, accompanied by tachycardia and arrhythmias. Most cases evolve into an asymptomatic chronic stage. The mortality rate is 10%. Congenital disease is characterized by low birth weight, hepatomegaly, and meningoencephalitis.

Chronic Trypanosomiasis. In the symptomatic chronic stage, inflammation and fibrosis result in myocarditis, cardiac failure, or enlargement of a hollow viscus, especially of the esophagus (megaesophagus) or the colon (megacolon). This occurs in 10–15% of cases.

Diagnosis. In acute disease, *T. cruzi* can be demonstrated in blood smears. EIA tests are available, and PCR techniques have been developed.

Treatment. Nifurtimox has been used successfully to treat acute trypanosomiasis.

Prevention. Insect control and adequately protected housing are keys to breaking the bug-human cycle. Blood donors in endemic areas must be screened by serology.

REFERENCES

Behrman RE, Kliegman RM, Jenson HB, editors: *Nelson textbook of pediatrics,* ed 16, Philadelphia, 2000, WB Saunders, Chapters 276–277.

Grant IH, Gold JWM, Wittner M, et al: Transfusion-associated acute Chagas disease acquired in the United States, *Ann Intern Med* 111:849–851, 1989.

Viotti R, Vigliano C, Armenti H, et al: Treatment of chronic Chagas' disease with benznidazole: clinical and serological evolution of patients with long-term follow-up, *Am Heart J* 127: 151–162, 1994.

Malaria

Etiology. Malaria is caused by one or more of four *Plasmodium* species: *P. falciparum, P. vivax, P. ovale,* and *P. malariae.*

Epidemiology. Malaria usually is acquired from the bite of an infected female *Anopheles* mosquito. Less commonly, it is acquired transplacentally or via an infected blood transfusion. Infection transmitted through blood transfusion or the transplacental route occurs without the preerythrocytic hepatic phase. In children with no preexisting immunity to malaria, the incubation period varies from 6–16 days, depending on the *Plasmodium* species involved. Indigenous malaria has been reported in the southern United States, but most often it is imported by travelers or immigrants.

Pathology. Infected red blood cells rupture, causing hemolytic anemia and pigment deposition in reticuloendothelial cells. The infected red cells also may sludge and stick in organs, interfering with circulation and inducing pneumonia, encephalitis, or enteritis. *P. falciparum* is associated with the heaviest degree of parasitemia and is the most lethal. Serum antibody production seems to be correlated with clearance of the erythrocyte (but not the hepatic) stage of parasites. Sickle cell anemia and glucose-6-phosphate dehydrogenase (G6PD) deficiency are associated with some protection against lethal malaria.

Clinical Manifestations. Malaria is most severe in children lacking antibody and is milder in children having survived initial attacks. The illness is characterized by a nonspecific prodrome prior to the onset of sudden high fevers with chills. An abrupt return to normal temperature occurs after 2–12 hours. Fever is associated with headache, abdominal and back pain, nausea, and, often, splenomegaly. In established *P. vivax* or *P. malariae* infection, fever may occur every 2 or 3 days, respectively. *P. falciparum* infection also may produce encephalitis, pneumonitis, enteritis, and nephritis. The most serious form of malaria is caused by severe and sudden intravascular hemolysis (blackwater fever), associated with heavy *P. falciparum* infection, as well as with the use of drugs that induce hemolysis in G6PD-deficient individuals.

Diagnosis. The diagnosis of malaria and the species of *Plasmodium* may be confirmed by examining thick and thin blood smears. These smears should be examined at 12-hour intervals because the level of parasitemia fluctuates. In convalescence there is an antibody response to the parasite.

Treatment. Specific therapy for malaria depends on the species acquired, the mode of acquisition, and the locale of acquisition. Chloroquine is the therapy for malaria acquired in locales that do not have chloroquine-resistant malaria, such as Mexico, Haiti, the Dominican Republic, most of the Northern Middle East, and west of the Panama Canal Zone. In areas with *P. falciparum* known to be chloroquine-resistant, including much of Africa, Oceania, Southeast Asia, the Indian subcontinent, and South America, therapy consists of quinine plus pyrimethamine/sulfadoxine or quinine plus doxycycline, tetracycline, or mefloquine. Severe illness may necessitate the intravenous use of quinine or quinidine. To prevent relapse of mosquito-transmitted *P. ovale* and *P. vivax* infection, primaquine is used to eradicate the hepatic phase of the parasite cycle. Because a hepatic phase does not occur with congenital or transfusion-acquired *P. malariae* or *P. falciparum* infection, primaquine is not indicated in these situations. Primaquine induces hemolysis in patients with G6PD deficiency. In severe disease, multisystem support, transfusion, and possibly exchange transfusion are necessary.

Prevention. Malaria can be prevented by administration of chemoprophylaxis, which includes the use of weekly dosages of chloroquine (which must also be taken for 6 weeks after leaving the endemic area) and possibly the use of primaquine for terminal prophylaxis in order to eradicate hepatic forms. In areas where *Plasmodium* species are chloroquine resistant, mefloquine or doxycycline may be used. Many regimens are possible, depending on the local resistance and the potential side effects of the drugs. Control of malaria relies on the prevention of mosquito bites by using special clothing, repellents, night netting, and mosquito eradication programs.

REFERENCES

Behrman RE, Kliegman RM, Jenson HB, editors: *Nelson textbook of pediatrics,* ed 16, Philadelphia, 2000, WB Saunders, Chapter 278.

Croft A: Malaria: prevention in travellers, *BMJ* 321:154, 2000.

Subramanian D, Moise KJ Jr, White AC Jr: Imported malaria in pregnancy: report of four cases and review of management, *Clin Infect Dis* 15:408–413, 1992.

Von Seidlein L, Milligan P, Pinder M, et al: Efficacy of artesunate plus pyrimethamine-sulphadoxine for uncomplicated malaria in Gambian children: a double-blind, randomized controlled trial, *Lancet* 355:352–357, 2000.

Weiss WR, Oloo AJ, Johnson A, et al: Daily primaquine is effective for prophylaxis against falciparum malaria in Kenya: a comparison with mefloquine, doxycycline, and chloroquine plus proguanil, *J Infect Dis* 171:1569–1575, 1995.

Toxoplasmosis

Etiology. *Toxoplasma gondii,* an intracellular protozoan parasite, causes toxoplasmosis.

Epidemiology. Newly infected cats excrete the infectious oocysts in their feces. The oocysts and tissue cysts are infectious when ingested. High frequency of human infection occurs in warm, humid climates. Infection also occurs from ingesting undercooked meat containing cysts. Less commonly, transmission occurs by blood transfusion or organ transplant, or transplacentally during acute infection of pregnant women. In the United States the incidence of congenital infection is 1–2:1000 live births. The incubation period for acquired infection is about 7 days.

Clinical Manifestations

Congenital Toxoplasmosis. Most maternal infection is asymptomatic. Among women infected during pregnancy, 40–60% give birth to an infected infant. The later in pregnancy that infection occurs, the more likely it is that the fetus will be infected but the less severe the illness. Severely affected fetuses will be stillborn. In infants, illness may occur at birth and become manifest by poor feeding, fever, rash, petechiae, lymphadenopathy, hepatomegaly, splenomegaly, jaundice, hydrocephalus or microcephaly, microphthalmia, seizures, cerebral calcifications, and chorioretinitis. This illness must be differentiated from other congenital infections included in the TORCH syndrome (rubella, CMV, HSV, syphilis, hepatitis, and VZV). In 67–75% of infants who are asymptomatic at birth, subsequent defects, such as chorioretinitis, retardation, and neurologic disability, will develop years after birth.

Acquired Toxoplasmosis. Acquired toxoplasmosis is usually an asymptomatic infection. Symptomatic infection is characterized as a heterophil-negative mononucleosis syndrome that includes lymphadenopathy, fever, and hepatosplenomegaly. Disseminated infection, including myocarditis, pneumonia, and encephalitis, is more common in immunosuppressed patients, especially those with AIDS. Localized lymphadenopathy that is difficult to differentiate from Hodgkin disease is one of the more common manifestations of toxoplasmosis. CNS toxoplasmosis is seen in patients after stem cell or other transplantations.

Diagnosis. In toxoplasmosis involving the CNS, the parasites may be visualized in CSF by cytocentrifuge preparations or by growth in inoculated infant mice. Typical histopathology or cysts may be identified in biopsy specimens of involved lung, brain, or lymph node.

Serologic diagnosis can be established by several different antibody tests. A fourfold rise in antibody titer or seroconversion from negative to positive indicates the presence of infection. In congenital infection the diagnosis is complicated by the presence of maternally derived transplacental antibody. If the maternal antibody status is negative, the diagnosis of congenital toxoplasmosis is excluded; if the maternal and neonate levels are positive, serial studies for several months are necessary to distinguish transplacental antibody (levels will fall) from congenital infection (levels will remain stable or rise). Several research laboratories can perform an IgM/anti-*Toxoplasma* antibody study or PCR to test for *T. gondii* in peripheral WBCs, CSF, serum, or amniotic fluid.

Treatment. Treatment includes both pyrimethamine and sulfadiazine, which act synergistically against *Toxoplasma* organisms. Because these compounds are folic acid inhibitors, they are used in conjunction with folinic acid. Spiramycin, which is not licensed in the United States, also is used in therapy of pregnant women with toxoplasmosis. Corticosteroids are reserved for patients with acute CNS or ocular infection.

Prevention. Ingesting only well-cooked meat and avoiding cats or soil in areas where cats defecate are prudent measures for pregnant or immunocompromised patients. Cat litter should be disposed of daily because oocysts are not infectious during the first 48 hour after passage. Administration of spiramycin to infected pregnant women has been associated with lower risks of congenital infection in their babies.

REFERENCES

Behrman RE, Kliegman RM, Jenson HB, editors: *Nelson textbook of pediatrics*, ed 16, Philadelphia, 2000, WB Saunders, Chapter 280.

Foulon W, Naessens A, Ho-yen D: Prevention of congenital toxoplasmosis, *J Perinat Med* 28:337–345, 2000.

Naessens A, Jenum PA, Pollak A, et al: Diagnosis of congenital toxoplasmosis in the neonatal period: a multicenter evaluation, *J Pediatr* 135:714–719, 1999.

Helminthiases

The helminths are divided into three groups: one group of roundworms, the nematodes, and two groups of flatworms, the trematodes (flukes) and the cestodes (tapeworms).

Infections Caused by Intestinal Nematodes

Infections are normally acquired by inadvertent ingestion of eggs or by larval forms from soil penetrating the skin.

Ascariasis

Etiology. Ascariasis is the most prevalent type of helminthiasis, involving 1 billion people. It is caused by *Ascaris lumbricoides*, a large nematode.

Epidemiology. After humans ingest the eggs, larvae are released and then penetrate the intestine, migrate to the lungs, ascend the trachea, and are reswallowed. On entering the intestines again, they mature and produce eggs that are excreted in the stool and are deposited in the soil, where they survive for prolonged periods. This is a ubiquitous parasite that generally occurs in warm areas. Human fecal soilage, use of human manure for agriculture, and hand-to-mouth spread are the major sources of ascariasis.

Clinical Manifestations. Manifestations may be the result of migration of the larvae to other sites of the body or the presence of adult worms in the intestine. Pulmonary ascariasis occurs as the larvae migrate through the lung. The manifestations of the condition are cough, blood-stained sputum, eosinophilia, and transient infiltrates on chest x-ray films. Adult larvae in the small intestine may cause abdominal pain and distention. It is rare that intestinal obstruction from adult worms occurs. Migration of worms into the bile duct may result in the rare occurrence of acute biliary obstruction. Steatorrhea and decreased vitamin A absorption may occur in heavily infected children. Asymptomatic infections are common.

Diagnosis. Results from examination of stool for characteristic eggs are diagnostic.

Treatment. Albendazole or mebendazole is currently considered the drug of choice; pyrantel pamoate is an alternative.

Prevention. Effective control of this worldwide parasite depends on adequate sanitary treatment and disposal of infected human feces, especially before it is used as fertilizer.

Enterobiasis (Pinworm)

Etiology. Pinworm is caused by *Enterobius vermicularis*, a nematode that is distributed worldwide.

Epidemiology. Enterobiasis affects individuals at all socioeconomic levels, especially children. Crowded living conditions predispose individuals to infection. Humans ingest the eggs carried on hands or present in house dust or on bedclothes. They hatch in the stomach, and the larvae migrate to the cecum and mature. At night the females migrate to the perianal area to lay their eggs, which are viable for 2 days.

Clinical Manifestations. The most common symptoms are nocturnal anal pruritus and sleeplessness, presumably resulting from the migratory female worms. Vaginitis and salpingitis can occur secondary to aberrant worm migration. *Enterobius* has been recovered from the appendix in several cases, although its role in appendicitis is doubtful.

Diagnosis. The eggs are detected by microscopically examining adhesive cellophane tape pressed against the anus in the morning to collect eggs. Less commonly, a worm may be seen in the perianal region.

Treatment. The drug of choice is pyrantel pamoate or mebendazole given as a single dose and repeated in 2 weeks. Alternatives include albendazole. Repeated therapy may be necessary because of reinfection. Therapy for all family members at once is also often used.

Hookworm Infections

Etiology. Hookworm infection is caused by several species of hookworms; *Ancylostoma duodenale* and *Necator americanus* are the most important. *A. duodenale* is the predominant species in Europe, the Mediterranean region, northern Asia, and the west coast of South America. *N. americanus* predominates in the western hemisphere, sub-Saharan Africa, Southeast Asia, and several Pacific islands.

Epidemiology. More than 9 million humans are infected with hookworms. Optimal soil conditions and fecal contamination are found in many agrarian tropical countries and in the southeastern United States. Infection typically occurs in young children, especially during the first decade of life. The larvae are found in warm, damp soil and infect humans by penetrating the skin. They migrate to the lungs, ascend the trachea, are swallowed, and reside in the intestine. The worms then mature and attach to the intestinal wall, where they suck blood and shed eggs.

Clinical Manifestations. Infections usually are asymptomatic. Intense pruritus ("ground itch"), which may include papules and vesicles, can occur at the site of larval penetration, usually the soles of the feet or between the toes. Migration of larvae through the lungs usually is asymptomatic. Symptoms of abdominal pain, anorexia, indigestion, fullness, and diarrhea occur with hookworm infestation. The major manifestation of infection is subsequent anemia. Chronic infection causes hypoalbuminemia and edema, which may lead to heart failure.

Diagnosis. Examination of fresh stool reveals hookworm eggs.

Treatment. Albendazole is the drug of choice. Therapy for anemia may involve iron therapy or, in severe cases, transfusion.

Prevention. Eradication depends on sanitation of the patient's environment and chemotherapy. Eradication essentially has been achieved in the southeastern United States.

Systemic Nematodes

Visceral Larva Migrans (Toxocariasis)

Etiology. Visceral larva migrans (VLM) is caused by ingestion of the eggs of the dog or cat tapeworms *Toxocara canis*, *Toxocara cati*, and *Toxascaris leonina*.

Epidemiology. VLM is most common in young children with pica who have dogs or cats as pets. Ocular toxocariasis occurs in older children. Approximately 2% of dogs in the United States excrete *Toxocara* eggs, and up to 25% of soil samples in public parks contain the eggs. The eggs of these roundworms are produced by adult worms residing in the dog and cat intestine. Ingested eggs hatch into larvae that penetrate the gastrointestinal tract and migrate to the liver, lung, eye, CNS, and heart, where they die and calcify.

Clinical Manifestations. Symptoms are the result of the number of migrating worms and the immune response they elicit. Most persons who are lightly infected are asymptomatic. Symptoms include fever, cough, wheezing, and seizures. Physical findings may include hepatomegaly, rales, rash, and adenopathy. Visual symptoms may include decreased acuity, strabismus, periorbital edema, or blindness. Eye examination may reveal granulomatous lesions near the macula or disc. These must be differentiated from retinoblastoma and other granulomatous infections.

Diagnosis. Eosinophilia and hypergammaglobulinemia associated with elevated isohemagglutinin levels suggest the diagnosis, which may be confirmed by serology (ELISA) or, less commonly, by biopsy.

Treatment. This is a self-limiting illness. In severe disease, albendazole or mebendazole is used.

Prevention. Avoiding pica and washing the hands after animal contact may help control the illness. Deworming puppies and kittens, the major excretors of eggs, decreases the risk of infection.

Infections Caused by Trematodes (Flukes)

Trematodes include flukes, which infect the intestine, liver, lung, and blood. Eosinophilia is a prominent clinical sign of trematode infection. These infections are uncommon in the United States.

Schistosomiasis

Etiology. The trematodes (flukes) include *Schistosoma haematobium*, *S. mansoni*, *S. japonicum*, and, rarely, *S. intercalatum* and *S. mekongi*.

Epidemiology. Schistosomiasis affects more than 2 million people, mainly children and young adults. (The maximum incidence of infection is between ages 10 and 20 years.) Humans are infected in contaminated water by cercariae that emerge in an infectious form from snails. They penetrate intact skin. Each adult worm migrates to specific sites: *S. haematobium* to the bladder plexus, and *S. intercalatum* and *S. mekongi* to the mesenteric vessels. The eggs are deposited by the adult flukes in urine (*S. haematobium*) or stool (*S. mansoni* and *S. japonicum*). Intermediate hosts for these complex parasites are freshwater snails that are infected by miracidia, which hatch from eggs in freshwater. *S. haematobium* is prevalent in Africa and the Middle East; *S. mansoni* in Africa, the Middle East, the Caribbean, and South America; *S. japonicum* in China, the Philippines, and Indonesia; *S. mekongi* in the Far East; and *S. intercalatum* in West Africa.

Clinical Manifestations. The pathogenesis of schistosomiasis is the result of eggs that are trapped at the site of depository or at metastatic locations. Within 3–12 weeks of infection, while the worms are maturing, a syndrome of fever, malaise, cough, abdominal pain, and rash can occur. This is followed by a resultant inflammatory response that leads to further symptoms. In infection with *S. haematobium,* bladder granulomas may lead to renal failure and cancer of the bladder. In the other schistosomal infections, intestinal and hepatic egg deposition and inflammation lead to ulceration of the intestine, colic, abdominal pain, and bloody diarrhea. Parasinusoidal liver obstruction causes hepatosplenomegaly, portal hypertension, ascites, and hematemesis. *Katayama fever* is an acute condition, with fever, weight loss, hepatosplenomegaly, and eosinophilia.

Diagnosis. Eggs may be found in the stool or urine (*S. haematobium*) of infected individuals. Biopsy of the bladder or rectal mucosa may be helpful but usually is not necessary.

Treatment. Praziquantel is the drug of choice for therapy of schistosomiasis in children.

Prevention. Sanitary measures, molluscicides, and therapy for infected individuals may help control the illness.

Tissue Tapeworms

Etiology. Canines become infected with tapeworms by eating infected sheep or cattle viscera. The larval stage of the canine tapeworm *Echinococcus granulosus* (hydatid disease) infects humans when *Echinococcus* eggs from dog feces or dog feces–contaminated material are ingested. Humans then become an intermediate host. The embryos pass through the intestine to the liver and other visceral organs, forming cysts up to 2 cm in diameter.

The cysticercus stage of *Taenia solium* (pork tapeworm) is responsible for *neurocysticercosis.* Humans are infected after consuming raw or undercooked larva-containing pork from pigs that were fed raw sewage contaminated with human feces containing *T. solium.* Fecal-hand contamination is a potential source of infection.

Epidemiology. E. granulosa has a worldwide distribution but is endemic in sheep-raising and cattle-raising areas of Australia, South America, South Africa, the Soviet Union, and the Mediterranean region. The prevalence is highest in children. *T. solium* is endemic in Asia, Africa, and Latin and South America.

Clinical Manifestations. Symptoms caused by *E. granulosa* result from space-occupying cysts and are most typical in adults. Pulmonary cysts may cause hemoptysis, cough, dyspnea, and respiratory distress. Brain cysts appear as tumors; liver cysts cause problems as they compress and obstruct blood flow.

Neurocysticercosis presents with generalized or focal seizures, variable eosinophilia, and calcification of cerebral cysts.

Diagnosis. Radiologic diagnosis is possible in endemic areas. Ultrasound confirms the cystic nature of the granulosa mass. Neurocysticercosis demonstrates CT findings of calcified cysts. Serologic tests also are helpful.

Treatment. Large or asymptomatic granulosa cysts are removed surgically. Treatment with albendazole has shown some benefit. Neurocysticercosis is treated with albendazole, praziquantel, steroids, and anticonvulsant drugs.

REFERENCES

Behrman RE, Kliegman RM, Jenson HB, editors: *Nelson textbook of pediatrics,* ed 16, Philadelphia, 2000, WB Saunders, Chapters 283, 296, 298, 299.

Despommier DD: Tapeworm infection: the long and the short of it, *N Engl J Med* 327:727–728, 1992.

Drugs for parasitic infections, *Med Lett* 37:99–108, 1995.

Hall A, Anwar KS, Tomkins AM: Intensity of reinfection with *Ascaris lumbricoides* and its implications for parasite control, *Lancet* 140:1253–1257, 1992.

Park SY, Barkovich AJ, Weintrub PS: Clinical implications of calcified lesions of neurocysticercosis, *Pediatr Infect Dis J* 19:581–583, 2000.

Singhi P, Ray M, Singhi S, et al: Clinical spectrum of 500 children with neurocysticercosis and response to albendazole therapy, *J Child Neurol* 15:207–213, 2000.

CHAPTER 11

The Gastrointestinal Tract

Barbara S. Kirschner ▾ Dennis D. Black

Gastrointestinal complaints are common pediatric problems. A careful history and physical examination are necessary to determine whether the symptoms are caused by a primary gastrointestinal illness or by systemic disease states that may produce abdominal complaints. For example, abdominal pain in patients with sickle cell anemia may indicate sickle cell pain crisis, transfusion-associated hepatitis, hemolysis-associated bilirubin stones and cholecystitis, renal papillary necrosis, or the usual causes of abdominal pain not associated with sickle cell anemia, such as gastroenteritis, appendicitis, and lactose malabsorption. Knowledge of the family history and questions that determine the relationship of symptoms to feeding, the color of emesis, the number and character of stools, the nature of defecation, and the location of maximum pain can help formulate a differential diagnosis and select laboratory tests or diagnostic (roentgenographic or endoscopic) procedures.

Recognizing diseases and their manifestations that are associated with particular age groups is important. Most patients with intestinal obstruction resulting from congenital anomalies of the esophagus, small intestine, and large bowel have symptoms in the first week of life, whereas the onset of inflammatory bowel disease usually occurs during adolescence. Common manifestations of many gastrointestinal illnesses, both benign and serious, are pain, diarrhea, emesis, constipation, and gastrointestinal hemorrhage.

CLINICAL MANIFESTATIONS OF GASTROINTESTINAL DISEASE
Abdominal Pain

Abdominal pain is the most frequent gastrointestinal complaint that brings children and adolescents to the physician. This pain is classified as visceral, somatic, or referred.

The sensation of pain from the abdominal viscera is produced in response to stretching or distending of the wall of a hollow organ or the capsule of a solid organ, inflammation, or ischemia. *Visceral pain* usually is dull or crampy and is poorly localized along the dermatomes that innervate the organ. Pain originating from the liver, pancreas, biliary tree, stomach, or proximal small intestine is felt in the epigastrium; pain from the distal small intestine, right side of the colon, and appendix is felt in the periumbilical region; and pain from the left side of the colon, urinary tract, or genital organs usually is felt in the suprapubic area.

Parietal or *somatic pain* represents peritoneal inflammation and is localized to the area of the involved viscera. Peritoneal pain is steady and sharp and associated with voluntary guarding or involuntary rigidity of the overlying abdominal muscles, with or without rebound pain.

Referred pain is caused by local irritation, with referral along the pathway of innervation of the organ. Pain that begins as dull and poorly localized but becomes more diffuse and severe suggests that a hollow viscus has ruptured and progressed to peritonitis.

Critical to the evaluation of abdominal pain is both "how ill" the child appears and whether the onset of the complaint is new or recent (*acute*) or is recurrent (*chronic*). As part of the history, it is necessary to determine the following (Table 11–1):
1. The age of onset, the location of the pain, its relation to feeding, its severity, time and frequency of occurrence, and duration and nature
2. The presence or absence of associated symptoms, such as weight loss, fever, vomiting, bloating, diarrhea, hematochezia, or urinary symptoms
3. Whether any intercurrent illness or recent trauma has occurred

Acute Abdominal Pain

In children, acute abdominal pain may be the result of extraabdominal diseases (e.g., lower lobe pneumonia;

TABLE 11–1
Distinguishing Features of Abdominal Pain in Children

Disease	Onset	Location	Referral	Quality	Comments
Functional: irritable bowel syndrome	Recurrent	Periumbilical splenic and hepatic flexures	None	Dull, crampy, intermittent; duration 2 hr	Family stress, school phobia, diarrhea and constipation; hypersensitive to pain from distention
Esophageal reflux	Recurrent, after meals, at bedtime	Substernal	Chest	Burning	Sour taste in mouth; Sandifer syndrome
Duodenal ulcer	Recurrent, before meals, at night	Epigastric	Back	Severe burning, gnawing	Relieved by food, milk, antacids; family history important
Pancreatitis	Acute	Epigastric-hypogastric	Back	Constant, sharp, boring	Nausea, emesis, marked tenderness
Intestinal obstruction	Acute or gradual	Periumbilical–lower abdomen	Back	Alternating cramping (colic) and painless periods	Distention, obstipation, bilious emesis, increased bowel sounds
Appendicitis	Acute	Periumbilical or epigastric; localizes to right lower quadrant	Back or pelvis if retrocecal	Sharp, steady	Nausea, emesis, local tenderness, ±fever, avoids motion
Meckel diverticulum	Recurrent	Periumbilical–lower abdomen	None	Sharp	Hematochezia; painless unless intussusception, diverticulitis, or perforation
Inflammatory bowel disease	Recurrent	Depends on site of involvement		Dull cramping, tenesmus	Fever, weight loss, ± hematochezia
Intussusception	Acute	Periumbilical–lower abdomen	None	Cramping, with painless periods	Guarded position with knees pulled up; "currant jelly" stools, lethargy
Lactose intolerance	Recurrent with milk products	Lower abdomen	None	Cramping	Distention, gaseousness, diarrhea
Urolithiasis	Acute, sudden	Back	Groin	Severe, colicky pain	Hematuria
Pyelonephritis	Acute, sudden	Back	None	Dull to sharp	Fever, costochondral tenderness, dysuria, urinary frequency, emesis
Cholecystitis and cholelithiasis	Acute	Right upper quadrant	Right shoulder	Severe, colicky pain	Hemolysis ± jaundice, nausea, emesis

Adapted from Andreoli TE, Carpenter CJ, Plum F, et al: *Cecil essentials of medicine*, Philadelphia, 1986, WB Saunders.

pharyngitis, especially when caused by group A streptococcus; otitis media; and upper respiratory tract infections), although acute gastroenteritis is one of the most common abdominal causes of acute abdominal pain. Pain that persists and brings the patient back to the physician is often the result of appendicitis, intussusception, urinary tract infections, pneumonia, or pharyngitis, as well as of gastroenteritis and viral syndromes. In infants younger than 2 years of age, trauma, incarcerated hernias, intestinal malrotation, and volvulus also must be considered. Between 2 and 5 years of age, sickle cell anemia, lower lobe pneumonia, and urinary tract infections may mimic intestinal disorders. In the older child and adolescent, appendicitis is more common and may be difficult to distinguish from gastroenteritis. In the adolescent girl, *mittelschmerz*, ectopic pregnancy, ovarian cysts, and pelvic inflammatory disease are important considerations. Less common causes of acute pain are pancreatitis, Henoch-Schönlein purpura, mesenteric adenitis, lead poisoning, diabetic ketoacidosis, renal stones, and cholecystitis. Sudden acute, excruciating pain suggests obstruction (stones), adhesions, perforation, or ischemia. A complete blood count (CBC) with differential, urinalysis, pregnancy test, bacterial cultures, serum amylase or lipase, ultrasonography or CT scans, and abdominal plain films support the findings of a careful history and physical examination. Reexamination several hours later may be necessary to help establish the diagnosis.

REFERENCES

Scholer S, PiTuch K, Orr D, et al: Clinical outcomes of children with acute abdominal pain, *Pediatrics* 98(4 Pt 1):680–685, 1996.

Chronic Abdominal Pain

Of all children between the ages of 5 and 15 years, 10–15% have chronic abdominal pain. *Chronic recurrent abdominal pain* is defined as three or more episodes of pain, severe enough to affect activities, occurring over a period of 3 months.

In a large percentage of children, no specific underlying organic cause is found. Recurrent abdominal pain can present as isolated paroxysmal abdominal pain or be associated with dyspepsia or altered bowel pattern. Dyspepsia involves nausea, vomiting, early satiety, epigastric pain, or repeated belching. Altered bowel patterns include constipation, diarrhea, or alternating periods of both. The latter pattern is referred to as irritable bowel syndrome. In most instances, these symptoms have a functional basis. Although the mechanisms of functional bowel disease are difficult to identify, it is felt that children with this disease have altered gastrointestinal motility and visceral hypersensitivity. It is not "all in their

heads." Disorders such as nocturnal enuresis, fears, and sleep disturbances are seen in 30% of those with this syndrome. The mother, the father, or other siblings often suffer from abdominal pain. Social factors, such as a new school, new teacher, examinations, peer group conflict, moving, family illness or death, sibling rivalry, or parental pressure for achievement, frequently precipitate or are associated with attacks of pain.

An unknown proportion of patients with chronic pain have lactose intolerance, also manifested by bloating, gaseousness, or diarrhea. In infants, chronic abdominal pain also may be caused by colic, gastroesophageal reflux and esophagitis, celiac disease, ingestion of nondigestible carbohydrates (e.g., fruit juices, chewing gum: sorbitol), malrotation, and intraabdominal tumors. Older children may have pain resulting from acid peptic disease (esophagitis, gastritis, gastric or duodenal ulcer), giardiasis, inflammatory bowel disease, sickle cell anemia, lead poisoning, and constipation; rarely, pain may result from porphyria, hereditary angioedema, systemic lupus erythematosus (SLE) (vasculitis, serositis), and familial Mediterranean fever. Menstruation-related pain is common in adolescence.

Diagnostic evaluation may include a CBC, measurement of erythrocyte sedimentation rate (ESR), urinalysis, evaluation of stools for occult blood and ova and parasites, abdominal ultrasound, and upper gastrointestinal series with small bowel follow-through. Breath hydrogen testing after a lactose challenge identifies lactose intolerance. An upper gastrointestinal series or a barium enema is indicated when malrotation or intussusception is suggested, respectively.

Treatment of the irritable bowel syndrome should be directed at explaining the functional and benign nature of this syndrome, identifying sources of stress and providing guidance on how to relieve them, and offering sympathetic reassurance. In some patients, short-term antispasmodic anticholinergic agents may relieve pain, and a high-fiber diet may be beneficial, especially when constipation is present.

Diarrhea and Malabsorption

The small intestinal mucosa is composed of villous epithelium, crypt epithelium, lamina propria, and muscularis mucosa (Fig. 11–1).

Pathophysiology of Diarrhea. Six mechanisms explain the pathophysiology of diarrhea (Table 11–2). More than one mechanism may be present at the same time. A number of disease processes directly affect the secretory and absorptive functions of the enterocyte. Some of these processes act by increasing cyclic adenosine monophosphate (cAMP) levels

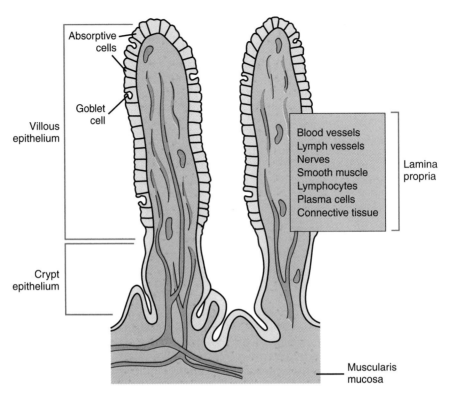

FIG. 11–1

Anatomy of the mucosa of the small intestine.

TABLE 11–2
Mechanisms of Diarrhea

Primary Mechanism	Defect	Stool Examination	Examples	Comment
Secretory	Decreased absorption, increased secretion; electrolyte transport	Watery, normal osmolality; osmols = 2 × $(Na^+ + K^+)$	Cholera, toxigenic *E. coli*; carcinoid, VIP, neuroblastoma, congenital chloride diarrhea, *Clostridium difficile*, cryptosporidiosis (AIDS)	Persists during fasting; bile salt malabsorption also may increase intestinal water secretion; no stool leukocytes
Osmotic	Maldigestion, transport defects, ingestion of unabsorbable solute	Watery, acidic, and reducing substances; increased osmolality; osmols >2 × $(Na^+ + K^+)$	Lactase deficiency, glucose-galactose malabsorption, lactulose, laxative abuse	Stops with fasting; increased breath hydrogen with carbohydrate malabsorption; no stool leukocytes

From Behrman RE, Kliegman RM, Jenson HB, editors: *Nelson textbook of pediatrics*, ed 16, Philadelphia, 2000, WB Saunders.
AIDS, Acquired immunodeficiency syndrome; *VIP,* vasoactive intestinal peptide; *WBC,* white blood cell.

TABLE 11–2
Mechanisms of Diarrhea—cont'd

Primary Mechanism	Defect	Stool Examination	Examples	Comment
Increased motility	Decreased transit time	Loose to normal-appearing stool, stimulated by gastrocolic reflex	Irritable bowel syndrome, thyrotoxicosis, postvagotomy dumping syndrome	Infection also may contribute to increased motility
Decreased motility	Defect in neuromuscular unit(s) Stasis (bacterial overgrowth)	Loose to normal-appearing stool	Pseudoobstruction, blind loop	Possible bacterial overgrowth
Decreased surface area (osmotic, motility)	Decreased functional capacity	Watery	Short bowel syndrome, celiac disease, rotavirus enteritis	May require elemental diet plus parenteral alimentation
Mucosal invasion	Inflammation, decreased colonic reabsorption, increased motility	Blood and increased WBCs in stool	*Salmonella, Shigella,* amebiasis, *Yersinia, Campylobacter*	Dysentery = blood, mucus, and WBCs

AIDS, Acquired immunodeficiency syndrome; *VIP,* vasoactive intestinal peptide; *WBC,* white blood cell.

(*Vibrio cholerae, Escherichia coli,* heat-labile toxin, vasoactive intestinal peptide-producing tumors); other processes (*Shigella* toxin, congenital chloridorrhea) cause secretory diarrhea by affecting ion channels or by unknown mechanisms. Activation of intestinal production of cAMP produces secretory diarrhea by inhibiting free mucosal sodium chloride absorption and stimulating mucosal chloride secretion. Stimulation of cyclic guanosine monophosphate by *E. coli* heat-stable toxin produces the same effect. Virulence factors for various enteropathogens are noted in Table 11–3. Intestinal resection, inflammation, and infection reduce mucosal surface area, which impairs both digestion and absorption. Abnormal intestinal motility reduces mucosal contact time, decreasing both digestion and absorption.

Acute Diarrhea

A *differential diagnosis* of acute diarrhea in children is presented in Table 11–4. In addition to a complete history, which includes epidemiologic data (day care, travel, single-source outbreak, and animal and food contact), antibiotic exposure, and a physical examination, the stool should be tested for occult blood and white blood cells (with methylene blue smear). If the stool test result is negative for both blood and white blood cells and there is no history to suggest contaminated food ingestion, the cause is most likely viral. Parasitic infestations other than giardiasis, cryptosporidiosis, and (where endemic) amebiasis are potential causes of acute diarrhea. Stool examinations for parasites usually are not helpful unless the diarrhea persists. If the stool test result is positive for blood and white blood cells, bacterial causes must be excluded first. The absence of bacterial pathogens and toxins suggests the diagnosis of inflammatory bowel disease, particularly in the adolescent patient who demonstrates weight loss, fever, and abdominal pain.

Specific Causes of Infectious Diarrhea

Viral Causes. Viruses associated with gastroenteritis in infants are the rotavirus, calicivirus, enteric adenovirus, astrovirus, and members of the Norwalk agent group. *Rotavirus* is the most frequent cause of diarrhea during the winter months. Primary infection with rotavirus in infancy may cause moderate to severe disease, whereas reinfection in adolescence leads to mild illness. Rotavirus invades the epithelium of the upper small intestine; in severe cases it may extend throughout the small bowel and colon, resulting in villous damage, secondary transient disaccharidase deficiency, and inflammation in the lamina propria. Vomiting may last for 3–4 days, and diarrhea may last for 7–10 days; dehydration is noted in younger patients.

TABLE 11–3
Virulence Characteristics of Enteropathogens

Organisms	Virulence Properties
Campylobacter jejuni	Invasion; enterotoxin
Clostridium difficile	Cytotoxin; enterotoxin
Cryptosporidium	Adherence
Cyclospora	Inflammation
Entamoeba histolytica	Cyst resistant to physical destruction; invasion; enzyme and cytotoxin production
Enteric adenovirus	Mucosal lesion
Escherichia coli	
Enteropathogenic	Adherence, effacement
Enterotoxigenic	Enterotoxins (heat stable or labile)
Invasive	Invasion
Enterohemorrhagic (O157:H7)	Adherence, effacement, cytotoxin
Enteroaggregative	Adherence, mucosal damage
Giardia lamblia	Cyst resistant to physical destruction; adheres to mucosa
Norwalk-like viruses	Mucosal lesion
Rotavirus	Damage to microvilli
Shigella	Invasion; enterotoxin; cytotoxin
Salmonella	Invasion; enterotoxin
Vibrio cholerae	Enterotoxin
Vibrio parahaemolyticus	Invasion; cytotoxin
Yersinia enterocolitica	Invasion; enterotoxin

The *diagnosis* may be confirmed by Rotazyme (enzyme-linked immunosorbent assay [ELISA]) testing of the stool. *Treatment* is supportive and consists of the supplying of fluid and electrolytes to prevent dehydration. Traditionally, therapy for 24 hours with oral rehydration solutions alone is quite effective in oral diarrhea. Addition of probiotics (*Lactobacillus* GG) or an enkephalinase inhibitor (racecadotril) may shorten the duration of the illness. Refractory cases featuring protracted diarrhea may benefit from oral immunoglobulins (IgG) or lactobacillus GG.

Bacterial Causes

E. COLI. Only certain strains of *E. coli* produce diarrhea. *E. coli* is classified by the mechanism of diarrhea: enteropathogenic (EPEC), enterotoxigenic (ETEC), enteroinvasive (EIEC), enteroadherent (EAEC), and enterohemorrhagic (EHEC) (Table 11–3). EPEC and ETEC adhere to the epithelial cells in the upper small intestine and produce disease by liberating toxins that induce intestinal secretion and limit absorption. EIEC invades the colonic mucosa, producing widespread mucosal damage with acute inflammation. EPEC is responsible for many of the epidemics of diarrhea in nurseries for neonates and in day care centers. ETEC plays a major role in **traveler's diarrhea.** EHEC, especially the *E. coli* O157:H7 strain, is responsible for a hemorrhagic colitis and most cases of the **hemolytic-uremic syndrome** (HUS). *Treatment* is indicated for infants under 3 months of age with EPEC and for patients who remain symptomatic (Table 11–5). Antibiotic treatment is not advised for patients with *E. coli* O157:H7 or HUS because release of toxin may precipitate or worsen the course of HUS. Toxin binding resins given early may prevent the development of HUS.

SALMONELLA. Salmonellae are transmitted through contact with infected animals (e.g., chickens, pet reptiles, or turtles) or from contaminated food products such as milk, eggs, and poultry. The organism produces disease by invading the intestinal mucosa. *Treatment* of mild illness does not shorten the clinical course but does prolong bacterial excretion. Antibiotic therapy is necessary only for high-risk patients who have symptoms of toxicity or in whom metastatic foci or *S. typhi* infection develops (Table 11–5).

SHIGELLA. Shigellae may cause disease by pro-

TABLE 11–4
Differential Diagnosis of Diarrhea

	Infant	Child	Adolescent
Acute			
Common	Gastroenteritis	Gastroenteritis	Gastroenteritis
	Systemic infection	Food poisoning	Food poisoning
	Antibiotic associated	Systemic infection	Antibiotic associated
	Overfeeding	Antibiotic associated	
Rare	Primary disaccharidase deficiency	Toxic ingestion	Hyperthyroidism
	Hirschsprung toxic colitis		
	Adrenogenital syndrome		
Chronic			
Common	Postinfectious secondary lactase deficiency	Postinfectious secondary lactase deficiency	Irritable bowel syndrome
	Cow's milk/soy protein intolerance	Irritable bowel syndrome	Inflammatory bowel disease
	Chronic nonspecific diarrhea of infancy	Celiac disease	Lactose intolerance
	Celiac disease	Lactose intolerance	Giardiasis
	Cystic fibrosis	Giardiasis	Laxative abuse (anorexia nervosa)
	AIDS enteropathy	Inflammatory bowel disease	AIDS enteropathy
		AIDS enteropathy	
Rare	Primary immune defects	Acquired immune defects	Secretory tumors
	Familial villous atrophy	Secretory tumor	Primary bowel tumor
	Secretory tumors	Pseudoobstruction	Gay bowel disease
	Congenital chloridorrhea	Factitious	
	Acrodermatitis enteropathica		
	Lymphangiectasia		
	Abetalipoproteinemia		
	Eosinophilic gastroenteritis		
	Short bowel syndrome		
	Intractable diarrhea syndrome		
	Autoimmune enteropathy		
	Factitious		

AIDS, Acquired immunodeficiency syndrome.

ducing toxin, either alone or in combination with tissue invasion. High fever and seizures may occur, in addition to diarrhea. Infection is spread by person-to-person contact or by the ingestion of contaminated food. The colon is selectively affected. Antibiotic *treatment* produces a bacteriologic cure in 80% of patients after 48 hours, thus reducing the spread of the disease. Many *S. sonnei*, the predominant strain affecting children, are ampicillin resistant. Treatment with trimethoprim/sulfamethoxazole generally is effective (Table 11–5).

CAMPYLOBACTER JEJUNI. *C. jejuni* may account for 15% of episodes of bacterial diarrhea. The infection is spread by person-to-person contact and by contaminated water and food. The organism invades the mucosa of the jejunum, ileum, and colon, producing enterocolitis. Most patients recover spontaneously before the diagnosis is established. *Treatment* speeds recovery and reduces the duration of the carrier state (Table 11–5).

YERSINIA ENTEROCOLITICA. *Yersinia enterocolitica* is transmitted by pets and contaminated food (e.g., chitterlings). Infants and young children character-istically have a diarrheal disease, whereas older children usually have acute lesions of the terminal ileum or acute mesenteric lymphadenitis resembling appendicitis or Crohn disease. Arthritis, rash, and spondylopathy may develop. The course usually is self-limited, lasting 3 days to 3 weeks. The efficacy of antibiotic *treatment* is questionable, but children with septicemia or infection in sites other than the gastrointestinal tract should be treated (Table 11–5).

CLOSTRIDIUM DIFFICILE. *Clostridium difficile* is a common cause of antibiotic-associated diarrhea.

TABLE 11–5
Antibiotic Therapy for Diarrhea

Organism	Treatment*	Comment
Salmonella typhi	Ampicillin,† chloramphenicol,† trimethoprim/sulfamethoxazole, cefotaxime, ciprofloxacin‡	Invasive, bacteremic disease
Other *Salmonella*	Usually none; amoxicillin, ampicillin, trimethoprim/sulfamethoxazole, cefotaxime, ciprofloxacin‡	Treatment indicated if less than 3 months of age, or if malignancy, sickle cell anemia, AIDS, or evidence of nongastrointestinal foci of infection is present
Shigella	Trimethoprim/sulfamethoxazole, ampicillin	Amoxicillin not recommended; treatment reduces infectivity and improves outcome
Escherichia coli		
Toxigenic	Usually none if endemic; trimethoprim/sulfamethoxazole or ciprofloxacin for traveler's diarrhea	Prevention of traveler's diarrhea with bismuth subsalicylate, doxycycline, or ciprofloxacin‡
Invasive or pathogenic	Trimethoprim/sulfamethoxazole, neomycin	No treatment if HUS is suspected
Campylobacter	Mild disease needs no treatment; erythromycin or azithromycin for diarrhea; aminoglycoside, meropenem, or imipenem for systemic illness	If started early (days 1–3), treatment reduces symptoms and fecal organisms
Yersinia	None for diarrhea; gentamicin, chloramphenicol, trimethoprim/sulfamethoxazole, or cefotaxime for systemic illness	Value of treatment of mesenteric adenitis with antibiotics is not established
Vibrio cholerae	Tetracycline, trimethoprim/sulfamethoxazole	Fluid maintenance is critical
Clostridium difficile	Oral vancomycin, metronidazole§	*C. difficile* is agent of antibiotic-associated diarrhea and pseudomembranous colitis
Giardia lamblia	Quinacrine, furazolidone, metronidazole§	Furazolidone is only preparation available in liquid form
Cryptosporidium	None; azithromycin or paromomycin and octreotide in AIDS	A serious infection in immunocompromised patients (AIDS)
Entamoeba histolytica	Metronidazole,§ tinidazole followed by iodoquinol	

AIDS, Acquired immunodeficiency syndrome; *HUS,* hemolytic-uremic syndrome.
*All treatment is predicated on knowledge of antimicrobial sensitivities.
†Often resistant.
‡Ciprofloxacin is not indicated for children with growing bones and uncomplicated infections.
§The safety of metronidazole in children is unknown.

Treatment includes discontinuation of the prior antibiotic and, if diarrhea is severe, oral vancomycin or metronidazole.

Many bacterial agents may be food contaminants and cause food poisoning. Sudden onset, a common source, epidemic vomiting, and diarrhea suggest food poisoning (Table 11–6).

Parasitic Causes. *Entamoeba histolytica* and *Giardia lamblia* are important parasites found in North America that produce disease. Amebiasis occurs in warmer climates, whereas giardiasis is endemic throughout the United States and is common among infants in day care centers.

ENTAMOEBA HISTOLYTICA. The site of infection with *E. histolytica* is the colon, although amebae may pass through the bowel wall and invade the liver, lung, and brain. Diarrhea is of acute onset, is bloody, and contains white blood cells. *Diagnosis* depends on identification of the organism in the stool and may be confirmed serologically. The drug of choice for *treatment* is metronidazole.

GIARDIA LAMBLIA. *G. lamblia* is transmitted through ingestion of cysts, either from contact with an infected individual or from food or fresh or well water contaminated with infected feces. The organism adheres to the microvilli of the duodenal and jejunal epithelium. The onset of the illness usually is insidious but may be acute. *Clinical manifestations* are anorexia,

---

TABLE 11–6
Common Causes of Food Poisoning

Agent	Mechanism	Source	Time of Onset	Signs
Salmonella*	Tissue invasion	Dairy and meat products, eggs	16–48 hr	Fever, cramps, vomiting, bloody diarrhea
Staphylococcus aureus*	Preformed toxin	Meat, egg salad, pastries	1–6 hr	Vomiting, diarrhea
Clostridium perfringens*	In vivo toxin production	Meat, gravy	8–16 hr	Cramps, diarrhea
Clostridium botulinum*	Preformed toxin	Canned food, honey, fish	18–36 hr	Nausea, vomiting, diarrhea, constipation, paralysis
Escherichia coli O157:H7	Attaching and effacing lesion Verotoxin	Undercooked meat, cider, water	24–72 hr	Watery, bloody diarrhea: HUS
Bacillus cereus				
Short incubation	Preformed toxin	Fried rice	1–6 hr	Nausea, vomiting
Long incubation	Toxin produced in vivo	Vegetables	8–16 hr	Vomiting, diarrhea, cramps
Cryptosporidiosis	Adherence	Apple cider, water	24–48 hr	Vomiting, diarrhea, cramps
Norwalk agent	Invasion	Waterborne, shellfish	16–48 hr	Watery diarrhea
Heavy metals†	Direct toxicity	Acidic juices in metal containers: lemonade, fruit punch	1–4 hr	Vomiting, cramps, diarrhea
Scombroid	Histamine	Tuna	Minutes	Flushing, dizziness, headache, vomiting, diarrhea
Ciguatera	Toxin	Mackerel	1–6 hr	Paresthesia of lips, tooth pain, cramps, vomiting, diarrhea
Paralytic shellfish	Neurotoxin	Dinoflagellates of mollusks	1–3 hr	Paresthesia of lips and extremities, dysphagia, ataxia

HUS, Hemolytic-uremic syndrome.
*Salmonella (23%), *S. aureus* (18%), *C. perfringens* (8%), and *C. botulinum* (8%) are the most common causes of food poisoning.
†Includes copper, zinc, tin, and cadmium.

nausea, gaseousness, abdominal distention, watery diarrhea, secondary lactose intolerance, and weight loss. The *diagnosis* may be made by identifying the organism in the stool, in duodenal aspirate, or in the mucosa of a small bowel biopsy. Table 11–5 provides a description of *treatment*.

CRYPTOSPORIDIUM. *Cryptosporidium* causes mild diarrhea in immunocompetent infants attending day care centers. In contrast to the severe diarrhea it produces in patients with acquired immunodeficiency syndrome (AIDS), cryptosporidiosis in normal children is a self-limited disease (Table 11–5).

Management of Diarrhea

Therapy must be directed to curing the initiating event, to correcting dehydration and ongoing fluid and electrolyte deficits, and to managing secondary complications resulting from mucosal injury. Antibiotic treatment is noted in Table 11–5. **Traveler's diarrhea** may be prevented by avoiding uncooked food and untreated drinking water; preventive medication with Pepto-Bismol, tetracycline (for children 8 years of age or older), or trimethoprim/sulfamethoxazole is controversial.

Treatment of fluid deficits requires an estimation of the degree of dehydration and the determination of any electrolyte imbalance, such as hypernatremia, hyponatremia, or metabolic acidosis (see Chapter 16). Acidosis is caused by stool bicarbonate losses, lactic acidosis resulting from fermentation of malabsorbed carbohydrate or shock, and phosphate retention resulting from transient prerenal-renal insufficiency. Therapy for severe fluid and electrolyte losses involves intravenous alimentation, whereas less severe degrees of dehydration ($<10\%$) in infants without excessive vomiting or shock may be managed with oral rehydration solutions containing glucose and electrolytes. Jejunal and ileal glucose absorption carries sodium into the enterocyte, thus also drawing in water. Oral rehydration solutions contain 2–2.5% glucose, 75–90 mEq/L Na^+, 20–25 mEq/L K^+, 45–80 mEq/L Cl^-, and 30 mEq/L bicarbonate or citrate.

Severe infections may damage the mucosa, producing a secondary lactase deficiency that causes osmotic diarrhea if a lactose-containing formula is given to an infant. Therefore, a formula that does not contain lactose may be needed during the immediate rehabilitation phase following episodes of *severe* diarrhea. Drugs such as loperamide, paregoric, and diphenoxylate are potentially dangerous and have no place in the management of acute infectious diarrhea in children.

REFERENCES

Behrman RE, Kliegman RM, Jenson HB, editors: *Nelson textbook of pediatrics*, ed 16, Philadelphia, 2000, WB Saunders, Chapters 176, 179, 196–202, 306.

Caprioli A, Pezzella C, Morelli R, et al: Enteropathogens associated with childhood diarrhea in Italy, *Pediatr Infect Dis J* 15(10):876–883, 1996.

Committee on Infectious Disease, American Academy of Pediatrics: *Red book 2000*, ed 25, Elk Grove Village, Ill, 2000, The Academy.

Guandalini S, Pensabene L, Zikri MA, et al: Lactobacillus GG administered in oral rehydration solution to children with acute diarrhea: a multicenter European trial, *J Pediatr Gastroenterol Nutr* 30(1):54–60, 2000.

Hansson T, Dahlbom I, Hall J, et al: Antibody reactivity against human and guinea pig tissue transglutaminase in children with celiac disease, *J Pediatr Gastroenterol Nutr* 30(4):379–384, 2000.

Provisional Committee on Quality Improvement, Subcommittee on Acute Gastroenteritis: Practice parameter: the management of acute gastroenteritis in young children, *Pediatrics* 97(3): 424–435, 1996.

Salazar-Lindo E, Santisteban-Ponce J, Chea-Woo E, et al: Racecadotril in the treatment of acute watery diarrhea in children, *N Engl J Med* 343(7):463–467, 2000.

Chronic Diarrhea

Clinical Manifestations. During infancy, chronic diarrhea may be a manifestation of specific genetic diseases, such as disaccharidase deficiencies, cystic fibrosis, or immunologically mediated diseases (Table 11–4). *Cow's milk-soy protein intolerance* should be considered in infants younger than 1 year of age when the stool contains erythrocytes, with or without eosinophils. This can occur even in breast-fed infants when cow's milk proteins enter maternal milk. The mechanism by which milk proteins result in mucosal injury is poorly understood. Immune-mediated disease against gluten (celiac disease) begins once the infant is exposed to solid foods containing this protein. Cereals composed of wheat, barley, rye, or oats produce the disease, which may necessitate a lifelong withdrawal from these foods.

Chronic diarrhea may also be the only manifestation of cystic fibrosis. Cystic fibrosis may also occur in association with meconium ileus, rectal prolapse, hypoalbuminemia, hyponatremic dehydration, and hypoprothrombinemia. The *diagnosis* of cystic fibrosis is confirmed by an elevated sweat chloride content. Primary metabolic disorders of absorption, such as *glucose-galactose malabsorption* and *congenital chloridorrhea*, appear in the neonatal period.

The most common cause of chronic diarrhea during infancy is **chronic nonspecific diarrhea of infancy, or toddler's diarrhea.** The onset is between 6 months and 3 years of age and is rarely accompanied by pain. Often the first stool in the morning is formed, but stools (four to six per 24 hours) progress during the day to greater liquidity, sometimes containing mucus and food. The infants do not demonstrate fluid and electrolyte abnormalities, dehydration, or failure to thrive. Often the family history includes similar intestinal problems in siblings or in parents. Symptoms may be precipitated by teething or common infectious illnesses. This disorder may be the result of ingestion of fruit juices containing large quantities of nonabsorbable sugars that produce diarrhea. In this same age group, a **lactase deficiency** following viral gastroenteritides also is common and may result in secondary lactose malabsorption that may persist for months. Increased breath hydrogen excretion following a standard oral lactose challenge, resulting from colonic bacterial fermentation of malabsorbed lactose, is diagnostic. Bloating, cramping, borborygmus, and flatus also are noted in lactose-intolerant patients during the lactose challenge. A lactose-free formula may be needed until lactase activity regenerates. **Congenital sucrose deficiency** is rare and occurs after sucrose-containing foods (e.g., fruits, juices, and vegetables) are added to the diet in sufficient quantities to exceed the digestive capacity of the brush border sucrase; treatment consists of avoiding sucrose sugar–containing foods.

Beyond infancy, lactase deficiency and parasitic infection, usually giardiasis, are important common causes of chronic diarrhea (Table 11–4). Diarrhea as the only manifestation of irritable bowel syndrome is unusual in older children and adolescents. During this older age period, **inflammatory bowel disease** should be considered, especially when diarrhea is associated with fever, oral aphthoid ulcers, anemia, hematochezia, abdominal pain, weight loss, rash, arthralgias or arthritis, and uveitis or episcleritis.

When chronic diarrhea persists and is associated with weight loss and global or specific nutritional deficiencies, a **malabsorption syndrome** exists. The usual early manifestations of malabsorption are frequent, bulky-oily, foul-smelling stools (steatorrhea); weight loss; and a ravenous appetite. Late manifestations include poor weight gain or weight loss, growth failure, muscle wasting, protuberant abdomen, secondary immune deficiency, and nutritional disorders. Malabsorption of specific nutrients (e.g., vitamin D, which results in rickets; vitamin K, which results in hemorrhage; vitamin B_{12}, folate, and iron, which result in anemia; and calcium, which results in hypocalcemic tetany, osteopenia, or fractures) may develop. Mechanisms of malabsorption include impaired digestion, reduced absorption, decreased surface area, lymphatic obstruction, drugs, infection, collagen-vascular disease, and endocrine abnormalities (Table 11–7). Cystic fibrosis, celiac sprue, short

---

TABLE 11–7
Malabsorption Syndromes

Reduced Digestion	
Pancreatic exocrine deficiency	Cystic fibrosis, pancreatitis, Shwachman syndrome, Pearson syndrome
Bile salt deficiency	Cholestasis, biliary atresia, hepatitis, cirrhosis, bacterial deconjugation
Enzyme defects	Lactase, sucrase, enterokinase, lipase deficiencies
Reduced Absorption	
Primary absorption defects	Glucose-galactose malabsorption, abetalipoproteinemia, cystinuria, Hartnup disease
Decreased mucosal surface area	Crohn disease, malnutrition, short bowel syndrome, antimetabolite chemotherapy, familial villous atrophy
Small intestinal disease	Celiac disease, tropical sprue, giardiasis, immune-allergic enteritis, Crohn disease, lymphoma, AIDS
Lymphatic Obstruction	Lymphangiectasia, Whipple disease, lymphoma, chylous ascites
Others	
Drugs	Antibiotics, antimetabolites, neomycin, laxatives
Collagen vascular	Scleroderma
Infestations	Hookworms, tapeworm, giardiasis, immune defects

AIDS, Acquired immunodeficiency syndrome.

bowel syndrome, and giardiasis are common causes of malabsorption. Immune deficiencies usually associated with enteritis include Wiskott-Aldrich syndrome, common variable immunodeficiency syndrome, agammaglobulinemia, and acquired immunodeficiency syndrome (AIDS). Certain AIDS-related opportunistic intestinal infections (*Isospora belli, Cryptosporidium, Entamoeba,* and cytomegalovirus) also cause malabsorption and failure to thrive.

Diagnosis. The *diagnosis* of chronic diarrhea in a patient begins with a careful history, including a family and dietary history as it relates to the onset of symptoms. It is important to remember that neither stool odor, which is usually unpleasant, nor stool color, unless blood is seen or pale (acholic), has any consistent relationship to the presence of gastrointestinal disease. Physical examination should include a careful assessment of the patient's nutritional status (see Chapter 2) and a check for signs of infection.

Stool should be tested for blood, white blood cells, fat content, and carbohydrate malabsorption. Carbohydrate malabsorption is assessed by identifying an acid stool pH and reducing substances. Fecal fat should not exceed 15% of intake in infants and 10% in older children. To exclude parasitic infection, the clinician must collect three fresh stool specimens for examination. Barium studies should not be done within several days of the stool collection because parasites adhere to the barium. *Roentgenographic findings* may be diagnostic for inflammatory bowel disease; however, for many of the small intestinal mucosal disorders, only a nonspecific "malabsorption pattern," characterized by thickened mucosal folds, edema of the bowel wall, and flocculation of the barium, is present.

A number of studies are available for assessment of specific types of malabsorption. The D-xylose test provides an index of mucosal carbohydrate absorption. Lactose and sucrose malabsorption can be measured by the breath hydrogen technique. A Sudan stain of the stool may be used as a qualitative assessment of fecal fat, but steatorrhea is best quantitated by a 72-hour fecal fat study. Measurement of the fecal alpha$_1$-antitrypsin level is a screening study for documenting enteric protein loss. Protein loss can be quantified by assessment of alpha$_1$-antitrypsin clearance with simultaneous measurement of serum and 24-hour stool concentrations. Serum calcium levels, prothrombin time, and vitamin A, 25-OH vitamin D, and vitamin E levels may be determined to assess fat-soluble vitamin deficiencies.

Peroral, *transpyloric biopsy* of the small intestinal mucosa during gastroduodenoscopy may be needed to document diseases such as celiac sprue, lymphangiectasia, giardiasis, abetalipoproteinemia, and tropical sprue.

Treatment. Treatment must be directed at the primary disease and at the correction of associated deficiency states, such as rickets and hypoprothrombinemia. Primary therapy for cystic fibrosis involves lifelong pancreatic enzyme replacement, whereas therapy for celiac disease requires strict adherence to a gluten-free diet. Hyperalimentation may be needed for familial enteropathies, short bowel syndrome, or refractory cases of chronic intractable diarrhea.

REFERENCES

Behrman RE, Kliegman RM, Jenson HB, editors: *Nelson textbook of pediatrics,* ed 16, Philadelphia, 2000, WB Saunders, Chapters 306, 340, 341.

Goulet O, Kedinger M, Brousse N, et al: Intractable diarrhea of infancy with epithelial and basement membrane abnormalities, *J Pediatr* 127(2):212–219, 1995.

Hyams J, Burke G, Davis P, et al: Abdominal pain and irritable bowel syndrome in adolescents: a community-based study, *J Pediatr* 129(2):220–226, 1996.

Constipation and Encopresis

Constipation is defined as infrequent passage of hard, dry stools. *Obstipation* is the absence of bowel movements. The causes of constipation are noted in Table 11–8. Beyond the neonatal period, the most common cause (90–95% of cases) of constipation is voluntary withholding (*functional constipation*), a problem often beginning with the attempt to toilet train the infant (Table 11–9). A family history of similar problems often is obtained. Stool retention may be the result of conflicts in toilet training but usually is caused by pain on defecation, which creates a fear of defecation and leads to further retention. Milk protein allergy–induced rectal inflammation and painful fissures may lead to stool avoidance. Voluntary withholding of stool increases distention of the rectum, which decreases rectal sensation, necessitating an even greater fecal mass to initiate the urge to defecate. Complications of stool retention include impaction, abdominal pain, overflow diarrhea resulting from leakage around the fecal mass, anal fissure, rectal bleeding, and urinary tract infection caused by extrinsic pressure on the urethra.

Encopresis, daytime or nighttime soiling by formed stools beyond the age of expected toilet training (4–5 years), is another complication of constipation (see Chapter 1). Older children should be asked specifically about soiling, since such information may not be expressed because of embarrassment. These children frequently are unable to sense the need to defecate because of stretching of the internal sphincter by the retained fecal mass.

TABLE 11–8
Causes of Constipation

Nonorganic (Functional)	Drugs—cont'd
Organic	Psychoactive drugs (e.g., chlorpromazine [Thorazine])
Intestinal	Chemotherapeutic agents (e.g., vincristine)
Milk protein allergy	Pancreatic enzymes (e.g., in fibrosing colonopathy)
Hirschsprung disease	Metabolic
Neuronal dysgenesis	Dehydration
Anal stenosis	Cystic fibrosis (meconium ileus equivalent)
Anal stricture	Hypothyroidism
Anterior dislocation of the anus	Hypokalemia
Pseudoobstruction	Hypercalcemia
Collagen-vascular diseases	Hypermagnesemia
Rectal abscess or fissure	Neuromuscular
Stricture post-NEC	Infant botulism
Drugs	Absent abdominal muscle
Lead	Myotonic dystrophy
Narcotics	Spinal cord lesions (tumors or spina bifida)
Antidepressants	Chagas disease

NEC, Necrotizing enterocolitis.

TABLE 11–9
Distinguishing Features of Hirschsprung Disease and Functional (Acquired) Constipation

	Functional Constipation	Hirschsprung Disease*
History		
Onset of constipation	After 2 yr of age	At birth or before 1 mo of age
Encopresis	Common	Very rare
Forced bowel training	Usual	None
Stool size	Very large	Small, ribbon-like
Enterocolitis	None	Possible
Abdominal pain	Common	Common
Failure to thrive	Uncommon	Common
Family history	Variable	Yes, but not always
Examination		
Abdominal distention	Variable	Common
Poor growth	Rare	Common
Anal tone	Patulous	Tight
Rectal examination	Stool in ampulla	Ampulla empty
Malnutrition	Absent	Possible
Laboratory		
Barium enema	Massive amounts of stool, no transition zone	Transition zone, delayed evacuation (greater than 24 hr)
Rectal biopsy	Normal	No ganglion cells; hypertrophied nerve fibers; ↑acetylcholinesterase staining
Anorectal manometry	Distention of the rectum causes relaxation of the internal sphincter	No sphincter relaxation

Modified from Behrman RE, Kliegman RM, Jenson HB, editors: *Nelson textbook of pediatrics*, ed 16, Philadelphia, 2000, WB Saunders, p 1140.
*Note that ultra-short-segment Hirschsprung disease may have clinical features of functional (acquired) megacolon (e.g., constipation).

In term infants, meconium should be passed within the first 24 hour of life; failure to pass meconium suggests an underlying disorder. The consistency and frequency of bowel movements vary greatly, both in the individual child and among different children. Breast-fed infants usually produce stool with every feeding but may produce stool only one to two times a day. Formula-fed infants usually produce stool daily but may produce stool once every 2 or 3 days. In general, the range of normal for infants is from five stools/day to as few as one every third day.

Stool is produced as the fecal fluid is moved through the colon by three to four mass-propulsive movements per day. Water and electrolytes are reabsorbed (95%) in the colon and rectosigmoid, resulting in formed stool. Stool is stored in the rectum until sufficient distention produces the urge to defecate. The internal anal sphincter then relaxes and stool enters the anal canal. The external anal sphincter is a voluntary muscle controlling fecal continence. Failure to defecate may be a result of decreased peristalsis (caused by aganglionic segment, a spinal cord defect), decreased expulsion (caused by a weakened abdominal muscle), and anatomic malformations (caused by anterior dislocation of the anus, neuronal dysgenesis, aganglionic Hirschsprung disease, or stenosis). The exclusion of Hirschsprung disease is critical in the *differential diagnosis* of constipation. This is especially critical in infants because of the risk of bacterial overgrowth, enterocolitis, and intestinal perforation (Table 11–9).

Functional constipation may be self-perpetuating, often becoming more severe with time; symptomatic treatment is indicated. In infants, increases in the intake of juices and fruits, malt extract, or lactulose are effective. For older children, either lactulose or mineral oil, 1–3 oz/24 hr given either in divided doses or as a single dose 2 hours after meals, and increased dietary fiber content usually are successful. If there is marked fecal retention, the rectum must be cleared of impacted stool with enemas, cathartics, or both. Once stools are softened, the oil is gradually tapered, but the fiber supplements must be continued on a regular basis for several months, during which time the dose gradually is reduced. Psychologic problems leading to or resulting from the constipation may need special attention (see Chapter 1).

Vomiting

Vomiting occurs in both gastrointestinal and nongastrointestinal diseases in childhood. The forceful ejection of gastric contents is often preceded by nausea and is caused by the coordination of gastric atony (except in pyloric stenosis), relaxation of the gastro-esophageal junction, and increased intragastric (abdominal) pressure from abdominal wall contractions. Vomiting is mediated by the medullary emesis center in the floor of the fourth ventricle, which is influenced by gastrointestinal (visceral afferent) or nongastrointestinal (chemoreceptive trigger zone) stimuli. The latter elements are affected by various stimuli, including drugs and motion sickness. *Regurgitation* is not vomiting but rather a passive, nonforceful ejection of gastric contents resulting from reflux through a relaxed lower esophageal sphincter. Most infants younger than 3 months of age regurgitate some formula with no apparent ill effects.

The *differential diagnosis* of vomiting should be approached by consideration of age-specific diseases. During the neonatal period, gastrointestinal obstruction often is a result of congenital malformations (Table 11–10). In infants, gastroenteritis, overfeeding, and gastroesophageal reflux are the most common causes of emesis and regurgitation. Food allergy and milk protein intolerance also are common. Nongastrointestinal diseases that produce emesis in the infant include systemic infections, hyperammonemia, other inborn errors of metabolism, adrenogenital syndrome, rumination, increased intracranial pressure, and subdural hemorrhage.

In children and adolescents, vomiting commonly is caused by gastroenteritis, systemic infection, toxic ingestions, and appendicitis. Less common causes are Reye syndrome, hepatitis, *Helicobacter pylori* gastritis, ulcers, pancreatitis, malrotation, brain tumor, increased intracranial pressure, cyclic vomiting or abdominal migraine, middle ear infection, and chemotherapy. Children also may have vomiting associated with pertussis syndrome and achalasia. Vomiting also may occur in adolescence as a result of bulimia and inflammatory bowel disease.

Cyclic vomiting often begins before 5 years of age and is characterized by repeated episodes (two or fewer per week) of intense vomiting (four or more episodes per hour). It may affect <1% of school-age children; 50% require intravenous therapy. Associated features are pallor, lethargy, anorexia, nausea, and abdominal pain. The disorder may be a migraine variant, but more serious disorders (e.g., intestinal obstruction, inborn errors of metabolism, increased intracranial pressure, or Addison disease) must be ruled out.

A careful history and physical examination are necessary to determine whether the source of vomiting is gastrointestinal or some other systemic disturbance. Neonates with polyhydramnios, drooling, a large amount of gastric aspirate (10–20 mL), persistent emesis, abdominal distention, or bile-stained or blood-stained vomitus may have an obstruction and should have a contrast study to determine the

TABLE 11–10
Causes of Gastrointestinal Obstruction

Esophagus		Small Intestine—cont'd	
Congenital	Tracheoesophageal fistula	Acquired	Postsurgical adhesions
	Isolated esophageal atresia		Trauma (hematoma)
			Crohn disease
Acquired	Caustic agent esophageal stricture		Intussusception
	Peptic stricture		Meconium ileus equivalent (cystic
	Chagas disease		fibrosis)
	Collagen-vascular disease		Superior mesenteric artery
			syndrome
Stomach			
Congenital	Antral webs	**Colon**	
	Pyloric stenosis	Congenital	Meconium plug
			Hirschsprung disease
Acquired	Bezoars/foreign body		Colonic atresia, stenosis
	Pyloric stricture (ulcer)		Imperforate anus
	Crohn disease		Rectal stenosis
	Eosinophilic gastroenteropathy		Malrotation/volvulus
	Prostaglandin induced		Pseudoobstruction
	Chronic granulomatous disease		
	Epidermolysis bullosa	Acquired	Ulcerative colitis (toxic megacolon)
			Crohn disease
Small Intestine			Chagas disease
Congenital	Duodenal atresia		Stricture post-NEC
	Annular pancreas		Fibrosing colonopathy (cystic
	Malrotation/volvulus		fibrosis)
	Malrotation/Ladd bands		
	Ileal atresia		
	Meconium ileus		
	Inguinal hernia		
	Pseudoobstruction		

NEC, Necrotizing enterocolitis.

site of the obstruction. Bile-stained emesis suggests obstruction distal to the ampulla of Vater. Persistent emesis in older children usually necessitates endoscopic evaluation, especially in the presence of dysphagia, gastrointestinal hemorrhage, or a foreign body. *Laboratory investigation* should be directed by the information obtained from the history and physical examination in order to determine the presence of infection (by culture), reflux (prolonged esophageal pH testing), metabolic disorders (testing for acidosis and hyperammonemia), pancreatitis (by testing for amylase and lipase), pyloric stenosis (by testing for alkalosis and ultrasound or a contrast radiograph), and inflammatory bowel disease (ESR, mucosal biopsy, roentgenographic contrast study).

Treatment of emesis is directed toward the underlying disorders and toward correction of dehydration and electrolyte disturbances. Short periods of small, frequent feedings of clear fluids may be all that is needed to stop emesis. Rarely, drugs such as promethazine, chlorpromazine, and prochlorperazine by rectal suppository may be useful, but these drugs may produce extrapyramidal side effects. Ondansetron, a serotonin antagonist, is effective treatment for chemotherapy-induced emesis and other causes of refractory vomiting.

REFERENCES

Behrman RE, Kliegman RM, Jenson HB, editors: *Nelson textbook of pediatrics,* ed 16, Philadelphia, 2000, WB Saunders, Chapters 306, 323, 329, 330, 332, 338.

Diseth T, Bjørnland K, Nøvik T, et al: Bowel junction, mental health, and psychosocial function in adolescents with Hirschsprung's disease, *Arch Dis Child* 76(2):100–106, 1997.

Li BU, Balint JP: Cyclic vomiting syndrome: evolution in our understanding of a brain-gut disorder, *Adv Pediatr* 47:117–160, 2000.

TABLE 11–11
Differential Diagnosis of Gastrointestinal Bleeding in Childhood

	Infant	Child	Adolescent
Common	Bacterial gastroenteritis Swallowed maternal blood Anal fissure Milk protein allergy Necrotizing enterocolitis Intussusception Lymphonodular hyperplasia	Bacterial gastroenteritis Anal fissure Intussusception Ulcer/gastritis (*Helicobacter pylori*) Swallowed epistaxis Juvenile polyp (colonic) Mallory-Weiss syndrome	Bacterial gastroenteritis Inflammatory bowel disease Ulcer/gastritis (*H. pylori*) Polyps (colonic) Anal fissure
Rare	Volvulus Hemorrhagic disease of newborn Meckel diverticulum Necrotizing enterocolitis Stress ulcer	Esophageal varices Esophagitis Coagulopathy Meckel diverticulum Lymphonodular hyperplasia Foreign body Hemangioma, AVM Sexual abuse Hemolytic-uremic syndrome Henoch-Schönlein purpura	Hemorrhoids Esophageal varices Esophagitis Coagulopathy Mallory-Weiss syndrome Telangiectasia (angiodysplasia) Gay bowel disease

AVM, Arteriovenous malformation.

Madoff RD, Williams JG, Caushaj PF: Fecal incontinence, *N Engl J Med* 326(15):1002–1009, 1992.

Partin JC, Hamill SK, Fischel JE, et al: Painful defecation and fecal soiling in children, *Pediatrics* 89(6 Pt 1):1007–1009, 1992.

Van der Plas R, Benninga M, Büller H, et al: Biofeedback training in treatment of childhood constipation: a randomized controlled study, *Lancet* 348(9030):776–780, 1996.

Gastrointestinal Hemorrhage

Hemorrhage may occur at any location in the gastrointestinal tract, and the differential diagnosis depends to a large extent on the patient's age. **Hematemesis,** blood-stained emesis, results from bleeding proximal to the ligament of Treitz. Less severe upper gastrointestinal bleeding results in a coffee-grounds appearance of the emesis. **Melena** refers to soft, usually black or dark-colored stool of a tarry consistency; it usually is suggestive of bleeding from the oropharynx to the proximal small intestine. With stasis of blood in the right colon, bleeding lesions in that area also may appear as melena. **Hematochezia** refers to bright red or maroon-colored stools. Although the lesion is typically colonic, massive upper gastrointestinal bleeding may cause bright red blood per rectum because blood is a cathartic and decreases transit time. *Bright red streaks* of blood coating the surface of a stool suggest a rectal or anal le-

sion. **Occult gastrointestinal bleeding** is defined as significant, ongoing blood loss in the absence of a discernible change in the color or texture of stools; such loss may produce iron-deficiency anemia if it persists.

Before the evaluation for gastrointestinal hemorrhage, it is important to be sure that the stool does indeed contain blood and that the blood is from the gastrointestinal tract. A number of commonly ingested substances may simulate hematochezia: noncarbonated drinks (e.g., Kool-Aid or Hawaiian Punch), colored gelatins, beets, fruit bars, clingstone peaches, and antibiotics. Similarly, melena is simulated by the ingestion of compounds containing bismuth (e.g., Pepto-Bismol), therapeutic iron supplements, charcoal, and spinach. Swallowed and subsequently regurgitated blood from a briskly bleeding nasopharyngeal or oral lesion also may be misinterpreted as upper gastrointestinal bleeding. Rarely, hemoptysis may be confused with hematemesis. Vaginal bleeding and hematuria have been mistakenly interpreted as hematochezia.

The *differential diagnosis* is based primarily on a careful history and a physical examination of the child (Table 11–11) and on the site of bleeding (Table 11–12). Abdominal pain that awakens the patient at night, is relieved by food, and is accompanied by he-

---

TABLE 11–12
Sites and Causes of Gastrointestinal (GI) Bleeding

Upper GI
Epistaxis
Esophagitis
Gastritis
Gastric ulcer
Duodenal ulcer
Esophageal varices
Mallory-Weiss syndrome
Foreign body
Caustic ingestion

Upper and Lower GI
Hemorrhagic disease of newborn
Hemangioma
Osler-Weber-Rendu syndrome
Arteriovenous malformation
Tumor

Lower GI
Milk/soy protein colitis
Eosinophilic colitis
Gastroenteritis (bacterial)
Intussusception
Henoch-Schönlein purpura
Polyps
Inflammatory bowel disease
Volvulus
Meckel diverticulum
Lymphonodular hyperplasia
Pseudomembranous colitis
Hemolytic-uremic syndrome

---

mine whether the blood is fetal or maternal. Swallowed maternal blood at the time of delivery or from a ruptured lacteal during breast feeding is a common cause of hematemesis or hematochezia in the newborn (see Chapter 6).

During the initial evaluation, an appropriately sized nasogastric tube should be placed in the stomach to determine whether the bleeding site is above the ligament of Treitz and to monitor the rate of upper gastrointestinal system hemorrhage. If the pylorus is closed, duodenal bleeding may not be detected with a nasogastric tube. If the gastric fluid return is clear, the source of the bleeding probably is below the ligament of Treitz. A small amount of hematemesis or melena may be misleading because a source of major blood loss may be concealed within the intestines. Furthermore, an initial normal hemoglobin and hematocrit value may give a false sense of security since reequilibration may take 2–4 hours to reflect blood losses.

To diagnose the specific cause of upper gastrointestinal bleeding, *endoscopy* should be performed after the hemorrhaging has decreased or stopped. An upper gastrointestinal tract–contrast roentgenographic study also may be helpful. Lower intestinal bleeding may be evaluated with proctosigmoidoscopy, colonoscopy, arteriography, or specific scans. The technetium-99m (^{99m}Tc) pertechnetate scan, preceded by pentagastrin stimulation or a histamine H_2-receptor antagonist, identifies the ectopic acid-secreting cells creating the hemorrhage in **Meckel diverticulum.**

When the site of bleeding is unclear, arteriography, ^{99m}Tc sulfur colloid, or ^{99m}Tc-labeled autologous red blood cells can be infused intravenously. Arteriography and ^{99m}Tc sulfur colloid detect rapid bleeding, whereas intermittent bleeding is more reliably identified by ^{99m}Tc-labeled red blood cells.

The goals of *management* of acute gastrointestinal hemorrhage, in order of importance, are as follows:
1. Correcting hypovolemia
2. Correcting anemia
3. Stopping the bleeding
4. Preventing recurrence
5. Diagnosing the cause
6. Applying specific therapy

The immediate approach to the patient includes:
1. Assessing pulse and blood pressure (both supine and orthostatic changes)
2. Establishing intravenous access for administration of fluids
3. Expanding the intravascular volume in the presence of hypovolemia by providing intravenous crystalloid fluids
4. Determining serial blood hemoglobin content

matemesis is highly suggestive of acid-peptic disease. Substernal pain suggests esophagitis. Infants and older children with chronic hepatic disease and cirrhosis who exhibit hematemesis probably have bleeding esophageal varices. A history of neonatal omphalitis and subsequent portal vein thrombophlebitis also suggests variceal bleeding secondary to portal vein obstruction. For many children who have acute gastrointestinal hemorrhage, no obvious diagnosis is evident at the time of the first episode of bleeding.

If hepatic disease is present, coagulation studies should be performed. If coagulopathy is present, therapy is initiated with parenteral vitamin K and fresh frozen plasma. In newborn infants with bright red, bloody emesis or bright red blood passed per rectum, an Apt test should be performed to deter-

5. Typing and cross-matching whole blood or packed cells for continued replacement of whole blood or erythrocyte losses

The *treatment* of gastrointestinal hemorrhage should be specific for the underlying disorder. Anion pump inhibitors (omeprazole), H_2-receptor–blocking drugs, and antacids are useful agents for gastritis, esophagitis, and peptic ulcer disease, whereas treatment of the Mallory-Weiss syndrome involves the above in addition to close inpatient observation. Acute abdominal crises, such as volvulus and intussusception, necessitate immediate contrast studies, which may be therapeutic for intussusception. Bleeding esophageal varices may be managed with intravenous somatostatin (octreotide), vasopressin, sclerotherapy, or banding. Rarely, emergency transjugular, intrahepatic portosystemic shunting or portosystemic shunts are needed to stop variceal hemorrhage in children. Persistent massive hemorrhage that is unresponsive to therapy may necessitate surgical exploration, whether or not a lesion has been identified. Techniques that may be used to avoid emergency surgery include direct intraarterial infusion of vasopressin, selective embolization of an arteriovenous malformation or isolated bleeding site, and electrocoagulation and laser photocoagulation for a bleeding ulcer or bleeding from angiodysplastic lesions.

Jaundice

Jaundice (icterus) is the yellow discoloration of the skin, mucous membranes, and sclera caused by increased serum bilirubin concentrations that are deposited in tissue. Although indirect hyperbilirubinemia appears on the skin as yellow-brown coloration and direct hyperbilirubinemia gives the skin a yellow-green appearance, laboratory evaluation is needed for diagnosis and classification of the jaundice. Hyperbilirubinemia may be caused by overproduction, decreased hepatic uptake or metabolism, and decreased hepatic excretion of bilirubin. Jaundice is the most common physical finding of hepatic dysfunction in children of all ages. Jaundice may be a result of a benign process (as in physiologic jaundice of the newborn), or it may be a sign of serious underlying disease, such as hepatitis. The production and excretion of bilirubin are discussed in Chapter 6.

Jaundice in the neonatal patient is discussed in Chapter 6. In older patients jaundice always is a sign of significant disease. Icterus in the young infant may not be visible until the bilirubin level is 10 mg/dL; older children and adolescents demonstrate jaundice when the bilirubin is 2.5 mg/dL. Additional signs of underlying hepatic disease are protuberant abdomen, ascites, edema, pruritus with excoriations, dark urine, and acholic, white-gray stools.

The *differential diagnosis* and *laboratory evaluation* of jaundice in an infant depend on whether there is indirect or direct hyperbilirubinemia (Fig. 11–2). Patients with indirect hyperbilirubinemia should be evaluated further for evidence of immune-mediated or non–immune-mediated hemolysis by a CBC, peripheral blood smear, and Coombs test. Nonhemolytic indirect hyperbilirubinemia is common in newborn infants and older children with **Gilbert syndrome.** The remaining patients with indirect hyperbilirubinemia should have an appropriate laboratory assessment based on the history and physical examination (e.g., constipation and a large anterior fontanel suggest hypothyroidism).

All patients with direct-reacting hyperbilirubinemia (direct bilirubin >1 mg/dL or 20% of total bilirubin), regardless of age, should have a comprehensive diagnostic evaluation to determine potentially serious causes of hepatic dysfunction. The laboratory studies should be based on the following:

- Family history (e.g., metabolic or hepatic disease)
- Exposure history (e.g., to toxins, drugs, and infectious agents)
- Age-related diseases (e.g., biliary atresia in infancy)
- Physical examination (e.g., look for unusual facies, splenomegaly, or psychomotor retardation)
- Screening liver function tests

Screening tests include tests of hepatic synthetic function (e.g., serum albumin level and prothrombin time); tests of biliary obstruction (e.g., direct bilirubin, serum alkaline phosphatase, 5'-nucleotidase, and gamma-glutamyl transpeptidase levels); and tests of hepatocellular injury (i.e., aspartate aminotransferase and alanine aminotransferase levels). In many infants, hepatic imaging with ultrasonography, radionucleotide, or CT scans also may be necessary, as may liver biopsy.

REFERENCES

Behrman RE, Kliegman RM, Jenson HB, editors: *Nelson textbook of pediatrics*, ed 16, Philadelphia, 2000, WB Saunders, Chapters 306, 336, 356.

Caulfield M, Wyllie R, Sivak M, et al: Upper gastrointestinal tract endoscopy in the pediatric patient, *J Pediatr* 115(3):339–345, 1989.

Doig C: Paediatric problems. II. Rectal bleeding, *BMJ* 305(6852): 511–513, 1992.

Khuroo M, Yattoo G, Javid G, et al: A comparison of omeprazole and placebo for bleeding ulcer, *N Engl J Med* 336(15):1054–1058, 1997.

Shields R, Jenkin S, Baxter J, et al: A prospective randomized controlled trial comparing the efficacy of somatostatin with injection sclerotherapy in the control of bleeding esophageal varices, *J Hepatol* 16(1-2):128–137, 1992.

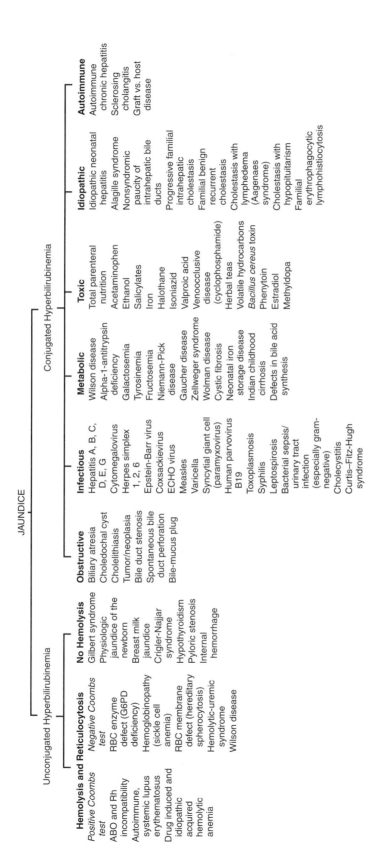

FIG. 11–2

Differential diagnosis of jaundice in childhood. *G6PD*, Glucose-6-phosphate dehydrogenase; *RBC*, red blood cell.

GASTROINTESTINAL DISORDERS BY ORGAN

Oral Cavity

Mastication, the primary function of the oral cavity, requires healthy teeth with proper approximation. Two sets of teeth include the 20 *primary*, or *deciduous*, and the 32 *secondary*, or *permanent* teeth. The schedule of dental eruption is indicated in Table 11–13. Disorders of tooth development include **enamel hypoplasia,** which appears as enamel fissures, pits, or grooves and may be caused by rickets, serious illness, amelogenesis imperfecta, or the intake of tetracycline. Because enamel formation of permanent teeth is complete between 8 and 10 years of age, tetracycline given after this age is not incorporated and thus does not stain the teeth. Abnormally shaped teeth are seen in congenital syphilis. Hypodontia (missing teeth) may be genetic or associated with syndromes (e.g., Down or ectodermal dysplasia). Natal, congenital, or prematurely erupted teeth are uncommon and usually are not a clinical problem. **Delayed eruption** of all teeth indicates impacted teeth or an endocrine, metabolic, genetic, or nutritional disturbance, such as hypopituitarism, hypothyroidism, osteopetrosis, Gaucher disease, Down syndrome, cleidocranial dysplasia, or rickets. Discoloration of the teeth may occur as a consequence of excessive fluoride (>5 ppm), prolonged neonatal hyperbilirubinemia, or the intake of tetracycline.

TABLE 11–13
Time of Eruption of the Primary and Permanent Teeth

Tooth Type	Primary Age (mo)		Permanent Age (yr)	
	Upper	Lower	Upper	Lower
Central incisor	6 ± 2	7 ± 2	7–8	6–7
Lateral incisor	9 ± 2	7 ± 2	8–9	7–8
Cuspids	18 ± 2	16 ± 2	11–12	9–10
First bicuspids	—	—	10–11	10–12
Second bicuspids	—	—	10–12	11–12
First molars	14 ± 4	12 ± 4	6–7	6–7
Second molars	24 ± 4	20 ± 4	12–13	11–13
Third molars	—	—	17–21	17–21

Early tooth loss may be a result of genetic causes (e.g., Down syndrome, juvenile periodontitis, Ehlers-Danlos, or Chédiak-Higashi), immunodeficiencies (e.g., neutropenia or neutrophil defects or human immunodeficiency virus [HIV]), enzyme deficiencies (e.g., acatalasia or hypophosphatasia), or tumors (e.g., eosinophilic granuloma or leukemia).

Dental Caries

The development of dental caries depends on the interaction of dietary carbohydrate and oral bacteria, specifically *Streptococcus mutans*, on the tooth surface. Organic acids produced by the bacterial fermentation of carbohydrate demineralize the tooth surface, leading to pit formation that progresses to cavity (caries) formation. If unchecked, the process erodes through the tooth, permitting a bacterial invasion of the pulp that becomes painful (toothache). Further spread of the inflammatory process to the alveolar bone results in a dental abscess. Caries in primary teeth may disrupt the development of the permanent teeth.

The best *treatment* for caries is *prevention*, and the most effective preventive measure is fluoridation of the water supply to 1 ppm. In fluoride-deficient areas, supplementation may be necessary. Reducing dietary carbohydrate intake also is important. To prevent the damaging effects of continuous bottle feeding (nursing bottle caries), bedtime bottles, if they are necessary, should contain only water. Brushing and flossing of teeth should begin by age 3, although most children under 10 years of age do not have the eye-to-hand coordination to perform either activity properly. The parents must assume this responsibility according to the child's ability. Regular dental visits should begin by age 3.

Early dental *treatment* can salvage most carious teeth. Dental infection confined to the tooth itself may be managed with filling or extraction. When the infection extends to the adjacent alveolar bone, oral antibiotics (e.g., penicillin) should be initiated. More serious spread of infection to the submandibular space **(Ludwig angina)** and to the buccal or orbital spaces, both of which may produce cellulitis, should be managed with intravenous penicillin. The diseased tooth can be identified by localized pain; local treatment (filling or extraction) is needed after the infection is treated.

Oropharyngeal Candidiasis (Thrush)

Oral candidiasis is common in young infants. The *diagnosis* is made by visual inspection of white plaques covering the oropharyngeal mucosa. Initial *treatment* consists of the topical application of nystatin. All toys and bottle nipples must be boiled daily to prevent reinfection. Refractory cases may require clotrimazole troches or, rarely, intravenous amphotericin. Fluconazole or itraconazole may be required in immunocompromised patients. Persistent candidiasis resistant to therapy or the presence of this lesion in older infants who are not receiving broad-spectrum antibiotics suggests an immune disorder, such as AIDS.

Ulcerating lesions of the oral cavity include infections (e.g., herpes simplex virus, herpangina, and hand-foot-mouth disease), bullous disease (e.g., dermatitis herpetiformis, pemphigus, erythema multiforme, and epidermolysis bullosa), and aphthous-like lesions (e.g., canker sore, SLE, inflammatory bowel disease, and Behçet, Reiter, and Sweet syndromes).

REFERENCES

Behrman RE, Kliegman RM, Jenson HB, editors: *Nelson textbook of pediatrics*, ed 16, Philadelphia, 2000, WB Saunders, Chapters 307–314.

Holt R, Roberts G, Scully C: Oral health disease, *BMJ* 320(7250): 1652–1655, 2000.

Roberts G, Scully C, Shotts R: Dental emergencies, *BMJ* 321(7260): 559–562, 2000.

Scully C, Shotts R: Mouth ulcers and other causes of orofacial soreness and pain, *BMJ* 321(7254):162–165, 2000.

Cleft Lip and Palate

Cleft Lip

Cleft lip, with or without cleft palate, occurs in 1:1000 births and is more common in males. Unilateral cleft lip is caused by failure of the ipsilateral maxillary prominence to fuse with the medial nasal prominence, a process that produces a persistent labial groove. Failure of bilateral fusion produces bilateral cleft lip. Multiple genetic and environmental factors appear to play a role in the etiology of cleft lip. The recurrence risk in siblings is 3–4%; the risk for a child of a mother with cleft lip is 14%. Associated malformations include hypertelorism and heart, foot, and hand anomalies. Most cleft lips are repaired shortly after birth or once the infant demonstrates steady weight gain. In general, feeding is not a problem with isolated cleft lip deformities.

Cleft Palate

Development of the palate proper, which includes the hard palate, soft palate, uvula, and maxillary teeth, is completed by the ninth week of gestation. This region develops from the maxillary bone plates that are initially separated by the tongue. As the tongue descends in the floor of the mouth and moves forward, the two plates fuse. Failure of the tongue to descend produces the midline palatal clefts. The incidence of cleft palate is 1:2500 births.

Genetic factors are important in the *etiology* of cleft palate. The recurrence risks are the same as those for cleft lip. Cleft palates are common in patients with chromosomal syndromes. Surgical repair usually is undertaken between 12 and 24 months of age. In the immediate newborn period, respiratory and feeding problems may occur. Repositioning the tongue and feeding the baby on his or her side should resolve respiratory difficulties. Most patients do well with a long, soft nipple that has a hole that is larger than usual. Patients with sucking or swallowing difficulty require gavage or gastrostomy feedings. The main problems after cleft palate repair are speech and tooth disturbances and recurrent otitis media. Although two thirds of these patients demonstrate acceptable speech, the voice may have a nasal quality or a muffled tone.

Pierre Robin syndrome is an identifiable sporadic or familial condition characterized by high arched or cleft palate, micrognathia, and glossoptosis. Glossoptosis is caused by the smallness of the mandible and results in airway obstruction and feeding problems during infancy. As the mandible grows, respiratory and feeding disturbances resolve.

Esophagus

Development

Tracheoesophageal Fistula. The esophagus develops as an elongation of the superior portion of the primitive foregut very early in the embryonic process. When the septation between the ventral tube and the dorsal esophagus develops abnormally, **esophageal atresia** results, a condition usually associated with tracheoesophageal fistula (TEF) (Fig. 11–3).

Forty percent of patients with TEF have associated anomalies; cardiovascular anomalies (e.g., patent ductus arteriosus, vascular ring, coarctation of the aorta, and ventricular septal defects) are the most frequent. The incidence of imperforate anus, intestinal malrotation, and duodenal anomalies is also increased. VATER syndrome describes the association between *v*ertebral defects (hemivertebra), *a*nal atresia, *T*EF, and *r*adial limb dysplasia.

Polyhydramnios and excessive salivation are early *clinical manifestations* of TEF, followed by choking, coughing, and cyanosis after the first feeding. The *diagnosis* may be made by passing a radiopaque catheter and observing coiling in the esophageal pouch on a chest roentgenogram or observing a pool of contrast dye collected in the atretic esophagus. Infants with TEF without esophageal atresia (H type) may have nonspecific symptoms for several months, but they usually exhibit chronic cough with feeding and recurrent pneumonia.

Primary surgical repair is the *treatment* of choice when the infant's condition is stable. Postoperative anastomotic leak occurs in 5–10% of these infants and

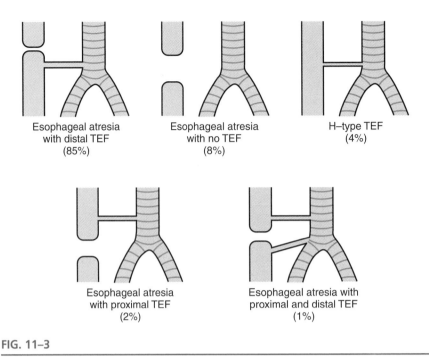

Esophageal atresia
with distal TEF
(85%)

Esophageal atresia
with no TEF
(8%)

H–type TEF
(4%)

Esophageal atresia
with proximal TEF
(2%)

Esophageal atresia with
proximal and distal TEF
(1%)

FIG. 11–3

Various types of trachoesophageal fistulas (TEF) with relative frequency (%).

necessitates parenteral or duodenal feedings. Strictures at the anastomotic site necessitate dilating bougienage. In patients with TEF, there is a persistent derangement of esophageal motility. Abnormal lower esophageal sphincter (LES) function leads to gastroesophageal reflux, which may lead to esophagitis, stricture formation, wheezing (associated tracheobronchomalacia), and recurrent pneumonia. The survival rate with this lesion in term infants without other anomalies or complications is greater than 90%.

Esophageal Disease. One *clinical manifestation* of esophageal diseases is a sensation that food is stuck in the esophagus (dysphagia), which may be the result of motility disorders or obstruction. Pain on swallowing (odynophagia), another manifestation, may be the result of high reflux of acidic stomach contents. *Regurgitation,* rather than forceful emesis, is the most common manifestation of esophageal disease in children.

Gastroesophageal Reflux (Chalasia)

Gastroesophageal reflux (GER) is a common problem during the first year of life. A number of factors alone or in combination may be responsible: reduced LES pressure, poor-amplitude esophageal contractions, inappropriate LES relaxation, large hiatal hernia, gastric distention, or delayed gastric emptying. Delayed gastric emptying may suggest distal intestinal obstruction.

In older patients GER is the result of neurally mediated episodes of transient relaxation of the lower esophageal sphincter and of the surrounding crural diaphragm. Gastric distention, pharyngeal stimulation, high-fat meals, and upright or right lateral decubitus postures stimulate transient relaxation of the sphincter. In infants, regurgitation, vomiting, and irritability are the most frequent complaints; if severe, these may result in failure to thrive, choking, aspiration pneumonia, wheezing, or esophagitis with bleeding and anemia. On rare occasions, especially in premature infants, GER may be associated with apnea or bradycardia. **Sandifer syndrome** is associated with GER, with the infant manifesting lateral head tilt and back arching resulting from esophagitis. GER in the older child or adolescent may present with regurgitation, retrosternal burning (esophagitis), dysphagia (stricture), or severe asthma.

The *diagnostic* evaluation of GER often includes a barium swallow with fluoroscopy, but at least 30% of infants have normal esophagram results because of the intermittent nature of GER. The study excludes anatomic causes such as a large hiatal hernia, antral web, duodenal web, pyloric stenosis, or annular pancreas. In patients with recurrent pneumonia, swallowing function should be assessed as part of the upper gastrointestinal series. The definitive test for establishing the presence of GER is the 24-hour esophageal pH probe study. This test measures the percent of time that the esophageal pH is less than 4.0, as well as duration of reflux episodes. Formula or food containing ^{99m}Tc can be used to assess gastric emptying. Esophageal manometry, which directly measures LES pressure, also may help determine the cause of GER. Finally, when blood loss, anemia, retrosternal burning, or dysphagia is present, endoscopy and esophageal biopsy detect the presence of peptic esophagitis, infection, or stricture formation.

Patients with mild to moderate reflux can be managed with medical *treatment,* which may involve feeding cereal-thickened formula and careful burping. Position therapy consisting of a 30° prone upright position after feeding has been recommended in the past but is now controversial because prone posturing increases the risk of **sudden infant death syndrome** (SIDS) (see Chapter 12). Most young infants outgrow reflux by 18 months of age. In cases complicated by esophagitis, H_2-blocking agents or omeprazole may help reduce acid reflux. Bethanechol, a parasympathomimetic drug, increases esophageal peristalsis and LES tone, whereas metoclopramide, a dopamine antagonist and cholinergic agonist, increases gastric emptying (reducing nausea) and LES tone. The use of both medications is limited by side effects, the most important being a dystonic type of extrapyramidal reaction with metoclopramide. Cisapride, a prokinetic agent, increases lower esophageal sphincter pressure, lower esophageal peristalsis, and gastrointestinal motility by enhancing the release of acetylcholine at the myenteric plexus. Cisapride is beneficial in the treatment of GER. However, bradycardia and nodal dysrhythmias have been described when this drug is given concomitantly with macrolide antibiotics or fluconazole-type medications. Cisapride is no longer available in the United States except through a limited access program from the manufacturer. Infants should receive medications other than theophylline for wheezing because this drug lowers LES pressure. Repeated episodes of pneumonia, failure to thrive, recurrent esophagitis with stricture, severe apnea, and failure to respond to 4–6 weeks of medical management are indications for surgery. The most common antireflux operation is the *Nissen fundoplication,* in which the fundus of the stomach is wrapped 270°–360° around the distal esophagus. Gastric distention after a feeding increases pressure around the wrap, preventing acid reflux.

Foreign Bodies

Coins, marbles, disc batteries, and pins are often swallowed and become lodged in the esophagus at one of three sites of narrowing: the cricopharyngeal muscle, the level of the aortic arch, and the LES at the diaphragm. Symptoms are cough, choking, stridor, odynophagia, retrosternal pain, and excessive salivation. However, many children are asymptomatic. If the foreign body is left in place, ulceration accompanied by bleeding and perforation may occur. Perforation with resultant mediastinitis is heralded by pain, fever, and shock. In experienced hands, smooth objects such as coins, buttons, or marbles may be removed by passing of a Foley catheter (8–12 Fr) into the distal esophagus, inflation of the balloon, and use of fluoroscopic guidance to slowly pull back until the object is obtained. Some physicians favor removing the objects endoscopically or pushing them into the stomach to prevent aspiration. For resistant smooth objects and sharp objects that might penetrate the mucosa, general anesthesia and removal through an esophagoscope or bronchoscope are required. Button batteries contain caustic substances that can cause burns or perforation if lodged in the esophagus; children with esophageal batteries should undergo endoscopic removal. Once batteries have reached the stomach, the vast majority are handled without endoscopic or surgical intervention if the child is asymptomatic.

Corrosive Burns

Corrosive burns are a common cause of esophageal stricture. The most common chemicals producing esophageal damage are the tasteless alkali caustics found in drain cleaners. Household bleaches and ammonia-containing cleaners are much weaker and produce less damage. Alkali agents cause full-thickness penetrating coagulation necrosis, whereas acid burns produce an eschar that coats the mucosa, preventing deeper penetration. Burns in the mouth suggest that the esophagus also is burned. However, the absence of burns on the oral mucosa does not preclude esophageal involvement.

Following a lye ingestion, vomiting should not be induced. Water or milk should be given to dilute the corrosive. Hospitalization, intravenous fluids, and endoscopy are recommended even if there is a doubt about the ingestion. The presence of a burn warrants follow-up with a barium swallow 3–4 weeks after the initial injury to check for stricture formation. Strictures must be treated with bougienage dilation. Steroids are of no benefit.

Esophageal injury may be caused by a variety of drugs, including tetracycline, doxycycline, slow-release potassium chloride, aspirin, and NSAIDs. Capsules are more likely to cause injury than tablets because of adherence of the gelatin to the esophageal wall.

REFERENCES

Behrman RE, Kliegman RM, Jenson HB, editors: *Nelson textbook of pediatrics*, ed 16, Philadelphia, 2000, WB Saunders, Chapters 319–327.

Glassman M, George D, Grill B: Gastroesophageal reflux in children: clinical manifestation, diagnosis, and therapy, *Gastroenterol Clin North Am* 24(1):71–98, 1995.

Lovejoy FJ: Corrosive injury of the esophagus in children: failure of corticosteroid treatment reemphasizes prevention, *N Engl J Med* 323(10):668–670, 1990.

Wilcox CM, Alexander LN, Contsonis GA, et al: Non-steroidal anti-inflammatory drugs are associated with both upper and lower gastrointestinal bleeding, *Dig Dis Sci* 42(5):990–997, 1997.

Stomach

Pyloric Stenosis

After inguinal hernia, hypertrophic pyloric stenosis is the most common condition requiring surgery during the first 2 months of life. The incidence is 1:150 in males and 1:750 in females. The condition occurs in 5% of siblings and 25% of offspring if the mother was affected. Pylorospasm secondary to reduced tissue nitric oxide levels (a mediator of relaxation) may lead to hypertrophic pyloric stenosis; exposure to erythromycin may also predispose the infant.

The typical *clinical manifestation* is nonbilious vomiting beginning between the second and fourth week of life. Emesis increases in frequency and eventually becomes projectile. Clear liquids or frequent feedings may lessen the severity of the vomiting temporarily, but weight loss becomes apparent as the obstruction becomes more complete. *Laboratory* abnormalities include hypokalemic metabolic alkalosis with paradoxic aciduria, and dehydration. Indirect hyperbilirubinemia also may be present.

The *diagnosis* may be made during or immediately after a feeding by palpating an olive-shaped mass to the right of the midline and witnessing marked peristaltic waves progressing from the left upper quadrant to the epigastrium. The diagnosis is confirmed by ultrasound demonstration of the thick hypoechoic ring in the region of the pylorus. Contrast roentgenographic studies are occasionally necessary.

Pyloromyotomy is the *treatment of choice* once dehydration and electrolyte abnormalities are corrected. Within 1–2 days, most infants can tolerate formula feeding.

Acid-Peptic Disease

The designation acid-peptic disease refers to a variety of disorders of the proximal gastrointestinal tract resulting from the action of gastric secretions. Included under acid-peptic disease are gastritis, gastric ulcer, duodenitis, and duodenal ulcer. Strictly speaking, gastritis and duodenitis refer to inflammatory processes in the mucosa, whereas ulcer implies a sharply circumscribed lesion. *Helicobacter pylori (H. pylori)* is the most common cause of duodenal ulcers in children. It can also cause a nodular chronic gastritis. The typical symptoms are epigastric pain, with or without vomiting, and hematemesis. Serologic tests reveal exposure to *H. pylori*, which is acquired in early childhood (perhaps from siblings) but may not coincide with active infection. The ^{13}C urea breath test can detect current *H. pylori* infection and can also be used to identify recurrence in previously treated patients.

Additional tests include a test for the presence of IgG to *H. pylori*, stool antigen detection, and direct tests of the gastric mucosa (culture, biopsy, urease assay, polymerase chain reaction). Most patients have chronic asymptomatic gastritis. Approximately 15% develop gastric or duodenal ulcers; a smaller subset are at risk for gastric adenocarcinoma in adulthood.

Gastritis. Acute gastritis may be localized or diffuse. Necrosis of the superficial mucosal cells and damage to the blood vessels of the lamina propria may cause extravasation of blood (acute hemorrhagic gastritis). If erosions form (erosive gastritis) and extend to the submucosa and muscularis, an ulcer may form. Acute gastritis may follow viral infections, the ingestion of aspirin or nonsteroidal antiinflammatory drugs, cancer chemotherapy, and the ingestion of corrosive agents, such as strong acids. Gastritis also may occur following severe trauma, major surgery, burns, or septic shock.

Hematemesis is the major *clinical manifestation*. Other symptoms include abdominal pain, nausea, and vomiting. Endoscopy is the *diagnostic* method of choice; barium studies usually are not helpful. *Treatment* is similar to that for peptic ulcer disease.

Gastric Ulcer–Duodenal Ulcer. Ulcers no longer are considered rare in children because increased rates have been detected by endoscopy. Primary ulcers occur in previously healthy individuals with no history of medication use. They are more duodenal than gastric and tend to have an insidious onset. Gastric ulcers occur in the antrum, whereas primary duodenal ulcers are found in the bulb and usually are solitary. The finding of multiple ulcers either in the third or fourth portion of the duodenum or in the jejunum should raise suspicion of the **Zollinger-Ellison syndrome.** Secondary ulcers are seen in association with underlying systemic disorders (e.g., sepsis, burns, and raised intracranial pressure) or occur as a consequence of drug therapy. They may hemorrhage or perforate without a history of pain, are more common in the stomach, and frequently are multiple.

The *etiology* of ulcer disease is closely related to

H. pylori infection, which is detected in 90% of children with duodenal ulcers and 60–80% of children with gastric ulcers. Drugs such as salicylates and nonsteroidal antiinflammatory drugs (NSAIDs), genetics, stress, alcohol abuse, and smoking may be contributing factors. In addition to gastritis, duodenitis, and ulcers, NSAIDs have been associated with inflammatory reactions, ulceration, and perforation in the small bowel (especially ileum) and colon.

Epigastric burning or gnawing abdominal pain relieved by food or antacids and recurring 1–3 hours after eating is the most common *clinical manifestation* of ulcer disease. Nocturnal pain that awakens a child from sleep is typical of peptic ulcer disease. This pain occurs in 30% of children with primary peptic ulcers but is rare in children with psychophysiologic disorders. Vomiting and nausea are other frequent symptoms. Discovery of an ulcer crater by an upper gastrointestinal roentgenographic series is sufficient to establish the *diagnosis* of peptic ulcer, but the ulcer may be undetected in up to 25% of cases. Endoscopy is often required to identify the lesion.

The goal of *treatment* is to reduce gastric acidity. Antacids are used but have a short duration of action. H_2-receptor–blocking agents, such as cimetidine and ranitidine, are effective for 6–12 hours and thus provide sustained relief. Drug interactions are common (see Appendix I). Anion pump inhibitors (omeprazole) effectively reduce acidity by preventing acid release from the parietal cell. Sucralfate has a local coating action and is not absorbed. Therapy should be continued for 6–8 weeks. Combination antimicrobial therapy (bismuth salts, amoxicillin or clarithromycin, and metronidazole) for 7–14 days is needed to eradicate *H. pylori*. Indications for surgical vagotomy with pyloroplasty include perforation, obstruction, uncontrolled bleeding, rebleeding in the hospital, and intractable pain.

Foreign Bodies and Bezoars

Most foreign bodies that reach the stomach pass through to the intestine and should be managed conservatively. Objects without sharp edges should be removed endoscopically if serial roentgenograms show no progress after 3–4 weeks. Objects with sharp points, such as safety pins, nails, or needles, and newer zinc-containing pennies, should be monitored roentgenographically and should be removed endoscopically if they do not move from the stomach after several days.

Three types of stomach bezoars occur in children: *trichobezoars* (composed primarily of hair), *phytobezoars* (composed of vegetable material), and *lactobezoars* (occurring from milk). Symptoms include abdominal pain, anorexia, vomiting, and weight loss. Children with trichobezoars may be retarded and may have alopecia. Lactobezoars, which may cause gastric outlet obstruction, usually are seen in neonates receiving high-caloric-density formulas by continuous drip.

REFERENCES

Behrman RE, Kliegman RM, Jenson HB, editors: *Nelson textbook of pediatrics,* ed 16, Philadelphia, 2000, WB Saunders, Chapters 329–334.

Goodman KJ, Correa P: Transmission of *Helicobacter pylori* among siblings, *Lancet* 355(9201):358–362, 2000.

Ni YH, Lin JT, Huang SF, et al: Accurate diagnosis of *Helicobacter pylori* infection by stool antigen test and six other currently available tests in children, *J Pediatr* 136(6):823–827, 2000.

Disorders of the Intestine and Colon
Congenital Malformations
Abdominal Wall Defects

OMPHALOCELE. When the abdominal viscera herniate through the umbilical and supraumbilical portions of the abdominal wall into a sac covered by peritoneum and amniotic membrane, the defect is called an omphalocele. The omphalocele results from a failure of migration of the bowel from the umbilical coelom, and its incidence is 1:6000 births. Large defects may contain the liver and spleen, as well as most of the gastrointestinal tract. The sac covering the defect is thin and may rupture in utero or during delivery. Ten percent of infants with omphaloceles are born prematurely; the incidence of associated malformations is high. Thirty-five percent have other gastrointestinal defects; 20% have congenital heart defects; and 10% have the **Beckwith-Wiedemann syndrome** (exophthalmos, macroglossia, gigantism, hyperinsulinemia, and hypoglycemia). Primary closure of small defects often is possible. Larger defects necessitate staged repairs that involve covering the sac with a prosthetic material. Survival rates vary and depend on the severity of associated anomalies.

UMBILICAL HERNIA. Umbilical hernia results from the incomplete closure of the fascia of the umbilical ring. Herniated omentum or bowel is covered by skin. Umbilical hernia is more common in premature infants and blacks; it is found in up to 40% of black children younger than 1 year of age. Fascial defects with a diameter of less than 0.5 cm heal spontaneously before the age of 2 years. With a ring between 0.5 and 1.5 cm, healing usually is complete by the age of 4 years. Surgical closure is advisable if the defect exceeds 1.5 cm at 2 years of age or if incarceration or symptoms such as abdominal pain have occurred. The practice of manually reducing the hernia and taping some device (such as a coin) over the ring does not accelerate the healing process.

Gastroschisis. Gastroschisis is the herniation, without a covering sac, of a variable length of small intestine, and occasionally of portions of the liver, through an abdominal wall defect located to the right of the umbilical cord. The eviscerated, uncovered mass of bowel is adherent, edematous, dark in color, and covered by a gelatinous matrix of greenish material. Sixty percent of these infants are born prematurely; 14% have associated jejunoileal malformations, usually stenosis or atresias; and 4% have nongastrointestinal malformations. There is little evidence to support the notion that genetic factors play a role, and the risk of congenital anomalies in future pregnancies is small. Gastroschisis is a surgical emergency, and a single-stage primary closure is possible in only 10% of patients. Postoperative hypomotility is common.

Intestinal Atresia

Duodenum. Duodenal obstruction may be complete (atresia), as the result of the failure of the lumen to recanalize, or partial (stenosis), as the result of a web, band, or annular pancreas. Intrinsic duodenal lesions are caused by a failure of the lumen to recanalize during the eighth to tenth week of gestation. Duodenal atresia is associated with other anomalies (in 30% of cases), prematurity (25%), and trisomy 21 (20%).

With complete obstruction, bile-stained vomiting begins within a few hours after the first feeding. In utero polyhydramnios may be present. Abdominal roentgenograms usually show gastric and duodenal gaseous distention, also called the "double bubble" sign, proximal to the atretic site. The presence of gas in the distal bowel suggests partial obstruction, and a contrast roentgenographic study should be performed.

Treatment is surgical. Mortality is related to prematurity and associated congenital anomalies.

Jejunum and Ileum. Jejunoileal atresias occur more frequently (2:1) than duodenal atresias and probably are caused by intrauterine infarction. Two thirds of cases involve complete obstruction of either the distal ileum or the proximal jejunum, with multiple atresias accounting for only 10–20%. **Meconium ileus** with atresia is the result of thick intestinal secretions from cystic fibrosis.

Polyhydramnios is present in 25% of cases. Vomiting of bile-stained material usually begins within 24–48 hours after birth. The abdomen becomes distended, and plain films show dilated loops of small bowel and an absence of colonic gas. Peritoneal calcifications signify **meconium peritonitis,** the result of intrauterine bowel perforation. A barium enema shows a narrowed unused colon **(microcolon).** Surgery is mandatory with meconium peritonitis and when meconium ileus does not respond to hypertonic Gastrografin enemas.

Malrotation and Volvulus. Anomalies of intestinal rotation result from failure of the midgut to appropriately reenter the fetal abdomen. The severity of the malrotation depends on the extent of the rotational arrest. Volvulus occurs when the small intestine is not fixed in the abdomen and becomes suspended by a stalk containing the superior mesenteric artery. Twisting of the bowel leads to arterial obstruction, midgut ischemia, and infarction. Further complicating the malrotation is the presence of peritoneal fixation bands (Ladd bands), which may result in partial duodenal obstruction.

Eighty percent of children with malrotation and volvulus have symptoms within the first month of life, although in some the condition is first diagnosed during adulthood. Abdominal distention and bilious vomiting suggest obstruction. If volvulus occurs, bloody stools may be followed by perforation and peritonitis. Children who are brought to the physician's attention after the neonatal period may manifest intermittent cramping, abdominal pain, vomiting, and diarrhea (often with hypoalbuminemia and secondary hypogammaglobulinemia) or constipation.

The *diagnosis* of malrotation can be made by demonstrating an abnormal position of the duodenum in an upper gastrointestinal roentgenographic series with small bowel follow-through. Midgut volvulus is a surgical emergency.

Meckel Diverticulum. Meckel diverticulum, the vestigial remnant of the omphalomesenteric duct, is the most frequent anomaly of the gastrointestinal tract. It is present in 2–3% of the population, is 2–3 cm long, and is located within 100 cm of the ileocecal valve along the antimesenteric border of the small intestine. The peak incidence is 2 years of age, and more males have the anomaly than do females (2:1). Heterotopic tissue occurs in 50% of cases; it is usually gastric and is 10 times more common in symptomatic cases because of acid secretion and ulceration.

The *clinical manifestations* include painless rectal bleeding (melena, in 84% of cases), intestinal obstruction (intussusception or volvulus, 10%), and painful diverticulitis mimicking appendicitis (6%). *Diagnosis* is discussed in the section on Gastrointestinal Hemorrhage. The definitive *treatment* is surgical resection.

Congenital Aganglionic Megacolon (Hirschsprung Disease). The failure of antegrade migration of neural crest–derived ganglion cells in the developing colon results in an aganglionic segment of variable length. This disorder is three times more common among males. It may be associated with syndromes such as trisomy 21 or Waardenburg, and it accounts for 20% of cases of neonatal intestinal obstruction. In 75% of cases, the aganglionic segment is limited to the rectosigmoid colon; 15% extend beyond the splenic flexure. **Neuronal intestinal dysplasia** (hyperganglionosis) demonstrates hyperplasia of the intramural plexus and clinically resembles Hirschsprung disease.

The *diagnosis* should be suspected in any infant who fails to pass meconium within the first 24 hours or who requires repeated rectal stimulation to induce bowel movements. Failure to thrive and abdominal distention may occur. Fever and diarrhea are ominous signs that suggest the presence of coexisting enterocolitis. In some cases, particularly those with short segment (<5 cm) involvement, the diagnosis goes undetected into childhood. These children often are poorly nourished and suffer from massive abdominal distention and anemia. The palpable presence of stool throughout the abdomen and an empty rectum on digital examination are most suggestive of the disease (Table 11–9).

The *treatment* of Hirschsprung disease is surgical and is usually performed in two stages. The first stage involves the creation of a colostomy through a section of bowel containing ganglion cells, thus permitting decompression of the dilated colon. In the second stage the aganglionic segment is removed by pulling the ganglionic segment through the rectum. This procedure is often postponed until the infant is 12–14 months old; the procedure is delayed for 3–6 months when the disease has been diagnosed in an older child. The mortality rate is low in the absence of enterocolitis, and the major complications include anal stenosis (in 5–10% of cases) and incontinence (1–3%).

Anorectal Malformation and Imperforate Anus. Anorectal anomalies arise either because of a failure of the urorectal septum to divide the cloaca completely or because of incomplete convergence of the anal tubercles around the termination of the hindgut. The incidence is 1:5000, and 50% of cases are associated with vertebral or genitourinary malformations.

The recognition of anorectal malformations depends on careful inspection of the perianal area at birth. Fig. 11–4 illustrates the various types of anomalies. Fistulization between the rectum and surrounding structures may occur. Rectourethral fistulas in males and rectovaginal fistulas in females are associated with "high" lesions, whereas fistulas through to the perineum are associated with "low" lesions. Contrast roentgenograms of a fistula or tube instillation of contrast into the rectum should allow delineation of the anatomy. Anal stenosis may be treated with simple dilation. Other lesions necessitate surgery. Bowel control is achieved in 90% of children with low lesions but in only 50% of those with high lesions.

Inguinal Hernia. During fetal development, a peritoneal sac precedes the testicle as it descends from the genital ridge into the scrotum. The lower portion of this sac (the processus vaginalis) envelops the testes and forms the tunica vaginalis, and the remainder of the sac atrophies. In 50% of patients, the processus vaginalis remains patent. If abdominal contents become trapped in the processus vaginalis, an **indirect hernia** exists. Indirect inguinal hernias are more common in males (4:1), in premature infants, and following increased intraabdominal pressure (ascites). The hernia becomes manifest as a painless swelling in the inguinal area. Contents of the hernia sac usually can be reduced with gentle pressure. When the contents of the sac cannot be reduced, the hernia is said to be **incarcerated,** necessitating immediate surgery to avoid bowel necrosis and testicular infarction. Repair of an asymptomatic, reducible hernia should be carried out as soon as possible unless other conditions preclude surgery.

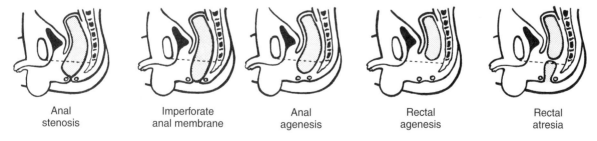

Anal stenosis   Imperforate anal membrane   Anal agenesis   Rectal agenesis   Rectal atresia

FIG. 11–4

Various types of anorectal anomalies. The stippled line is a projection of the puborectalis sling. On a roentgenogram, it is drawn from the lower part of the pubis to the sacrococcygeal junction. (Modified from Silverman A, Roy CE, editors: *Pediatric clinical gastroenterology,* St. Louis, 1983, Mosby.)

REFERENCES

Behrman RE, Kliegman RM, Jenson HB, editors: *Nelson textbook of pediatrics*, ed 16, Philadelphia, 2000, WB Saunders, Chapters 330–336.

Ford EG, Senac MO, Srikanth MS, et al: Malrotation of the intestine in children, *Ann Surg* 215(2):172–178, 1992.

Martin LW, Torres AM: Hirschsprung's disease, *Surg Clin North Am* 65(5):1171–1180, 1985.

St-Vil D, Brandt ML, Panic S, et al: Meckel's diverticulum in children: a 20-year review, *J Pediatr Surg* 26(11):1289–1292, 1991.

Disaccharidase Deficiencies

Primary congenital disaccharidase deficiencies are rare. Sucrase-isomaltase deficiency is the most common form occurring in infancy and is inherited as an autosomal recessive trait. Osmotic diarrhea begins with the introduction of sucrose-containing foods or drinks and may be associated with vomiting, dehydration, abdominal cramping, bloating, and growth failure. The *diagnosis* may be confirmed by breath hydrogen testing and quantitative determination of sucrase-isomaltase activity in a jejunal mucosal biopsy. The *treatment* consists of excluding from the diet any foods that contain more than 2% sucrose.

Congenital **lactase deficiency** is rare, but late-onset lactase deficiency is common. This inherited form has a striking ethnic variation; it is present in 5–10% of whites, in contrast to 70% of blacks. The absence of brush border lactase activity causes lactose malabsorption and osmotic diarrhea within hours of lactose ingestion. Symptoms begin between 8 and 15 years of age and include crampy abdominal pain, bloating, and acidic diarrhea (containing reducing substances). The *diagnosis* may be based on breath hydrogen or less often on the results of lactose tolerance testing. Because the deficiency is relative rather than absolute, some lactose restriction from the diet usually is sufficient to prevent symptoms. Transient secondary lactase deficiency often occurs as a consequence of damage to the small intestinal mucosa following severe viral gastroenteritis. Mucosal recovery occurs in 4–6 weeks. *Treatment* consists of a formula that does not contain lactose. For older children, lactase-hydrolyzed milk or lactase-containing tablets or capsules can be ingested concurrently with dairy products to reduce symptoms.

Protein Intolerance and Sensitivity Syndromes: Cow's Milk and Soy Milk

The proteins in cow's milk and soy milk may cause an immune-mediated inflammatory injury of the small bowel, with villous atrophy. The proteins may also cause an injury of the large bowel, producing colitis (inflammation with or without ulceration). The precise immune mechanisms are undetermined. Systemic signs, such as anaphylaxis, wheezing, rhinitis, pulmonary hemosiderosis, and urticaria, are less common and may be mediated by IgE antibody. Approximately 6–8% of all infants are intolerant to cow's milk proteins, and 20–30% of these also are intolerant to soy protein. Milk protein intolerance syndrome usually has an onset within the first month of life. Premature infants may be at increased risk. When the syndrome causes **enterocolitis,** this leads to vomiting, diarrhea, enteric blood loss, and anemia. Rectal biopsy findings include inflammation, eosinophilic infiltration of the lamina propria and mucosa, ulceration, and crypt abscesses. Another form of this syndrome, **enteropathy,** begins by 2–3 months of age, and clinical manifestations include prolonged diarrhea, protein-losing enteropathy (edema, hypoproteinemia), malabsorption, and failure to thrive. Small intestinal villous atrophy, at times associated with inflammatory colitis, is present.

The *diagnosis* of cow's or soy milk protein intolerance is usually made by history but may require laboratory tests and mucosal biopsy if the diagnosis is in doubt. Improvement with protein hydrolyzed formula and recurrence of symptoms when milk proteins are reintroduced confirm the diagnosis. Most infants eventually tolerate bovine or soy proteins by 2–3 years of age. Infants with severe reactions (e.g., anaphylaxis) should not undergo challenge. Breast-fed infants may manifest similar symptoms because of the presence of dietary bovine proteins in human breast milk. *Treatment* of the breast-fed infant requires elimination of dairy products from the mother's diet and supplementation of the mother's diet with calcium and vitamin D.

Eosinophilic gastroenteropathy is not usually associated with cow's milk sensitivity. It is characterized by eosinophilic infiltration of the intestinal mucosa, muscularis, or serosal layers; elevated IgE levels; and peripheral eosinophilia. Protein-losing enteropathy, pyloric obstruction (muscular involvement), gastrointestinal bleeding with anemia (mucosal involvement), and ascites (serosal involvement) also may be present. The cause is unknown, but it is a chronic condition that shows a variable response to corticosteroids or oral disodium cromolyn. The *differential diagnosis* includes intestinal parasite infestation. Elemental formulas may be necessary in some patients.

Gluten-Sensitive Enteropathy (Celiac Disease)

Celiac disease, an immunologically mediated intolerance to gluten-containing grains (wheat, rye, barley, and possibly oats), results in small intestinal villous atrophy with lymphocytic and plasma cell infiltration. The incidence in the United States is 1:2000 births. A genetic predisposition is involved in the disease: 98% of affected individuals have human leukocyte antigen (HLA)-DQW2, and 80% are HLA-

B8 positive. The prevalence of celiac disease is increased in patients with IgA deficiency, diabetes mellitus, thyroiditis, and Down syndrome. Children with these conditions should be screened for celiac disease by serologic assays.

Clinical manifestations usually begin between 6 and 18 months and include apathy, irritability, pain, vomiting, chronic diarrhea, steatorrhea, abdominal distention, and failure to thrive. Some infants are asymptomatic. A wasted skeletal muscle mass, finger clubbing, and peripheral edema also may occur. Older children may exhibit unexplained growth failure or anemia or may be asymptomatic.

The *diagnosis* is confirmed by results of two biopsies: an initial, abnormal biopsy specimen of the small bowel showing partial or subtotal villous atrophy, and a second specimen, taken after administration of a gluten-free diet, showing improvement. Mild or early cases may show only an increase in intraepithelial lymphocytes, without villous atrophy. When the diagnosis is in doubt, especially in infants younger than 1 year of age, a subsequent biopsy showing reappearance of disease after gluten challenge may be necessary.

The most accurate screening tests are commercial assays of endomysial (IgA and IgG) and transglutaminase antibodies. Since the IgA assay is the test of choice and 10% of affected patients are IgA deficient, the level of total IgA should also be obtained. Confirmation of the diagnosis requires a small bowel biopsy (as already described) that shows increased numbers of intraepithelial lymphocytes and variable degrees of villous atrophy. *Treatment* consists of permanent elimination of gluten-containing foods. Older patients may not have signs when rechallenged with cereals; mucosal atrophy does develop, however, which may place the patients at increased risk for intestinal lymphoma.

Inflammatory Bowel Disease

Inflammatory bowel disease (IBD) includes **ulcerative colitis, Crohn disease,** and **indeterminate colitis.** These conditions result from a genetic predisposition, with associated alterations in immunoregulatory action of the gut. They are more common among whites, Jews, and family members and occur equally in males and females. Most pediatric patients are adolescents, but both diseases have been reported in infancy. Crohn disease may involve any part of the gastrointestinal tract (mouth to anus), whereas ulcerative colitis produces only colonic disease (Table 11–14). Both may have common extraintestinal manifestations, including arthralgias, mono-, pauci- or polyarticular arthritis; primary sclerosing cholangitis (ulcerative colitis primarily); chronic active hepatitis; sacroiliitis; pyoderma gangrenosum; erythema nodosum; nephro-

lithiasis; and uveitis or episcleritis. The pathology of Crohn disease involves transmural inflammation in a discontinuous pattern (skipped lesions); granulomas are present in some specimens. Ulcerative colitis produces superficial, diffuse colonic acute and chronic inflammation, ulceration, and crypt abscesses. It involves the rectum in 95% of patients, with or without contiguous extension higher in the colon.

Clinical Manifestations. Most children with ulcerative colitis exhibit blood in the stool (100%), abdominal pain (95%), and tenesmus (75%) (Table 11–14). Ninety percent of patients exhibit mild (less than four stools per day, with no fever, anemia, or hypoalbuminemia) to moderate (more than six stools a day, with fever, anemia, and hypoalbuminemia) disease. Severe disease may be a fulminant illness accompanied by high fever, abdominal tenderness, distention, tachycardia, leukocytosis, hemorrhage,

TABLE 11–14
Comparison of Crohn Disease and Ulcerative Colitis

Feature	Crohn Disease	Ulcerative Colitis
Malaise, fever, weight loss	Common	Common
Rectal bleeding	Sometimes	Usual
Abdominal mass	Common	Rare
Abdominal pain	Common	Common
Perianal disease	Common	Rare
Ileal involvement	Common	None (backwash ileitis)
Strictures	Common	Unusual
Fistula	Common	Very rare
Skip lesions	Common	Not present
Transmural involvement	Usual	Not present
Crypt abscesses	Variable	Usual
Intestinal granulomas	Common	Rarely present
Risk of cancer*	Increased	Greatly increased
Erythema nodosum	Common	Less common
Mouth ulceration	Common	Rare
Osteopenia at onset	Yes	No
Autoimmune hepatitis	Rare	Yes
Sclerosing cholangitis	Rare	Yes

*Colonic cancer, cholangiocarcinoma.

more than 10 stools a day, and severe anemia. Toxic megacolon and subsequent intestinal perforation are rare complications. Peripheral arthritis, erythema nodosum, uveitis, and thromboembolism actively are related to the activity of the colitis; sclerosing cholangitis, sacroiliitis, and pyoderma gangrenosum are not related to colitis activity.

The onset of Crohn disease often is subtle. Cramping abdominal pain, fever of unknown origin, weight loss, and diarrhea are common manifestations. Arthritis may precede gastrointestinal or other extraintestinal manifestations. Perianal disease may produce skin tags, fissures, fistulas, or abscesses. Severe disease is characterized by complications (e.g., fever, arthritis, iritis-uveitis, erythema nodosum, abscesses, or fistulas), an abdominal mass, abdominal pain, severe weight loss, anemia, and hypoalbuminemia.

Diagnosis. The differential diagnosis involves chronic bacterial or parasitic causes of diarrhea such as *Clostridium difficile, Campylobacter jejuni, Yersinia enterocolitica*, amebiasis, and giardiasis. Because ulcerative colitis involves the rectum in 95% of patients, proctosigmoidoscopy or colonoscopy and biopsy are indicated. Visualization of the mucosa in ulcerative colitis reveals diffuse superficial ulceration and easy bleeding. In Crohn disease direct visualization and biopsy of the affected area are not always possible.

Roentgenographic examination with a double (air)-contrast barium enema demonstrates diffuse colonic lesions and loss of haustration in ulcerative colitis. This study should not take the place of endoscopic evaluation (the initial diagnostic procedure of choice) or be performed in patients with severely active disease, to prevent precipitation of toxic megacolon. In Crohn disease radiologic studies often reveal focal small bowel (especially ileal) lesions or colonic involvement with skipped lesions, rectal sparing, segmental narrowing (string sign), and longitudinal ulcers.

Treatment. General management includes drug therapy combined with nutritional support (enteral or parenteral); dietary modifications as needed for control of diarrhea, narrowing due to stenotic segments, or lactose intolerance; and transfusion for anemia.

Therapy for ulcerative colitis depends on the severity of the illness. Mild disease may be treated with oral sulfasalazine, which is poorly absorbed and is split by colonic bacteria into sulfapyridine and the active 5-aminosalicylate. Sulfasalazine is active against lipoxygenase and may reduce the elevated mucosal prostaglandin levels. Sulfapyridine may cause headache, hemolytic anemia, and gastrointestinal discomfort. Topical 5-aminosalicylate or hydrocortisone enemas also may be used in mild left-sided disease. These medications hasten healing but may be refused by children and adolescents. Oral mesalamine (5-aminosalicylate) should be tried in patients who do not tolerate sulfasalazine. Moderate ulcerative colitis is managed with the addition of 1–2 mg/kg/day of prednisone (maximum 60 mg/day) to the above regimen. Sulfasalazine helps maintain remission. Patients with severe disease require intravenous alimentation; systemic corticosteroids; and close monitoring for hypokalemia, acidosis, anemia, and intestinal dilatation or perforation. Cyclosporine or tacrolimus may be efficacious in severe refractory disease. Emergency colectomy is indicated for refractory toxic megacolon or severe, persistent hemorrhage. Colectomy also is indicated for chronic refractory disease, persistent growth failure, and the presence of any dysplasia on biopsy. The risk of colon carcinoma is increased in patients with extensive disease of greater than 10 years' duration. Colonoscopic surveillance is mandatory to determine the presence of dysplasia.

Prednisone is the most effective drug for Crohn disease of the small bowel, although mesalamine is often used concurrently. Colonic involvement also may be ameliorated by the addition of sulfasalazine, whereas perianal disease and fistula formation may respond to metronidazole. Azathioprine and 6-mercaptopurine (6-MP) usually permit reduction of corticosteroid dose in children who are dependent on or whose condition is refractory to prednisone. Methotrexate may induce remission and reduce corticosteroid requirement in children who are intolerant or refractory to azathioprine or 6-MP. Other therapies include antibodies to tumor necrosis factor-α (infliximab) for Crohn disease; this therapy heals fistulas and is effective in moderate to severe disease. Concomitant azathioprine, 6-MP, or methotrexate prolongs the remission. Surgery eventually is needed in approximately 25% of children with ulcerative colitis and 70% of children with Crohn disease because of failure of medical management, intestinal fistula or obstruction, and growth failure.

Polyps

Most polyps in children are of the juvenile type, although some may occur in association with familial syndromes. Polyps associated with familial syndromes include **Peutz-Jeghers syndrome,** which has mucocutaneous pigmentation and is autosomal dominant; **Gardner syndrome,** which has soft tissue or bone tumors and rectal cancer and is autosomal dominant; and **familial polyposis coli,** which has carcinoma and is autosomal dominant. Juvenile polyps are usually solitary, pedunculated hamartomas, which have a peak incidence between 3 and 5 years. Seventy percent occur in the rectum or sigmoid colon, and the majority are solitary. The usual presenting symptom is painless rectal bleeding. If the polyp is in the rectum, the *diagnosis* may be based on digital examination; otherwise, the diagnosis depends on a carefully performed air-contrast enema or colonoscopy. Colonoscopy affords the opportunity for removal of the polyp at the time of the procedure.

Juvenile polyposis coli, defined by >10 polyps or a positive family history, is associated with rectal bleeding, iron deficiency, and adenomatous changes with an increased risk for carcinoma. Solitary hamartomatous polyps are not premalignant or malignant lesions.

Appendicitis

Appendicitis is the most common cause of an acute abdomen in older children and adolescents (4:1000 children <16 years of age). The cause may be obstruction of the appendiceal lumen by a fecalith or by inflammatory edema produced by lymphatic hyperplasia from a nonspecific infection. Meconium ileus equivalent or ileus-producing drugs (e.g., vincristine) are rarer causes of obstruction.

Clinical manifestations include a history of 1–2 days of periumbilical dull or crampy pain, *followed by* anorexia and nausea, with or without vomiting. The pain remains constant but then localizes in the right lower quadrant (McBurney point) as a result of irritation of the parietal peritoneum. With rupture the pain initially may subside but then is followed by signs of peritonitis, such as high fever, abdominal wall muscle rigidity resulting from voluntary guarding, and involuntary spasm. Unfortunately, atypical presentations are common among children or patients with retrocecal (less peritoneal irritation and a positive psoas sign) or pelvic (less peritoneal irritation and tender rectal examination) appendices. Fever is often 38°–38.5°C (100°–102° F), and the peripheral white blood cell count usually is normal unless perforation has occurred or peritonitis is present. Urinalysis occasionally may reveal proteinuria and mild pyuria. Abdominal *roentgenograms* may demonstrate a fecalith or acute scoliosis as a result of psoas muscle spasm. Ultrasonography reveals a noncompressible, enlarged appendix surrounded by fluid (donut or target sign) but also excludes ovarian or pelvic disease, mesenteric adenitis, and calculi. The CT scan may reveal an appendicolith, a mass or fluid collection, extraluminal gas, a cross sectional area greater than 6 mm, and incomplete filling by gas or contrast media.

The *differential diagnosis* includes those age-related and sex-related diseases listed in Table 11–1. **Mesenteric adenitis** caused by *Yersinia* species also may mimic appendicitis, whereas **primary peritonitis** may be confused with a ruptured appendix. Primary peritonitis is noted in patients with ascites or nephrotic syndrome; rarely, patients have no underlying illness, and the peritonitis is caused by *Streptococcus pneumoniae* or *E. coli.*

Treatment is surgical excision of the acutely inflamed appendix. Peritoneal drainage and broad-spectrum antibiotics effective against anaerobic and gram-negative enteric organisms are added if perforation is present.

Intussusception

Intussusception occurs when one segment of bowel telescopes into a distal segment. Idiopathic intussusception usually occurs between 6 and 18 months of age, with only 10% of cases occurring after 3 years of age. The cause is unknown, but lymphoid hyperplasia (Peyer patches) may form a lead point of the proximal intussusception segment. A lead point is seen in 5% of cases. In older children Meckel diverticulum, lymphosarcoma, and polyps may form lead points. Intussusception also is seen in cystic fibrosis and Henoch-Schönlein purpura. The ileocolic form is the most frequent, followed by ileoileal and colocolic. Intussusception causes an acute onset of colicky, intermittent abdominal pain. During the episodes of pain, the infant will cry, draw up the knees, and vomit. Lethargy and fever are late findings, as is the passage of currant jelly–colored stools. On physical examination, a sausage-shaped mass may be found in the upper abdomen. The KUB x-ray examination may reveal a mass, obstruction, or visualization of the actual intussusception. Barium enema not only confirms the diagnosis, but with appropriate hydrostatic pressure, may also reduce the intussusception in 75% of patients. Surgical reduction should be performed if there are clinical signs of perforation, peritonitis, or shock; if medical reduction is unsuccessful; or if there is a high likelihood of finding a pathologic lead point.

REFERENCES

Behrman RE, Kliegman RM, Jenson HB, editors: *Nelson textbook of pediatrics,* ed 16, Philadelphia, 2000, WB Saunders, Chapters 333, 337, 343.

Bell S, Kamm MA: Antibiotics to tumour necrosis factor K as treatment for Crohn's disease, *Lancet* 355(9207):858–860, 2000.

Ghosh S, Shand A, Ferguson A: Ulcerative colitis, *BMJ* 320(7242):1119–1123, 2000.

Hoffenberg EJ, Haas J, Drescher A, et al: A trial of oats in children with newly diagnosed celiac disease, *J Pediatr* 137(3):361–366, 2000.

Hyams JS: Crohn's disease in children, *Pediatr Clin North Am* 43(1):255–277, 1996.

Kerner JA: Formula allergy and intolerance, *Gastroenterol Clin North Am* 24(1):1–25, 1995.

Kirschner BS: Ulcerative colitis in children, *Pediatr Clin North Am* 43(1):235–254, 1996.

Kirschner BS: Safety of azathioprine and 6-mercaptopurine in pediatric patients with inflammatory bowel disease, *Gastroenterology* 115(4):815–821, 1998.

Kuppermann N, O'Dea T, Pinckney L, et al: Predictors of intussusception in young children, *Arch Pediatr Adolesc Med* 154(3):
250–255, 2000.

Picarelli A, Sabbatella L, Di Tola M, et al: Celiac disease diagnosis
in misdiagnosed children, *Pediatr Res* 48(5):590–592, 2000.

Sivit CJ, Applegate KE, Stallion A, et al: Imaging evaluation of
suspected appendicitis in a pediatric population: effectiveness
of sonography versus CT, *AJR* 175(4):977–980, 2000.

Wagner J, McKinney P, Carpenter J: Does this patient have appendicitis? *JAMA* 276(19):1589–1594, 1996.

Liver

Manifestations of hepatic disease may include abnormalities of any or all of the specific liver functions.
The most common manifestations are jaundice (Fig.
11–2), hepatomegaly, metabolic disturbances (e.g.,
hypoglycemia, hyperammonemia, encephalopathy,
metabolic acidosis, and hyperaminoacidemia), portal hypertension (cirrhosis, ascites, varices), and hemorrhage (varices, hypoprothrombinemia).

Laboratory tests of hepatic function (Table 11–15)
can be divided into two categories: those that suggest the presence of hepatobiliary disease and those
that assess "liver function." Most liver function tests
do not quantitatively measure function but instead
provide clinical information about the course or
severity of disease. In interpreting these tests, the
physician should remember that the liver has a large
reserve capacity, with the capability for regeneration.

Acute Viral Hepatitis

A number of agents cause acute hepatic injury (Table
11–16). Characteristics of hepatitis viruses are listed
in Table 11–17. The delta agent produces disease
only in patients with hepatitis B infection. Community or parenteral viral hepatitis not caused by the
agents listed in Tables 11–16 and 11–17 should be
considered non-A to non-G hepatitis.

The *clinical course* for the hepatitis A virus (HAV),
hepatitis B virus (HBV), and hepatitis C virus (HCV)
is shown in Figure 11–5. A prodromal phase, which
lasts approximately 1 week, is characterized by
headaches, anorexia, malaise, nausea, and vomiting
and usually precedes the onset of clinically detectable disease. Infants with HBV may have immune complexes accompanied by urticaria and
arthritis prior to the onset of icterus. Jaundice and a
large, tender liver are the most common physical

TABLE 11–15
Liver Evaluation Tests

Test	Mechanism	Significance
Hepatic Function		
Albumin	Decreased synthesis	Decreased hepatic synthesis; increased loss by protein-losing enteropathy or nephrotic syndrome; increased volume of distribution (edema, ascites)
Prothrombin time	Decreased synthesis of factors II, VII, IX, and X	Hepatic dysfunction: unresponsive to vitamin K; malabsorption: responsive to vitamin K
Ammonia	Decreased ureagenesis; increased portosystemic shunting; increased ammonia load (GI bleeding)	Increased ammonia associated with hepatic encephalopathy; inborn errors of metabolism
Indocyanine green clearance	Low dose: indicator of liver blood flow; high dose: indicator of hepatic processing	Particularly sensitive for detecting cirrhosis
Galactose elimination test	Hepatic uptake and metabolism	Reflective of functional liver cell mass; useful for following declining hepatic function
Aminopyrine breath test	Hepatic uptake; demethylation by cytochrome P_{450}; measurement of breath excretion of radiolabel from methyl group	Index of hepatic excretion; useful for detection of cirrhosis; a prognostic indicator in patients with cirrhosis
Lidocaine clearance test	Measurement of appearance of MEGX, a major hepatic metabolite	Useful to evaluate liver dysfunction, especially in liver transplantation (before and after)

TABLE 11–15
Liver Evaluation Tests—cont'd

Test	Mechanism	Significance
Cellular Injury		
Aspartate aminotransferase (AST/SGOT)	Released from damaged hepatocytes	Also in heart, skeletal muscle, kidney, pancreas, RBCs, and brain
Alanine aminotransferase (ALT/SGPT)	Released from damaged hepatocytes	More specific for liver injury than AST
Cholestasis		
Alkaline phosphatase	Greatest elevation usually in extrahepatic obstruction	Also in bone, intestine, placenta, kidney—may need to be fractionated for liver-specific isozyme
γ-Glutamyl transpeptidase (GGTP)	Sensitive, but not specific, index of biliary tract disease	Inducible by ethanol, phenobarbital, and other drugs; elevated in diabetes, myocardial infarction, renal failure, and other conditions
5'-Nucleotidase	More specific for liver disease than alkaline phosphatase or GGTP	Biliary disease
Direct bilirubin	Decreased hepatic excretion in cholestasis	May also be elevated with hepatocellular injury; may be normal to slightly elevated with cholestasis (primary biliary cirrhosis, chronic cholestatic syndromes)
Bile acids	Decreased extraction from portal blood; decreased hepatic excretion in cholestasis	Do not discriminate hepatocellular from obstructive cholestasis
Other		
α-Fetoprotein	Derepressed fetal gene	Hepatic tumor
Anti–smooth muscle, antinuclear, anti–liver-kidney microsomal autoantibodies	Autoimmunity	Autoimmune chronic active hepatitis
Imaging		
Ultrasonography	Gross anomalies and blood flow using Doppler study	For gallstones, larger masses; can assess hepatic vein or artery, and portal vein thrombosis/obstruction
Computed tomography (CT scan)	Greater resolution than with ultrasound	Particularly useful for detecting abscesses and tumors
Angiography	Definition of hepatic vessels by contrast injection	Particularly useful for better definition of hepatic vein/portal vein thrombosis/obstruction; defining blood supply to tumors
Cholangiography	Definition of biliary tree by contrast injection	Defining biliary tract anatomy for source/site of obstruction
^{99m}Tc-sulfur colloid scan	Kupffer cell uptake	Large focal lesions
^{99m}Tc-DISIDA scan	Hepatic uptake and biliary excretion	Discriminating hepatocellular from obstructive cholestasis; confirming presence of choledochal cyst
Magnetic resonance imaging (MRI)	Greater resolution than CT	Evaluation of focal lesions (especially hemangiomas) and detecting excess hepatic iron; new applications in hepatic angiography and cholangiography
Liver Biopsy		
Percutaneous, transjugular, laparoscopic, surgical	Obtaining liver tissue for histology, electron microscopy, immunostaining, measurement of copper or iron, and specific enzyme assays	May provide specific diagnosis and prognosis (degree of necrosis/fibrosis) for liver diseases

TABLE 11–16
Causes of Acute Liver Disease in Childhood

Viral	**Toxic—cont'd**
Hepatitis A, B, C, E, G	Chlorpromazine
Hepatitis D (with B)	Allopurinol
Epstein-Barr virus	Acetaminophen
Cytomegalovirus	Salicylates
Enterovirus	Hydralazine
Human parvovirus B19	Halothane
Herpes simplex 1, 2, 6, 7	"Ecstasy" drug use
Adenovirus	Iron
Lassa fever virus	Erythromycin estolate
Dengue	Alcohol
Yellow fever	Mushroom poisoning (*Amanita phalloides*)
Ebola virus	Valproic acid
Measles	Phenytoin
Varicella-zoster virus	Carbamazepine
Undefined paramyxovirus (syncytial giant cells)	Methotrexate
	6-Mercaptopurine
Bacterial	Herbal teas
Syphilis	
Leptospirosis	
Bacterial sepsis	**Other**
Coxiella burnetii	Wilson disease
Miliary tuberculosis	Inborn errors of metabolism (e.g., galactosemia,
Gonococcus (perihepatitis)	tyrosinemia)
Chlamydia trachomatis (perihepatitis)	Chronic active hepatitis
	Venoocclusive disease
	Tumor
Toxic	Infarction
Isoniazid	Shock
Oral contraceptives	Heart failure
Androgens	Anoxia
Carbon tetrachloride	

From Behrman RE, editor: *Nelson textbook of pediatrics*, ed 14, Philadelphia, 1992, WB Saunders, p 1018.

findings. However, infants and young children with HAV, HBV, or HCV may not become icteric and may be mistakenly diagnosed as having the flu. Liver enzymes may increase 15- to 20-fold. Resolution of the hyperbilirubinemia and normalization of the transaminases may take 6–8 weeks. Whereas chronic hepatitis develops in approximately 10% of patients with acute HBV hepatitis, chronic liver disease or asymptomatic viremia develops in 80% or more of HCV-infected individuals (from blood transfusions) (Fig. 11–5). Note the fluctuating transaminase levels characteristic of chronic HCV hepatitis.

A number of *serologic markers* are available to detect the presence of hepatitis A, B, or C. Their appearance and time course are shown in Fig. 11–5. The pres-

ence of high-titer, IgM-specific antibody to HAV and low or absent IgG antibody titer to the same virus is presumptive evidence of hepatitis A infection. The presence of hepatitis B virus surface antigen (HB$_s$Ag) signifies infection with HBV. Antigenemia may appear early in the illness and may be transient. The presence of HB$_s$Ag also is diagnostic of the carrier state, and maternal HB$_s$Ag status always should be determined when hepatitis B infection is diagnosed in infants less than 1 year of age. Hepatitis B "e" antigen (HB$_e$Ag) appears in the serum with HB$_s$Ag. The continued presence of HB$_s$Ag and HB$_e$Ag in the absence of antibody to e antigen (anti-HB$_e$) is predictive of a high risk of transmission and is associated with ongoing viral replication. Clearance of HB$_s$Ag from

TABLE 11-17
Characteristics of the Agents Causing Acute Viral Hepatitis

	Hepatitis A Virus (HAV) (Enterovirus 72)	Hepatitis B* Virus (HBV)	Hepatitis C† Virus (HCV) (Formerly Posttransfusion Non-A, Non-B Virus)	Hepatitis D Virus (HDV)	Hepatitis E Virus (HEV) (Formerly Enteral, Non-A, Non-B Virus)	Hepatitis F Virus (HFV)	Hepatitis G Virus (HGV)/(HGBV-C)
Agent	27-nm RNA virus	42-nm DNA virus	30–60-nm RNA virus; similar to flaviviruses	36-nm circular RNA hybrid particle with HBsAg coat	27–34-nm RNA virus; similar to Norwalk-type viruses	27–37-nm DNA virus-like particles	RNA virus; similar to flaviviruses, 25% homology with HCV
Transmission	Fecal-oral, food-water, rarely parenteral	Transfusion, sexual, inoculation, vertical	Parenteral, transfusion, vertical (sexual?)	Similar to HBV	Enteral—endemic and epidemic	Enteral	Parenteral, transfusion
Incubation period	15–30 days	60–180 days	30–60 days	Similar to HBV	35–60 days	Unknown	Unknown
Serum markers	Anti-HAV	Antigens,* anti-HBs, anti-HBc	Anti-HCV‡ (IgG, IgM), RIBA, HCV-RNA PCR	Anti-HDV, RNA	Anti-HEV	None	RNA by RT-PCR
Fulminant liver failure	Rare	Uncommon unless with δ agent§	Uncommon	Yes	Yes in pregnancy	Unknown	Probably no
Chronic liver disease	No	Yes	Yes	Yes	Uncommon	Unknown	Persistent infection common; chronic liver disease rare
Carrier state	No	Yes‖	Yes	Yes	No	Unknown	Yes
Risk of hepatocellular cancer	No	Yes	Yes	No	No	Unknown	Unknown
Prophylaxis against	Immune serum globulin, vaccine; hygiene	Hepatitis B immune globulin, vaccine; Screen blood products for HBsAg	Screen blood for antibody appearing 4 mo postinfection (6 mo posttransfusion)	Screen blood for HBV markers	Screen blood for IgM, IgG antibody	None	None

PCR, Polymerase chain reaction; *RT*, reverse transcription.
*Hepatitis B whole virus particle is the Dane particle, which consists of a surface-antigen HBsAg, a core-antigen HBcAg, an e-antigen HBeAg, and DNA with a DNA polymerase. Mutant HBV also may produce severe hepatitis.
†An unknown number of posttransfusion hepatitis cases are the result of viruses other than HBV, HCV or cytomegalovirus, Epstein-Barr virus, human herpesvirus-6, or known agents and remain designated as caused by a non-A, non-B hepatitis agent.
‡May be measured by enzyme-linked immunosorbent assay (ELISA) and confirmed by the more specific recombinant immunoblot assay (RIBA) or RT-PCR for HCV RNA.
§Agent or hepatitis D virus requires hepatitis B virus coinfection or superinfection of a chronic HBV carrier for replication.
‖Chronic carrier state common in African-Asian, Haitian, Inuit, and South Pacific immigrants; drug abusers; individuals with Down syndrome; multiply transfused patients; homosexuals; patients on hemodialysis; and dental workers.

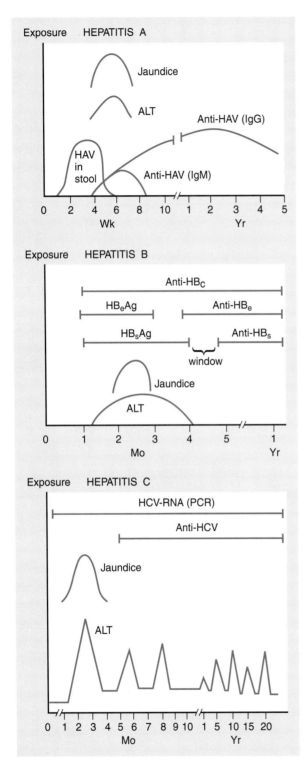

FIG. 11–5

Clinical course and laboratory findings associated with hepatitis A, B, and C. *ALT,* Alanine aminotransferase; *HAV,* hepatitis A virus; *HB,* hepatitis B; *HCV,* hepatitis C virus; *IgG,* immunoglobulin G; *PCR,* polymerase chain reaction; *RNA,* ribonucleic acid.

the serum precedes a variable "window" period followed by the emergence of the antibody to surface antigen (anti-HB_s), which confers lifelong immunity. Antibody to core antigen (anti-HB_c) is a useful marker for recognizing HBV infection during the window phase (i.e., when HB_sAg has disappeared but before the appearance of anti-HB_s). Anti-HB_e is useful in predicting a low degree of infectivity during the carrier state. Seroconversion following HCV infection may occur up to 6 months after illness. A positive result on HCV enzyme-linked immunosorbent assay (ELISA) should be followed with the more specific recombinant immunoblot assay (RIBA), which detects antibodies to multiple HCV antigens. Detection of HCV RNA by polymerase chain reaction (PCR) is a sensitive marker for active infection, and results of this test may be positive as early as 3 days after inoculation.

Recovery is the rule in most cases of acute viral hepatitis. Less than 1:1000 cases progress to fulminant hepatic necrosis, encephalopathy, and death (this is discussed in this chapter under Fulminant Hepatic Failure). The virus-specific risks for chronic hepatitis, carrier state, and hepatocellular carcinoma are noted in Table 11–17.

The *treatment* of acute hepatitis is largely supportive and involves rest, hydration, and adequate dietary intake. Hospitalization is indicated for patients with severe vomiting and dehydration, a prolonged prothrombin time, or evidence of early hepatic encephalopathy. Once the *diagnosis* of viral hepatitis is made, attention should be directed toward preventing its spread. For HAV, careful hygienic measures include hand washing and the careful disposal of excreta, contaminated diapers or clothing, needles, and other blood-contaminated items. As soon as the diagnosis is established, immune serum globulin should be given to all immediate family contacts and, in the case of infants and toddlers, to all close playmates and children at day care centers. Similar hygienic measures are necessary for hepatitis B and C.

The *prevention* of hepatitis may be accomplished by immunization and isolation (Table 11–18). Immune globulin is recommended after exposure to hepatitis A and B. High-risk groups should receive immunization against HBV (e.g., parenteral drug abusers; male homosexuals; prisoners; sexual partners of HBV-infected individuals; infants born to HBsAg-positive mothers; patients and staff in hemodialysis and oncology units; patients requiring frequent blood or clotting factor concentrates and health care personnel who handle these products; physicians, dentists, and morticians; household contacts of HB_sAg carriers; and patients with Down syndrome). The current recommendation is that all neonates and infants, as well as all unvaccinated adolescents, be immunized against HBV regardless

TABLE 11–18
Prevention of Hepatitis

Etiology	Clinical Situation	Prevention
HAV	Before and 1 wk following jaundice	Enteric isolation
	Household contacts	IG within 2 wk of exposure
	School outbreak	IG only in day care or custodial institutions with high risk of fecal-oral spread
	Travel, military, Native Alaskans, Native Americans, homosexuals, IV drug users, epidemics, other underlying liver disease, inhabitants of states with high incidence of infection	Vaccination
HBV	Perinatal exposure	Vaccination + HBIG
	Sexual: acute infection	HBIG ± vaccination
	Sexual: chronic carrier	Vaccination
	Household contact: chronic carrier	Vaccination
	Household contact: acute case	None unless known exposure
	Household contact: acute case, known exposure	HBIG + vaccination
	Infant (<12 mo): acute case in primary caregiver	HBIG + vaccination
	Inadvertent: percutaneous or permucosal exposure	HBIG + vaccination
	All unvaccinated infants and children up to 18 years of age	Vaccination
HCV	Inadvertent: percutaneous exposure	None

HAV, Hepatitis A virus; *HBIG,* hepatitis B immune globulin; *HBV,* hepatitis B virus; *HCV,* hepatitis C virus.

of risk (see Chapter 10). HAV vaccine may be used in the clinical settings listed in Table 11–18.

Fulminant Hepatic Failure

Fulminant hepatic failure may occur in patients who have had no preexisting pathologic conditions of the liver. Massive hepatic necrosis in many cases may be the result of viral agents, fatty acid oxidation defects, or hepatotoxins. Most cases of fulminant liver failure in childhood are of unknown etiology, although an infectious agent is suspected. Impending acute liver failure should be suspected when transaminase values that initially were elevated 15- to 20-fold fall rapidly as the prothrombin time becomes prolonged (often >100 sec) and unresponsive to parenteral vitamin K. The direct bilirubin level continues to rise (often >15 mg/dL). In severe liver failure, the total bilirubin level continues to rise while the direct fraction decreases as a result of loss of conjugating function. Hepatic encephalopathy is the most dramatic sign of fulminant hepatic failure, and progression to cerebral edema with brainstem herniation is often the cause of death. Other complications are hypoglycemia, gastrointestinal hemorrhage, hyponatremia, renal insufficiency (hepatorenal syndrome), and sepsis.

Treatment is supportive and involves the following steps:

1. Oral feedings should be discontinued, and lactulose should be administered by nasogastric tube to trap ammonia in the intestinal lumen as ammonium ion for elimination in the feces.
2. Endotracheal intubation should be considered early to allow control of the airway and pulmonary toilet.
3. Central venous alimentation should be used to provide quantities of glucose and fluid sufficient to prevent hypoglycemia and hypovolemia.
4. Central venous pressure should be monitored.
5. Intracranial pressure should be monitored and, in selected patients with elevated intracranial pressure, mannitol should be administered (hyperventilation is not effective in reducing intracranial pressure in these patients).
6. Antacids, H_2 receptor antagonists, or proton pump inhibitors should be administered to keep the gastric pH above 4.
7. Intravenous vitamin K or fresh frozen plasma should be administered to improve or maintain clotting status.

Liver transplantation is an effective therapy. In patients with high serum ammonia levels and worsening encephalopathy, exchange transfusion or plasmapheresis may result in transient improvement while transplantation is awaited.

The short-term *prognosis* is poor, with mortality rates of 80–90%. However, for those who survive, the long-term prognosis is excellent, with full recovery of normal liver function following hepatic regeneration. However, aplastic anemia may develop in approximately one third of survivors of non-A to non-G fulminant hepatitis, even after successful transplantation.

Chronic Liver Disease

Chronic hepatitis is an inflammatory process that lasts more than 6 months and may become manifest as hepatic failure or chronic liver disease. Viral infections with HBV and HCV are the most frequently identifiable infectious causes. Other causes are drugs (e.g., alpha-methyldopa, isoniazid, and methotrexate), Wilson disease, alpha$_1$-antitrypsin deficiency, cystic fibrosis, and inflammatory bowel disease. Autoimmune disease is an important cause of chronic liver disease in older children, particularly females.

Chronic hepatitis may be classified as either persistent or active, based on the histologic appearance of the liver. In patients with **chronic persistent hepatitis** the liver architecture is normal and the inflammatory process is confined to the portal area, without extension into the periportal region. Patients are usually asymptomatic. Laboratory studies demonstrate fluctuating transaminase levels, minimal or no hyperbilirubinemia, normal prothrombin time, and HBV or HCV seropositivity in most patients. Chronic persistent hepatitis is the most common cause of chronic hepatitis and is a self-limited condition that necessitates reassurance of the child and family but no specific treatment. Recovery is the rule, but the pathologic lesion and mild biochemical abnormalities may persist for years.

Chronic active hepatitis is a more serious form of the disease; the inflammatory process of lymphocytes and plasma cells not only involves the portal area but also extends into the adjacent lobule (interface hepatitis, piecemeal necrosis). Fibrosis may extend between portal areas (bridging fibrosis). Chronic active hepatitis may progress to cirrhosis and hepatic failure. The *diagnosis* should be considered in any child with persistent or relapsing jaundice 6 months after an episode of HBV or HCV hepatitis. However, most patients have no evidence of antecedent acute hepatitis. The most common form of chronic active hepatitis in children is the autoimmune form, which may have an indolent course. Many patients already have cirrhosis when the diagnosis is made.

The classification of chronic hepatitis as chronic persistent or chronic active hepatitis with or without cirrhosis is being replaced with a histologic scoring system that quantifies the degree of inflammation and fibrosis. This system seems to be more clinically useful in staging the severity of liver disease and assessing the response to treatment.

Clinical manifestations include hepatosplenomegaly, jaundice, malaise, anorexia, and right upper quadrant pain. In addition to the aforementioned features of liver disease, patients with autoimmune chronic active hepatitis also may have extrahepatic manifestations such as amenorrhea, arthritis, arthralgia, low-grade fever, and thyroiditis. Patients with autoimmune hepatitis have circulating autoimmune markers. The presence of antinuclear antibodies (ANAs) along with smooth muscle antibodies (SMAs) and antiasialoglycoprotein receptor antibodies suggests the diagnosis of type I autoimmune chronic hepatitis. The isolated presence of liver-kidney microsomal antibodies (LKMs) with anti-liver cytosol I antibodies identifies a group of patients with type II autoimmune chronic hepatitis with a worse outcome. In chronic active hepatitis the serum transaminase level is variable, but it may not reflect the severity of the liver disease and usually is accompanied by hypergammaglobulinemia. The *diagnosis* is based on results of a liver biopsy, which is a prerequisite for treatment with immunosuppressive agents.

In cases of autoimmune hepatitis, *treatment* with prednisone alone or in combination with azathioprine may lead to a dramatic improvement in the clinical, laboratory, and histologic features and a decrease in the mortality rate. The response in type I is much better than in type II autoimmune hepatitis (>95% versus 65%). Azathioprine is of value because of its steroid-sparing effect. Corticosteroids are contraindicated in patients with viral chronic active hepatitis. In autoimmune chronic active hepatitis, most children respond to therapy, but 50% relapse with discontinuation of prednisone. Progression to cirrhosis may occur despite a good response to initial immunosuppression. Patients who are LKM positive have a poor response to therapy and are unlikely to remain in remission when immunosuppressive drugs are discontinued. Treatment of HBV and HCV chronic active hepatitis with interferon-α shows promise, but relapse may occur when therapy is discontinued. New treatment regimens using long-acting pegylated interferon and additional antiviral therapy with lamivudine (for HBV) and ribavirin (for HCV) may prove more effective.

Cirrhosis

Cirrhosis is the end result of destructive processes producing irreversible fibrosis, scarring, and hepatocellular regeneration, which lead to the formation of regenerative nodules. The nodules cause irreversible distortion of the hepatic vasculature and biliary system. Nodules may be small (<3 mm in micronodular cirrhosis) or large (>3 mm in macronodular cirrhosis). This distortion of the vascular bed leads to portal hypertension and portosystemic shunting. In childhood and adolescence, the *etiology* of cirrhosis includes biliary malformations (atresia), alpha$_1$-antitrypsin deficiency, Wilson disease, galactosemia, tyrosinemia, chronic active hepatitis, and prolonged total parenteral nutrition.

Clinical manifestations of cirrhosis include palmar erythema, spider angiomata, gynecomastia, splenomegaly, ascites, hemorrhoids, cutaneous excoriations from pruritus, and jaundice. The liver may be large and hard (in biliary cirrhosis) or small, scarred, and shrunken (in postnecrotic cirrhosis). *Laboratory findings* depend on the cause and severity of the process. The major *complications* of cirrhosis in children are portal hypertension with variceal bleeding and hypersplenism, ascites, liver failure with encephalopathy, hepatorenal syndrome, and, rarely, hepatocellular carcinoma.

Portal Hypertension

Although cirrhosis is an important cause of portal hypertension, any process leading to an increased resistance to portal blood flow into the liver (prehepatic or presinusoidal [e.g., portal vein thrombosis, omphalitis, or schistosomiasis]), through the liver (intrahepatic or sinusoidal), or from above the liver (suprahepatic or postsinusoidal [e.g., Budd-Chiari syndrome, venoocclusive disease, or pericarditis]) results in portal hypertension. Prehepatic and suprahepatic causes are more likely in children younger than 5 years of age with no history of liver disease. Although rare, lesions such as an arteriovenous malformation, which increases hepatic blood flow, also result in portal hypertension. Portal hypertension leads to the formation of collaterals between the portal and systemic venous circulations. The most important of these connections is that between the portal vein and the azygos vein via submucosal veins (varices) in the stomach and esophagus.

Hemorrhage from *esophageal varices* is associated with hematemesis or melena (discussed in this chapter under Gastrointestinal Hemorrhage). In children the bleeding often stops spontaneously, but rebleeding may occur. Impaired synthesis of clotting factors, resulting from severe hepatocellular dysfunction or hypersplenism-induced thrombocytopenia, can result in uncontrollable hemorrhage.

Treatment of portal hypertension consists of replacing blood losses and of intravenous infusion of vasopressin or octreotide (somatostatin analog), which causes constriction of the splanchnic arterioles and a reduction of portal pressure and flow, respec-

tively. Endoscopic sclerotherapy can be used to arrest acute bleeding and prevent rebleeding. Repeated sclerosing injections lead to variceal obliteration. Endoscopic banding of varices is another effective technique. Portosystemic shunt surgery may decompress the entire portal system (portocaval anastomosis) or only the varices (distal splenorenal shunt). Transjugular intrahepatic portosystemic shunting (TIPS) is an emergency shunt procedure to avoid surgery and is used to prevent rebleeding of esophageal varices. Portal hypertension also produces *hypersplenism* that becomes manifest by anemia, neutropenia, and thrombocytopenia.

Ascites

Ascites is the accumulation of abnormal amounts of fluid in the peritoneal cavity. It is caused by hypoalbuminemia; portal hypertension; and increased hepatic and splanchnic lymph production, accompanied by impaired renal sodium and water excretion secondary to hyperaldosteronism and increased levels of antidiuretic hormone. Ascites is clinically detectable as a shifting dullness to percussion when at least 300 mL of fluid is present in an adult. Ascites caused by liver disease has the characteristics of a transudate (<3 g protein/dL).

Treatment of ascites consists of the administration of spironolactone and the restriction of sodium intake. The administration of furosemide may be necessary in refractory cases. Diuresis usually should be accomplished slowly over several days, but aggressive diuresis with abdominal paracentesis or intravenous albumin followed by furosemide is indicated when respiratory function is compromised. The latter approach may lead to plasma volume depletion, hypokalemia, hepatorenal syndrome, and encephalopathy. Spontaneous bacterial peritonitis may be a complication of ascites and should be considered if fever and abdominal pain are present (discussed further under Peritoneal Cavity). However, abdominal symptoms may be minimal or absent in infants.

Hepatic Encephalopathy

Progressive deterioration of liver function results in impaired detoxification of metabolic products. This process, along with portosystemic shunting, leads to hepatic encephalopathy. Encephalopathy may be acute, as seen in fulminant hepatic failure, or chronic, as seen in slowly progressive liver disease with cirrhosis.

The *etiology* is unknown but may be related to disturbances in neuronal function resulting from the presence of false neurotransmitters in the central nervous system. Ammonia and bacterial products, such as octopamine, mercaptan (odor of fetor hepaticus), or endogenous benzodiazepines and gamma-aminobutyrate, may play important roles. Serum ammonia levels often correlate poorly with the degree of encephalopathy.

The *clinical manifestations* of hepatic encephalopathy are described as four stages: (1) impaired mentation; (2) lethargy, disorientation, and asterixis ("liver flap"); (3) arousable stupor; and (4) coma. *Treatment* of chronic encephalopathy should focus on identification of the precipitating causes, such as intestinal bleeding, infection, central nervous system–depressant drugs, and complications of diuretic therapy. Therapy involves maintaining adequate nutrition and reducing ammonia production. Some protein restriction may be needed, but at least 1 g/kg/24 hr must be provided to meet metabolic requirements and prevent endogenous protein breakdown. During acute encephalopathy, no protein should be given; however, glucose infusions are needed to prevent hypoglycemia and proteolysis. Neomycin (oral) reduces the number of bacteria in the intestine that are available for producing ammonia. Lactulose also should be given to reduce ammonia absorption; it lowers stool pH, trapping ammonia in the form of the nondiffusible ammonium ion, and is a cathartic, reducing intestinal stasis. Flumazenil, a benzodiazepine antagonist, may reverse hepatic encephalopathy.

Neonatal Cholestasis

Direct hyperbilirubinemia during the first month of life signifies significant pathologic conditions resulting from hepatobiliary structural anomalies, infections, metabolic and genetic disease, drug and nutritional toxicity, and disorders of unknown cause (see Fig. 11–2 and Chapter 6). Except for parenteral alimentation–induced cholestasis in premature infants, the most common disorders in full-term infants that are associated with neonatal cholestasis are extrahepatic biliary atresia and idiopathic neonatal hepatitis. The usual *clinical manifestations* of cholestatic diseases during infancy are jaundice, hepatomegaly, dark urine, and acholic (white) stools.

After specific diagnostic tests are performed, the supportive *treatment* of patients with neonatal cholestasis depends on the extent of the hepatocellular dysfunction and the severity of the cholestasis. Hepatocellular dysfunction predisposes the patient to complications such as bleeding, encephalopathy, and hepatorenal syndrome, whereas bile salt deficiency in the intestinal lumen may lead to fat-soluble vitamin deficiencies, rickets, hypocalcemia (vitamin D deficiency), hemorrhage (vitamin K deficiency), and peripheral neuropathy (vitamin E deficiency). Retention of bile salts may produce pruritus.

Supportive therapy involves medium-chain triglyceride and fat-soluble vitamin supplementation; administration of cholestyramine to decrease reabsorption of bile salts from the gut; and administration of phenobarbital to increase the hepatic excretion of bile. The administration of oral ursodeoxycholic acid may improve bile secretion. *Definitive treatment* depends on the underlying process and may involve an exclusion diet (lactose in galactosemia), surgery (in extrahepatic biliary atresia or choledochal cyst), or liver transplantation.

Biliary Atresia

Biliary atresia is seen in 1:10,000 births and typically involves the extrahepatic bile ducts. In some patients, however, both intrahepatic and extrahepatic biliary structures are affected as a result of an inflammatory process beginning in the perinatal period. The condition is more common in girls, and the *etiology* is unknown. Bile duct injury and obliteration may be caused by toxic, infectious, or autoimmune processes that so far have not been identified. All infants with jaundice at 2 months of age must be evaluated for biliary atresia because surgery is most effective before 3 months of age.

Clinical manifestations usually present in a full-term infant in whom jaundice develops during the second or third week of life. The stools often are acholic, although the shedding of bilirubin-laden intestinal mucosal cells may color the stool. The liver enlarges and becomes quite hard. Splenomegaly usually is detectable by 8 weeks. Other than these physical findings, the infants usually appear healthy. An association exists with the polysplenia (biliary splenic) syndrome and with trisomy 13 and 18.

Laboratory tests demonstrate conjugated hyperbilirubinemia and elevated levels of serum alkaline phosphatase, GGTP, and transaminases. Ultrasound examination is helpful in excluding a choledochal cyst. A biliary scan following 5 days of phenobarbital administration (5 mg/kg/day) demonstrates normal hepatocyte uptake but a failure to excrete the isotope into the intestine after 24 hours. This test is less reliable in infants with serum bilirubin levels above 10 mg/dL. Percutaneous liver biopsy shows bile duct proliferation with bile plugging and confirms the diagnosis in 95% of patients.

Ultimately, patients with suspected biliary atresia require exploratory laparotomy. If biliary atresia is found, a *Kasai procedure* (hepatoportoenterostomy) is used to connect the bowel lumen and the porta hepatis containing bile duct remnants. Without surgery, patients usually die from cirrhosis before 2 years of age. Surgical success is judged by improvement in bile drainage; the earlier the operation (<2 months of age), the greater the chance of establishing bile flow. Jaundice clears in only 55% of Kasai procedures. Over 90% of patients survive 5 years after a successful Kasai procedure, but complications of the procedure include progressive biliary cirrhosis and ascending cholangitis. The treatment for infants with unresolving jaundice is liver transplantation, which has a 70–90% survival rate.

Biliary Hypoplasia

Patients with intrahepatic biliary hypoplasia may be classified as either "syndromic" (e.g., **Alagille syndrome,** arteriohepatic dysplasia) or "nonsyndromic." In addition to intrahepatic biliary hypoplasia, infants with Alagille syndrome have facial, cardiac (e.g., valvular or peripheral pulmonic stenosis), vertebral (e.g., butterfly vertebra), ocular (e.g., posterior embryotoxon), and renal (e.g., dysplastic kidneys) anomalies. Patients have hypercholesterolemia and associated cutaneous xanthomata. Many of the children have growth failure, and some are mildly mentally impaired.

Alagille syndrome is inherited as an autosomal dominant trait with variable penetrance. The syndrome is associated with microdeletions on the short arm of chromosome 20. Mutations in the *Jagged-1* gene on this chromosome have been found in families with the Alagille syndrome. This gene product is involved in intercellular signaling during development and differentiation.

Treatment is directed at controlling hypercholesterolemia with diet and cholestyramine and at preventing manifestations of vitamin E deficiency (e.g., ataxia, areflexia, loss of vibratory and position sensation, and ophthalmoplegia) with aggressive vitamin E supplementation. Phenobarbital and ursodeoxycholic acid therapy also may help lower serum bilirubin and bile acid levels.

The *prognosis* for hepatic disease of the "syndromic" form is better than that for the nonsyndromic form. Cirrhosis and liver failure usually occur in the nonsyndromic form before adolescence.

Idiopathic Neonatal Hepatitis

Idiopathic neonatal hepatitis is responsible for most of the cases of intrahepatic cholestasis in infants who are not receiving parenteral nutrition. It usually presents at birth, is more common in boys, and may be associated with growth retardation. Idiopathic neonatal hepatitis probably represents more than one disease resulting from infectious or familial causes. It is unusual to have acholic stools and a very high alkaline phosphatase or GGTP level. Patency of bile ducts may be confirmed by a biliary scan, although severe cholestasis may cause a false-positive scan result. Liver biopsy shows numerous giant cells, lobular disorganization, necrosis, and inflam-

mation without the neoductular proliferation and fibrosis characteristic of extrahepatic atresia.

The *differential diagnosis* includes TORCH (*t*oxoplasmosis, *o*ther, *r*ubella, *c*ytomegalovirus, *h*erpes simplex) infections, biliary atresia (which may be difficult to exclude without biopsy), and other causes of conjugated hyperbilirubinemia (Fig. 11–2). *Treatment* is as described for Alagille syndrome, and most patients recover within 6–8 months.

Progressive Familial Intrahepatic Cholestasis

Progressive familial intrahepatic cholestasis (PFIC), originally known as Byler's disease, was first described in an Amish kindred. Several distinct phenotypes of PFIC have been described. The molecular defects for three of these phenotypes have been determined. All appear to involve defective hepatocyte transporters for either bile acids or phospholipids. All appear to be inherited in an autosomal recessive manner and result in progressive cholestasis and pruritus progressing to cirrhosis and end-stage liver disease. PFIC type I was originally described in an Amish kindred, the Byler family. Biochemically, this type of PFIC is characterized by normal serum GGTP and cholesterol levels and high serum concentrations of primary bile acids. The defect in Byler's disease is in the gene *FICI*, which encodes a P-type ATPase that may be involved in the transport of aminophospholipids in the hepatocyte. Several homozygous mutations in the *FICI* gene have been identified in children with PFIC type 1. Interestingly, this same gene also appears to be defective in a milder form of cholestatic liver disease, benign recurrent intrahepatic cholestasis. Patients with PFIC type 2 also exhibit cholestasis, normal serum GGTP and cholesterol levels, and high levels of serum primary bile acids. However, these patients are unrelated to the original Byler family and have a defect in an ATP-dependent canalicular bile acid transporter or bile salt export pump (BSEP). Several mutations of the gene for this transporter have been identified in families with PFIC type 2. Patients with PFIC type 3 are distinguishable from those with the other two types by high serum GGTP and cholesterol levels. Patients with PFIC type 3 generally demonstrate symptoms later in life and reach end-stage liver disease at a later age. PFIC type 3 is caused by a defect in the *MDR3* gene, which encodes a phospholipid lipase in the canalicular membrane. Mutations of this gene associated with low biliary phospholipid levels have been identified in affected patients. Other than in cases necessitating liver transplantation, chronic biliary diversion and ursodeoxycholic acid therapy may reduce pruritus and improve liver function in some patients.

Reye Syndrome

Reye syndrome is characterized by encephalopathy and the noninflammatory fatty infiltration of the liver and kidney. It has been associated with epidemics of influenza A or B virus and varicella. The administration of aspirin predisposes the patient to this condition. The peak incidence is in children 6 years of age, with most cases occurring between 4 and 12 years of age.

The *clinical manifestations* begin with intractable vomiting during or immediately following recovery from an upper respiratory tract infection. Over a period of 2–24 hours, the child becomes confused, combative, agitated, stuporous, and finally comatose. In addition to the altered level of consciousness, physical findings include dilated pupils, hyperactive deep tendon reflexes, and Kussmaul respirations. Jaundice and fever are absent, and the liver may be normal to moderately enlarged in size. The serum transaminase and ammonia levels are elevated, and the prothrombin time may be prolonged. Hypoglycemia and acidosis also may be present. Cerebrospinal fluid examination is normal, and toxicologic findings of the blood and urine are negative.

The *diagnosis* is based on results of a liver biopsy. Histologic findings include a diffuse microvesicular steatosis, without necrosis or inflammation. The mitochondria are swollen. Infants under 2 years of age should be evaluated for underlying inborn errors of metabolism, such as medium-chain acyl-coenzyme A dehydrogenase deficiency.

Treatment is supportive and similar to that outlined for fulminant hepatic failure. Careful monitoring and treatment of increased intracranial pressure are mandatory.

The *prognosis* correlates best with the depth of coma. Death from Reye syndrome usually is the result of increased intracranial pressure because liver regeneration is often present at the time of autopsy.

Prevention may be possible by avoidance of salicylates during viral respiratory illnesses.

Nonalcoholic Steatohepatitis

Fatty infiltration of the liver may be seen in a variety of clinical settings. However, with the increasing prevalence of obesity and insulin resistance in children and adolescents, as well as in the population in general, this disorder is being seen more frequently in pediatric patients. The spectrum of hepatic steatosis, or fatty liver, may range from simple fatty infiltration to fatty infiltration with inflammation and fibrosis, which in some cases may progress to cirrhosis. The term nonalcoholic steatohepatitis (NASH) should probably be applied only to those cases with steatosis and inflammation. Mallory bodies, balloon-

ing degeneration of hepatocytes, and some degree of fibrosis are also usually present. Lipid accumulation may result from both increased influx of fatty acids and impaired triglyceride secretion.

NASH appears to represent the hepatic component of a metabolic syndrome characterized by obesity, hyperinsulinemia, peripheral insulin resistance, diabetes, hypertriglyceridemia, and hypertension. Although obesity is clearly associated with NASH, most patients are only moderately overweight. NASH may also be associated with other conditions, such as malnutrition, abetalipoproteinemia, hypobetalipoproteinemia, hepatotoxins, total parenteral nutrition, and jejunoileal bypass for morbid obesity. The current theory of the pathogenesis of NASH is the "two-hit" hypothesis. The first insult is the accumulation of lipid in the liver in the setting of a predisposition, such as type II diabetes, insulin resistance, and obesity. The liver injury is initiated during a second insult, with free radical generation causing membrane lipid peroxidation and hepatocyte injury. Over half of obese children may have some degree of hepatic steatosis or full progression to NASH. This disorder usually presents with hepatomegaly in the setting of obesity, occasionally associated with right upper quadrant discomfort. The most common biochemical abnormality is a modest elevation of the serum transaminase levels.

Although cirrhosis from NASH has been reported in adults, it has not been described in children. Treatment for NASH involves strategies to decrease fatty acid delivery to the liver, with carefully supervised weight loss and control of type II diabetes. Other treatment interventions that may protect the hepatocyte from oxidative injury include vitamin E, ursodeoxycholic acid, and selenium therapy. Iron overload has been associated with accelerated hepatic fibrosis in NASH, and if iron overload is present, induction of marginal iron deficiency may be beneficial.

Alpha₁-Antitrypsin Deficiency

The glycoprotein alpha$_1$-antitrypsin is produced by hepatocytes under the influence of two autosomally inherited, codominant alleles and makes up 80% of the serum alpha$_1$-globulin fraction. It functions as an inhibitor of trypsin, pancreatic elastase, neutral proteases of leukocytes, and acid proteases of alveolar macrophages. Uninhibited proteolytic activity by these enzymes may cause hepatic or pulmonary injury. There are more than 175 different alleles of this protease inhibitor (Pi) system. The normal phenotype is MM; Pi ZZ is associated with liver or lung disease. The incidence of the ZZ phenotype is 1:1600–1800, but only 10–15% of patients with the ZZ phenotype have neonatal cholestasis. The liver disease may be a result of the accumulation of an abnormally folded protein within the hepatocyte. Variability in the severity of the liver disease may be related to variations of the endoplasmic reticulum degradative pathway, which removes the abnormal protein.

Cholestatic jaundice that is indistinguishable from neonatal hepatitis during the first 1–3 months of life may be the initial presenting sign of alpha$_1$-antitrypsin deficiency. Hepatosplenomegaly also may be present. Cirrhosis develops in 30–50% of patients, leading to hepatic failure; progression may be extremely variable, spanning months to years. Pulmonary emphysema may develop in older patients, and hepatocellular cancer has developed following cirrhosis. Pancreatitis also may develop.

The *diagnosis* is made by quantifying levels of circulating alpha$_1$-antitrypsin and phenotyping. Liver biopsy reveals the presence of eosinophilic cytoplasmic granules that stain intensely with periodic acid–Schiff (PAS) stain and are resistant to digestion with diastase.

There is no specific *treatment*. Plasma-derived or recombinant alpha$_1$-antitrypsin infusions restore plasma levels but have not yet been demonstrated to cure the hepatic complications. Therapy for cholestasis and the complications of cirrhosis are similar to those previously outlined. In severe cases, transplantation may be necessary.

Wilson Disease (Hepatolenticular Degeneration)

Wilson disease is an autosomal recessive disorder caused by the accumulation of copper in the liver, brain, eyes, kidney, and bone. The defective gene is on chromosome 13 and appears to encode a P-type membrane adenosine triphosphatase (ATPase) involved in copper transport. More than 40 mutations in this gene have been described. Most patients are compound heterozygotes. *Clinical manifestations* are unusual before 5 years of age and include hepatosplenomegaly and jaundice resembling chronic active hepatitis, hemolytic anemia, deterioration of neurologic function (e.g., worsening school performance and handwriting, intention tremor, clumsiness, and personality changes), renal tubular acidosis, and the appearance of corneal Kayser-Fleischer rings. Liver disease is common in younger patients, and neuropsychiatric problems are noted in older patients. Wilson disease may present with fulminant liver failure and should be considered in this case, particularly when severe hemolysis is also present.

Low serum copper and low serum ceruloplasmin levels suggest the *diagnosis,* but normal copper values may be found early in the course of the disease. Quantitation of urinary copper output, with or without penicillamine administration or quantitation of hepatic copper levels, usually confirms the diagnosis.

The goal of *treatment* is to lower tissue copper levels. This has been successfully accomplished with the copper chelating agent D-penicillamine and trientine. Oral zinc therapy interferes with absorption of copper from the intestine. Foods high in copper, such as chocolate, nuts, and dried fruits, should be avoided. The *prognosis* depends on early diagnosis and successful chelation of the copper.

Liver Transplantation

Liver transplantation is considered accepted therapy for end-stage liver disease in infants and children. The current (since 1993) 1- and 5-year survival rates for children after orthotopic liver transplantation are 88% and 85%, respectively. Extrahepatic biliary atresia is the most frequent indication, followed by metabolic liver disease and fulminant hepatic necrosis. Improved survival in pediatric liver transplant recipients is the result of several factors, including better pretransplant care, with particular emphasis on nutrition and treatment of complications of end-stage liver disease; refinements in surgical technique; and advances in posttransplant immunosuppression. A major problem, especially for infants requiring liver transplantation, is the paucity of donor organs in this age group. The advent of reduced-size and split grafts and living donor transplantation has greatly contributed to the expansion of the donor pool for this group of patients. Posttransplant immunosuppression involves corticosteroids and either cyclosporine (Sandimmune or Neoral) or tacrolimus (Prograf or FK-506). Azathioprine (Imuran) and mycophenolate mofetil (CellCept) are also sometimes used as adjunctive therapy. Posttransplant complications include primary graft failure, hepatic artery thrombosis, infection (bacterial, viral, and fungal), and graft rejection. One serious posttransplant complication, associated most often with the use of tacrolimus, is posttransplant lymphoproliferative disease (PTLD). This disorder is caused by an uncontrolled proliferation of B cells, triggered by either a new Epstein-Barr viral infection or reactivation of a previous infection in the face of immunosuppression. However, the monoclonal form generally has a poor outcome, even with chemotherapy. In most transplant centers now, children are eventually weaned to very low doses or are completely weaned from corticosteroids and maintained on monotherapy with either cyclosporine or tacrolimus. The long-term prognosis after orthotopic liver transplantation in children is encouraging. Generally, growth catch-up occurs after transplantation, and most children return to a relatively normal lifestyle.

REFERENCES

Balistreri W: Mechanisms and management of pediatric hepato-biliary disease, *J Pediatr Gastroenterol Nutr* 10(1):138–147, 1990.

Behrman RE, Kliegman RM, Jenson HB, editors: *Nelson textbook of pediatrics,* ed 16, Philadelphia, 2000, WB Saunders, Chapters 354–367.

Fong DG, Nehra V, Lindor KD, et al: Metabolic and nutritional considerations in nonalcoholic fatty liver, *Hepatology* 32(1):3–10, 2000.

Hardie R, Newton L, Bruce J, et al: The changing clinical pattern of Reye's syndrome, 1982–1990, *Arch Dis Child* 74(5):400–405, 1996.

Heyman MB, Laberge JM, Somberg KA, et al: Transjugular intra-hepatic portosystemic shunts (TIPS) in children, *J Pediatr* 131(6): 914–919, 1997.

Hussein M, Howard E, Mieli-Vergani G, et al: Jaundice at 14 days of life: exclude biliary atresia, *Arch Dis Child* 66(10):1177–1179, 1991.

Jonas MM: Viral hepatitis: from prevention to antivirals, *Clin Liver Dis* 4(4):849–877, 2000.

Laner GM, Walker BD: Hepatitis E virus infection, *N Engl J Med* 345(1):41–52, 2001.

Mas A, Rodes J: Fulminant hepatic failure, *Lancet* 349(9058): 1081–1085, 1997.

McDiarmid SV: Liver transplantation: the pediatric challenge, *Clin Liver Dis* 4(4):879–927, 2000.

McFarlane IG: Lessons about antibodies in autoimmune hepatitis, *Lancet* 355(9214):1475–1476, 2000.

McKiernan PJ, Baker AJ, Kelly DA: The frequency and outcome of biliary atresia in the UK and Ireland, *Lancet* 355(9179):25–29, 2000.

Mieli-Vergani G, Vergani D: Immunological liver diseases in chil-dren, *Semin Liver Dis* 18(3):271–279, 1998.

Miltenberg DM, Schaffer R III, Breslin T, et al: Changing indica-tions for pediatric cholecystectomy, *Pediatrics* 105(6):1250–1253, 2000.

Miyakawa Y, Mayumi M: Hepatitis G virus: a true hepatitis virus or an accidental tourist? *N Engl J Med* 336(11):795–796, 1997.

Mousseau DD, Butterworth RF: Current theories on the patho-genesis of hepatic encephalopathy, *Proc Soc Exp Biol Med* 206(4): 329–344, 1994.

Novy MA, Schwarz KB: Nutritional considerations and manage-ment of the child with liver disease, *Nutrition* 13(3):177–184, 1997.

Orozco H, Mercado MA, Chan C, et al: A comparative study of the elective treatment of variceal hemorrhage with beta-blockers, transendoscopic sclerotherapy, and surgery, *Ann Surg* 232(2): 216–219, 2000.

Shneider B: Genetic cholestasis syndromes, *J Pediatr Gastroenterol Nutr* 28(2):124–131, 1999.

Teckman J, Perlmutter DH: Conceptual advances in the patho-genesis and treatment of childhood metabolic liver disease, *Gastroenterology* 108(4):1263–1279, 1995.

Zeuzem S, Feinman SV, Rasenack J, et al: Peginterferon Alfa-2a in patients with chronic hepatitis C, *N Engl J Med* 343(23):1666–1672, 2000.

Pancreas

Isolated disease of the exocrine pancreas is uncom-mon in children. Pancreatic exocrine insufficiency of-ten is part of a genetic or systemic illness. Cystic fi-brosis (see Chapter 12) and severe malnutrition are the leading causes of pancreatic disease. **Shwachman syndrome** (involving neutropenia and dysostosis), an autosomal recessive disorder, accounts for 3–5% of pancreatic insufficiency in childhood. **Pearson syn-drome,** a mitochondrial DNA disorder, manifests as macrocytic anemia, ring sideroblasts in the bone mar-row, and variable thrombocytopenia that may pro-duce both bone marrow and pancreatic insufficiency.

Pancreatic function tests include determination of the levels of serum amylase and lipase (which are in-creased when pancreatitis is present) and trypsino-gen (which is increased in cystic fibrosis); examina-tion of stool for fat droplets or meat fibers (indicating fat and protein maldigestion); and analysis of urine for reduced *para*-aminobenzoic acid (PABA) excre-tion (which is a result of deficient pancreatic chy-motrypsin) following ingestion of N-benzoyl-L-tyrosyl-PABA. Cannulation of the pancreatic duct and collection of fluid for enzyme analysis, with and without secretagogue stimulation (endoscopic retro-grade cholangiopancreatoduodenoscopy), also may be helpful in evaluating pancreatic insufficiency.

Annular Pancreas

The annular pancreas is a rare malformation caused by a failure of rotation and fusion of the ventral and dorsal pancreatic buds. A complete pancreatic ring may obstruct the duodenum.

Pancreas divisum is caused by failure of fusion of the dorsal and ventral embryonic pancreas that drains through an accessory papilla. Pancreas divi-sum is a cause of recurrent pancreatitis.

Pancreatitis

Pancreatic duct obstruction or nonspecific parenchy-mal inflammation results in tissue injury from diges-tive enzymes, which leads to autodigestion and fur-ther inflammation and edema. Fat necrosis and hemorrhage are additional complications of acute pancreatitis. The *etiology* is idiopathic in as many as 25% of cases. Other causes are infectious agents (e.g., mumps, coxsackievirus, hepatitis virus, influenza virus, and *Mycoplasma*), drugs (e.g., alcohol, thiazide diuretics, valproic acid, L-asparaginase, aceta-minophen, corticosteroids, sulfonamides, azathio-prine, 6-mercaptopurine, and tacrolimus), cystic fi-brosis, alpha$_1$-antitrypsin deficiency, gallstones, biliary "sludge," shock, pancreas divisum, hyper-triglyceridemia, hypercalcemia, trauma, renal failure, familial disease, and vasculitis. Idiopathic chronic pancreatitis is associated with mutations in the cystic fibrosis gene in 30–40% of patients who have no other sign of cystic fibrosis and a normal sweat chlo-ride test.

The *clinical manifestations* include intense epigas-tric pain (occasionally radiating to the back), nausea, and vomiting. The abdomen may be tender and rigid, and a mass may be palpable if a pseudocyst has formed. Hemorrhagic pancreatitis may cause shock and produce a blue discoloration around the umbilicus (Cullen sign) or around the flank (Grey Turner sign). Left-sided pleural effusion and ascites are less common manifestations. Poor prognostic features include hyperglycemia (>200 mg/dL), leukocytosis (>16,000), elevated lactic dehydrogenase (>700 IU) and serum glutamic oxaloacetic transaminase (>250 U) levels, the development of anemia, hypocalcemia, azotemia (blood urea nitrogen >50 mg/dL), metabolic acidosis, hypoxia, and the need for continuous fluid resuscitation.

Laboratory findings include elevated serum amylase and lipase levels. Diabetic ketoacidosis, renal failure, parotid gland disease, perforated gastric ulcer, or acidosis may produce false elevations of the serum amylase level. Pleural or ascitic fluid amylase levels are elevated. Hyperglycemia and hypocalcemia may be present. Abdominal roentgenograms may demonstrate a sentinel loop, pancreatic calcification, or a mass. Ultrasonography demonstrates a swollen pancreas, pseudocyst, or both.

Treatment includes fluid replacement for hypovolemic shock, bowel rest, nasogastric decompression, and pain medication. Management is also directed toward the relief of complications such as anemia and hypocalcemia. Pseudocysts that persist beyond 6 weeks may necessitate surgery. Endoscopic retrograde cholangiopancreoduodenoscopy to define anatomic abnormalities may have a role in the management of recurrent pancreatitis. Slow refeeding should be encouraged once the vomiting and severe pain stop.

REFERENCES

Behrman RE, Kliegman RM, Jenson HB, editors: *Nelson textbook of pediatrics*, ed 16, Philadelphia, 2000, WB Saunders, Chapters 348–352.
Dugernier T: Severe acute pancreatitis. The therapeutic dilemma: medical or surgical intensive care, *Intensive Crit Care Digest* 10:47, 1991.
Weizman Z, Durie P: Acute pancreatitis in childhood, *J Pediatr* 113(1 Pt 1):24–29, 1988.
Windsor JA: Search for prognostic markers for acute pancreatitis, *Lancet* 355(9219):1924–1925, 2000.

Peritoneal Cavity

Primary peritonitis is an acute inflammatory process in the peritoneal cavity that is attributable to a perforated viscus. It usually occurs in children after splenectomy or in children who have chronic ascites, such as that seen in nephrotic syndrome or cirrhosis.

Clinical manifestations include the acute onset of fever, severe abdominal pain, and vomiting. The *diagnosis* may be based on the result of abdominal paracentesis. The fluid is an exudate, Gram stain reveals organisms, and many polymorphonucleated leukocytes are present. The responsible bacteria are *Pneumococcus* and gram-negative enteric pathogens. All patients at risk should receive the pneumococcal vaccine. Peritonitis in patients receiving chronic ambulatory peritoneal dialysis includes that caused by *Staphylococcus epidermidis*.

Secondary peritonitis is an inflammatory response to bacteria, bile, or pancreatic enzymes in the abdominal cavity resulting from a ruptured viscus. Necrotizing enterocolitis, appendicitis, and penetrating wounds are common causes. *E. coli, Klebsiella, Proteus, Enterobacter,* and *Bacteroides fragilis* are frequently found pathogens. Combined therapy for anaerobic and gram-negative organisms and appropriate surgery are the treatments of choice.

REFERENCES

Behrman RE, Kliegman RM, Jenson HB, editors: *Nelson textbook of pediatrics*, ed 16, Philadelphia, 2000, WB Saunders, Chapters 369, 370.

CHAPTER 12

The Respiratory System

Carolyn M. Kercsmar

Disorders of the respiratory system—for example, viral upper respiratory infections, otitis media, pneumonia, asthma, and cystic fibrosis—constitute a substantial part of the pediatrician's clinical practice. Respiratory disease may be insidious because normally a large lung reserve capacity exists and more than half the total lung tissue (or function) may be lost before an individual complains of dyspnea. In addition, the typical symptoms (dyspnea, cough, and chest pain) or signs (tachypnea, rales, and wheezing) may be overlooked or may be subtle in young children. Fever may be the only symptom of pneumonia, tachypnea the only manifestation of asthma, and cough the only symptom of foreign body aspiration. During a child's development, the pediatrician also must consider genetic (e.g., cystic fibrosis), anatomic (e.g., congenital anomalies), iatrogenic (e.g., oxygen toxicity), immunologic (e.g., immunosuppression or immunodeficiency), and extrapulmonary (e.g., heart failure) conditions as etiologic variables contributing to pulmonary pathology.

The lung has a tremendous capacity for growth. At birth, the full-term infant has approximately 25 million alveoli; this number increases to nearly 300 million in adulthood. Most of this growth occurs by 8 years of age; the greatest growth is in the first 3–4 years.

ANATOMY OF THE RESPIRATORY SYSTEM

Air enters the nostrils and passes over three turbinates (bony protrusions into the nasal cavity), which are covered by ciliated respiratory epithelium and which increase the total surface area within the nostril. The large surface area and the convoluted patterns the airflow takes as it passes over the turbinates create a high resistance but serve to warm, humidify, and filter the inspired air. Secretions draining from the paranasal sinuses are carried from the nasal cavity to the pharynx by the mucociliary action of the epithelium. The eustachian tubes open from the middle ear into the posterior aspect of the nasopharynx. Lymphoid tissue at this location (the adenoids) may obstruct the orifice of the eustachian tubes.

The epiglottis helps protect the larynx during swallowing by deflecting swallowed material toward the esophagus. The epiglottis of children has a contour somewhat like the Greek letter *omega* (Ω) and usually is shaped differently from that of adults. The arytenoid cartilages, which assist in opening and closing the glottis, usually are not very prominent in children. The vocal cords form a V-shaped opening (the glottis), with the apex of the V being anterior, at the base of the epiglottis. Beneath the cords, the walls of the subglottic space converge toward the cricoid ring, a complete ring of cartilage. In children younger than 2 or 3 years of age, the cricoid ring (in effect, the first tracheal ring) is the narrowest portion of the airway; in older children and adults, the glottis is the smallest part of the airway.

The trachea and main bronchi are supported by rings of cartilage that extend about 320 degrees around the airway circumference; the posterior wall is membranous. Beyond the lobar bronchi, the cartilaginous support for the airways becomes discontinuous. The more peripheral airways are supported entirely by elastic forces within the lung parenchyma.

The right lung normally has three lobes (upper, middle, and lower) and occupies about 55% of the total lung volume. The left lung normally has two lobes. The left upper lobe has an inferior division (the lingula) that is analogous to the middle lobe on the right.

PULMONARY PHYSIOLOGY
Pulmonary Mechanics

The major function of the lungs is to exchange oxygen (O_2) and carbon dioxide (CO_2) between the atmosphere and the blood. Factors that influence this function are the anatomy and mechanics of the airways, the mechanics of the respiratory muscles and rib cage, the structure of the blood-gas interface (i.e., the alveolar surface), the pulmonary circulation, and the central mechanisms for neuromuscular control of ventilation.

Air enters the lungs via the upper airway whenever the pressure in the thorax is less than that of the surrounding atmosphere. During inspiration at rest, the negative intrathoracic pressure is caused by contraction (and lowering) of the diaphragm. Accessory muscles of respiration may be recruited during labored breathing. The external intercostal, scalene, and sternocleidomastoid muscles lift the rib cage and thus function as muscles of inspiration. During quiet breathing, most exhalation is passive, but during forced exhalation, intrathoracic pressure is increased by the abdominal muscles and by the internal intercostal muscles, which pull the ribs together.

Airway resistance is determined by the diameter of the conducting airway, its length, the viscosity of the gas, and the nature of the airflow. During quiet breathing, airflow (especially in the smaller airways) may be laminar, in which case the resistance is inversely proportional, to the fourth power, of the radius of the airway. At higher flow rates (as during exercise), the flow becomes turbulent and the resistance increases even more. Thus relatively small changes in airway diameter (e.g., increases with normal growth or decreases resulting from mucosal edema or bronchoconstriction) may produce large changes in airway resistance. This phenomenon is more dramatically demonstrated in infants because the same degree of airway narrowing in the smaller airways of an infant produces proportionately greater physiologic effects than it does in the larger airways of an older child or an adult.

When all mechanical forces acting on the lung are at equilibrium (e.g., at the end of a normal relaxed breath), the lung contains a volume of gas known as the *functional residual capacity* (FRC) (Fig. 12–1). This gas volume is important in maintaining exchange of oxygen across the alveolar surface during exhalation. Alterations in pulmonary homeostasis that lead to decreased FRC include surfactant deficiency (neonatal respiratory distress syndrome), acute respiratory distress syndrome (ARDS), and restrictive lung diseases. Obstructive lung disease, such as cystic fibrosis, increases FRC.

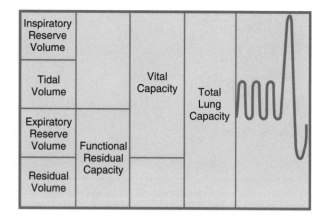

FIG. 12–1

Lung volumes and capacities. Although vital capacity and its subdivisions can be measured by spirometry, calculation of residual volume requires measurement of functional residual capacity by body plethysmography, helium dilution technique, or nitrogen washout. (From Andreoli TE, Bennett JC, Carpenter CJ, et al, editors: *Cecil essentials of medicine*, ed 4, Philadelphia, 1997, WB Saunders, p 127.)

Normal tidal breathing uses the middle range of lung volumes, reaching neither residual volume nor total lung capacity (Fig. 12–1). Residual volume (RV) is the volume of gas in the lungs at the end of a maximal exhalation, whereas total lung capacity (TLC) is the volume of gas in the lungs at the end of a maximal inhalation. Vital capacity (VC) is the difference between TLC and RV.

With *partial airway obstruction,* airways collapse during exhalation, preventing normal emptying and thus increasing RV and decreasing VC. An increase in degree of obstruction eventually increases FRC. Another manifestation of obstruction is decreased expiratory flow rates. A useful technique for clinically defining airway obstruction is to measure the volume of air exhaled during the first second of a forced vital capacity maneuver (forced expiratory volume in 1 second [FEV_1]). The forced expiratory flow rate (FEF_{25-75}) is the volume of air exhaled per second during the forced expiratory maneuver between 25% and 75% of forced vital capacity. It is more sensitive to obstruction in peripheral airways than is FEV_1. VC, FEV_1, and FEF_{25-75} are clinically useful measures and can be determined with a simple spirometer. Peak expiratory flow rate (PEFR) measures the most rapid rate of airflow (in liters/second or minute) during a forced expiratory maneuver. It is largely a measure of airflow in central airways and is highly dependent on patient effort. PEFR is best measured with a peak flowmeter, a simple hand-held device readily available in the office or emergency department setting.

Not all the air inspired during each breath reaches the alveoli. Normally, about 30% of each tidal breath fills the anatomic dead space (non–gas-exchanging parts of the respiratory system). The efficiency of ventilation therefore can be enhanced by increasing the tidal volume (because dead space is relatively constant). If tidal volume is decreased (as with central depression of respiratory drive or neuromuscular disease), the ratio of dead space to tidal volume will increase, and alveolar ventilation will decrease.

The most common forms of lung disease in children result in airway obstruction. Excess secretions, bronchospasm, mucosal edema, inflammation, stenosis, and airway compression (intraluminal or extraluminal masses or blood vessels) all may produce symptomatic airway obstruction. *Restrictive disease* is less common and is characterized by normal to low FRC and RV, low total lung capacity and VC, decreased lung compliance, and relatively normal flow rates.

Respiratory Gas Exchange

Gas exchange depends on alveolar ventilation and pulmonary capillary blood flow, as well as on the ability of the gases to diffuse across the alveolar-capillary surfaces. Carbon dioxide diffuses 20 times more readily than oxygen. Thus hypercapnia is a relatively late manifestation of disordered gas exchange, whereas hypoxemia occurs earlier. Under normal circumstances, physiologic matching of ventilation ($\dot{V}_A$) and blood flow ($\dot{Q}$) is maintained by anatomic mechanisms and local constriction of the pulmonary vessels in areas that are hypoventilated. The flow to the pulmonary circulation is capable of increasing at least fivefold. A significant percentage of the capillary bed is not open under normal resting conditions, and blood normally is shunted away from underventilated areas of the lung. However, if hypoxic pulmonary vasoconstriction fails for any reason, the underventilated lung continues to be perfused, and the blood returning from that area is unoxygenated, producing an intrapulmonary shunt with hypoxemia. Under normal circumstances, the hypoxemia leads to an increased minute volume and a fall in the arterial carbon dioxide partial pressure ($PaCO_2$) as the shunt increases. Additionally, disorders of unequal ventilation-perfusion matching are much more common causes of hypoxemia than are abnormalities of diffusion, especially in children (Table 12–1).

Control of Ventilation

Ventilation is controlled by central chemoreceptors in the medulla that respond to the intracellular pH (and, therefore, to the partial pressure of CO_2 [PCO_2]) (Fig. 12–2). To a lesser extent, ventilation also is controlled by peripheral receptors in the carotid and aortic bodies, which respond predominantly to the partial pressure of oxygen (PO_2). The central receptors are quite sensitive; small changes in $PaCO_2$ normally result in significant changes in minute ventilation. If $PaCO_2$ is elevated for some time, however, equilibration of the cerebral intracellular space to a higher bicarbonate level may result in relative hypoventilation for the degree of carbon dioxide elevation. The peripheral receptors do not affect ventilation until the arterial oxygen partial pressure (PaO_2) falls to approximately 50 torr. These receptors may become quite important when lung disease results in chronic elevation of $PaCO_2$.

The output of the central respiratory center also is modulated by reflex mechanisms. Full lung inflation inhibits inspiratory effort (the Hering-Breuer reflex) through vagal afferent fibers. Other reflexes from the airways and intercostal muscles may influence the depth and frequency of respiratory efforts (Fig. 12–2).

Lung Defense Mechanisms

The airways are a direct connection between the lungs and the atmosphere, which is not typically clean or sterile. Large particles are filtered primarily by the nose. The paranasal sinuses and the nasal turbinates are lined with ciliated epithelium, which carries these filtered particles to the pharynx. Particles smaller than 10 μm in diameter may reach the trachea and bronchi, where they are deposited on the mucosa. Particles smaller than 1 μm may reach the alveoli, where they either remain or are exhaled without being deposited. Ciliated cells line the airways from the larynx to the bronchioles; the cilia continuously move a thin layer of mucus toward the mouth, carrying inhaled particulates. Normally, mucociliary transport in the larger airways is fast, with rates averaging 10 mm/min. Alveolar macrophages and polymorphonuclear cells can engulf particles or pathogens opsonized by locally secreted immunoglobulin A (IgA) antibodies or transudated serum antibodies. Additional immunologically active proteins include the collectins (surfactant associated proteins), β defensins, and cathelicidins.

Reflex mechanisms also protect the lungs. The most important of these mechanisms is cough, a forceful expiration that removes foreign or infected

TABLE 12–1
Differentiation of Mechanisms of Hypoxia

Etiology	Example	Pao_2	$Paco_2$	A-aDO_2 (gradient)* Room Air	A-aDO_2 (gradient)* 100% O_2	$\dot{Q}s/\dot{Q}T$ (shunt)† Room Air	$\dot{Q}s/\dot{Q}T$ (shunt)† 100% O_2
Hypoventilation	Narcotic overdose, neuromuscular disease	↓	↑	N	N	N	N
Altitude	Mountain climbing	↓	↓	N	N	N	N
Intrapulmonary shunt	Atelectasis	↓	N or ↓	↑	↑	↑	↑
Cyanotic heart disease	Tetralogy of Fallot	↓	N or ↓	↑	↑	↑	↑
Pulmonary edema	Cardiomyopathy	↓	↓ N ↑	↑	N or ↑	↑	N or ↑
Acute respiratory distress syndrome	Sepsis, shock	↓	N to ↑	↑	N or ↑	↑	↑
Pneumonia	Lobar pneumococcal pneumonia	N or ↓	↓ or N	N or ↑	N	↑	↑
Pure $\dot{V}_A/\dot{Q}$ mismatch	Bronchopulmonary dysplasia, cystic fibrosis	↓	N or ↑	↑	N	↑	N
Diffusion defect	Scleroderma	↓	N	↑	N or ↑	↑	N

N, Normal; *Paco₂*, arterial carbon dioxide partial pressure; *Pao₂*, arterial oxygen partial pressure.
*A-aDO_2 = alveolar-arterial O_2 gradient, which is not influenced by changes in minute ventilation and is a measure of gas exchange. The A-aDO_2 can be determined by the *alveolar gas equation:* A-aDO_2 = $(P_B - pH_2O) \times Fio_2 - Paco_2/R$, where P_B = atmospheric pressure (usually 760 mm Hg); pH_2O = partial pressure of H_2O (~ 47 mm Hg); R = respiratory exchange ratio (0.8); Fio_2 = inspired O_2 (21% for room air). Normal value of A-aDO_2 = 30–50 mm Hg (while breathing 100% O_2). Under normal conditions, alveolar or inspired O_2 should be close to arterial O_2.
†$\dot{Q}s/\dot{Q}T$ = the calculation of venous admixture or shunt. $\dot{Q}s$ = flow through the shunt (area of perfusion but no ventilation). $\dot{Q}T$ = total cardiac output to well-ventilated and poorly ventilated (shunt) areas of the lung. An increased $\dot{Q}s/\dot{Q}T$ is the result of shunting or ventilation-perfusion inequality ($\dot{V}_A/\dot{V}Q$). With 100% O_2, $\dot{V}_A/\dot{V}Q$ is eliminated and the $\dot{Q}s/\dot{Q}T$ represents shunting.

FIG. 12–2

Schematic representation of the respiratory control system. The respiratory neurons in the brainstem receive information from the chemoreceptors, peripheral sensory receptors, and cerebral cortex. This information is integrated, and the resulting neural output is transmitted to the chest bellows and lungs. +, Stimulation; −, inhibition. (From Andreoli TE, Bennett JC, Carpenter CJ, et al, editors: *Cecil essentials of medicine,* ed 4, Philadelphia, 1997, WB Saunders, p 171.)

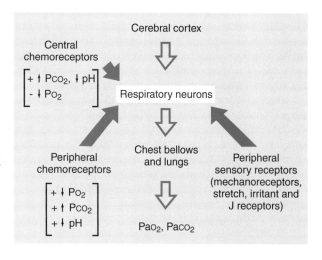

material from the airways. A cough may be voluntary or may be generated by reflex irritation of the nose, sinus, pharynx, larynx, trachea, bronchi, or bronchioles. During a cough, the person inspires deeply, to 60–80% of total lung capacity (~ 100 cm H_2O); the glottis closes, the expiratory muscles contract to increase intrathoracic pressure, and the glottis opens suddenly, forcefully releasing air from the system. Loss of the cough reflex leads to aspiration and pneumonia. In young infants secretions may be swallowed rather than expectorated. Nasal irritation may produce reflex bronchoconstriction to limit the penetration of noxious vapors.

REFERENCES

Behrman RE, Kliegman RM, Jenson HB, editors: *Nelson textbook of pediatrics*, ed 16, Philadelphia, 2000, WB Saunders, Chapters 373–375.
Maturation of the respiratory system. In Loughlin GM, Eigen H, editors: *Respiratory disease in children: diagnosis and management*, Baltimore, 1994, Williams & Wilkins.
West JB: *Respiratory physiology: the essentials*, ed 5, Baltimore, 1997, Williams & Wilkins.

DIAGNOSTIC MEASURES
Patient Evaluation, History-Taking, and Physical Examination

The diagnostic evaluation begins with a careful and complete history and physical examination. Much can be learned by seemingly casual observation of the child during the formal history-taking with the parents. The physician should also question the child because children as young as 3–4 years of age

often know things their parents do not ("last week I choked on a peanut"). The signs or symptoms in children with airway disease often appear quite different during sleep, and therefore the physician should inquire specifically about observations of the sleeping child.

To avoid producing anxiety in the child, the physician might recommend that the parent hold the child in his or her lap during the physical examination. For the observation of the respiratory pattern, rate, depth, and retractions, the child should be quiet and not crying. Clothing should be removed from the upper half of the child's body so that the thorax may be clearly inspected. The observations made during auscultation of the chest may be misleading in young children because they may not take a breath deep enough to produce audible **crackles (rales)** or **rhonchi** (described later in this section), despite the presence of fluid in the alveoli and small airways. With patience, however, most infants can be observed during at least one deep inspiration. The physician may induce older children to take a deep breath by asking them to pretend to blow out a candle.

The *respiratory rate* is an important indicator of respiratory status. Any factor that impairs respiratory mechanics is likely to result in more rapid breathing. Because anxiety or excitement also increases respiratory rates, the sleeping respiratory rate is most reliable. Infants younger than 1 year of age have sleeping rates ranging from 25–35 breaths/min; while awake, the same infants may take from 40–60 breaths each minute. With increasing maturity, sleeping rates gradually decline toward the adult range of 10–15 breaths/min (Table 12–2).

TABLE 12–2
Breathing Patterns

Pattern	Features
Normal rate (breaths/min)	*Preterm:* 40–60 *Term:* 30–40 *5 yr:* 25 *10 yr:* 20 *15 yr:* 16 *Adult:* 12
Obstructed	
Mild	Reduced rate, increased tidal volume
Severe	Increased rate, increased retraction of accessory muscles, anxiety, cyanosis
Restrictive	Rapid rate, decreased tidal volume
Kussmaul respiration	Increased rate, increased tidal volume, regular deep respiration; consider metabolic acidosis or diabetes mellitus
Cheyne-Stokes respiration	Gradually increasing tidal volume followed sequentially by gradually decreasing tidal volume and apnea; consider central nervous system injury, depressant drugs, heart failure, uremia, or prematurity
Biot respiration	Ataxic or periodic breathing with a respiratory effort followed by apnea; consider brainstem injury or posterior fossa mass
Gasping	Slow rate, variable tidal volume; consider hypoxia, shock, sepsis, or asphyxia

In addition to the rate of respiration, its *pattern* or depth and the degree of effort required for its maintenance are important points to note. *Hyperpnea* (increased depth of respiration) may occur with fever, metabolic acidosis, salicylism, pulmonary and cardiac disease, or extreme anxiety (as in hyperventilation syndrome or panic attack). Hyperpnea without signs of respiratory distress suggests a nonpulmonary etiology (acidosis, fever, and salicylism). When the degree of effort is increased because of airway obstruction or decreased pulmonary compliance, the intrathoracic pressure may be more negative than usual, and intercostal retractions can be observed (Table 12–2). Use of accessory muscles such as the sternocleidomastoids should be apparent on physical examination and should alert the physician to the presence of a pathologic pulmonary condition. In children, increased inspiratory effort also results in flaring of the alae nasi, which is a relatively reliable sign of dyspnea. **Grunting** (forced expiration against a partially closed glottis) suggests hypoxia, atelectasis, pneumonia, or pulmonary edema.

The *sounds of breathing* deserve careful documentation. **Stridor,** usually heard on inspiration, is a harsh sound that emanates from the upper airway and is caused by a partially obstructed extrathoracic airway. If stridor is accompanied by signs of respiratory distress or if it is present at rest, immediate investigation and intervention are required. Stridor also may be chronic or congenital in nature, in which case it may be of less importance physiologically unless infection further compromises the airway.

A **wheeze** is produced by partial obstruction of the lower airway and is heard on exhalation. Wheezes may be harsh and low-pitched (usually from large, central airways) or high-pitched and almost musical (from small, peripheral airways). Secretions in the intrathoracic airways may result in wheezing, but more commonly they result in irregular sounds called **rhonchi.** Fluid or secretions in the alveolar spaces or terminal airways may produce a sound that is characteristic of crumpling cellophane **(rales** or **crackles).** This sound may disappear after a few deep inspirations or a cough, but its persistence suggests pneumonitis or pulmonary edema. The quality of breath sounds may be **bronchial,** normally heard over the trachea, with inspiration and expiration clearly auscultated. More peripheral breath sounds are **vesicular,** with a greater proportion of inspiration heard as the expiratory component lessens. Bronchial breath sounds in the lung periphery suggest consolidation or the interface of a pleural effusion.

The physical findings discussed here, when combined with inspection for tracheal or cardiac deviation, chest wall motion, percussion, fremitus, voice signs, and the presence or absence of breath sounds, help identify the intrathoracic pathology (Table 12–3). **Digital clubbing** is a sign of chronic pulmonary disease, but it also may be noted in other chronic diseases (cyanotic congenital heart disease, endocarditis, celiac disease, inflammatory bowel disease, chronic active hepatitis, biliary cirrhosis, thalassemia, and Hodgkin disease) or, rarely, as a benign familial trait.

Imaging Techniques

Chest roentgenograms are extremely useful in diagnosing respiratory disease in children, but they must be performed in a technically correct manner and be properly interpreted. Failure to obtain satisfactory inspiration, the most common problem, may lead to the erroneous impression of cardiomegaly or of the presence of infiltrates. External skinfolds, rotation or other improper position of the chest, or motion also may produce a distorted or unclear image. Whenever possible, chest roentgenograms should be obtained in both the posteroanterior and the lateral projections. Lesions may be apparent on only one of the two views. Expiratory views or fluoroscopy is helpful in detecting the presence of partial bronchial obstruction; a lung or lobe that does not empty on expiration appears hyperinflated.

A *barium esophagram* frequently is of great value in the diagnosis of chest disease in children. Disorders of swallowing or esophageal motility, vascular rings, tracheoesophageal fistulas, or gastroesophageal reflux may lead to aspiration and recurrent or persistent pulmonary disease. When the esophagram reveals that abnormal vascular structures are compressing the esophagus, this may be a major clue that those same vessels are compressing the airways. When the examination involves the search for an H-type tracheoesophageal fistula, the contrast material should be injected into the esophagus under pressure through a catheter while the injection sites are observed in the lateral projection. Simple barium swallows are much less likely to demonstrate the often small connection between the trachea and esophagus.

Computed tomography (CT) is quite useful in diagnosing chest disease in children, especially in evaluating lesions in the mediastinum or hilum. Rapid, fine-cut, high-resolution CT provides information about the lumen size or presence of masses within the central intrathoracic airways; bronchiectasis also may be detected. Chest CT may also be useful in the evaluation of pulmonary embolism, pleural effusion, pulmonary abscess, and interstitial pneumonitis.

Magnetic resonance imaging (MRI) can identify

TABLE 12–3
Physical Signs of Pulmonary Disease

Disease Process	Mediastinal Deviation	Chest Motion	Vocal Fremitus	Percussion	Breath Sounds	Adventitious Sounds	Voice Signs
Consolidation	No	Reduced over area	Increased	Dull	Bronchial or reduced	Rales	Egophony,* whispering, pectoriloquy increased†
Bronchospasm	No	Hyperexpansion with limited motion	Normal or decreased	Hyperresonant	Normal to decreased	Wheezes, rales	Normal to decreased
Atelectasis	Shift toward lesion	Reduced over area	Decreased	Dull	Reduced	None or rales	None
Pneumothorax	Tension deviates trachea and PMI to opposite side	Reduced over area	None	Resonant	None	None	None
Pleural effusion	Deviation to opposite side	Reduced over area	None or reduced	Dull	None	Friction rub; splash if hemopneumothorax	None
Interstitial process	No	Reduced	Normal to increased	Normal	Normal	Rales	None

Adapted from Andreoli TE, Bennett JC, Carpenter CJ, et al, editors: *Cecil essentials of medicine*, ed 4, Philadelphia, 1997, WB Saunders, p 115.
PMI, Point of maximum impulse.
*Egophony is present when *e* sounds like *a*.
†Whispering pectoriloquy produces clearer-sounding whispered words.

pathologic conditions in the trachea and large central airways. MRI also may visualize the relationships between the great vessels and central airways.

Ultrasonography can determine the nature of some intrathoracic masses and the presence of pleural fluid and can identify loculated fluid collections, such as those occurring with empyema or complicated pleural effusion. Diaphragmatic dysfunction (e.g., paralysis or paresis) may also be assessed by ultrasound examination.

Measures of Respiratory Gas Exchange

A properly performed *arterial blood gas analysis* is one of the most useful measures of lung function, but it is nonspecific in terms of the etiology of dysfunction. Because of the shape of the oxyhemoglobin dissociation curve, oxygen saturation does not fall appreciably until the PaO_2 reaches approximately 60 torr. The arterial pH and PCO_2 also are important measures of respiratory function; PCO_2 is regulated almost entirely by ventilation (given a constant carbon dioxide production). Bicarbonate concentration is regulated chiefly by the kidneys. The distinction should be made between metabolic and respiratory causes of acidosis or alkalosis. At the normal pH of 7.4, the $PaCO_2$ should be about 40 torr, and the bicarbonate about 25 mEq/L. This relationship is governed by the Henderson-Hasselbalch equation:

$$pH = 6.1 + \log ([HCO_3]/0.03 \, PCO_2)$$

Thus it is the ratio of bicarbonate to PCO_2 that governs pH. Metabolic acidosis, which exhibits low bicarbonate, can be compensated by hyperventilation, which lowers the PCO_2, whereas respiratory acidosis, which is due to elevated PCO_2, can be compensated by renal retention of bicarbonate. Respiratory compensation is a much faster process than renal compensation, which generally requires several days to reach equilibrium.

Noninvasive methods of assessing oxygenation and ventilation are available; however, the information provided, although useful, has more limited value than arterial blood gas measurement. *Pulse oximetry* (measurement of oxygen saturation using light absorption) provides a painless, relatively easy, and reliable means of measuring oxygenation. A small probe consisting of a light source and sensor is clipped to a finger or toe, and either continuous or single oxygen saturation measurements are obtained. *Capnography* (measurement of carbon dioxide by gas analysis) permits a measure of ventilation. Monitoring the content of carbon dioxide in expired air (sampled at end-expiration or averaged over the respiratory cycle) provides an approximate measure of alveolar PCO_2. Although they are most com-

monly used in intubated and mechanically ventilated patients, capnography units that monitor carbon dioxide content in expired air at the nares are now available. Similarly, transcutaneous electrodes may be used to monitor PO_2 and PCO_2 at the skin surface, but these techniques are best suited for continuous monitoring in an intensive care unit and for detecting trends rather than for providing absolute numbers.

Pulmonary Function Testing

The simplest clinically useful measures of ventilatory function are *vital capacity* and *expiratory flow rates*, which can be measured with a spirometer. Simple spirometry can be performed in most children 6 years of age or older. Even an older child cannot be expected to perform reproducibly without training and experience with the technique, and great care must be taken in interpreting the results of testing. Predicted values for lung functions are based on the patient's height and gender. Airway resistance, FRC, and RV (among other measures) require the use of a plethysmograph and a spirometer. Flow rates at lower lung volumes are relatively independent of effort and reflect the function of more peripheral airways. Full forced expiratory maneuvers in sedated infants using an inflatable jacket to produce a rapid thoracoabdominal compression can be obtained.

Pulmonary function studies may be useful in evaluating an older child's functional status, although they rarely yield an etiologic diagnosis. Abnormal results may be described in terms of **obstructive disease** (e.g., low flow rates and increased RV or FRC) or **restrictive disease** (e.g., low VC and TLC, with relative preservation of flow rates and FRC); in addition, the extent of functional impairment often can be estimated.

Pulmonary function testing also can be used to detect reversible airway obstruction characteristic of asthma. A significant increase in pulmonary function after the inhalation of a bronchodilator indicates reactive airway disease. These tests are useful not only for determining the diagnosis but also for managing therapy. Inhalational *challenge testing* with methacholine or cold, dry air is another useful test for the diagnosis of reactive airway disease, but such tests require more sophisticated equipment and special expertise and can be performed only in a formal pulmonary function laboratory.

Endoscopic Evaluation of the Airways

Diagnostic *bronchoscopy* is indicated whenever necessary information about the lungs or airways can be most definitively, safely, or rapidly obtained by this method. Airway structure can be examined, the dynamics of the airways during breathing can be documented, and specimens can be obtained for a variety of diagnostic purposes. For patients of any age, no absolute contraindications to bronchoscopy exist, provided that the proper equipment is available and the physician's skill is adequate. Flexible instruments are advantageous for most diagnostic purposes, whereas rigid instruments must be used for foreign body extraction and for most operative procedures. An airway mucosal biopsy is also possible through pediatric-sized flexible bronchoscopes. Bronchoscopy accompanied by bronchoalveolar lavage assists in the diagnosis of pulmonary infection, particularly in the immunocompromised patient.

Laryngoscopy often is useful in the diagnosis of stridor and should be performed carefully under appropriate conditions and with the use of sedation, anesthesia, or both. The common technique of *direct* laryngoscopy at the bedside or in the treatment room in an unsedated infant or young child is traumatic to the child, and the results often are misleading. Mirror *(indirect)* laryngoscopy usually can be performed in children 4–5 years of age or older; in infants and younger children, however, transnasal laryngoscopy using a flexible bronchoscope yields much better diagnostic information.

Examination of Sputum

Sputum specimens, although important in evaluating inflammatory processes in the lower airways, are often difficult to obtain in young children. An expectorated specimen may not provide a representative sample of the lower airway secretions, but microscopic examination helps determine the source of a putative sputum specimen. Sputum should contain macrophages; often ciliated cells also are seen. Material containing large numbers of squamous epithelial cells either is most likely not from the lower airways or is heavily contaminated, so that diagnostic tests performed on such a specimen may yield misleading results. Infected sputum should have many polymorphonucleated leukocytes and one predominant organism in large numbers present on Gram stain. If sputum cannot be obtained, obtaining lung washings by bronchoscopy for microbiologic or cytologic diagnosis may be useful in selected situations (bronchoalveolar lavage).

Lung Biopsy

When less invasive methods have failed in the diagnosis of pulmonary disease, lung biopsy may be re-quired. Although transbronchial lung biopsy through a bronchoscope is useful in adults, a thoracotomy with open biopsy has major advantages in most pediatric patients; thoracotomy allows the surgeon to inspect and palpate the lung and initially to choose the best site for performing the biopsy, and open biopsy provides sufficient material for a variety of diagnostic tests. The site of biopsy should be chosen after inspection of the involved lobe on roentgenogram. In most cases, infants and children tolerate open lung biopsy well.

REFERENCES

Behrman RE, Kliegman RM, Jenson HB, editors: *Nelson textbook of pediatrics,* ed 16, Philadelphia, 2000, WB Saunders, Chapter 377.

Castile R, Filbrun D, Flucke R, et al: Adult type pulmonary function tests in infants without respiratory disease, *Pediatr Pulmonol* 30(3):215–227, 2000.

Effman EL: Basic concepts of lung imaging. In Chernik V, Mellins RB, editors: *Basic mechanisms of pediatric respiratory disease,* Philadelphia, 1991, BC Decker.

McLoud TC: CT and MR in pleural disease, *Clin Chest Med* 19(2):261–276, 1998.

Moyle JT: Uses and abuses of pulse oximetry, *Arch Dis Child* 74(1):77–80, 1996.

Naidich DP, Harkin TJ: Airways and lung: correlation of CT with fiberoptic bronchoscopy, *Radiology* 197(1):1–12, 1995.

Wood RE: Bronchoscopy. In Loughlin GM, Eigen H, editors: *Respiratory disease in children: diagnosis and management,* Baltimore, 1994, Williams & Wilkins.

THERAPEUTIC MEASURES
Oxygen Administration

Any child in respiratory distress should be given supplemental oxygen as soon as feasible. Although depressing the respiratory drive is possible if the patient's central chemoreceptors are blunted by chronic hypercapnia, patients in such a state are rare in pediatric practice and should be readily recognized as having chronic, severe respiratory disease (e.g., cystic fibrosis or bronchopulmonary dysplasia). Even in these patients, oxygen therapy may be lifesaving without producing apnea.

In the acute situation, an appropriately sized mask is often the most useful technique for administering oxygen, although some children may become frightened. For a frightened child, a high-flow oxygen source may be held near the child's face until a more satisfactory method can be arranged. For chronic administration of oxygen, a nasal cannula may be helpful because it frees the face and mouth, allowing the patient to eat and speak unhindered by the oxygen delivery system.

The concentration of oxygen administered should be high enough to relieve hypoxemia, yet as low as feasible to prevent oxygen toxicity. In general, inspired oxygen concentrations below 40% are safe for long-term use. Determining the concentration of inspired oxygen is more difficult in patients receiving oxygen by nasal cannula; titrating the delivery (in liters/min) according to measurements of PaO_2 or by pulse oximetry is best. The safe, acceptable range of oxygen saturation is 92–95%. It is unnecessary to achieve 100% saturation, especially because this may require potentially toxic levels of inspired oxygen. Oxygen, as obtained from tanks or wall sources, is dry and must be humidified to avoid dehydration of the mucosa of the upper respiratory tract.

Aerosol Therapy

Delivering therapeutic agents to the lower respiratory tract often is accomplished by having the patient inhale the agents in aerosol form. The use of aerosol generators that deliver relatively small particles (2–5 μm) is necessary to achieve optimum deposition in the lower airways. The pattern of the patient's breathing greatly influences deposition of the particles. Slow, deep inspirations are needed for maximal effect, but most children, especially infants, cannot perform in this fashion. However, inhaling aerosols from a face mask or mouthpiece for a period of several minutes during quiet tidal breathing will usually achieve the desired therapeutic effect. Metered-dose inhalers produce a high-pressure stream of particles and with proper technique deposit an amount of medication in the lower airways equivalent to that with an aerosol generator. Infants and children should use spacer devices that trap the respirable aerosol particles issuing from the inhaler into a chamber from which the patient then breathes more slowly.

The drugs most often given by aerosol are bronchodilators. In certain situations, antibiotics may be given by aerosol.

Physical Therapy

When disease processes impair clearance of pulmonary secretions, physical therapy may help maintain airway patency. Percussion of the thorax over the pulmonary segments while the patient is positioned so that the airways of the percussed segments are directed downward may move secretions toward the central airways, from which they can be expectorated. Chest physiotherapy may also be effectively performed with techniques and devices such as autogenic drainage, the flutter valve, and percussive vests. A typical therapy session may require 15–30 minutes; most children with lung disease requiring chest physiotherapy need one to four such sessions daily. In older children, sustained exercise (for 5–15 minutes) that produces hyperpnea also can be helpful. Chest physiotherapy is most beneficial for children with cystic fibrosis but also may be useful for individuals with neuromuscular disease and atelectasis. It generally is not beneficial for pneumonia or asthma.

Intubation

When the natural upper airway is obstructed because of disease or when assisted ventilation is needed because of disease or anesthesia, providing an artificial airway for the patient may be necessary. Intubation alters the physiology of the respiratory tract in a number of ways, not all of which are beneficial: it interferes with the humidification, warming, and filtration of inspired air; with phonation; and with transport of secretions by mucociliary escalation and through cough. Intubation also stimulates increased production of secretions. Depending on the reason for the intubation, the airway resistance may be increased or decreased and the physiologic dead space may be increased.

Endotracheal tubes can easily damage the larynx and the airways if the tubes are of improper size or are not carefully maintained. Because the cricoid ring is the smallest portion of the airway in children and is completely surrounded by cartilage, it is vulnerable to damage, which results in subglottic stenosis. If the tube pressure exceeds capillary filling pressure (roughly 35 cm H_2O) against the airway mucosa, mucosal ischemia develops and, within hours, mucosal necrosis results. An endotracheal tube should allow a small air leak at the larynx.

Artificial airways of all types must be kept clear of secretions. Mucous plugs in artificial airways can be fatal. Providing adequate humidification of the inspired air and suctioning the tube will help reduce the probability of occlusion by secretions.

Tracheostomy

Tracheostomy is the surgical placement of an artificial airway into the trachea below the larynx. If prolonged intubation is anticipated, elective tracheostomy should be considered to prevent laryngeal trauma and subsequent subglottic stenosis and to increase the patient's comfort and the ease of nursing care. Unfortunately, no clear guidelines are available as to how long a particular patient is likely to tolerate an endotracheal tube or when a tracheostomy is necessary. Once laryngeal damage has occurred, the probability of subglottic stenosis is much higher.

Children with **subglottic stenosis** may require a tracheostomy for a prolonged period. Because the tracheostomy tube typically prevents the child from effectively phonating and thus from communicating distress, the child must be monitored carefully at all times. As with endotracheal tubes, tracheostomy tubes must be kept clear and clean, and vigilant care must be taken to reduce complications. Occlusion of the tube with secretions or accidental dislodgment of the tube can be fatal. Children with tracheostomies may be successfully cared for at home if the caretakers are well trained and adequately equipped.

Mechanical Ventilation

Patients who are unable to maintain an adequate gas exchange because of airway obstruction, an intrapulmonary pathologic condition, neuromuscular disease, or other factors are candidates for mechanical ventilation. Techniques for mechanical ventilation involve inflation of the lungs with compressed gas. Exhalation is always passive. No method accurately mimics the natural breathing mechanisms, and all methods have their drawbacks and complications.

Positive pressure ventilation requires intubation or tracheostomy. Positive pressure is transmitted to the entire thorax and may impede venous return to the heart during inspiration (venous return increases during spontaneous inspiration). The airways and lung parenchyma may be damaged by high inflation pressures, as well as by high inspired oxygen concentrations. In general, inflation pressures should be limited to those necessary to provide sufficient lung expansion for adequate ventilation and prevention of atelectasis. Other modes of ventilation are high-frequency jet ventilation and very-high-frequency oscillation; these techniques are used to reduce mean airway pressure and thus the probability of barotrauma (see Chapter 6).

Pressure-cycled ventilators frequently are used in infants and deliver an indefinite volume of gas at a fixed inflation pressure. A major disadvantage of this system is that the pressure is sensed in the ventilator circuit rather than in the lung, and increasing degrees of airway resistance (e.g., occlusion of the endotracheal tube) will result in decreasing delivered volumes. *Volume-cycled ventilators* deliver a fixed volume of gas at whatever inflation pressure is necessary, up to a preset maximum. These instruments are more often used in children and adolescents. In either case, the response of the patient must be as-

sessed carefully and frequently. Regardless of the method chosen for ventilation, alveolar ventilation (assessed by breath sounds, chest wall excursion, and arterial blood gas measurements) and oxygenation (assessed by arterial blood gas measurements or oximetry) must be adequate.

The normal tidal volume is 5–7 mL/kg body weight; values less than this usually result in hypoventilation and hypercapnia. Patients with lung disease and uneven distribution of ventilation often require larger tidal volumes; most volume-cycled ventilators are operated at tidal volumes of 8–10 mL/kg body weight. Continuous ventilation at smaller volumes results in redistribution of surfactant and atelectasis. Low tidal volume ventilation with permissive hypercarbia reduces the risk of barotrauma. An occasional full lung inflation may be provided by a "sigh" on some ventilators or by inflation with an Ambu bag to prevent atelectasis.

REFERENCES

Behrman RE, Kliegman RM, Jenson HB, editors: *Nelson textbook of pediatrics,* ed 16, Philadelphia, 2000, WB Saunders, Chapter 377.

Chatburn RL: Mechanical ventilators. In Branson RD, Hess DR, Chatburn RL, editors: *Respiratory care equipment,* ed 2, Philadelphia, 1999, Lippincott, Williams & Wilkins.

MAJOR PEDIATRIC PULMONARY SYMPTOM COMPLEXES
Upper Airway Obstruction

An upper airway obstruction is defined as blockage of the portion of the airways located above the thoracic inlet. A blockage is manifested during inspiration because the pressure within the upper airway is negative relative to the atmosphere. This negative pressure tends to collapse the upper airway, producing the characteristic sounds associated with upper airway obstruction. Upper airway obstruction ranges from nasal obstruction associated with the common cold to life-threatening obstruction of the larynx or upper trachea. Nasal obstruction is usually more of a nuisance than a danger because the mouth can be used as an airway; however, it may be a serious problem for neonates, who breathe predominantly through the nose. The etiology of airway obstruction varies with the age of the child (Tables 12–4 and 12–5), and a careful history and physical examination are necessary for the diagnosis.

The *clinical manifestation* most commonly associated with upper airway obstruction is inspiratory **stridor,** a harsh sound produced usually at or near the larynx by the vibration of upper airway

---

TABLE 12–4
Age-Related Differential Diagnosis of Airway Obstruction

Newborn
Foreign material (e.g., meconium or amniotic fluid)
Congenital subglottic stenosis (uncommon)
Choanal atresia
Micrognathia (Pierre Robin syndrome, Treacher Collins syndrome, DiGeorge syndrome)
Macroglossia (Beckwith-Wiedemann syndrome, hypothyroidism, Pompe disease, trisomy 21, hemangioma)
Laryngeal web, clefts, atresia
Laryngospasm (intubation, aspiration, transient)
Vocal cord paralysis (weak cry; unilateral or bilateral, with or without increased intracranial pressure from Arnold-Chiari malformation or other CNS pathology)
Tracheal web, stenosis, malacia, atresia
Pharyngeal collapse (cause of apnea in preterm infant)
Dislocated nasal cartilage
Nasal pyriform aperture stenosis
Nasal encephalocele

Infancy
Laryngomalacia (most common etiology)
Subglottic stenosis (congenital, acquired after intubation)
Hemangioma
Tongue tumor (dermoid, teratoma, ectopic thyroid)
Laryngeal dyskinesis

Infancy—cont'd
Laryngeal papillomatosis
Vascular rings
Rhinitis

Toddlers
Viral croup (most common etiology in children 6 months to 4 years of age)
Bacterial tracheitis (toxic, high fever)
Foreign body (sudden cough; airway or esophageal)
Spasmodic (recurrent) croup
Laryngeal papillomatosis
Retropharyngeal abscess
Hypertrophied tonsils and adenoids
Diphtheria (rare)

Above 2–3 Years Old
Epiglottitis (infection, aryepiglottic folds; uncommon)
Inhalation injury (burns, toxic gas, hydrocarbons)
Foreign bodies
Rhinitis medicamentosa
Angioedema (familial history, cutaneous angioedema)
Anaphylaxis (allergic history, wheezing, hypotension)
Trauma (tracheal or laryngeal fracture)
Peritonsillar abscess (adolescents)
Mononucleosis
Ludwig angina
Diphtheria (rare)

CNS, Central nervous system.

---

structures. Less commonly, stridor also may be an expiratory noise. Hoarseness suggests involvement of the vocal cords, whereas stridor that changes with position of the child's head or neck suggests a supraglottic etiology. Children with laryngomalacia or pharyngeal hypotonia may exhibit much less stridor while crying because their parapharyngeal muscle tone increases. In contrast, an obstructing lesion below the glottis usually produces more stridor during crying because the inspiratory flow rates increase. In many children stridor decreases during sleep because inspiratory flow rates are lowest at that time. Positional stridor suggests an anatomic problem.

A child with upper airway obstruction usually has some degree of suprasternal retraction as a result of the pressure gradient between the trachea and the atmosphere. Obstruction below the thoracic inlet seldom leads to suprasternal retraction because the major pressure drop occurs below the sternal notch.

Radiographic evaluation of the child with stridor should include views of the lateral neck and nasopharynx and an anteroposterior (AP) view of the neck taken with the head in extension. The subglottic space on the AP view should be symmetric, and the lateral walls of the airway should fall away steeply. Asymmetry suggests subglottic stenosis or a mass lesion, whereas narrow tapering suggests subglottic edema. An important differential diagnosis is the diagnosis between supraglottic and subglottic obstruction (Table 12–6).

Lower Airway Obstruction

In contrast to upper airway obstruction, obstruction of the airways below the thoracic inlet produces more expiratory symptoms than inspiratory symptoms. During inspiration, intrathoracic pressure becomes negative relative to the atmosphere. Therefore, the airways tend to increase their diameter during inspiration, and unless substantial, relatively fixed obstruction (or increased airway secretion) is present, few or no abnormal noises may be generated during inspiration. Intrathoracic pressure is increased relative to atmospheric pressure during exhalation, which tends to collapse the intrathoracic airways and produce wheezing. A **wheeze** is a relatively continuous expiratory sound, generally with a more musical quality than stridor, that is produced by turbulent airflow. Partial airway obstruction may produce wheezing only during the later phase of exhalation.

The *etiology* of wheezing involves multiple causes (Table 12–7), the most common of which is diffuse bronchial obstruction resulting from constriction of bronchial smooth muscle, airway inflammation, or excessive secretions. However, the importance of the aphorism "All that wheezes is not asthma" cannot be overemphasized. Although it often is useful to administer a bronchodilator to determine whether the wheezing is acutely reversible, mere reversibility does not establish a diagnosis of asthma, nor does it eliminate anatomic causes of wheezing. Conversely, the most common cause of wheezing in childhood is reactive airway disease (asthma). Wheezing that begins in the first weeks or months of life or that is persistent despite maximal bronchodilator therapy is more likely to be the result of some other cause, and more extensive diagnostic evaluation may be warranted. Because of their small airways, children younger than 2–3 years of age are more likely to wheeze in response to viral infections. Wheezing that is localized to one area of the chest deserves especially close diagnostic attention (e.g., foreign body or compressing lymph node).

Although children known to have asthma certainly do not need *roentgenographic evaluation* with each episode of wheezing, other children with significant respiratory distress, fever, history of aspiration, localizing signs, or persistent wheezing should have chest films included as part of their diagnostic evaluation. Both posteroanterior and lateral views should be obtained. Generalized hyperinflation, with flattening of the diaphragm and an increased AP diameter of the chest, suggests diffuse obstruction of small airways. Localized hyperinflation, especially on expiratory films, suggests localized bronchial obstruction, such as with a foreign body or anatomic anomalies.

Cough

Cough is one of the most common (and sometimes most vexing) respiratory symptoms at all ages. Cough results from stimulation of irritant receptors in the airway mucosa or in other respiratory locations, including the ear. It may have many different characteristics, depending on anatomic factors and the cause of the irritation, and significant diagnostic information usually may be derived from the history and physical examination.

Most cases of *acute cough* are associated with respiratory infections (e.g., pneumonia, rhinitis, tracheobronchitis, bronchitis, sinusitis, or pertussis), and the cough subsides with resolution of the infection. A history of the sudden onset of choking and coughing is often described after aspiration of a foreign body. Other causes include pulmonary edema, thermal or chemical inhalation injury (smoke), and pulmonary embolism or hemorrhage.

Chronic cough (daily cough for greater than 6 weeks), however, has a more diverse etiology, including allergy (e.g., asthma, postnasal drip syndrome, or rhinitis), anatomic abnormalities (e.g., tracheoesophageal fistula, cysts, or gastroesophageal reflux), chronic infection (e.g., cystic fibrosis, sinusitis, recurrent aspiration pneumonia, abscess, tuberculosis, fungal pneumonia, histoplasmosis, or acquired immunodeficiency syndrome [AIDS]–related infection), environmental exposure to irritants (e.g., smoking, hypersensitivity pneumonitis, or drug abuse), foreign body aspiration, psychogenic causes (habit, cough tic, or Tourette syndrome), and neurologic dysfunction.

Children in the first several years of life often have frequent viral respiratory infections, especially if they are exposed to many other children, as in day care centers. Cough that resolves promptly and clearly is associated with a viral infection and does not require further diagnostic evaluation. However, cough that persists beyond 4–6 weeks and is not associated with classic viral upper respiratory tract infection symptoms may necessitate investigation.

The circumstances under which chronic cough occurs are important to consider in diagnosis. Nocturnal cough suggests allergy (especially to antigens in the child's bedroom), asthma, gastroesophageal reflux, or drainage from sinuses. Cough associated with exercise suggests reactive airway disease or bronchitis and bronchiectasis. Cough on first arising in the morning frequently is associated

TABLE 12–5
Differential Diagnosis of Acute Upper Airway Obstruction

	Laryngotracheobronchitis (Croup)	Laryngitis	Spasmodic Croup	Epiglottitis	Membranous Croup (Bacterial Tracheitis)
Age	6 mo–3 yr	5 yr–teens	3 mo–3 yr	2–6 yr	Any age (3–10 yr)
Location	Subglottic	Subglottic	Subglottic	Supraglottic	Trachea
Etiology	Parainfluenza virus, influenza virus, RSV; rarely *Mycoplasma*, measles, adenovirus	As per croup	Unknown	*Haemophilus influenzae* b and a	Prior croup or influenza virus with secondary bacterial infection by *Staphylococcus aureus*, *Moraxella catarrhalis*, *H. influenzae*
Prodrome onset	Insidious, URI	As per croup	Sudden onset at night; prior episodes	Rapid, short prodrome	Biphasic illness with sudden deterioration
Stridor	Yes	None	Yes	Yes—soft inspiratory	Yes
Retractions	Yes	None	Yes	Yes	Yes
Voice	Hoarse	Hoarse; whispered	Hoarse	Muffled	Normal or hoarse
Position and appearance	Normal	Normal	Normal	Tripod sitting leaning forward; agitation	Normal
Swallowing (dysphagia)	Normal	Normal	Normal	Drooling	Normal
Barking cough	Yes	Rare	Yes	No	Yes
Toxicity	Rare	No	No	Severe	Severe; may also manifest toxic shock syndrome
Fever	<101° F	<101° F	None	>102° F	>102° F
X-ray	Subglottic narrowing; steeple sign	Normal	Subglottic narrowing	Thumb sign of thickened epiglottis	Ragged irregular tracheal border; as per croup
WBC count	Normal	Normal	Normal	Leukocytosis with left shift	Leukocytosis with left shift
Therapy	Racemic epinephrine aerosol, systemic steroids, aerosolized steroids, cold mist	None	Cool mist; occasionally as for croup	Endotracheal intubation, ceftriaxone	Ceftriaxone; intubation if needed
Prevention	None	None	None	*H. influenzae* b conjugated vaccine	None

Modified from Arnold JE: Airway obstruction in children. In Kliegman RM, Nieder ML, Super DM, editors: *Practical strategies in pediatric diagnosis and therapy*, Philadelphia, 1996, WB Saunders, p 126.
FFP, Fresh frozen plasma; *HPV,* human papilloma virus; *RSV,* respiratory syncytial virus; *URI,* upper respiratory tract infection, coryza, sneezing; *WBC,* white blood cell.

Retropharyngeal Abscess	Foreign Body	Angioedema	Peritonsillar Abscess	Laryngeal Papillomatosis
<6 yr Posterior pharynx	6 mo–5 yr Supraglottic, subglottic, variable	All ages Variable	>10 yr Oropharynx	3 mo–3 yr Larynx, vocal cords, trachea
S. aureus, anaerobes	Small objects, vegetables, toys, coins	Congenital C1-esterase deficiency; acquired anaphylaxis	Group A streptococci, anaerobes	HPV
Insidious to sudden	Sudden	Sudden	Biphasic with sudden worsening	Chronic
None	Yes	Yes	No	Possible
Yes Muffled	Yes—variable Complete obstruction—aphonic; other variable	Yes Hoarse, may be normal	No "Hot potato," muffled	No Hoarse
Arching of neck or normal	Normal	Normal; may have facial edema, anxiety	Normal	Normal
Drooling	Variable, usually normal	Normal	Drooling, trismus	Normal
No	Variable; brassy if tracheal	Possible	None	Variable
Severe	No, but dyspnea	No, unless anaphylactic shock or severe anoxia	Dyspnea	None
>101° F Thickened retropharyngeal space	None Radiopaque object may be seen	None As per croup	>101° F None needed	None May be normal
Leukocytosis with left shift	Normal	Normal	Leukocytosis with left shift	Normal
Nafcillin; ampicillin-sulbactam; ceftriaxone; surgical drainage if abscess	Endoscopic removal	Anaphylaxis; epinephrine, IV fluids, steroids; C1-esterase deficiency—danazol, C1-esterase infusion	Penicillin; aspiration	Laser therapy, repeated excision, interferon
None	Avoid small objects; supervision	Avoid allergens; FFP for congenital angioedema; danazol	Treat group A streptococci early	Treat maternal genitourinary lesions; possible cesarean section?

TABLE 12–6
Differentiating Supraglottic from Subglottic Causes of Airway Obstruction

	Supraglottic	Subglottic
Example	Epiglottitis, peritonsillar and retropharyngeal abscess	Croup, angioedema, foreign body, tracheitis
Stridor	Quiet	Loud
Voice	Muffled	Hoarse
Dysphagia	Yes	No
Sitting-up or arching posture	Yes	No
Barking cough	No	Yes
Fever	High (40° C [104° F])	Low grade (38°–39° C [100.4°–102.2° F])
Toxic	Yes	No, unless tracheitis is present
Trismus	Yes	No
Drooling	Yes	No
Facial edema	No	No, unless angioedema is present

Adapted from Davis H, Gartner JC, Galvis AG, et al: *Pediatr Clin North Am* 28:859–880, 1981.

TABLE 12–7
Causes of Wheezing in Childhood

Acute
Reactive Airway Disease
Asthma
Exercise-induced asthma
Hypersensitivity reactions
Bronchial Edema
Infection
Inhalation of irritant gases or particulates
Increased pulmonary venous pressure
Bronchial Hypersecretion
Infection
Inhalation of irritant gases or particulates
Cholinergic drugs
Aspiration
Foreign body
Aspiration of gastric contents

Chronic or Recurrent
Reactive Airway Disease
(see under Acute)
Hypersensitivity Reactions, Allergic Aspergillosis
Dynamic Airway Collapse
Bronchomalacia
Vocal cord adduction

Airway Compression by Mass or Blood Vessel
Vascular ring
Anomalous innominate artery
Pulmonary artery dilation (absent pulmonary valve)
Bronchial or pulmonary cysts
Lymph nodes or tumors
Aspiration
Foreign body
Gastroesophageal reflux
Tracheoesophageal fistula
Bronchial Hypersecretion or Failure to Clear Secretions
Bronchitis, bronchiectasis
Cystic fibrosis
Dysmotile cilia syndrome
Intrinsic Airway Lesions
Endobronchial tumors
Endobronchial granulation tissue
Bronchial or tracheal stenosis
Bronchiolitis obliterans
Sequelae of bronchopulmonary dysplasia
Congestive Heart Failure

with excessive production of tracheobronchial secretions, such as occurs in asthma, bronchitis,
bronchiectasis, or cystic fibrosis. Paroxysmal cough
suggests pertussis syndrome, foreign body aspiration, or cystic fibrosis. Chlamydial infections characteristically produce a repetitive, staccato cough.
Children with a harsh, brassy cough often have
an anatomic problem, such as subglottic edema
(croup), tracheomalacia, or tracheal compression,
but also may have habit cough. Habit cough disappears with sleep. Cough that arouses a child from
sleep is usually the result of a pathologic process.
Unfortunately, the sound or timing of the cough is
not always diagnostically valuable. Tumors, mediastinal or parabronchial lymphadenopathy, and
pulmonary vasculitis are uncommon causes of
chronic cough.

Severe coughing may result in complications such
as rib fractures; chest wall pain; pneumothorax; rupture of conjunctival, nasal, or anal veins; syncope;
hernias; emesis; urinary incontinence; or rectal prolapse. Severe, repeated episodes of coughing, as seen
in pertussis, may interfere with oral intake and produce malnutrition or may result in cyanosis.

The *diagnostic evaluation* of the child with chronic
cough should involve a chest roentgenogram and,
if possible, an examination of sputum. In children
too young to expectorate, a specimen often may be
obtained with a throat swab placed deep into the
posterior pharynx during coughing. Children with
allergies most often produce clear mucoid sputum,
although microscopic examination should be performed (discussed earlier in this chapter under Diagnostic Measures). Some children with allergies
produce apparently purulent sputum that contains
numerous eosinophils. Purulent sputum (containing many white blood cells) suggests infection, and
a specimen should be obtained for culture. A variety of rapid diagnostic tests (e.g., immunofluorescence or enzyme-linked immunosorbent assay
[ELISA] using nasal washings or serum) are available to help reach a diagnosis of certain viral pulmonary infections.

REFERENCES

Behrman RE, Kliegman RM, Jenson HB, editors: *Nelson textbook
   of pediatrics*, ed 16, Philadelphia, 2000, WB Saunders, Chapter
   377.
Irwin RS, Bochet LP, Cloutier MM, et al: Managing cough as a defense mechanism and as a symptom: a consensus panel report
   of the American College of Chest Physicians, *Chest* 114(2 Suppl
   Managing):133S–181S, 1998.
Irwin RS, Madison JM: The diagnosis and treatment of cough, *N
   Engl J Med* 343(23):1715–1721, 2000.

STRUCTURAL AND DYNAMIC ABNORMALITIES

The Upper Airway

Adenoidal Tonsillar Hypertrophy

The major abnormalities of the upper airway involve
obstructive lesions. The most common is adenoidal
tonsillar hypertrophy. The adenoids consist of lymphoid tissue arising from the posterior and superior
wall of the nasopharynx in the region of the choanae.
Lymphoid hyperplasia may result from recurrent infection, allergy, or nonspecific stimuli and may cause
partial or total obstruction of the nasopharynx. The
signs of adenoidal hypertrophy are persistent mouth
breathing, snoring, and in some patients, obstructive
sleep apnea. The eustachian tube enters the nasopharynx at the choanae and may be obstructed by
enlarged adenoids, promoting recurrent or persistent otitis media.

The *diagnosis* of adenoidal hypertrophy is confirmed by a lateral roentgenogram of the nasopharynx or by nasopharyngoscopy; *treatment* of airway
obstruction is by surgical excision. Because the adenoids are not a discrete organ but consist merely of
lymphoid tissue, regrowth following adenoidec-
tomy is not uncommon. Tonsils also may enlarge to
the point of producing airway obstruction. Obstruction sufficient to produce sleep apnea, retractions, or
cor pulmonale may necessitate tonsillectomy.

Choanal Stenosis (Atresia)

Choanal stenosis (atresia) may be bilateral or unilateral and is a relatively rare cause of respiratory distress in the newborn. The neonate is generally an obligate nose breather; thus nasal obstruction may be
fatal. Crying relieves the obstruction, which is worse
during quiet activity. Inability to pass a small catheter through the nostrils easily should raise the suspicion of choanal atresia. An oral airway may be lifesaving, but the definitive *treatment* is surgery. The
diagnosis is confirmed by CT or roentgenographically by instilling a small amount of contrast material or
by inspecting the area directly with a nasopharyn-
goscope or bronchoscope.

Laryngomalacia

Stridor beginning at birth or shortly thereafter should
raise the suspicion of laryngomalacia (Table 12–4).
This relatively common condition involves the collapse of the epiglottis or arytenoid cartilages during
inspiration and usually is benign and self-limiting. In
some infants the epiglottis alone is involved; these
patients tend to become asymptomatic during the
first year of life. Other infants have very large arytenoid cartilages that prolapse into the glottis during

inspiration; in these patients stridor tends to last longer, sometimes for several years.

Establishing a definitive *diagnosis* in suspected laryngomalacia is important both for its appropriate management and to exclude other, more serious lesions. The *differential diagnosis* includes vocal cord paralysis, laryngeal cysts or other mass lesions (especially when the stridor begins several weeks after birth), congenital subglottic stenosis, tracheomalacia, and compression of the upper trachea by an anomalous, innominate artery (Table 12–4). The child with laryngomalacia has **inspiratory stridor** but should have no evidence of significant expiratory obstruction. The stridor typically is loudest when the child is feeding or quietly relaxing or is in a supine or neck flexion position. Stridor usually diminishes during sleep or when the child is crying (when increased muscle tone may hold the supraglottic structures out of the air stream). Viral infections may exacerbate laryngomalacia.

No *treatment* is needed unless the infant has hypoxia or growth failure resulting from the airway obstruction; tracheostomy or epiglottoplasty then may be required. Symptoms usually disappear by 18–24 months of age.

Subglottic Stenosis

Subglottic stenosis may be congenital or, more commonly, iatrogenic. Aggressive management of premature infants with intubation and mechanical ventilation may produce residual damage to the larynx. Infants with Down syndrome appear to have a smaller larynx than normal and are more susceptible to subglottic stenosis. Subglottic obstruction produces stridor, and evidence of obstruction will be present on expiration and on inspiration. With increasing degrees of respiratory effort, the stridor will worsen (in contrast to laryngomalacia, in which the stridor may lessen with increasing respiratory efforts). Viral infection may exacerbate subglottic stenosis. Definitive *diagnosis* requires endoscopic evaluation.

Treatment may necessitate tracheostomy and reconstructive surgery; however, milder congenital cases improve with age as the larynx grows.

Mass Lesions

A number of mass lesions affect the larynx, but the most common laryngeal tumor in childhood is the **hemangioma,** which usually is found in the subglottic space. Infants with stridor should be examined carefully for cutaneous hemangiomas, which may occur in 50% of children with a laryngeal hemangioma. Most patients who have subglottic hemangioma come to the physician's attention before 6 months of age. Subglottic lesions produce asymmetric narrowing of the subglottic space and may be detected on AP roentgenograms of the larynx. Definitive diagnosis requires endoscopy. The airway obstruction, which usually worsens with crying, may eventually produce pulmonary hypertension and cor pulmonale.

Treatment of hemangiomas is controversial, but in many patients tracheostomy is required. Laser therapy and steroids have been used with moderate success. As with cutaneous hemangiomas, spontaneous regression is the rule, but this may require many months to several years.

Juvenile laryngeal papillomatosis, benign tumors caused by human papilloma virus acquired at birth from maternal genital warts, occurs in infants younger than 2 years of age. *Treatment* involves laser therapy and interferon, but response to therapy is often poor.

The Lower Airway

Tracheomalacia

The most common anomaly of tracheal structure and dynamics, although a less common cause of upper airway obstruction, is tracheomalacia. The tracheal cartilage rings normally extend through an arc of approximately 300 degrees, maintaining rigidity of the trachea during changes in intrathoracic pressure. In tracheomalacia the cartilage rings do not extend nearly so far around the circumference, and thus a larger portion of the tracheal wall is membranous. Therefore, the lumen of the intrathoracic portion of the trachea tends to collapse during expiration. This collapse may be apparent in most patients only during forced exhalation or with cough, but coarse, persistent wheezing may be a prominent symptom in other patients. The voice is normal, as is inspiratory effort. Tracheomalacia localized to the cervical trachea may lead to inspiratory obstruction. Tracheomalacia almost invariably is present in children who have had esophageal atresia and a tracheoesophageal fistula. Tracheomalacia must be differentiated from extrinsic compressing lesions. In some patients localized tracheomalacia may persist after the trachea has been relieved of compression by a mass lesion or an abnormal blood vessel. Viral infections may exacerbate the airway obstruction of tracheomalacia. Treatment usually is not necessary; rarely, patients may require long-term tracheostomy and ventilatory support.

Tracheoesophageal Fistula

Tracheoesophageal fistula is another relatively common anomaly of the trachea, occurring in 1:3000–4500 live births (see Chapter 11).

Tracheal Compression

Compression of the trachea by abnormal vessels may produce persistent wheezing, stridor, or both, as well as cough and dyspnea. The most common cause of an aberrant vessel is anterior compression resulting from an **anomalous innominate artery,** which arises more distally than normal along the arch of the aorta. Surgical treatment generally is required only for the most severe cases, especially those complicated by apnea.

A more serious lesion involves complete **encirclement of the trachea** at and just above the carina by a vascular ring. This anomaly may be caused by a double aortic arch or by a right aortic arch with a persisting left-sided ligamentum arteriosum and an aberrant left subclavian artery (most common). Both lesions have a right-sided aortic arch visible on chest x-ray examination. The rarest lesion is the pulmonary sling (aberrant left pulmonary artery arising from the right pulmonary artery). In addition to respiratory symptoms, emesis or dysphagia may be present as a result of esophageal compression. Complications include tracheomalacia, complete tracheal rings (stenosis), and lower airway compression.

The *definitive diagnosis* often can be made by barium swallow, although vascular dye contrast study or magnetic resonance angiography (MRA) may be required before surgical repair. Less common causes of extrinsic tracheal compression are mediastinal masses and cystic hygromas.

Endobronchial Mass Lesions

Endobronchial mass lesions are relatively uncommon in children, but when they occur, they most commonly consist of granulation tissue and are the result of localized inflammatory lesions. Partial obstruction of an airway by either an intrinsic or an extrinsic mass may result in wheezing or obstructive emphysema if there is more obstruction during exhalation than during inspiration. If the airways become totally obstructed, atelectasis results.

Chest roentgenograms, CT scans, bronchoscopy, or vascular contrast studies may be required for *diagnosis*. Primary tumors of the lungs and airways, such as nonsecreting carcinoid tumor and congenital bronchial cysts, are rare in children. Metastatic tumors, such as osteogenic sarcoma, may spread to the endobronchial airways from other areas of the body.

Bronchial Stenosis

Bronchial stenosis may be congenital or acquired and may lead to localized wheezing, air trapping, atelectasis, or infection. Acquired stenosis is usually the result of a chronic inflammatory process or localized trauma. *Diagnosis* usually requires bronchoscopy or high-resolution CT scan.

Emphysema

Emphysema, a condition that results when alveolar septa are disrupted or destroyed, is relatively uncommon in children, but generalized or localized overinflation is common and is the result of airway obstruction from a variety of causes. Although the term "emphysema" often is used somewhat inaccurately to refer to overinflation or to leakage of air into the interstitial tissues of the lung or into the subcutaneous tissue, this use of the term has become accepted.

Congenital lobar emphysema consists of overinflation of one lobe, most often the left upper lobe, which may produce respiratory distress because the surrounding lung tissue has become compressed, shifting the mediastinum. Lobectomy may be required if respiratory distress is severe and progressive. True emphysema develops in the absence of antiproteases (alpha$_1$-antitrypsin deficiency) but rarely appears before the third decade of life.

Chest Wall and Pleura

Scoliosis

Scoliosis, when severe, may result in respiratory dysfunction (see Chapter 19). Marked curvature of the thoracic spine is associated with chest wall deformity and limitation of chest wall movement, which decreases lung volumes (restrictive lung disease). In advanced scoliosis bronchial obstruction may develop when the bronchi become kinked or compressed by the great vessels that shift to abnormal positions in relation to the airways. Significant loss of inspiratory capacity often leads to pulmonary hypertension, recurrent infection, atelectasis, and respiratory insufficiency.

Pneumothorax

Pneumothorax is the accumulation of air in the pleural space that may result from external trauma or from leakage of air from the lungs or airways (see Chapter 6, Fig. 6–8). It may occur spontaneously in teenagers and young adults, more commonly in tall, thin males and smokers. Predisposing conditions include mechanical ventilation, asthma, cystic fibrosis, trauma, disorders of collagen (e.g., **Marfan syndrome),** idiopathic subpleural bullae (common and often bilateral), and exertion with a Valsalva maneuver. The symptoms of pneumothorax often begin while the patient is at rest (if spontaneous). Symptoms are pain, dyspnea, and cyanosis; if the air leak communicates with the mediastinum, subcutaneous emphysema may become apparent. Physical findings may include decreased breath sounds, a tympanitic percussion note, signs of mediastinal shift, and subcutaneous crepitance (Table 12–3). Few or no physical signs of pneumothorax may be present if the amount of air collection is small, but symptoms may progress rapidly if the air in the pleural space is under pressure (known as tension pneumothorax), with death resulting if the tension is not relieved.

The *diagnosis* is confirmed by chest roentgenogram. In infants, transillumination of the chest wall may help in the rapid diagnosis of pneumothorax.

Treatment depends on the amount of intrapleural air and the nature of the underlying disease. Small (<20%) pneumothoraces often resolve spontaneously; inhaling high-concentration oxygen for 12–24 hours can speed reabsorption. Larger pneumothoraces (and certainly tension pneumothoraces) necessitate immediate drainage of the air. In an emergency situation a simple needle aspiration may suffice, but placement of a chest tube may be required for resolution. Sclerosing the pleural surfaces to obliterate the pleural space may benefit patients with recurrent pneumothoraces.

Pneumomediastinum

Pneumomediastinum results from the dissection of air from a leak in the pulmonary parenchyma into the mediastinum. The most common cause in children is acute asthma. Symptoms are pain and dyspnea. Physical findings may be absent or may include a crunching noise over the sternum on auscultation. Frequently, subcutaneous emphysema is present in the neck.

The *diagnosis* is confirmed by roentgenogram. *Treatment* is directed toward the underlying lung disease.

Pleural Effusion

Pleural effusion commonly accompanies inflammatory processes in the lungs and may be heralded by pain, dyspnea, and signs of respiratory insufficiency resulting from compression of the underlying lung. Physical findings include dullness to percussion, decreased breath sounds, mediastinal shift, and decreased tactile fremitus (Table 12–3).

The *diagnosis* is confirmed roentgenographically; decubitus views, ultrasonography, or CT scan may help distinguish fluid collections from other densities in the thorax.

Fluid accumulates in the pleural space whenever the local hydrostatic forces pushing fluid out of the vascular space exceed osmotic forces pulling fluid back into the vascular space. The underlying causes of pleural effusion are congestive heart failure, hypoproteinemia, obstruction of lymphatic drainage, malignancy, collagen-vascular disease, and inflammation or infection of the pleura. Infection producing a reactive parapneumonic effusion or a more serious purulent **empyema** is the most common cause of pleural effusion in children. Empyema often is caused by *Streptococcus pneumoniae*, streptococci, or *Staphylococcus aureus* (and rarely by *Mycobacterium tuberculosis*, *Mycoplasma*, or adenovirus), whereas anaerobic bacteria produce empyema associated with aspiration pneumonia and dental, lung, or subdiaphragmatic abscesses. *Haemophilus influenzae* frequently causes parapneumonic effusion but is rare in immunized populations.

Diagnostic thoracentesis is necessary to establish the cause of the effusion and to exclude infection. Patients with effusion should undergo diagnostic thoracentesis unless the underlying causes for the effusion are clearly evident (e.g., systemic lupus erythematosus [SLE]), the patient does not have significant respiratory distress, and infection is not suspected. In the absence of inflammation, the fluid should have a low specific gravity (<1.015) and protein content (<2.5 g/dL), low lactic dehydrogenase activity (<200 IU/L), and a low cell count with few polymorphonuclear cells. In contrast, exudative pleural effusions resulting from inflammation have a high specific gravity, high protein (>3 g/dL) and lactic dehydrogenase (>250) content, low pH (<7.2) and glucose (<40 mg/dL) level, and a high cell count with many polymorphonuclear leukocytes.

Treatment is directed at the underlying condition that caused the effusion and at relief of the mechanical consequences of the fluid collection. For small effusions, especially if they are transudative, usually no therapy is required. For large effusions, drainage with a chest tube, especially if the fluid is purulent (empyema), is often needed. In this latter case the fluid is often very thick and may be loculated, which makes simple drainage difficult. All patients with empyema require tube drainage. Drainage of loculated fluid may be facilitated by instillation of streptokinase or urokinase into the pleural space via a catheter placed under CT guidance. Surgical removal of organized fibrinous parapneumonic effusions is rarely necessary.

If the underlying condition is treated successfully, the *prognosis* for patients with pleural effusions, including empyema, is excellent.

REFERENCES

Behrman RE, Kliegman RM, Jenson HB, editors: *Nelson textbook of pediatrics*, ed 16, Philadelphia, 2000, WB Saunders, Chapters 385, 418–420.

Heffner JE, Brown LK, Barbieri C, et al: Pleural fluid analysis in parapneumonic effusions: a meta-analysis, *Am Rev Respir Crit Care Med* 151(6):1700–1708, 1995.

Kravitz RM: Congenital malformations of the lung, *Pediatr Clin North Am* 41(3):453–472, 1994.

Peek GJ, Morcos S, Cooper G: The pleural cavity, *BMJ* 320(7245): 1318–1321, 2000.

Richardson MA, Cotton RT: Anatomic abnormalities of the pediatric airway, *Pediatr Clin North Am* 31(4):821–834, 1984.

Sahn SA, Heffner JE: Spontaneous pneumothorax, *N Engl J Med* 342(12):868–874, 2000.

Tan TQ, Mason EO, Barson WJ, et al: Clinical characteristics and outcome of children with pneumonia attributable to penicillin-susceptible and penicillin-nonsusceptible *Streptococcus pneumoniae, Pediatrics* 102(6):1369–1375, 1998.

GENETIC DISORDERS
Cystic Fibrosis

Cystic fibrosis (CF), an autosomal recessive disorder, is the most common lethal genetic disease affecting Caucasians (1:2500 live births). The gene for cystic fibrosis has been localized to the long arm of chromosome 7 and has been characterized as a large gene (>250 kb) of genomic deoxyribonucleic acid (DNA) that encodes a polypeptide of 1480 amino acids, termed *cystic fibrosis transmembrane regulator* (CFTR). The most common mutation, which occurs in approximately 70% of the CF chromosomes, is a specific deletion of three base pairs resulting in a deletion of phenylalanine at position ΔF 508. However, more than 800 other different mutations also have been reported to result in the CF phenotype. Heterozygote detection and prenatal diagnosis of individuals with ΔF 508 deletion and over 70 other deletions is readily accomplished. Many mutations occur at low frequency; present testing identifies over 90% of carriers.

Etiology. The major organs involved in CF are epithelial; the secretory and absorptive characteristics of these tissues are affected. The CFTR protein is involved in Cl^- conductance, consistent with the observation that 99% of patients with CF have elevated levels of sweat Cl^-. The CFTR is a chloride channel and substantially regulates epithelial Cl^- and possibly Na^+ transport. How the abnormal Cl^- conductance accounts for the clinical manifestations of CF is as yet uncertain. It may reduce the function of airway defenses or promote bacterial adhesion to the airway epithelium.

Clinical Manifestations. The respiratory epithelium of patients with CF exhibits marked impermeability to chloride and an excessive reabsorption of sodium. These alterations in the bioelectric properties of the epithelium lead to a relative dehydration of the airway secretions, resulting in impaired mucociliary transport and airway obstruction. **Chronic bronchial infection** then develops. Most patients are colonized with *H. influenzae, Staphylococcus aureus,* and/or *Pseudomonas aeruginosa* (which predominates in older patients with advanced disease). Chronic bronchial infection leads to cough, which is the most common initial pulmonary manifestation; sputum production; hyperinflation; bronchiectasis; and, eventually, pulmonary insufficiency and death. Digital clubbing is nearly universal in patients with significant lung disease.

Most patients with CF (90%) have exocrine **pancreatic insufficiency** early in life (if not at birth) as a result of inspissation of mucus in the pancreatic ducts and consequent autodigestion of the pancreas. Maldigestion with secondary malabsorption results in steatorrhea (large, fatty, floating, foul-smelling stools) and a number of secondary deficiency states (of vitamins K, D, A, and E) in the untreated patient. Nutrient malabsorption also results in failure to thrive despite a ravenous appetite. Approximately 10% of patients are born with intestinal obstruction resulting from inspissated meconium (meconium ileus). In older patients, intestinal obstruction may occur because of maldigestion and thick mucus in the intestinal lumen (distal intestinal obstruction syndrome). Such events may occur after dietary indiscretions or with inadequate pancreatic enzyme replacement. In adolescent or adult patients, relative insulin deficiency may develop; **hyperglycemia** and CF-related diabetes may become symptomatic, although ketoacidosis is rare.

As in the respiratory and gastrointestinal tracts, inspissation of mucus in the *reproductive tract* leads to dysfunction. Female fertility is low and the cervical mucus is abnormal, but a number of patients have given birth. Secondary amenorrhea often is present as a result of chronic illness and markedly reduced body weight. Males almost universally are azoospermic, with atrophy or absence of the vas deferens.

The failure of the *sweat ducts* to conserve salt may lead to heat exhaustion or to unexplained hypochloremic alkalosis in infants but has relatively little clinical consequence otherwise. CF is a chronic, insidiously progressive disease exhibiting multiple *complications* related to viscous mucus, malabsorption, and infection (Table 12–8).

Diagnosis. The diagnosis of CF should be considered seriously in any patient with chronic or recurring respiratory or gastrointestinal symptoms. Indications for sweat testing are shown in Table 12–9. For the diagnosis to be established, the following criteria must be met: one or more typical phenotypic features of CF (chronic sinopulmonary disease, characteristic gastrointestinal and nutritional abnormalities, salt loss syndromes, and obstructive azoospermia) must be present, a sibling must have a history of CF, or a positive result must be obtained from a newborn screening test; and a positive result must be obtained from a sweat test on two or more occasions (60 mEq/L with adequate sweat collection of

TABLE 12–8
Complications of Cystic Fibrosis

Pulmonary
Bronchiectasis, bronchitis, bronchiolitis, pneumonia
Atelectasis
Hemoptysis
Pneumothorax
Nasal polyps
Sinusitis
Reactive airway disease
Cor pulmonale
Respiratory failure
Mucoid impaction of the bronchi
Allergic bronchopulmonary aspergillosis

Gastrointestinal
Meconium ileus
Meconium peritonitis
Distal intestinal obstruction syndrome (nonneonatal obstruction)
Rectal prolapse
Intussusception
Volvulus
Fibrosing colonopathy (strictures)
Appendicitis
Intestinal atresia

Gastrointestinal—cont'd
Pancreatitis
Biliary cirrhosis (portal hypertension: esophageal varices, hypersplenism)
Neonatal obstructive jaundice
Hepatic steatosis
Gastroesophageal reflux
Cholelithiasis
Inguinal hernia
Growth failure (malabsorption)
Vitamin deficiency states (vitamins A, K, E, D)
Insulin deficiency, symptomatic hyperglycemia, diabetes
Malignancy (rare)

Other
Infertility
Delayed puberty
Edema-hypoproteinemia
Dehydration–heat exhaustion
Hypertrophic osteoarthropathy–arthritis
Clubbing
Amyloidosis

TABLE 12–9
Indications for Sweat Testing

Pulmonary
Chronic or recurrent cough
Chronic or recurrent pneumonia
Recurrent bronchiolitis
Atelectasis
Hemoptysis
Staphylococcal pneumonia
Pseudomonas aeruginosa in the respiratory tract (in the absence of such circumstances as tracheostomy or prolonged intubation)
Mucoid *P. aeruginosa* in the respiratory tract

Gastrointestinal
Meconium ileus
Neonatal intestinal obstruction (meconium plug, atresia)
Steatorrhea, malabsorption
Hepatic cirrhosis in childhood (including any manifestations such as esophageal varices or portal hypertension)

Gastrointestinal—cont'd
Pancreatitis
Rectal prolapse
Vitamin deficiency states (A, D, E, K)
Prolonged, direct-reacting neonatal jaundice

Miscellaneous
Digital clubbing
Failure to thrive
Family history of cystic fibrosis (sibling or cousin)
Salty taste when kissed; salt crystals on skin after evaporation of sweat
Heat prostration, especially under seemingly inappropriate circumstances
Hyponatremic hypochloremic alkalosis in infants
Nasal polyps
Pansinusitis
Aspermia
Absent vas deferens

at least 75 mg), two mutations known to cause CF must be identified, or a characteristic abnormality in ion transport across nasal epithelium must be demonstrated in vivo. Although highly specific for CF, the sweat test is subject to numerous technical problems and is reliable only in laboratories that perform the test frequently and with scrupulous quality control. False-positive and false-negative sweat test results occur in a few well-defined clinical states (Table 12–10). A few patients may have typical but mild symptoms and borderline or even normal sweat Cl⁻ levels. Other supportive tests, such as measurement of bioelectrical potential differences across respiratory epithelium, low levels of stool trypsin, and detection of a known CF mutation by DNA analysis, may be useful. Prenatal detection of a known CF genotype may be accomplished by amniotic fluid or chorionic villus sampling.

Treatment. The complex management of CF is best coordinated by a tertiary referral center. As in the treatment of any chronic disease, physicians, patients, families, and other caretakers must work together to maintain an optimistic, aggressive approach to life and treatment. Efforts to prevent the occurrence of complications and the progression of lung disease are vital, and immunization against influenza virus and other diseases should be kept up to date. Unfortunately, no universally accepted protocol for treatment exists, and many measures are controversial.

The **electrolyte loss** resulting from the sweat defect is treated by adding more salt to the patient's diet.

Lung disease is treated by combining physical measures to help remove mucus from the airways (e.g., chest physiotherapy, exercise), pharmacologic measures to clear mucus and improve airway patency (e.g., bronchodilators and aerosolized DNAase), and antibiotic therapy to control chronic infection. Monitoring pulmonary bacterial flora and providing aggressive therapy with appropriate antibiotics in full therapeutic doses (oral, aerosolized, and parenteral) help slow the progression of the lung disease. Intermittent treatment (bid × 4 weeks) with inhaled tobramycin improves pulmonary function tests and reduces infections with *Pseudomonas*. Patients are hospitalized for high-dose intravenous antibiotic therapy whenever necessary, especially when they are infected with organisms resistant to oral agents (e.g., *Pseudomonas*). Under normal circumstances, therapy should last for at least 2 weeks; even when the most aggressive therapy is used, it is difficult to sterilize the lungs. Infection with certain virulent strains of *Burkholderia cepacia* is particularly difficult to treat and may be associated with an accelerated clinical deterioration. **Allergic bronchopulmonary aspergillosis** also may complicate CF and necessitate treatment with steroids and antifungal agents (e.g., itraconazole). Pulmonary complications such as pneumothorax, hemoptysis (check vitamin K status), and atelectasis are treated as they are in other patients.

Pancreatic insufficiency is treated by replacing pancreatic enzymes, preferably in enteric-coated form, and by encouraging higher caloric intake than normal. Even with the best enzyme replacement, stool losses of fat and protein may be relatively high. Fat is not withheld from the diet, even when significant steatorrhea exists. Instead, enzyme doses are increased to normalize the stools as much as possible; however, lipase concentrations exceeding 2500 U/ kg/meal have been associated with intestinal obstruction caused by fibrosing colonopathy. Fat-soluble vitamins are given in twice-normal doses, preferably in water-miscible form. Meconium ileus often necessitates surgical intervention but may respond to enemas of hyperosmolar roentgenographic contrast material. Intestinal obstruction in older patients is treated similarly or with oral laxatives.

Therapies under ongoing investigation and showing some benefit are directed toward thinning mucus with inhaled DNAase; antiinflammatory medications (antiproteases and nonsteroidal antiinflammatory agents); agents that improve Cl⁻ lung transplantation; and ultimately gene therapy.

TABLE 12–10
Causes of False-Positive and False-Negative Sweat Test

False Positive
Adult age
Adrenal insufficiency
Ectodermal dysplasia
Nephrogenic diabetes insipidus
Hypothyroidism (?)
Fucosidosis
Mucopolysaccharidosis
Malnutrition
Poor technique
Type I glycogen storage disease
Panhypopituitarism
Pseudohypoaldosteronism
Hypoparathyroidism
Prostaglandin E_1 administration

False Negative
Edema
Poor technique
Atypical cystic fibrosis (uncommon)

Prognosis. Pulmonary disease is the major cause of morbidity in CF and is influenced by the inherent severity of disease and by therapy. Patients with meconium ileus have the same prognosis as others with CF if they survive the first year of life. Current data from the Patient Registry of the Cystic Fibrosis Foundation indicate that the median survival age for patients with CF is approximately 27 years, but patients vary greatly in the severity of their disease.

Immotile (Dysmotile) Cilia Syndrome

Immotile (dysmotile) cilia syndrome is an inherited disorder in which ultrastructural abnormalities in the cilia result in absent or disordered movement. The disorder affects 1:19,000 persons. The most classic form of the syndrome, **Kartagener syndrome,** is an autosomal recessive disorder characterized by situs inversus, pansinusitis, and bronchiectasis. Otitis media also is common, and male infertility is universal (as a result of immotile sperm). The cilia lack dynein arms, an ultrastructural feature that represents an ATPase necessary for ciliary motility. Many other variants of the syndrome exist that have a variety of ultrastructural abnormalities of the cilia. In some patients cilia may move, but their beat is abnormal, usually uncoordinated, and ineffective.

Because respiratory tract cilia fail to beat normally, secretions accumulate in the airways and bacterial infection occurs. Chronic infection leads to bronchiectasis by early adulthood. The *diagnosis* should be suspected in individuals with early-onset chronic bronchitis or bronchiectasis; in patients with chronic, recurrent, or persistent pneumonia; and especially in patients with pansinusitis or chronic otitis media. Cystic fibrosis should be excluded by sweat testing. The diagnosis is confirmed by electron microscopy of respiratory cilia; the cilia may be obtained from nasal scrapings. Because chronic infection and inflammation may lead to ultrastructural abnormalities in nasal cilia, care must be taken in confirming the diagnosis.

Treatment is similar to the pulmonary therapy in cystic fibrosis and is directed toward improving clearance of respiratory secretions and controlling infection. Chest physiotherapy, immunoprophylaxis of viral infections (e.g., influenza), and prompt treatment of bacterial infection are helpful, but the course of the disease tends to be slowly progressive.

ALPHA₁-ANTITRYPSIN DEFICIENCY

Alpha$_1$-antitrypsin deficiency is an inherited absence (relative or absolute) of antiprotease activity. In the respiratory tract, the proteases (especially elastase) released by the normal turnover of phagocytic cells thus are not inhibited, and over a period of time (usually two or more decades), emphysema develops. In some forms of the disorder, liver disease appears early in life, but in most children with alpha$_1$-antitrypsin deficiency little evidence for lung disease exists in the first decade. In children or adolescents, dyspnea is the first *clinical manifestation.* Chest roentgenograms may reveal hyperinflation; often the disease may be confused with late-onset asthma. Progressive emphysema or pulmonary cyst formation may be associated with previous pulmonary infection or with exposure to cigarette smoke.

The *diagnosis* is confirmed by demonstration of reduced total alpha$_1$-antitrypsin levels and a ZZ phenotype. Recombinant alpha$_1$-antitrypsin is now available and has some efficacy in *treatment* and *prevention* of the lung disease.

REFERENCES

Behrman RE, Kliegman RM, Jenson HB, editors: *Nelson textbook of pediatrics,* ed 16, Philadelphia, 2000, WB Saunders, Chapters 407, 416, 417.

Lai HC, Fitzsimmons SC, Allen DB: Risk of persistent growth impairment after alternate-day prednisone treatment in children with cystic fibrosis, *N Engl J Med* 342(12):851–859, 2000.

Marshall BC, Liou TG: Elusiveness of ideal approach to *Pseudomonas aeruginosa* infection complicating cystic fibrosis, *Lancet* 356(9230):613–614, 2000.

Rosenstein BJ, Cutting GR: The diagnosis of cystic fibrosis: a consensus statement, *J Pediatr* 132(4):589–595, 1998.

INFECTIOUS DISORDERS
The Upper Airway
Otitis Media

See Chapter 10.

Sinusitis

See Chapter 10.

Croup

The most common syndrome of infectious upper airway obstruction is croup, or acute infectious laryngotracheobronchitis (Table 12–5; see Chapter 10). Croup is predominantly of viral etiology; parainfluenza types 1 and 2 viruses are the most common agents.

Clinical Manifestations. The typical episode of croup begins with a child between 6 months and 3 years of age having symptoms of an upper respiratory infection (the common cold) and lasts less than 5 days. A brassy cough (typically characterized as sounding like the barking of a seal), inspiratory stridor, and respiratory distress may develop slowly or acutely. Signs of upper airway obstruction, such as labored breathing and marked suprasternal, intercostal, and subcostal retractions, are evident on examination. Associated lower airway disease accompanied by wheezing and a productive cough may be present. Although the majority of such children are not seriously ill, the airway obstruction may become severe, necessitating placement of an artificial airway. The subglottic space is the major site of obstruction, which is caused by edema resulting from the viral inflammation (Table 12–6). Roentgenogram reveals the "steeple" sign of a narrowed subglottic space.

Treatment. Administration of aerosolized racemic (or L-) epinephrine may reduce the edema temporarily, producing marked clinical improvement, but the edema and obstruction soon return, and the disease runs its course over several days. Epinephrine aerosol treatment may need to be repeated as often as every 20 minutes (for no more than 1–2 hours) in severe cases. During inspiration the walls of the subglottic space are drawn together, aggravating the obstruction (and probably also the edema); children should be kept as calm as possible to reduce their respiratory efforts. The best calming method for a child with croup is to sit in the parent's lap. Sedatives should be used cautiously and only in the setting of an intensive care unit. Cool mist administered by tent or face mask may help prevent drying of the secretions around the larynx.

Children with severe croup requiring hospitalization should be monitored carefully. The subsidence of symptoms may indicate that the patient either is improving or is becoming fatigued and is in respiratory failure. Because aerosolized epinephrine has a short duration of action, most authorities believe that children requiring such therapy should be hospitalized (or observed for several hours), even if their obstructive signs clear completely with the first aerosol treatment. Systemically administered corticosteroids are beneficial in treating croup but generally are reserved for more significantly ill patients. Topically active inhaled corticosteroids may also be of benefit. If the patient is very young (<4 months of age) or if symptoms continue for more than 1 week, the patient should undergo careful laryngoscopy because there is an increased probability that another lesion exists (subglottic stenosis or hemangioma). Sudden worsening (e.g., fever, respiratory distress, or leukocytosis) suggests a complicating *bacterial tracheitis*. This is a serious and potentially life-threatening condition (Table 12–5).

Some children have acute episodes of croup-like symptoms without exhibiting evidence of a viral infection. These episodes may be severe but usually are of short duration. This acute "spasmodic croup" is not well understood but may involve allergic mechanisms in some patients. It tends to recur and to respond to relatively simple therapies, such as exposure to cool or moist air.

Epiglottitis

Acute epiglottitis, another syndrome of upper airway obstruction, typically occurs in older children (ages 2–7 years). The causative agent is predominantly bacterial (*H. influenzae* type b). Immunization of infants and children to *H. influenzae* has made epiglottitis extremely rare.

Clinical Manifestations. Epiglottitis is characterized by sudden onset, high fever, respiratory distress, fulminant progression, severe dysphagia, and a muffled voice (Tables 12–5 and 12–6). Patients usually find it easier to breathe sitting erect, and they drool because of the dysphagia. Acute epiglottitis is a true pediatric emergency because the inflamed airway suddenly may become totally obstructed, leading to death.

Diagnosis. In typical cases, epiglottitis should be suspected on observing the patient's clinical presentation. The *differential diagnosis* includes severe croup, bacterial tracheitis, foreign body aspiration, Ludwig angina, and retropharyngeal and peritonsillar abscess (Table 12–5). Confirmation of the diagnosis is based on direct observation of the inflamed and swollen supraglottic structures and cherry-red enlarged epiglottis, but this procedure should be performed only in the operating room with a competent surgeon and anesthesiologist prepared to place an endotracheal tube or perform a tracheostomy. *H. influenzae* may be recovered from the surface of the epiglottis or from blood culture. Epiglottitis may be distinguished from severe croup on the basis of a lateral neck film if there is doubt as to the clinical diagnosis (the "thumb sign" of swollen epiglottis). A physician should accompany the patient to the radiology department and be prepared to manage the airway.

Treatment. Endotracheal intubation is currently the preferred method of treatment, but the intubated patient requires constant supervision and restraint to decrease the probability of accidental extubation. Antibiotics (ceftriaxone) suitable for *H. influenzae* should be given at once. With effective therapy, clinical recovery is rapid, and most patients can be safely extubated within 48–72 hours.

The Lower Airway
Bronchiolitis

Bronchiolitis is an acute respiratory illness of young children resulting from inflammation of small airways and characterized by wheezing. Respiratory syncytial virus (RSV) is the principal agent, although other viruses, such as parainfluenza, adenovirus, influenza, rhinovirus, and, infrequently, *M. pneumoniae*, have been associated with the illness.

Epidemiology. Bronchiolitis is a common illness of young children; approximately 50% of children have this illness during the first 2 years of life, and 95% of children have serologic evidence of previous infection by the age of 3 years. Children generally acquire the infection when exposed to family members who typically have symptoms of an upper respiratory tract infection or from infected children in a day care setting. Most cases occur during the winter and early spring, when the associated viral agents are most prevalent in the community.

Clinical Manifestations. The affected infant usually has rhinorrhea, sneezing, cough, and low-grade fever, followed in several days by the onset of rapid breathing and wheezing. The child may feed poorly. Results of *physical examination* are notable for signs of acute respiratory distress, including nasal flaring, tachypnea, intermittent cyanosis, retractions, a prolonged expiratory phase, and wheezes and crackles in the chest. The white blood cell count usually is normal. Chest roentgenograms typically reveal air trapping and may show peribronchial thickening, atelectasis, and infiltrates. Hypoxemia is not universal but is secondary to mismatching of ventilation and perfusion. Hypercapnia does not usually develop, but it can occur in the severely affected infant with significant airway obstruction or in infants who become fatigued. Acute symptoms last 5–6 days; recovery is complete in 10–14 days.

Diagnosis. The diagnosis of bronchiolitis is based on clinical findings and on knowledge of the epidemiology of viral illnesses prevalent in the community. RSV may be identified on nasopharyngeal secretions by PCR, culture, or antigen assay. Many other diagnoses should be considered in the young child who exhibits an acute **wheezing-associated respiratory illness.** Asthma typically has a recurrent pattern and is responsive to bronchodilators. Pneumonia usually is associated with an infiltrate demonstrated on a chest roentgenogram and, if bacterial infection is present, with a high white blood cell count. In heart failure, an enlarged heart usually is seen on the chest roentgenogram, and either related structural cardiac abnormalities or viral myocarditis may be present. Children with foreign body aspiration often have a history of aspirating an object and may exhibit localized wheezing or air trapping. Wheezing associated with gastroesophageal reflux is likely to be chronic or recurrent, and the patient may have a history of frequent emesis. Cystic fibrosis may be associated with poor growth, chronic diarrhea, or a family history of the disease.

Treatment. The management of the child with bronchiolitis depends on the severity of the illness. Most children have mild symptoms and can be managed with supportive measures at home. Approximately 5% of children with bronchiolitis require hospitalization. *Indications for hospitalization* include young age (<6 months), moderate to marked respiratory distress (sleeping respiratory rates of 50–60 breaths/min or higher), hypoxemia (Po$_2$ <60 mm Hg or oxygen saturation <92% on room air), the occurrence of apnea, inability to tolerate oral feeding, and lack of appropriate care available at home. Children with chronic lung disease such as bronchopulmonary dysplasia, with congenital heart disease (particularly with associated pulmonary hypertension), with neuromuscular weakness, and with immunodeficiency are at increased risk of having severe, potentially fatal disease. Consideration should be given to the hospitalization of all of these high-risk children.

Supportive measures appropriate to the care of the child with bronchiolitis include administration of adequate oral or (in the hospitalized child) parenteral fluids to ensure maintenance of normal hydration in the presence of increased insensible water losses associated with tachypnea. Fever, if high or associated with increased respiratory distress, may be treated with antipyretic agents. Supplemental humidified oxygen should be provided for the hospitalized child in a sufficient concentration to maintain a Pao$_2$ of 70–90 mm Hg (oxygen saturation ≥93%). The use of *bronchodilators,* such as aerosolized beta$_2$-agonists or racemic epinephrine, may be beneficial in selected patients and should be tried in severely affected children. Corticosteroids offer little benefit.

Administration of *ribavirin aerosol,* a specific antiviral agent, to children with RSV infection has been demonstrated to be mildly efficacious in clinical trials. This should be considered in severely affected infants and in those at high risk for development of severe, protracted disease (e.g., chronic lung disease and congenital heart disease). Antibacterial therapy is not indicated unless evidence suggests the existence of a concomitant bacterial infection. *Intubation* and *mechanical ventilation* are required to treat respiratory failure or severe apnea. Monthly injections (IM) of RSV-specific monoclonal antibodies confer some protection from severe disease to infants and toddlers under the age of 2 years (e.g., those with bronchopulmonary dysplasia or very low birth weight).

Prognosis. Complications of bronchiolitis include apnea, respiratory failure, atelectasis, otitis media (RSV ± bacteria), secondary bacterial infection, and pneumothorax or pneumomediastinum (in the child requiring mechanical ventilation). However, the immediate prognosis of most children with bronchiolitis is excellent, with symptoms resolving in 7–10 days. Several studies suggest that some children who have an episode of bronchiolitis (particularly if they needed to be hospitalized) may be prone to further episodes of wheezing, manifest allergic symptoms, have lower average levels of lung function, and have a modestly higher prevalence of increased airway reactivity later in life. Factors other than the occurrence of bronchiolitis, such as underlying increased bronchial reactivity and exposure to environmental pollutants like cigarette smoke, may contribute to the apparent sequelae of bronchiolitis. Mortality caused by RSV bronchiolitis is 1–4%; the higher figure is associated with high-risk groups.

Bronchiolitis Obliterans

Bronchiolitis obliterans is an uncommon form of chronic bronchiolitis in which endobronchiolar granulation tissue and peribronchiolar fibrosis are seen. Most reported cases in young infants have been related to the occurrence of severe viral infection, most commonly adenovirus. Association with influenza, pertussis, measles, and *M. pneumoniae* has been reported. In adults bronchiolitis obliterans also has been associated with toxic inhalational exposures, connective tissue disorders, and drug administration (such as penicillamine). An interstitial pneumonia may be present. Abnormalities may be diffuse or localized.

Clinical Manifestations. The typical illness begins with fever, cough, tachypnea, and wheezing. Notable physical findings include retractions, wheezes, and rales. Chest roentgenograms typically show a nonspecific diffuse infiltrate exhibiting areas of atelectasis, but the roentgenograms may reveal a more miliary pattern. The course of the illness differs from that of acute, uncomplicated bronchiolitis in that the symptoms progress, often after a brief period of improvement, and are accompanied by an increasing shortness of breath, the development of productive cough, hypoxia, and persistent wheezing. Clinically there is fixed airway obstruction that is poorly responsive to bronchodilators. Increased symptoms can occur as acute exacerbations or more insidiously over a prolonged period. CT scan reveals obstruction of small airways; arteriography reveals a reduction of the pulmonary bed.

Complications include progressive respiratory failure, atelectasis, secondary bacterial infection, and the development of the **unilateral hyperlucent lung syndrome** in those in whom the disease appears to be confined to one lung. Some patients die early in the course of the disease; others experience a more chronic course.

Diagnosis. Bronchiolitis obliterans should be considered in the child who has significant recurrent or persistent respiratory symptoms and evidence of fixed airway obstruction following a severe viral lung infection. Typical bronchographic findings support the diagnosis; confirmation requires lung biopsy. Other diagnoses to consider in a child with recurrent or persistent cough and wheezing with an infiltrate or atelectasis on chest roentgenographic examination are cystic fibrosis, asthma, gastroesophageal reflux, and foreign body aspiration.

Treatment. No specific therapy is available, although corticosteroids often are used in an attempt to mitigate the progressive fibrosis. Appropriate supportive measures are supplemental oxygen, chest physiotherapy, a trial of bronchodilator therapy, and early, aggressive treatment of further lung infections.

Pneumonia

Pneumonia refers to the inflammation of pulmonary tissue. It is associated with consolidation of the alveolar spaces. **Pneumonitis** is a general term for lung inflammation that may or may not be associated with consolidation. **Lobar pneumonia** describes pneumonia localized to one or more lobes of the lung in which the affected lobe or lobes are completely consolidated.

Bronchopneumonia refers to inflammation of the lung that is centered in the bronchioles and leads to the production of a mucopurulent exudate that obstructs some of these small airways and causes patchy consolidation of the adjacent lobules. Bronchopneumonia is usually a generalized process involving multiple lobes of the lung. The distinction between bronchopneumonia and bronchiolitis can be somewhat arbitrary.

Interstitial pneumonitis refers to inflammation of the interstitium, which is composed of the walls of the alveoli, the alveolar sacs and ducts, and the bronchioles. Interstitial pneumonitis may be seen acutely with viral infections but also may be a chronic process.

Anatomic respiratory system malformations, altered systemic or local immunity, and exposure to cigarette smoke predispose the patient to infectious pneumonia. The cause of pneumonia depends on the age, immune status, presence of CF or other chronic lung disease, exposure history, and nosocomial versus community acquisition.

Etiology. Pneumonia may be caused by a variety of infectious agents (e.g., bacterial, viral, fungal, rickettsial, and parasitic organisms), inflammatory processes (e.g., SLE, sarcoidosis, and histiocytosis), and toxic substances (e.g., hydrocarbons, smoke, molds, dusts, chemicals, gases, and gastric contents) that are inhaled or aspirated. The most common cause of pneumonia in children is viral infections; bacterial infections account for only 10–30% of all pediatric pneumonias. Certain infectious pneumonias are more common at a particular age (Table 12–11).

Microorganisms gain access to the lung by hematogenous dissemination or local spread descending through the respiratory bronchial tree. Although aspiration pneumonia may be seen following seizures or in patients with altered mental status, neuromuscular disease, and gastroesophageal reflux, most cases of pediatric pneumonia are not related to these causes. *Streptococcus pneumoniae* is the most common cause of bacterial pneumonia. *H. influenzae* type b pneumonia often is associated with bacteremia, meningitis, and other sites of infection but is rarely seen in immunized children. *S. aureus* is a rare cause of pneumonia in infants; when it is present, the child is acutely ill with empyema, pneumatoceles, and respiratory failure. Staphylococcal skin infection may precede bacteremia and pneumonia. RSV, influenza viruses, and parainfluenza virus are common causes of viral pneumonia. Adenovirus and measle virus may produce severe disease. Viral respiratory infections may precede bacterial pneumonias. Infants between 1 and 3 months of age often have an **afebrile pneumonia,** which typically is caused by congenitally or environmentally acquired agents such as *Ureaplasma urealyticum, Chlamydia trachomatis* (with or without conjunctivitis), cytomegalovirus (CMV), *Pneumocystis carinii,* or RSV. Pneumonia in immunocompromised patients may be caused by *P. carinii,* gram-negative enteric bacteria, fungi (aspergillosis or histoplasmosis), mycobacteria (*M. tuberculosis* or *M. avium*), or CMV, whereas disease in patients with CF usually is caused by *S. aureus* (in infancy), *P. aeruginosa,* or *B. cepacia* (in older patients).

Children with immune system dysfunction, malnutrition, or defects in the normal defense mechanisms of the lung are quite susceptible to pulmonary infections. The causative agents often are unusual, opportunistic organisms, including gram-negative enteric bacteria, anaerobes, CMV, measles, varicella, *P. carinii,* or fungi.

Clinical Manifestations. The typical clinical patterns of viral and bacterial pneumonias usually differ, although the distinction is not always clear for a particular patient. Tachypnea, cough, malaise, fever, pleuritic chest pain, and retractions are common to both.

Viral pneumonias more often are associated with cough, wheezing, or stridor; fever is less prominent than in bacterial pneumonia. The chest roentgenogram shows diffuse, streaky infiltrates of bronchopneumonia, and the white blood cell count often is not elevated (lymphocytes are the predominant cell type).

Bacterial pneumonias typically are associated with cough, high fever, chills, dyspnea, and auscultatory findings of lung consolidation (e.g., decreased

TABLE 12–11
Common Causes of Pneumonia at Different Ages*

Age	Bacterial	Viral	Others
Neonate	Group B streptococci, coliform bacteria	CMV, herpesvirus, enterovirus	*Mycoplasma hominis, Ureaplasma urealyticum*
4–16 wk	*Staphylococcus aureus, Haemophilus influenzae,*† *Streptococcus pneumoniae*	CMV, RSV, influenza virus, parainfluenza virus	*Chlamydia trachomatis, U. urealyticum*
Up to 5 yr	*S. pneumoniae, S. aureus, H. influenzae,* group A streptococcus	RSV, adenovirus, influenza virus	
Over 5 yr	*S. pneumoniae, H. influenzae*†	Influenza virus, varicella, adenovirus	*Mycoplasma pneumoniae, Chlamydia pneumoniae, Legionella pneumophila*

CMV, Cytomegalovirus; *HIV,* human immunodeficiency virus; *RSV,* respiratory syncytial virus.
*An increasingly important consideration is *Mycobacterium tuberculosis. Pneumocystis carinii* should always be considered in HIV-infected patients.
†Invasive *H. influenzae* type b is now rare in immunized populations.

or tubular breath sounds, dullness to percussion, and egophony in a localized region) (Table 12–3). The chest roentgenogram often shows lobar consolidation (or a round pneumonia) and pleural effusion (10–30%), and the peripheral white blood cell count is elevated (>15,000–20,000/mm³), with a predominance of neutrophils.

Many cases of pneumonia have characteristics that fall between these two typical patterns of viral and bacterial pneumonia. Lower lobe pneumonia may present with abdominal pain.

Diagnosis. The definitive diagnosis of pneumonia requires identification of the causative organism. Sputum for culture is not easily obtained from children. Certain viral agents (RSV, influenza, parainfluenza, and adenovirus) may be identified by culture, polymerase chain reaction (PCR), or immunofluorescent staining of infected epithelial cells washed from the nasopharynx. CMV and enterovirus can be cultured from the nasopharynx, urine, or bronchoalveolar lavage fluid. *M. pneumoniae* may be suspected if cold agglutinins are present in peripheral blood samples; this may be confirmed if the presence of *Mycoplasma*-specific IgM is detected or by PCR. Bacterial agents may be cultured or identified by antigen detection (for pneumococcus or *H. influenzae*) from blood or from an associated pleural effusion. The diagnosis of *M. tuberculosis* may be made by tuberculin skin tests and analysis of sputum or gastric aspirates (by culture, antigen detection, or PCR).

Invasive procedures such as bronchoscopy and bronchoalveolar lavage or lung biopsy may be necessary to obtain culture specimens. These invasive procedures are not used in typical pneumonias, but they may be used in special instances, such as pneumonia in the immunocompromised host or when the clinical picture is unusual.

Treatment. The management of pneumonia depends on the age of the patient and the clinical presentation (i.e., whether the presentation is more consistent with viral or with bacterial pneumonia). Neonatal or congenital pneumonia is life threatening; therefore, infants younger than 2 months of age with pneumonia should be hospitalized and treated with intravenous antibiotics. If bacterial pneumonia is suspected at birth, antibiotics effective against group B streptococcus and coliform bacteria should be used (see Appendix I). After the first week of life, antibiotic coverage for *S. aureus* should be included if the roentgenogram demonstrates effusions or pneumatoceles. In older children, drugs effective against *S. pneumoniae* should be used. Appropriate antibiotic choices in older children are amoxicillin, ceftriaxone, clarithromycin, or trimethoprim-sulfamethoxazole for 10 days. Newer

fluoroquinolones, such as levofloxacin, may also be considered. Pneumonia in children 5–10 years of age frequently is caused by *M. pneumoniae* or *S. pneumoniae* and may be treated with erythromycin or clarithromycin; the latter may be better tolerated. Penicillin-resistant pneumococcus is now common in many communities. These organisms often are resistant to multiple antibiotics and require initial therapy with ceftriaxone. Vancomycin should be added with fulminant life-threatening disease or if the patient does not improve in 24–48 hours. A small percentage of children with pneumonia require hospitalization. Most children beyond early infancy may be managed as outpatients. Indications for hospitalization include the following:

- Moderate to severe respiratory distress
- Failure to respond to oral antibiotics
- Inability to take oral antibiotics at home because of vomiting or poor compliance
- Lobar consolidation in more than one lobe
- Immunosuppression
- Empyema
- Abscess or pneumatocele
- Underlying cardiopulmonary disease (e.g., bronchopulmonary dysplasia or pulmonary hypertension)

Prognosis. Most children recover from pneumonia rapidly and completely, and the roentgenographic findings should return to normal within 6–8 weeks. In a few children pneumonia may persist longer than 1 month or may be *recurrent*. In such cases the possibility of underlying disease must be investigated further (Table 12–12). Evaluation then may include the tuberculin skin test, sweat chloride determination, serum immunoglobulin and IgG subclass determinations, bronchoscopy, and barium swallow.

Bronchiectasis

Bronchiectasis, or the dilation of bronchi, may be either *congenital* or *acquired* but most often results from long-standing localized bronchial infection.

Etiology. Cystic fibrosis, immotile cilia syndrome, foreign body aspiration, immunodeficiency states, and certain postinfectious conditions (e.g., adenovirus, pertussis, measles, and tuberculosis) are the most common causes of bronchiectasis. Chronic sinusitis, allergic bronchopulmonary aspergillosis, and (rarely) asthma are other etiologic factors. Chronic infection and inflammation lead to destruction of the bronchial wall, with dilation, loss of mucociliary transport, and chronic mucus hypersecretion with obstruction. In its early stages bronchiectasis may be reversible if the underlying problem can be corrected and the infection controlled.

Clinical Manifestations. The presentation of bronchiectasis may be subtle, but it often includes pro-

TABLE 12–12
Differential Diagnosis of Recurrent Pneumonia

Hereditary Disorders
Cystic fibrosis
Sickle cell disease

Disorders of Immunity
AIDS
Bruton agammaglobulinemia
Selective IgG subclass deficiencies
Common variable immunodeficiency syndrome
Severe combined immunodeficiency syndrome

Disorders of Leukocytes
Chronic granulomatous disease
Hyperimmunoglobulin E syndrome (Job syndrome)
Leukocyte adhesion defect

Disorders of Cilia
Immotile cilia syndrome
Kartagener syndrome

Anatomic Disorders
Sequestration
Lobar emphysema
Esophageal reflux
Foreign body
Tracheoesophageal fistula (H type)
Gastroesophageal reflux
Bronchiectasis
Aspiration (oropharyngeal incoordination)

AIDS, Acquired immunodeficiency syndrome; *Ig,* immunoglobulin.

ductive cough, fever, hemoptysis, digital clubbing, and persistent moist rales over the affected area. Bronchiectasis leads to the development of a rich bronchial blood supply to the affected area; thus **hemoptysis** is a frequent *complication.* Atelectasis is common and is caused by obstruction of the affected bronchus. Wheezing is infrequent.

Diagnosis. Chest roentgenograms may reveal dilated airways that usually are manifested as parallel densities ("tram tracks"), and high-resolution CT scans may show dilated airways appearing as ring shadows. Fusiform dilation (cylindrical bronchiectasis) may be reversible when the disease is managed aggressively, but saccular dilation usually is irreversible.

Treatment. Therapy for bronchiectasis involves antibiotics and chest physiotherapy. Underlying conditions should be treated if possible. When evidence of localized, irreversible bronchiectasis is present, pulmonary resection should be considered because a focus of infection may spread to other, uninvolved areas of the lung. Additional indications for surgery are hemorrhage and resectable disease accompanied by failure to thrive that does not respond to medical therapy.

Lung Abscess

Lung abscess is an uncommon but serious problem in children and usually is caused by aspiration of foreign material into the lung or by infection behind an obstructed bronchus. Occasionally an abscess develops from hematogenous spread of infection. The most commonly involved sites are the posterior segments of the upper lobes and the superior segments of the lower lobes (into which aspirated material will drain when the child is recumbent). A lung abscess results when there is localized infection that destroys lung tissue, leaving a cavity containing pus and debris. Anaerobic bacteria most often are isolated from abscess cavities, but other organisms also may cause abscesses, including *S. aureus, Klebsiella pneumoniae,* fungi, and mycobacteria.

The *clinical manifestations* of lung abscess initially are fever and other systemic symptoms; cough usually develops later in the course of the disease. Symptoms may be like those of typical pneumonia (from which abscesses sometimes evolve). Chest roentgenograms or CT scan reveal a cavitary lesion, often with an air-fluid level, surrounded by parenchymal inflammation. If the cavity communicates with the bronchi, organisms may be isolated from sputum.

Diagnostic bronchoscopy may be indicated to rule out a foreign body and to obtain microbiologic specimens, especially if the patient does not produce sputum. In almost all cases the lesion will regress when appropriate antimicrobial therapy is administered. Antibiotics should be chosen to cover the most likely organisms (clindamycin, penicillin, or ampicillin-sulbactam will cover the majority of anaerobic flora) and should be continued for several weeks until all signs of infection have cleared. In most patients clinical and roentgenographic resolution is complete within several months. Occasionally a patient with previously undiagnosed diaphragmatic hernia is suspected of having a lung abscess because air-fluid levels are present on a chest film. If the patient's symptoms do not correspond to the roentgenographic picture, an upper gastrointestinal series may help in the diagnosis.

Pulmonary Tuberculosis

See Chapter 10.

Pertussis

See Chapter 10.

REFERENCES

Behrman RE, Kliegman RM, Jenson HB, editors: *Nelson textbook of pediatrics*, ed 16, Philadelphia, 2000, WB Saunders, Chapters 175, 393, 410, 411.

Britto J, Habibi P, Walters S, et al: Systemic complications associated with bacterial tracheitis, *Arch Dis Child* 74(3):249–250, 1996.

Dowell SF, Kupronis BA, Zell ER, et al: Mortality from pneumonia in children in the United States, 1939 through 1996, *N Engl J Med* 342(19):1399–1407, 2000.

Epler GR, Colby TV, McLoud TC, et al: Bronchiolitis obliterans organizing pneumonia, *N Engl J Med* 312(3):152–158, 1985.

Fitzgerald D, Mellis C, Johnson M, et al: Nebulized budesonide is as effective as nebulized adrenaline in moderately severe croup, *Pediatrics* 97(5):722–725, 1996.

Lewiston NJ: Bronchiectasis in childhood, *Pediatr Clin North Am* 31(4):865–878, 1984.

Owayed AF, Campbell DM, Wang EE: Underlying causes of recurrent pneumonia in children, *Arch Pediatr Adolesc Med* 154(2): 190–194, 2000.

Palafox M, Guiscafre H, Reyes H, et al: Diagnostic value of tachypnoea in pneumonia defined radiologically, *Arch Dis Child* 82(1):41–45, 2000.

Perlstein PH, Kotagal UR, Schoettker PJ, et al: Sustaining the implementation of an evidence-based guideline for bronchiolitis, *Arch Pediatr Adolesc Med* 154(10):1001–1007, 2000.

Rowe P, Klassen T: Corticosteroids for croup, *Arch Pediatr Adolesc Med* 150(4):344–346, 1996.

Tan T, Seilheimer D, Kaplan S: Pediatric lung abscess: clinical management and outcome, *Pediatr Infect Dis J* 14(1):51–55, 1995.

HYPERSENSITIVITY DISEASES
Asthma

See Chapter 8.

Hypersensitivity Pneumonitis

Nonasthmatic allergic pulmonary disease, also known as **extrinsic allergic alveolitis,** is caused by inhalation of a variety of organic antigens found in dust and may occur as an acute syndrome or as a chronic, progressive disease. The most common antigens are from fungal organisms (such as thermophilic actinomycetes) and avian danders. The antigens are associated with occupational or agricultural exposure and include thermophilic bacteria found in moldy hay, grain, mushrooms, sugar cane, home or automobile air conditioners, heated humidifiers, *Bacillus subtilis* and amebae found in water, and animal proteins derived from feathers, serum, or excrement.

Clinical Manifestations. *Acute symptoms,* which usually begin within 4–8 hours after exposure, are dyspnea, coughing, malaise, fever, and chills. Physical examination reveals tachypnea and diffuse rales without wheezing. Marked leukocytosis and elevation of serum immunoglobulins other than IgE are often present. The immune mechanism is similar to a type III or Arthus-like immune response because antigen-antibody complexes are present and the polymorphonuclear leukocytes become activated (see Chapter 8). Chest roentgenograms reveal a diffuse interstitial infiltrate without hyperinflation.

The *chronic form* of hypersensitivity pneumonitis is characterized by persistent and progressive respiratory symptoms (e.g., dyspnea and exercise intolerance) without the fever and chills of the acute form. Anorexia and weight loss may be prominent. Fine basilar crackles are heard on physical examination, and the roentgenogram reveals diffuse interstitial fibrosis. Type III and type IV immune responses may be activated in chronic allergic alveolitis.

Pulmonary function testing reveals decreased vital capacity, which may be reversible in the acute form but becomes irreversible in the chronic form. PaO_2 is decreased as a result of reduced diffusion of oxygen; $PaCO_2$ usually is decreased because of hyperventilation. Precipitating IgG antibodies to the inciting antigen usually are found in the serum but also may be seen in asymptomatic patients.

Diagnosis. The diagnosis depends on a high index of suspicion and a careful history and epidemiologic investigation. Often symptoms subside after hospitalization, only to recur on the patient's return home. Serologic tests for precipitins and cultures of airborne fungi may be helpful; inhalational challenge testing may be necessary for some patients. If a humidifier or air conditioning unit is the source of disease, Legionnaire disease may need to be excluded from the diagnosis.

Treatment. Therapy consists of administering steroids and helping the patient avoid exposure to the inciting agent. Proper cleaning of water sources is important. In severe cases, drastic measures to prevent environmental exposure may be necessary. The *prognosis* is usually good if the patient can prevent further exposure.

Allergic Bronchopulmonary Aspergillosis

See Chapter 8.

REFERENCES

Amin RS, Wilmott RW: Hypersensitivity pneumonitis and eosinophilic pulmonary diseases. In Chernick V, Boat TF, Kendig EL, editors: *Disorders of the respiratory tract in children,* ed 6, Philadelphia, 1998, WB Saunders.

Behrman RE, Kliegman RM, Jenson HB, editors: *Nelson textbook of pediatrics,* ed 16, Philadelphia, 2000, WB Saunders, Chapters 396, 397.

NEUROLOGIC DISORDERS AFFECTING RESPIRATORY FUNCTION

Apnea

Apnea is defined as the cessation of breathing resulting from the lack of respiratory effort (**central apnea**) or total airway obstruction (**obstructive apnea**). In many patients, apneic episodes may have both central and obstructive components (**mixed apnea**). Brief respiratory pauses usually lasting up to 10 seconds, during which no respiratory effort can be detected, are common in normal infants and children, especially after a sigh. Pauses lasting longer than 15 seconds, however, are considered abnormal. Normally when a child whose airway is occluded tries to breathe, respiratory centers in the brain recruit a progressively greater amount of motor output from the respiratory center until the obstruction is overcome; however, if this output fails to overcome the obstruction, an arousal impulse is triggered in the brain that causes the child to involuntarily move his or her head or body in order to relieve the obstruction. If any individual component of this final arousal response system fails, the apneic child will die.

The *etiology* of apnea is diverse and not well understood (Table 12–13). Premature infants commonly exhibit episodes of apnea, which may be associated with cyanosis and bradycardia (see Chapter 6). Apnea occurring in older infants warrants thorough investigation. Surgical therapy (removal of adenoids, tonsils, or other obstructing tissue or bypass of the obstruction by tracheostomy) may be necessary in children who are symptomatic with obstructive apnea.

Obstructive sleep apnea syndrome (OSAS) affects 1–2% of children and presents with snoring and distress during sleep because of complete or partial upper airway obstruction. Episodes of respiratory pauses, gasping, and hypoxia may lead to cor pulmonale, failure to thrive, and poor school performance. Tonsil and adenoid hypertrophy, obesity, craniofacial malformations, glossoptosis, and neuromuscular diseases are risk factors. Polysomnography is required because not all children who snore have OSAS.

Central alveolar hypoventilation leads to apnea and respiratory arrest, usually during sleep if primary. Secondary causes are Arnold-Chiari malformation, obesity, dysautonomia, increased intracranial pressure, and mitochondrial metabolic disorders.

Sudden Infant Death Syndrome

Sudden infant death syndrome (SIDS) is defined as the unexpected death of an infant less than 1 year of age, the cause of which remains unexplained after an autopsy, death scene investigation, and review of clinical history. The incidence of SIDS has fallen dramatically in the past 20 years, with a current incidence of 0.74/1000 births. The rates are highest in black and American Indian populations; in children of young, impoverished mothers who smoke cigarettes; in premature infants; in infants whose mothers have abused drugs; and during the winter. SIDS is rare before 4 weeks or after 6 months of age.

A variety of mechanisms have been proposed to explain SIDS, although none have been proven. Leading theories include cellular brainstem abnormalities or maturational delay related to neural or cardiorespiratory control. A portion of SIDS deaths may be attributed to prolongation of the QT interval; abnormal central nervous system control of respiration; CO_2 rebreathing from sleeping face down, especially in soft bedding; and possibly vascular compression of the vertebral arteries in some positions of the infant head.

The risk of SIDS is increased three to five times in siblings of infants who have died of SIDS. The etiology of the increased risk is unknown. Monitoring of siblings may be indicated. Because infants who sleep in the prone position are at increased risk for SIDS, current recommendations are that otherwise normal infants sleep supine. The decline in SIDS deaths seen in recent years is correlated with supine sleeping. Other preventive measures are prevention of maternal cigarette smoking and avoidance of use of polystyrene and other soft cushions for infant bedding.

Because SIDS strikes without warning in an infant previously thought to be healthy, the effect on families is especially devastating, and psychologic support is needed. Inappropriate investigation for possible child abuse should be avoided. The *differential diagnosis* is noted in Table 12–14.

Acute Life-Threatening Events (Near-Miss SIDS)

An acute life-threatening event is defined as an unexpected and frightening change in behavior characterized by apnea, color change, limpness, choking, and gagging. The incidence of such events is 0.05–1%. Specific causes can be identified in over 50% of the cases; central nervous system causes account for 15% of cases, and cardiovascular, metabolic, airway obstruction, and child abuse a smaller percentage. Numerous possible *etiologies* (Table 12–14) warrant diagnostic evaluation, which should include an electroencephalogram; chest

TABLE 12–13
Categories of Apnea

Disease	Example	Mechanism	Signs	Treatment
Apnea of prematurity	Premature (<36 wk)	Central control, airway obstruction	Apnea, bradycardia	Theophylline, caffeine, nasal CPAP, intubation
Ondine curse	Congenital central hypoventilation syndrome	Central control	Apnea	Mechanical ventilation
Obesity hypoventilation	Obesity, Prader-Willi syndrome	Airway obstruction, central control	Obesity, somnolence, polycythemia, cor pulmonale	Theophylline, weight loss
Obstructive sleep apnea	Chronic tonsil hypertrophy, Pierre Robin syndrome, Down syndrome, cerebral palsy, myotonic dystrophy, myopathy	Airway obstruction by enlarged tonsils or adenoids, choanal stenosis or atresia, large tongue, temporomandibular joint dysfunction, micrognathia, velopharyngeal incompetence; also may be central	Daytime sleepiness, snoring, night insomnia and enuresis, hyperactivity, poor school performance, behavior problems, mouth breathing, inspiratory stridor	Tonsillectomy, adenoidectomy, nasal trumpets, CPAP, uvuloveloplasty
Cyanotic "breath-holding spells"	Breath holder younger than 3 yr of age	Prolonged expiratory apnea; hyperventilation; cerebral anoxia	Cyanosis, syncope, brief tonic-clonic movements	Reassurance that the condition is self-limiting; must exclude seizure disorder
Pallid "breath-holding spells"	Breath holder	Asystole; reflex anoxic seizures	Rapid onset, with or without crying; pallor; bradycardia; opisthotonos; seizures; follows painful stimuli	Atropine (?); must exclude seizure disorder; less benign than cyanotic breath holding
SIDS	Previously normal child; increased incidence with prematurity, SIDS in sibling, maternal drug abuse, cigarette smoking, males; may have preceding minor URI	Central respiratory control; cardiac arrhythmia (prolonged QT syndrome) (?); central cardiac control (?); prolonged expiratory apnea (?) Rebreathing (?) *Other:* 1. Parental-induced airway obstruction–suffocation (accidental or abuse) 2. Chemoreceptor dysfunction 3. Overheating	2–3-month-old child found cyanotic, apneic, and pulseless in bed	No treatment; prevention with home apnea monitor unproven; supine sleep position reduces risk

Data from Southall D: *Pediatrics* 80:73, 1988; Mark J, Brooks J: *Pediatr Clin North Am* 31:907, 1984; Gordon N: *Dev Med Child Neurol* 29:805, 1987.
(?), Unproven contributing factor; *CPAP,* continuous positive airway pressure by facial mask or nasal prongs; *SIDS,* sudden infant death syndrome; *URI,* upper respiratory infection.

TABLE 12–14
Differential Diagnosis of Sudden Infant Death Syndrome

Fulminant infection*
Infant botulism†
Seizure disorder
Brain tumor*
Hypoglycemia†
Medium-chain acyl-coenzyme A dehydrogenase deficiency†
Carnitine deficiency*†
Urea cycle defect†
Child abuse*
Hemosiderosis/pulmonary hemorrhage syndrome
Exposure to toxic environmental fungus
Drug intoxication†
Cardiac arrhythmia
Gastroesophageal reflux*
Midgut volvulus/shock*
Laryngospasm

---

*Obvious or suspected at autopsy.
†Diagnostic test required.

roentgenogram; electrocardiogram; blood gas analysis; blood chemistry evaluations, including measurements of glucose, calcium, blood urea nitrogen, and electrolytes; an evaluation for gastroesophageal reflux (e.g., barium swallow or pH probe study); and a 12–24-hour recording of heart and respiratory activity (pneumogram).

Parents of infants ascertained to be at high risk for recurrence of such events may be offered home monitoring with an electronic monitor. No objective guidelines exist for instituting or terminating the monitoring. The ability to predict which infant is at high risk for SIDS on the basis of a pneumogram is not established, but infants with a high percentage of periodic breathing or with apneic spells lasting longer than 15 seconds may be at high risk. However, many infants with previously normal pneumograms have subsequently died of SIDS, whereas most infants with abnormal pneumograms have not. The parents of infants who have had acute life-threatening events should be instructed in basic cardiac pulmonary resuscitation.

Vocal Cord Paralysis

Vocal cord paralysis is an important cause of laryngeal dysfunction. Paralysis may be unilateral or bilateral and more often is caused by damage to the recurrent laryngeal nerves than by a central lesion. The left recurrent laryngeal nerve passes around the arch of the aorta and thus is more susceptible to damage than the right laryngeal nerve. Trauma, such as neck traction during delivery, and lesions in the mediastinum are common causes of vocal cord paralysis. Central causes are the Arnold-Chiari malformation, hydrocephalus, intracranial hemorrhage, and dysgenesis of the nucleus ambiguus.

The symptoms of vocal cord paralysis are stridor, a weak cry (in infants), hoarseness, and aphonia. Unilateral paralysis may be relatively asymptomatic. Rarely, the cords are paralyzed in the abducted position, and aspiration results. Patients with such a condition, as well as those with bilateral abductor paralysis resulting in severe airway obstruction, may require tracheostomy. No specific treatment exists. However, patients with traumatic injury to the recurrent laryngeal nerve may have spontaneous improvement over time, in part as a result of compensatory movement by the nonparalyzed cord.

The *prognosis* for return of vocal cord function depends on the nature of the injury and whether or not the recurrent laryngeal nerve has been disrupted.

REFERENCES

American Academy of Pediatrics Task Force on Infant Positioning and SIDS: Positioning and SIDS: update, *Pediatrics* 98(6 Pt 1):1216–1218, 1996.
Behrman RE, Kliegman RM, Jenson HB, editors: *Nelson textbook of pediatrics*, ed 16, Philadelphia, 2000, WB Saunders, Chapters 383, 714.
Cote A, Russo P, Michaud J, et al: Sudden unexpected deaths in infancy: what are the causes? *J Pediatr* 135(4):437–443, 1999.
Donnelly LF, Strife JL, Myer CM III: Glossoptosis (posterior displacement of the tongue) during sleep: a frequent cause of sleep apnea in pediatric patients referred for dynamic sleep fluoroscopy, *AJR* 175(6):1557–1560, 2000.
Nieminen P, Tolonen U, Löppönen H: Snoring and obstructive sleep apnea in children, *Arch Otolaryngol Head Neck Surg* 126(4):481–486, 2000.
Southall DP, Plunkett MC, Bunts MW, et al: Covert video recordings of life-threatening child abuse: lessons for child protection, *Pediatrics* 100(5):735–760, 1997.

CARDIOVASCULAR DISORDERS
Pulmonary Hypertension and Cor Pulmonale

Diffuse lung disease, upper airway obstruction (such as hypertrophied tonsils or adenoids), pulmonary thromboembolism, or exposure to high altitude may produce pulmonary hypertension. Pulmonary hypertension also may result from excessive pulmonary blood flow when there is a left-to-right cardiac shunt (see Chapter 13). With prolonged hypertension, resulting from either increased flow or hypoxic vasoconstriction, permanent changes occur in the intima and media of the pulmonary artery, making the increased vascular resistance irreversible. Primary pulmonary hypertension is idiopathic, occurs in the absence of parenchymal lung or cardiac disease, may be associated with autoimmune disease (e.g., SLE or scleroderma) or anorectic antiobesity drugs, or may be inherited (autosomal dominant with incomplete penetrance and a female predominance) because of mutations in the bone morphogen receptor gene. Pulmonary hypertension responds poorly to therapy.

Pulmonary hypertension resulting from *lung disease* leads to hypertrophy and eventually to dilation of the right ventricle, a condition known as cor pulmonale. In advanced states, right heart failure may occur, with limitation of exercise capacity, hepatic congestion, fluid retention, and signs of tricuspid insufficiency. In severe disease the ventricular septum may be displaced toward the left ventricle, reducing its volume and thus also reducing left ventricular function.

The most common causes of cor pulmonale in children are diffuse chronic lung diseases such as CF and bronchopulmonary dysplasia. In these conditions airway obstruction leads to alveolar hypoxia, and parenchymal scarring may increase pulmonary vascular resistance.

The *diagnosis* of pulmonary hypertension should be suspected whenever there is prolonged hypoxemia or severe left-to-right shunting (see Chapter 13). In addition to the other physical findings associated with pulmonary or cardiac disease, an accentuated pulmonic component of the second heart sound may be heard in the left second interspace. Definitive diagnosis is made by cardiac catheterization, but echocardiography may confirm the presence of significant right ventricular hypertrophy, ventricular dysfunction, and tricuspid insufficiency indicative of increased pulmonary artery pressure.

Treatment is directed at the underlying condition. The relief of hypoxemia is essential and usually requires supplemental oxygen therapy. Heart failure may necessitate administration of diuretics and restriction of salt and fluid intake. Vasodilator therapy (calcium channel blockers) are helpful in approximately 25–35% of patients. Intravenous infusions of prostacyclin, either acutely or chronically, can help reduce pulmonary artery pressures. Lung or heart-lung transplantation is the treatment for end-stage cor pulmonale.

The *prognosis* is poor once chronic cor pulmonale is present; if left ventricular failure is evident, the prognosis is even worse.

Pulmonary Edema

Pathophysiology. At the alveolar-capillary interface, capillary hydrostatic forces and tissue osmotic pressures tend to push fluid into the air spaces, whereas plasma osmotic pressures and tissue mechanical forces tend to force fluid away from the air spaces. Under normal circumstances the vectorial sum of these forces favors absorption, so that the alveolar spaces remain dry. Any fluid entering the alveolus normally is removed by the pulmonary lymphatics. Pulmonary edema forms when transcapillary fluid flux exceeds lymphatic drainage. Reduced left ventricular function accompanied by pulmonary venous hypertension increases capillary hydrostatic pressure, which floods the interstitial spaces and alveoli with fluid, producing pulmonary edema. Fluid initially enters the interstitial space around the terminal bronchioles, alveoli, and arteries **(interstitial edema),** causing increased lung stiffness, premature closure of bronchioles on expiration, and dyspnea and tachypnea as a result of stimulation of lung receptors. If the process continues, fluid enters the alveolar space, reducing compliance and creating a perfused but unventilated area called a *shunt.* Shunting, not the presence of fluid in the alveoli, produces hypoxia.

Pulmonary hypertension as occurs in cor pulmonale rarely produces pulmonary edema, because the site of increased vascular resistance is proximal to the capillary bed. However, pulmonary edema may be seen when intrathoracic pressure becomes excessively negative (e.g., in upper airway obstruction from hypertrophied tonsils). Pulmonary edema also may occur in patients having decreased serum oncotic pressure; receiving large volumes of intravenous fluid following capillary damage (e.g., from smoke inhalation or hydrocarbon aspiration); with ascent to high altitude; and having a history of central nervous system injury (neurogenic).

Clinical Manifestations. Pulmonary edema typically produces dyspnea, cough (often with frothy, pink-tinged sputum), tachypnea, signs of increased respiratory effort, and diffuse rales. Chest roentgenograms reveal a diffuse infiltrate that classically is in a perihilar pattern but may be obscured by underlying lung disease. Signs of interstitial edema (Kerley B lines) may be seen, especially at the lung bases.

Treatment. Treatment should include positioning of the patient in an upright posture and administration of oxygen but otherwise is directed toward relieving the underlying problem. Morphine may relieve dyspnea and, by dilating central veins, reduce venous return to the heart. Diuretic therapy (furosemide) and rapid-acting intravenous positive inotropic agents also are helpful. In severe cases, mask continuous positive airway pressure (CPAP) or intubation with positive end-expiratory pressure (PEEP) may be required.

The *prognosis* for patients with pulmonary edema depends on the nature of the underlying cause and on the response to therapy.

Acute (Adult) Respiratory Distress Syndrome

ARDS is a syndrome of acute and persistent lung inflammation with increased vascular permeability that results from injury to the alveolar-capillary interface. Profound hypoxemia and bilateral infiltrates are characteristic findings, but there is no demonstrable increase in pulmonary capillary wedge pressure. Inflammatory mediators (tumor necrosis factor, interleukin-1, and interleukin-6) increase vascular permeability and produce chemotactic factors that recruit inflammatory cells to the site of injury. Preformed and newly synthesized mediators (proteases, kinins, and prostaglandins) and oxygen free radicals cause further vascular and parenchymal damage, leading to hypoxia and hypercapnia, which produce acute pulmonary hypertension. Therefore, ARDS becomes manifested as a composite condition of a pulmonary shunt, decreased pulmonary compliance, and pulmonary hypertension.

The *etiology* of ARDS is varied, but the condition often results from shock (especially septic shock), aspiration (of hydrocarbons), inhalation of toxic fumes (e.g., smoke, nitrogen dioxide, sulfur dioxide, and ammonia), pancreatitis, or trauma (e.g., burns, near-drowning, head injury, or fat emboli from fractures). ARDS also may be associated with pneumonia, pulmonary emboli, disseminated intravascular coagulation, drug overdose, uremia, and multiple transfusions. ARDS is one organ manifestation of **multiple organ dysfunction syndrome** (MODS), which is usually initiated by one of the above etiologic factors during the development of **systemic inflammatory response syndrome** (SIRS) (see Chapter 3).

Patients with ARDS have severe hypoxemia and respiratory distress. Chest roentgenograms reveal diffuse alveolar infiltrates, although only interstitial edema may be seen in the early stages. Often a period of hours to even days may elapse between the original insult and the development of overt respiratory failure.

Treatment consists of mechanical ventilation allowing for lung-protective permissive hypercarbia (low tidal volume ventilation), accompanied by the application of PEEP, oxygen, and therapy for the underlying problem. Surfactant and inhaled nitric oxide may also be of some benefit. Unresolving ARDS (>7 days) may improve with high-dose and pro-longed (32 days) methylprednisolone therapy. The mortality rate in patients with ARDS ranges from 35–50%, reflecting the severity of the insult to the lungs and other organ systems that issues both from ARDS itself and from its underlying diseases.

Pulmonary Embolism

Pulmonary embolism is rare in childhood and may be associated with indwelling vascular catheters, oral contraceptives, lupus anticoagulant or other hypercoagulable states (see Chapter 14), trauma, abortion, or malignancy. Because the pulmonary vascular bed is very distensible, small emboli, even if multiple, usually are not detected unless they are infected and cause pulmonary infection. However, large emboli may lead to acute dyspnea, pleuritic chest pain, cough, hemoptysis, and even death. Hypoxia is common, as are nonspecific ST segments and T-wave changes on the electrocardiogram, an increased P_2 heart sound or presence of a fourth heart sound, and atelectasis or cardiomegaly on chest radiograph. Usually the chest x-ray is negative.

Ventilation-perfusion scans are useful in *diagnosis* by revealing defects in perfusion without matching ventilation defects. Other diagnostic tests, such as measurement of D-dimers in circulating blood, helical chest CT scan, and venous ultrasonography for patients with leg symptoms can be useful adjuncts. For *definitive diagnosis*, however, a pulmonary angiogram is the procedure of choice.

Treatment of proven pulmonary embolism is supportive (oxygen administration) and also should be directed toward the predisposing factors. Heparin may be useful in preventing the development of further emboli. Thrombolytic therapy or surgery may be helpful in treating massive embolization.

REFERENCES

Arcasoy SM, Kreit JW: Thrombolytic therapy of pulmonary embolism, *Chest* 115(6):1695–1707, 1999.

Beck C, Dubois J, Grignon A, et al: Incidence and risk factors of catheter-related deep vein thrombosis in a pediatric intensive care unit: a prospective study, *J Pediatr* 133(2):237–241, 1998.

Behrman RE, Kliegman RM, Jenson HB, editors: *Nelson textbook of pediatrics,* ed 16, Philadelphia, 2000, WB Saunders, Chapters 64, 65, 408, 409.

Ware LB, Matthay MA: The acute respiratory distress syndrome, *N Engl J Med* 342(18):1334–1349, 2000.

Wyncoll DL, Evans TW: Acute respiratory distress syndrome, *Lancet* 354(9177):497–501, 1999.

ASPIRATION SYNDROMES

Aspiration of material into the lungs is common in children and may be asymptomatic or fatal. When children with depressed levels of consciousness aspirate gastric contents from emesis, it may lead to severe pneumonia or to ARDS. The most common aspiration syndromes include the following:

- Foreign body aspiration
- Aspiration associated with gastroesophageal reflux
- Near-drowning

Foreign Body Aspiration

Aspiration of foreign bodies into the tracheobronchial tree is more common than usually is recognized. The majority of patients are younger than 4 years of age; most of the deaths also occur in this age group. Such children often put virtually anything into their mouths and frequently are out of sight of even the most diligent caretaker. Younger children most commonly aspirate food, balloons, small toys, and other small objects. Older children also may aspirate objects that they have held in their mouths.

Clinical Manifestations. A high percentage of children who aspirate foreign bodies exhibit either a clear-cut history of choking (or witnessed aspiration) or physical or roentgenographic evidence of the foreign body. However, a small percentage of patients with foreign body aspiration have a negative history because events have gone unobserved or unrecognized. Physical findings consistent with acute foreign body aspiration include unilateral absence of breath sounds, localized wheezing, stridor, and bloody sputum. Roentgenographic studies may reveal the presence of a radiopaque object or evidence of air trapping on exhalation. When aspiration is suspected, expiratory or lateral decubitus chest films should be requested, although fluoroscopy may be more helpful.

Because the right main bronchus is a more direct continuation of the trachea than the left main bronchus, foreign bodies tend to enter the right lung preferentially. However, they also may be coughed out more readily from the right side; in many large reported series nearly as many foreign bodies were found on the left as on the right. Some foreign bodies, especially nuts or seeds, may migrate from place to place in the airways and even lodge in the larynx on coughing, totally occluding the airway. Such migratory foreign bodies often are not associated with roentgenographic abnormalities and are difficult to detect.

Foreign bodies also may lodge in the esophagus and compress the trachea, producing respiratory symptoms. An esophageal foreign body should be included in the *differential diagnosis* of infants or young children with persistent stridor or wheezing, particularly if the conditions are associated with dysphagia.

Diagnosis. Most foreign bodies are small and quickly coughed out, but many may remain in the lung for long periods before diagnosis and may come to medical attention because of symptoms of fever, cough, sputum production, or chest pain. In patients with persistent wheezing unresponsive to bronchodilator therapy, with persistent atelectasis, with recurrent or persistent pneumonia, or with persistent cough without other explanation, the presence of a foreign body should be suspected. If good evidence exists (in history or in physical or roentgenographic examination) for a bronchial foreign body, the patient should undergo rigid bronchoscopy. Flexible bronchoscopy may be a useful diagnostic technique when the presentation is not straightforward.

Prevention and Treatment. The best approach to foreign body aspiration is to educate parents and caretakers in preventing the event. Before their molar teeth have developed, infants and children should not have nuts, uncooked carrots, and other foods that may be easily broken into small pieces and aspirated. Toys should be free of small parts that may be aspirated.

Gastroesophageal Reflux

See Chapter 11.

Near-Drowning

Near-drowning is a frequent emergency in children that may lead to hypoxic organ damage and pulmonary dysfunction. In some cases, laryngospasm prevents the victim from aspirating water into the lungs, and the damage results from hypoxia alone. Usually, however, the victim aspirates water, which disturbs ventilation-perfusion relationships, causes loss of surfactant, and produces pulmonary edema.

The primary goal in *treatment* is the correction of acidosis and hypoxia as rapidly as possible. In children, cardiac activity persists long after ventilation ceases, and the most urgent priority is provision of effective ventilation. Under most circumstances water is absorbed from the lungs quickly, and ventilation should be initiated without delay and without attempting to clear water from the airways. Rewarming the severely hypothermic patients (core temperature <33° C) should be initiated promptly. Closed-chest cardiac massage is used, if necessary. Intubation and PEEP often are very helpful in reducing intrapulmonary shunting and improving oxygenation. Once effective ventilation is established, metabolic acidosis often corrects itself, but judicious administration of bicarbonate may be necessary in the presence of profound acidosis.

Cerebral edema often results from the hypoxic insult and must be managed aggressively. Hyperventilation (to maintain PCO_2 in the range of 35–38 torr), fluid restriction, and mild osmotic diuresis may be necessary to prevent or treat intracranial hypertension.

The *prognosis* for victims of near-drowning is variable and depends chiefly on the degree of initial hypoxic insult. Children who regain consciousness after they are resuscitated have an excellent prognosis. Submersion for longer than 10 minutes, hypothermia, elapse of more than 10 minutes before initiation of effective basic life support, and cardiopulmonary resuscitation for longer than 25 minutes in the emergency room are associated with a high mortality rate and severe neurologic impairment. Exceptions to this latter observation may occur, however, in persons who have nearly drowned in very cold water, because the cold temperature slows metabolism, activates the diving reflex, and limits hypoxic damage.

REFERENCES

Behrman RE, Kliegman RM, Jenson HB, editors: *Nelson textbook of pediatrics*, ed 16, Philadelphia, 2000, WB Saunders, Chapters 69, 386.

Metrangelo S, Monetti C, Meneghini L, et al: Eight years' experience with foreign body aspiration in children: what is really important for timely diagnosis? *J Pediatr Surg* 34(8):1229–1231, 1999.

Sachdeva RC: Near drowning, *Crit Care Clin* 15(2):281–296, 1999.

HEMOSIDEROSIS

Pulmonary hemosiderosis is characterized by the accumulation of hemosiderin in the lungs as a result of bleeding into the lungs. Red blood cells are phagocytosed by alveolar macrophages, and the hemoglobin is converted to hemosiderin; with the use of special iron-staining techniques, the hemosiderin within the alveolar macrophages can be identified microscopically. Hemosiderin-laden macrophages may be found in sputum, gastric aspirate, bronchoalveolar lavage fluid, or a lung biopsy.

Etiology. Hemosiderosis may result from bleeding anywhere in the lung, airway, pharynx, nasopharynx, or mouth, but it usually occurs as a result of diffuse alveolar bleeding, which may be of low grade and transient or brisk and massive.

Clinical Manifestations. The presentation of hemosiderosis is variable but often includes iron-deficiency anemia with a history of cough, tachypnea, and wheezing. Occasionally, acute, frank hemoptysis or hematemesis is seen. At the time of acute pulmonary bleeding, fever, leukocytosis, and an elevated erythrocyte sedimentation rate (ESR) may occur. Some cases are associated with eosinophilia. Chest roentgenograms usually reveal transient infiltrates, but massive infiltrates, atelectasis, and hyperinflation may occur. In the chronic stages an interstitial pattern suggestive of interstitial fibrosis has been seen.

Many patients are given an incorrect diagnosis of bacterial pneumonia. Iron-deficiency anemia or the presence of guaiac-positive stools in a child with pneumonia (particularly if eosinophilia is present) suggests pulmonary hemosiderosis, and sputum, gastric aspirate, or bronchoalveolar lavage samples should be obtained to confirm the presence of hemosiderin-laden macrophages.

The *classification* of pulmonary hemosiderosis reflects the associated findings and presumed etiology of the alveolar hemorrhage. In the majority of pediatric cases, no etiology can be identified (**"idiopathic pulmonary hemosiderosis"**). Some of these idiopathic cases are later found to have autoimmune diseases (e.g., SLE, celiac disease, juvenile rheumatoid arthritis, and polyarteritis). Cases of pulmonary hemosiderosis associated with glomerular basement membrane disease (glomerulonephritis) may be subdivided into those with circulating antigen-antibody complexes and those with antibody deposited along the basement membrane of the kidney or lung (Goodpasture syndrome). These antigen-antibody complexes may be associated with a number of collagen-vascular diseases or systemic vasculitis (e.g., **Henoch-Schönlein purpura** or **Wegener granulomatosis**); occasionally lung involvement with collagen-vascular diseases occurs without or before renal involvement. Many of these cases have a positive result in tests for antineutrophil cytoplasm antibodies (ANCAs); this finding is associated with a poor prognosis. Pulmonary hemosiderosis in infants also can be associated with precipitating serum antibodies to cow's milk (**Heiner syndrome**). These infants may exhibit wheezing, eosinophilia, high IgE levels, and failure to thrive. The role of the milk sensitivity is unclear, but elimination of cow's milk from the diet often decreases the frequency and severity of the alveolar hemorrhage. Certain forms of **heart disease** associated with increased pulmonary venous and capillary pressures also may cause alveolar bleeding and pulmonary hemosiderosis. Acute fulminant pulmonary hemorrhage occurring largely in black male infants currently has an unknown etiology.

Treatment. Management of the acute episodes of bleeding should involve administration of oxygen, blood transfusions, intratracheal epinephrine, and, if necessary, mechanical ventilation accompanied by PEEP to tamponade the bleeding. Attempts should be made to identify the cause of the bleeding; often an open lung biopsy is necessary (Table 12–15). Idiopathic pulmonary hemosiderosis may respond to

TABLE 12-15
Differential Diagnosis of Hemoptysis–Pulmonary Hemorrhage

Cardiovascular
Heart failure
Eisenmenger syndrome
Arteriovenous fistula (Osler-Weber-Rendu syndrome)
Pulmonary embolism

Pulmonary
Respiratory distress syndrome
Bronchogenic cyst
Sequestration
Pneumonia (bacterial, mycobacterial, fungal, or
  parasitic)
Cystic fibrosis
Tracheobronchitis
Bronchiectasis
Toxic fungus (*Stachybotrys atra*) exposure
Abscess
Tumor (adenoma, carcinoid, hemangioma, metastasis)
Foreign body retention
Contusion-trauma

Immune
Henoch-Schönlein purpura
Heiner syndrome
Goodpasture syndrome
Wegener granulomatosis
Systemic lupus erythematosus
Allergic bronchopulmonary aspergillosis

Other
Hyperammonemia
Kernicterus
Intracranial hemorrhage (preterm infant)
Toxins

corticosteroids. Other immunosuppressant agents, such as azathioprine and cyclophosphamide, have been used when the condition has not responded to the administration of corticosteroids over 2–3 months. A trial period on a milk-free diet may be useful, and removal of mold-infested home materials is advised.

Prognosis. The outlook depends on the underlying cause of the bleeding. In some children the course of idiopathic hemosiderosis may be relentless, whereas other children bleed only once. Repeated hemorrhage often leads to chronic pulmonary fibrosis and respiratory insufficiency.

RESPIRATORY FAILURE

Respiratory failure occurs when the lungs are unable to deliver sufficient oxygen to the blood to meet metabolic demands. It may develop insidiously or may have an abrupt onset. The *etiology* of respiratory failure is legion. Common causes in children include bronchopulmonary dysplasia, respiratory distress syndrome, ARDS, end-stage cystic fibrosis, neuromuscular disorders, and status asthmaticus. These disorders produce respiratory failure by impairing normal respiratory muscle function as a result of abnormal metabolic states, nutritional deficiencies, or disease of the pulmonary parenchyma, airways, chest wall, or respiratory muscles. Among the *clinical manifestations* is usually increased respiratory drive, leading to tachypnea, dyspnea, retractions, and the use of accessory muscles. Auscultatory findings vary with the etiology of the problem and may include diminished or absent breath sounds, wheezing or prolonged expiration, crackles and rhonchi, and grunting on exhalation. Because approximately 5 g/dL of circulating deoxygenated hemoglobin is normally required for cyanosis to be evident clinically, patients who are anemic may have seriously impaired oxygen transport without obvious cyanosis. Early in the course of the condition, tachycardia is common. Bradycardia is a late and especially ominous sign and usually is followed rapidly by hypotension and cardiac arrest. Hypoxemia may produce restlessness and irritability that may progress to confusion, decreased levels of consciousness, seizures, and eventually coma. Hypercapnia leads to cerebral vasodilation and often severe headache and, in later stages, profound depression of the central nervous system.

Respiratory failure in children with chronic neuromuscular diseases is associated with restrictive lung disease (inspiratory weakness), ineffective cough as the result of expiratory weakness, atelectasis, chronic aspiration, and pneumonia (poor inspiration and poor cough). In addition, thoracoabdominal asynchrony and scoliosis may be present. Sleep apnea may also be present.

Diagnosis. The diagnosis of respiratory insufficiency and failure depends on careful observation of the patient, suspicion heightened by knowledge of the history and underlying clinical circumstances, and appropriate laboratory evaluation. The single most useful laboratory study is an arterial blood gas determination. However, when clinical evidence of respiratory insufficiency or failure is present, oxygen therapy should never be withheld while results of a blood gas study are being awaited.

Treatment. Treatment of respiratory failure should be directed immediately to relieve hypoxemia and hypercapnia. In pediatric patients it rarely is harmful to administer 100% oxygen for short periods, although the patient should be monitored carefully. Rarely, children with chronic respiratory insufficiency have blunted respiratory responses to hypercapnia and function chiefly on their hypoxic drive. In such instances the administration of high concentrations of oxygen can result in paradoxic respiratory depression.

A careful and systematic search should be made for the underlying (and potentially reversible) causes of the respiratory failure, and appropriate treatment should be instituted. In the presence of refractory hypoxia or significant hypercapnia ($PaCO_2$ >60 mm Hg), institution of mechanical ventilation or noninvasive positive-pressure ventilation should be considered.

Patients in respiratory failure often are very unstable and must be monitored carefully. Only a few minutes separate apnea from cardiac arrest. In children most cardiac arrests are the direct result of hypoxemia rather than of a primary cardiac abnormality. If respiratory failure cannot be reversed promptly by specific therapy (e.g., relief of pneumothorax or upper airway obstruction, and treatment of bronchospasm), intubation and mechanical ventilation usually will be necessary. In end-stage disease, lung transplantation may be indicated.

Patients with chronic neuromuscular disease require therapies that improve cough and mucociliary clearance (chest physiotherapy, external and internal vibration, cough assist devices) and, if these are un-successful, tracheostomy. Bilevel positive-pressure ventilation by nasal mask can provide IPPB of 9–14 cm H_2O and PEEP of 4–5 cm H_2O.

Prognosis. The outcome for patients with respiratory failure depends almost entirely on the nature of the underlying cause of the failure and the rapidity and efficacy of the therapy initiated. In patients with acute disease the prognosis should be good. However, in patients with chronic disease such as CF, respiratory failure has an ominous prognosis, although most patients can survive several episodes if treated vigorously.

REFERENCES

Behrman RE, Kliegman RM, Jenson HB, editors: *Nelson textbook of pediatrics,* ed 15, Philadelphia, 2000, WB Saunders, Chapters 424, 425.

Boat TF: Pulmonary hemorrhage and hemoptysis. In Chernic V, Boat TF, Kendig EL, editors: *Disorders of the respiratory tract in children,* Philadelphia, 1998, WB Saunders.

Kiper N, Goemen A, Ozcelik U, et al: Long-term clinical course of patients with idiopathic pulmonary hemosiderosis (1979–1994): prolonged survival with low-dose corticosteroid therapy, *Pediatr Pulmonol* 27(3):180–184, 1999.

LeClainche L, Le Bourgeois M, Fauroux B, et al: Long-term outcome of idiopathic pulmonary hemosiderosis in children, *Medicine* 79(5):318–326, 2000.

Montana E, Etzel RA, Allan T, et al: Environmental risk factors associated with pediatric idiopathic pulmonary hemorrhage and hemosiderosis in a Cleveland community, *Pediatrics* 99(1 Suppl 5):E51–E58, 1997.

CHAPTER 13

Cardiovascular System

Michael M. Brook*

The physiologic diagnosis and initial treatment of heart disease in children can usually be determined by a careful history and physical examination. Echocardiography is used to determine the exact features of cardiac defects before surgery. Cardiac catheterization and angiography are used when specific physiologic or anatomic information is needed or when therapeutic catheter interventions are indicated.

The origin of heart disease in children is a combination of genetic and environmental causes. Congenital heart disease (CHD) may be either genetic (e.g., Down and DiGeorge syndromes) or acquired (e.g., through maternal rubella) (Table 13–1). Acquired heart disease, such as rheumatic fever or atherosclerosis, may have genetic predispositions or may be the result of systemic diseases that directly or indirectly affect the heart or vasculature (Table 13–2). CHD is present in about 8 of every 1000 babies. It is slightly more common in premature infants and even more common in fetuses. About half of congenital heart defects are relatively insignificant, but half may result in infant death or disability if left untreated. Fortunately, current treatment methods allow the vast majority of even severely affected infants to survive into adolescence. Defects such as small ventricular septal defects (VSDs) and bicuspid aortic valves cause little or no disability, but the associated murmurs or clicks may cause substantial parental concern.

Although clinical evaluation is helpful and usually diagnostic in *symptomatic infants,* many other infants, even those with serious cardiac disease, can initially be asymptomatic in the immediate neonatal period. The same mechanism that allows fetuses with cardiac disease to thrive—the patent ductus arteriosus (PDA)—can obscure clinical manifestations in the infant. The PDA can supply blood to either the systemic or the pulmonary circulation as needed. For example, coarctation of the aorta can be missed because the pulses and leg blood pressures may be normal for the first day or so until the ductus arteriosus closes and completes the coarctation. A PDA in severe tetralogy of Fallot can supply pulmonary blood flow and increase the oxygen saturation. Even lethal defects such as hypoplastic left heart syndrome may be inapparent at birth because of the palliative effects of the PDA. Tests performed at the primary level in the newborn nursery, such as electrocardiography and chest radiography, may be nonspecific. Results may be normal for the first week or two of life. Many but not all serious congenital cardiac defects are associated with a lower than normal oxygen saturation. However, a normal oxygen saturation ($\geq$95%), as determined by pulse oximetry, does not guarantee a normal heart. Stenotic valve lesions often have normal oxygen saturation, even if they are severe. Other physical signs, such as tachypnea, hyperpnea, and tachycardia, also are important. Because many nonpathologic heart murmurs are heard at birth, the physician must use good judgment in deciding which require further evaluation by a pediatric cardiologist. Conversely, the absence of a heart murmur in a neonate is not evidence of the absence of CHD.

It is vital that the diagnosis of serious congenital cardiac defects be made as early as possible because virtually every congenital cardiac defect can be treated at least by palliation. If the defect is unrecognized, death, permanent damage, or serious complications (such as stroke) may occur before medical or surgical palliation can be provided. The physician caring for the infant in the newborn nursery must have a high index of suspicion regarding minor signs and symptoms. It is not the pediatrician's job

---

*Some material in this chapter was originally written by Paul C. Gillette, M.D.

TABLE 13–1
Congenital Malformation Syndromes Associated with Congenital Heart Disease

Syndrome	Cardiac Features
Trisomy 21 (Down syndrome)	Endocardial cushion defect
Trisomy 18	VSD, ASD, PDA, PS
Trisomy 13	VSD, ASD, PDA, dextrocardia
XO (Turner syndrome)	Coarctation of aorta, aortic stenosis
CHARGE association (coloboma, heart, atresia choanae, retardation, genital and ear anomalies)	TOF, endocardial cushion defect, VSD, ASD
22q11 (DiGeorge) syndrome	Aortic arch anomalies, conotruncal anomalies*
VACTERL association† (vertebral, anal, cardiac, tracheoesophageal, radial and/or renal, limb anomalies)	VSD
Congenital rubella	PDA, peripheral pulmonic stenosis, mitral regurgitation (in infancy)
Marfan syndrome	Dilated and dissecting aorta, aortic valve regurgitation, mitral valve prolapse
Williams syndrome	Supravalvular aortic stenosis, peripheral pulmonary stenosis
Infant of diabetic mother	Hypertrophic cardiomyopathy, VSD, conotruncal anomalies
Holt-Oram syndrome	ASD, VSD
Asplenia syndrome	Complex cyanotic heart lesions, anomalous pulmonary venous return, dextrocardia, single ventricle, single AV valve
Polysplenia syndrome	Azygos continuation of inferior vena cava, pulmonary atresia, dextrocardia, single ventricle
Fetal alcohol syndrome	VSD, ASD
Ellis–van Creveld syndrome	Single atrium
Zellweger syndrome	PDA, VSD, ASD

ASD, Atrial septal defect; *AV*, atrioventricular; *PDA*, patent ductus arteriosus; *PS*, pulmonic stenosis; *TOF*, tetralogy of Fallot; *VSD*, ventricular septal defect.
Conotruncal, Tetralogy of Fallot, pulmonary atresia, truncus arteriosus, transposition of great arteries.
†VACTERL association is also known as VATER (*v*ertebral, *a*nal, *t*racheoesophageal, *r*adial, *r*enal anomalies) association.

TABLE 13–2
Cardiac Manifestations of Systemic Diseases

Systemic Disease	Cardiac Complications
Hunter-Hurler syndrome	Valvular insufficiency, heart failure, hypertension
Fabry disease	Mitral insufficiency, coronary artery disease with myocardial infarction
Pompe disease	Short PR interval, cardiomegaly, heart failure, arrhythmias
Friedreich ataxia	Myocardiopathy, arrhythmias
Duchenne dystrophy	Myocardiopathy, heart failure
Juvenile rheumatoid arthritis	Pericarditis
Systemic lupus erythematosus	Pericarditis, Libman-Sacks endocarditis; congenital AV block
Marfan syndrome	Aortic and mitral insufficiency; dissecting aortic aneurysm
Homocystinuria	Coronary thrombosis
Kawasaki disease	Coronary artery aneurysm, thrombosis, myocardial infarction, myocarditis
Lyme disease	Arrhythmias, myocarditis
Graves disease (hyperthyroidism)	Tachycardia, arrhythmias, heart failure
Tuberous sclerosis	Cardiac rhabdomyoma

AV, Atrioventricular.

to make the detailed anatomic or physiologic diagnosis but rather to suspect heart disease, perform initial rapid stabilization, and obtain consultation of a pediatric cardiology team. The pediatric cardiologist then determines the physiologic diagnosis and uses echocardiography to make the exact anatomic diagnosis. Magnetic resonance imaging (MRI) or cardiac catheterization and angiography may be used to clear up details before surgical or catheter palliation or cure.

DIAGNOSTIC EVALUATION

CHD is the major cause of pediatric cardiovascular disease. The diagnostic evaluation of a child suspected of having CHD should proceed in an organized manner and usually includes the following:

1. Careful history
2. Physical examination
3. Pulse oximetry
4. Electrocardiography
5. Chest radiography
6. Echocardiography and Doppler studies
7. Cardiac catheterization
8. Exercise testing

History

In obtaining a history, the examiner must take into account the age of the patient. For example, in the infant, congestive heart failure usually becomes manifest through feeding difficulties (very common), easy fatigability, vomiting, lethargy, increased perspiration, and rapid respirations. In the older child congestive heart failure causes easy fatigability, shortness of breath, and dyspnea on exertion, which is usually best described in terms of specific activities such as walking on level ground, walking up steps, and bicycle riding. Orthopnea, paroxysmal nocturnal dyspnea, and edema are uncommon manifestations of heart failure in children. Congenital malformation syndromes (Table 13–1) and systemic illnesses must be considered (Table 13–2). The family history of congenital cardiac defects also is important, because almost all forms of CHD have a genetic component and can recur within a family. Certain lesions, such as tetralogy of Fallot, are more likely to recur than others.

Physical Examination

A thoughtful, thorough, and careful cardiac examination may provide significant clues to the presence of heart disease. The normal *heart rate* varies considerably according to age (Fig. 13–1). Tachycardia may be seen as a manifestation of heart failure or as a

dysrhythmia. Bradycardia is seen as a normal finding in patients with high vagal tone, particularly athletes, but may be a manifestation of second-degree or third-degree atrioventricular (AV) block.

The *respiratory rate* in pediatric patients with heart disease may be increased when there is a large left-to-right shunt or pulmonary venous congestion (caused by poor LV function or by venous obstruction). The increased pulmonary blood flow produces greater interstitial fluid, and this fluid increases lung stiffness (decreased compliance). The patient's *height, weight,* and *head circumference* (in infants) always should be assessed. Failure to thrive is frequently seen in infants with congestive heart failure and may be an important indication for surgery if medical management proves unsuccessful. In general, growth failure from congestive heart failure affects the weight first, then length, and, last, the head circumference.

The patient's *blood pressure* should be measured in the upper and lower extremities to identify coarctation of the aorta. If the pressure in only one arm is measured, it should be the right arm because the coarctation may involve the left subclavian artery. The appropriate-size cuff for the size of the arm should be used because a cuff that is too small (bladders that encircle less than 90% of the arm and cover less than 75% of the length) will produce a blood pressure measurement that is higher than the true intravascular reading. Blood pressure may be measured by the auscultation, oscillometric (Dynamap), or Doppler method. The pulse pressure, determined by subtracting the diastolic pressure from the systolic pressure, normally is less than 50 mm Hg or half the systolic pressure, whichever is less. A wide pulse pressure, as assessed by palpation, is usually seen with aortopulmonary connections (PDA, aortopulmonary window, truncus arteriosus), aortic insufficiency, fever, anemia, arteriovenous malformations (AVMs), or complete AV block. A narrow pulse pressure is recognized in congestive heart failure, severe aortic stenosis, or pericardial tamponade.

The level of the *jugular vein venous pulsations* in the neck provides a rough assessment of the right atrial pressure. This sign is difficult to ascertain in infants and young children but may be very helpful in the school-aged or older child. The veins are observed with the child sitting or lying in a relaxed manner on an examining table raised to 30 degrees. Greatly increased venous distention then can be recognized because normally pulsations are not visible above the clavicle in the sitting position. In complete AV block, the venous pulsations are variable and depend on the position of the tricuspid valve at the time of atrial systole; if the right atrium contracts when the tricuspid valve is closed, a large venous pulsation (cannon wave) will occur.

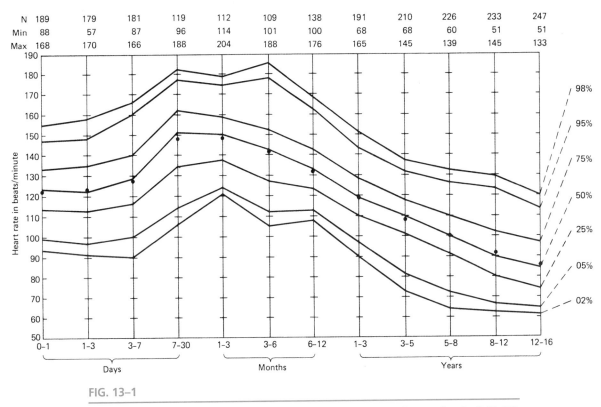

N	189	179	181	119	112	109	138	191	210	226	233	247
Min	88	57	87	96	114	101	100	68	68	60	51	51
Max	168	170	166	188	204	188	176	165	145	139	145	133

FIG. 13–1

Heart rate versus age (• = mean). (From Davignon A, Rautaharju P, Boiselle E: *Pediatr Cardiol* 1:123, 1980.)

The presence of *rales (crackles)* in the chest may be a sign of pulmonary edema caused by increased pulmonary venous pressure; rales also may indicate infection. The absence of rales is nonspecific because the patient in congestive heart failure may take shallow breaths. *Hepatomegaly* is one of the cardinal signs of heart failure in the infant and child. The liver is quite distensible in young children and thus provides a good measure of the intravascular volume and does not necessarily imply increased venous pressure. The liver should be palpated lightly so as not to create a tense abdomen. *Splenomegaly* may be present in some children with congestive heart failure and may be seen in children with infective endocarditis.

Cyanosis, a bluish discoloration of the skin, nails, and mucous membranes, is apparent in infants and children with hypoxemia who have 3–5 g/dL of unsaturated hemoglobin (discussed later in this chapter under Pulse Oximetry). *Clubbing,* a rounding or convexity of the nails, may begin in infancy; it may become very prominent in hypoxemic adolescents and young adults. *Edema* of the lower extremities is an uncommon characteristic of heart failure in infants but may be seen in older children or adolescents.

On inspection, *prominence of the precordial chest wall* frequently is seen in infants and children with cardiomegaly and is especially prominent when the right ventricle is involved. A *hyperdynamic precordium* suggests a volume load, usually caused by a large left-to-right shunt or semilunar or AV valve regurgitation. A *thrill,* the palpable manifestation associated with a loud *murmur,* is felt where the accompanying murmur is loudest.

Auscultation

The art of auscultation can be improved by a careful, systematic approach, with the examination carried out in a quiet room and without distractions. The infant should be examined in whatever position will quiet him or her, and the stethoscope bell should be used first to avoid the startle reaction. The examiner should listen first to the entire cardiac cycle, determining the first *heart sound* (S_1), systole, the second sound (S_2), and diastole. The examiner then should listen carefully for each and every type of sound and *murmur* possible, concentrating so hard on the sound or murmur in question that nothing else is heard. This technique is called "dissection" and is used at each location over the precordium.

Heart Sounds

The *first heart sound,* caused by AV valve closure (Fig. 13–2), is best heard at the lower left sternal border or apex. It may be split, with the second component soft and best recognized at the lower left sternal border. Anomalies (other than splitting) of the first heart sound are unusual. The sound can vary in intensity in complete AV block and can be muffled with a pericardial effusion or tamponade.

The *second heart sound,* produced by semilunar valve closure, is best heard at the second intercostal space. During inspiration, filling of the right side of the heart is increased, and the right ventricular ejection time is increased. This leads to wider splitting of the aortic and pulmonic components of the second heart sound in inspiration than in expiration. Widening of the splitting is seen with right ventricular volume overload, which occurs in an atrial septal defect (ASD) and in pulmonic stenosis or right bundle-branch block. The pulmonary component of the second heart sound is accentuated when the pulmonary artery pressure is increased, and it is decreased in intensity when low pulmonary artery diastolic pressure is present, as in pulmonary stenosis. The higher the pulmonary artery diastolic pressure, the earlier the closure of the pulmonic valve. Therefore, when pulmonary hypertension is present, the split is narrow or may be absent. It is obviously single in the presence of pulmonic or aortic valve atresia. The second heart sound is also increased when the aortic valve, which is normally the louder component, is closer to the chest than normal. This occurs in transposition of the great arteries. In aortic stenosis left ventricular systole may be prolonged enough to delay aortic valve closure, causing a narrow split, a single S_2, or rarely a paradoxical split. Advanced left bundle-branch block also may cause a paradoxical split.

The *third heart sound* (Fig. 13–2) is best heard with the stethoscope bell placed at the apex of the heart that is one third into diastole, but a right ventricular third heart sound is best heard at the lower left sternal border. The third heart sound is most commonly caused by increased flow through an AV valve as the result of a left-to-right shunt. A *fourth heart sound* (Fig. 13–2) just before the first heart sound, best heard at the third or fourth interspace, may be a sign of poor ventricular compliance.

Clicks

Ejection clicks are heard early in systole and are related to dilation of the ascending aorta or pulmonary artery. *Pulmonary ejection clicks* are heard best at the upper

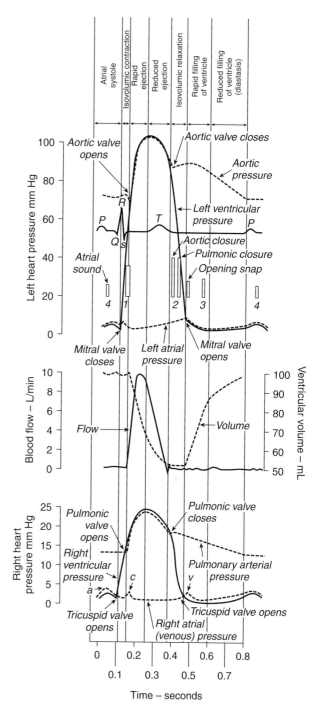

FIG. 13–2

Idealized diagram of temporal events of a cardiac cycle. (From Behrman RE, Kliegman RM, Jenson HB, editors: *Nelson textbook of pediatrics,* ed 16, Philadelphia, 2000, WB Saunders.)

left sternal border and may occur as late as 0.08 sec after the first sound; they also may be heard much earlier, even simultaneous with the first sound. They are louder on expiration and may disappear on inspiration. Because S_1 normally is soft at the upper left sternal border, an apparent S_1 that is loud at the upper left sternal border, especially on expiration, is a clue that the sound is a pulmonary ejection click, not S_1. Valvular pulmonic stenosis almost always is associated with a pulmonary ejection click, and pulmonary vascular disease frequently is associated with the condition. In contrast, *aortic ejection clicks* usually are well separated from the first sound, do not vary in intensity with respiration, and usually are heard best at the apex or mid–left sternal border. They usually are associated with a bicuspid aortic valve, valvular aortic stenosis, truncus arteriosus, and tetralogy of Fallot with pulmonary atresia.

Murmurs

Murmurs are described with regard to their intensity, timing, position, pitch, and distinguishing characteristics (such as variability). The intensity of the heart sounds can be used as a reference guide for the loudness of a murmur:

A grade 1 murmur is softer than the heart sounds and is difficult to hear.

A grade 2 murmur is equal to the heart sounds, and a grade 3 murmur is louder than the heart sounds. Grade 2 and 3 murmurs are easily heard but are not associated with a thrill.

A grade 4 murmur is associated with a precordial thrill.

A grade 5 murmur is heard with only the edge of the stethoscope on the chest.

A grade 6 murmur is heard either with the stethoscope off the chest or with the naked ear.

Systolic ejection murmurs (Fig. 13–3) typically are associated with obstruction to flow through abnormal semilunar valves or increased flow through normal semilunar valves. The murmurs begin after isovolumic contraction, about 0.08 sec after the first heart sound. In contrast, *holosystolic* or *regurgitant murmurs* typically are heard with a VSD with left-to-right shunt or mitral regurgitation. They begin during isovolumic contraction, obscuring the first heart sound. Ejection murmurs tend to have a crescendo and decrescendo (diamond) shape. Regurgitant murmurs may continue at the same intensity throughout systole, may be decrescendo, may peak late, or may even be of diamond shape. A late systolic murmur, usually crescendo, beginning after a midsystolic nonejection click, frequently is heard with mitral valve prolapse, indicating mitral regurgitation.

Diastolic murmurs (see Fig. 13–3) are heard when regurgitation occurs across the semilunar valves or when stenosis (real or relative from high flow) of the AV valves is present. The murmur of aortic regurgitation usually is very high pitched, the decrescendo beginning with the second heart sound, and located along the left sternal border. Pulmonary regurgitation can begin with the second heart sound or may be slightly after it (particularly with right bundle-branch block) but is usually of a lower pitch, unless pulmonary hypertension is present, in which case it sounds very much like aortic regurgitation. Stenotic murmurs across the AV valves usually are middiastolic and rumbling (very low pitch); the murmur of mitral stenosis occurs at the apex, and that of tricuspid stenosis occurs along the lower left sternal border. Murmurs of relative stenosis with anatomically normal AV valves may be associated with an ASD or with high flow across either the tricuspid valve or the mitral valve; these murmurs occur in children with large left-to-right shunts at the level of either the ventricle or the great artery.

Continuous murmurs usually peak in intensity near the end of systole and decrease in intensity a variable time into diastole. This murmur is characteristic of a persistent PDA after the newborn period. The murmur is loudest under the left clavicle and frequently is very harsh and uneven in systole. Other causes of continuous murmurs are cerebral AV fistula, aortopulmonary collateral vessels, and aortopulmonary shunts. These latter continuous murmurs tend to be of similar pitch in both systole and diastole, and they have a higher pitch than that of the PDA murmur.

A variety of normal murmurs may be heard throughout childhood. The most common is the *vibratory systolic ejection murmur (Still murmur)*. This left lower–sternal border ejection systolic murmur is heard most frequently in preschool-aged children but also can be heard in children near the age of puberty. The murmur rarely is louder than grade 2 or 3, usually lasts about two thirds the length of systole, is heard well in the neck, and rarely is heard in the back. It is believed to originate in the root of the aorta, where people of all ages have a normal ejection systolic murmur. The still murmur decreases with inspiration or the Valsalva maneuver and is often less prominent or less vibratory when an individual is sitting or standing. Also, a systolic murmur in the root of the pulmonary artery is present, projected onto the chest as the most common normal murmur in adolescents and adults (the normal pulmonary ejection murmur). Another type of common, benign murmur is the *venous hum* heard at the right upper or, less commonly, left upper sternal border, with particular radiation into the neck. This continuous, medium-pitched murmur disappears when the patient is placed in a supine position, when the jugular vein is compressed, or when the patient looks sharply to the left.

Newborn infants usually do not have any of the aforementioned normal murmurs. For reasons not completely clear, the *patent ductus arteriosus murmur*, present because the infant is premature or has a

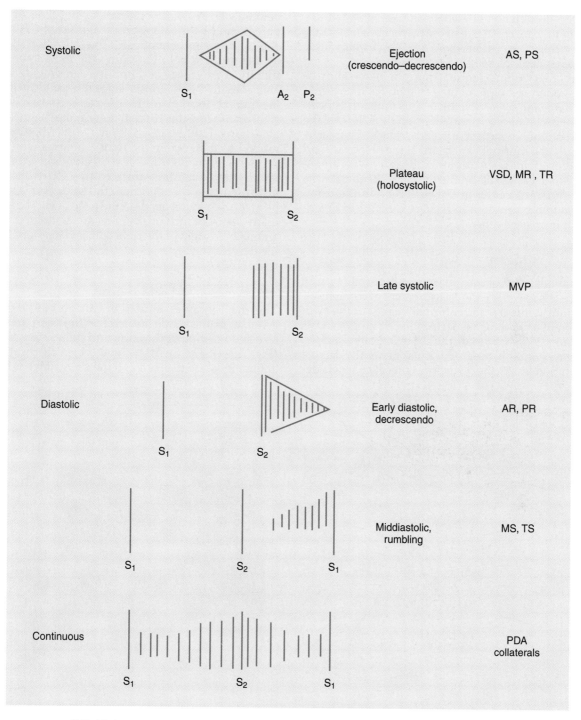

FIG. 13–3

Types of murmurs. *AR*, Aortic regurgitation; *AS*, aortic stenosis; *MR*, mitral regurgitation; *MS*, mitral stenosis; *MVP*, mitral valve prolapse; *PDA*, patent ductus arteriosus; *PR*, pulmonary regurgitation; *PS*, pulmonary stenosis; *TR*, tricuspid regurgitation; *TS*, tricuspid stenosis; *VSD*, ventricular septal defect.

low PO₂ from lung disease, often does not sound like that of the congenital patent ductus that becomes manifest weeks later. The newborn's PDA murmur is usually a nondescript, soft systolic murmur.

Another common normal murmur in newborn infants, often lasting 6 months or more, is the *peripheral pulmonic stenosis murmur.* This murmur is present because of a normal sharp angle between the main pulmonary artery and each branch. Characteristically the murmurs are heard at the first or second intercostal spaces, both left and right, with transmission to each axilla and to the back. Frequently the murmurs are louder in the back than in the front. These two murmurs can be very difficult to distinguish from each other.

Pulse Oximetry

The availability of inexpensive and portable pulse oximeters has made the measurement of oxygen saturation an integral and informative part of the evaluation of a child for suspected CHD. Since cyanosis requires 3–5 g of desaturated hemoglobin, a child with a normal hemoglobin must generally have a saturation less than 85% before clinical cyanosis de-

velops. Mild desaturation (85–90%) not clinically apparent can be the only sign of significant CHD, including complex heterotaxies. The saturation should be measured in both the right arm and a lower extremity. A difference in saturation can provide valuable clues to the diagnosis, since it reflects the effect of shunting through a PDA. If the saturation in the right arm is less than that in the leg, the diagnosis is almost invariably transposition. A lower-body saturation less than that in the right arm implies an aortic arch obstruction (lower oxygen blood from the RV to the descending aorta from a PDA). If both measurements are abnormal, the saturation should be measured in the head (in the nose or ear) because many forms of arch obstruction are associated with anomalous origin of the right subclavian artery from the descending aorta.

Chest Radiography

The chest x-ray examination can provide a good estimate of the shape and size of the heart and the size and position of the aorta and pulmonary artery (Fig. 13–4). Frequently clues to specific cardiac anomalies also are present. If the x-ray film has been

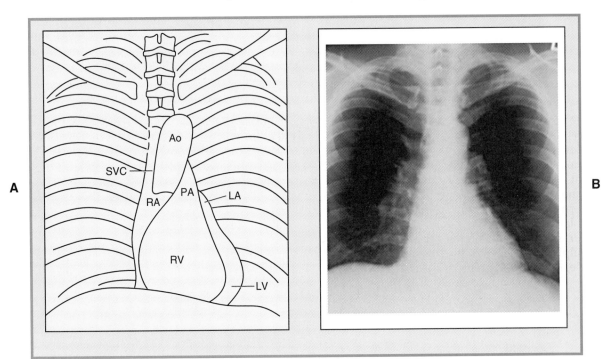

FIG. 13–4

A, Schematic illustration of the parts of the heart whose outlines can be identified on a routine chest x-ray **(B)**. *Ao,* Aorta; *SVC,* superior vena cava; *RA,* right atrium; *PA,* pulmonary artery; *LA,* left atrium; *RV,* right ventricle; *LV,* left ventricle. **B,** Routine posteroanterior x-ray of the normal cardiac silhouette. (From Andreoli TE, Carpenter CCJ, Plum F, et al: *Cecil essentials of medicine,* ed 2, Philadelphia, 1990, WB Saunders.)

obtained during maximal inspiration, the cardiothoracic ratio should be less than 55% in infants younger than 1 year of age and less than 50% in older children and adolescents. Interpretation of specific ventricular chamber enlargement is unreliable, but right atrial and left atrial enlargement frequently can be recognized.

Cardiac enlargement can be seen with any lesion that causes increased volume load to the heart or can be secondary to the presence of myocardial dysfunction. The normal large pulmonary arteries are seen in the central one third of the lung fields, with smaller vessels seen in the middle third and no pulmonary vessels seen in the lateral third of the lung fields. In the presence of a large left-to-right shunt (in VSD, PDA, truncus arteriosus, or single ventricle without pulmonary stenosis), the increased pulmonary flow allows visualization of medium-sized vessels in the middle third and of small vessels (frequently "end-on") in the most lateral third of the lung fields. Conversely, congenital cardiac lesions that are associated with a *right-to-left shunt,* in which blood destined for the pulmonary circulation is diverted into the systemic circulation, result in diminished pulmonary blood flow. The diminished flow is seen by a reduction in size of pulmonary arteries in the middle third of the lung fields (so-called black lung fields).

Elevated pulmonary venous pressure secondary to left-sided congestive heart failure or obstructed pulmonary venous return, which occurs in newborns with total anomalous pulmonary venous connection, results in increased lung water. In the older child this increase in lung water results in prominence of the pulmonary veins and redistribution of pulmonary flow, so that the upper lobe pulmonary arteries are fuller than the lower lobe vessels. In the infant and neonate, however, these signs are absent, and the usual pattern is a diffuse haziness or "fluffy" pattern that results from an increased amount of alveolar water.

Certain other signs on the chest x-ray films may be helpful in the diagnosis of heart disease. For example, *rib notching,* an indentation on the underside of the ribs, may be seen in older children with coarctation of the aorta as a result of large and tortuous intercostal arteries. It may also be seen in children with tetralogy with pulmonary atresia, in which collateral vessels from the aorta to the intraparenchymal pulmonary arteries provide pulmonary blood flow.

Several characteristic radiographic patterns are associated with specific cardiac conditions. Severe tetralogy of Fallot is associated with the "boot-shaped" heart. The right ventricular hypertrophy causes the apex of the heart to be lifted from the diaphragm, creating the "toe," and the small main pulmonary artery results in a scooped-out left heart border, creating the top of the boot. Anomalous drainage of the pulmonary veins without obstruction results in a "snowman" appearance. The upper circle (the "head") is caused on the left by the vertical vein draining the pulmonary veins and on the right by the enlarged superior vena cava. The lower circle (the "body") is produced by the enlarged heart. When the venous drainage is obstructed, a very small heart with severe pulmonary venous congestion is usually present. d-Transposition of the great arteries can be associated with an "egg-on-a-string" pattern. The string is the narrowed upper mediastinum, since the aorta and pulmonary artery are aligned on the posteroanterior projection. The egg is represented by the heart, with a left ventricular apex. Ebstein anomaly of the tricuspid valve often produces a large cardiac shadow that fills the entire chest.

Electrocardiography

The standard 12-lead electrocardiogram (ECG) is a recording of the electrical activity from cardiac muscle cells onto each lead on the surface of the torso. The ECG is a useful screening test when used along with the chest x-ray and a careful physical examination. The ECG also provides insight into the metabolic state of the cardiac cell (e.g., hyperkalemia). Analysis of the ECG includes the rate, rhythm, P wave, PR interval, QRS complex, QT interval, and ST segment (Fig. 13–5).

P Wave

The P wave represents atrial depolarization (Figs. 13–2 and 13–5). The first part of the P wave is caused by right atrial depolarization. The best criterion for right atrial enlargement is an increase of the amplitude of the P wave, reflected best in lead II. The diagnosis of left atrial enlargement is best made by prolongation of the second portion of the P wave, exhibited best in the chest leads.

PR Interval

The PR interval is measured from the beginning of the P wave to the beginning of the QRS complex and represents the time it takes for electricity to travel from the high right atrium to the ventricular myocardium (Figs. 13–2 and 13–5). The greatest time is spent in the AV node. The PR interval increases with age. The conduction time is shortened when conduction velocity is increased, as in glycogen storage disease, or when the AV node is bypassed, as in the Wolff-Parkinson-White syndrome. A prolonged PR interval usually indicates prolonged conduction through the AV node, but disease in the atrial myocardium, bundle of His, or Purkinje system could contribute to this abnormality.

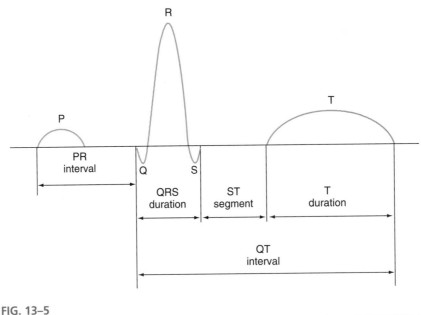

FIG. 13–5

Nomenclature of electrocardiogram waves and intervals.

QRS Complex

The QRS complex represents ventricular depolarization. Unlike in the atrium, right and left ventricular activation begins virtually simultaneously in the right and left septa, halfway to two thirds down, as well as in the contiguous left ventricular free wall and right ventricular endocardium. To interpret the ventricular ECG properly, it is necessary to understand a number of major concepts:

- A sequence of activation is present, so that what is being depolarized (and when) must be known.
- A greater volume of the ventricle causes greater magnitude, as does a greater mass of right or left ventricular muscle.
- Proximity of the right ventricular wall to the chest surface accentuates that ventricle's contribution.
- Continued changes occur in the normal ECG with time, beginning with that of the premature or full-term infant and continuing throughout childhood. The spatial magnitudes are quite low in the premature infant, become higher in the full-term infant, rise sharply until the age of 2–3 months, stabilize until puberty, and then decrease throughout life.
- Normative data for each age group must be known to make diagnoses.

In the fetus and full-term newborn the right and left ventricular masses are approximately equal, although the right ventricle may be up to one third thicker. In the premature infant, compared with the full-term infant, less right ventricular dominance is exhibited. By the age of 3–6 months the left ventricular mass is about twice that of the right ventricle, and when the child reaches school age, the ratio is similar to that of the adult, about 2.5:1 in favor of the left ventricle.

QT Interval

The QT interval is measured from the beginning of the QRS complex to the end of the T wave (Fig. 13–5). The corrected QT interval (corrected for rate) should be less than 0.45 second ($QT_c = QT/\sqrt{RR}$). The interval may be prolonged in children with hypocalcemia or hypokalemia (although the latter condition may involve a *QU interval*). It also is prolonged in a group of children at risk for severe ventricular arrhythmias and sudden death (i.e., the prolonged QT syndrome); drugs such as quinidine also may prolong the QT interval.

Echocardiography and Doppler Ultrasonography

Echocardiography, especially with Doppler and color flow ultrasonography, is the most important noninvasive tool for the evaluation of congenital and acquired heart disease. The majority of children with CHD undergo both palliative and corrective surgery solely on the basis of echocardiographic assessment of the anatomy and physiology. The two-dimensional

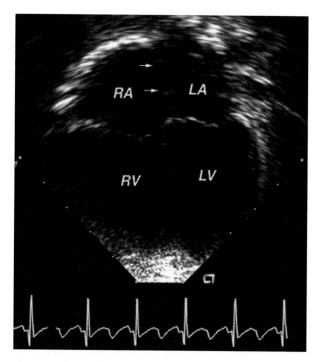

FIG. 13–6

Four-chamber echocardiogram of an atrial septal defect. The defect margins are identified by the two arrows. *LA,* Left atrium; *LV,* left ventricle; *RA,* right atrium; *RV,* right ventricle.

echocardiogram allows visualization of spatial relationships of the cardiac structures in the beating heart (Fig. 13–6). Anatomic details previously requiring angiography are easily visualized noninvasively, with little or no risk to the patient. All pertinent details can generally be ascertained, including the presence of intracardiac and extracardiac shunts, valve stenosis and insufficiency, and cardiac function. The magnitude of shunts, severity of valve gradients, and cardiac outputs can be calculated.

Doppler echocardiography is an adaptation of ultrasound that displays flow in cardiac chambers and vascular structures. The change in frequency imparted to sound waves caused by moving blood can be used to calculate cardiac output, valve and orifice pressure gradients, and directionality of flow within structures. Color flow Doppler encodes the flow direction and velocity in color superimposed on the two-dimensional image, allowing easy detection of small septal defects and valve regurgitation. Fetal echocardiography may delineate normal and abnormal function and structure before birth (discussed later in the chapter under Prenatal Detection).

Transesophageal echocardiography has become the standard for intraoperative assessment of the results of surgical procedures. A specialized transducer is placed in the esophagus before surgery, where it provides excellent anatomic detail without interfering with the surgical field. Immediate assessment of the surgical procedure can be made and any residual defects can be immediately corrected, alleviating potential postoperative instability.

Cardiac Catheterization and Angiography

Catheterization is now reserved for children in whom echocardiography is either unclear or unable to provide the necessary specific anatomic information or whose defect is amenable to transcatheter intervention. Children with complicated pulmonary artery anatomy or in whom precise physiologic information (e.g., pulmonary artery pressure) is needed require diagnostic catheterization. Postoperative patients, particularly those doing poorly, may require catheterization for complete determination of the anatomy and physiology. A growing percentage of cardiac catheterizations are performed for therapeutic purposes (thus reducing the need for surgery), such as balloon catheter dilatation of stenotic semilunar valves or pulmonary arteries and closure of PDAs, ASDs, VSDs, and aortopulmonary collateral vessels.

Access to the vascular system is usually gained by percutaneous femoral vein catheterization, with the right-sided chambers entered sequentially. The presence of a patent foramen ovale, especially in infants, frequently allows entrance to the left side of the heart. The left side of the heart also can be entered by a transseptal technique or via retrograde arterial catheterization.

Catheterization data include analysis of the pressures in cardiac structures and blood vessels, calculations derived from the aforementioned data, and the findings on cineangiography. The normal values are shown in Fig. 13–7. The oxygen saturation of the entire right side of the heart reflects the mixed venous saturation and is normally 70–75%; a significant increase in oxygen saturation in a chamber or vessel on the right side indicates a *left-to-right shunt.* The left side of the heart should have a saturation of above 95%; significant decreases below the pulmonary veins suggest the presence of a *right-to-left shunt* resulting from systemic venous blood entering the left side of the heart. A decreased pulmonary venous saturation may be the result of hypoventilation, pulmonary disease, or pulmonary venous congestion.

The pressures should be measured in all chambers and vessels entered. Normally the systolic pressure in the ventricles equals the systolic pressure in the great arteries, and the end-diastolic pressures in

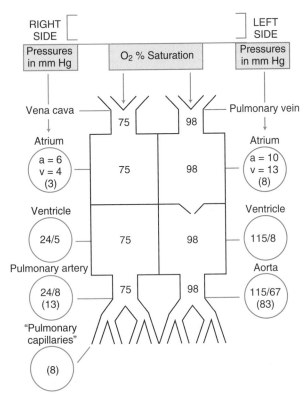

FIG. 13–7

Normal data from cardiac catheterization.

the atria are equal to the end-diastolic pressure in the ventricles. If a "gradient" in pressure exists, it suggests obstruction across the valve. Analysis of the severity of the obstruction requires measurement of both the pressure gradient and the flow across that valve.

Systemic and pulmonary outputs can be measured by the Fick equation: the cardiac output is equal to the measured oxygen consumption divided by the arteriovenous oxygen content differences between the systemic and pulmonary circulations. The pulmonary-to-systemic flow ratio can be measured by the ratio between the pulmonary and systemic arteriovenous differences, because the same oxygen consumption is in the numerator for both calculations.

Evaluation of the anatomy and physiology of the patient rarely is complete without selective angiocardiograms using a biplane system. Contrast material is injected rapidly into the cardiac chambers or vessels.

Exercise Testing

Evaluation of the cardiovascular system normally is performed with the patient at rest. However, infor-

mation on cardiac reserve and the adaptation of the normal or abnormal heart to exercise can provide important data on the cardiac status that more closely approximate everyday living. It can also be used to evaluate for the presence of arrhythmias and to measure coronary reserve after coronary manipulation (as in the arterial switch procedure).

REFERENCES

Behrman RE, Kliegman RM, Jenson HB, editors: *Nelson textbook of pediatrics*, ed 16, Philadelphia, 2000, WB Saunders, Chapters 427–430.

Braden DS, Strong WF: Cardiovascular responses to exercise in children, *Am J Dis Child* 144(11):1255–1260, 1990.

Brook MM, Silverman NH, Villegas M: Cardiac ultrasound in structural abnormalities and arrhythmias: recognition and treatment, *West J Med* 159(3):286–300, 1993.

Davignon A, Rautaharju P, Boisselle E, et al: Normal ECG standards for infants and children, *Pediatr Cardiol* 1:123, 1979-80.

Frommelt MA, Frommelt PC: Advances in echocardiographic diagnostic modalities for the pediatrician, *Pediatr Clin North Am* 46(2):427–439, 1999.

Higgins CB et al: Magnetic resonance imaging in patients with congenital heart disease, *Circulation* 70(5):851–860, 1984.

Pelech AN: Evaluation of the pediatric patient with a cardiac murmur, *Pediatr Clin North Am* 46(2):167–188, 1999.

Stümpflen I, Stümpflen A, Wimmer M, et al: Effect of detailed fetal echocardiography as part of routine prenatal ultrasonographic screening on detection of congenital heart disease, *Lancet* 348(9031):854–857, 1996.

PRENATAL AND NEONATAL CIRCULATION

See Chapter 6.

MYOCARDIAL FUNCTION AND HEART FAILURE

Myofibril contraction is summated and translated into cardiac work or pump performance. The force generated by the muscle fiber depends on its contractile status and its basal length, which is equivalent to the preload, as noted in the normal Starling curve of Fig. 13–8. As the preload (fiber length, left ventricular filling pressure, or volume) increases, the myocardial performance (stroke volume and wall tension) increases up to a point. The relationship is the ventricular function curve; alterations in the contractile state of the muscle lower the relative position of the curve but retain the relationship of fiber length to muscle work. Heart rate is another important determinant of cardiac work because the cardiac output equals stroke volume times the heart rate. Additional factors that affect cardiac performance are noted in Table 13–3.

Heart failure results when the cardiac output does not meet the metabolic needs (in terms of oxygen delivery and other factors) of the body. The term *con-*

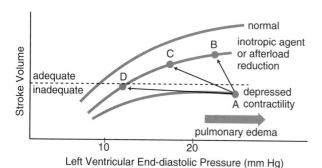

FIG. 13-8

Ventricular function curve illustrating the effect of inotropic agents or arterial vasodilators. Unlike diuretics, the effect of digitalis or arterial vasodilator therapy in a patient with heart failure is movement onto another ventricular function curve intermediate between the normal and depressed curves. When the patient's ventricular function moves from *A* to *B* by the administration of one of these agents, the left ventricular end-diastolic pressure also may decrease because of improved cardiac function; further administration of diuretics or venodilators may shift the function further to the left along the same curve from *B* to *C* and eliminate the risk of pulmonary edema. A vasodilating agent that has both arteriolar and venous dilating properties (e.g., nitroprusside) would shift this function directly from *A* to *C*. If this agent shifts the function from *A* to *D* because of excessive venodilation or administration of diuretics, the cardiac output may fall too low, even though the left ventricular end-diastolic pressure would be normal (10 mm Hg) for a normal heart. Thus left ventricular end-diastolic pressures of between 15 and 18 mm Hg are usually optimal in the failing heart to maximize cardiac output but to avoid pulmonary edema. (From Andreoli TE, Carpenter CCJ, Griggs RC, Loscalzo J: *Cecil essentials of medicine*, ed 5, Philadelphia, 2001, WB Saunders.)

TABLE 13-3
Factors Affecting Cardiac Performance

Preload (left ventricular diastolic volume)
Total blood volume
Venous tone (sympathetic tone)
Body position
Intrathoracic and intrapericardial pressure
Atrial contraction
Pumping action of skeletal muscle

Afterload (impedance against which the left ventricle must eject blood)
Peripheral vascular resistance
Left ventricular volume (preload, wall tension)
Physical characteristics of the arterial tree (for example, elasticity of vessels or presence of outflow obstruction)

Contractility (cardiac performance independent of preload or afterload)
Sympathetic nerve impulses*
Circulating catecholamines*
Digitalis, calcium, other inotropic agents*
Increased heart rate or postextrasystolic augmentation*
Anoxia, acidosis†
Pharmacologic depression†
Loss of myocardium†
Intrinsic depression†

Heart Rate
Autonomic nervous system
Temperature, metabolic rate

From Andreoli TE, Carpenter CCJ, Griggs RC, Loscalzo J: *Cecil essentials of medicine*, ed 5, Philadelphia, 2001, WB Saunders.
*Increases contractility.
†Decreases contractility.

gestive heart failure refers to increased venous pressure in the pulmonary (left heart failure) or the systemic (right heart failure) veins. Myofibrillar failure is the result of a decline of the myofibril contractility, as noted by a shift of the normal Starling curve (Fig. 13-8). The compensatory mechanisms used to improve cardiac output include augmented endogenous sympathetic activity (which increases inotropy and chronotropy) and the response of the kidney to a perceived reduction of effective plasma volume, leading to salt and water retention. These compensatory mechanisms have beneficial and adverse effects (Table 13-4).

The *etiology* of heart failure is different in various ages of development (Table 13-5). Fetal causes of heart failure include arrhythmias (e.g., supraventricular tachycardia or heart block) or severe anemia secondary to hemolysis or blood loss. In the neonate, CHD, AVMs, cardiomyopathy, and myocarditis are common causes of heart failure; in the older child,

myocarditis, acute hypertension (in glomerulonephritis or hemolytic-uremic syndrome), and rheumatic fever are important causes of heart failure.

The *treatment* of heart failure is directed toward improving myocardial contractility, preload, and reducing afterload (Table 13-6 and Fig. 13-8).

REFERENCES

Behrman RE, Kliegman RM, Jenson HB, editors: *Nelson textbook of pediatrics*, ed 16, Philadelphia, 2000, WB Saunders, Chapter 448.
Cohn J: The management of chronic heart failure, *N Engl J Med* 335(7):490–498, 1996.

TABLE 13–4
Compensatory Mechanisms in Heart Failure

Mechanism	Favorable Effects	Unfavorable Effects
↑Sympathetic activity	↑Heart rate ↑Contractility ↑Venoconstriction →↑venous return (preload)	↑Arteriolar constriction →↑afterload ↑O_2 requirements
Cardiac hypertrophy	↑Working muscle mass	↑Wall tension ↓Coronary flow ↑O_2 requirements Abnormal systolic and diastolic properties of hypertrophic muscle
Frank-Starling mechanism	↑Stroke volume for any given amount of venous return	Pulmonary and systemic congestion: ↑LV size →↑ wall tension and O_2 requirements
Renal salt and water retention	↑Venous return	Pulmonary and systemic congestion: ↑Renin-angiotensin →↑ vasoconstriction (afterload)
Increased peripheral O_2 extraction	↑O_2 delivery per unit cardiac output	

From Andreoli TE, Carpenter CCJ, Plum F: *Cecil essentials of medicine,* ed 4, Philadelphia, 1997, WB Saunders.
LV, Left ventricle.

TABLE 13–5
Etiology of Heart Failure

Fetus
Severe anemia (hemolysis, fetal-maternal transfusion, hypoplastic anemia)
Supraventricular tachycardia
Ventricular tachycardia
Complete heart block
Atrioventricular valve insufficiency
High-output cardiac failure (arteriovenous malformation, teratoma)

Premature Neonate
Fluid overload
PDA
VSD
Cor pulmonale (BPD)

Full-Term Neonate
Asphyxial cardiomyopathy
Arteriovenous malformation (vein of Galen, hepatic)
Left-sided obstructive lesions (coarctation of aorta, hypoplastic left heart)
Transposition of great arteries
Large mixing cardiac defects (single ventricle, truncus arteriosus)
Viral myocarditis

Infant-Toddler
Left-to-right cardiac shunts (VSD)
Hemangioma (arteriovenous malformation)
Anomalous left coronary artery
Metabolic cardiomyopathy
Acute hypertension (hemolytic-uremic syndrome)
Supraventricular tachycardia
Kawasaki disease
Postoperative repair of congenital heart disease

Child-Adolescent
Rheumatic fever
Acute hypertension (glomerulonephritis)
Viral myocarditis
Thyrotoxicosis
Hemochromatosis-hemosiderosis
Cancer therapy (radiation, Adriamycin)
Sickle cell anemia
Endocarditis
Cor pulmonale (cystic fibrosis)
Arrhythmias
Chronic upper airway obstruction (cor pulmonale)
Unrepaired or palliated congenital heart disease
Cardiomyopathy

BPD, Bronchopulmonary dysplasia; *PDA,* patent ductus arteriosus; *VSD,* ventricular septal defect.

TABLE 13–6
Treatment of Heart Failure

Therapy	Mechanism
General Care	
Rest	Reduces cardiac output
Oxygen	Improves oxygenation in presence of pulmonary edema
Sodium, fluid restrictions	Decreases vascular congestion; decreases preload
Diuretics	
Furosemide	Salt excretion by ascending loop of Henle; reduces preload; afterload reduced if hypertension improves; also may cause venodilation
Combination of distal tubule and loop diuretics	Greater sodium excretion
Inotropic Agents	
Digitalis	Inhibits membrane Na^+, K^+-ATPase and increases intracellular Ca^{2+}, improves cardiac contractility, increases myocardial oxygen consumption
Dopamine	Releases myocardial norepinephrine plus direct effect on beta receptor, may increase systemic blood pressure; at low infusion rates, dilates renal artery, facilitating diuresis
Dobutamine	Beta (β_1)-receptor agent; often combined with dopamine
Amrinone/milrinone	Nonsympathomimetic, noncardiac glycosides with inotropic effects; may produce vasodilation
Afterload Reduction	
Hydralazine	Arteriolar vasodilator
Nitroprusside	Arterial and venous relaxation; venodilation reduces preload
Captopril/enalapril	Inhibition of angiotensin-converting enzyme; reduces angiotensin II production
Other	
Mechanical counterpulsation	Improves coronary flow, afterload
Transplantation	Remove diseased heart
Extracorporeal membrane oxygenation (ECMO)	Bypasses heart

O'Laughlin MP: Congestive heart failure in children, *Pediatr Clin North Am* 46(2):263–273, 1999.
Park M: Use of digoxin in infants and children with specific emphasis on dosage, *J Pediatr* 108(6):871–877, 1986.
Schneeweiss A: Cardiovascular drugs in children: angiotensin-converting enzyme inhibitors, *Pediatr Cardiol* 9(2):109–115, 1989.

CONGENITAL HEART DISEASE

Epidemiology. Congenital heart disease affects 8:1000 births. If congenital dysrhythmias (e.g., Wolff-Parkinson-White syndrome) are included, the ratio is 1:100. Most of these lesions occur between days 18 and 50 of gestation. At birth, VSD is the most common lesion, followed in order of decreasing frequency by PDA, tetralogy of Fallot, ASD, coarctation of the aorta, transposition of the great arteries, atrioventricular canal defects (endocardial cushion), and heterotaxies (right and left isomerism). The remaining individual lesions each represent 1–4% of congenital heart defects. Most affected neonates are full-term, appropriate-sized infants of normal pregnancies.

Approximately 30% of infants with heart lesions have extracardiac malformations that also affect their morbidity and mortality (Table 13–1). Most cases of CHD (90%) are not associated with single-gene defects or teratogens. A certain number are associated with chromosomal disorders (deletions or trisomies), congenital anomaly syndromes (e.g., VATER or CHARGE), or maternal metabolic disorders (e.g., phenylketonuria or diabetes).

The *inheritance* in most patients is multifactorial (polygenic). The recurrence risk for CHD in the sibling of an affected infant varies from 2–4%. The risk is greater for the child of a parent with CHD; in this case, the risk increases to 4–5%.

Heart Disease Resulting from Abnormal Embryonic Development

The heart begins to develop in the very early embryo and circulates blood by the third week. The initial heart is a straight tube without valves. Because the heart tube grows faster than the organs around it, it loops. Abnormal looping leads to abnormal cardiac position, such as dextrocardia, or other anomalies, such as congenitally corrected transposition. When a major abnormality occurs, such as looping in the wrong direction, usually one or several other abnormalities occur, such as a VSD.

As the heart divides itself into four chambers and as valves develop, many other abnormalities may occur. Abnormalities of connection (e.g., dTGA or tetralogy of Fallot) or valve formation (e.g., HLHS or AV canal) occur at these stages. Most defects cause no prenatal hemodynamic abnormality. However, some defects can cause fetal decompensation or death. In addition, some defects alter the blood flow, causing secondary problems (e.g., mitral atresia causing a hypoplastic left ventricle).

Fetal cardiac diseases also may be iatrogenic. For example, maternal treatment with indomethacin to prevent premature labor may prematurely close the ductus arteriosus, resulting in right ventricular failure.

Abnormal Development of Venous and Arterial Systems

The development of the venous and arterial systems in the fetus is at least as complex as that of the cardiac chambers themselves. The single mature aorta and aortic arch develop from multiple paired aortic arches. Abnormalities in their development, such as a complete interruption of the aorta, may occur at any one of a number of sites. The fact that genetics plays a great role in development is underscored by the marked difference in the incidence and site of aortic arch interruption in patients of Chinese or Japanese ancestry versus that in Caucasians or Filipinos. The influence of fetal hemodynamics on the development of congenital cardiovascular defects is shown by the fact that coarctation of the aorta and interruption of the aortic arch are associated with "upstream lesions" such as aortic or mitral stenosis and certain VSDs that cause less aortic blood flow.

An understanding of *fetal blood flow* is critical to an understanding of fetal and neonatal physiology and of the development of congenital cardiovascular defects. The fetus is dependent on placental blood flow. The fetus receives oxygenated, nutrient-loaded blood by way of the umbilical vein. This blood preferentially shunts across the foramen ovale to the left atrium, the left ventricle, and out the aorta to the upper body and brain. The superior vena cava blood preferentially directs blood to the right ventricle, the pulmonary artery, and through the ductus arteriosus to the lower half of the body and the umbilical arteries to the placenta. Only a small amount of blood perfuses the lungs during fetal life. The patent foramen ovale and ductus arteriosus cause the ventricles to work in parallel rather than in series, as they do after birth.

Fetal cardiovascular physiology explains why certain devastating defects, such as transposition of the great arteries, have no effect on the fetus. A similar quantity of blood with a similar oxygen concentration will reach the same organs at the same pressure, no matter which chambers and vessels it passes through. Children with transposition of the great arteries are often large for gestational age. This is partly because the left ventricle, with higher blood glucose, supplies the misplaced pulmonary artery and thus the lower body. The insulin produced in response acts as a growth factor for the infant. Subvalvular or valvular aortic stenosis, particularly in association with a VSD, results in decreased flow through the aortic arch, impairing arch growth and increasing the incidence of coarctation. An anomalous left coronary artery from the pulmonary artery will have the same pressure and a similar oxygen concentration in utero but a markedly lower pressure and lower oxygen saturation shortly after birth. In this situation the fetal heart does not infarct, but the neonatal or infant heart usually does.

At birth and shortly afterward, major changes in the circulation occur. The manifestation of congenital cardiovascular defects and their timing are dependent on these changes. The umbilical venous and arterial flows are obliterated immediately at birth. The pulmonary blood flow must increase immediately and support the entire organism. It is aided in doing this by the expansion of the lungs, which greatly reduces resistance to pulmonary blood flow. Systemic vascular resistance increases as a result of loss of the low-resistance placental circuit.

Sometimes, because of lung problems such as meconium aspiration, the pulmonary vascular resistance does not decrease. The fetal circulatory pathways may persist in part. Right-to-left shunting may continue to occur at the ductus arteriosus and/or foramen ovale level, resulting in extreme cyanosis. Persistent increase in pulmonary vascular resistance also may severely compromise infants with congenital cardiac defects. Children with anatomic defects that usually would allow a left-to-right shunt will have a large right-to-left shunt. Children with an anatomically tenuous pulmonary blood flow may have an even further diminished flow. Early aggressive management of this physiology may reverse it or prevent its progression (see Chapter 6).

Abnormal Positions of the Heart

The location of the heart within the chest may be quite abnormal, and the relationships of the chambers may be very confusing. A systematic classification simplifies analysis. In this classification the heart may be in the right (*dextrocardia*) or the left side of the chest (*levocardia*). The cardiac chambers are described in terms of their relationship to each other. The atrium may be *solitus,* with the right atrium to the right of the left atrium; *inversus,* with the anatomic right atrium to the left of the anatomic left atrium; or *ambiguous,* when abnormalities of systemic and pulmonary venous return make identification of the two atrial chambers impossible. The ventricles may be in their normal position (*d*) with the right ventricle to the right of the left ventricle, or they may be positioned with the anatomic right ventricle to the left of the anatomic left ventricle (*l*). The great arteries may be normally related, with the pulmonary artery anterior to and to the left of the aorta; *d*-transposed, with the aorta anterior to but still to the right of the pulmonary artery; or *l*-transposed, if the aorta is anterior to and to the left of the pulmonary artery.

Classification of Congenital Cardiac Defects

Congenital cardiac defects can be classified into four groups based on their presentation and physiology (Tables 13–7 and 13–8). This classification is an oversimplification, and many variations occur. The severity of each lesion is extremely variable. The timing and nature of the clinical presentation in a patient are controlled by the physiology of the lesions. In each case, however, there are modifiers. An example is the size of the foramen ovale in complete *d*-transposition of the great arteries. Transposition presents early with cyanosis and tachypnea, but a very small foramen ovale makes it present even earlier.

The simplest lesions are the stenoses in which usually only one valve or artery is stenotic. In children it is usually the aortic or pulmonic valve, although the mitral and tricuspid valves (rarely) can be stenotic. Valve stenosis usually is isolated, although syndromes (such as **Shone syndrome**) of multiple left heart obstruction occur uncommonly. The right-to-left shunt lesion involves much more complex anatomy and physiology. In most cases there must also be a left-to-right shunt, which occurs as a simple defect in the septa or arterial walls. Because pulmonary vascular resistance is high at birth,

TABLE 13–7
Classification of Congenital Cardiac Defects

| Stenotic | Shunting | | Mixing |
	Right→Left	Left→Right	
Aortic stenosis	Tetralogy	Patent ductus arteriosus	Truncus
Pulmonic stenosis	Transposition	Ventricular septal defect	TAPVR
Coarctation of the aorta	Tricuspid atresia	Atrial septal defect	HLH

HLH, Hypoplastic left heart syndrome; *TAPVR,* total anomalous pulmonary venous return.

neonates with congenital cardiac defects may have no shunting and thus no physical findings. The "mixing" lesions are those in which both right-to-left and left-to-right shunts are present without significant stenosis, resulting in an arterial saturation in the upper 80th percentile.

Hemodynamic Measurements

Representative oxygen saturations and pressures from catheterization of a child are presented in Figure 13–7. The formulas for calculating pulmonary and systemic *cardiac outputs* are as follows:

$$\text{Pulmonary output} = \frac{O_2 \text{ consumption in (mL/min)}}{\text{Pulmonary arteriovenous difference (mL/L)}}$$

and

$$\text{Systemic output} = \frac{O_2 \text{ consumption (mL/L)}}{\text{Systemic arteriovenous difference (mL/L)}}$$

where

Pulmonary arteriovenous difference =
    Pulmonary vein − Pulmonary artery oxygen content

and

Systemic arteriovenous difference =
    Systemic artery − Mixed venous oxygen content

Because cardiac output increases with the size of the child, it is related to the patient's surface area in square meters. For the resting child normal cardiac output is about 4 L/min/m². In the absence of

TABLE 13–8
Categories of Presenting Symptoms in the Neonate

Symptom	Physiologic Category	Anatomic Cause	Lesion
Cyanosis with respiratory distress	Increased pulmonary blood flow	Transposition	*d*-Transposition with or without associated lesions
Cyanosis without respiratory distress	Decreased pulmonary blood flow	Right heart obstruction	Tricuspid atresia Ebstein anomaly Pulmonary atresia Pulmonary stenosis Tetralogy of Fallot
Hypoperfusion	Poor cardiac output	Left heart obstruction	Total anomalous pulmonary venous return with obstruction Aortic stenosis Hypoplastic left heart syndrome
	Poor cardiac function	Normal anatomy	Cardiomyopathy Myocarditis
Respiratory distress with desaturation (not visible cyanosis)	Bidirectional shunting	Complete mixing	Truncus arteriosus AV canal Complex single ventricle (including heterotaxias) without pulmonary stenosis
Respiratory distress with normal saturation	Left-to-right shunting	Simple intracardiac shunt	ASD VSD PDA Aortopulmonary window AVM

ASD, Atrial septal defect; *AVM,* arteriovenous malformation; *PDA,* patent ductus arteriosus; *VSD,* ventricular septal defect.

cardiac failure the body's homeostatic mechanisms tend to keep the systemic output near normal, whatever the congenital defect. In the presence of heart failure the systemic output usually is lowered.

The cardiac outputs and pressures in each side of the heart are critically related to each other. Thus an elevated systolic pressure of 60 mm Hg in the pulmonary artery in the presence of a VSD is indicative of a greater degree of pulmonary hypertension when the aortic pressure is 90 mm Hg systolic than when the aortic pressure is 120 mm Hg. In the former case pulmonary hypertension is said to be at two thirds of the systemic level, whereas in the latter it is one half of the systemic level. When the pressure in the pulmonary artery is equal to that in the aorta, it is referenced as "systemic level" pulmonary hypertension; when it is higher than that of the aorta, it is characterized as "suprasystemic" pulmonary artery pressure.

Systemic (SVR) and *pulmonary* (PVR) *vascular resistance* also can be calculated. These measures are the resistances to flow across the resistance vessels,

which are mainly small muscular arteries and arterioles. This calculation requires knowledge of the pressures on each side of these resistance vessels. On the systemic side, ΔP is systemic artery pressure (P_{sa}) − right atrial pressure (P_{ra}). On the pulmonary side, P is pulmonary artery pressure (P_{pa}) − left atrial pressure (P_{la}). The calculation is made from a modification of the Poiseuille equation:

$$\text{PVR} = \frac{P_{pa} - P_{la} \text{ [pulmonary } \Delta P]}{\text{Pulmonary flow}}$$

and

$$\text{SVR} = \frac{P_{sa} - P_{ra} \text{ [systemic } \Delta P]}{\text{Systemic flow}}$$

If the pressure drop is measured in mm Hg and the flow in L/min/m², the calculated resistance is in Wood units. (One Wood unit is equal to 80 dynes sec/cm⁵/m².) The normal PVR is 2–3 units, whereas the normal SVR is 15–20 units.

An important concept to remember is that *blood flow goes where resistance is least.* Of course, other types of resistance are present besides vascular resistance: at valves, where obviously a narrowed valve has a greater resistance to flow than does a wide-open valve; at septal defects, where a small septal defect has a greater resistance to flow than does a large defect; and at ventricles, where a thick-walled, less compliant ventricle has a greater resistance to flow into it than does a thinner-walled, more compliant ventricle.

Acyanotic Congenital Heart Lesions

Left-to-Right Shunt Acyanotic Lesions

Acyanotic conditions are those in which the systemic arterial saturation is normal. Left-to-right shunt lesions have communication between the two sides of the heart through which extra blood traverses from the left to the right side. The result is an increase in pulmonary blood flow. A moderate-sized left-to-right shunt has approximately twice as much pulmonary blood flow as systemic blood flow (i.e., a 2:1 pulmonary-to-systemic [P/S] flow ratio). Assuming a normal systemic output of 4 L/min/m², the pulmonary flow is 8 L/min/m².

Hemodynamics of Common Left-to-Right Shunts

ATRIAL SEPTAL DEFECT. Flow from all four pulmonary veins streams through the ASD in both systole and diastole (Fig. 13–9). The result is that very little increase in volume occurs in the left atrium (LA). The right atrium (RA) and the right ventricle (RV) handle twice the normal flow. X-ray examination reveals increased pulmonary artery vascularity, and the ECG and echocardiogram reveal pure right ventricular enlargement (RVE).

No murmur is present from the low-velocity flow across the ASD, but twice the normal flow occurs across the normal tricuspid valve and normal pulmonic valve. The result is that, on the physical examination, in addition to the abnormal right ventricular impulse and widely persistently split S_2, a middiastolic rumbling murmur is exhibited at the lower left sternal border and a soft systolic ejection murmur is exhibited at the upper left sternal border.

PATENT DUCTUS ARTERIOSUS. Fig. 13–10 shows normal flow through the right heart until after the blood has reached the pulmonary artery. Twice the normal flow is present in the pulmonary veins, LA, left ventricle (LV), the aorta proximal to the PDA, and in the pulmonary arteries distal to the PDA. X-ray examination reveals increased pulmonary artery vascularity and may also reveal increased pulmonary vein size. The ECG and echocardiogram reveal left atrial enlargement (LAE) and left ventricular hypertrophy (LVH), excluding any effects of increased pulmonary artery pressure.

If the pulmonary artery diastolic pressure is less

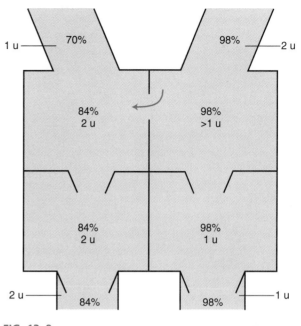

FIG. 13–9

Atrial septal defect with 2:1 pulmonary-to-systemic (P/S) flow ratio. One unit (u) of cardiac output is 4 L/min/m². "%" is percent saturation.

than the aortic diastolic pressure, a continuous runoff from aorta to pulmonary artery occurs. The result is a continuous murmur. Also, twice the normal flow occurs through the normal mitral and aortic valves. The result of this is that in addition to the abnormal left ventricular impulse and hyperdynamic upper left sternal edge and apex, a middiastolic rumble is present at that apex and a soft systolic ejection murmur is present at the upper right sternal border. If the caliber of the PDA is wide, greater transmission of systemic pressure into the pulmonary artery occurs. The wider and shorter the PDA is, the higher the right ventricular pressure is and the greater is the right ventricular hypertrophy (RVH) than the LVH.

VENTRICULAR SEPTAL DEFECT. Fig. 13–11 shows twice as much flow as normal in the pulmonary veins, LA, and LV. The LV sends as much blood through the VSD as into the aorta, so the RV and pulmonary artery also have twice the normal flow. X-ray examination reveals increased pulmonary artery vascularity and may show increased pulmonary vein size. The ECG and echocardiogram show LAE and both LVH and RVH.

A holosystolic murmur is present because of the left-to-right blood flow through the VSD. Because LV pressure rises slightly before RV pressure, the left-

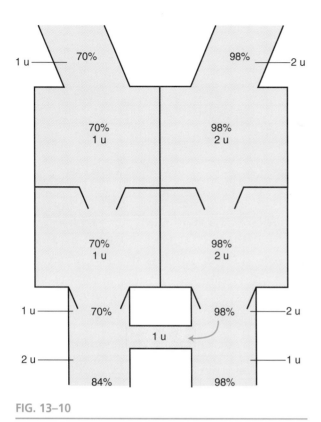

FIG. 13–10

Patent ductus arteriosus with 2:1 pulmonary-to-systemic (P/S) flow ratio (see Fig. 13–9). *u*, Unit.

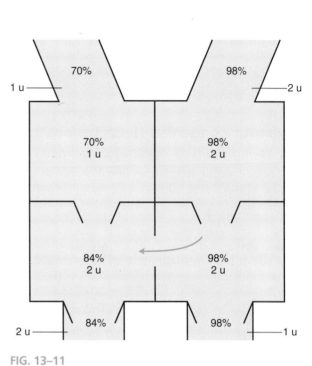

FIG. 13–11

Ventricular septal defect with 2:1 pulmonary-to-systemic (P/S) flow ratio (see Fig. 13–9). *u*, Unit.

to-right shunt begins before mitral valve closure, resulting in S_1 being obscured by the murmur. Twice the flow occurs through the normal mitral and pulmonic valves, so that in addition to the combined ventricular impulse and the hyperdynamic left sternal edge and apex, a middiastolic rumble is exhibited at the apex and a soft systolic ejection murmur is exhibited at the upper left sternal border.

The Natural History of Acyanotic Lesions with Left-to-Right Shunts

ATRIAL SEPTAL DEFECT. The most common ASD (6.4:10,000 live births) is of the secundum type, which makes up approximately 7% of all cases of CHD. The ratio of females to males is 2:1. The PVR is lower than normal throughout childhood, and heart failure is infrequent. In adulthood, however, heart failure, atrial flutter, or both develop in a significant number of individuals, as well as pulmonary vascular disease. Therefore, surgery or catheter closure, which is of extremely low risk, should be performed electively at what is judged the appropriate psychologic age for the particular child. In most children this is between 2 and 5 years of age (Tables 13–9 and 13–10).

VENTRICULAR SEPTAL DEFECT. Ventricular septal defects are the most common congenital cardiac lesions, making up at least 30% of all cases of CHD.

The incidence in males equals that in females. The most common position of the defect is perimembranous and subaortic, although many muscular defects may be present. VSDs in the endocardial cushion area are not rare, but supracristal (or doubly committed subarterial) defects are quite uncommon except in children of Asian or Hispanic descent, in whom they are the most common type. VSD is usually a benign disease. The majority of the defects are small, most of which close spontaneously. VSDs small enough to have normal pulmonary artery pressures and pulmonary-to-systemic flow ratios of less than 1.5–2:1 do not necessitate surgery, even if closure does not occur. Infants with moderate to large defects are at risk for development of both congestive heart failure and pulmonary hypertension. Infants who go into heart failure almost always do so by 2 months of age.

Management is directed toward symptomatology and the prevention of pulmonary vascular disease. Children with significant pulmonary hypertension are often asymptomatic because the high PVR decreases shunting and lessens symptoms. However, the presence of significant pulmonary hypertension at 4–6 months of age is generally an indication for surgery, regardless of the presence of symptoms, in order to

TABLE 13-9
Therapy of Congenital Heart Disease: Palliative Procedures

Procedure	Lesion	Comments
Blalock-Taussig Teflon tube graft or shunt (subclavian artery to ipsilateral pulmonary artery, usually right-sided)	TOF, pulmonary valve atresia	Improves pulmonary blood flow; most common shunting procedure
Balloon atrial septostomy (Rashkind procedure)	TGA	Improves oxygenation with increased atrial mixing
Catheter balloon dilating valvotomy (balloon valvuloplasty)	Pulmonary valve stenosis; aortic valve stenosis	Increases valve patency
Operative valvotomy	As above for balloon plus pulmonary atresia	Increases valve patency
Prostaglandin E$_1$ infusion	Pulmonary atresia, tricuspid atresia, TOF, coarctation of aorta, interrupted aortic arch, TGA	Maintains pulmonary blood flow via PDA, improves mixing
Pulmonary artery banding	Single ventricle	Decreases pulmonary blood flow, prevents heart failure
Device occlusion (embolization, umbrella); correction/closure	PDA, VSD, ASD, arteriovenous malformations	Nonsurgical, catheter closure, curative

ASD, Atrial septal defect; *PDA*, patent ductus arteriosus; *TGA*, transposition of great arteries; *TOF*, tetralogy of Fallot; *VSD*, ventricular septal defect.

TABLE 13–10
Therapy of Congenital Heart Disease: Corrective Procedures

Procedure	Lesion	Effect
Repair of septal defects (patching)	ASD, VSD, endocardial cushion defects	Complete repair
Valve replacement, repair	Aortic, mitral, pulmonic stenosis; Ebstein anomaly	Repair but prosthetic valve complications
Aortic patch, subclavian flap or end-to-end aortic anastomosis	Interrupted arch, coarctation of aorta	Repair but possible late recoarctation
Total correction possible	TOF; anomalous venous return; PDA	Complete repair
Jatene procedure (arterial switch)	TGA	Anatomic correction
Fontan procedure (inferior vena cava–to–pulmonary artery anastomosis)	Tricuspid atresia, single ventricle, pulmonary atresia	Alleviates shunting, enhances pulmonary blood flow
Norwood procedure	Hypoplastic left heart	Three-staged procedure with variable success
Heart transplant	Hypoplastic left heart	Normal heart with risk of immune rejection, coronary vasculopathy
Heart-lung transplant	Eisenmenger syndrome; cor pulmonale?	Normal organs with risk of rejection

ASD, Atrial septal defect; *PDA*, patent ductus arteriosus; *TGA*, transposition of great arteries; *TOF*, tetralogy of Fallot; *VSD*, ventricular septal defect.

prevent the development of pulmonary vascular disease, which can occur as early as 9–12 months of age.

In individuals with less severe or no pulmonary hypertension but a large shunt, symptoms of congestive heart failure are more likely to develop. Anticongestive therapy (Table 13–6) is indicated for respiratory symptoms or failure to thrive. Because feeding is the most strenuous activity for most infants, symptoms usually involve poor feeding. Caloric supplementation with increased density formula or nasogastric supplementation can increase caloric intake without increasing caloric expenditure. However, because surgical closure is safe, it is being used earlier in the management of symptomatic patients, with the goal of preventing delay in head growth.

PATENT DUCTUS ARTERIOSUS. The natural history of the congenital PDA is poorly defined because surgery has been available for a long time. However, three major observations should be noted. First, at the same pulmonary artery pressure, the risk of developing pulmonary vascular disease is greater in PDA than in VSD. Second, at the same age, the risk of developing infective endocarditis is greater in PDA than in VSD because of jet stream–induced intimal damage. Third, the incidence of spontaneous closure of the congenital PDA is very small. Therefore, because treatment is simple and low risk, all simple congenital PDAs with a left-to-right shunt should be closed. Although surgery is safe and effective, coil embolization during cardiac catheterization has become the procedure of choice for most patients outside the neonatal period. This procedure involves a slightly higher risk of a tiny residual defect, but the procedure is less invasive and less expensive than surgery (Tables 13–9 and 13–10). Infants who have congestive heart failure or large left-to-right shunts with increased pulmonary artery pressure should be operated on at the time of diagnosis.

ENDOCARDIAL CUSHION DEFECT (ATRIOVENTRICULAR CANAL). A broad spectrum of endocardial cushion defects have been observed, from varieties of the complete AV canal (including marked deficiency in the ventricular and atrial septa, as well as medial portions of tricuspid and mitral valves making a common AV valve) to several varieties of the partial AV canal. The simplest forms are the VSD in the endocardial cushion position and the ostium primum ASD with varying deficiencies of the anteromedial leaflet, which causes mitral regurgitation. Equal numbers of males and females are affected. The more complete the defect is, the more likely it is that the child has Down syndrome. Approximately one half of children with Down syndrome have some form of AV canal; therefore, all Down syndrome children should receive a cardiac evaluation if symptomatic or before 6 months of age.

The natural history of the various partial AV canal defects depends on the size of the various atrial and ventricular defects and the amount of mitral regurgitation. The large ostium primum ASD with no mitral regurgitation has the same benign natural history as that of the simple secundum ASD. With a complete AV canal, severe heart failure or pulmonary vascular disease is the rule. The clinical and echocardiographic diagnosis depends on the specific anatomy. Characteristically, an ECG shows an abnormally left superior vector (formerly termed "left axis deviation"). A congenital abnormality of the anterior branch of the left bundle leads to initial QRS conduction inferiorly, followed by the remainder of the conduction sequence superiorly.

In complete AV canal, left ventricular to right atrial communication is present in addition to the large VSD, leading to an early increase in pulmonary blood flow. If mitral regurgitation is present, early left ventricular failure may occur. The high left ventricular end-diastolic pressure causes the pulmonary venous pressure to be elevated. Thus three of the four major factors that slow maturation of the pulmonary resistance vessels are present. In addition, continued high pulmonary blood flow at systemic-level pulmonary artery pressure and high pulmonary venous pressure may be exhibited. Therefore, even when heart failure can be managed, the pulmonary vascular resistance eventually increases, and pulmonary vascular disease occurs. Early complete surgical repair, preferably by 3 months of age, is strongly recommended.

Obstructive Lesions

Right-Sided Lesions. The most common pure right-sided obstructive lesion is **valvular pulmonic stenosis.** Peripheral pulmonic stenosis that is not part of other congenital cardiac lesions (e.g., tetralogy of Fallot) occurs most commonly in association with such entities as congenital rubella, Williams syndrome, Noonan syndrome, Alagille syndrome, cutis laxa, and Ehlers-Danlos syndrome. Isolated pulmonary infundibular stenosis may exist only when a VSD is present or has been present and closed.

The majority of stenotic pulmonic valves have three leaflets with varied leaflet fusion. A less common variety is pulmonary valvular dysplasia, in which the pathology is not of fusion but of a myxomatous tissue that is disorganized, thickened, and immobile. Most patients with dysplastic pulmonary valves have Noonan syndrome.

The *diagnosis* is suggested by a pulmonary ejection click that is maximal on expiration at the upper left sternal border, followed by an ejection systolic murmur and a widely split S_2. The more severe the stenosis, the longer the murmur; full-length murmurs are associated with the right ventricular pressures near systemic level. With mild stenosis, the S_2 split is not much above normal and pulmonary closure may be of increased intensity. With increasing severity, the split widens and the pulmonary closure softens. In many severe cases, with suprasystemic right ventricular pressure, the murmur may extend across the aortic closure, so that no second sound is heard at the upper left sternal border. The ECG shows pure RVH, and the chest x-ray films reveal no significant cardiomegaly and a large dilated (poststenotic) pulmonary artery. In some severe cases the elevated right atrial pressure may cause the flap of the foramen ovale to open, resulting in a significant right-to-left shunt. Thus this "acyanotic lesion" would be associated with cyanosis.

Cases have been observed, especially in infancy, in which the pulmonic stenosis is so severe that marked right ventricular failure occurs, associated with venous distention, a large liver, and a large right-to-left shunt at the atrial level. In other infants the severe stenosis leads to cyanosis very shortly after birth from inadequate pulmonary blood flow. These children are dependent on a patent ductus arteriosus for oxygenation. This condition is termed **critical pulmonic stenosis.**

Treatment of valvular pulmonic stenosis is straightforward. Mild pulmonic stenosis with right ventricular pressure of less than 50 mm Hg is very common; it is known not to increase in severity over the years and is associated with normal life expectancy. When the right ventricular pressure is above 60 mm Hg, the treatment is balloon valvuloplasty (Tables 13–9 and 13–10). The success rate is very high, and the risk is very low. Surgery is performed only in cases in which valvuloplasty has been unsuccessful.

Left-Sided Lesions

VALVULAR AORTIC STENOSIS. Left-sided lesions are quite common, particularly if *bicuspid aortic valve without stenosis* is included in this category. It is not known how common this latter lesion is, although it is known to occur in about two thirds of patients with coarctation of the aorta. The recognition of bicuspid aortic valve (with two sinuses) is important because patients with this abnormality are susceptible to infective endocarditis. The *diagnosis* is readily made by identifying a sharp sound well separated from S_1 and usually maximal at the apex, not varying with respiration, and less well heard at the lower left sternal border and anterior axillary line. This sound is an aortic ejection click.

VALVULAR AORTIC STENOSIS WITH SYSTOLIC GRADIENT. Valvular aortic stenosis with systolic gradient is a major lesion with tremendous variation in severity. In most cases surgery is not required in childhood. Although it is a potentially progressive lesion, mild cases do not progress until adulthood.

The systolic murmur usually is maximal at the upper right sternal border or over the sternum and often is associated with suprasternal notch and carotid systolic thrills. When the murmur is significantly less than full length and the split of S_2 is normal, indicating no significant prolongation of left ventricular systole, the condition almost certainly is mild. Such patients usually have ECGs that are normal. When the murmur is full length and the split of S_2 is narrow, indicating prolongation of left ventricular systole, the condition is significant. Important clues to severity are the initial QRS vector being situated to the left; LVH; and the development of ST-segment and T-wave abnormalities with exercise. Echo-Doppler techniques for predicting severity have become reliable, and thus baseline catheterization is usually not necessary.

If no ST or T abnormalities are present at rest and if the systolic gradient is less than 60 mm Hg, most cardiologists agree that no intervention is indicated (Tables 13–9 and 13–10). (The presence of ST and T abnormalities at rest, however, provides a clear indication for intervention.) Most cardiologists advise that children with significant aortic stenosis should not participate in competitive athletics. When exercise requiring sustained strength is involved (e.g., weightlifting and competitive wrestling), the end-diastolic pressure increases significantly, reducing coronary perfusion. Therefore, this type of exercise especially should be avoided. Sudden unexpected death caused by valvular aortic stenosis in childhood or young adulthood is rare. Both surgery and balloon aortic valvuloplasty are palliative and equally successful procedures. For most patients, balloon valvuloplasty is the procedure of choice. Surgery is reserved for those patients unresponsive to balloon dilation or who have severe valve dysplasia or aortic insufficiency. Even after successful intervention, the stenosis tends to recur over time, with reintervention needed. Repeated interventions often lead to the development of aortic insufficiency, which necessitates valve replacement. Prosthetic valve replacement has traditionally been the procedure of choice. The autologous transfer of the pulmonary root (Ross procedure) is another option.

The infants who have *critical aortic stenosis*, sometimes recognized in the first week of life, are quite ill. They have very stenotic valves and sometimes abnormal left ventricles. All would die without intervention (Tables 13–9 and 13–10).

COARCTATION OF THE AORTA. Simple coarctation of the aorta is almost always at the level of the ductus arteriosus (or ligamentum arteriosum) and just below the origin of the left subclavian artery. (Occasionally, the origin of the left subclavian is at or below the coarctation.) Because of the position of the ductus, there is no obstruction to flow in the aorta in utero or while the ductus is open in the newborn period. Therefore, simple coarctation often is not recognized in newborns.

The murmur is usually systolic, with a late peak, and can be located anywhere in the anterior chest. The murmur usually is heard well at the apex, left axilla, and left back, but often it is maximal over the left back. An ECG early in infancy may show pure RVH, although later in childhood LVH is expected.

Rarely, coarctation causes heart failure in the first month of life, but often the children are asymptomatic throughout childhood. Eventually most children have upper extremity systolic hypertension. Because of the position of the left subclavian artery, the right arm pressure may be higher than that of the left arm. Because the pulse pressure is low below the coarctation, renal endocrine factors work to raise the pressure, both above and below the coarctation.

Treatment of *simple* coarctation of the aorta is indicated in Table 13–10. Previously it had been recommended to wait until 4–5 years of age for surgery in asymptomatic children because of a higher risk of recoarctation. Advances in surgical techniques have decreased this risk. Therefore, most children should be considered for surgery at the time of diagnosis. Children who are hypertensive should be treated to normalize their blood pressure before surgery, which decreases the risk of malignant postoperative hypertension. Special problems arise when the diagnosis is missed or if surgery is not performed until later in life. First, more collateral vessels may be present, leading to increased bleeding during surgery. In addition, by adolescence the aorta may have stiffened, so that end-to-end anastomosis cannot be done. Also, the incidence of essential hypertension and death may be significantly higher in later life.

Complicated coarctation of the aorta, a coarctation in association with another lesion (e.g., PDA arising above the coarctation or, more commonly, a VSD), commonly leads to heart failure by the second week of life. After treatment of heart failure, surgery must be performed within a few days. For those infants with a PDA, operating on both lesions successfully alleviates the problem. For the more common cases with a VSD, the decision regarding the appropriate approach must be individualized and based upon the VSD size. Often only the coarctation is operated on because it is difficult to determine the size of the VSD. If the infant remains very ill, a second operation soon may be necessary to close the VSD.

When a coarctation is corrected, the area of repair may not grow. Consequently, a situation called "restenosis" may develop. However, newer surgical techniques, such as the end-to-side anastomosis, have significantly decreased the incidence of restenosis. Balloon arterioplasty, often with placement of an intravascular stent, is often recommended instead of surgery for relief of restenosis. Balloon arterioplasty is also performed as a treatment for primary coarctation, but the long-term risk of restenosis and aortic aneurysm formation is not yet known.

TABLE 13–11
Cyanotic Congenital Heart Disease with Decreased Pulmonary Blood Flow

Right Ventricular Hypertrophy
Pulmonary stenosis (severe) with atrial septal defect
Pulmonary atresia (with or without ventricular septal defect)
Tetralogy of Fallot

Left Ventricular Hypertrophy
Tricuspid atresia
Pulmonary atresia and hypoplastic right ventricle

Right, Left, or Combined Ventricular Hypertrophy
Transposition of great arteries with pulmonary stenosis
Truncus arteriosus with hypoplastic pulmonary arteries

Neither Ventricle Predominant
Ebstein anomaly

TABLE 13–12
Cyanotic Congenital Heart Disease with Increased Pulmonary Blood Flow

Right Ventricular Hypertrophy
Total anomalous venous return
Transposition of great arteries

Right, Left, or Combined Ventricular Hypertrophy
Transposition of great arteries ± ventricular septal defect
Single ventricle without pulmonary stenosis
Tricuspid atresia with transposition
Truncus arteriosus

Cyanotic Congenital Heart Disease

Cyanotic CHD can be divided into lesions that have decreased (Table 13–11) or increased (Table 13–12) pulmonary blood flow. Because of persistent cyanosis or right-to-left shunts, these patients often have characteristic extracardiac complications (Table 13–13).

TABLE 13–13
Extracardiac Complications of Cyanotic Congenital Heart Disease

Problem	Etiology	Therapy
Polycythemia	Persistent hypoxia	Phlebotomy
Relative anemia	Nutritional deficiency	Iron replacement
CNS abscess	Right-to-left shunting	Antibiotics, drainage
CNS thromboembolic stroke	Right-to-left shunting or polycythemia	Phlebotomy
Gum disease	Polycythemia, gingivitis, bleeding	Dental hygiene
Gout	Polycythemia, diuretic agents	Allopurinol
Arthritis, clubbing	Hypoxic arthropathy	None
Pregnancy	Poor placental perfusion, poor ability to increase cardiac output	Bed rest
Infectious disease	Associated asplenia, DiGeorge syndrome	Antibiotics
	Fatal RSV pneumonia with pulmonary hypertension	Ribavirin, RSV immune globulin
Growth	Failure to thrive, increased oxygen consumption, decreased nutrient intake	Treat heart failure; correct defect early
Psychosocial adjustment	Limited activity, peer pressure; chronic disease, multiple hospitalizations	Counseling

CNS, Central nervous system; *RSV,* respiratory syncytial virus.

Tetralogy of Fallot

The four components of tetralogy of Fallot are a large nonrestrictive VSD, severe right ventricle outflow tract obstruction, overriding of the aortic root over the ventricular septum, and RVH. The RVH is secondary. Embryologically, there is one defect—anterior malalignment of the conus. Because conal tissue provides the major portion of the tissue that closes the membranous ventricular septum and because the conus is hypoplastic, the result is a nonrestrictive VSD and severe infundibular pulmonic stenosis. Flow through the small conus is restricted in utero, resulting in a small annulus and small pulmonary arteries.

Although the location and size of the VSD are relatively constant, the severity of the pulmonary stenosis varies considerably and accounts for the varying ages at presentation and the varying clinical courses. In a few infants the pulmonary stenosis may be less severe, associated initially with a left-to-right shunt. A true tetralogy, however, has a right-to-left shunt.

Occasionally the narrowing is located almost exclusively at the infundibular level, associated with a normal pulmonary valve annulus, normal valve leaflets, and normal distal pulmonary arteries. More commonly, obstruction at the infundibular level is associated with a hypoplastic pulmonary valve annulus and a dysplastic, stenotic pulmonary valve.

The main pulmonary artery and distal pulmonary arteries may be hypoplastic, and occasionally discrete stenoses are noted at the takeoff of the right and left pulmonary arteries or even more distally. In the most severe form, complete atresia of the infundibulum, the pulmonary valve, and even sometimes the main pulmonary artery occurs. Other intracardiac anomalies are not commonly associated with tetralogy, except that a right aortic arch is present in 25% of the patients.

Pathophysiology. Because of the large size of VSD, blood passing through the tricuspid and mitral valves may flow to either the aorta or the pulmonary artery; the degree of intracardiac shunting is a function of the relative outflow resistances (Fig. 13–12). The systemic resistance is composed primarily of the systemic arteriolar resistance, but the pulmonary resistance is a result of the anatomic pulmonary stenosis. Because the pulmonary stenosis is severe, there is primarily or exclusively a right-to-left shunt, with blood bypassing the pulmonary artery and going to the aorta.

Although the severity of the anatomic abnormality is the primary determinant of the degree of cyanosis, changes in systemic venous oxygen saturation or pulmonary or systemic resistances also influence the degree of right-to-left shunting. For example, exercise or crying, by reducing the systemic arteriolar resistance and increasing systemic venous

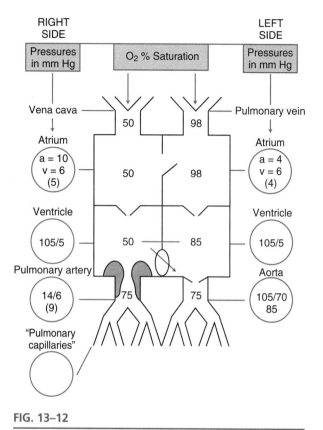

FIG. 13–12

Tetralogy of Fallot.

return, is associated with a larger right-to-left shunt, more cyanosis, and a decrease in oxygen saturation. Any agent that increases systemic resistance has the opposite effect, by decreasing systemic and increasing pulmonary blood flow and therefore reducing the right-to-left shunt. The child inherently learns to decrease cyanosis by assuming a squatting position. Squatting increases systemic venous return, making more blood available to the pulmonary artery, and increases systemic resistance, driving more venous blood into the lungs.

Clinical Manifestations. The clinical findings vary, depending on the degree of right ventricular outflow obstruction. Children with a less severe degree of outflow obstruction may not be cyanotic at birth and initially may have a left-to-right shunt. Usually the right ventricular outflow tract obstruction is progressive, leading to increasing hypoxemia and cyanosis over the first few months and years of life. Such children usually do well clinically except for dyspnea and increased cyanosis on exertion. Occasionally children younger than 5 years of age assume a squatting position.

Hypoxic ("tet") spells can occur and are usually progressive. During such spells the child typically becomes quite restless and agitated and may cry inconsolably. The child is hyperpneic, with gradually increasing cyanosis, which then often leads to a deep sleep. In severe spells, prolonged unconsciousness and even convulsions, hemiparesis, or death may occur. Treatment of these spells consists of administering oxygen (to increase the oxygen delivery), placing the child in the knee-chest position (to increase venous return), and giving morphine sulfate (to relax the pulmonary infundibulum and for sedation). If necessary, the SVR can be acutely increased by intravenous administration of an alpha-adrenergic agonist such as phenylephrine or methoxamine. Muscular spasm of the infundibulum can be a component of spells and can be decreased by the beta-adrenergic antagonist propranolol. If acidosis is present, intravenous sodium bicarbonate should be given. In refractory cases emergency surgery, either systemic–to–pulmonary artery shunt or total correction, may be necessary. It is not unusual for the family to be unaware of the presence of mild spells. All children with tetralogy will become somewhat more cyanotic with crying. The association of a period of crying followed by sleep is often overlooked as a spell, so it should be elicited by a careful history. Although medical management can decrease the frequency of spells, their presence is generally considered an indication for surgery.

The volume work of the heart in tetralogy of Fallot is less than normal. Therefore, heart failure does not occur.

On *physical examination*, cyanosis and digital clubbing (in older children) are evident. A quiet heart with a right ventricular impulse is noted. Because of the severe pulmonic stenosis, pulmonary closure is not heard. The audible second sound is that of a loud aortic closure at the lower left sternal border resulting from transmission down the descending aorta. Because no murmur occurs from a right-to-left shunt through the VSD, the only murmur heard is that of blood flowing through the pulmonic stenosis. With more severe stenosis, less blood goes through the stenotic right ventricular outflow tract and more goes through the VSD, resulting in a softer, shorter murmur. In tetralogy with pulmonary atresia no systolic murmur is present, although a loud aortic ejection click may be. Also, a continuous murmur from either a PDA or large collateral artery off the descending aorta (best heard in the back) may be present. In the patient who has a hypoxic spell, the previously heard systolic murmur softens or disappears, returning when the spell is over.

On the *chest x-ray* film, the heart is not enlarged. Often a concavity is found in the area usually occupied by the main pulmonary artery ("boot-shaped" heart), and the ascending aorta is large. A right aortic arch may be present.

The *ECG* shows RVH and often right atrial enlargement, although in the first weeks of life the ECG may be normal. Echocardiography can define the important features in most patients with tetralogy of Fallot. The extent and anatomy of right ventricular outflow obstruction, the VSD, the proximal branch pulmonary arteries, and the coronary arteries are visualized. Coronary anomalies, specifically a left coronary artery (either left anterior descending or large conal branch) crossing the anterior surface of the right ventricular outflow tract, are present in 5% of patients.

Cardiac catheterization usually is not necessary in the infant, and it is not necessary to take the risk of producing hypoxic spells. On *cardiac catheterization,* equal systolic pressures in the RV and LV and ascending aorta are noted (Fig. 13–12). The oxygen saturation on the right side of the heart usually is lower than normal because of systemic hypoxemia; however, the pulmonary venous and left atrial saturations are normal.

Angiography of the RV, LV, and ascending aorta identifies the anatomy of the VSD(s) and pulmonary arteries. An aortogram can help identify the coronary artery pattern, the presence of a patent ductus arteriosus, or aortopulmonary collateral vessels, which can develop in older children with prolonged cyanosis.

Complications. A *cerebrovascular accident* is a devastating complication of cyanotic CHD (Table 13–13). In children younger than 2 years of age, this complication almost invariably is secondary to hypoxemia and anemia rather than to polycythemia, sludging, and in situ thrombosis, and it occurs most commonly in children who are quite hypoxemic, with a relative anemia for the degree of oxygen saturation. Iron deficiency makes the red blood cells somewhat stiffer and leads to less oxygen delivery. In older children, in particular, the hematocrit may rise above 65%. Even in this situation, considerable iron deficiency may be present, a diagnosis that cannot be made by examination of the red cells on the blood smear. Serum iron and iron-binding capacity must be measured. When iron therapy is given, the hemoglobin level may rise, but the hematocrit value usually does not. Conversely, if the iron saturation is normal, the administration of iron can raise the hematocrit to dangerous levels.

Although the viscosity of the blood may increase significantly when the hematocrit is above 55%, this involves a tradeoff of improved delivery of oxygen to the tissue at the higher hematocrit level. A large number of patients with congenital defects resulting in chronic cyanosis need to maintain their hematocrit levels between 60% and 65% for optimal well-being. However, if questions of symptoms of polycythemia at that hematocrit level have arisen or if the hematocrit level has risen above 65%, partial exchange transfusion is necessary. Withdrawal of blood without continuous exchange is dangerous, the risks being the acute lowering of systemic resistance, more right-to-left shunt, and a cerebrovascular accident.

Brain abscess is a less common complication than a cerebrovascular accident. Patients usually are older than 2 years of age and exhibit headaches and localizing signs. Any central nervous system event in a cyanotic child over the age of 2 years should be considered a brain abscess until proven otherwise, because of the drastic implications of the condition. CT scans are diagnostic. Antibiotic therapy occasionally may keep the infection localized, but surgical drainage of the abscess often is needed.

Bacterial endocarditis is always a risk before complete repair in children with tetralogy of Fallot, particularly in patients with systemic-to-pulmonary shunts.

Treatment. The treatment of tetralogy of Fallot is surgical (Tables 13–9 and 13–10), and complete repair is recommended before the child is 6 months of age. Earlier surgery is indicated if the affected child is significantly symptomatic, hypoxemic with an arterial oxygen saturation of less than 75%, or having hypercyanotic spells. Surgery can be delayed if the child has required a palliative procedure earlier in life. *Palliative operations* are becoming much less frequent because total correction can be performed for most patients at any age, even in the neonatal period. Palliation is performed in patients deemed inappropriate for total correction, such as those with unusual anatomy in which the small size makes correction difficult. The *Blalock-Taussig shunt* connecting the subclavian artery to the pulmonary artery is the preferred systemic-to-pulmonary shunt. The Blalock-Taussig shunt is an excellent temporizing procedure, but it does not eliminate right-to-left shunting and does have the potential of distorting the pulmonary arteries, making later repair more difficult. Balloon pulmonary valvuloplasty is a palliative option for patients with primarily valvular stenosis.

Total correction of tetralogy of Fallot is performed under cardiopulmonary bypass. It involves closure of the VSD with a pericardial patch and excision of muscle in the right ventricular outflow tract. A right ventriculotomy may be necessary to adequately resect the infundibular muscle, but this procedure can lead to later arrhythmias. Transatrial resection is the preferred method for most patients. When hypoplasia of the pulmonary annulus, main pulmonary artery, or distal pulmonary arteries is significant, a patch may be required to enlarge the outflow tract, but this increases the likelihood of insufficiency (discussed later in this section). In institutions in which complete repair is done before the age of 1 year, the surgical mortality rate is lower than 5%.

Short-term complications include a residual VSD and residual right ventricular outflow tract obstruction because of incomplete relief of the pulmonary stenosis. Pulmonary regurgitation also is common even with excellent surgical results and is the most common cause of late reoperation. Late complications are ventricular ectopy and sudden death resulting from ventricular tachycardia. Although long-term data are not available, most children do quite well and remain asymptomatic at least throughout childhood and into young adulthood.

d-Transposition of the Great Arteries

Complete transposition of the great arteries (TGA), although less common than tetralogy of Fallot, is the most common cardiac lesion seen in the cyanotic infant in the newborn period. In children with this lesion the great arteries arise off the inappropriate ventricle, the aorta from the right and the pulmonary artery from the left. The systemic venous drainage and pulmonary venous drainage are usually normal, and the right and left atria and the right and left ventricles are in their normal positions. Therefore, desaturated blood from the systemic venous return passes through the RA and RV and out to the aorta, whereas oxygenated pulmonary venous blood passes through the LA and LV and then out through the pulmonary artery (Fig. 13–13). Survival is dependent on mixing of blood between the circulations.

Associated abnormalities of the atrial and ventricular septum, AV valves, and coronary arteries are common and may alter the physiology significantly. The clinical presentation and hemodynamics vary significantly in relation to the presence or absence of significant associated defects.

d-Transposition of the Great Arteries with an Intact Ventricular Septum. In children with this anomaly, the most common variant, no other intracardiac or extracardiac anomalies are present. Before birth the oxygenation of the fetus is normal; after delivery, however, mixing between the parallel circulations diminishes as the ductus arteriosus closes, and severe hypoxemia, acidosis, and death can occur rapidly.

Clinical Manifestations. Cyanosis usually is noted within the first day of life and progresses rapidly as the ductus arteriosus closes. Differential cyanosis may be present. Because the RV supplies blood to the ascending aorta, the upper body will have a lower saturation than the lower. d-TGA is the only

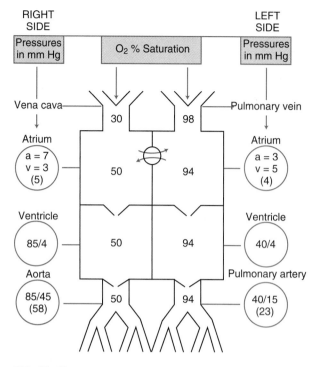

FIG. 13–13

Transposition of the great arteries.

condition that leads to preferential desaturation of the upper body.

The remainder of the cardiac examination may be normal, with no murmur or only a grade 2/6 ejection systolic murmur present. The chest x-ray results may be normal but may reveal mild cardiac enlargement with normal or increased pulmonary blood flow. The base of the heart is narrower than usual because of the frequent absence of a significant thymus and the more anterior-posterior relationship of the aorta and pulmonary arteries, causing an egg shape. The ECG usually is normal. The two-dimensional echocardiogram and Doppler study are diagnostic by showing the anterior great vessel branching into innominate, carotid, and subclavian arteries and the posterior great vessel branching into the right and left pulmonary arteries. The coronary artery origins, which can vary widely, must also be identified.

Cardiac catheterization is usually not necessary, but it shows the right ventricular pressure to be at systemic levels because the RV is connected to the aorta. The left ventricular pressure may be high in the perinatal period because of elevated pulmonary vascular resistance, but it usually drops to a level of 30 or 40 mm Hg by the first or second week of life. This is the only congenital cardiac lesion in which the left ventricular pressure is less than the aortic pressure. Angiography in the RV and LV shows the great vessels arising inappropriately and rules out associated cardiac anomalies.

Treatment. The finding of cyanosis in the perinatal period in the child with *d*-TGA is a true medical emergency. As the ductus arteriosus closes, severe hypoxemia, acidosis, and death occur unless another intracardiac connection is present for mixing. The child should be started on a prostaglandin (PGE_1) infusion immediately on diagnosis. When patency of the ductus arteriosus is maintained, more blood goes from the aorta into the pulmonary artery, increasing pulmonary venous and left atrial flow. Thus more blood is available to go left to right at the atrial level. Almost any cyanotic full-term infant will benefit from administration of PGE_1, and very few have adverse reactions. Because apnea does occur after PGE_1 administration, close observation, intubation, or both are necessary.

The initial palliation of newborn infants who have TGA and an intact ventricular septum involves improving intracardiac mixing by tearing the fossa ovalis with a balloon catheter developed by William Rashkind (Table 13–9). This can be performed either under fluoroscopic control or in the intensive care unit using two-dimensional echocardiography to guide the balloon catheter into the LA. A successful *Rashkind procedure* is signaled by improvement in oxygenation and elimination of the interatrial pressure gradient.

The surgical treatment of choice is the arterial switch operation (ASO), which provides both an anatomic and a physiologic correction. (Previously an "atrial switch" was accomplished by a *Mustard* or *Senning procedure.* A pantaloon-shaped baffle was inserted within the atrium to divert pulmonary venous return anteriorly through the tricuspid valve, into the RV and aorta.) The inferior and superior vena caval blood then can go through the mitral valve into the LV and pulmonary artery. Both atrial techniques provide a physiologic but not an anatomic repair because the RV continues pumping to the systemic circulation. Long-term complications may occur, such as obstruction at either the pulmonary venous or the systemic venous portion of the baffle and a variety of interatrial arrhythmias. The most common arrhythmias are together described as the **sick sinus syndrome.** This includes sinus bradycardia or no sinus activity with atrial or junctional bradycardia, together with supraventricular tachycardia or atrial flutter. The syndrome occurs in 50% of cases. This disturbing combination of tachyarrhythmias and bradyarrhythmias makes pharmacologic treatment difficult without insertion of a pacemaker.

Complications with the "atrial switch" procedure and improvements in intraoperative techniques have led to total repair of transposition by the ASO (Table 13–10). This technique involves removing the coronary arteries along with a button of tissue from the base of the aorta and moving them posteriorly onto the base of the pulmonary artery. The great arteries then are divided and switched so that the anterior aortic valve arises from the RV and is connected to the pulmonary arterial tree, and the posterior pulmonary valve arises from the LV and is connected to the aorta. This operation can be done only with an LV that is able to maintain a systemic pressure. This is possible in the perinatal period because with transposition both ventricles have been generating systemic pressure in utero. The left ventricular pressure decreases to 30 or 40 mm Hg within a few days to one week. Therefore, in most centers the arterial switch is performed in the first 10–14 days of life. It can, however, be performed up to 6 weeks of age. In these older children the likelihood of postoperative low cardiac output increases because the LV must reacclimate to the systemic pressure. Therefore, it should be performed at this age only when a temporary means of ventricular support is available, such as mechanical ventricular assist or ECMO.

Prognosis. If the lesion is left untreated, the prognosis for TGA is poor; 30% of the infants die in the first week, 50% in the first month, and more than 90% in the first year. This outcome has been improved markedly, first with balloon atrial septostomy and more recently by early correction. The mortality after the ASO is 5%, and late mortality is rare; 10–15-year survival is greater than 90%. Late coronary complications and supravalvular stenosis are the primary concerns, but they occur in fewer than 5% of patients 10 years after surgery. Aortic insufficiency is a rare late complication.

d-Transposition of the Great Arteries with a Ventricular Septal Defect. The presence of a large VSD dramatically improves intracardiac mixing, so cyanosis is not the major problem. In infants with this abnormality, pulmonary blood flow increases as the pulmonary vascular resistance drops; these infants exhibit heart failure after a few weeks of life.

Clinical Manifestations. The clinical manifestations in the newborn who has TGA and a large VSD are dominated by signs and symptoms of heart failure. The infant usually is tachypneic and tachycardic, with increased perspiration and poor feeding. The heart is very hyperdynamic, with prominent right and left ventricular impulses. The second heart sound is single, and frequently a grade 3 or louder systolic murmur is present, obscuring S_1 at the third or fourth left interspace, as a result of the VSD.

Radiographic examination of the chest reveals the heart to be enlarged, with increased pulmonary blood flow and a haziness consistent with increased interstitial fluid from elevated pulmonary venous pressure. The base of the heart sometimes is narrow because of the more anterior-posterior relationship of the great arteries and the small thymus. The ECG shows combined ventricular hypertrophy or occasionally pure RVH.

The two-dimensional echocardiogram and Doppler study are diagnostic, showing the great vessels arising off the inappropriate ventricle and a large VSD. At cardiac catheterization, left atrial pressure usually is greater than the right, but both are increased; the pressures in each ventricle are equal, and usually bidirectional shunting (right to left in systole; left to right in diastole) is found at the ventricular level. Nonetheless, left-to-right shunting at the atrial level and right-to-left shunting at the ventricular level predominate. The left and right ventricular angiograms show the great arteries arising off the inappropriate ventricles, as well as the presence of a VSD.

Treatment. In infants with heart failure the usual anticongestive measures, including digoxin, diuretics, increased caloric density of the formula, and afterload reduction, are useful as a temporizing measure (Table 13–6). Surgery is usually recommended within the first 2–3 weeks and is required by 3 months of age because systemic-level pulmonary artery hypertension in the presence of high pulmonary blood flow invariably leads to pulmonary vascular disease. The ASO with closure of the VSD is the preferred approach.

Pulmonary Atresia with an Intact Ventricular Septum and a Hypoplastic Right Ventricle

Pulmonary atresia with an intact ventricular septum and a hypoplastic right ventricle is an uncommon but very important condition because all affected infants die without urgent treatment. The pulmonary valve is atretic as a result of an obstructing diaphragm or fusion of the commissures. The RV is markedly hypoplastic. The tricuspid valve is appropriate for the size of the RV and therefore is small. Connections between sinusoids of the RV and the coronary arteries occasionally result in flow from the ventricle to the coronary artery in systole because of high intracavitary pressure in the RV.

Because of the atretic right ventricular outflow tract, all the systemic venous return passes through the RA into the LA, where it mixes with the pulmonary venous return. The LV pumps blood to the systemic circulation and to the lungs via the ductus arteriosus. As the ductus arteriosus closes soon after birth, hypoxemia becomes progressively severe. Without intervention, death occurs rapidly.

Clinical Manifestations. Newborn infants may appear normal at birth, but as the ductus narrows, progressive cyanosis develops. On physical examination, the second heart sound is single. The precordium is quiet, although some children have a murmur of tricuspid insufficiency at the lower left sternal border. Chest x-ray examination reveals decreased pulmonary vascular markings. The heart may be normal in size or may show dilation from right atrial enlargement. The ECG shows right atrial enlargement and LVH with a normal inferior vector.

The two-dimensional echocardiogram and Doppler study shows absence of the pulmonary valve, hypoplasia of the right ventricular cavity, and, frequently, significant tricuspid regurgitation. Coronary communications can be difficult to delineate by echocardiography. The diagnosis can be confirmed by cardiac catheterization and angiography. The oxygen saturation data show right-to-left shunting at the atrial level. The degree of hypoxemia depends on the pulmonary blood flow. The right ventricular pressure usually exceeds the left ventricular and aortic systolic pressures. Angiography of the RV shows the hypoplasia of the cavity and tricuspid valve and, most important, illuminates right ventricular sinusoid–to–coronary artery connections.

Treatment and Prognosis. Because hypoxemia becomes worse as the ductus arteriosus closes, PGE_1 infusion, by dilating the ductus, improves the oxygen saturation and is lifesaving. When the right ventricle is of reasonable size and significant coronary communications are not present, the valve can be percutaneously punctured with a wire, a laser, or a radiofrequency catheter; this is followed by balloon dilation. In most cases, however, an artificial connection between the aorta and pulmonary artery (e.g., a Blalock-Taussig shunt) is necessary because the poor compliance of the RV forces most right atrial blood into the LA. At a later age (>2 years), if the RV is large and the hemodynamics is appropriate, the Blalock-Taussig connection can be ligated and the foramen ovale closed. Both of these can be done surgically or by catheter intervention.

When significant coronary communications are present, valvuloplasty is not indicated because the decrease in RV pressure can steal blood from the coronary circulation, causing ischemia or arrhythmias. In this instance or when the right ventricle is severely hypoplastic, a Blalock-Taussig shunt alone is indicated in preparation for an eventual *modified Fontan procedure.* This procedure connects the systemic venous return to the pulmonary artery. The surgery usually is staged, beginning with a bidirectional superior vena cava–to–pulmonary artery shunt (*Glenn procedure*) at 2–6 months of age, followed by connection of the inferior vena cava to the pulmonary artery at 2–4 years. The operative risk of a Glenn procedure is less than 10%, and postoperative mortality is minimal. Pulmonary arteriovenous fistulas are a long-term complication of the bidirectional Glenn procedure and can lead to severe oxygen desaturation or death. The Fontan procedure carries a 5–10% mortality. Over the long term, there is a late mortality rate of 0.5–1% per year from arrhythmias, ventricular failure, or protein-losing enteropathy.

The long-term prognosis for infants with pulmonary atresia with an intact ventricular septum is mixed. For infants with a reasonable-sized right ventricular cavity, the prognosis is good. For infants with severe hypoplasia, the cumulative mortality rate from the operations and waiting period is on the order of 20–30% in early childhood.

Tricuspid Atresia

Tricuspid atresia is more common than hypoplastic RV with pulmonary atresia, but it is less likely to be recognized in the first days of life. The tricuspid valve is atretic (usually with hardly a dimple on the floor of the right atrium), and the right ventricular cavity is hypoplastic. Tricuspid atresia is different embryologically from pulmonary atresia. In tricuspid atresia (without TGA) a VSD always is present, almost always posterior, in the position of an endocardial cushion defect.

All the systemic venous return passing into the RA goes across the foramen ovale into the LA, where it mixes with pulmonary venous return and then passes into the LV. The amount of pulmonary blood flow then depends mostly on the size of the VSD, through which all pulmonary blood must flow. The LV must handle increased volume despite diminished pulmonary blood flow (Fig. 13–14). Occasionally the VSD is large and the pulmonary blood flow almost unimpeded. In this instance pulmonary blood flow increases as the PVR decreases after birth, and may become excessive enough to cause heart failure. The VSD tends to get smaller with age; thus even in these cases, eventually diminished pulmonary blood flow occurs.

Clinical Manifestations. The age of the patient and findings on presentation are primarily related to the size of the VSD and thus dependent on the pulmonary blood flow. In those infrequent cases in which the VSD is very small from birth, pulmonary blood flow depends on the ductus arteriosus, so that marked hypoxemia occurs when the ductus closes. In most cases, however, the VSD is large enough so that the infants do well in the first 1–3 months. In the infant with a small VSD, the chest x-ray reveals a

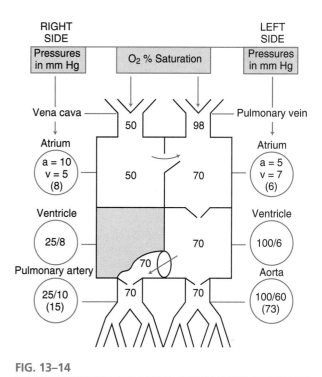

FIG. 13–14

Hypoplastic right ventricle with tricuspid atresia and ventricular septal defect.

normal-sized heart with diminished pulmonary vascularity. The ECG reveals considerable LVH because of the hypoplastic RV and the increased volume work of the LV. Because the VSD is in the endocardial cushion position, conduction of the left anterior branch of the left bundle is abnormal, resulting in an abnormally superior vector. In the newborn this latter ECG finding is a strong clue in distinguishing this lesion from a hypoplastic RV with pulmonary atresia.

After 2–3 years of life, inverted T waves over the left precordium are common, which suggests a more severe LVH and fibrosis as part of left ventricular cardiomyopathy. Also, right atrial enlargement is present. The echocardiogram describes the anatomy, and at catheterization (necessary only before consideration of Fontan types of procedures) all right atrial blood goes across the atrial opening to the LA. The catheter is easily passed into the LV and usually the aorta. Cineangiography shows the large LV, the hypoplastic RV, and the VSD. The pulmonary arteries usually are well visualized past the bifurcation into right and left branches.

Treatment and Prognosis. In the newborn period for the child with markedly diminished pulmonary blood flow, PGE_1 infusion maintains patency of the ductus arteriosus and thus may be lifesaving until a Blalock-Taussig shunt can be performed. Usually the administration of PGE_1 is not necessary; for those infants who have a good VSD murmur and whose systemic arterial saturation is above 80%, administration of PGE_1 and creation of a shunt are not indicated. For those few infants with excessive pulmonary blood flow who go into heart failure in the first month of life, the usual anticongestive measures are indicated (Table 13–6). Later, after the VSD becomes smaller, administration of digoxin and diuretics is discontinued.

For safe performance of a *physiologic repair,* the PVR must be low, the pulmonary arteries must not have been badly distorted, and the LV must be compliant. The long-term "corrective" operation is a Fontan procedure, described earlier in the section on pulmonary atresia.

Truncus Arteriosus

In children with truncus arteriosus a single arterial trunk from the base of the heart gives rise to the aorta, pulmonary arteries, and coronary arteries. A large VSD invariably is present, and the single semilunar valve has a variable number of leaflets, between two and six. The valve may be stenotic, regurgitant, or both. The pulmonary arteries may arise as a single trunk before bifurcating (type 1) or may arise separately from the posterior wall of the aorta (type 2).

Because there is a common exit to the aorta and pulmonary artery, the saturation of blood in the systemic arteries is approximately equal to that in the pulmonary arteries. The level of arterial saturation depends on the amount of pulmonary blood flow. If the PVR is high, moderate hypoxemia may result. When the PVR is low, pulmonary blood flow may be torrential, cyanosis minimal, and heart failure severe.

Clinical Findings. Initially after birth, the PVR is high and the newborn may do well. As the PVR drops, the pulmonary blood flow increases, and the signs and symptoms of heart failure develop. The runoff of blood from truncus into the pulmonary artery in diastole leads to a wide pulse pressure. The heart is hyperdynamic, with loud first and second heart sounds, and an aortic ejection click almost always is present. A grade 2 to 3/6 systolic ejection murmur usually is noted at the upper left or right sternal border from increased flow across the semilunar valve; however, if the truncal valve is stenotic, the murmur may be grade 4 and associated with a thrill. An early, high-frequency diastolic murmur is present if the truncal valve is regurgitant, and a mid-diastolic rumble at the apex may be present if the pulmonary blood flow (and therefore flow across the mitral valve) is increased. The combination of stenosis and regurgitation results in the characteristic to-and-fro ("washing machine") murmur. In the older child with an increased PVR, progressive cyanosis, polycythemia, and clubbing may occur.

Chest x-ray examination usually reveals the heart to be large, with increased pulmonary vascularity and pulmonary venous congestion; in 40% of patients a right aortic arch is found. Because of the association with **DiGeorge syndrome,** the thymus shadow may be absent. When an elevated PVR and diminished pulmonary blood flow are present, the ECG shows RVH. In the more usual cases with very increased pulmonary blood flow, biventricular hypertrophy is expected.

On echocardiogram the anatomy is seen well, with no demonstrable infundibulum present. At cardiac catheterization and angiography, the catheter usually can pass into the pulmonary arteries from the truncus arteriosus. Right-to-left and left-to-right shunts at the ventricular level are present, with systolic pressures equal in both ventricles.

Treatment and Prognosis. Affected children should be evaluated for hypocalcemia and T-cell deficiencies associated with DiGeorge syndrome. Children with persistent truncus arteriosus usually exhibit the condition early in life, within the first few weeks. The use of vigorous anticongestive measures in an attempt to get the children to grow are usually unsuccessful. A modified *Rastelli procedure* preferably is performed at diagnosis or before 2–3 months of age. The VSD is closed so that the LV passes unimpeded into the truncal valve. The pulmonary artery is removed from the back of the aorta, usually using a button of aortic tissue; the aortic opening is closed, and the RV is connected to the pulmonary arteries with a pulmonary or aortic homograft. Successful surgery necessitates a later reoperation because the children outgrow the conduit.

Total Anomalous Pulmonary Venous Connection

In children with a total anomalous pulmonary venous connection, there is a failure of incorporation of the common pulmonary vein into the posterior wall of the LA. During embryogenesis the pulmonary venous return is diverted into one of the early embryonic channels returning to the right side of the heart.

If the left cardinal system persists, pulmonary venous return is to the left superior vena cava, which may drain into the innominate vein or into the coronary sinus and then into the RA. If the right cardinal system persists, the pulmonary veins drain into the right superior vena cava, usually by way of a persistent ascending LV vein. Drainage directly into the RA is rare.

If the umbilical-vitelline system persists, the common pulmonary veins drain inferiorly through the diaphragm, usually into the portal system of the liver. Severe obstruction is present in the liver, and thus right atrial flow is diminished and pulmonary venous hypertension and congestion are severe. Also, severe pulmonary hypertension is present as a result of a very high PVR. When the drainage is above the diaphragm, pulmonary venous obstruction is less common, and PVR usually becomes low. Rarely, children exhibit this condition late and in a manner similar to infants who have an ASD; heart failure and cyanosis are milder than in those infants who exhibit the condition earlier.

Clinical Manifestations. Infants with obstructed pulmonary veins exhibit the condition in the newborn period with severe cyanosis and tachypnea in the first hours of life. Usually no murmurs are present, and the electrocardiogram shows marked RVH. On the chest x-ray film, the heart is small, and the amount of interstitial fluid is increased as a result of the marked pulmonary venous congestion, often quite similar in appearance to that of respiratory distress syndrome. For children with only mild or no obstruction who exhibit the condition after the newborn period, cyanosis is subtle but may increase with crying or other exertion. Heart failure may be quite severe, with a hyperactive right ventricular impulse and a widely split second heart sound that moves little with respiration. The ECG shows severe RVH; cardiac enlargement and increased pulmonary vascularity are apparent on the chest x-ray film. Rarely, infants in this group are asymptomatic, with the abnormality resembling a simple large ASD.

The echocardiogram is diagnostic and usually sufficient for the decision of surgical repair. Cardiac catheterization shows common mixing at the right atrial level, with approximately equal saturations in the RA, RV, and pulmonary artery, as well as in the LA, LV, and aorta. Cineangiocardiograms reveal the sites of drainage by injections either directly into the pulmonary artery or into the common pulmonary vein, entered by way of its anomalous connection. Catheterization is contraindicated in infants with obstructed venous return; the angiographic contrast exacerbates the pulmonary edema, increasing the respiratory distress.

Treatment and Prognosis. For the newborn with obstructed pulmonary veins, emergency surgery is necessary. For those who exhibit the condition later in infancy or childhood, elective surgery is recommended. The usual operation involves opening a wide connection between the common pulmonary vein and the back wall of the LA, after which the previously useful anomalous connection is ligated.

For the infant or older child with low PVR, the prognosis is excellent, with a low surgical risk (under 2%) and a low incidence of postoperative complications. For the newborn with obstructed total veins, surgery is more hazardous (5–15% mortality rate) because of difficult anatomic problems and serious cardiovascular decompensation before and after (persistent pulmonary hypertension) surgery. Rapid identification and diagnosis lead to a lower mortality rate because the surgery is not technically difficult.

Hypoplastic Left Heart Syndrome

Hypoplastic left heart syndrome (HLHS) includes a number of closely related anomalies that are part of hypoplasia and the underdevelopment of the LV. The mitral and aortic valves usually are hypoplastic, and one or both of them may be atretic. The ascending aorta usually is small, although coronary arteries are in the normal position. Discrete coarctation of the aorta is usually present. After birth, the pulmonary venous return from the LA passes across the atrial septum into the RA and then to the RV and the pulmonary artery. The systemic blood flow is via the ductus arteriosus to the ascending and descending aorta. Affected fetuses do well in utero, but after birth the infants become ill very quickly. After birth, the pulmonary venous return comes back to the LA and must go across the atrial septum. If the atrial defect is small, as is usually the case, pulmonary venous pressure increases and the signs and symptoms of left-sided heart failure appear. The entire systemic cardiac output must pass through the ductus arteriosus, so that when this vessel constricts, systemic cardiac output is reduced. Eventually acidosis, hypotension, and death occur.

Clinical Manifestations. The usual manifestations are a combination of heart failure, resulting from excessive pulmonary blood flow, and obstructed pulmonary venous return. Low cardiac output and acidosis occur after constriction of the ductus arteriosus. All peripheral pulses are weak or absent. Cyanosis usually is not prominent, but low cardiac output gives a grayish color to the cool, mottled skin. The cardiac impulse usually is hyperdynamic. Murmurs are not prominent but may be present as a result of increased flow across the tricuspid and pulmonic valves. Because children with HLHS or other left heart obstructive lesions (e.g., coarctation, interrupted aortic arch, or aortic stenosis) can be asymptomatic before the ductus arteriosus closes, the infant may be discharged from the nursery without the diagnosis being suspected. These children then exhibit profound cardiovascular collapse within the first weeks of life when the ductus arteriosus closes. PGE_1 should be considered in any infant who exhibits shock, particularly if the child has hepatomegaly or poor response to fluid resuscitation.

The ECG reveals severe RVH because of the systemic right ventricular pressure, torrential pulmonary blood flow, and hypoplastic LV. On the chest x-ray films, the heart usually is enlarged, and increased pulmonary vascularity and pulmonary venous congestion are seen. The echocardiogram is diagnostic. The right side of the heart is large. A cardiac catheterization is not necessary because it merely adds undue risk for the infant.

Treatment and Prognosis. Without surgery, early death is inevitable. A three-stage palliative approach is most common. The first stage, developed by Norwood, involves creating a large atrial opening by an atrial septectomy, dividing the pulmonary artery, connecting the proximal segment to the ascending aorta, reconstructing the aortic arch, and placing a Blalock-Taussig shunt to provide pulmonary blood flow. Thus the RV serves as the systemic ventricle, pumping blood through the pulmonary valve into the aorta, with pulmonary blood flow supplied via a systemic-to-pulmonary artery shunt. The second stage consists of a bidirectional cavopulmonary (Glenn) shunt at 2–6 months, followed by a Fontan operation at 2–4 years of age.

After the first stage, most major centers achieve an 80–90% survival rate. The second and third stages have low (5–10%) mortality, but the long-standing problems of a systemic right ventricle and the underlying difficulties of a Fontan palliation lead to an overall survival rate of approximately 50% to late childhood. Cardiac transplantation is an alternative approach. Major transplantation centers report a 15–30% mortality in neonates awaiting transplantation and a 75–85% 5-year survival rate for these children. Because of the magnitude of the long-term commitment and relatively poor outcome, some families choose to refuse any surgery.

High-Risk Newborn

Many congenital heart diseases are exhibited in the neonatal period, often causing great diagnostic confusion. Despite the large varieties of possible diagnoses, approximately 75% of infants affected by these diseases have one of seven lesions:

- Transposition of the great arteries
- Tetralogy of Fallot
- Tricuspid atresia
- Pulmonary atresia with intact ventricular septum
- Coarctation of the aorta with VSD
- Hypoplastic left heart syndrome
- Total anomalous pulmonary venous return with obstruction

By systematically assessing the predominant symptoms, the physician can usually make the physiologic diagnosis from the history, physical examination, chest x-ray examination, and ECG, generating a fairly small differential diagnosis. The important presenting symptoms (Table 13-8) are the following:

- *Cyanosis,* with or without respiratory distress
- *Hypoperfusion* with respiratory distress
- *Respiratory distress* without cyanosis or hypoperfusion

Treatment is summarized in Tables 13–9 and 13–10.

Prenatal Detection and Treatment of Congenital Cardiac Effects

Congenital heart defects can be diagnosed prenatally. Cardiac ultrasound scans usually are performed first by obstetricians. An abnormal four-chamber view of the heart prompts referral to the pediatric cardiac center. Primary pediatric cardiac fetal ultrasound examinations often are performed if the mother or father has had CHD or if the parents have had a previous child with a congenital heart defect. Other indications are maternal diabetes (associated with TGA and hypertrophic cardiomyopathy), certain drugs (e.g., lithium or phenytoin), major chromosomal anomalies (e.g., Down syndrome or other trisomies), and nonimmune hydrops (dysrhythmias, atrioventricular valve regurgitation, or cardiomyopathy).

Fetal echocardiography is accurate in diagnosis of the most severe types of congenital cardiac defects, such as valve atresia and severe stenosis. It cannot diagnose mild defects, such as PDA or ASD, that are normal in the fetus. It can usually diagnose VSDs or coarctation of the aorta. It has taught us that fetal CHD is more common than once thought, that fetal wastage is common, and that the defects progress throughout fetal life. Although the usual earliest time at which fetal echocardiography can be performed is now about 16 weeks, this time will decrease with improved techniques and technology.

Fetal ultrasonography is useful in the diagnosis of arrhythmias and in following the progression and response to treatment. Both tachyarrhythmias and bradyarrhythmias occur in the fetus and may lead to fetal congestive heart failure and death. Other arrhythmias, such as premature atrial contractions, are common and probably benign. Congenital complete AV block usually is well tolerated in the fetus. The ventricles are able to compensate for the slow rate by increasing their stroke volume. If associated CHD is present, however, **fetal hydrops** (congestive heart failure) may occur. This diagnosis is made by fetal scalp edema or ascites or by other fetal edema noted by echocardiography. Congenital complete AV block without associated heart defects often is associated with maternal lupus.

Fetal supraventricular tachycardias cause hydrops more frequently than do bradycardias. Hydrops can occur within 24 hours or less. Thus rapid, effective treatment is necessary. Initial treatment may be delivery if the fetus is mature. For less mature fetuses, drug treatment through the mother is used. Different antiarrhythmics pass through the placenta to the fetus with different fetal-maternal ratios. Digitalis has the advantages of a virtual 1:1 ratio, increasing contractility and slowing conduction in the AV node in the attempt to stop the tachycardia. The drug has the disadvantage of a relatively slow onset of action and a small therapeutic-toxic ratio in the fetus and mother. If digitalis fails, other drugs may be administered orally to the mother. If the fetus has hydrops, the drugs do not pass the placenta as well. The fetal umbilical vein may be cannulated and drugs given directly to the fetus. Amiodarone is particularly useful in this regard because it has a long half-life even when given intravenously. Frequent follow-up using fetal ultrasound helps control therapy.

The diagnosis of a severe congenital cardiac defect presents a bioethical dilemma. Most congenital cardiac defects now can at least be well palliated after birth, and for some lesions (such as HLHS) prenatal detection can lead to improved outcome by optimizing the perinatal management. This includes delivery at a cardiac center to prevent the complications of transport, prompt administration of PGE_1 before acidosis or severe cyanosis develops, and intensive respiratory support. The decision between fetal termination and delivery of the infant and treatment of the heart defect is a difficult and individual one.

REFERENCES

Behrman RE, Kliegman RM, Jenson HB, editors: *Nelson textbook of pediatrics*, ed 16, Philadelphia, 2000, WB Saunders, Chapters 384–387.

Brook MM, Silverman NH, Villegas M: Cardiac ultrasound in structural abnormalities and arrhythmias: recognition and treatment, *West J Med* 159(3):286–300, 1993.

Castaneda AR, Jonas RA, Mayer JE, et al: *Cardiac surgery of the neonate and infant*, Philadelphia, 1994, WB Saunders.

Grifka RG: Cyanotic congenital heart disease with decreased pulmonary blood flow in children, *Pediatr Clin North Am* 46(2): 405–425, 1999.

Morgan BC: Incidence, etiology, and classification of congenital heart disease, *Pediatr Clin North Am* 25(4):721–723, 1978.

O'Kelly SW, Bove EL: Hypoplastic left heart syndrome, *BMJ* 314(7074):87–88, 1997.

Pihkala J, Nykanen D, Freedom RM, et al: Interventional cardiac catheterization, *Pediatr Clin North Am* 46(2):441–464, 1999.

Radford DJ, Thong YH: The association between immunodeficiency and congenital heart disease, *Pediatr Cardiol* 9(2):103–108, 1988.

Reddy VM, Liddicoat JR, Brook MM, et al: Results of a protocol of routine primary repair of tetralogy of Fallot in neonates and infants under 3 months of age, *Ann Thorac Surg* 60(6 Suppl): S592–S596, 1995.

CARDIOMYOPATHIES

The primary cardiomyopathies are conditions involving the myocardium. Invariably the problem for the patient is left ventricular dysfunction; however, biopsy data indicate that the RV also is involved. Most of these cardiomyopathies are of the dilated type, often referred to as *congestive cardiomyopathy*. *Restrictive cardiomyopathies* are rare, as is the slightly more common *hypertrophic cardiomyopathy*.

Although many cases are considered idiopathic, specific etiologic factors are increasingly being discovered. Almost all the dilated cardiomyopathies can be categorized into three types (Table 13–14):
- Myocarditis
- A primary cardiomyopathy, often familial, caused by various abnormalities of mitochondrial energy metabolism
- Those induced by drugs, particularly doxorubicin

Myocarditis can occur at any age, including during the newborn period; it frequently is found to be related to a viral infection, such as echovirus or coxsackie B virus. The diagnosis is confirmed during the acute episode by a dilated large heart; severe heart failure, sometimes with shock; and marked ST segment abnormalities on the ECG. Before the era of intensive care units, children often died within 24 hours; if they survived when treated with digitalis and diuretics, they frequently recovered. Today many patients survive as a result of intensive care with intubation, mechanical ventilation, positive inotropes, and various afterload-reducing drugs (Table 13–6).

No specific *treatment* is available. Various antiinflammatory regimens, including steroids, intravenous gamma globulin, and specific autoimmune therapy (such as antithymocyte globulin), have met with mixed success. Antiviral therapy may have a role, with the use of pleconaril against enteroviruses. Most of these children also appear to recover completely, but some develop severe, chronic (dilated) cardiomyopathy. Some patients in whom congestive (dilated) cardiomyopathy gradually develops may have had asymptomatic viral myocarditis in the past, but others with this disorder have mitochondrial abnormalities and metabolic and familial disorders; fewer cases are being called idiopathic. After appropriate metabolic testing, carnitine therapy should be started empirically.

Another related concept is **endocardial fibroelastosis** (EFE); it is usually a secondary rather than a primary disorder. Occasionally it is associated with a small LV and small, very abnormal aortic and mitral valves. However, it is also a nonspecific response to some cardiomyopathies. In rare instances, primary endocardial fibroelastosis may be seen in certain families and in infants with an anomalous left coronary artery arising from the pulmonary artery.

TABLE 13–14
Etiology of Myocardial Disease

Familial-Hereditary
Duchenne muscular dystrophy
Other muscular dystrophies (Becker, limb girdle)
Myotonic dystrophy
Kearns-Sayre syndrome (progressive external
    ophthalmoplegia)
Friedreich ataxia
Hemochromatosis
Fabry disease
Pompe disease (glycogen storage)
Carnitine deficiency syndromes
Endocardial fibroelastosis
Mitochondrial myopathy syndromes
Familial restrictive cardiomyopathy
Familial hypertrophic cardiomyopathy
Familial dilated cardiomyopathy (dominant, recessive,
    X-linked)

Infections (Myocarditis)
Viral (e.g., coxsackievirus, mumps, Epstein-Barr virus,
    influenza, parainfluenza, measles, varicella, HIV)
Rickettsiae (e.g., psittacosis, *Coxiella*, Rocky Mountain
    spotted fever)
Bacterial (e.g., diphtheria, *Mycoplasma*, meningococcus,
    leptospirosis, Lyme disease)
Parasitic (e.g., Chagas disease, toxoplasmosis, *Loa loa*)

Metabolic, Nutritional, Endocrine
Beriberi (thiamine deficiency)
Keshan disease (selenium deficiency)
Hypothyroidism
Hyperthyroidism
Carcinoid
Pheochromocytoma

Metabolic, Nutritional, Endocrine—cont'd
Mitochondrial myopathies and oxidative respiratory
    chain defects
Type II, X-linked 3-methylglutaconic aciduria

Connective Tissue—Granulomatous Disease
SLE
Scleroderma
Churg-Strauss syndrome
Rheumatoid arthritis
Rheumatic fever
Sarcoidosis
Amyloidosis
Dermatomyositis

Drugs-Toxins
Doxorubicin (Adriamycin)
Ipecac
Iron overload (hemosiderosis)
Irradiation
Cocaine
Amphetamines

Coronary Arteries
Anomalous left coronary artery
Kawasaki disease

Other
Sickle cell anemia
Hypereosinophilic syndrome
Endomyocardial fibrosis
Asymmetric septal hypertrophy
Right ventricular dysplasia
Idiopathic

HIV, Human immunodeficiency virus; *SLE*, systemic lupus erythematosus.

Patients with acute myocarditis may die. However, if they survive the difficult early period, they have an excellent chance for complete recovery. In contrast, patients with cardiomyopathy not caused by myocarditis have a poorer prognosis and are not likely to recover. Although some children may stabilize, others rapidly deteriorate. A heart transplant is the only useful therapy after unsuccessful treatment with regimens to manage congestive heart failure.

REFERENCES

Behrman RE, Kliegman RM, Jenson HB, editors: *Nelson textbook of pediatrics*, ed 16, Philadelphia, 2000, WB Saunders, Chapters 392–396.
Burch M, Runciman M: Dilated cardiomyopathy, *Arch Dis Child* 74(6):479–481, 1996.
Guenthard J, Wyler F, Fowler B, et al: Cardiomyopathy in respiratory chain disorders, *Arch Dis Child* 72(3):223–226, 1995.
Towbin JA: Pediatric myocardial disease, *Pediatr Clin North Am* 46(2):289–312, 1999.

ACUTE RHEUMATIC FEVER

Rheumatic fever was quite common in the United States until the late 1960s and early 1970s, when a sharp decline in the incidence was reported; since the mid-1980s, multiple small outbreaks have been reported. Furthermore, acute rheumatic fever (ARF) remains very common in many developing nations.

TABLE 13-15
Major Criteria in the Jones System for Acute Rheumatic Fever*†

Sign	Comments
Polyarthritis	Common; swelling, limited motion, very tender, erythema
	Migratory; involves large joints but rarely small or unusual joints, such as vertebrae
Carditis	Common; pancarditis, valves, pericardium, myocardium
	Tachycardia greater than explained by fever; new murmur of mitral or aortic insufficiency; Carey-Coombs middiastolic murmur; heart failure
Chorea (Sydenham disease)	Uncommon; presents long after infection has resolved; more common in females; antineuronal antibody positive
Erythema marginatum	Uncommon; pink macules on trunk and proximal extremities, evolving to serpiginous border with central clearing; evanescent, elicited by application of local heat; nonpruritic
Subcutaneous nodules	Uncommon; associated with repeated episodes and severe carditis; present over extensor surface of elbows, knees, knuckles, and ankles or scalp and spine; firm, nontender

*Minor criteria include fever (101°–102° F [38.2°–38.9° C]), arthralgias, previous rheumatic fever, leukocytosis, elevated erythrocyte sedimentation rate/C-reactive protein, and prolonged PR interval.
†One major and two minor, or two major, criteria with evidence of recent group A streptococcal disease (e.g., scarlet fever, positive throat culture, or elevated antistreptolysin O or other antistreptococcal antibodies) strongly suggest the diagnosis of acute rheumatic fever.

The most commonly affected group is children between 5 and 15 years of age, but infants and adults also can be affected.

The *pathogenesis* is related to an immune reaction to untreated group A beta-hemolytic streptococcus infection. The serotype of the streptococcus and the genetically determined immune response of the host play a role in the development of ARF.

Clinical Manifestations. The wide variety of manifestations of the disease and the similarity to many other diseases may lead to difficulty in diagnosis. The Jones criteria are an attempt to improve diagnosis (Table 13–15). Typically, a child exhibits the disease 2–6 weeks after a pharyngitis with one or more of the major or minor manifestations of ARF, as described in these criteria. Arthritis may be difficult to establish. Chorea and erythema marginatum usually are easy to identify, but subcutaneous nodules are not likely to be present unless the disease is obvious and chronic. Evidence of carditis is very reliable in the hands of experienced physicians. Widening of the PR interval is a weak minor criterion because it is nonspecific; if it varies with time (e.g., hourly), it is helpful. Varying QRS voltage in the chest leads provides a strong minor criterion if the voltages are measured daily. The presence of a new murmur is strong evidence for carditis, although overdiagnosis is common because auscultation is not always specific.

For carditis of acute rheumatic fever to be diagnosed on the basis of heart murmur, the murmur must be one of the following:

- The murmur of mitral regurgitation, a murmur that may be as soft as grade 2, is high frequency, does not necessarily start with S_1, usually is almost full length, peaks late, and is best heard at the apex
- The murmur of aortic regurgitation, a high-frequency diastolic decrescendo murmur at the third to fifth left interspace of any intensity or length, with or without a wide pulse pressure
- A mid-diastolic rumbling murmur at the apex—the Carey-Coombs murmur, believed to result from edema of the mitral valve

Finally, the erythrocyte sedimentation rate (ESR) usually is elevated in ARF. Proof of streptococcal infection is critical to the diagnosis. The echocardiographic delineation of mild mitral regurgitation is not diagnostic.

Chronic rheumatic heart disease produces a specific type of lesion: mitral regurgitation, mitral stenosis, mitral stenosis with mitral regurgitation, aortic regurgitation, or aortic regurgitation with aortic stenosis. Rarely, the tricuspid valve is involved. The pulmonary valve is not known to be involved, and pure or dominant aortic stenosis does not occur.

In pure mitral regurgitation the middiastolic low-frequency murmur does not extend into late diastole. When pure mitral stenosis (and sinus rhythm) is present, the diastolic low-frequency murmur extends into late diastole, often with presystolic accentuation. If mitral regurgitation with stenosis is present, a long diastolic murmur extending into late diastole also is present. Aortic regurgitation may distort the anterior leaflet of the mitral valve as the blood leaks back into the LV, leading to the low-frequency middiastolic murmur called the *Austin Flint murmur.*

Treatment. Management consists almost entirely of nonspecific measures: bed rest, penicillin to eradicate the beta-hemolytic streptococcus, and aspirin for the arthritic pain. Steroids have not proved effective in minimizing valve damage, and they should not be used except for patients with severe, life-threatening carditis.

Once the diagnosis is made, whether or not valvulitis is present, permanent penicillin prophylaxis is essential. Intramuscular penicillin G benzathine (Bicillin) given every 28 days is more reliable than low-dose oral penicillin given twice a day. Patients following a continuous Bicillin regimen for 10 years usually improve; only 30% of patients with mitral regurgitation on initial evaluation still have a murmur, although fewer patients with aortic regurgitation lose the murmur. Mitral stenosis develops only in a few treated patients, although this condition is associated with poor compliance. The development of a stenotic valvular lesion probably is usually the result of repeated episodes of ARF. Prevention of such attacks with penicillin should eliminate this late sequela.

Treatment of valve disease involves balloon valvotomy, valve replacement, and vigilant antimicrobial prophylaxis to prevent bacterial endocarditis.

REFERENCES

American Heart Association, Special Writing Group of the Committee on Rheumatic Fever, Endocarditis, and Kawasaki Disease of the Council on Cardiovascular Disease in the Young: Guidelines for the diagnosis of rheumatic fever. Jones criteria, 1992 update, *JAMA* 268(15):2069–2073, 1992.

Behrman RE, Kliegman RM, Jenson HB, editors: *Nelson textbook of pediatrics,* ed 16, Philadelphia, 2000, WB Saunders, Chapter 392.

Markowitz M: Rheumatic fever in the eighties, *Pediatr Clin North Am* 33(5):1141–1150, 1986.

Veasy L, Wiedmeier S, Orsmond G, et al: Resurgence of acute rheumatic fever in the intermountain area of the United States, *N Engl J Med* 316(8):421–427, 1987.

PERICARDITIS

Pericardial diseases and inflammatory responses of the pericardium may be caused by common and uncommon disorders. Inflammatory processes such as viral or bacterial infections and immune-mediated disease (e.g., postinfectious immune complexes, connective tissue diseases, and the presence of autoantibody) are the most common pathogenic mechanisms in pediatric patients. Other causes are uremia, hypothyroidism, trauma, postpericardiotomy, and malignancy (Table 13–16).

The *clinical manifestations* of pericarditis as it progresses from a simple inflammatory response of the pericardium with no cardiovascular compromise to cardiac tamponade and constrictive pericarditis are noted in Table 13–17. *Laboratory diagnosis* is obtained by evaluation of the ECG and chest x-ray examination but is confirmed by echocardiography and eventually by examination of the pericardial fluid obtained by pericardiocentesis (Table 13–18).

Treatment is directed at the underlying disease process, alleviation of pericardial fluid accumulation by pericardiocentesis or pericardial drainage, or surgical stripping of the pericardium in patients with constrictive pericarditis.

REFERENCES

Behrman RE, Kliegman RM, Jenson HB, editors: *Nelson textbook of pediatrics,* ed 16, Philadelphia, 2000, WB Saunders, Chapter 397.

Brook I, Frazier E: Microbiology of acute purulent pericarditis, *Arch Intern Med* 156(16):1857–1860, 1996.

Sinzobahamvya N, Ikeogu MO: Purulent pericarditis, *Arch Dis Child* 62(7):696–699, 1987.

INFECTIVE ENDOCARDITIS

(See Chapter 10)

Bacterial endocarditis is infrequent in pediatric patients and occurs on native valves, valves damaged by rheumatic fever, congenitally abnormal valves, acquired valvular lesions (mitral valve prolapse), and prosthetic replacement valves. The condition is a potential consequence of jet streams of turbulent blood (from PDA, VSD, or systemic-to-pulmonary shunts). A listing of predisposing factors for the preceding bacteremia, laboratory tests, and *clinical manifestations* of bacterial endocarditis is presented in Table 13–19. Because of the endovascular nature of endocarditis, bacteremia is usually of a continuous nature, may be low grade (few bacteria per milliliter of blood), and is not necessarily altered during episodes of fever or chills. Therefore, the volume of the blood culture probably is more important than the frequency or timing of obtaining specimens for culture. The pathogens responsible for endocarditis depend on the status of the heart valve and the presence or absence of a predisposing procedure. Because some bacterial agents have unusual nutritional requirements and others may need longer than the usual incubation period to demonstrate growth in vitro, the blood samples should be labeled when endocarditis is suspected; the sample then can be ob-

TABLE 13–16
Etiology of Pericarditis and Pericardial Effusion

Idiopathic (Presumed Viral)
Infectious Agents
Bacteria
Group A streptococcus
Staphylococcus aureus
Pneumococcus, meningococcus*
Haemophilus influenzae*
Salmonella species
Mycoplasma pneumoniae
Borrelia burgdorferi
Mycobacterium tuberculosis
Rickettsia
Tularemia
Viral†
Coxsackievirus (group A, B)
Echovirus
Mumps
Influenza
Epstein-Barr
Cytomegalovirus
Herpes simplex
Herpes zoster
Hepatitis B
Fungal
Histoplasma capsulatum
Coccidioides immitis
Blastomyces dermatitidis
Cryptococcus neoformans
Candida species
Aspergillus species
Parasitic
Toxoplasma gondii
Entamoeba histolytica
Schistosomes

Collagen-Vascular–Inflammatory and Granulomatous
Diseases
Rheumatic fever
Systemic lupus erythematosus (idiopathic and drug-
   induced)
Rheumatoid arthritis
Kawasaki disease
Scleroderma
Mixed connective tissue disease
Reiter syndrome

Collagen-Vascular–Inflammatory and Granulomatous
Diseases—cont'd
Inflammatory bowel disease
Wegener granulomatosis
Dermatomyositis
Behçet syndrome
Sarcoidosis
Vasculitis
Familial Mediterranean fever
Serum sickness
Stevens-Johnson syndrome

Traumatic
Cardiac contusion (blunt trauma)
Penetrating trauma
Postpericardiotomy syndrome
Radiation

Contiguous Spread
Pleural disease
Pneumonia
Aortic aneurysm (dissecting)

Metabolic
Hypothyroidism
Uremia
Gaucher disease
Fabry disease
Chylopericardium

Neoplastic
Primary
Contiguous (lymphoma)
Metastatic
Infiltrative (leukemia)

Others
Drug reaction
Pancreatitis
After myocardial infarction
Thalassemia
Central venous catheter perforation
Heart failure
Hemorrhage (coagulopathy)
Biliary-pericardial fistula

From Sigman G: Chest pain. In Kliegman RM, Nieder ML, Super DM, editors: *Practical strategies in pediatric diagnosis and therapy*, Philadelphia, 1996, WB Saunders.
*Infectious or immune complex.
†Common (viral pericarditis or myopericarditis is probably the most common cause of acute pericarditis in a previously normal host).

TABLE 13–17
Manifestations of Pericarditis

Symptoms
Chest pain (worsened if lying down or with
inspiration)
Dyspnea
Malaise
Patient assumes sitting position

Signs
Nonconstrictive
Fever
Tachycardia
Friction rub (accentuated by inspiration, body position)
Enlarged heart by percussion and x-ray examination
Distant heart sounds
Tamponade
As above, plus:
Distended neck veins

Tamponade—cont'd
Hepatomegaly
Pulsus paradoxus (greater than 10 mm Hg with
inspiration)
Narrow pulse pressure
Weak pulse, poor peripheral perfusion
Constrictive Pericarditis
Distended neck veins
Kussmaul sign (inspiratory increase of jugular venous
pressure)
Distant heart sounds
Pericardial knock
Hepatomegaly
Ascites
Edema
Tachycardia

TABLE 13–18
Laboratory Evidence of Pericarditis

Test	Evidence Seen
ECG	Elevated ST segments, T-wave inversion (late), tachycardia, reduced QRS voltage, electrical alternans (variable QRS amplitudes)
Chest x-ray	Cardiomegaly ("water bottle heart")
Echocardiogram	Pericardial fluid
Pericardiocentesis	Gram and acid-fast stains, culture, PCR (virus, bacteria, mycobacteria, fungus), cytology, cell count, glucose, protein, pH
Blood tests	ESR, viral titers, ANA, ASO titers, EBV titers

ANA, Antinuclear antibodies; *ASO*, antistreptolysin O; *EBV*, Epstein-Barr virus; *ECG*, electroencephalogram; *ESR*, erythrocyte sedimentation rate.

TABLE 13–19
Manifestations of Infective Endocarditis

History	Signs—cont'd
Prior congenital or rheumatic heart disease	Embolic phenomena (Roth spots, petechiae, Osler nodes, and CNS lesion)
Preceding dental, urinary, or intestinal procedure	Janeway lesions
Intravenous drug abuse	New or changing murmur
Central venous catheter	Splenomegaly
Prosthetic heart valve	Arthritis
	Heart failure
Symptoms	Arrhythmias
Fever	
Chills	
Chest pain	**Laboratory Tests**
Arthralgia and myalgia	Positive blood culture
Dyspnea	Elevated ESR, C-reactive protein
Malaise	Leukocytosis
	Immune complexes
	Rheumatoid factor
Signs	Hematuria
Fever	Echocardiographic evidence of valve vegetations
Tachycardia	

CNS, Central nervous system; *ESR,* erythrocyte sedimentation rate.

served for a longer time. Despite adequate blood culture techniques, 10–15% of cases of endocarditis are culture negative.

Treatment of a culture-negative patient requires knowledge of the epidemiology and historical risk factors for that patient. Treatment of a culture-positive patient is directed against the particular bacteria (e.g., *Staphylococcus aureus,* viridans streptococcus, enterococcus, or HACEK group bacteria), using bactericidal antibiotics. Therapy is continued for 4–8 weeks. Surgery is indicated if medical treatment is unsuccessful or for an unusual pathogen, myocardial abscess formation, refractory heart failure, serious embolic complications, or refractory prosthetic valve disease.

Antibiotic prophylaxis to *prevent* endocarditis is becoming somewhat controversial. Although prophylaxis has not been proven to be of benefit, the practice has a pathophysiologic justification, carries a very low risk, and prevents a potentially life-threatening disease. Prophylaxis is recommended for all patients with most structural CHD, including unoperated, palliated or repaired defects; rheumatic valve lesions; prosthetic heart valves; mitral valve prolapse with a regurgitant valve; idiopathic hypertrophic subaortic stenosis; transvenous pacemaker leads; or previous endocarditis. Antimicrobial prophylaxis is not indicated for an isolated secundum ASD, a repaired secundum ASD or VSD 6 months after patch placement, or a divided and ligated PDA 6 months after repair. The antibiotic regimen to prevent endocarditis during dental or respiratory procedures is oral amoxicillin. Preventive treatment for gastrointestinal or genitourinary manipulation includes oral amoxicillin or parenteral ampicillin and gentamicin. The latter recommendation is for high-risk patients, such as those with prosthetic heart valves, systemic-to-pulmonary shunts, or previous endocarditis. Clindamycin is indicated for most patients allergic to penicillin.

REFERENCES

Behrman RE, Kliegman RM, Jenson HB, editors: *Nelson textbook of pediatrics,* ed 16, Philadelphia, 2000, WB Saunders, Chapter 390.
Brook MM: Pediatric bacterial endocarditis: treatment and prophylaxis, *Pediatr Clin North Am* 46(2):275–287, 1999.

DYSRHYTHMIAS

Cardiac dysrhythmias frequently occur in children. A dysrhythmia is an abnormal rhythm; the term *arrhythmia* often is used as a synonym. The diverse causes are presented in Table 13–20, and the common types and their treatment are presented in Table 13–21. Many pediatric dysrhythmias do not present a risk to the patient and are normal variants.

Some cardiac abnormalities are subtle, such as the prolonged QT interval, arrhythmogenic right ven-

TABLE 13–20
Etiology of Arrhythmias

Drugs
Intoxication (e.g., cocaine, tricyclic antidepressants, and others)
Antiarrhythmic agents (e.g., proarrhythmic agents, [quinidine])
Sympathomimetic agents (e.g., caffeine, theophylline, ephedrine, and others)
Digoxin

Infection and Postinfection
Endocarditis
Lyme disease
Diphtheria
Myocarditis
Guillain-Barré syndrome
Rheumatic fever

Metabolic-Endocrine
Cardiomyopathy
Electrolyte disturbances ($\downarrow\uparrow K^+$, $\downarrow\uparrow Ca^{2+}$, $\downarrow Mg^{2+}$)
Uremia

Metabolic-Endocrine—cont'd
Thyrotoxicosis
Pheochromocytoma
Porphyria
Mitochondrial myopathies

Structural Lesions
Mitral valve prolapse
Ventricular tumor
Ventriculotomy
Preexcitation and aberrant conduction system (Wolff-Parkinson-White syndrome)
Congenital heart defects
Arrhythmogenic right ventricle (dysplasia)

Other Causes
Adrenergic-induced
Prolonged QT interval
Maternal SLE
Idiopathic
Central venous catheter

SLE, Systemic lupus erythematosus.

TABLE 13–21
Arrhythmias in Children

Type	ECG Characteristics	Treatment
Complete heart block	Atria and ventricles have independent pacemakers; atrioventricular (AV) dissociation; escape-pacemaker is at atrioventricular junction if congenital	Awake rate <55 beats/min in neonate or <40 beats/min in adolescent or hemodynamic instability requires permanent pacemaker
First-degree heart block	Prolonged PR interval for age	Observe, obtain digoxin level if on therapy
Mobitz type I (Wenckebach) second-degree heart block	Progressive lengthening of PR interval until P wave is not followed by conducted QRS complex	Observe, correct underlying electrolyte or other abnormalities
Mobitz type II second-degree heart block	Sudden nonconduction of P wave with loss of QRS complex without progressive PR interval lengthening	Consider pacemaker
Sinus tachycardia	Rate less than 240 beats/min	Treat fever, remove sympathomimetic drugs

TABLE 13–21
Arrhythmias in Children—cont'd

Type	ECG Characteristics	Treatment
Supraventricular tachycardia	Rate usually greater than 200 beats/min (180–320); abnormal atrial rate for age; ventricular rate may be slower because of AV block; P waves usually present and are related to QRS complex; normal QRS complexes unless aberrant conduction is present	Increase vagal tone (bag of ice water to face, Valsalva maneuver); adenosine; digoxin; sotalol; electrical cardioversion if acutely ill; catheter ablation
Atrial flutter	Atrial rate usually 300 beats/min, with varying degrees of block; sawtooth flutter waves	Digoxin, sotalol, cardioversion
Premature ventricular contraction (PVC)	Premature, wide, unusually shaped QRS complex, with large inverted T wave	None if normal heart and if PVCs disappear on exercise; lidocaine, procainamide
Ventricular tachycardia	Three or more premature ventricular beats; AV dissociation; fusion beats, blocked retrograde AV conduction; sustained if longer than 30 sec; rate 120–240 beats/min	Lidocaine, procainamide, propranolol, amiodarone, cardioversion
Ventricular fibrillation	No distinct QRS complex or T waves; irregular undulations with varied amplitude and contour; no conducted pulse	Nonsynchronized cardioversion

TABLE 13–22
Classification of Drugs for Antiarrhythmia

Class	Action	Examples
I	Depresses phase O depolarization (velocity of upstroke of action potential); sodium channel blockers	
Ia	Prolongs QRS complex and QT interval	Quinidine, procainamide, disopyramide
Ib	Significant effect on abnormal conduction	Lidocaine, mexiletine, phenytoin, tocainide
Ic	Prolongs QRS complex and PR interval	Flecainide, propafenone, moricizine?
II	Beta-blockade, slows sinus rate, prolonged PR interval	Propranolol, atenolol, acebutolol
III	Prolonged action potential; prolonged PR, QT intervals, QRS complex; sodium and calcium channel blocker	Bretylium, amiodarone, sotalol
IV	Calcium channel blockade; reduced sinus and AV node pacemaker activity and conduction; prolonged PR interval	Verapamil and other calcium channel blocking agents

tricular dysplasia, and mild cardiomyopathy or myocarditis. Ventricular dysrhythmias that necessitate treatment usually are treated with antiarrhythmic drugs (Table 13–22). A specific, treatable etiology rarely is found. Infants and young children (≤4 years) are the exception; they may have small tumors that can be treated with surgery.

Sinus Arrhythmia and Wandering Atrial Pacemaker

Sinus arrhythmia and wandering atrial pacemaker are phasic variations with respiration that are heard in virtually all normal children. These variations are accentuated in athletic children and diminished during most illnesses. Sinus arrhythmia is differentiated from wandering atrial pacemaker by the continuous normal morphology of the P wave preceding each QRS complex in the former, compared with the continuously changing P wave morphology in the latter (Fig. 13–5). These two arrhythmias are thought to be controlled by an interaction of the vagal and sympathetic divisions of the autonomic nervous system.

Premature Beats

Premature atrial contractions (PACs) are common in fetuses, neonates, and infants, and are less common in children. They often are of little concern. If they are extremely frequent or early in the cardiac cycle, they may predispose the neonate to atrial flutter. PACs often decrease in frequency quite rapidly after birth; thus a short period of observation and parental counseling about the presentation and significance of atrial flutter in a neonate may be all that is necessary. If a PAC occurs after each sinus beat and if it fails to conduct to the ventricle (a blocked PAC), a relative bradycardia develops. Thus the ST segment and T wave should be searched for blocked PACs in bradycardic neonates. If the PACs do not stop or decrease, treatment with digoxin may suppress them. In any case, it does not worsen the bradycardia.

Premature ventricular contractions (PVCs) are more common in adolescents and are found infrequently in neonates or infants. Benign PVCs are single (i.e., not two or three consecutively) and uniform. They disappear with exercise and occur in patients with normal hearts. Any deviations necessitate extensive evaluation. Bigeminal patterns and frequent PVCs are not considered deviations from benignness, nor is the R-on-T phenomenon. Benign PVCs of childhood do not cause serious dysrhythmias but are present at 5-year follow-up in 50% of patients. Multiform PVCs, triplets or longer runs, and any types of cardiac abnormality are associated with more sustained dysrhythmias and with symptoms, syncope, and death.

Supraventricular Tachycardia

Supraventricular tachycardia (SVT) is the most frequent sustained dysrhythmia in pediatrics. Although SVT is not immediately life threatening, it can lead to serious symptoms if it persists. It most commonly occurs in neonates and infants but also is common in fetuses and older children. The mechanism is usually reentry, although enhanced automaticity accounts for 5–10% of cases. Reentry most often involves an accessory connection (e.g., bundle of Kent) but may occur in the AV node, sinus node, or atrial muscle (i.e., atrial flutter).

Pediatric SVT is characterized by a rate of greater than 210 beats/min, a normal narrow QRS complex, and extreme regularity. If the QRS complex is even slightly wide or abnormal in morphology, the diagnosis is likely ventricular tachycardia. The relationship between the atrium and the ventricle is usually 1:1, but the atrium can be either faster (atrial flutter) or slower (junctional automaticity).

The initial *treatment* of pediatric SVT involves enhancing vagal tone by the diving reflex (Table 13–21). This involves applying a cold (ice water bag) stimulus to the entire face. If this fails to convert, intravenous adenosine usually is effective at a dose of 100–250 µg/kg. In patients in whom the AV node or sinus node is not part of the reentry circuit, adenosine may only temporarily (for 5–10 seconds) slow the rate by creating AV block. Atrial overdrive pacing (intraatrial or transesophageal) often is effective in atrial reentry tachycardia. Pacing also can be used to create temporary AV block and stabilize the blood pressure. Direct-current synchronized cardioversion at 0.25–1 Watt sec/kg is the gold standard for converting resistant reentrant tachycardias.

Once SVT is converted in a child, there is an approximately 90% chance it will recur; therefore, prophylactic pharmacologic therapy is warranted for 6–12 months. In patients with manifest **Wolff-Parkinson-White syndrome,** digitalis often is not used for fear of precipitating a worse dysrhythmia; otherwise, it is the drug of choice. Propranolol and verapamil also may be used orally in older children.

In older children, cases of SVT that are resistant to medical therapy or have life-threatening components (Wolff-Parkinson-White syndrome), or cases in which the patient does not want to take medication, the dysrhythmogenic substrate frequently (90%) can be ablated by catheter ablation.

Bradydysrhythmias

Bradydysrhythmias may be congenital, surgically acquired, or (rarely) caused by infection (Table 13–20). The surgically acquired type is by far the most common. Despite improving knowledge of the location of the heart's electrical system in various heart defects and improving surgical results, both acute and chronic abnormalities of the conduction system and the sinus node occur. Modern pacemakers and leads have greatly improved treatment of these problems.

Congenital complete AV block is often the result of maternal systemic lupus erythematosus, with antibodies to the fetal cardiac conduction system crossing the placenta. Association with morphologic cardiac defects is the other common etiologic factor.

REFERENCES

Behrman RE, Kliegman RM, Jenson HB, editors: *Nelson textbook of pediatrics,* ed 16, Philadelphia, 2000, WB Saunders, Chapters 388–389.

Case CL: Diagnosis and treatment of pediatric arrhythmias, *Pediatr Clin North Am* 46(2):347–354, 1999.

Committee on Sports Medicine and Fitness: Cardiac dysrhythmias and sports, *Pediatrics* 95(5):786–788, 1995.

Dick M, Scott WA, Serwer GS, et al: Acute termination of supraventricular tachyarrhythmias in children by transesophageal atrial pacing, *Am J Cardiol* 61(11):925–927, 1988.

Kugler J, Danford D: Management of infants, children, and adolescents with paroxysmal supraventricular tachycardia, *J Pediatr* 129(3):324–338, 1996.

SUDDEN DEATH

Sudden death is a rare but important problem in pediatrics. Most pediatric sudden deaths occur in patients with known heart disease. Unoperated CHD used to be a prime cause. Because most congenital heart defects now are repaired or palliated early in life, postoperative dysrhythmias are assuming increasing importance. Also, more precise repairs with improved myocardial protection and postoperative screening for dysrhythmias, together with pacemakers and medical treatment, have improved the outlook for postoperative patients.

Infrequently a child without known heart disease dies suddenly because of anomalous coronary arteries, aortic stenosis, arrhythmias, myocarditis, or cardiomyopathy (usually hypertrophic). This often occurs in relation to athletics. Many of these deaths probably could be prevented by including a screening ECG with a proper preparticipation history (e.g., syncope, dizziness, chest pain, and external dyspnea) and physical examination, although this would be expensive. Attention to the symptoms of exercise-related symptoms could prevent many other deaths. Drug use (e.g., cocaine, alcohol, tricyclic antidepressants, or heroin) must also be considered. Immediate defibrillation at the site of arrest is critical to a successful resuscitation.

CHEST PAIN IN CHILDHOOD AND ADOLESCENCE

Chest pain among pediatric patients usually does not represent serious cardiovascular disease, as it does in adult patients. Many patients are preadolescents or adolescents who have pain at rest of noncardiac origin (Table 13–23). A careful history (including family history), physical examination, and screening laboratory tests are indicated to reassure the patient and family. These tests should be based on the history and physical findings and should be directed to musculoskeletal, pulmonary, gastrointestinal, or cardiac signs and symptoms. Chest pain suggestive of cardiac pain that is associated with syncope, exertional dyspnea, or an irregular pulse necessitates more detailed evaluation, such as 24-hour continuous ECG monitoring (Holter monitor).

Chest pain is a frequent symptom in children, as it is in adults. The most frequent cause of **cardiac chest pain** is pericarditis. It usually is associated with a febrile illness, and the young age of a patient may result in the chest pain being expressed nonspecifically. Exercise-induced chest pain may indicate exercise-induced asthma, but it also (rarely) may indicate cardiac disease, including coronary artery anomalies. The chest wall is a common source of chest pain in children. The diagnosis of **costochondritis** may be confirmed by a finding of tenderness of one or more costochondral joints. Esophagogastritis is another frequent cause of chest pain in children. The "pleuritic catch" may be the most frequent benign cause of chest pain in children; it is brief but may recur for years. The popularization of this important symptom in the mass media in an attempt to help recognize coronary artery disease also may confuse children and their parents. Children with chest pain may be mimicking their parents or grandparents.

Cardiac Pain in Infancy

Cardiac pain may be the result of an **anomalous origin of the left coronary artery** from the pulmonary artery.

The *clinical manifestations* are marked irritability, pallor, diaphoresis, apnea, or shock during or after nursing. These paroxysmal episodes of discomfort are similar to attacks of angina pectoris in adults. Heart failure may develop as a result of poor myocardial performance. Usually no murmur is heard unless mitral regurgitation is present as a result of papillary muscle ischemia. If there are large collateral vessels (a left-to-right shunt through the coronary artery to the pulmonary arteries), a continuous murmur may be present, but children with this condition usually are not ill. Thus the *diagnosis* often is made after infancy.

Laboratory evidence reveals ECG signs of myocardial ischemia or infarction. Cardiomegaly is present on chest x-ray examination, and the echocardiogram and angiography reveal the anomalous coronary artery. The *differential diagnosis* includes SVT, myocarditis, and cardiomyopathy.

Treatment of the acute condition involves administration of oxygen, intravenous inotropic agents, and morphine. Transplantation of a cuff of the pulmonary artery with the coronary ostium to the subclavian artery or aorta is the procedure of choice. The *prognosis* is mixed. Many patients can have near-

TABLE 13–23
Differential Diagnosis of Pediatric Chest Pain

Musculoskeletal (Common)	Gastrointestinal (Rare)—cont'd
Trauma (accidental or by abuse)	Cholecystitis
Exercise, overuse injury (e.g., strain or bursitis)	Subdiaphragmatic abscess
Tietze syndrome	Perihepatitis (Fitz-Hugh–Curtis syndrome)
Costochondritis	Peptic ulcer disease
Herpes zoster (cutaneous)	Pancreatitis
Pleurodynia	
Sickle cell anemia vasoocclusive crisis	**Cardiac (Rare)**
Osteomyelitis (rare)	Pericarditis (Table 13–16)
Primary or metastatic tumor (rare)	Postpericardiotomy syndrome
Fibrositis	Endocarditis
Slipping rib	Mitral valve prolapse (uncertain cause)
	Aortic stenosis (angina)
Pulmonary (Common)	Arrhythmias
Pneumonia	Hypertrophic cardiomyopathy
Pleurisy	Marfan syndrome (dissecting aortic aneurysm)
Asthma	Anomalous coronary artery (angina)
Chronic cough	Kawasaki disease (angina)
Pneumothorax, pneumomediastinum	Cocaine, sympathomimetic ingestion (angina)
Infarction (sickle cell anemia)	Familial hypercholesterolemia (angina)
Foreign body	
Embolism (rare)	**Idiopathic (Common)**
Pulmonary hypertension (rare)	Anxiety, hyperventilation
Tumor (rare)	Panic disorder
Gastrointestinal (Rare)	**Other (Rare)**
Esophagitis (gastroesophageal reflux)	Spinal cord or nerve root compression
Esophageal foreign body	Breast-related pathology
Esophageal spasm	Castleman disease (lymph node neoplasm)
Esophageal rupture	

From Sigman G: Chest pain. In Kliegman RM, editor: *Practical strategies in pediatric diagnosis and therapy,* Philadelphia, 1996, WB Saunders.

complete recovery of ventricular function, but some develop a chronic ischemic cardiomyopathy. Therefore, prompt diagnosis and treatment are critical.

SYNCOPE

Syncope is an increasingly important symptom in cardiologic and neurologic evaluation. It has been estimated that two thirds of children will have syncope. Most important, it can be a precursor to sudden death. In this instance, associated diagnosable heart disease is usually present. The second type of important syncope is *vasodepressor (neurocardiogenic) syncope,* which, although it does not lead to death, is quite frequent. Many other causes of syncope exist

(e.g., dehydration, viral illness), and the presence of heart disease and exercise induction of the syncope are helpful to distinguish the rare patient who needs treatment from the common patient with benign transient syncope (Table 13–24).

When the heart ceases effective function, either syncope or seizures may develop. Thus some pediatric patients with seizures also should be evaluated for syncope. Several cardiologic diseases, including the *long QT syndrome* and *hypertrophic cardiomyopathy,* frequently cause syncope. The evaluation of syncope should involve a detailed history, including family history. Physical examination may reveal signs of heart disease. ECG and echocardiography are useful in diagnosing electrical and structural heart disease.

TABLE 13–24
Syncope and Dizziness: Etiology

Diagnosis	History	Symptoms	Description	Heart Rate/ Blood Pressure	Duration	Postsyncope	Recurrence
Neurocardiogenic (Vasodepressor)	At rest	Pallor, nausea, visual changes	Brief ± convulsion	↓/↓	<1 min	Residual pallor, sweaty, hot; recurs if child stands	Common
Other Vagal							
Vasovagal	Needle stick	Pallor, nausea	Brief ± convulsion	↓/↓	<1 min	Residual pallor; may recur if child stands	Situational
Micturition	Postvoiding	Pallor, nausea	Brief; convulsions rare	↓/↓	<1 min	Fatigue or baseline	(+)
Cough (deglutition)	Paroxysmal cough	Cough	Abrupt onset	May not change	<5 min	Fatigue or baseline	(+)
Carotid sinus	Tight collar, turned head	Vague, visual changes	Sudden onset, pallor	Usually ↓/↓	<5 min	Fatigue or baseline	(+)
Metabolic							
Hypoglycemia	Fasting, insulin use	Gradual hunger	Pallor, sweating, loss of consciousness rare	No change or mild tachycardia	Variable	Relieved by eating only	(+)
Neuropsychiatric							
Hyperventilation	Anxiety	SOB, fear, claustrophobia	Agitated, hyperpneic ± Pallor	Mild ↓/↓	<5 min	Fatigue or baseline	(+)
Syncopal migraine	Headache	Aura, migraine, nausea	No change	No change	<10 min	Headache, often occipital	(+)

From Lewis DA: Syncope and dizziness. In Kliegman RM, editor: *Practical strategies in pediatric diagnosis and therapy*, Philadelphia, 1996, WB Saunders.
LVOT, Left ventricular outflow obstruction; *SOB*, shortness of breath; ±, with or without.

Continued

TABLE 13–24
Syncope and Dizziness: Etiology—cont'd

Diagnosis	History	Symptoms	Description	Heart Rate/ Blood Pressure	Duration	Postsyncope	Recurrence
Seizure disorder	Anytime	± Aura	Convulsion ± incontinence	No change or mild tachycardia	Any duration	Postictal lethargy + confusion	(+)
Hysterical	Always an "audience" present	Psychologic distress	Gentle, graceful swoon	No change	Any duration	Normal baseline	(+)
Breath-holding (hypoxic)	Agitation or injury	Crying	Cyanosis ± brief convulsion	↓/↓ Frequent asystole	<10 min	Fatigue, residual pallor	(+)
Cardiac Syncope							
LVOT obstruction	Exercise	± Chest pain, SOB	Abrupt during or after exertion, pallor	↑/↓	Any duration	Fatigue, residual pallor, and sweating	(+)
Pulmonary hypertension	Anytime, especially exercise	SOB	Cyanosis and pallor	↑/↓	Any duration	Fatigue, residual cyanosis	(+)
Myocarditis	Postviral exercise	SOB, chest pain, palpitations	Pallor	↑/↓	Any duration	Fatigue	(+)
Tumor or mass	Recumbent, paroxysmal	SOB ± chest pain	Pallor	↑/↓	Any duration	Baseline	(+)
Coronary artery disease	Exercise	SOB ± chest pain	Pallor	↑/↓	Any duration	Fatigue, chest pain	(+)
Dysrhythmia	Anytime	Palpitations ± chest pain	Pallor	↑ or ↑/↓	Usually <10 min	Fatigue or baseline	(+)

From Lewis DA: Syncope and dizziness. In Kliegman RM, editor: *Practical strategies in pediatric diagnosis and therapy,* Philadelphia, 1996, WB Saunders.
LVOT, Left ventricular outflow obstruction; *SOB,* shortness of breath; ±, with or without.

In the patient having recurrent syncope with a normal heart, testing of the response of the autonomic nervous system to assuming the upright posture is useful. If a cardiac cause of syncope is found, it should be treated directly. If vasodepressor syncope is diagnosed by autonomic testing, it may be treated by salt and fludrocortisone or beta-blockers. Treatment of vasodepressor syncope usually is temporary. The rare form of autonomic syncope, *cardioinhibitory syncope,* may necessitate a combination of pacemaker and medical treatment.

REFERENCES

Berger S, Dhala A, Friedberg DZ: Sudden cardiac death in infants, children, and adolescents, *Pediatr Clin North Am* 46(2):221–234, 1999.

Erickson CC, Jones CS: Pediatric sudden cardiac death: what the pediatrician needs to know, *Pediatr Ann* 29(8):509–518, 2000.

Johnsrude CL: Current approach to pediatric syncope, *Pediatr Cardiol* 21(6):522–531, 2000.

Kocis KC: Chest pain in pediatrics, *Pediatr Clin North Am* 46(2):189–203, 1999.

CHAPTER 14

Hematology

J. Paul Scott

Hematologic disorders are caused by quantitative or qualitative abnormalities of the formed elements of the blood, of the circulating proteins, or of the vascular wall. Diseases of the blood are either congenital or acquired. Hereditary abnormalities in molecular structure may lead to decreased stem cell production (Fanconi anemia), abnormal cell membrane function (hereditary spherocytosis or Glanzmann thrombasthenia), deficiency of an essential enzyme (glucose-6-phosphate dehydrogenase [G6PD] deficiency, chronic granulomatous disease), or dysfunction of a cytosolic (sickle cell anemia) or plasma (hemophilia) protein. Advances in molecular biology and genetic therapy allow us to envision the correction of many of these fundamental defects in the next generation. Secondary causes of hematologic disease include infiltration of normal structures (e.g., leukemia or neuroblastoma), nutritional deficiency (e.g., iron, folate, and vitamins K, E, and B_{12}), autoimmune disease (immune thrombocytopenic purpura), exogenous drugs (e.g., antimetabolites, penicillin, or antiinflammatory agents), and altered vascular matrix (thrombosis with vasculitis).

Hematologic disorders have characteristic clinical presentations related to the specific affected blood component or factor (Table 14–1). These manifestations are not diagnostic of the cause of the disorder, but certain characteristic signs and symptoms point to a likely diagnosis. These signs and symptoms include spoon-shaped nails or pica with iron deficiency, deteriorating neurologic findings with anemia in vitamin B_{12} deficiency, vasoocclusive crises in sickle cell anemia, and progressive pancytopenia in association with congenital abnormalities in Fanconi anemia.

DEVELOPMENTAL HEMATOPOIESIS

Hematopoiesis begins by the third week of gestation with erythropoiesis in the yolk sac. By 2 months' gestation, the primary site of hematopoiesis has migrated to the liver; red blood cells (RBCs), platelets, and leukocytes are synthesized at this site. By 5–6 months' gestation, the process of hematopoiesis shifts from the liver to the bone marrow. Therefore, an extremely premature infant may have significant **extramedullary hematopoiesis** with limited bone marrow hematopoiesis. During infancy, virtually all marrow cavities are actively hematopoietic, and the proportion of hematopoietic to stromal elements is quite high. As the child grows, hematopoiesis moves to the central bones of the body (the vertebrae, sternum, ribs, and pelvis), and the marrow of the extremities and the skull is replaced with fat. This replacement of marrow with fat is a gradual and partially reversible process. Hemolysis or marrow damage may lead to marrow repopulation of cavities where hematopoiesis had previously ceased or may cause a delay in the shift of hematopoiesis. Children with thalassemia and other chronic hemolytic diseases may have large head circumferences and prominent skull bones as a result of increased erythropoiesis within the medullary cavities of the skull. Furthermore, hepatosplenomegaly in patients with chronic hemolysis may signify extramedullary hematopoiesis. Because of the extensive use of all bone marrow cavities, very young children do not have the marrow reserves of older children and adults. When a patient with cytopenia is being evaluated, a bone marrow examination provides valuable information about processes that lead to underproduction of circulating cells. Additionally, bone marrow infiltration by neoplastic elements or storage cells often occurs in concert with similar infiltration in the spleen, liver, and lymph nodes.

The hematopoietic cells consist of (1) a small compartment of pluripotential progenitor stem cells that morphologically resemble small lymphocytes and are capable of forming all myeloid elements; (2) a

TABLE 14–1
Presentation of Hematologic Disorders

Condition	Symptoms and Signs	Common Examples
Anemia	Pallor, fatigue, heart failure, jaundice	Iron deficiency, hemolytic anemia
Polycythemia	Irritability, cyanosis, seizures, jaundice, stroke, headache	Cyanotic heart disease, infant of diabetic mother
Neutropenia	Fever, pharyngitis, oral ulceration, cellulitis, lymphadenopathy, bacteremia	Congenital or drug-induced agranulocytosis, leukemia
Thrombocytopenia	Petechiae, ecchymosis, gastrointestinal hemorrhage, epistaxis	ITP, leukemia
Coagulopathy	Bruising, hemarthrosis, mucosal bleeding	Von Willebrand disease, hemophilia, DIC
Thrombosis	Pulmonary embolism, deep venous thrombosis	Lupus anticoagulant; protein C, protein S, or antithrombin III deficiency, factor V Leiden, prothrombin 20210

DIC, Disseminated intravascular coagulation; *ITP,* thrombocytopenic purpura.

large compartment of committed, proliferating cells of myeloid, erythroid, and megakaryocytic lineage; and (3) a large compartment of postmitotic maturing cells (Fig. 14–1). Hematopoiesis is controlled by a large number of cytokines (Fig. 14–1). In the following paragraph only those shown to be of major clinical importance are noted. The bone marrow is the major storage organ for mature neutrophils and contains about seven times the intravascular pool of neutrophils; it contains 2.5–5 times as many cells of myeloid lineage as those of erythroid lineage. In addition, smaller numbers of megakaryocytes and plasma cells, histiocytes, lymphocytes, and stromal cells are stored in the marrow.

Erythropoiesis (RBC production) is controlled by erythropoietin, a hormone made by the juxtaglomerular apparatus of the kidney in response to local tissue hypoxia (Fig. 14–1). Control of erythropoiesis by erythropoietin begins at the time of hepatic hematopoiesis in early gestation. The normally high hemoglobin level of the fetus is a result of fetal erythropoietin production in the liver in response to low PO_2 in utero. Erythropoietin is a glycoprotein that stimulates the primitive pluripotent stem cell to differentiate along the erythroid line, leading to production of what is recognized in vitro as the erythroid colony-forming unit (CFU-E). The earliest recognizable erythroid cell in vivo is the erythroblast, which forms eight or more daughter cells. During maturation, the immature red cell nucleus becomes gradually pyknotic as the cell matures and eventually is extruded before the cell is released from the marrow as a reticulocyte. The reticulocyte maintains residual mitochondrial and protein synthetic capac-

ity. These highly specialized red cell precursors are engaged primarily in the production of globin chains, glycolytic enzymes, and heme. Iron is taken up via transferrin receptors and incorporated into the heme ring, which then combines with globin chains synthesized within the immature RBC. Once the messenger ribonucleic acid (mRNA) and mitochondria are gone from the red cell, it is no longer capable of heme or protein synthesis; however, it continues to function for its normal life span of about 120 days in older children and adults.

During embryonic and fetal life, the globin genes are sequentially activated and inactivated. The control mechanism of globin chain switching remains incompletely understood. Embryonic hemoglobins are produced during yolk sac erythropoiesis and then are replaced by fetal hemoglobin (hemoglobin F-$\alpha_2\gamma_2$) during the hepatic phase. During the third trimester, γ-chain production gradually diminishes and is replaced by β chains, resulting in hemoglobin A ($\alpha_2\beta_2$). Some fetal factors (e.g., being an infant of a diabetic mother) delay onset of β-chain production, but premature birth does not affect its timing. Just after birth, with the expansion of the lungs and establishment of normal neonatal cardiorespiratory function, the oxygen saturation rapidly rises from 65% in utero to nearly 100%. Erythropoietin production ceases and shuts down erythropoiesis. In addition, fetal RBCs have a short survival time compared with that of RBCs of older children (60 versus 120 days). Fetal red cells have less deformable membranes and have enzymatic differences from the cells of older children. Senescent red cells are destroyed in the liver and spleen, where they are recognized as

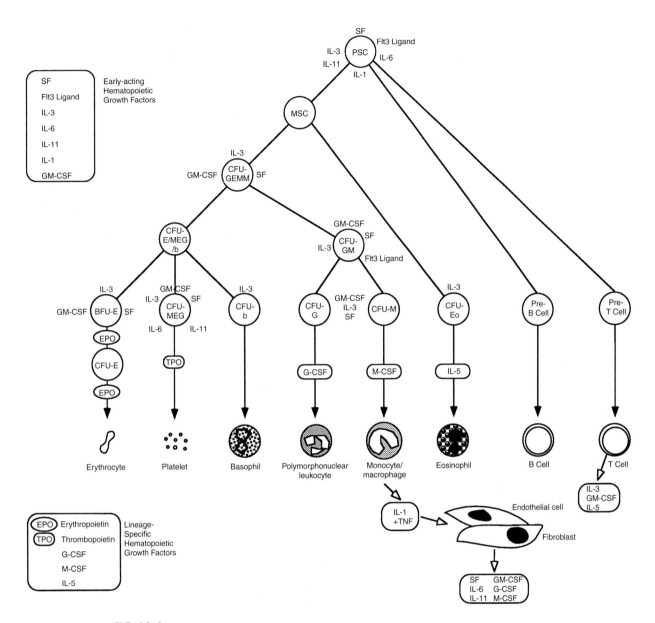

FIG. 14–1

Major cytokine sources and actions to promote hematopoiesis. Cells of the bone marrow microenvironment, such as macrophages (ma), endothelial cells (ec), and reticular fibroblasts (fb) produce macrophage colony–stimulating factor (M-CSF), granulocyte-macrophage colony–stimulating factor (GM-CSF), granulocyte colony–stimulating factor (G-CSF), interleukin-6 (IL-6), and probably steel factor (SF). T cells produce IL-3, IL-5, and GM-CSF after stimulation. These cytokines and others as listed in the text have overlapping interactions during hematopoietic differentiation, as indicated; for all lineages, optimal development requires a combination of early- and late-acting factors. *BFU,* Burst-forming unit; *CFU,* colony-forming unit; *EPO,* erythropoietin; *MSC,* myeloid stem cells; *PSC,* pluripotent stem cells; *TNF,* tumor necrosis factor; *TPO,* thrombopoietin. (From Sieff CA, Nathan DG, Clark SC: The anatomy and physiology of hematopoiesis. In Orkin SH, Nathan DG, editors: *Hematology of infancy and childhood,* ed 5, Philadelphia, 1998, WB Saunders.)

abnormal by changes in their membrane sialic acid content and by the metabolic depletion that occurs as they age. During the first few months of postnatal life, rapid growth, shortened RBC survival, and shutting down of erythropoiesis cause a gradual decline in hemoglobin levels, with a nadir at 6–8 weeks of life. This so-called physiologic nadir is accentuated in premature infants. In response to the fall in Hg and decreased oxygen delivery, erythropoietin is produced; erythropoiesis subsequently resumes, with a rise in the reticulocyte count. The hemoglobin level gradually rises, accompanied by the synthesis of increasing amounts of hemoglobin A. By 6 months of age in healthy infants, only trace γ-chain synthesis occurs.

Production of neutrophil precursors is controlled predominantly by two different colony-stimulating factors (Fig. 14–1). The most immature neutrophil precursors are controlled by granulocyte-monocyte–colony–stimulating factor (GM-CSF), which is produced by monocytes and lymphocytes. GM-CSF increases the entry of primitive precursor cells into the myeloid line of differentiation. Granulocyte colony–stimulating factor (G-CSF) augments the production of more mature granulocyte precursors. Both, working in concert, can augment production of neutrophils, shorten the usual baseline 10–14-day production time from stem cell to mature neutrophil, and stimulate functional activity. The rapid increase in neutrophil count that occurs with infection is caused by release of stored neutrophils from the bone marrow; this is also under the control of GM-CSF. During maturation, a mitotic pool of neutrophil precursors exists: myeloblasts, promyelocytes, and myelocytes possessing primary granules. The postmitotic pool consists of metamyelocytes, bands, and mature polymorphonuclear leukocytes containing secondary or specific granules that define the cell type. Only bands and mature neutrophils are fully functional with regard to phagocytosis, chemotaxis, and bacterial killing. Eosinophil production is under the control of a related glycoprotein hormone, interleukin-3 (IL-3).

Neutrophils migrate from the bone marrow, circulate for 6–7 hours, and then enter the tissues, where they become end-stage cells that do not recirculate (Fig. 14–2). The ability to adhere to endothelium is controlled by the interaction of adhesive molecules/receptors on the endothelial and leukocyte membrane modulated by cytokines. Neutrophils respond to chemotactic stimuli, especially C5a, and then migrate toward inflammatory stimuli, where they ingest and kill invading microorganisms. Monocytes migrate into tissues, where they become macrophages and may live from months to years. Eosinophils, which play a role in host defense against parasites, also are capable of living in tissues for prolonged periods.

Megakaryocytes are giant, multinucleated cells that derive from the primitive stem cell and are polyploid (16–32 times the normal deoxyribonucleic acid [DNA] content) because of nuclear but not cytoplasmic cell division. Platelets form by invagination of the megakaryocytic cell membrane and bud off from the periphery. Thrombopoietin (TPO) is the primary regulator of platelet production. Platelets function by adhering to damaged endothelium and subendothelial surfaces via specific receptors for the adhesive proteins, von Willebrand factor, and fibrinogen. Platelets also have specific granules that readily release their contents following stimulation and trigger the process of platelet aggregation. Platelets circulate for 7–10 days and, like red cells, have no nucleus.

Lymphocytes are particularly abundant in the bone marrow of young children, although they are a significant component of normal bone marrow at all ages. These are primarily B lymphocytes arising in the spleen and lymph nodes, but T lymphocytes also are present (see Chapter 8).

The stroma of the bone marrow is of major importance for the marrow's normal function. Less is known about details of its function than about the function of the other hematopoietic components because of difficulties in growing these cells in culture.

An essential element in the understanding of the hematology of pediatric patients is a detailed knowledge of normal hematologic values during infancy and childhood. These values vary according to age and, after puberty, according to sex (Table 14–2).

The *coagulation factors* and *anticoagulant proteins* are synthesized primarily in the liver, except for factor VIII and von Willebrand factor, which are also synthesized at other sites. Levels of most of these factors increase throughout gestation; levels of factor VIII, von Willebrand factor, and fibrinogen reach adult normal values by the second trimester.

ANEMIA

Anemia may be defined either quantitatively or functionally (physiologically). The presence of anemia usually is determined by comparison of the patient's hemoglobin level with age-specific and sex-specific normal values. The data presented in Table 14–2 provide the normal ranges, and hemoglobin values below those ranges represent a perfectly acceptable definition of anemia in most circumstances. However, in certain pathologic states, anemia may be present when the hemoglobin level is within the "normal range," such as in cyanotic cardiac or pulmonary disease or when a hemoglobin with an

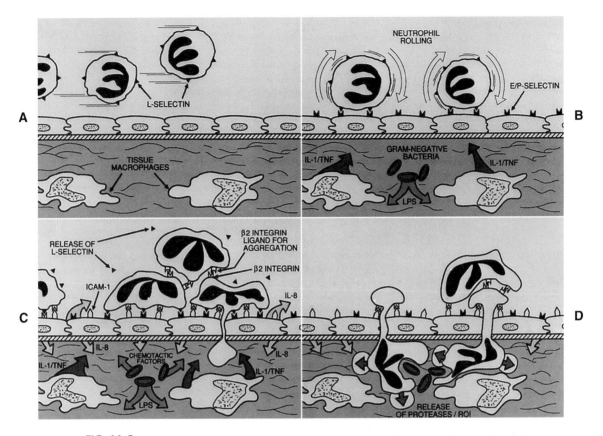

FIG. 14–2

The neutrophil-mediated inflammatory response. **A,** Unstimulated neutrophils expressing L-selectin enter a postcapillary venule. **B,** Gram-negative bacteria invade the subendothelium, release lipopolysaccharide, and stimulate macrophages to secrete inflammatory cytokines IL-1 and TNF, which then activate endothelial cells to express E-selectins and P-selectins. Selectins have a high affinity for sugar molecules (Lewis X) on neutrophils and cause low-avidity neutrophil rolling. **C,** Activated endothelial cells express ICAM-1, which serves as a counter-receptor for neutrophil β2-integrin receptors, leading to high-avidity leukocyte spreading and the start of transendothelial migration. Transendothelial migration is stimulated by chemotactic factors that promote neutrophil activation with release of L-selectin and an increase in β2-integrin affinity for ICAM-1 and other counter-receptors. **D,** Neutrophils invade through the vascular basement membranes with release of proteases and reactive oxidative intermediates. (Redrawn from Smolen JE, Boxer LA: Functions of neutrophils. In Williams WJ, Beutler E, Erslev AJ, et al, editors: *Hematology,* ed 5, New York, 1994, McGraw-Hill. Reprinted in Bennett JC, Plum F, editors: *Cecil textbook of medicine,* ed 20, Philadelphia, 1994, WB Saunders.)

TABLE 14–2
Hematologic Values During Infancy and Childhood

Age	Hemoglobin (g/dL) Mean	Range	Hematocrit (%) Mean	Range	Reticulocytes (%) Mean	Leukocytes (per mm³) Mean	Range	Differential Counts Neutrophils (%) Mean	Range	Lymphocytes (%) Mean	Eosinophils (%) Mean	Monocytes (%) Mean	Nucleated Red Cells/ 100 WBCs
Cord blood	16.8	13.7–20.1	55	45–65	5.0	18,000	9000–30,000	61	40–80	31	2	6	7
2 wk	16.5	13.0–20.0	50	42–66	1.0	12,000	5000–21,000	40		48	3	9	3–10
3 mo	12.0	9.5–14.5	36	31–41	1.0	12,000	6000–18,000	30		63	2	5	0
6 mo–6 yr	12.0	10.5–14.0	37	33–42	1.0	10,000	6000–15,000	45		48	2	5	0
7–12 yr	13.0	11.0–16.0	38	34–40	1.0	8000	4500–13,500	55		38	2	5	0
Adult Female	14.0	12.0–16.0	42	37–47	1.6	7500	5000–10,000	55	35–70	35	3	7	0
Male	16.0	14.0–18.0	47	42–52									

From Behrman RE, editor: *Nelson textbook of pediatrics*, ed 14, Philadelphia, 1992, WB Saunders.
WBCs, White blood cells.

abnormally high affinity for oxygen is present. In these circumstances the physiologic definition is more appropriate. It should be recognized that anemia is not a disease per se, but rather a manifestation of some other primary process. Anemia is a common complication that may accentuate other organ dysfunction. The easiest quantitative definition of anemia is any value for the hemoglobin or hematocrit that is two standard deviations (95% confidence limits) below the mean for age and sex. Thus the diagnosis of anemia in children frequently requires reference to tables providing age-dependent normal values. The normal hemoglobin concentration is higher in males after puberty because high levels of androgen lead to greater red cell synthesis.

Pathophysiology. The physiologic consequences of anemia can be determined from the history and physical examination. Acute onset of anemia is often poorly compensated for and may be manifested as an elevated pulse rate, hemic flow murmur, poor exercise tolerance, headache, excessive sleeping (especially in infants), poor feeding, and syncope. Chronic anemia often is exceptionally well tolerated in children because of their cardiovascular reserve. Anemia that would induce angina in an adult may not produce symptoms in a young child. The extent of cardiovascular or functional impairment, more so than the absolute level of hemoglobin, should dictate the urgency of diagnostic and therapeutic intervention, especially the use of packed RBC transfusion to correct a low hemoglobin level.

Etiology. Common etiologies and mechanisms leading to anemia and an approach to their organization are presented in Fig. 14–3. The causes of anemia can often be suspected from a careful history and physical examination. Often the focus of the history is dictated by the patient's age (Table 14–3). In a newborn a history of jaundice, pallor, previously affected siblings, drug ingestion by the mother, or excessive blood loss at the time of birth provides important clues to the diagnosis. When the patient is a young infant, a careful *dietary history* is crucial. A history of jaundice, blood loss, drug ingestion, or acute or chronic illnesses also indicates probable causes of anemia. In later childhood and in teenagers the presence of constitutional symptoms, unusual diets, drug ingestion, or blood loss, especially from menstrual bleeding, often point to a diagnosis. Congenital red cell disorders (e.g., enzyme deficiencies and membrane problems) often present in the first 6 months of life and frequently are associated with neonatal jaundice, although these disorders often go undiagnosed. A careful drug history is essential for detecting problems that may be drug induced (e.g., hemolysis in G6PD deficiency, bone marrow sup-

pression, or antibody-mediated hemolysis). Pure dietary iron deficiency is rare except in infancy, when cow's milk protein intolerance causes gastrointestinal blood loss and further complicates an inadequate iron intake. A supportive history justifies providing replacement therapy without performing an extensive search for blood loss (Table 14–3).

Clinical Manifestations. The *physical examination* also suggests the presence of anemia and may point to the potential causes of the anemia (Table 14–4). The presence of jaundice suggests hemolysis. Petechiae and purpura indicate a bleeding tendency. Hepatosplenomegaly and adenopathy suggest infiltrative disorders. Growth failure or poor weight gain suggests an anemia of chronic disease or organ failure. An essential element of the physical examination in a patient with anemia is the investigation of the stool for the presence of occult blood.

The initial *laboratory evaluation* of anemia involves a hemoglobin or hematocrit test to indicate the severity of the anemia. Once the diagnosis of anemia has been substantiated, the workup should include a complete blood count with differential, platelet count, indices, and reticulocyte count. The blood smear should be studied for morphologic abnormalities (Fig. 14–4). Using data obtained from the indices and reticulocyte count, the workup for anemia can be organized on the basis of whether red cell production is adequate or inadequate and whether the cells are microcytic, normocytic, or macrocytic (Fig. 14–3). Examination of the peripheral blood smear is critical for assessing the number and morphology of red cells, white blood cells (WBCs), and platelets. All cell lines should be scrutinized to determine whether anemia is the result of a process limited to the erythroid line or of a process that affects other marrow elements.

The reticulocyte production index (RPI), which corrects the reticulocyte count (retic ct) for the degree of anemia, indicates whether the bone marrow is responding appropriately to the anemia. Reticulocytes routinely are counted per 1000 red cells; hence a reduction in the denominator, which occurs in anemia, will falsely increase the reticulocyte count. The formula for calculating the RPI is as follows:

$$RPI = retic\ ct \times Hgb_{observed} / Hgb_{normal} \times 0.5$$

An RPI greater than 3 suggests increased production and implies either hemolysis or blood loss, whereas an index less than 2 suggests decreased production or ineffective production for the degree of anemia. Reticulocytopenia signifies that the anemia is so acute in onset that the marrow has not had adequate time to respond, or that reticulocytes are being destroyed (antibody-mediated), or that intrinsic bone marrow disease is present.

ANEMIA

↓

**HEMOGLOBIN AND INDICES
RETIC COUNT AND MORPHOLOGY**

Inadequate Response (RPI < 2)

**Adequate Response (RPI > 3)
R/O Blood loss**

Hypochromic, Microcytic

Iron deficiency
- Chronic blood loss
- Poor diet
- Cow's milk protein intolerance
- Menstruation

Thalassemia
- β major, minor
- α minor

Chronic inflammatory disease

Copper deficiency

Sideroblastic anemia

Aluminum, (?) lead intoxication

Normochromic, Normocytic

Chronic inflammatory disease
- Infection
- Collagen-vascular disease
- Inflammatory bowel disease

Recent blood loss

Malignancy/marrow infiltration

Chronic renal failure

Transient erythroblastopenia of childhood

Marrow aplasia/hypoplasia

HIV infection

Hemophagocytic syndrome

Macrocytic

Vitamin B$_{12}$ deficiency
- Pernicious anemia
- Ileal resection
- Strict vegetarian
- Abnormal intestinal transport
- Congenital intrinsic factor or transcobalamin deficiency

Folate deficiency
- Malnutrition
- Malabsorption
- Antimetabolite
- Chronic hemolysis
- Phenytoin
- Trimethoprim/sulfa

Hypothyroidism
Oroticaciduria
Chronic liver disease
Lesch-Nyhan syndrome
Down syndrome

Marrow failure
- Myelodysplasia
- Fanconi anemia
- Aplastic anemia
- Pearson syndrome (mitochondrial disorder)

Drugs
- Alcohol
- Azidothymidine (zidovudine)

Hemolytic Disorders

Hemoglobinopathy
- Hemoglobin SS, S-C, S-β thalassemia

Enzymopathy
- G6PD deficiency
- Pyruvate kinase deficiency

Membranopathy
- Hereditary spherocytosis
- Elliptocytosis
- Ovalocytosis

Extrinsic factors
- DIC, HUS, TTP
- Abetalipoproteinemia
- Burns
- Wilson disease
- Vitamin E deficiency

Immune hemolytic anemia
- Autoimmune
- Isoimmune
- Drug-induced

FIG. 14–3

Use of the complete blood count, reticulocyte count, and blood smear in the diagnosis of anemia. *DIC,* Disseminated intravascular coagulation; *HIV,* human immunodeficiency virus; *HUS,* hemolytic-uremic syndrome; *R/O,* rule out; *RPI,* reticulocyte production index; *TTP,* thrombotic thrombocytopenic purpura.

TABLE 14-3
Historical Clues in Evaluation of Anemia

Variable	Comments
Age	Iron deficiency rare in the absence of blood loss prior to 6 mo in term or prior to doubling birth weight in preterm infants
	Neonatal anemia with reticulocytosis suggests hemolysis or blood loss; with reticulocytopenia, suggests bone marrow failure
	Sickle cell anemia and β-thalassemia appear as fetal hemoglobin disappears (4–8 mo of age)
Family history and genetic considerations	X-linked: G6PD deficiency
	Autosomal dominant: spherocytosis
	Autosomal recessive: sickle cell, Fanconi anemia
	Family member with early age of cholecystectomy (bilirubin stones) or splenectomy
	Ethnicity (thalassemia in individuals of Mediterranean origin; G6PD deficiency in blacks, Greeks, and Middle Eastern individuals)
	Race (β-thalassemia in individuals of Mediterranean, African, or Asian descent; α-thalassemia in blacks and those of Asian descent; SC and SS in blacks)
Nutrition	Cow's milk diet: iron defiency
	Strict vegetarian: vitamin B_{12} deficiency
	Goat's milk: folate deficiency
	Pica: plumbism, iron deficiency
	Cholestasis, malabsorption: vitamin E deficiency
Drugs	G6PD: oxidants (e.g., nitrofurantoin, antimalarials)
	Immune-mediated hemolysis (e.g., penicillin)
	Bone marrow suppression (e.g., chemotherapy)
	Phenytoin increasing folate requirements
Diarrhea	Malabsorption of vitamins B_{12} or E or iron
	Inflammatory bowel disease and anemia of chronic disease with or without blood loss
	Milk protein intolerance–induced blood loss
	Intestinal resection: vitamin B_{12} deficiency
Infection	*Giardia:* iron malabsorption
	Intestinal bacterial overgrowth (blind loop): vitamin B_{12} deficiency
	Fish tapeworm: vitamin B_{12} deficiency
	Epstein-Barr virus, cytomegalovirus: bone marrow suppression, hemophagocytic syndromes
	Mycoplasma: hemolysis
	Parvovirus: bone marrow suppression
	Human immunodeficiency virus
	Chronic infection
	Endocarditis
	Malaria: hemolysis
	Hepatitis: aplastic anemia

G6PD, Glucose-6-phosphate dehydrogenase.

TABLE 14–4
Physical Findings in the Evaluation of Anemia

System	Observation	Significance
Skin	Hyperpigmentation	Fanconi anemia, dyskeratosis congenita
	Café-au-lait spots	Fanconi anemia
	Vitiligo	Vitamin B_{12} deficiency
	Partial oculocutaneous albinism	Chédiak-Higashi syndrome
	Jaundice	Hemolysis
	Petechiae, purpura	Bone marrow infiltration, autoimmune hemolysis with autoimmune thrombocytopenia, hemolytic-uremic syndrome
	Erythematous rash	Parvovirus, Epstein-Barr virus
	Butterfly rash	SLE antibodies
Head	Frontal bossing	Thalassemia major, severe iron deficiency, chronic subdural hematoma
	Microcephaly	Fanconi anemia
Eyes	Microphthalmia	Fanconi anemia
	Retinopathy	Hemoglobin SS, SC disease
	Optic atrophy	Osteopetrosis
	Blocked lacrimal gland	Dyskeratosis congenita
	Kayser-Fleischer ring	Wilson disease
	Blue sclera	Iron deficiency
Ears	Deafness	Osteopetrosis
Mouth	Glossitis	Vitamin B_{12} deficiency, iron deficiency
	Angular stomatitis	Iron deficiency
	Cleft lip	Diamond-Blackfan syndrome
	Pigmentation	Peutz-Jeghers syndrome (intestinal blood loss)
	Telangiectasia	Osler-Weber-Rendu syndrome (blood loss)
	Leukoplakia	Dyskeratosis congenita
Chest	Shield chest or wide-spread nipples	Diamond-Blackfan syndrome
	Murmur	Endocarditis: prosthetic valve hemolysis; severe anemia
Abdomen	Hepatomegaly	Hemolysis, infiltrative tumor, chronic disease, hemangioma, cholecystitis, extramedullary hematopoiesis
	Splenomegaly	Hemolysis, sickle cell disease, (early) thalassemia, malaria, lymphoma, Epstein-Barr virus, portal hypertension
	Nephromegaly	Fanconi anemia
	Absent kidney	Fanconi anemia
Extremities	Absent thumbs	Fanconi anemia
	Triphalangeal thumb	Diamond-Blackfan syndrome
	Spoon nails	Iron deficiency
	Beau line (nails)	Heavy metal intoxication, severe illness
	Mees line (nails)	Heavy metals, severe illness, sickle cell anemia
	Dystrophic nails	Dyskeratosis congenita
Rectal	Hemorrhoids	Portal hypertension
	Heme-positive stool	Gastrointestinal bleeding
Nerves	Irritable, apathy	Iron deficiency
	Peripheral neuropathy	Deficiency of vitamins B_1, B_{12}, and E, lead poisoning
	Dementia	Deficiency of vitamins B_{12} and E
	Ataxia, posterior column signs	Vitamin B_{12} deficiency
	Stroke	Sickle cell anemia, paroxysmal nocturnal hemoglobinuria
General	Small stature	Fanconi anemia, human immunodeficiency virus, malnutrition

SLE, Systemic lupus erythematosus.

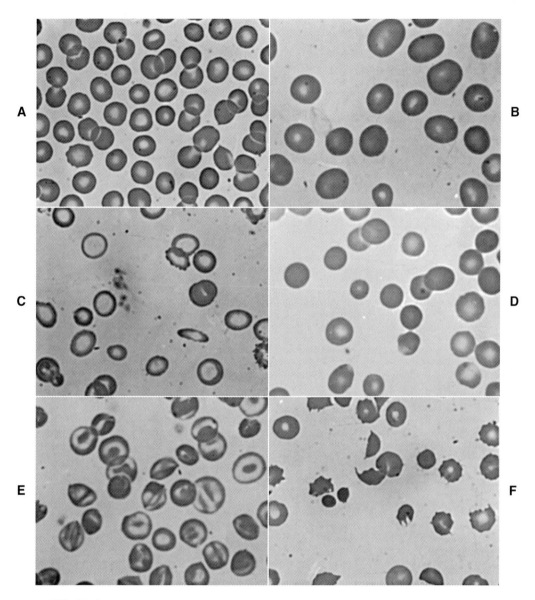

FIG. 14–4

Morphologic abnormalities of the red cell. **A,** Normal. **B,** Macrocytes (folic acid deficiency). **C,** Hypochromic microcytes (iron deficiency). **D,** Spherocytes (hereditary spherocytosis). **E,** Target cells (Hgb CC disease). **F,** Schistocytes (hemolytic-uremic syndrome). (From Behrman RE, editor: *Nelson textbook of pediatrics,* ed 14, Philadelphia, 1992, WB Saunders.)

Hypochromic, Microcytic Anemia with Inadequate Red Cell Production

Hypochromic, microcytic anemia is caused by an inadequate production of hemoglobin (Table 14–5).

Iron-Deficiency Anemia

Dietary iron-deficiency anemia is most common in bottle-fed infants who are receiving large volumes of cow's milk. They ingest little in the way of dietary substances high in iron, such as meat and green vegetables (see Chapter 2). Iron deficiency is the most common cause of anemia in the world.

Breast-fed infants have iron deficiency less commonly than bottle-fed infants because, although there is less iron in breast milk, this iron is more effectively absorbed. Menstruating adolescents are also at increased risk of iron deficiency. The sequence of events in the development of iron-deficiency anemia is noted in Table 14–6. In addition to the manifestations of anemia, central nervous system (CNS) abnormalities (e.g., apathy, irritability, and poor concentration) have been linked to iron-deficiency, presumably resulting from alterations of iron-containing enzymes (e.g.,

---

TABLE 14–5
Differentiating Feature of Microcytic Anemias*

Tests	Iron-Deficiency Anemia	Thalassemia Minor†	Anemia of Chronic Disease‡
Serum iron	Low	Normal	Low
Serum iron–binding capacity	High	Normal	Low or normal
Serum ferritin	Low	Normal or high	Normal or high
Marrow iron stores	Low or absent	Normal or high	Normal or high
Marrow sideroblasts	Decreased or absent	Normal or increased	Normal or increased
Free erythrocyte protoporphyrin	High	Normal or slightly increased	High
Hemoglobin A_2 or F	Normal	High β-thalassemia; normal α-thalassemia	Normal
Red cell distribution width (RDW)§	High	Normal	Normal/↑

*See Table 14–6 for definition of microcytosis.
†Alpha thalassemia minor can be diagnosed by the presence of Bart hemoglobin on newborn screening.
‡Usually normochromic; 25% are microcytic.
§RDW quantitates the degree of anisocytosis (different sizes) of red blood cells.

TABLE 14–6
Stages in Development of Iron-Deficiency Anemia

Hemoglobin (g/dL)	Peripheral Smear	Serum Iron (μg/dL)	Bone Marrow	Serum Ferritin (ng/mL)
13+ (normal)	nc/nc	50/150	Fe^{2+}	40–340 (male) 40–150 (female)
10–12	nc/nc	↓	Fe^{2+} absent, erythroid hyperplasia	<12
8–10	hypo/nc	↓	Fe^{2+} absent, erythroid hyperplasia	<12
<8	hypo/micro*	↓	Fe^{2+} absent, erythroid hyperplasia	<12

From Andreoli TE, Bennett JC, Carpenter CC, et al: *Cecil essentials of medicine*, ed 4, Philadelphia, 1997, WB Saunders.
Hypo/micro, Hypochromic, microcytic; *Hypo/nc*, hypochromic, normocytic; nc/nc, normochromic, normocytic.
*Microcytosis, determined by a mean corpuscular volume (in fL) less than two standard deviations below the mean, must be adjusted for age (e.g., −2 SD at 3–6 months = 74; at 0.5–2 years = 70; at 2–6 years = 75; at 6–12 years = 77; and at 12–18 years = 78).

monoamine oxidase) and cytochromes. Poor muscle endurance, gastrointestinal dysfunction, and impaired white blood cell and T-cell function also have been noted in association with iron deficiency. Some studies suggest that iron deficiency in infancy may be associated with later cognitive deficits.

A detailed dietary history usually discloses the child's poor diet. If the dietary history suggests iron deficiency, a therapeutic trial of iron is appropriate with or without laboratory confirmation. In an otherwise healthy child a therapeutic trial is the best diagnostic study for iron deficiency as long as the child is reexamined and a response is documented. The response to oral iron includes rapid subjective improvement, especially in neurologic function (in 24–48 hours) and reticulocytosis (in 48–72 hours); an increase in hemoglobin levels (in 4–30 days); and repletion of iron stores (in 1–3 months). A usual therapeutic dose of 3–6 mg/day of elemental iron will induce an increase in hemoglobin of 0.25–0.4 g/dL/day (a 1%-per-day rise in hematocrit). If the hemoglobin level fails to rise within 2 weeks after the institution of iron treatment, the clinician should carefully reevaluate the patient for ongoing blood loss, development of infection, poor compliance, or other causes of microcytic anemia (Fig. 14–3 and Table 14–5).

Thalassemia Minor

The thalassemia minor syndromes are characterized by a mild hypochromic, microcytic anemia with a low RPI (Table 14–7; Fig. 14–3). **Alpha-thalassemia** occurs in 1.5% of African-Americans and is a common cause of microcytosis, either without anemia or with a mild hypochromic, microcytic anemia. Alpha-thalassemia is common in Southeast Asia; individuals of Southeast Asian descent also are at risk of having homozygous alpha-thalassemia cause fetal hydrops with all Bart hemoglobin in the newborn (γ_4 tetramers) or with hemoglobin H (β_4 tetramers) in older children. The blood smear is normal with the alpha-thalassemia trait, except for microcytosis. No basophilic stippling is present. Outside of the neonatal period, when Bart hemoglobin is detectable, hemoglobin electrophoresis usually is normal in alpha-thalassemia minor (Fig. 14–5).

Beta-thalassemia minor is prevalent throughout the Mediterranean region, the Middle East, India, and Southeast Asia. The peripheral blood smear shows hypochromic, microcytic red blood cells; target cells and basophilic stippled red cells may also be present. The stippling is caused by precipitation of alpha-chain tetramers. The diagnosis is based on an elevation of hemoglobin A_2 and F levels.

Lead Poisoning

Lead poisoning may be associated with a hypochromic, microcytic anemia, although most patients have concomitant iron deficiency. The history of a child with pica who lives in an older home with chipped paint or lead dust should raise suspicion of lead poisoning. Basophilic stippling on the blood smear is common. Detection by routine screening, removal from exposure, chelation therapy, and correction of iron deficiency are of utmost importance to the potential development of affected children (see Chapter 3). Lead intoxication may rarely also cause hemolytic anemia.

Normocytic Anemia with Inadequate Red Cell Production

Normocytic anemias include a wide variety of red cell disorders in which the marrow fails to synthesize adequate numbers of red blood cells as a result of a systemic illness. Red cell synthesis fails because of fibrosis, tumor, storage cells, transient or prolonged marrow failure (in transient erythroblastopenia of childhood or aplastic anemia), or failure to synthesize erythropoietin (e.g., in renal failure). Normocytic anemias also occur in the presence of acute blood loss before the marrow has had time to respond. The site of blood loss usually is obvious, commonly in the gastrointestinal tract (see Chapter 11).

Anemia is a common component of **chronic inflammatory disease.** Elevated cytokine levels cause a reticuloendothelial blockade within the marrow, wherein iron is taken up by the reticuloendothelial cells but is not released for erythroid synthesis. The anemia may be normocytic or, less often, microcytic. At times this poses a clinical challenge, when children with inflammatory disorders that may be associated with blood loss (e.g., inflammatory bowel disease) exhibit a microcytic anemia. In these circumstances the only specific diagnostic test that can clearly differentiate the two entities is a bone marrow aspiration with staining of the sample for iron (Table 14–5). Serum ferritin levels also may be helpful. A trial of iron therapy is not indicated without a specific diagnosis in children who appear to be systemically ill.

Bone marrow **infiltration by malignant cells** commonly leads to a normochromic, normocytic anemia. The mechanism by which neoplastic cells interfere with red cell and other marrow cell synthesis is multifactorial. The reticulocyte count is low. Immature myeloid elements may be released into the peripheral blood as a result of the presence of the offending tumor cells. An examination of the peripheral blood may reveal lymphoblasts; when solid tumors metastasize

TABLE 14–7
Comparison of the Thalassemia Syndromes

Genetic Abnormality	Percent Hemoglobin			Other	Clinical Syndrome
	Hb A	Hb A$_2$	Hb F		
Normal αβ	90–98	2–3	2–3		None
Beta-Thalassemias					
Thalassemia Major					
β⁰ β⁰	0	2–5	95	—	Severe anemia, abnormal growth, iron overload, needs transfusion, Cooley anemia
β⁰ β⁺	Very low	2–5	20–80	—	
Thalassemia Intermedia					
β⁺ β⁺	20–40		60–80		Severe hypo/micro anemia with Hb 7–9 g/dL, hepatosplenomegaly, bone changes, iron overload, less need for transfusion
Thalassemia Minor					
β β⁰ or β β⁺	90–95	5–7	2–10	Stippled RBCs	Hypo/micro blood smear, mild to no anemia
Alpha-Thalassemias					
Homozygous α-thalassemia − −/− −	—	—	—	Hb H (B4) Hb Bart (γ4)	Hydrops fetalis, stillborn
Hemoglobin H disease − −/− α	60–70	2–5	2–5	Hb H 30–40	Hypo/micro anemia, Hb 7–10 g/dL, Heinz bodies
α-Thalassemia trait − α/− α , α α/− −	90–98	2–3	2–3		Hypo/micro smear, no anemia
Silent carrier − α/α α	90–98	2–3	2–3		Normal
Hemoglobin Lepore (δβ fusion)					
Heterozygote	70–80	1–2	5–20	Hb Lepore 5–15	Mild hypo/micro anemia
Homozygote	0	0	70–90	Hb Lepore 10–30	Severe thalassemia major

From Andreoli TE, Bennett JC, Carpenter CC, et al: *Cecil essentials of medicine*, ed 4, Philadelphia, 1997, WB Saunders.
Hypo/micro, Hypochromic, microcytic; *RBCs,* red blood cells.

FIG. 14–5

Schematic illustration of alpha-globin gene deletions and their clinical consequences. *Hb,* Hemoglobin; *MCV,* mean corpuscular volume. (From Beutler E: *JAMA* 259[16]:2433, 1988.)

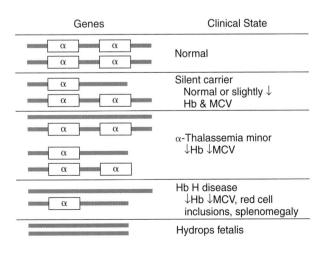

to the marrow, these cells seldom are seen in the peripheral blood. Teardrop cells may be seen in the peripheral blood. Performance of a bone marrow examination frequently is necessary in the face of normochromic, normocytic anemia.

Congenital pure red cell aplasia (Diamond-Blackfan syndrome) usually presents in the first few months of life or even at birth (Table 14–8). This is a lifelong disorder. Congenital anomalies are common. Most patients respond to corticosteroid treatment but must receive therapy indefinitely. At the time of presentation, the patient may have mild macrocytosis or may be normocytic. Patients who do not respond to steroid treatment are transfusion dependent and are at risk of the multiple complications of chronic transfusion therapy, including blood-borne, virus-associated illnesses and iron overload.

In contrast to the congenital hypoplastic anemias, **transient erythroblastopenia of childhood** (TEC) usually appears after 6 months of age (Table 14–8). This is a normocytic anemia caused by bone marrow suppression. Viral infections are thought to be the major cause of TEC, but no specific etiology has been identified. The onset is gradual; however, the anemia may become severe. Recovery usually is spontaneous; transfusion of packed red cells may be necessary, pending recovery. The key to the diagnosis of TEC is a gradual onset of normocytic anemia in a child over 6 months of age with a normal physical examination. Differentiation from Diamond-Blackfan syndrome, in which erythroid precursors also are absent or diminished in the bone marrow, is noted in Table 14–8.

Aplastic crises, which may complicate any chronic hemolytic anemia, are periods of reticulocytopenia during which the usual high rate of red cell destruction leads to an acute exacerbation of the anemia, potentially precipitating cardiovascular decompensation. Human parvovirus B19 (the cause of fifth disease) infects erythroid precursors and shuts down erythropoiesis. Transient erythroid aplasia is without consequence in individuals with normal red cell survival. Recovery from parvovirus infection in hemolytic disease is spontaneous, but patients may need transfusion if the anemia is severe.

Macrocytic Anemia

Vitamin B_{12} and folic acid deficiencies lead to macrocytic anemia (Figs. 14–3 and 14–4); these deficiencies are discussed in Chapter 2. *Pearson syndrome,* sideroblastic anemia in association with pancreatic insufficiency, is a mitochondrial disorder (Chapter 11) associated with progressive macrocytic anemia. Examination of the bone marrow reveals vacuolated precursor cells and ring sideroblasts.

Hemolytic Anemias

Hemolytic diseases are mediated either by intrinsic disorders of the red blood cell or by disorders extrinsic to the red blood cell itself. The best indicators of the severity of hemolysis are the hemoglobin level and the elevation of the reticulocyte count.

Hemolytic Anemia Caused by Intrinsic Red Cell Disorders

Membrane Disorders. The most common red cell membrane disorders are **hereditary spherocytosis (HS)** and **hereditary elliptocytosis (HE).** These disorders frequently are associated with neonatal jaundice, although the disorder often goes undiagnosed in the neonate. In both of these disorders, abnormalities of proteins within the cytoskeleton lead to abnormal red cell shape and function.

HEREDITARY SPHEROCYTOSIS. Hereditary spherocytosis varies greatly in clinical severity, ranging from a severe hemolytic anemia with growth failure, splenomegaly, and chronic transfusion requirements in infancy necessitating early splenectomy to an asymptomatic, well-compensated, mild hemolytic anemia that may be discovered incidentally. The biochemical bases of both HS and HE probably are similar and appear to have in common a defect in the protein lattice (spectrin, ankyrin, protein 4.2, band 3) that underlies the red cell lipid bilayer and provides stability of the membrane shape. In HS because of abnormal vertical interaction of the cytoskeletal proteins and uncoupling of the lipid bilayer from the cytoskeleton, pieces of membrane bud off as microvesicles. When the red cell loses membrane, the shape changes from a biconcave disc to a spherocyte; the spherocyte shape has the lowest ratio of surface area to volume. Therefore, the red cell is less deformable when passing through narrow passages in the spleen. The transmission of this disorder usually is autosomal dominant but occasionally is recessive. Spontaneous mutations causing HS are common. The *diagnosis* should be suspected in patients with even a few spherocytes exhibited on the blood smear because the spherocytes are removed preferentially by the spleen. An incubated osmotic fragility test confirms the presence of spherocytes and increases the likelihood of the diagnosis of hereditary spherocytosis. However, the osmotic fragility test result is abnormal in any hemolytic disease in which spherocytes are present, especially antibody-mediated hemolysis.

Splenectomy corrects the anemia and normalizes the red cell survival, but the morphologic abnormalities persist. Splenectomy should be considered for any child with symptoms referable to anemia or growth failure but should be deferred until the age of 5 years, if at all possible, to minimize the risk of

TABLE 14–8
Differentiation of Red Cell Aplasias and Aplastic Anemias

Disorder	Age of Onset	Characteristics	Treatment
Congenital			
Diamond-Blackfan syndrome (congenital hypoplastic anemia)	Newborn–1 mo; 90% are younger than 1 yr of age	Pure red cell aplasia, autosomal recessive trait, elevated fetal hemoglobin, fetal i antigen present, macrocytic, short stature, web neck, cleft lip, triphalangeal thumb; late-onset leukemia	Prednisone, transfusion
Acquired			
Transient erythroblastopenia	6 mo–5 yr of age; 85% are older than 1 yr of age	Pure red cell defect; no anomalies, fetal hemoglobin, or i antigen; spontaneous recovery, normal MCV	Expectant transfusion for symptomatic anemia
Idiopathic aplastic anemia (s/p hepatitis, drugs, unknown)	All ages	All cell lines involved; exposure to chloramphenicol, phenylbutazone, radiation	Bone marrow transplant, antithymocyte globulin, cyclosporine, androgens
Familial			
Fanconi syndrome	Before 10 yr of age; mean is 8 yr	All cell lines; microcephaly, absent thumbs, café-au-lait spots, cutaneous hyperpigmentation, short stature; chromosomal breaks, high MCV and hemoglobin F; horseshoe or absent kidney; leukemic transformation; autosomal recessive trait	Androgens, corticosteroids, bone marrow transplant
Paroxysmal nocturnal hemoglobinuria	After 5 yr	Initial hemolysis followed by aplastic anemia; increased complement-mediated hemolysis; thrombosis; iron deficiency	Iron, bone marrow transplant, androgens, steroids
Dyskeratosis congenita	Mean 10 yr for skin; mean 17 yr for anemia	Pancytopenia; hyperpigmentation, dystrophic nails, leukoplakia; X-linked recessive; lacrimal duct stenosis; high MCV and fetal hemoglobin	Androgens, splenectomy, bone marrow transplant
Familial hemophagocytic lymphohistiocytosis	Before 2 yr	Pancytopenia; fever, hepatosplenomegaly, hypertriglyceridemia, CSF pleocytosis	Transfusion; often lethal; VP-16, bone marrow transplantation, IVIG, cyclosporine
Infectious			
Parvovirus	Any age	Any chronic hemolytic anemia, typically sickle cell; new-onset reticulocytopenia	Transfusion
Epstein-Barr virus (EBV)	Any age; usually younger than 5 yr of age	X-linked immunodeficiency syndrome, pancytopenia	Transfusion, bone marrow transplantation
Viral-associated hemophagocytic syndrome (CMV, HHV-6, EBV)	Any age	Pancytopenia; hemophagocytosis present in marrow, fever, hepatosplenomegaly	Transfusion, antiviral therapy (see Chapter 10), IVIG

CMV, Cytomegalovirus; *CSF*, cerebrospinal fluid; *HHV-6*, human herpesvirus-6; *IVIG*, intravenous immunoglobulin; *MCV*, mean corpuscular volume.

overwhelming postsplenectomy sepsis and maximize the antibody response to the polyvalent pneumococcal vaccine. In several reports, partial splenectomy appears to improve the hemolytic anemia and maintain splenic function in host defense. Before splenectomy, vaccinations against pneumococcus and *Haemophilus influenzae* type b should be given according to current recommendations. Gallstones (bilirubinate), a result of chronic hemolysis, may be asymptomatic or may be the cause of vague abdominal pain.

HEREDITARY ELLIPTOCYTOSIS. Hereditary elliptocytosis is a disorder of spectrin dimer interactions that occurs primarily in individuals of African descent. The most common variant is a clinically insignificant, morphologic abnormality without shortened red cell survival. The less common variant is associated with spherocytes, ovalocytes, and elliptocytes and with a moderate, usually compensated, hemolysis. Both variants are transmitted as autosomal dominant traits. Far more significant hemolysis occurs in a very small percentage of patients with elliptocytes, spherocytes, fragmented red cells, and striking microcytosis. This disorder is termed *hereditary pyropoikilocytosis* and is the result of a structural abnormality of spectrin. The term "pyropoikilocytosis" refers to the unusual instability of the erythrocytes when they are exposed to heat (45° C).

Red Cell Enzyme Deficiencies. Numerous red cell enzyme deficiencies exist, but only two are common: glucose-6-phosphate dehydrogenase deficiency and pyruvate kinase deficiency.

GLUCOSE-6-PHOSPHATE DEHYDROGENASE DEFICIENCY. Glucose-6-phosphate dehydrogenase deficiency is an abnormality in the hexose monophosphate shunt pathway of glycolysis that results in the depletion of NADPH and the inability to regenerate reduced glutathione. Reduced glutathione protects SH groups in the red cell membrane from oxidation. When a patient with G6PD is exposed to significant oxidant stress, hemoglobin is oxidized, forming precipitates of sulfhemoglobin (so-called Heinz bodies). Heinz bodies are visible on specially stained preparations. As a result, episodes of hemolysis develop in children with G6PD deficiency when they are exposed to oxidant stress.

The severity of the hemolysis depends on the enzyme variant. In many G6PD variants the enzymes become unstable with aging. Young red cells have normal G6PD activity that is lost as the cell ages; the activity cannot be replaced because the cell is anucleated. Older cells are most susceptible to oxidant-induced hemolysis. In other variants the enzyme is kinetically abnormal. The most common variants of G6PD have been found in areas where malaria is endemic. G6PD deficiency protects against parasitism

of the erythrocyte. The most common variant with normal activity is termed type B and is defined by its electrophoretic mobility. The approximate gene frequencies in African-Americans are 70% type B, 20% type A⁺, and 10% type A⁻. Only the A⁻ variant is unstable. The A⁻ variant is termed the "African" variant; 10% of black males are affected. A group of variants found in Sardinians, Sicilians, Greeks, Sephardic and Oriental Jews, and Arabs is termed the "Mediterranean" variant and is associated with chronic hemolysis and potentially life-threatening hemolytic disease. The gene for G6PD is carried on the X chromosome. Clinical hemolysis is most common in males; affected males possess a single abnormal X chromosome. Heterozygous females who have randomly inactivated a higher percentage of the normal gene may become symptomatic, as may homozygous females with the A⁻ variant, which occurs in 0.5–1% of females of African descent.

Clinically, G6PD deficiency has two common presentations. Individuals with the A⁻ variant often exhibit acute hemolysis triggered by significant acute infection or ingestion of an oxidant drug. Outside of these episodes no evidence of chronic hemolysis exists. Individuals with the chronic hemolyzing variants have lifelong chronic hemolysis that is exacerbated by oxidant stress. The RBC morphology during episodes of acute hemolysis is striking. Red cells appear to have "bites" (cookie cells) taken out of them. These are areas of absent hemoglobin that are produced by phagocytosis of Heinz bodies by splenic macrophages; as a result, the red cells appear blistered. Jaundice, dark urine resulting from both bilirubin pigments, hemoglobinuria when hemolysis is intravascular, and decreased haptoglobin levels are common during hemolytic episodes. Because 5% of African-Americans lack haptoglobin, absent haptoglobin is meaningful only in the context of the other abnormalities. Early on, the hemolysis usually exceeds the ability of the bone marrow to compensate, so the reticulocyte count may be low for 3–4 days.

The *diagnosis* of G6PD deficiency is based on decreased NADPH formation. However, G6PD levels may be normal in the setting of acute, severe hemolysis because the most deficient cells have been destroyed. Repeating the test at a later time when the patient is in a steady-state condition, testing the mothers of boys with suspected G6PD deficiency, or performing electrophoresis to identify the precise variant present facilitates diagnosis.

The *treatment* of G6PD deficiency is supportive, including transfusion when significant cardiovascular compromise is present and protecting the kidneys against damage from precipitated free hemoglobin by maintaining hydration and urine alkalization. Hemolysis is prevented by avoiding known oxidants,

particularly long-acting sulfonamides, nitrofurantoin, primaquine, and dimercaprol; fava beans (fav-
ism) have triggered hemolysis, particularly in patients with the Mediterranean variant. Infection also
is a major precipitant of hemolysis in G6PD-deficient
young children.

PYRUVATE KINASE DEFICIENCY. Pyruvate kinsase
deficiency is much less common than G6PD deficiency and also represents a clinical spectrum of disorders caused by the functional deficiency of pyruvate kinase (PK). Some individuals have a true
deficiency state, and others have abnormal enzyme
kinetics. This enzyme in the Embden-Meyerhof
pathway of glycolysis is important for the production of two moles of adenosine triphosphate (ATP)
per mole of glucose metabolized. The metabolic consequence of PK deficiency is ATP depletion, which
impairs red cell survival.

PK deficiency is an autosomal disorder, and most
children who are affected (and are not products of
inbreeding) are double heterozygotes for two abnormal enzymes. Hemolysis is not aggravated by oxidant stress because patients with this condition tend
to have a profound reticulocytosis. Aplastic crises
potentially are life threatening. The spleen is the site
for red cell removal in PK deficiency. Most patients
have amelioration of the anemia and a reduction of
transfusion requirements after splenectomy.

Major Hemoglobinopathies. Because alpha chains
are needed for fetal erythropoiesis and production
of hemoglobin F ($\alpha_2\beta_2$), alpha-chain hemoglobinopathies present in utero. Four alpha genes are
present on the two number-16 chromosomes (Fig.
14–5 and Table 14–7). Single-gene deletions produce
no disorder (the silent carrier state) but can be detected by measuring the rates of alpha and beta synthesis or by using molecular biologic techniques.
Deletion of two genes produces alpha-thalassemia
minor with mild or no anemia and microcytosis. In
individuals of African origin the gene deletions occur on different chromosomes *(trans)* and the disorder is benign because few individuals of African descent have more than two genes deleted. In the
Oriental (Asian descent) population, deletions may
occur on the same chromosome *(cis)*, and therefore
infants may inherit two number-16 chromosomes
lacking three or even four genes. Deletion of all four
genes leads to hydrops fetalis, severe intrauterine
anemia, and death unless intrauterine transfusions
are administered. Deletion of three genes produces
moderate hemolytic anemia with γ_4 tetramers (Bart
hemoglobin) in the fetus and β_4 tetramers (hemoglobin H) in older children and adults (Table 14–7).

A greater number of disorders occur in beta-chain
hemoglobinopathies because these abnormalities
are not symptomatic in utero. In contrast, severe

gamma-chain abnormalities would be expected to be
lethal. The major group of beta-hemoglobinopathies
includes those that alter hemoglobin function, including hemoglobins S, C, E, D, and G, and those that
alter beta-chain production, the beta-thalassemias.
Because each red cell has two copies of chromosome 11 and the beta-globin genes are both expressed, most of the disorders of beta chains are
not clinically severe unless both beta chains are
abnormal. By convention, when describing β-
thalassemia genes, "β^0" indicates a thalassemic
gene resulting in absent β-chain synthesis, whereas
"β^+" indicates a thalassemic gene that permits reduced but not absent synthesis of normal β chains.
Disorders of the beta chain usually manifest themselves clinically between 6 and 12 months of age
unless they have been detected prenatally or by
cord blood screening.

BETA-THALASSEMIA MAJOR (COOLEY ANEMIA). Beta-
thalassemia major is a hemoglobinopathy caused by
mutations that impair beta-chain synthesis (Table
14–7); excess gamma and beta chains do not damage
the red cells, whereas excess alpha chains are toxic. Because of unbalanced synthesis of alpha and beta
chains, alpha chains precipitate within the cells, resulting in red cell destruction either in the bone marrow or in the spleen once the cell is released. The clinical severity of the illness varies, partly on the basis of
the molecular defect. Nevertheless, most patients are
transfusion dependent from early infancy when they
demonstrate severe anemia and hepatosplenomegaly.

Clinical manifestations of beta-thalassemia major
result from the combination of chronic hemolytic
disease, decreased or absent production of normal
hemoglobin A, and ineffective erythropoiesis in the
marrow. The anemia is severe and leads to growth
failure and heart failure. Ineffective erythropoiesis
causes increased expenditure of energy and expansion of the bone marrow cavities of all bones, leading to osteopenia, pathologic fractures, extramedullary erythropoiesis, and an increase in the rate of
iron absorption. Patients usually are transfusion dependent from the end of the first year of life. Adolescents are subject to complications from iron overload *(hemochromatosis)*, including nonimmune
diabetes mellitus, cirrhosis, heart failure, bronzing of
the skin, and multiple endocrine abnormalities (e.g.,
of the thyroid or gonad). The amount of iron the patient acquires from transfusion may be estimated by
the formula stating that each milliliter of packed
RBCs contains approximately 1 mg of iron.

Treatment of beta-thalassemia major is based on a
hypertransfusion program that corrects the anemia
and suppresses the patient's own inadequate erythropoiesis, thus limiting the stimulus for increased iron
absorption. This suppression permits the bones to

heal, decreases the metabolic expenditures, increases growth, and limits dietary iron absorption. Splenectomy may reduce the transfusion volume but adds to the risk of serious infection. Chelation therapy with deferoxamine, which removes excess iron and prolongs life, should start when laboratory evidence of iron overload is present and before occurrence of clinical manifestations. Bone marrow transplantation in childhood prior to organ dysfunction induced by iron overload has had a high success rate in beta-thalassemia major and is the treatment of choice.

An uncommon mutation that leads to deletion of both beta and delta chains results in **hereditary persistence of fetal hemoglobin** (HPFH), in which gamma-chain synthesis represents about 30% of non–alpha-chain synthesis in adult life. HPFH usually is asymptomatic.

SICKLE CELL DISEASE. The common sickle cell syndromes are hemoglobin SS disease, hemoglobin S-C disease, hemoglobin S-beta thalassemia, and rare variants (Table 14–9). The specific hemoglobin phenotype must be identified because the clinical complications differ in frequency, type, and severity.

Sickle cell disease is a chronic hemolytic anemia complicated by sudden, occasionally severe, and life-threatening events caused by the acute intravascular sickling of the red cells, with resultant pain or organ dysfunction (so-called crisis).

Pathophysiology. As a result of a single amino acid substitution (valine for glutamic acid at the β6 position), hemoglobin S cells change from a normal biconcave disc (when oxygenated) to a sickled form, with resultant decreased deformability in deoxygenated conditions. Sickle hemoglobin crystallizes and forms a gel in the deoxy state. When reoxygenated, the sickle hemoglobin is normally soluble. The so-called reversible sickle cell is capable of entering the microcirculation. However, as the oxygen saturation falls, sickling may occur, with resultant occlusion of the microvasculature. The surrounding tissue undergoes infarction, inducing pain and dysfunction. This sickling phenomenon is accentuated by hypoxia, acidosis, increased or decreased temperature, and dehydration (from increased concentration of erythrocyte hemoglobin S). The clinical manifestations may be the result of infection, anemia, or vasoocclusion (Table 14–10).

Clinical Manifestations. The child with sickle cell anemia is vulnerable to life-threatening infection as early as 4 months of age because of splenic dysfunction caused by sickling of the red cells within the spleen and the resultant inability of the spleen to filter microorganisms from the bloodstream. Splenic dysfunction is followed eventually by splenic infarction, usually by 2–4 years of age. In the absence of normal splenic function, the patient is susceptible to overwhelming infection by encapsulated organisms,

---

TABLE 14–9
Comparison of Sickle Cell Syndromes

| Genotype | Clinical Condition | Percent Hemoglobin | | | | | Other Findings |
		Hb A	Hb S	Hb A_2	Hb F	Hb C	
SA	Sickle cell trait	55–60	40–45	2–3	—	—	Usually asymptomatic
SS	Sickle cell anemia	0	85–95	2–3	5–15	—	Clinically severe anemia; Hb F heterogeneous in distribution
S-β^0 thalassemia	Sickle cell-beta^0 thalassemia	0	70–80	3–5	10–20	—	Moderately severe anemia; splenomegaly in 50%; smear: hypochromic, microcytic anemia
S-β^+ thalassemia	Sickle cell-beta$^+$ thalassemia	10–20	60–75	3–5	10–20		Hb F distributed heterogeneously; mild microcytic anemia
SC	Hb SC disease	0	45–50	—	—	45–50	Moderately severe anemia; splenomegaly; target cells
S-HPFH	Sickle-hereditary persistence of Hb F	0	70–80	1–2	20–30	—	Asymptomatic; Hb F is uniformly distributed

From Andreoli TE, Bennett JC, Carpenter CC, et al: *Cecil essentials of medicine,* ed 4, Philadelphia, 1997, WB Saunders.

TABLE 14-10
Clinical Manifestations of Sickle Cell Anemia*

Manifestation	Comments
Anemia	Chronic, onset 3–4 mo of age; may require folate therapy for chronic hemolysis; hematocrit usually 18–26%
Aplastic crisis	Parvovirus infection, reticulocytopenia; acute and reversible; may need transfusion
Sequestration crisis	Massive splenomegaly (may involve liver), shock; treat with transfusion
Hemolytic crisis	May be associated with G6PD deficiency
Dactylitis	Hand-foot swelling in early infancy
Painful crisis	Microvascular painful vasoocclusive infarcts of muscle, bone, bone marrow, lung, intestines
Cerebrovascular accidents	Large- and small-vessel occlusion → thrombosis/bleeding (stroke); requires chronic transfusion
Acute chest syndrome	Infection, atelectasis, infarction, fat emboli, severe hypoxemia, infiltrate, dyspnea, absent breath sounds
Chronic lung disease	Pulmonary fibrosis, restrictive lung disease, cor pulmonale
Priapism	Causes eventual impotence; treated with transusion, oxygen, or corpora cavernosa–to–spongiosa shunt
Ocular	Retinopathy
Gallbladder disease	Bilirubin stones; cholecystitis
Renal	Hematuria, papillary necrosis, renal-concentrating defect; nephropathy
Cardiomyopathy	Heart failure (fibrosis)
Skeletal	Osteonecrosis (avascular) of femoral or humeral head
Leg ulceration	Seen in older patients
Infections	Functional asplenia, defects in properdin system; pneumococcal bacteremia, meningitis, and arthritis; deafness from meningitis in 35%; *Salmonella* and *Staphylococcus aureus* osteomyelitis; severe *Mycoplasma* pneumonia
Growth failure, delayed puberty	May respond to nutritional supplements
Psychologic problems	Narcotic addiction (rare), dependence unusual; chronic illness, chronic pain

CMV, Cytomegalovirus; *EBV*, Epstein-Barr virus; *G6PD*, glucose-6-phosphate dehydrogenase; *HIV*, human immunodeficiency virus.
*Clinical manifestations with sickle cell trait are unusual but include renal papillary necrosis (hematuria), sudden death on exertion, intraocular hyphema extension, and sickling in unpressurized airplanes.

especially *Streptococcus pneumoniae* and other pathogens (Table 14–10). The hallmark of infection is fever. The patient with a sickle cell syndrome who has a temperature greater than 38.5° C (101.5° F) must be evaluated immediately (see Chapter 10). Current precautions to prevent infections include prophylactic daily oral penicillin begun at diagnosis and vaccinations against pneumococcus, *H. influenzae* type b, hepatitis B virus, and influenza virus.

The anemia of SS disease is usually a chronic, moderately severe, compensated anemia that is not routinely transfusion dependent. The severity depends in part on the patient's phenotype (Table 14–9). Decisions about transfusion should be made on the basis of the patient's clinical condition, the he-

moglobin level, and the reticulocyte count. Manifestations of chronic anemia include jaundice, pallor, variable splenomegaly in infancy, a cardiac flow murmur, and delayed growth and sexual maturation (Table 14–10).

In three different clinical situations an acute, potentially life-threatening decline in the hemoglobin level may be superimposed on the chronic compensated anemia. *Splenic sequestration crisis* is a life-threatening, hyperacute fall in the hemoglobin level (blood volume) secondary to splenic pooling of the patient's red cells and sickling within the spleen. The spleen is moderately to markedly enlarged, and the reticulocyte count is elevated. In an *aplastic crisis*, parvovirus B19 infects red cell precursors in the bone marrow and induces transient red cell aplasia with reticulocytopenia and a rapid worsening of anemia. In the *hyperhemolytic crisis*, there may be an acute fall in hemoglobin, associated with medications or infection. The level of bilirubin increases, and reticulocytosis and accentuated jaundice may also occur. Patients with these conditions usually have G6PD deficiency. For sequestration, aplastic, and hemolytic crises, simple transfusion therapy is indicated when the anemia is symptomatic.

Vasoocclusive crises may occur in any organ of the body, where they are manifested by pain or significant dysfunction (Table 14–10). The *acute chest syndrome* is a vasoocclusive crisis within the lungs, often in association with infection and infarction. The patient may first complain of pain but within a few hours has cough, increasing respiratory and heart rates, hypoxia, and progressive respiratory distress. Physical examination of the chest reveals areas of decreased breath sounds and dullness to percussion. Treatment involves early recognition and prevention of arterial hypoxemia. Oxygen, fluids, judicious use of analgesic medications, antibiotics, and blood transfusion (occasionally exchange transfusion) usually are indicated in therapy for acute chest syndrome. Incentive spirometry reduces the incidence of acute chest crisis in patients having pain in the chest or abdomen.

Vasoocclusive events may also develop in patients within the central nervous system, causing clinical or "silent" *stroke*. These events may present as the sudden onset of an altered state of consciousness, seizures, or focal paralysis. *Priapism* occurs most typically in boys between 6 and 20 years of age. The child experiences sudden, painful onset of a tumescent penis that will not relax. Therapeutic steps for stroke, priapism, and other potentially life-threatening complications are the administration of oxygen, fluids, transfusion to achieve a hemoglobin S less than 30% (often by partial exchange transfusion), and analgesia when appropriate. Fluid management requires recognition that renal medullary infarction results in loss of the ability to concentrate urine. Vasoocclusive crises may lead to *avascular necrosis of the femoral head* and chronic hip disease.

Pain crisis is the most common type of vasoocclusive event. The pain usually localizes to the long bones of the arms or legs but may occur in smaller bones of the hands or feet in infancy. These painful crises usually last 2–7 days. The treatment of a pain crisis includes administration of fluids, analgesia (usually with narcotics or nonsteroidal antiinflammatory agents), oxygen if the patient is hypoxic, and monitoring of arterial oxygen saturation. The clinician must maintain a sympathetic attitude toward the patient in pain crisis because pain is impossible to quantitate and the risk for drug dependency is highly overrated.

Diagnosis. The diagnosis is made by identifying the precise amount and type(s) of hemoglobin present using hemoglobin electrophoresis, isoelectric focusing, or HPLC. Every member of an at-risk population should have a precise hemoglobin phenotype performed at birth (preferably) or during early infancy. Most states perform newborn screening for sickle cell disease.

Treatment. Direct therapy of sickle cell anemia is evolving. Hydroxyurea has been shown in adults and children to decrease the number and severity of vasoocclusive events. Bone marrow transplantation has cured a number of children with sickle cell disease.

METHEMOGLOBINEMIA. Methemoglobinemia, in which ferrous (Fe^{+2}) iron has been oxidized to the ferric (Fe^{+3}) state, may be either congenital or acquired. Congenital methemoglobinemia may be a result of abnormalities in either the alpha or beta chain. Homozygosity is lethal, whereas heterozygotes usually have a level of 20–30% methemoglobin and are cyanotic in the face of normal PaO_2. Homozygous deficiency of NADH reductase (diaphorase) is common in Navajo Indians and results in chronic methemoglobinemia. Infants under the age of 3 months, whose antioxidant mechanisms are poorly developed, are especially vulnerable.

Acquired methemoglobinemia is seen with ingestion of certain oxidants. Nitrates and nitrites, derived from fertilizer and disinfectants in well water and foods or from enteric bacteria during diarrhea, are major etiologic factors. If sufficiently severe, this condition may be life threatening. Methemoglobinemia should be suspected in a deeply cyanotic infant without cardiopulmonary disease in whom metabolic acidosis, a high PaO_2, and unsaturated hemoglobin are present. When drawn to measure methemoglobin levels, blood is often described as chocolate colored. Treatment with methylene blue or ascorbate usually rapidly reduces Fe^{3+} to Fe^{2+}, correcting this condition.

Hemolytic Anemia Caused by Disorders Extrinsic to the Red Cell

Immune-mediated hemolysis may be extravascular when red cells coated with antibodies or complement are phagocytosed by the reticuloendothelial system; the hemolysis may be intravascular when antibody binding leads to complement fixation and lysis of red blood cells.

Isoimmune hemolysis is caused by active maternal immunization against fetal antigens that the mother's erythrocytes do not express (see Chapter 6). Examples are antibodies to the A, B, and Rh D antigens, other Rh antigens, and the Kell, Duffy, and other blood groups. Anti-A and anti-B hemolysis is caused by the placental transfer of naturally occurring maternal antibodies from mothers who lack A or B antigen (usually blood type O). Positive results of the direct antiglobulin (Coombs) test on the baby's red cells (Fig. 14–6) and the indirect antiglobulin test on the mother's serum and the presence of spherocytes and immature erythroid precursors (erythroblastosis) on the infant's blood smear confirm this diagnosis. Isoimmune hemolytic disease is highly variable in its clinical severity. No clinical manifestations may be present, or the infant may exhibit jaundice, severe anemia, and hydrops fetalis.

Autoimmune hemolytic anemia (AIHA) is usually an acute, self-limited process that develops after an infection (e.g., *Mycoplasma,* Epstein-Barr, or other viral infections). More than 80% of children with AIHA spontaneously recover. AIHA also may be the presenting symptom of a chronic autoimmune disease (e.g., systemic lupus erythematosus [SLE], lymphoproliferative disorders, or immune deficiency). Transfusion is challenging because cross-matching is difficult, since the autoantibodies react with virtually all red cells. The peripheral blood smear usually reveals spherocytes and, occasionally, nucleated red cells. The reticulocyte count is variable because some patients have relatively low reticulocyte counts as a result of autoantibody that cross-reacts with red cell precursors. In addition to transfusion, which may be lifesaving, management of AIHA depends on antibody type. Management may involve administration of corticosteroids and, at times, intravenous immunoglobulin (IVIG). The corticosteroids reduce the clearance of the sensitized red cells in the spleen.

Drugs also may induce a Coombs-positive hemolytic anemia. Withdrawal of the drug usually leads to resolution of the hemolytic process. Drugs may form a hapten on the red cell membrane (such as with penicillin). Alternatively, drugs may form immune complexes (such as with quinidine) that attach to the red cell membrane. Antibodies then activate complement-induced intravascular hemolysis. The third type of drug-induced immune hemolysis occurs during treatment with alpha-methyldopa and a few other drugs. In this type, prolonged exposure to the drug alters the red blood cell membrane, inducing neoantigen formation. Antibodies are produced that bind to the neoantigen; this produces a positive antiglobulin test result far more commonly than it actually induces hemolysis. In each of these conditions the erythrocyte acts as an "innocent bystander."

A second form of acquired hemolytic disease that is not antibody mediated is caused by mechanical damage to the membrane of the red cells during circulation. In **microangiopathic hemolytic anemia** (MAHA) the red cells are trapped by fibrin strands in the circulation and physically broken by shear stress as they pass through these strands. Hemolytic-uremic syndrome (HUS), disseminated intravascular coagulation (DIC), thrombotic thrombocytopenic purpura, malignant hypertension, toxemia, and hyperacute renal graft rejection all produce MAHA.

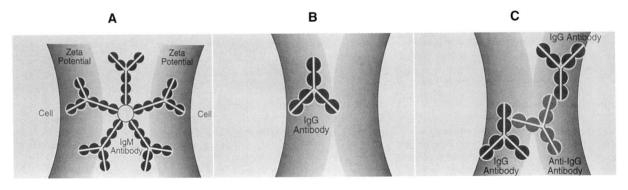

FIG. 14–6

Coombs or direct antiglobulin test (DAT). In the DAT, so-called Coombs sera that recognizes human immunoglobulin (Ig) or complement (C) is used to detect the presence of antibody or C on the surface of the red blood cells by agglutination. **A,** An IgM antibody can simultaneously bind two RBCs because of its multiple antigen-binding sites. The great size of the IgM allows it to bridge the surface repulsive forces (zeta potential) between RBCs and cause agglutination. **B,** An IgG antibody is too small to bridge the zeta potential and cause agglutination. **C,** On the addition of Coombs sera , the zeta potential is successfully bridged and RBCs agglutinate. (Modified from Ware RE, Rosse WF: Autoimmune hemolytic anemia. In Orkin SH, Nathan DG, editors: *Hematology of infancy and childhood,* ed 5, Philadelphia, 1998, WB Saunders.)

The platelets usually are large, indicating that they are young. These platelets have a decreased survival even if the numbers are normal. Consumption of clotting factors is more prominent in DIC than in the other forms of MAHA. The smear shows red cell fragments (schistocytes), microspherocytes, teardrop forms, and polychromasia. The red cells also may be damaged by exposure to nonendothelialized surfaces (e.g., as in artificial heart valves [the "Waring blender" syndrome]) or as a result of high flow and shear rates in giant hemangiomas **(Kasabach-Merritt syndrome).**

Alterations in the plasma lipids, especially cholesterol, may lead to damage to the red cell membrane and shorten red cell survival. Lipids in the plasma are in equilibrium with those in the red cell membrane; high cholesterol levels increase the membrane cholesterol and the total membrane surface without affecting the volume of the cell. This condition produces spur cells. The spur cells are seen in abetalipoproteinemia and liver diseases. Hemolysis occurs in the spleen, where poor red cell deformability results in erythrocyte destruction. *Circulating toxins* such as snake venoms and heavy metals (e.g., copper or arsenic) that bind sulfhydryl groups may damage the red cell membrane and induce hemolysis. Irregularly spiculated red cells (burr cells) are seen in renal failure. *Vitamin E deficiency* also can cause an acquired hemolytic anemia as a result of abnormal sensitivity of membrane lipids to oxidant stress. Vitamin E deficiency may occur in premature infants who are not being supplemented with vitamin E or who have insufficient nutrition, in severe malabsorption syndromes (including cystic fibrosis), and in transfusional iron overload, which can lead to severe oxidant exposure.

PANCYTOPENIA

Pancytopenia is a quantitative decrease in the formed elements of the blood—erythrocytes, leukocytes, and platelets. Patients more often exhibit symptoms of infection or bleeding than anemia because of the relatively short life span of white cells and platelets compared with that of red cells. Causes of pancytopenia include failure of production (implying intrinsic bone marrow disease), sequestration (as in hypersplenism), or increased peripheral destruction.

Features that suggest bone marrow failure and mandate an examination of bone marrow are a low reticulocyte count, teardrop forms of red cells (implying marrow replacement, not just failure), the presence of abnormal forms of leukocytes or myeloid elements less mature than band forms, small platelets, and an elevated mean corpuscular volume in the face of a low reticulocyte count. Pancytopenia re-

sulting from bone marrow failure is usually a gradual process. Patients may initially have one or two involved cell lines, but later progress to involvement of all three cell lines.

Features suggesting increased destruction are reticulocytosis, jaundice, immature erythroid or myeloid elements on the blood smear, large platelets, and increased serum bilirubin and lactic dehydrogenase.

APLASTIC ANEMIA

In the child with aplastic anemia, pancytopenia evolves as the hematopoietic elements of the bone marrow disappear and the marrow is replaced by fat. A biopsy is crucial to determine the extent of depletion of the hematopoietic elements. In developed countries, aplastic anemia is most often idiopathic. Alternatively, this disorder may be induced by such drugs as chloramphenicol and felbamate or by such toxins as benzene. Aplastic anemia also may follow infections, particularly hepatitis and infectious mononucleosis (Table 14–8).

Immune suppression of hematopoiesis is postulated to be an important mechanism in patients with postinfectious and idiopathic aplastic anemia. For children with severe aplastic anemia—defined by an RPI less than 1%, absolute neutrophil count less than 500/mm^3, platelet count less than 20,000/mm^3, and bone marrow cellularity on biopsy less than 10%—the *treatment* of choice is bone marrow transplantation from a human leukocyte antigen (HLA)–identical, mixed lymphocyte–compatible sibling. With supportive care alone, survival is only about 20% in severe aplastic anemia, although the duration of survival may be years when vigorous blood product and antibiotic support is provided. When bone marrow transplantation takes place before the recipient is sensitized to blood products, the survival rate is in excess of 80%. The treatment of aplastic anemia without an HLA-matched donor for transplantation is evolving, with two major options: potent immunosuppressive therapy or either unrelated or partially matched bone marrow transplantation (Table 14–8). Results of trials using antithymocyte globulin, cyclosporine, and corticosteroids in combination with hematopoietic growth factors have been encouraging. Such therapy is often toxic, and relapses do occur.

Fanconi anemia, a constitutional aplastic anemia, usually presents in the latter half of the first decade of life and may evolve over a period of years. A group of genetic defects in proteins involved in DNA repair have been identified in Fanconi anemia. A diagnosis of Fanconi anemia is based on demonstration of increased chromosomal breakage after exposure of cells to agents that damage DNA. The repair mechanism for DNA damage is abnormal in all cells in Fanconi anemia, which may contribute to the development of malignancies (terminal acute leukemia develops in 10% of cases). Patients with Fanconi anemia have a number of characteristic clinical findings (Table 14–8). Most patients with Fanconi anemia and about 20% of children with aplastic anemia appear to respond for a time to androgenic therapy, which unfortunately induces masculinization and may cause liver injury and liver tumors. Androgenic therapy increases red cell synthesis and may diminish transfusion requirements. The effect on granulocytes, and especially the platelet count, is less impressive.

Marrow Replacement

Marrow replacement may occur as a result of leukemia, solid tumors (especially neuroblastoma), storage diseases, osteopetrosis in infants, and myelofibrosis, which is rare in childhood. The mechanisms by which malignant cells impair marrow synthesis of normal hemopoietic elements are unclear. Bone marrow aspirate and biopsy are needed for precise diagnosis that then determines appropriate therapy.

Pancytopenia Resulting From Destruction of Cells

Pancytopenia resulting from destruction of cells may be caused by intramedullary destruction of hemopoietic elements (as occurs in myeloproliferative disorders and in deficiencies of folic acid and vitamin B_{12}) or by the peripheral destruction of mature cells. The usual site of peripheral destruction of blood cells is the spleen, although the liver and other parts of the reticuloendothelial system may participate. *Hypersplenism* may be the result of anatomic causes such as portal hypertension or splenic hypertrophy from thalassemia, infections (including malaria), storage diseases such as Gaucher disease, lymphomas, or histiocytosis. Splenectomy is indicated only when the pancytopenia is of clinical significance. An example of this is seen when the condition causes the patients to have increased susceptibility to bleeding or infection or produces high transfusion requirements.

REFERENCES

Alter BP: Arms and the man or hands and the child: congenital anomalies and hematologic syndromes, *J Pediatr Hematol Oncol* 19(4):287–291, 1997.
Ball SE: The modern management of severe aplastic anaemia, *Br J Haematol* 110(1):41–53, 2000.
Behrman RE, Kliegman RM, Jenson HB, editors: *Nelson textbook of pediatrics*, ed 16, Philadelphia, 2000, WB Saunders, Chapters 452–475.
Beutler E: Glucose-6-phosphate dehydrogenese deficiency, *N Engl J Med* 324(3):169–174, 1991.
Boutry M, Needlman R: Use of diet history in the screening of iron deficiency, *Pediatrics* 98(6 Pt 1):1138–1142, 1996.
Cherrick I, Karayalcin G, Lanzkowsky P: Transient erythroblastopenia of childhood, *Am J Pediatr Hematol Oncol* 16(4):320–324, 1994.
Delhommeau F, Cynober T, Schischmanoff PO, et al: Natural history of hereditary spherocytosis during the first year of life, *Blood* 95(2):393–397, 2000.
Ehlers KH, Giardina PJ, Lesser ML, et al: Prolonged survival in patients with beta-thalassemia major treated with deferoxamine, *J Pediatr* 118(4 Pt 1):540–545, 1991.
Embury SH, Hebbel RP, Mohandas N, et al, editors: *Sickle cell disease: basic principles and clinical practice,* ed 1, New York, 1994, Raven Press.
Goodnough L, Mark T, Andriole G: Erythropoietin therapy, *N Engl J Med* 336(13):933–938, 1997.
Kaushansky K: Thrombopoietin: the primary regulator of platelet production, *Blood* 86(2):419–431, 1995.
Kwiatkowski JL, West TB, Heidary N, et al: Severe iron deficiency anemia in young children, *J Pediatr* 135(4):514–516, 1999.
Miller ST, Sleeper LA, Pegelow CH, et al: Prediction of adverse outcomes in children with sickle cell disease, *N Engl J Med* 342(2):83–89, 2000.
Sears DA: Anemia of chronic disease, *Med Clin North Am* 76(3):567–579, 1992.
Steinberg MH: Management of sickle cell disease, *N Engl J Med* 340(13):1021–1030, 1999.
Walters MC, Patience M, Leisenring W, et al: Bone marrow transplantation for sickle cell disease, *N Engl J Med* 335(6):369–376, 1996.
Weatherall D: The hereditary anemias, *BMJ* 314(7079):492–496, 1997.

DISORDERS OF LEUKOCYTES

The major function of phagocytic cells is to ingest and kill pathogens (see Chapters 8 and 10). The major manifestation of neutropenia or neutrophil dysfunction is increased susceptibility to infection with bacteria, fungi, or both.

Neutropenia

The normal neutrophil count varies with age (Table 14–2). Neutropenia is defined as an absolute neutrophil count (ANC) less than $1500/mm^3$ for Caucasian children older than 1 year of age. Black children normally have somewhat lower total white count and neutrophil counts.

The effect of neutropenia depends on its severity. The susceptibility to infection is unaffected until the (ANC) is less than $1000/mm^3$. Patients do quite well as long as the ANC is greater than $500/mm^3$. At these levels of circulating neutrophils, localized infections are more common than generalized bacteremia. With an ANC less than $200/mm^3$, serious bacterial infections are common. Episodes of bacteremia also are associated with the presence of indwelling catheters, mucosal injury secondary to cytotoxic agents, and immunosuppressive agents. The presence of an underlying malignancy, treatment with chemotherapy, or immunodeficiency disorder also increases the risk for serious bacterial or fungal infection. In the absence of an adequate neutrophil count, migration of neutrophils to areas of damage in the skin and mucous membrane is delayed. The major types of infection associated with neutropenia are cellulitis, pharyngitis, gingivitis, lymphadenitis, abscesses (cutaneous or perianal), enteritis (typhlitis), and pneumonia. The sites of the infection usually are colonized heavily with normal bacterial flora that become invasive in the presence of neutropenia. Meticulous attention to oral and skin hygiene and prevention of colonization with fungi are helpful in minimizing such infections.

Neutropenia may be congenital or acquired. Neutropenia may be classified mechanistically (Table 14–11) and commonly may be associated with specific diseases, especially infections (Table 14–12), or drugs (Table 14–13).

Congenital Neutropenia

Most congenital neutropenias are caused by an inadequate production of cells. Severe congenital neutropenia **(Kostmann syndrome)** is inherited as an autosomal recessive disorder and may present in infancy. In severe congenital neutropenia, myeloid cells within the marrow fail to mature beyond the very early stages of the promyelocyte. The peripheral blood may show an impressive monocytosis. G-CSF levels are increased;

TABLE 14–11
Mechanisms of Neutropenia

Abnormal Bone Marrow
Marrow Injury
Drugs: idiosyncratic, cytotoxic (myelosuppressive)
Radiation
Chemicals: DDT, benzene
Hereditary
Immune-mediated: T and B cell and immunoglobulin
Infection: HIV, hepatitis
Infiltrative processes: tumor, storage disease
Maturation Defects
Folic acid deficiency
Vitamin B_{12}
Glycogen storage disease type Ib
Shwachman syndrome
Organic acidemias
Clonal disorders: congenital
Cyclic neutropenia

Peripheral Circulation
Pseudoneutropenia: Shift to Bone Marrow
Hereditary
Severe infection
Intravascular
Destruction: neonatal isoimmune, autoimmune, hypersplenism
Leukoagglutination: lung, after cardiac bypass surgery

Extravascular Mechanisms
Increased utilization: severe infection, anaphylaxis
Destruction: antibody-mediated, hypersplenism

Adapted from Bagby G: In Andreoli TE, Bennett JC, Carpenter CC, et al, editors: *Cecil essentials of medicine*, ed 4, Philadelphia, 1997, WB Saunders.
DDT, Chlorophenothane; *HIV*, human immunodeficiency virus.

TABLE 14–12
Infections Associated with Neutropenia

Bacterial
Typhoid-paratyphoid
Brucellosis
Neonatal sepsis
Meningococcemia
Overwhelming sepsis
Congenital syphilis
Tuberculosis

Viral
Measles
Hepatitis A and B
HIV
Rubella
CMV
Influenza A and B
Epstein-Barr virus

Rickettsial
Rocky Mountain spotted fever
Typhus
Ehrlichiosis
Rickettsialpox

CMV, Cytomegalovirus; *HIV*, human immunodeficiency virus.

TABLE 14–13
Drugs Associated With Neutropenia

Cytotoxic
Myelosuppressive, chemotherapeutic agents
Immunosuppressive agents

Idiosyncratic
Chloramphenicol
Sulfonamides
Propylthiouracil
Penicillins
Trimethoprim and sulfamethoxazole
Carbamazepine
Phenytoin
Cimetidine
Methyldopa
Indomethacin
Chlorpromazine
Penicillamine
Gold salts

---

nevertheless, exogenous G-CSF (filgrastim) produces a rise in the neutrophil count. Treatment with G-CSF has revolutionized the care of these children. Acute myeloid leukemia has developed in a few patients who have survived into adolescence. Bone marrow transplantation may be curative.

Severe congenital neutropenia that may be either persistent or cyclic is also a component of the syndrome of *pancreatic insufficiency accompanying bone marrow dysfunction* (**Shwachman-Diamond syndrome**). This is a panmyeloid disorder in which neutropenia is the most prominent manifestation. In this autosomal recessive condition patients may have all the common complications of neutropenia. A major complication is gingivitis, which may be severe and lead to serious oral infections and alveolar bone destruction. Patients may become edentulous at an early age. Metaphyseal dysostosis and dwarfism also may occur. Patients usually respond to G-CSF.

Other congenital neutropenias caused by deficient production of neutrophils vary in severity and are poorly characterized. *Benign congenital neutropenia* is a functional diagnosis for patients with significant neutropenia in whom major infectious complications do not develop. Many patients whose ANC ranges from 100–500/mm^3 have an increased frequency of infections, particularly respiratory infections, but the major problem is the slow resolution of the infections that develop. These disorders may be sporadic or familial and in some instances are transmitted as an autosomal dominant disorder. Se-

vere congenital neutropenia may also be associated with immune deficiency in *reticular dysgenesis* or congenital anomalies in *cartilage-hair hypoplasia.*

Cyclic neutropenia may be transmitted as an autosomal dominant, recessive, or sporadic disorder. This is a stem cell disorder in which all marrow elements cycle. However, the only clinically significant abnormality is neutropenia because of the short half-life of neutrophils (6–7 hours) in comparison with platelets (10 days) and red cells (120 days). The usual neutropenic cycle is 21 days, with agranulocytosis lasting 4–6 days, accompanied by monocytosis and often by eosinophilia. Clinical manifestations are stomatitis or oral ulcers, pharyngitis, lymphadenopathy, fever, and cellulitis at the time of neutropenia. Severe, debilitating bone pain is common in these patients when the neutrophil count is low. Cyclic neutropenia responds to G-CSF with a reduced number of days of neutropenia and an overall increase of neutrophils.

Acquired Neutropenia

Neutropenia may be caused by either decreased marrow production or peripheral neutrophil destruction. *Isoimmune neutropenia* occurs in up to 3% of neonates and is the result of transplacental transfer of maternal antibodies to fetal neutrophil antigens. In isoimmune neonatal neutropenia the mother is sensitized to specific neutrophil antigens (NA1, NA2, NB1, and NC1) on fetal leukocytes that are inherited from the father and not present on maternal cells. Isoimmune neonatal neutropenia, like isoimmune anemia and thrombocytopenia (see Chapter 6), is a transient process. Early treatment of infection (cutaneous is most common; sepsis is rarer) while the infant is neutropenic is the major goal of therapy. Administration of IVIG may decrease the duration of neutropenia.

Autoimmune neutropenia usually develops early in childhood (5–24 months of age) and often persists for prolonged periods. Neutrophil autoantibodies may be immunoglobulin (IgG, IgM, IgA, or a combination of these). Usually the condition resolves in 6 months to 4 years. Clinical symptoms may dictate treatment. Although IVIG or corticosteroids have been used in the past, most patients respond to G-CSF. Most patients do not progress to more generalized autoimmune disorders; however, rarely autoimmune neutropenia may be an early manifestation of SLE or rheumatoid arthritis. The marrow in autoimmune neutropenia and SLE shows myeloid hyperplasia, except that if antibody is directed against myeloid precursors, it reveals hypoplasia. The *differential diagnosis* of autoimmune neutropenia includes SLE, rheumatoid arthritis (Felty syndrome), immune deficiency, or drug-induced neutropenia.

Neutropenia is common in *stressed neonates*. Virtually any major illness, including asphyxia, may precipitate transient neonatal neutropenia. Maternal conditions such as hypertension and eclampsia can induce neonatal neutropenia. Significant neutropenia may develop in infected neonates, at least in part on the basis of depletion of bone marrow stores. The bone marrow stores, which are seven times as great as the circulating pool of neutrophils in adults, are far less extensive in neonates. Therefore, infectious processes readily deplete their marrow reserve.

Diagnosis. Neutropenia is confirmed by a complete blood count and differential. The evaluation of the neutropenic child depends on associated clinical abnormalities, such as signs of infection, family and medication history, age of the patient, cyclic or persistent nature of the condition, signs of bone marrow infiltration (e.g., malignancy or storage disease), and evidence of involvement of other cell lines. An algorithm for the workup of the child with neutropenia is presented in Fig. 14–7.

Treatment. Therapy for neutropenia depends on the underlying cause. Patients with severe bacterial infections require broad-spectrum antibiotics; the resolution of neutropenia during an infection is a good prognostic sign. Most patients with severe congenital neutropenia or autoimmune neutropenia respond to therapy with G-CSF. Granulocyte transfu-

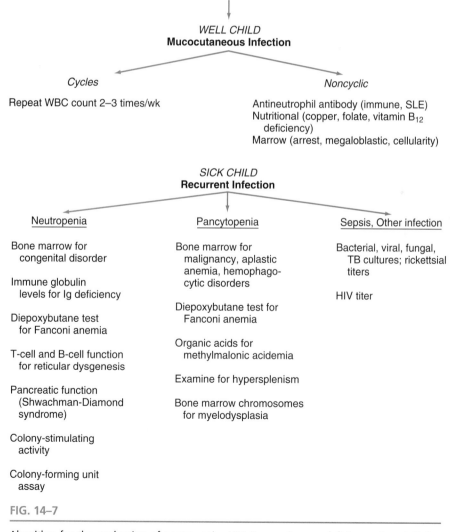

FIG. 14–7

Algorithm for the evaluation of neutropenia. *HIV,* Human immunodeficiency virus; *IgG,* immunoglobulin G; *SLE,* systemic lupus erythematosus; *TB,* tuberculosis; *WBC,* white blood cell.

sion should be reserved for life-threatening infection; even with transfusion, the results of these cases have been disappointing. Chronic mild neutropenia not associated with immunosuppression can be managed expectantly with prompt antimicrobial treatment of soft tissue infections (e.g., *Staphylococcus aureus* or *Streptococcus*).

Leukocytosis (Neutrophilia)

Leukocytosis most often is associated with infection (>15,000 WBCs/mm³). When acute infection occurs, particularly bacterial infection, neutrophils are released from bone marrow stores to induce a rapid increase in the circulating WBC count. Chronic infection, such as tuberculosis, osteomyelitis, and abscesses, also may cause neutrophilia. A shift in the distribution of the cells, with a greater number circulating than adhering to blood vessel walls, is a common mechanism for neutrophilia associated with drugs, including corticosteroids and epinephrine. Certain disorders of neutrophil function, especially the lack of the adhesion receptor CD18, are associated with a marked leukocytosis. Leukocytosis also may be a normal variant in some families in which several members have an increase in total neutrophil counts without an apparent underlying pathologic condition. Chronic myelogenous leukemia also is characterized by neutrophilia. However, immature forms of granulocytes usually are present.

Defects In Neutrophil Function

Defects in neutrophil function are relatively rare inherited disorders and tend to be associated with a marked susceptibility to bacterial infection (see Chapter 8). Congenital functional defects in neutrophil adhesion, intracellular signaling, interaction with cytokines, intracellular killing, and granule formation have been discovered recently and characterized on a molecular and functional basis. Acquired disorders of neutrophil function also occur and may be quite severe.

Neutrophils normally adhere to endothelium and migrate to areas of inflammation by the interaction of membrane proteins called integrins and selectins with endothelial cell adhesion molecules. In *leukocyte adhesion deficiency,* infants lacking the β₂ integrin CD18 exhibit the condition early in infancy with failure of separation of the umbilical cord, often until as late as 2 months after birth, with attendant omphalitis and sepsis. The neutrophil count usually is greater than 20,000/mm³ because of failure of the neutrophils to adhere normally to vascular endothe-

lium and to migrate out of blood to the tissues. Cutaneous, respiratory, and mucosal infections occur, and children with this condition usually have severe gingivitis. Sepsis usually leads to death in early childhood. This disorder is transmitted as an autosomal recessive trait that has an unknown frequency. Bone marrow transplantation may be lifesaving.

Defective bacterial killing of catalase-positive organisms, because the phagocytes are unable to generate reactive oxygen species such as hydrogen peroxide, hydroxyl radical, and superoxide anion, is the major feature of **chronic granulomatous disease** (see Chapter 8). Nonoxidative killing is abnormal in *secondary granule deficiency,* a rare disorder in which bacterial killing also is delayed. An acquired form of secondary granule deficiency occurs in patients with severe burn injuries; it occurs about 2 weeks after the original trauma. This poor killing ability may contribute to the increased susceptibility to bacterial infection of burn patients (see Chapter 3). The acquired defect is reversible.

Another abnormality of secondary granules is **Chédiak-Higashi syndrome,** an autosomal recessive disorder caused by a mutation in a cytoplasmic protein involved in protein transport, resulting in fusion of the primary and secondary granules of the neutrophil. Giant granules are present in many cells, including lymphocytes, platelets, and melanocytes. Patients usually have partial oculocutaneous albinism. Although most patients have frequent fevers in infancy and early childhood, documented bacterial infection is not common. Infection with the Epstein-Barr virus (EBV) produces a loss of natural killer cells and results in a **lymphoproliferative syndrome,** characterized by hepatomegaly, adenopathy, and pancytopenia. This may lead to an accelerated phase, which usually is rapidly fatal. Children who avoid EBV infection may live into adulthood without major clinical problems, except for gingivitis.

A variety of conditions also are associated with chemotactic defects in neutrophils. **Job syndrome** usually is acquired and may be seen in childhood. The major manifestations are eczema, hyperimmunoglobulinemia E, an extrinsic chemotactic defect, a T-cell defect with reduced interferon production, and recurrent "cold" boils (from *S. aureus*) that do not become markedly red or drain. In some patients, identifying offending allergens or removing the allergens has resulted in resolution of the chemotactic defect, as well as resolution of the eczema and boils. Several systemic disorders, including uremia, SLE, Hodgkin disease, liver disease, and poorly controlled diabetes mellitus, also have associated chemotactic defects.

REFERENCES

Behrman RE, Kliegman RM, Jenson HB, editors: *Nelson textbook of pediatrics*, ed 16, Philadelphia, 2000, WB Saunders, Chapters 127–132.

Bernini JC: Diagnosis and management of chronic neutropenia in childhood, *Pediatr Clin North Am* 43(3):773–792, 1996.

Bux J, Behrens G, Jaeger G, et al: Diagnosis and clinical course of autoimmune neutropenia in infancy: analysis of 240 cases, *Blood* 91(1):181–186, 1998.

Carr R: Neutrophil production and function in newborn infants, *Br J Haematol* 110(1):18–28, 2000.

Jonsson OG, Buchanan GR: Chronic neutropenia during childhood: a 13-year experience in a single institution, *Am J Dis Child* 145(2):232–235, 1991.

Lekstrom–Himes JA, Gallin JI: Immunodeficiency disease caused by defects in phagocytes, *N Engl J Med* 343(23):1703–1714, 2000.

HEMOSTATIC DISORDERS

Normal Hemostasis

Hemostasis is the dynamic process by which coagulation occurs on areas of vascular injury. Hemostasis is limited to areas of injury; the clot does not extend beyond the initial site of vascular damage. This process involves the carefully modulated interaction of platelets, vascular wall, and procoagulant and anticoagulant proteins. After an injury to the vascular endothelium, subendothelial collagen induces a conformational change in von Willebrand factor, an adhesive protein to which platelets bind via their glycoprotein Ib receptor. After adhesion, platelets undergo activation and release a number of intracellular contents, including adenosine diphosphate (ADP), that subsequently induce aggregation of additional platelets. Simultaneously tissue factor, collagen, and other matrix proteins in the tissue activate the coagulation cascade, leading to the formation of the enzyme thrombin (Fig. 14–8). Thrombin has multiple effects on the coagulation mechanism, such as further aggregation of platelets, a positive feedback activation of factors V and VIII, the conversion of fibrinogen to fibrin, and the activation of factor XIII. Thrombin also contributes to the eventual limitation of clot size by binding to the endothelial cell protein thrombomodulin, thereby converting protein C into activated protein C. Thrombin contributes to the eventual lysis of the thrombus by activating plasminogen to plasmin (Fig. 14–9). The platelet plug forms and bleeding ceases, usually within 3–7 minutes. The generation of thrombin leads

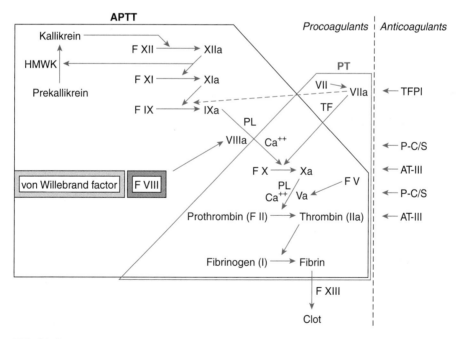

FIG. 14–8

Simplified pathways of blood coagulation. The area inside the solid black line is the intrinsic pathway, measured by the activated partial thromboplastin time (APTT). The area inside the green line is the extrinsic pathway, measured by the prothrombin time (PT). The area encompassed by both lines is the common pathway. *AT-III*, Antithrombin III; *F*, factor; *HMWK*, high-molecular-weight kininogen; *P-C/S*, protein C/S; *TFPI*, tissue factor pathway inhibitor. (Adapted from Montgomery RR, Scott JP. In Behrman RE, Kliegman RM, Jenson HB, editors: *Nelson textbook of pediatrics*, ed 16, Philadelphia, 2000, WB Saunders.)

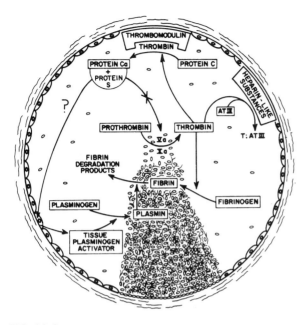

FIG. 14–9

Formation of the hemostatic plug at the site of vascular injury. Three major physiologic anticoagulant mechanisms, antithrombin III (AT III), protein C, and the fibrinolytic system, are activated to limit clot formation to the site of damage and to prevent generalized thrombosis. *T*, Thrombin. (From Schafer A: *Ann Intern Med* 102[6]:814–828, 1985.)

to formation of a permanent clot by the activation of factor XIII, which cross-links fibrin and results in a stable thrombus. These two processes are closely interwoven and occur on the biologic surfaces that mediate coagulation: the platelet, the endothelial cell, and the subendothelium. As a final element to this process, contractile elements within the platelet mediate clot retraction.

Although it is convenient to think of coagulation as having "intrinsic" and "extrinsic" pathways, the reality is that these pathways are closely interactive and do not react independently (Fig. 14–8). In vivo, factor VII autocatalyzes, forming small amounts of VIIa. When tissue is injured, tissue factor is released and causes a burst of VIIa generation. In vivo, tissue factor, in combination with calcium and factor VIIa, activates both factor IX and X. The major physiologic pathway is the activation of factor IX by factor VIIa, with eventual generation of thrombin. Thrombin then feeds back on factor XI, generating factor XIa, and accelerates thrombin formation. This explains why deficiency of factor VIII or IX leads to severe bleeding disorders, whereas deficiency of factor XI is usually mild, and deficiency of factor XII is asymptomatic.

As the procoagulant proteins are activated, a series of inhibitory factors serve to tightly regulate the activation of coagulation (Fig. 14–9). Antithrombin

III inactivates thrombin and factors Xa, IXa, and XIa. The protein C and protein S system inactivates the activated factors V and VIII, which are cofactors localized in the "tenase" and "prothrombinase" complexes. The tissue factor pathway inhibitor (TFPI), an anticoagulant protein, limits the activation of the coagulation cascade by factors VIIa and Xa. *Fibrinolysis* is initiated by the action of tissue plasminogen activator (TPA) on plasminogen, producing plasmin, the active enzyme that degrades fibrin into split products (Fig. 14–9). Fibrinolysis eventually dissolves the clot and allows normal flow to resume.

Approach to the Patient with a Hemostatic Disorder

Patients with hemostatic disorders may have complaints of either bleeding or clotting. A careful history and physical examination are crucial to the diagnosis of a bleeding or clotting disorder. Age at onset of bleeding indicates whether the problem is congenital or acquired. The sites of bleeding (mucocutaneous or deep) and degree of trauma (spontaneous or significant) required to induce injury suggest the type and severity of the disorder. Finally, certain medications (e.g., aspirin and valproic acid) are known to exacerbate preexisting bleeding disorders by interfering with platelet function.

A detailed *family history* is quite important. In the investigation of thrombotic disorders a personal and family history of early-onset stroke, heart attack, cutaneous thrombosis, and blood clots in the legs or lungs suggests a hereditary predisposition to thromboses. *Physical examination* should characterize the presence of cutaneous, synovial, and mucosal bleeding, in addition to deeper sites of hemorrhage. Evidence of malignancy (e.g., lymphadenopathy or hepatosplenomegaly) or chronic hepatic or renal disease also should be sought. The term *petechiae* refers to a nonblanching lesion less than 2 mm in size. *Purpura* is a group of adjoining petechiae, *ecchymoses* are isolated lesions larger than petechiae, and *hematomas* are raised ecchymoses.

Screening laboratory studies after the history and physical examination should include those in Table 14–14. No single laboratory test can screen for all bleeding disorders. Common causes of bleeding are shown in Fig. 14–10, and a brief differential diagnosis of hemostatic disorders is outlined in Fig. 14–11.

Disorders of Platelets
Thrombocytopenia
(Figs. 14–10 and 14–11)
Platelet counts below 150,000/mm³ constitute thrombocytopenia. Mucocutaneous bleeding is the hallmark of platelet disorders, including thrombocytopenia.

TABLE 14–14
Screening Tests for Bleeding Disorders

Test	Mechanism Tested	Normal Values	Disorder
Prothrombin time (PT)	Extrinsic and common pathway	<12 sec beyond neonate; 12–18 sec in term neonate	Defect in vitamin K–dependent factors; hemorrhagic disease of newborn, malabsorption, liver disease, DIC, oral anticoagulants, ingestion of rat poison
Activated partial thromboplastin time (APTT; PTT)	Intrinsic and common pathway	25–40 sec beyond neonate; 70 sec in term neonate	Hemophilia; von Willebrand disease, heparin; DIC; deficient factors XII and XI; lupus anticoagulant
Thrombin time (TT)	Fibrinogen to fibrin conversion	10–15 sec beyond neonate; 12–17 sec in term neonate	Fibrin split products, DIC, hypofibrinogenemia, heparin, uremia
Bleeding time (BT)	Hemostasis, capillary and platelet function	3–7 min beyond neonate	Platelet dysfunction, thrombocytopenia, von Willebrand disease, aspirin
Platelet count	Platelet number	150,000–450,000/mm^3	Thrombocytopenia differential diagnosis (Fig. 14-10)
Blood smear	Platelet number and size; RBC morphology	—	Large platelets suggest peripheral destruction; fragmented, bizarre RBC morphology suggests microangiopathic process (e.g., hemolytic-uremic syndrome, hemangioma, DIC)

DIC, Disseminated intravascular coagulation; *RBC,* red blood cell.

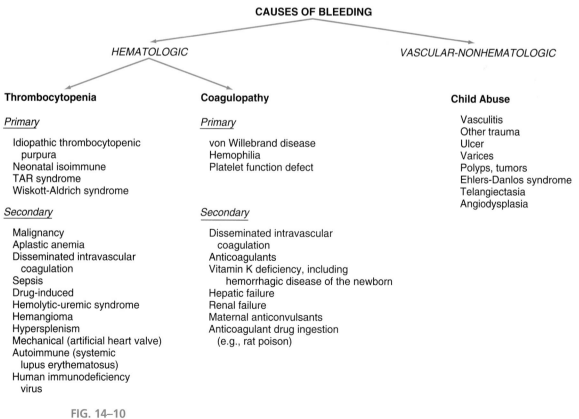

CAUSES OF BLEEDING

HEMATOLOGIC

Thrombocytopenia

Primary

Idiopathic thrombocytopenic purpura
Neonatal isoimmune
TAR syndrome
Wiskott-Aldrich syndrome

Secondary

Malignancy
Aplastic anemia
Disseminated intravascular coagulation
Sepsis
Drug-induced
Hemolytic-uremic syndrome
Hemangioma
Hypersplenism
Mechanical (artificial heart valve)
Autoimmune (systemic lupus erythematosus)
Human immunodeficiency virus

Coagulopathy

Primary

von Willebrand disease
Hemophilia
Platelet function defect

Secondary

Disseminated intravascular coagulation
Anticoagulants
Vitamin K deficiency, including hemorrhagic disease of the newborn
Hepatic failure
Renal failure
Maternal anticonvulsants
Anticoagulant drug ingestion (e.g., rat poison)

VASCULAR-NONHEMATOLOGIC

Child Abuse

Vasculitis
Other trauma
Ulcer
Varices
Polyps, tumors
Ehlers-Danlos syndrome
Telangiectasia
Angiodysplasia

FIG. 14–10

Common causes of bleeding. *TAR,* Thrombocytopenia with absence of radius.

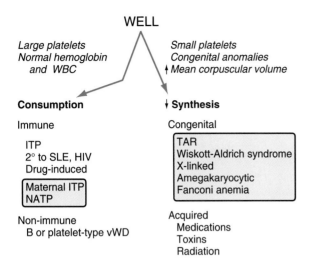

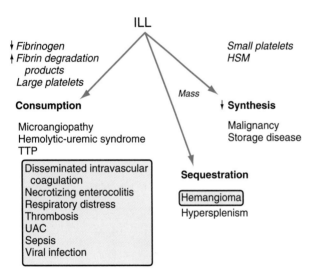

FIG. 14–11

Differential diagnosis of childhood thrombocytopenic syndromes. The syndromes are initially separated by their clinical appearances. Clues leading to the diagnosis are presented in italics. The mechanisms and common disorders leading to these findings are shown in the lower part of the figure. Disorders that commonly affect neonates are listed in the shaded boxes. *HIV,* Human immunodeficiency virus; *HSM,* hepatosplenomegaly; *ITP,* idiopathic immune thrombocytopenic purpura; *NATP,* neonatal alloimmune thrombocytopenic purpura; *SLE,* systemic lupus erythematosus; *TAR,* thrombocytopenia–absent radius (syndrome); *TTP,* thrombotic thrombocytopenic purpura; *UAC,* umbilical artery catheter; *WBC,* white blood cell. (From Scott JP: Bleeding and thrombosis. In Kliegman RM, Nieder ML, Super DM, editors: *Practical strategies in pediatric diagnosis and therapy,* Philadelphia, 1996, WB Saunders.)

However, the risk of bleeding correlates imperfectly with the platelet count. In general, children with platelet counts greater than 80,000/mm³ are able to withstand all but the most extreme hemostatic challenges, such as surgery or major trauma. In contrast, children with platelet counts less than 20,000/mm³ are at risk for spontaneous bleeding. These generalizations are modified by factors such as the age of the platelets (young, large platelets usually function better than old ones) and the presence of inhibitors of platelet function such as antibodies, drugs (especially aspirin), fibrin degradation products, and toxins in hepatic or renal disease.

The *etiology* of thrombocytopenia may be organized into disorders of (1) decreased platelet production, (2) increased destruction, and (3) sequestration.

Thrombocytopenia Resulting from Decreased Platelet Production. Primary disorders of megakaryopoiesis are rare in childhood, other than as part of an aplastic syndrome. **Thrombocytopenia with absent radii (TAR) syndrome** is characterized by severe thrombocytopenia in association with orthopedic abnormalities, especially of the upper extremity. The thrombocytopenia usually improves over time.

Acquired thrombocytopenia as a result of decreased production is rarely an isolated finding. It is more often seen in the context of *pancytopenia resulting from bone marrow failure* caused by infiltrative or aplastic processes. Certain chemotherapeutic agents may selectively affect megakaryocytes more than other marrow elements. *Cyanotic congenital heart disease with polycythemia* often is associated with thrombocytopenia, but this is rarely severe or associated with significant clinical bleeding. Both congenital (TORCH) and acquired *viral infections* (e.g., human immunodeficiency virus [HIV], EBV, and measles) and some *drugs* (e.g., anticonvulsants, antibiotics, cytotoxic agents, heparin, and quinidine) may induce thrombocytopenia. Postnatal infections and drug reactions usually cause transient thrombocytopenia, whereas congenital infections may produce prolonged suppression of bone marrow function.

Thrombocytopenia Resulting from Peripheral Destruction. In a child who appears well, immune-mediated mechanisms are the most common cause of thrombocytopenia. Thrombocytopenia results from increased rates of antibody-dependent platelet destruction. **Neonatal alloimmune thrombocytopenic purpura** (NATP) occurs as a result of sensitization of the mother to antigens present on fetal platelets during gestation. Antibodies cross the placenta and attack the fetal platelet (see Chapter 6). Many platelet alloantigens have been identified and sequenced, permitting prenatal diagnosis of the condition in an at-risk fetus. Mothers with **idiopathic thrombocytopenic purpura** (ITP) or with a history of ITP may have passive transfer of antiplatelet antibodies that react with fetal platelets, with resultant neonatal thrombocytopenia (see Chapter 6). The maternal platelet count is sometimes a useful indicator of the probability that the infant will be affected. If the mother has had a splenectomy, the maternal platelet count may be normal and is a poor predictor of the likelihood of severe neonatal thrombocytopenia, because maternal antibody will trigger destruction of the fetal platelets in the fetal spleen. The infant with NATP is at risk for intracranial hemorrhage, both in utero and during the immediate delivery process. In ITP the greatest risk appears to be present during passage through the birth canal, during which molding of the head may induce intracranial hemorrhage. Fetal scalp sampling or percutaneous umbilical blood sampling may be performed to measure the fetal platelet count. Administration of IVIG before delivery has been shown to be effective in raising fetal platelet counts and may alleviate thrombocytopenia in the infant in both NATP and ITP. Delivery by cesarean section is recommended to prevent CNS bleeding (see Chapter 6). Those neonates with severe thrombocytopenia (platelet counts <20,000) may be treated with IVIG or corticosteroids until the period of thrombocytopenia remits. If necessary, infants with NATP may receive washed maternal platelets.

The **Wiskott-Aldrich syndrome** is an X-linked disorder characterized by hypogammaglobinemia, eczema, and thrombocytopenia caused by a molecular defect in a cytoskeletal protein common to both lymphocytes and platelets (see Chapter 8). The platelets are seen to be small on a peripheral blood smear. Nevertheless, thrombocytopenia is often improved by splenectomy. Bone marrow transplantation results in a complete cure of the immunodeficiency and thrombocytopenia. Familial X-linked thrombocytopenia is a variant of Wiskott-Aldrich syndrome.

Autoimmune thrombocytopenic purpura of childhood (childhood ITP) is a common disorder in children that usually follows an acute viral infection. Childhood ITP is caused by an antibody (IgG or IgM) that binds to the platelet membrane. The condition results in splenic destruction of antibody-coated platelets. Rarely, ITP may be the presenting symptom of an autoimmune disease such as SLE. Approximately 80% of children have a spontaneous resolution of ITP within 6 months after diagnosis. Young children typically exhibit the condition 1–4 weeks after viral illness, with abrupt onset of petechiae, purpura, and epistaxis. The thrombocytopenia usually is severe. Significant adenopathy or hepatosplenomegaly is unusual, and the red cell and white cell counts are normal. Diagnosis of ITP

usually does not require a bone marrow examination. If atypical findings are noted, however, marrow examination is indicated to rule out an infiltrative disorder (e.g., leukemia) or an aplastic process (e.g., aplastic anemia). In ITP an examination of the bone marrow reveals increased megakaryocytes and normal erythroid and myeloid elements.

Serious bleeding, especially intracranial bleeding, occurs in fewer than 1% of patients with ITP. Therapy is seldom indicated for platelet counts greater than 30,000/mm³. Therapy does not affect the long-term outcome of ITP but is intended to raise the platelet count acutely. For clinical bleeding or severe thrombocytopenia (platelet count <20,000/mm³), therapeutic options include prednisone 2–4 mg/kg/24 hr for 2 weeks, IVIG 1 g/kg/24 hr for 1–2 days, or IV anti-D (WinRho-SD) 50 µg/kg/dose for Rh-positive individuals. All of these approaches appear to work by decreasing the rate of clearance of sensitized platelets rather than decreasing production of antibody. The optimal choice for therapy is controversial. Splenectomy is indicated in acute ITP only for life-threatening bleeding.

The *diagnosis of chronic ITP* is confirmed by 6–12 months of persistent thrombocytopenia. Repeated treatments with IVIG or IV anti-D or high-dose pulse steroids have been effective in delaying the need for splenectomy. Secondary causes of chronic ITP, especially SLE and infection with HIV, should be ruled out. Splenectomy is effective in inducing a remission in 70–80% of childhood chronic ITP cases. The risks of splenectomy (e.g., surgery or sepsis from encapsulated bacteria such as pneumococcus) must be weighed against the risk of severe bleeding.

Microangiopathic hemolytic anemia (MAHA) generally is associated with thrombocytopenia, anemia secondary to intravascular red cell destruction, and depletion of clotting factors. Children with MAHA usually are quite ill (discussed in this chapter under Anemia). In the child with **DIC,** the deposition of fibrin strands within the vasculature and activation of both thrombin and plasmin result in a wide-ranging hemostatic disorder with activation and clearance of platelets. **Hemolytic-uremic syndrome** occurs as a result of exposure to a toxin that induces endothelial injury, fibrin deposition, and platelet activation and clearance (see Chapter 16). In **thrombotic thrombocytopenic purpura,** platelet consumption precipitated or aggravated by a plasma factor or lack of an inhibitory factor appears to be the primary process, with a modest deposition of fibrin and red cell destruction.

Disorders of Platelet Function

Disorders of platelet function present with mucocutaneous bleeding and a prolonged bleeding time and may be primary or secondary. Primary disorders of platelet function may involve receptors on the platelet membrane for the adhesive proteins. Deficiency of glycoprotein (GP) Ib (the von Willebrand factor receptor) causes **Bernard-Soulier syndrome.** A deficiency of GPIIb-IIIa (the fibrinogen receptor) causes **Glanzmann thrombasthenia.** Mild abnormalities of platelet aggregation and release, detectable by platelet aggregometry, are far more common. Secondary disorders caused by toxins and drugs (e.g., uremia, valproic acid, salicylates, nonsteroidal anti-inflammatory drugs, and infections) may cause a broad spectrum of platelet dysfunction. The bleeding time is an insensitive screen for mild and moderate platelet function disorders.

Disorders of Clotting Factors

Hereditary deficiencies of procoagulant proteins lead to bleeding. Only deficiencies of the so-called contact factors (prekallikrein, high-molecular-weight kininogen [HMWK], and Hageman factor [XII]) are not associated with a predisposition to bleeding. The genes for factors VIII and IX are on the X chromosome, whereas virtually all the other clotting factors are coded on autosomal chromosomes and therefore are inherited autosomally. Factor VIII and factor IX deficiencies are the most common severe inherited bleeding disorders. Von Willebrand disease is the most common congenital bleeding disorder.

Hemophilia

Hemophilia A (factor VIII deficiency) occurs in 1 in 5000 males. *Hemophilia B* (factor IX deficiency) occurs approximately one fifth as often. Clinically, the two disorders are indistinguishable other than in their therapy. Because of a lack of factor VIII or IX, a delay occurs in the generation of thrombin, which is crucial to forming a normal, functional fibrin clot and solidifying the platelet plug that has formed in areas of vascular injury. The severity of the disorder is determined by the degree of clotting factor deficiency. Patients with less than 1% (severe hemophilia) factor VIII or factor IX may have spontaneous bleeding or bleeding with very minor trauma. Patients with 1–5% (moderate hemophilia) factor VIII or factor IX usually require moderate trauma to induce bleeding episodes. In mild hemophilia (>5% factor VIII or IX) significant trauma is necessary to induce bleeding; spontaneous bleeding does not occur. Mild hemophilia may go undiagnosed for many years, whereas severe hemophilia manifests in infancy when the child reaches the toddler stage. In severe hemophilia, spontaneous bleeding occurs, usually in the muscles or joints (hemarthroses).

Prevention of long-term crippling orthopedic ab-

normalities is a major goal of care. Early institution of factor replacement and continuous prophylaxis beginning in early childhood should prevent the chronic joint disease associated with hemophilia.

Diagnosis. The diagnosis of hemophilia is based on a prolonged activated partial thromboplastin time (APTT). In the APTT a surface-active agent activates the intrinsic system of coagulation, of which factors VIII and IX are critical components. In factor VIII or IX deficiency the APTT is quite prolonged but should correct to normal when the patient's plasma is mixed 1:1 with normal plasma. Once an abnormal APTT is obtained, specific factor assays are needed to make a precise diagnosis, which is critical for deciding on the appropriate factor replacement therapy (Table 14–15). Both prenatal diagnosis and carrier diagnosis now are possible, using either coagulation-based methods or (preferably) molecular techniques.

Treatment. Early, appropriate replacement treatment is the aim of optimal hemophilia care. Acute bleeding episodes are best treated in the home once the patient has attained the appropriate age and the parents have learned home treatment. Bleeding associated with surgery, trauma, or dental extraction often can be anticipated, and excessive bleeding can be prevented with appropriate replacement therapy (Table 14–16). For life-threatening bleeding, levels of 80–100% of normal factor VIII or IX are necessary. For mild to moderate bleeding episodes (e.g., hemarthroses), a 40% level for factor VIII or a 30–40% level for factor IX is appropriate. The dose can be calculated using the knowledge that 1 unit/kg body weight of factor VIII will raise the plasma level 2%, whereas 1.5 unit/kg of recombinant factor IX will raise the plasma level 1%. Therefore,

Dose = Desired level (%) × Weight (kg) × 0.5

(for factor VIII)

or

Dose = Desired level (%) × Weight (kg) × 1.5

(for recombinant factor IX)

Aminocaproic acid and tranexamic acid are inhibitors of fibrinolysis that may be useful for oral bleeding. Desmopressin acetate (DDAVP) is a synthetic vasopressin analog with minimal vasopressor effect. DDAVP triples or quadruples the initial factor VIII level of a patient with mild or moderate (not severe) hemophilia A but has no effect on factor IX levels. When adequate hemostatic levels can be attained, DDAVP is the treatment of choice for individuals with mild and moderate hemophilia A.

Patients treated with older factor VIII or IX concentrates were at high risk for hepatitis B, C, and D and HIV. Recombinant factor VIII and factor IX concentrates are safe from virally transmitted illnesses.

TABLE 14–15
Comparison of Hemophilia A, Hemophilia B, and von Willebrand Disease

	Hemophilia A	Hemophilia B	Von Willebrand Disease
Inheritance	X-linked	X-linked	Autosomal dominant
Factor deficiency	Factor VIII	Factor IX	Von Willebrand factor and VIIIC
Bleeding site(s)	Muscle, joint, surgical	Muscle, joint, surgical	Mucous membranes, skin, surgical, menstrual
Prothombin time (PT)	Normal	Normal	Normal
Activated partial thromboplastin time (APTT)	Prolonged	Prolonged	Prolonged or normal
Bleeding time	Normal	Normal	Prolonged or normal
Factor VIII coagulant activity (VIIIC)	Low	Normal	Low or normal
Von Willebrand factor antigen (vWF:Ag)	Normal	Normal	Low
Von Willebrand factor activity (vWF:Act)	Normal	Normal	Low
Factor IX	Normal	Low	Normal
Ristocetin-induced platelet agglutination	Normal	Normal	Normal, low, or increased at low-dose ristocetin
Platelet aggregation	Normal	Normal	Normal
Treatment	DDAVP* or recombinant VIII	Recombinant IX	DDAVP* or vWF concentrate

*Desmopressin (DDAVP) for mild to moderate hemophilia A or type 1 von Willebrand disease.

TABLE 14–16
Commonly Used Transfusion Products

Component	Content	Indication	Dose	Expected Outcome
Packed RBCs	250–300 cc RBCs/unit	↓ O_2 carrying capacity*	10–15 mL/kg	4 cc/kg →1 g/dL ↑ in Hg
Platelet concentrate	$5–7 \times 10^{10}$ platelets/unit	Severe thrombocytopenia ± bleeding	1 unit/10 kg	↑ Platelet count by 50,000/μL
Fresh frozen plasma	1 cc/kg of each clotting factor	Multiple clotting factor deficiency	10–15 mL/kg	Improvement in prothrombin and partial thromboplastin times
Cryoprecipitate	Fibrinogen, factor VIII, vWF, factor XIII	Hypofibrinogenemia, factor XIII deficiency	1 bag/5 kg	↑ Fibrinogen by 50–100 mg/dL
Recombinant factor concentrates	Units as labeled	Hemophilic bleeding or prophylaxis	FVIII: 20–50 units/kg* FIX: 40–120 units/kg*	FVIII: 2%/unit/kg FIX: 0.7/unit/kg

RBCs, Red blood cells; *vWF*, von Willebrand factor.
*Should be clinically significant.

Older patients who were exposed to factor concentrates or, less often, to cryoprecipitate before the use of HIV testing have a high prevalence of HIV infection. Acquired immunodeficiency syndrome (AIDS) is the most common cause of death in older patients with hemophilia. Many older patients also have chronic hepatitis C.

Inhibitors are IgG antibodies directed against transfused factor VIII or IX in congenitally deficient patients. Inhibitors arise in 15% of severe factor VIII hemophiliacs and less commonly in factor IX hemophiliacs. They may be high or low titer and demonstrate an anamnestic response to treatment. The *treatment* of bleeding patients with an inhibitor is difficult. For low-titer inhibitors, options include continuous factor VIII infusions or administration of porcine factor VIII. For high-titer inhibitors, it usually is necessary to administer a product that bypasses the inhibitor, such as recombinant factor VIIa or activated prothrombin complex concentrates. The use of frequent high doses of prothrombin complex concentrates, and especially the activated products, paradoxically increases the risks of thrombosis, which has resulted in fatal complications such as myocardial infarction. Induction of immune tolerance with continuous antigen exposure plus immunosuppression may be beneficial.

Von Willebrand Disease

Von Willebrand disease (vWD) is a common disorder (found in up to 1% of the population) caused by a deficiency of von Willebrand factor (vWF). vWF is an adhesive protein that serves two functions: to act as a bridge between subendothelial collagen and platelets, and to bind circulating factor VIII and thus protect factor VIII from rapid clearance from circulation. Von Willebrand disease usually is inherited as an autosomal dominant trait and rarely as an autosomal recessive trait. vWF may be either quantitatively deficient (partial = type 1 or absolute = type 3) or qualitatively abnormal (type 2 = dysproteinemia).

The *clinical manifestations* of vWD are mucocutaneous bleeding, epistaxis, gingival bleeding, cutaneous bruising, and menorrhagia. In severe von Willebrand disease, factor VIII deficiency may be profound and the patient also may have manifestations similar to hemophilia A (e.g., hemarthrosis). Approximately 80% of patients with von Willebrand disease have classic (type 1) disease (i.e., a mild to moderate deficiency of vWF). Several other subtypes are clinically important, each requiring somewhat different therapy. vWF testing involves measurement of the amount of protein, usually measured immunologically as the von Willebrand factor antigen (vWF:Ag). vWF activity (vWF:Act) is measured functionally in the ristocetin cofactor assay (vWFR:Co)

that uses the antibiotic ristocetin to induce vWF to bind to platelets. In Table 14–15 the findings in classic von Willebrand disease are compared with those in hemophilia A and B.

The *treatment* of von Willebrand disease depends on the severity of the bleeding. DDAVP is the treatment of choice for the majority of bleeding episodes in patients with type 1 disease and some patients with type 2 disease. When high levels of vWF are needed and the patient cannot be satisfactorily treated with DDAVP, treatment with a virally attenuated, vWF-containing concentrate (e.g., Humate P) may be appropriate, and the dosage can be calculated as for factor VIII in hemophilia. Cryoprecipitate should not be used because it is not virally attenuated. Hepatitis B vaccine should be given before the patient is exposed to plasma-derived products. As in all bleeding disorders, aspirin should be avoided for patients with von Willebrand disease.

Vitamin K Deficiency

See Chapters 2 and 6.

Disseminated Intravascular Coagulation

The term DIC refers to a disorder in which a severely ill patient sustains widespread activation of the coagulation mechanism, usually associated with shock. Bleeding and clotting manifestations may be present. Normal hemostasis is a balance between hemorrhage and thrombosis. In DIC this balance is altered by the severe illness, so the patient has activation of both coagulation mediated by thrombin and fibrinolysis mediated by plasmin. Coagulation factors, especially platelets, fibrinogen, and factors II, V, and VIII, are consumed, as are the anticoagulant proteins, especially antithrombin, protein C, and plasminogen. Endothelial injury, tissue release of thromboplastic procoagulant factors, or, rarely, exogenous factors (e.g., snake venoms) directly activate the coagulation mechanism (Table 14–17).

The *diagnosis* is clinical and is sustained by laboratory findings (Table 14–18). In some patients DIC may evolve more slowly, and there may be a degree of compensation. In an acutely ill patient the sudden occurrence of bleeding from a venipuncture or incision site, gastrointestinal or pulmonary hemorrhage, petechiae, or ecchymosis or evidence of peripheral gangrene or thrombosis suggests the diagnosis of DIC.

The *treatment* is problematic. The disorder inducing DIC should be treated effectively, and hypoxia, acidosis, and poor perfusion should be corrected. Depleted blood clotting factors, platelets, and anticoagulant proteins then should be replaced. Heparin may be useful in the presence of significant arterial

TABLE 14–17
Causes of Disseminated Intravascular Coagulation

Infectious
Meningococcemia (purpura fulminans)
Other gram-negative bacteria (*Haemophilus, Salmonella, Escherichia coli*)
Rickettsia (Rocky Mountain spotted fever)
Virus (cytomegalovirus, herpes, hemorrhagic fevers)
Malaria
Fungus

Tissue Injury
Central nervous system trauma (e.g., massive head injury)
Multiple fractures with fat emboli
Crush injury
Profound shock or asphyxia
Hypothermia or hyperthermia
Massive burns

Malignancy
Acute promyelocytic leukemia
Acute monoblastic or myelocytic leukemia
Widespread malignancies (neuroblastoma)

Venom or Toxin
Snake bites
Insect bites

Microangiopathic Disorders
"Severe" thrombotic thrombocytopenic purpura or hemolytic-uremic syndrome
Giant hemangioma (Kasabach-Merritt syndrome)

Gastrointestinal Disorders
Fulminant hepatitis
Severe inflammatory bowel disease
Reye syndrome

Hereditary Thrombotic Disorders
Antithrombin III deficiency
Homozygous protein C deficiency

Newborn
Maternal toxemia
Group B streptococcal infections
Abruptio placentae
Severe respiratory distress syndrome
Necrotizing enterocolitis
Congenital viral disease (e.g., cytomegalovirus or herpes)
Erythroblastosis fetalis

Miscellaneous
Severe acute graft rejection
Acute hemolytic transfusion reaction
Severe collagen-vascular disease
Kawasaki disease
Heparin-induced thrombosis
Infusion of "activated" prothrombin complex concentrates
Hyperpyrexia/encephalopathy, hemorrhagic shock syndrome

From Scott JP: Bleeding and thrombosis. In Kliegman RM, Nieder ML, Super DM, editors: *Practical strategies in pediatric diagnosis and therapy,* Philadelphia, 1996, WB Saunders.

TABLE 14–18
Differential Diagnosis of Coagulopathies That Can Be Confused with Disseminated Intravascular Coagulation

	Prothrombin Time	Partial Thromboplastin Time	Fibrinogen	Platelets	Fibrinogen Degradation Products	Clinical Keys
DIC	↑	↑	↓	↓	↑	Shock
Liver failure	↑	↑	↓	Normal or ↓	↑	Jaundice
Vitamin K deficiency	↑	↑	Normal	Normal	Normal	Malabsorption, liver disease
Sepsis without shock	↑	↑	Normal	Normal	↑ or normal	Fever

From Scott JP: Bleeding and thrombosis. In Kliegman RM, Nieder ML, Super DM, editors: *Practical strategies in pediatric diagnosis and therapy,* 1996, Philadelphia, WB Saunders.

TABLE 14–19
Common Hypercoagulable States

Congenital Disorders
Factor V Leiden (activated protein C resistance)
Prothrombin 20210
Protein C deficiency
Protein S deficiency
Antithrombin III deficiency
Plasminogen deficiency
Dysfibrinogenemia
Homocystinuria

Acquired Disorders
Indwelling catheters
Lupus anticoagulant/antiphospholipid syndrome
Nephrotic syndrome
Malignancy
Pregnancy
Birth control pills
Autoimmune disease
Immobilization/surgery
Trauma
Infection
Inflammatory bowel disease

From Scott JP: Bleeding and thrombosis. In Kliegman RM, Nieder ML, Super DM, editors: *Practical strategies in pediatric diagnosis and therapy,* Philadelphia, 1996, WB Saunders.

or venous thrombotic disease unless sites of life-threatening bleeding coexist. In addition, heparin may be useful for the treatment of DIC induced by meningococcemia, purpura fulminans, or acute promyelocytic leukemia. The use of concentrates containing protein C appears promising in treatment of DIC, especially for purpura fulminans.

Thrombosis

A hereditary predisposition to thrombosis (Table 14–19) may be caused by a deficiency of an anticoagulant protein (e.g., protein C or S, antithrombin, or plasminogen), by an abnormality of a procoagulant protein that makes such protein resistant to proteolysis by its respective inhibitor (factor V Leiden), or by a mutation resulting in an increased level of a procoagulant protein (prothrombin 20210). The functions of the anticoagulant proteins are outlined in Fig. 14–9. Deficiency syndromes may present in neonates, especially homozygous protein C deficiency, which presents with purpura fulminans or arterial thrombosis in the major vessels and necessi-

tates plasma replacement therapy. Most individuals with an inherited predisposition to thrombosis usually exhibit symptoms in adolescence or early adulthood. Protein C deficiency that presents in adulthood usually is inherited as an autosomal dominant trait, whereas the homozygous form usually is autosomal recessive. Protein S and AT-III deficiencies are inherited as autosomal dominant traits. Factor V Leiden is the most common hereditary cause of a predisposition to thrombosis, appearing in 3–5% of Caucasians. Acquired antiphospholipid antibodies (anticardiolipin and lupus anticoagulant) also predispose to thrombosis.

Clinical manifestations of thromboembolic disease in pediatrics occur most frequently in neonates or in adolescents. Indwelling catheters, vasculitis, sepsis, immobilization, nephrotic syndrome, coagulopathy, trauma, infection, surgery, inflammatory bowel disease, oral contraceptive agents, pregnancy, and abortion all predispose to thrombosis (Table 14–19). The *diagnosis* of venous thrombosis can be made noninvasively by Doppler flow compression studies or plethysmography; however, the gold standard remains the venogram. The manifestations of pulmonary emboli may be highly variable, from no findings to those of chest pain, diminished breath sounds, increased pulmonic component of the second heart sound, cyanosis, tachypnea, and hypoxemia. Findings on a chest roentgenogram vary, but an abnormal ("high probability") ventilation-perfusion scan (V-Q mismatch) or, more recently, detection of an intravascular thrombus on helical CT is diagnostic of pulmonary emboli.

Treatment of thrombotic disorders depends on the underlying condition and usually involves heparin and then longer-term anticoagulation with coumarin. Major vessel thrombosis or life-threatening thrombosis may necessitate treatment with fibrinolytic agents (e.g., streptokinase, urokinase, or tissue plasminogen activator). In the newborn, inherited deficiency syndromes may present as emergencies and necessitate replacement with plasma, AT-III concentrates, or protein C concentrates. Symptomatic individuals with an inherited predisposition to thrombosis are usually chronically anticoagulated with coumarin.

BLOOD COMPONENT THERAPY

Transfusion of red blood cells, granulocytes, platelets, and coagulation factors can be lifesaving or life maintaining (Table 14–16). Whole blood is indicated only when acute hypovolemia and reduced oxygen carrying capacity are present. Otherwise, packed red blood cells are indicated to treat anemia by increasing oxygen carrying capacity. Blood cell transfusions

TABLE 14–20
Evaluation of Transfusion Reactions

Type of Reaction	Clinical Signs	Management of Problems
Major hemolytic (1:100,000) (incompatibility)	Acute shock, back pain, flushing, early fever, intravascular hemolysis, hemoglobinemia, hemoglobinuria; may be delayed 5–10 days and less severe if anamnestic response is present	1. Stop transfusion; return blood to bank with fresh sample of patient's blood. 2. Hydrate IV; support BP, maintain high urine flow, alkalinize urine. 3. Check for hemoglobinemia, hemoglobinuria, hyperkalemia. 4. Jaundice, anemia if delayed.
Febrile (1:100)	Fever at end of transfusion, urticaria (usually because of sensitization to WBC HLA antigens), chills	Pretreat with hydrocortisone, antipyretics, diphenhydramine HCl (Benadryl), or all three; use leukocyte-poor RBCs, washed RBCs, filtered or frozen RBCs.
Allergic	Fever, urticaria, anaphylactoid reaction (often because of sensitivity to donor plasma proteins)	Benadryl, hydrocortisone; use washed RBCs or frozen RBCs.

Adapted from Andreoli TE, Bennett JC, Carpenter CC, Plum F, et al: *Cecil essentials of medicine*, ed 4, Philadelphia, 1997, WB Saunders. *BP*, Blood pressure; *HLA*, human leukocyte antigen; *RBCs*, red blood cells; *WBC*, white blood cell.

should not be used to treat asymptomatic nutritional deficiencies that can be corrected by administering the appropriate deficient nutrient (e.g., iron or folic acid). Blood component therapy requires proper anticoagulation of the blood, screening for a variety of infectious agents, and blood group compatibility testing before administration. Commonly used blood components are listed in Table 14–16. Typical transfusion reactions are listed in Table 14–20. Febrile reactions may be prevented by filtering of blood products to remove white cells. Long-term complications of transfusions are iron overload, alloimmunization to red and white blood cells or platelets and plasma proteins (1:100), graft-versus-host disease, and infectious diseases (e.g., hepatitis [1:250], HIV [<1:250,000], malaria, syphilis, babesiosis, brucellosis, or Chagas disease). Transfusion therapy also may result in circulatory overload, especially in the presence of chronic cardiopulmonary deficiency.

REFERENCES

Andrew M, Michelson AD, Bovill E, et al: Guidelines for antithrombotic therapy in pediatric patients, *J Pediatr* 132(4): 575–588, 1998.

Beardsley DS: Platelet abnormalities in infancy and childhood. In Nathan DG, Orkin SH, editors: *Hematology of infancy and childhood*, ed 5, Philadelphia, 1998, WB Saunders.

Behrman RE, Kliegman RM, Jenson HB, editors: *Nelson textbook of pediatrics*, ed 16, Philadelphia, 2000, WB Saunders, Chapters 481–490.

Blanchette VS, Imbach P, Andrew M, et al: Randomised trial of intravenous immunoglobulin G, intravenous anti-D, and oral prednisone in childhood acute immune thrombocytopenic purpura, *Lancet* 344(8294):703–707, 1994.

Bussel JB, Zabusky MR, Berkowitz RL, et al: Fetal alloimmune thrombocytopenia, *N Engl J Med* 337(1):22–26, 1997.

Dubansky AS, Boyett JM, Falletta J, et al: Isolated thrombocytopenia in children with acute lymphoblastic leukemia: a rare event in a pediatric oncology group study, *Pediatrics* 84(6): 1068–1071, 1989.

Ehrenforth S, Junker R, Koch HG, et al: Multicentre evaluation of combined prothrombotic defects associated with thrombophilia in childhood: Childhood Thrombophilia Study Group, *Eur J Pediatr* 158(Suppl 3):S97–S104, 1999.

George JN, Woolf SH, Raskob GE, et al: Idiopathic thrombocytopenic purpura: a practice guideline developed by explicit methods for The American Society of Hematology, *Blood* 88(1): 3–40, 1996.

Liesner R, Machin S: Platelet disorders, *BMJ* 314(7083):809–812, 1997.

Medeiros D, Buchanan GR: Major hemorrhage in children with idiopathic thrombocytopenic purpura: immediate response to therapy and long-term outcome, *J Pediatr* 133(3):334–339, 1998.

Montgomery RR, Gill JC, Scott JP: Hemophila and von Willebrand disease. In Nathan DG, Orkin SH, editors: *Hematology of infancy and childhood*, ed 5, Philadelphia, 1998, WB Saunders.

Nichols W, Ginsburg D: Von Willebrand disease, *Medicine* 76(1): 1–20, 1997.

Schreiber GB, Busch MP, Kleinman SH: The risk of transfusion-transmitted viral infections, *N Engl J Med* 334(26):1685–1690, 1996.

Scott JP: Bleeding and thrombosis. In Kliegman RM, Nieder ML, Super DM, editors: *Practical strategies in pediatric diagnosis and therapy*, Philadelphia, 1996, WB Saunders.

Strauss RG: Blood and blood component transfusions. In Behrman RE, Kliegman RM, Jenson HB, editors: *Nelson textbook of pediatrics*, ed 16, Philadelphia, 2000, WB Saunders.

CHAPTER 15

Oncology

James B. Nachman ▼ Herbert T. Abelson

Each year in the United States, approximately 12,400 individuals 0–20 years of age are given a diagnosis of cancer. Approximately 2300 children and adolescents die from cancer each year, making cancer the most common cause of disease-related death in the 1–19-year-old age group. Although the incidence of childhood cancer has increased slowly with time, mortality rates have declined in a dramatic fashion (Fig. 15–1). A coordinated, multidisciplinary team effort is needed for diagnosing and managing childhood malignancies. Patients should be cared for in specialized cancer centers by a staff that includes oncologists, surgeons, radiotherapists, pathologists, psychiatrists, psychologists, social workers, nutritionists, and specialized oncology nurses.

GENERAL CONSIDERATIONS

Epidemiology. The types of cancer that occur in childhood differ significantly from those that occur in adults. Carcinomas that develop in solid organs are the most common adult cancer, whereas carcinomas are rarely seen in individuals younger than 20 years of age. Acute leukemias, lymphomas, and brain tumors are the most common pediatric and young adult cancers. Fig. 15–2 shows incidence figures for the most common types of childhood cancer, and Fig. 15–3 shows the incidence of childhood cancer in various ethnic groups. The annual incidence of cancer in white children is higher than that seen in black children. Cancer incidence rates for Hispanics and Asian Americans are intermediate to those for white and black children. Leukemia and various embryonal tumors such as Wilms tumor, neuroblastoma, retinoblastoma, and hepatoblastoma are more common in infancy and early childhood, whereas Hodgkin disease, bone cancers, and gonadal malignancies are more common in adolescents. Rarely does cancer develop in newborns and

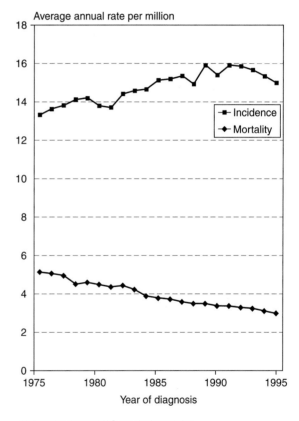

Average annual rate per million

*Adjusted to the 1970 U.S. standard population.

FIG. 15–1

Trends in age-adjusted* SEER incidence and United States mortality rates for all childhood cancers age <20, all races, both sexes, 1975–1995. (From Ries LA, Smith MA, Guaney JC, et al: Cancer incidence and survival and adolescents. United States SEER program 1975-1995. National Cancer Institute SEER program. NIH Publication No 99-4649, Bethesda, Md, 1999.)

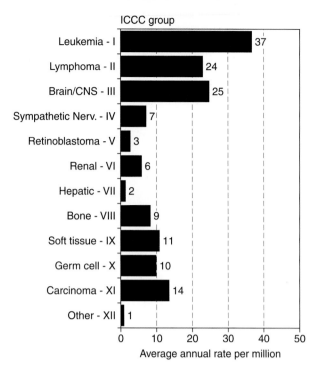

FIG. 15–2

Age-adjusted* incidence rates for childhood cancer by ICCC group, age <20, all races, both sexes, SEER, 1975–1995. (From Ries LA, Smith MA, Guaney JC, et al: Cancer incidence and survival and adolescents. United States SEER program 1975-1995. National Cancer Institute SEER program. NIH Publication No 99-4649, Bethesda, Md, 1999.)

*Adjusted to the 1970 U.S. standard population.

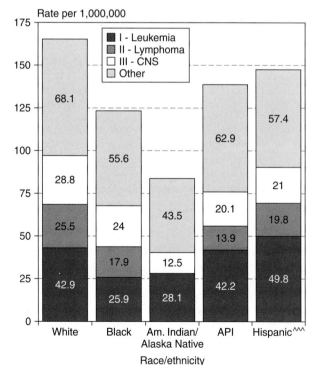

FIG. 15–3

Age-adjusted* incidence rates for childhood cancer by ICCC group and race/ethnicity, age <20, both sexes, SEER, 1990–1995. (From Ries LA, Smith MA, Guaney JC, et al: Cancer incidence and survival and adolescents. United States SEER program 1975–1995. National Cancer Institute SEER program. NIH Publication No 99-4649, Bethesda, Md, 1999.)

^^^Hispanic is not mutually exclusive from whites, blacks, Asian/Pacific Islanders, and American Indians/Alaskan Natives.
Data Source: SEER 11 (San Francisco, Conneticut, Detroit, Hawaii, Iowa, New Mexico, Seattle, Utah, Atlanta, San Jose-Monterey, and Los Angeles) and Alaska.

*Age adjusted to 1970 U.S. standard population.

infants younger than 1 year of age. Leukemias that develop in young infants tend to be very undifferentiated and often show a 4;11 translocation. Solid tumors seen in neonates include a specific type of neuroblastoma (4S), teratomas (most commonly in the sacrococcygeal region), retinoblastoma, and Wilms tumor. Benign tumors such as hemangiomas and mesoblastic nephromas also occur in neonates.

Certain childhood tumors are associated with germline mutations. Individuals with bilateral retinoblastoma invariably carry a germline retinoblastoma gene mutation. Individuals who carry a germline mutation for the p53 gene have a significantly increased risk for the development of certain types of tumors, such as rhabdomyosarcoma, adrenal cortical carcinoma, and breast cancer (Li-Fraumeni syndrome). It is important to determine which patients have hereditary conditions associated with an increased risk for malignancy (Table 15–1), because careful screening, examinations, and counseling can lead to the early detection of cancer and improve the chance for successful treatment. For example, in individuals with the Beckwith-Wiedemann syndrome,

frequent abdominal ultrasound examinations may lead to the early detection of Wilms tumor.

In utero exposure to ionizing radiation (e.g., Chernobyl) is associated with an increased incidence of cancer in childhood. No evidence exists that living near high-power lines leads to an increase in the incidence of childhood cancer. Many studies have examined in utero exposure to certain potential carcinogens (e.g., alcohol, smoke, pesticides, hair dyes, and organic solvents) and the risk for development of childhood cancer. The results of most of these studies have been equivocal. However, recent studies indicate that individuals showing certain genetic polymorphisms for the enzyme systems responsible for detoxifying potential carcinogens may be at increased risk for the development of a cancer.

Etiology. Two types of genes are generally involved in the regulation of normal and abnormal cell growth. Certain normal human genes that promote the process of cell growth are homologous to the genetic material of transforming ribonucleic acid (RNA) tumor viruses; these genes are called protooncogenes. Another set of human genes is responsible for the

TABLE 15–1
Familial or Genetic Susceptibility to Malignancy

Disorder	Tumor or Cancer	Comment
Chromosomal Syndromes		
Chromosome 11p− (deletion) with sporadic anemia	Wilms tumor	Associated with genitourinary anomalies, mental retardation
Chromosome 13q− (deletion)	Retinoblastoma	Associated with mental retardation, skeletal malformations
Trisomy 21	Lymphocytic or nonlymphocytic leukemia	Risk is 15 times normal
Klinefelter syndrome (47, XXY)	Breast cancer	
Gonadal dysgenesis (XO/XY)	Gonadoblastoma	Gonads must be removed; 25% chance of gonadal malignancy
DNA Fragility		
Xeroderma pigmentosum	Basal, squamous cell skin cancers	Autosomal recessive; failure to repair solar-damaged DNA
Fanconi anemia	Leukemia	Autosomal recessive; 10% risk for AML; chromosome fragility, positive diepoxybutane test
Bloom syndrome	Leukemia, lymphoma	Autosomal recessive; chromosome fragility, immunodeficiency; high risk for malignancy
Ataxia-telangiectasia	Lymphoma, leukemia	Autosomal recessive; sensitive to x-radiation, radiomimetic drugs; chromosome fragility, immunodeficiency
Dysplastic nevus syndrome	Melanoma	Autosomal dominant

Continued

TABLE 15–1
Familial or Genetic Susceptibility to Malignancy—cont'd

Disorder	Tumor or Cancer	Comment
Immunodeficiency Syndromes		
Wiskott-Aldrich syndrome	Lymphoma	Immunodeficiency; X-linked recessive
X-linked immunodeficiency (Duncan syndrome)	Lymphoma	Epstein-Barr virus is inciting agent
Severe combined immunodeficiency	Leukemia, lymphoma	Immunodeficiency; X-linked recessive
Other Single-Gene Defects		
Neurofibromatosis	Neurofibroma, peripheral nerve sheath, optic glioma, acoustic neuroma, astrocytoma, meningioma, pheochromocytoma	Autosomal dominant
Tuberous sclerosis	Fibroangiomatous nevi, myocardial rhabdomyoma	Autosomal dominant
Retinoblastoma, genetic form	Sarcoma	Autosomal dominant
Wilms tumor, genetic form	Wilms tumor	Autosomal dominant
Familial adenomatous polyposis coli	Adenocarcinoma of colon	Autosomal dominant
Gardner syndrome	Adenocarcinoma of colon; skull and soft tissue tumors	Autosomal dominant
Peutz-Jeghers syndrome	Gastrointestinal carcinoma	Autosomal dominant
Tyrosinemia, galactosemia	Hepatic carcinoma	Nodular cirrhosis; autosomal recessive
Multiple endocrine neoplasia (MEN) syndrome I (Werner syndrome)	Parathyroid adenoma, pancreatic islet tumor, pituitary adenoma carcinoid	Autosomal dominant; Zollinger-Ellison syndrome
Multiple endocrine neoplasia syndrome II (Sipple syndrome)	Medullary carcinoma of the thyroid, hyperparathyroidism, pheochromocytoma	Autosomal dominant; monitor calcitonin and calcium levels
Multiple endocrine neoplasia III (multiple mucosal neuroma syndrome)	Mucosal neuroma, pheochromocytoma, medullary thyroid carcinoma; Marfan habitus; neuropathy	Autosomal dominant
von Hippel-Lindau disease	Hemangioblastoma of the cerebellum and retina, pheochromocytoma	Autosomal dominant; mutation of tumor suppressor gene
Cancer family syndrome	Colonic, uterine carcinoma	Autosomal dominant
Li-Fraumeni syndrome	Bone, soft tissue sarcoma, breast	Autosomal dominant mutation of p53
Other Congenital Conditions		
Hemihypertrophy ± Beckwith syndrome	Wilms tumor, hepatoblastoma, adrenal carcinoma	25% develop tumor, most in first 5 yr of life

regulation of protooncogene function. These genes are referred to as antioncogenes or tumor suppressor genes. Carefully orchestrated activation and deactivation of these two types of genes lead to normal, orderly cell proliferation. Any event that produces un-

regulated expression of an oncogene could conceivably lead to the development of cancer. For example, a mutation in an oncogene could be present and could lead to a new gene not susceptible to regulation by tumor suppressor genes. Amplification of an oncogene occurs in certain childhood cancers such as neuroblastoma. Neuroblastoma cells may contain multiple extra copies of the n–*myc* oncogene. Overexpression of the n–*myc* oncogene is an adverse prognostic factor in neuroblastoma. Chromosomal translocation may move an oncogene from its normal site to a new, unregulated site, leading to increased expression. For example, in Burkitt's lymphoma, translocation occurs between chromosome 8 (c–*myc* oncogene) and the immunoglobulin gene locus on chromosome 2, 8, or 14, such that the c–*myc* oncogene comes to reside next to an immunoglobulin gene. The c–*myc* gene turns on the immunoglobulin gene, leading to a malignant B-cell lymphoma.

Insights into the function of tumor suppressor genes have been gained through the study of childhood retinoblastoma. Retinoblastoma exists in both a familial and a sporadic form. Familial cases tend to be bilateral and occur at an earlier age than cases with unilateral tumors. Retinoblastoma is associated with deletions or mutations in the RB gene, a known tumor suppressor gene. Knudson proposed that inactivation of both copies of a tumor suppressor gene is necessary for tumor formation (the "two-hit theory"). Genetic analysis of patients with familial retinoblastoma has shown that all somatic cells have a deletion of one allele of the RB gene. In this case it would take only one additional mutational event, the deletion of the remaining normal RB gene allele, to cause tumor formation. A second hit could occur in a number of different cells, leading to early-onset bilateral tumors. In patients with two normal germline RB alleles it would take two mutational events in the same somatic cell to produce a tumor, a more statistically improbable occurrence.

A translocation may lead to the formation of a new gene, whose expression may lead to a novel protein with transforming capabilities. In chronic myelogenous leukemia (CML) a translocation between chromosome 9 and 22 results in a fusion gene incorporating parts of two genes, *bcr* and *abl*. The protein formed by this novel gene plays an important role in the development of CML. Events preceding oncogene activation, tumor suppressor gene inactivation, or translocations are not well understood.

Clinical Manifestations and Diagnosis. Pediatric leukemias tend to present with manifestations related to bone marrow failure that is caused by replacement of normal marrow elements with undifferentiated blast cells. The classic triad of findings in acute leukemia is fever, pallor, and bruising. Occasionally leukemia may present as generalized or localized bone or joint pain. Patients who have bone pain may have relatively normal blood counts. The likely diagnosis of the particular type of leukemia (e.g., lymphoid or nonlymphoid) can often be made

by evaluating blast morphology on either a peripheral smear or a bone marrow aspirate. In all cases evaluation of surface markers should be performed to allow lineage assignment. Patients with solid tumors usually have a palpable mass lesion or symptoms related to a mass lesion (e.g., pain, respiratory distress, and abdominal obstruction). In the case of a suspected solid tumor, a biopsy should be obtained to determine the type of tumor. A number of pediatric solid tumors (e.g., neuroblastoma, non-Hodgkin lymphoma, Ewing sarcoma, and rhabdomyosarcoma) may have very similar appearances on light microscopic examination. This group of tumors is referred to as small, round blue cell tumors. To adequately diagnose the particular tumor type, additional pathologic studies, such as surface marker analysis, immunohistochemistry, and electron microscopy, may be required. Cytogenetic evaluations should be carried out in all cases of childhood cancer. Many types of leukemia and certain solid tumors show either specific chromosomal translocations or other recurring cytogenetic abnormalities that can lead to the correct diagnosis. Therefore, it is crucial that the oncologist, surgeon, and pathologist consult before the biopsy to determine the amount of tissue required and the appropriate distribution of the tissue, so that all necessary studies may be performed. Malignancy may produce nonspecific systemic effects, such as anorexia, weight loss, fever, and malaise. Specific manifestations of various malignancies are shown in Table 15–2. Chemical products produced by certain tumors may produce neuroendocrine effects such as hypertension (neuroblastoma or pheochromocytoma), diarrhea (neuroblastoma), hypoglycemia (pancreatic islet cell tumor), or Cushing syndrome (adrenal or pituitary tumors).

Following the diagnosis of a malignant solid tumor, a staging workup should be undertaken to identify any sites of metastasis. Such studies as computed tomography (CT), magnetic resonance imaging (MRI), plain x-ray films or ultrasound examination, nuclear scans such as bone or gallium, bone marrow aspiration and biopsy, and lumbar puncture may be used. Pediatric patients with a malignancy may manifest abnormalities in immune function as a result of the cancer itself or cancer treatment. Therefore, patients with a new diagnosis of cancer should undergo a basic immune system workup, including quantitative immunoglobulin levels, immune status determination for varicella, cytomegalovirus (CMV), Epstein-Barr virus (EBV), and herpes simplex virus (HSV), and a TB test with controls. Infectious complications are common in pediatric oncology patients (Table 15–3). Renal and hepatic function should be assessed. In addition, any organ that might be damaged by chemotherapy

TABLE 15–2
Common Manifestations of Childhood Malignancies

Signs and Symptoms	Significance	Example
Hematologic		
Pallor, anemia	Bone marrow infiltration	Leukemia, neuroblastoma
Petechiae, thrombocytopenia	Bone marrow infiltration	Leukemia, neuroblastoma
Fever, pharyngitis, neutropenia	Bone marrow infiltration	Leukemia, neuroblastoma
Systemic		
Bone pain, limp, arthralgia	Primary bone tumor, metastasis to bone	Osteosarcoma, Ewing sarcoma, leukemia, neuroblastoma
Fever of unknown origin, weight loss, night sweats	Lymphoreticular malignancy	Hodgkin disease, non-Hodgkin lymphoma
Painless lymphadenopathy	Lymphoreticular malignancy, metastatic solid tumor	Leukemia, Hodgkin disease, non-Hodgkin lymphoma, Burkitt lymphoma, thyroid carcinoma
Cutaneous lesion	Primary or metastatic disease	Neuroblastoma, leukemia, Langerhans cell histiocytosis, melanoma
Abdominal mass	Adrenal-renal tumor	Neuroblastoma, Wilms tumor, lymphoma
Hypertension	Sympathetic nervous system tumor	Neuroblastoma, pheochromocytoma, Wilms tumor
Diarrhea	Vasoactive intestinal polypeptide (VIP)	Neuroblastoma, ganglioneuroma
Soft tissue mass	Local or metastatic tumor	Ewing sarcoma, osteosarcoma, neuroblastoma, thyroid carcinoma, rhabdomyosarcoma, eosinophilic granuloma
Diabetes insipidus, galactorrhea, poor growth	Neuroendocrine involvement of hypothalamus or pituitary gland	Adenoma, craniopharyngioma, prolactinoma, Langerhans cell histiocytosis
Emesis, visual disturbances, ataxia, headache, papilledema, cranial nerve palsies	Increased intrathecal pressure	Primary brain tumor; metastasis
Ophthalmologic Signs		
Leukokoria	White pupil	Retinoblastoma
Periorbital ecchymosis	Metastasis	Neuroblastoma
Miosis, ptosis, heterochromia	Horner syndrome: compression of cervical sympathetic nerves	Neuroblastoma
Opsoclonus/ataxia	Neurotransmitters? Autoimmunity?	Neuroblastoma
Exophthalmos, proptosis	Orbital tumor	Rhabdomyosarcoma, lymphoma
Thoracic Mass		
Anterior mediastinal	Cough, stridor, pneumonia, tracheal-bronchial compression	Germ cell tumor, T-cell lymphoma, Hodgkin disease
Posterior mediastinal	Vertebral or nerve root compression; dysphagia	Neuroblastoma, neuroenteric cyst

TABLE 15–3
Infectious Complications of Malignancy

Predisposing Factor	Etiology	Site of Infection	Infectious Agents
Neutropenia	Chemotherapy, bone marrow infiltration	Sepsis, shock, pneumonia, soft tissue, proctitis, mucositis	*Staphylococcus aureus, Staphylococcus epidermidis, Escherichia coli, Pseudomonas aeruginosa, Candida, Aspergillus,* anaerobic oral and rectal bacteria
Immunosuppression, lymphopenia, lymphocyte-monocyte dysfunction	Chemotherapy, prednisone	Pneumonia, meningitis, disseminated viral infection	*Pneumocystis carinii, Cryptococcus neoformans, Mycobacterium, Nocardia, Listeria monocytogenes, Candida, Aspergillus, Strongyloides, Toxoplasma,* varicella-zoster, cytomegalovirus, herpes simplex
Splenectomy	Staging of Hodgkin disease	Sepsis, shock, meningitis	Pneumococcus, *Haemophilus influenzae*
Indwelling central venous catheter	Nutrition, administration of chemotherapy	Line sepsis, tract of tunnel infection, exit site infection	*S. epidermidis, S. aureus, Candida albicans, P. aeruginosa, Aspergillus, Corynebacterium* JK, *Streptococcus faecalis, Mycobacterium fortuitum, Propionibacterium acnes*

Data from Bodey GP: *Am J Med* 81(Suppl 1A):11–26, 1986; Engelhard D, Marks MI, Good RA: *J Pediatr* 108(3):335–346, 1986; Johnson PR, Decker MD, Edwards KM, et al: *J Infect Dis* 154(4):570–578, 1986; Pizzo PA: *Rev Infect Dis* 9(1):214–219, 1987; Whimbey E, Kiehn TE, Brannon P, et al: *Am J Med* 82(4):723–730, 1987.

should have its function assessed before the beginning of treatment. Certain cancers may produce metabolic, hematologic, or other abnormalities that may be life threatening if not recognized and treated (Table 15–4).

Principles of Cancer Treatment

Treatment for children with cancer may involve surgery, radiation therapy, or chemotherapy (Table 15–5). Surgery and radiation are local treatment modalities, whereas chemotherapy has both local and systemic effects. More recently, certain children with cancer have received treatment with cytokines, biologic response modifiers, or monoclonal antibodies in addition to standard treatments. Because most pediatric solid tumors have a high risk for micrometastatic disease at the time of diagnosis, chemotherapy is often used as the initial form of treatment. For patients with localized solid tumors, chemotherapy administered after removal of the primary tumor is referred to as adjuvant therapy. The administration of chemotherapy while the primary tumor is still present is referred to as neoadjuvant chemotherapy. Neoadjuvant chemotherapy has a number of potential benefits, including an early attack on presumed micrometastatic disease and shrinkage of the primary tumor to facilitate local control. For example, in patients with osteosarcoma who undergo surgical removal of the primary tumor following neoadjuvant chemotherapy, the degree of necrosis induced in the primary tumor can be used to assess the efficacy of the particular chemotherapy regimen used and to plan postoperative therapy.

Tumor growth is governed by the typical cell cycle. The cell cycle is divided into stages:
1. M phase: cell division
2. GI phase: protein and RNA synthesis
3. S phase: DNA synthesis and chromosome replication
4. G2 phase: preparation for the next cell division in M phase

Many types of normal cells are quiescent and not involved in the cell cycle at any given time. These cells are referred to as G0 cells. Pediatric

TABLE 15–4
Oncologic Emergencies

Condition	Manifestations	Etiology	Malignancy	Treatment
Metabolic				
Hyperuricemia	Uric acid nephropathy; gout	Tumor lysis syndrome	Lymphoma, leukemia	Allopurinol, alkalinize urine; hydration and diuresis
Hyperkalemia	Arrhythmias, cardiac arrest	Tumor lysis syndrome	Lymphoma, leukemia	Kayexalate; sodium bicarbonate, glucose, and insulin; check for pseudohyperkalemia from leukemic cell lysis in test tube
Hyperphosphatemia	Hypocalcemic tetany; metastatic calcification, photophobia, pruritus	Tumor lysis syndrome	Lymphoma, leukemia	Hydration, forced diuresis; stop alkalinization; oral aluminum hydroxide to bind phosphate
Hyponatremia	Seizure, lethargy, asymptomatic	Syndrome of inappropriate ADH (SIADH) secretion; fluid, sodium losses in vomiting	Leukemia, CNS tumor	Restrict free water for SIADH; replace sodium if depleted
Hypercalcemia	Anorexia, nausea, polyuria, pancreatitis, gastric ulcers; prolonged PR, shortened QT interval	Bone resorption; ectopic parathormone, vitamin D, or prostaglandins	Metastasis to bone rhabdomyosarcoma	Hydration and furosemide diuresis; corticosteroids; mithramycin; calcitonin, diphosphonates
Hematologic				
Anemia	Pallor, weakness, heart failure	Bone marrow suppression or infiltration; blood loss	Any with chemotherapy	Packed red blood cell transfusion
Thrombocytopenia	Petechiae, hemorrhage	Bone marrow suppression or infiltration	Any with chemotherapy	Platelet transfusion
Disseminated intravascular coagulation	Shock, hemorrhage	Sepsis, hypotension, tumor factors	Promyelocytic leukemia, others	Fresh frozen plasma; platelets; correct infection, etc.
Neutropenia	Infection	Bone marrow suppression or infiltration	Any with chemotherapy	If febrile, give broad-spectrum antibiotics and G-CSF if appropriate

Condition	Clinical features	Cause/Site	Tumor	Management
Hyperleukocytosis (>50,000/mm³)	Hemorrhage, thrombosis; pulmonary infiltrates, hypoxia; tumor lysis syndrome	Leukostasis; vascular occlusion	Leukemia	Leukapheresis; chemotherapy
Graft-versus-host disease	Dermatitis, diarrhea, hepatitis	Immunosuppression and nonirradiated blood products; bone marrow transplantation	Any with immunosuppression	Corticosteroids; cyclosporine; antithymocyte globulin
Space-Occupying Lesions				
Spinal cord compression	Back pain ± radicular *Cord above T10:* symmetric weakness, increased deep tendon reflex; sensory level present; toes up *Conus medullaris (T10–L2):* symmetric weakness, increased knee reflexes, decreased ankle reflexes; saddle sensory loss; toes up or down *Cord equina (below L2):* asymmetric weakness, loss of deep tendon reflex and sensory deficit; toes down	Metastasis to vertebra and extramedullary space	Neuroblastoma; medulloblastoma	Magnetic resonance imaging (MRI) or myelography for diagnosis; corticosteroids; radiotherapy; laminectomy; chemotherapy
Increased intracranial pressure	Confusion, coma, emesis, headache, hypertension, bradycardia, seizures, papilledema, hydrocephalus; III and VI nerve palsies	Primary or metastatic brain tumor	Neuroblastoma, astrocytoma; glioma	Computed tomography (CT) or MRI for diagnosis; corticosteroids; phenytoin; ventricular-peritoneal shunt; radiotherapy; chemotherapy
Superior vena cava syndrome	Distended neck veins, plethora, edema of head and neck, cyanosis, proptosis; Horner syndrome	Superior mediastinal mass	Lymphoma	Chemotherapy; radiotherapy
Tracheal compression	Respiratory distress	Mediastinal mass compressing trachea	Lymphoma	Radiation, steroids

ADH, Antidiuretic hormone; *G-CSF,* granulocyte colony–stimulating factor.

TABLE 15–5
Cancer Chemotherapy

Drug*	Action	Metabolism	Excretion	Indication	Toxicity
Antimetabolites					
Methotrexate	Folic acid antagonist; inhibits dihydrofolate reductase	Hepatic	Renal, 50–90% excreted unchanged; biliary	ALL, lymphoma, medulloblastoma, osteosarcoma	Myelosuppression (nadir 7–10 days), mucositis, stomatitis, dermatitis, hepatitis, renal and CNS with high-dose administration; prevent with leucovorin, monitor levels
6-Mercaptopurine	Purine analog	Hepatic; allopurinol inhibits metabolism	Renal	ALL	Myelosuppression; hepatic necrosis; mucositis; allopurinol increases toxicity
Cytosine arabinoside (Ara-C)	Pyrimidine analog; inhibits DNA polymerase	Hepatic	Renal	ALL, lymphoma, sarcoma	Myelosuppression, conjunctivitis, mucositis, CNS dysfunction
Alkylating Agents					
Cyclophosphamide	Alkylates guanine; inhibits DNA synthesis	Hepatic	Renal	ALL, lymphoma, sarcoma	Myelosuppression; hemorrhagic cystitis; pulmonary fibrosis, inappropriate ADH secretion, bladder cancer, anaphylaxis
Ifosfamide	Similar to Cytoxan	Hepatic	Renal	Lymphoma, Wilms tumor, sarcoma, germ cell and testicular tumors	Similar to Cytoxan; CNS dysfunction, cardiac toxicity
Antibiotics					
Doxorubicin (Adriamycin) and daunorubicin (Cerubidine)	Binds to DNA, intercalation	Hepatic	Biliary, renal	ALL, AML, osteosarcoma, Ewing sarcoma, lymphoma, neuroblastoma	Cardiomyopathy, red urine, tissue necrosis on extravasation, myelosuppression, conjunctivitis, radiation dermatitis, arrhythmia
Dactinomycin	Binds to DNA, inhibits transcription	—	Renal, stool, 30% excreted unchanged drug	Wilms tumor, rhabdomyosarcoma, Ewing sarcoma	Tissue necrosis on extravasation, myelosuppression, radiosensitizer, stomatitis
Bleomycin	Binds to DNA, cuts DNA	Hepatic	Renal	Hodgkin disease, lymphoma, germ cell tumors	Pneumonitis, stomatitis, Raynaud phenomenon, pulmonary fibrosis, dermatitis

Vinca Alkaloids

Drug	Mechanism	Metabolism	Excretion	Indications	Toxicity
Vincristine (Oncovin)	Inhibits microtubule	Hepatic	Biliary	ALL, lymphoma, Wilms tumor, Hodgkin disease, Ewing sarcoma, neuroblastoma, rhabdomyosarcoma, brain tumors	Local cellulitis, peripheral neuropathy, constipation, ileus, jaw pain, inappropriate ADH secretion, seizures, ptosis, minimal myelosuppression
Vinblastine (Velban)	Inhibits microtubule formation	Hepatic	Biliary	Hodgkin disease, Langerhans cell histiocytosis	Local cellulitis, leukopenia
Enzymes					
L-Asparaginase	Depletion of L-asparagine	—	Reticuloendothelial system	ALL	Allergic reaction; pancreatitis, hyperglycemia, platelet dysfunction and coagulopathy, encephalopathy
Hormones					
Prednisone	Direct lymphocyte cytotoxicity	Hepatic	Renal	ALL; Hodgkin disease, lymphoma	Cushing syndrome, cataracts, diabetes, hypertension, myopathy, osteoporosis, infection, peptic ulceration, psychosis
Miscellaneous					
BCNU (carmustine, nitrosourea)	Carbamylation of DNA; inhibits DNA synthesis	Hepatic; phenobarbital increases metabolism, decreases activity	Renal	CNS tumors, lymphoma, Hodgkin disease	Delayed myelosuppression (4–6 wk); pulmonary fibrosis, carcinogenic, stomatitis
Cisplatin	Inhibits DNA synthesis	—	Renal	Gonadal tumors; osteosarcoma, neuroblastoma, CNS tumors, germ cell tumors	Nephrotoxic; myelosuppression, ototoxicity, tetany, neurotoxicity, hemolytic-uremic syndrome; aminoglycosides may increase nephrotoxicity, anaphylaxis
Carboplatin	Inhibits DNA synthesis	—	Renal	Same as cisplatin	Myelosuppression
Etoposide (VP-16)	Topoisomerase inhibitor	—	Renal	ALL, lymphoma, germ cell tumor	Myelosuppression, secondary leukemia
Etretinate (vitamin A analog) and tretinoin	Enhances normal differentiation	Liver	Liver	Some leukemias; neuroblastoma	Dry mouth, hair loss, pseudotumor cerebri, premature epiphyseal closure

Data from *Med Lett* 37(3):25–32, 1995; Bleyer WA: *Pediatr Clin North Am* 32(3):557–574, 1985.
ADH, Antidiuretic hormone; *ALL*, acute lymphocytic leukemia; *AML*, acute myelogenous leukemia; *CNS*, central nervous system; *DNA*, deoxyribonucleic acid.
*Many drugs produce nausea and vomiting during administration, and many cause alopecia with repeated doses.

cancers are generally characterized by high cell proliferation rates; therefore, they tend to be particularly sensitive to chemotherapeutic agents that act as cellular toxins. Normal cells that also have high proliferative rates, such as those found in skin, the lining of the gastrointestinal tract, hair, and bone marrow, are adversely affected by these chemotherapeutic drugs. At any particular time, cancer cells in a particular malignancy may be in different cell phases. Most chemotherapeutic agents affect a particular cell cycle phase, most commonly S phase.

Resistance to a particular chemotherapeutic agent can develop in a number of ways. These include decreased influx or increased efflux of the chemotherapeutic agent from the malignant cell; mutation in the target of a chemotherapeutic drug, so that it cannot be inhibited by the drug; amplification of a drug target to overcome inhibition; and blockade of normal cellular processes, which leads to programmed cell death or apoptosis. Since mutation is an ongoing process in a malignant tumor, it follows that certain subpopulations of tumor cells within a tumor may be more or less sensitive to any particular chemotherapy drug. Given this fact, combinations of chemotherapy drugs are used (as opposed to sequential single agents) to treat the various forms of childhood cancer.

It has been shown that certain areas of the body may be inaccessible to chemotherapeutic agents given either orally, intravenously, or intramuscularly. The best example of this is the so-called blood-brain barrier that prevents the penetration of chemotherapeutic drugs administered in standard doses orally, intravenously, or intramuscularly into the central nervous system. In this case, instillation of the chemotherapeutic agent directly into the cerebrospinal fluid may be necessary. Because chemotherapy agents are cellular toxins, a number of side effects are associated with their use. Cells that normally show a high proliferation rate are most affected because most chemotherapeutic drugs are highly effective against cells in S phase. Bone marrow suppression, nausea and vomiting, and alopecia are general side effects of commonly used chemotherapy drugs. In addition, each chemotherapy drug has specific toxicities associated with its use. For example, adriamycin can cause cardiac damage, and cisplatin can cause renal damage and ototoxicity. Radiation therapy can produce a number of side effects, such as mucositis, growth retardation, organ dysfunction, and the later development of secondary cancers. Significant therapy-related late effects may develop in pediatric cancer patients (Table 15–6).

Leukemia

Each year, 2000–2500 new cases of childhood leukemia occur in the United States. The disease affects

---

TABLE 15–6
Long-Term Sequelae of Cancer Therapy

Problem	Etiology
Infertility	Alkylating agents; radiation
Second cancers	Genetic predisposition; radiation, alkylating agents, VP-16, topoisomerase II inhibitors
Sepsis	Splenectomy
Hepatotoxicity	Methotrexate, 6-mercaptopurine, radiation
Hepatic venoocclusive	High-dose, intensive chemotherapy (busulfan, cyclophosphamide) ± bone marrow transplant
Scoliosis	Radiation
Pulmonary (pneumonia, fibrosis)	Radiation, bleomycin, busulfan
Myocardiopathy, pericarditis	Adriamycin (doxorubicin), daunomycin, radiation
Leukoencephalopathy	Cranial irradiation ± methotrexate
Cognition/intelligence	Cranial irradiation ± methotrexate
Pituitary dysfunction (isolated growth hormone deficiency, panhypopituitary)	Cranial irradiation
Psychosocial	Stress, anxiety, death of peers; conditioned responses to chemotherapy
Thyroid dysfunction	Radiation
Osteonecrosis	Steroids

about 40 children per million under the age of 15 years. Acute lymphoblastic leukemia accounts for approximately 75% of cases. The various subtypes of nonlymphoblastic acute leukemia (Table 15–7) account for 15–20%. Chronic leukemias are quite rare in childhood.

Etiology. There are few instances of familial leukemia. Little is known concerning the etiology of individual cases of childhood acute leukemias. An identical twin of a leukemic patient under the age of 4 years has an increased risk for the development of leukemia. Other predisposing factors for leukemia include Down syndrome, Fanconi anemia, Bloom syndrome, and ataxia-telangiectasia. Children exposed to ionizing radiation or chemotherapy drugs (particularly to topoisomerase II inhibitors) are at a higher risk for developing leukemia. Recently it has been shown in certain patients with leukemia that the unique antigen receptor gene rearrangement or the specific chromosomal translocation characterizing the patient's leukemic clone can be demonstrated in cord blood cells and neonatal blood spots used for screening for metabolic diseases.

Clinical Manifestations. Signs and symptoms of acute leukemias are related to the infiltration of leukemic cells into normal tissues, resulting in either bone marrow failure (e.g., anemia, neutropenia, or thrombocytopenia), or specific tissue infiltration (e.g., lymph nodes, liver, spleen, brain, bone, skin, gingiva, or testes). Common presenting symptoms are fever, pallor, petechiae or ecchymoses, lethargy, malaise, anorexia, and bone or joint pain. Physical examination frequently reveals lymphadenopathy and hepatosplenomegaly. Symptomatic central nervous system involvement is rare at the time of presentation of acute leukemias. In patients with acute myeloid leukemia, extramedullary soft tissue tumors may be found in various sites. The presence of myeloperoxidase in these tumors may impart a greenish hue; such tumors are known as chloromas. The testicle is a common extramedullary site for acute lymphoblastic leukemia (ALL); a painless enlargement of one or both testes may be seen.

Diagnosis. The diagnosis of acute leukemia is made based on the findings of immature blast cells on either the peripheral blood smear, bone marrow aspirate, or both. In most cases morphologic examination of the blast cells reveals whether they belong to the lymphoid or nonlymphoid lineage. Analysis of markers on the blast cell surface identifies proteins restricted to either lymphoid or nonlymphoid cells. Cytogenetic analysis should be undertaken in all cases of acute leukemia. Certain types of both lymphoid and nonlymphoid acute leukemias have specific chromosomal abnormalities. A lumbar puncture should always be performed at the time of diagnosis to evaluate the possibility of central nervous system involvement.

Prognosis. For ALL, patients are divided into two general risk groups based on age and initial white blood cell count (Table 15–8). Standard-risk patients are patients 1–9 years of age with a white blood cell count <50,000 and no 9;22 translocation or hypodiploid (N ≤ 44) karyotype. All other patients fall into the high-risk group. Infants with ALL have a highly undifferentiated immunophenotype and have a worse outcome than other patients. Young infants with ALL who show a 4;11 translocation have a particularly poor prognosis. Once chemotherapy has been initiated, patients with ALL undergo an early assessment of response to chemotherapy. Measurement of either peripheral blood blast levels on day 7 or bone marrow blast levels on day 7 and/or 14 has significant prognostic importance. Switching patients with slow early response to induction therapy to a more aggressive treatment has resulted in improvement in outcome. The cure rate for childhood ALL in the year 2000 is approximately 50%. Acute myelogenous leukemia (AML) has a significantly worse outcome compared with ALL. The cure rate for childhood AML is approximately 50%. Certain studies have suggested that patients showing an 8;21 translocation, inversion of chromosome 16, or the presence of Auer rods may have a better outcome than other patients. A high white blood cell count is an adverse prognostic feature in AML.

Treatment. Patients with ALL generally receive three- or four-agent induction chemotherapy based on their initial risk-group assignment (Table 15–9). Standard-risk patients receive vincristine, prednisone, and L-asparaginase; high-risk patients also receive an anthracycline.

TABLE 15–7
Acute Nonlymphoblastic Leukemia Subtypes

	FAB Classification
Myeloblastic without maturation	M1
Myeloblastic with some maturation	M2
Hypergranular promyelocytic	M3
Myelomonocytic	M4
Monocytic	M5
Erythroleukemia	M6
Megakaryocytic	M7

FAB, French-American-British.

TABLE 15–8
Prognostic Factors in Acute Lymphoblastic Leukemia in Childhood

Factor	Favorable (Lower Risk)	Unfavorable (Higher Risk)
Demographic		
Age	1–9 yr	<1 yr or >10 yr
Race	White	Black
Sex	Female	Male
Leukemic Burden		
Initial WBC count	$<50 \times 10^9$/L	$\geq 50 \times 10^9$/L
Adenopathy	Absent	Present
Hepatosplenomegaly	Absent to mild (<3 cm)	Marked (>3 cm)
CNS disease at diagnosis	Absent	Absent
Morphology, Histochemistry, Cytogenetics,* and Biochemistry		
Lymphoblasts†	L1*	L2* or L3*
DNA index	>1,16	≤1,16
Cytogenetics	t(12;21)	t(4;11): t(8;22)
Immunologic Factors		
Immunoglobulins	Normal IgG, IgA, IgM	Decreased IgG, IgA, IgM
Glucocorticoid receptors	High number	Lower number
Response to Induction Therapy		
	Rapid	Slow

Modified from Miller DR: *Pediatr Clin North Am* 27(2):269–291, 1980.
LDH, Lactic dehydrogenase; *WBC*, white blood cell.
*Cytogenetics refers to chromosome changes; t is translocation (see Chapter 4).
†FAB classification: L1 typical (85%) = small cells, little cytoplasm; L2 undifferentiated (15%) = large cells, large cytoplasm; L3 Burkitt type (1%) = cytoplasmic vacuoles.

TABLE 15–9
Initial Treatment of Childhood Acute Lymphoblastic Leukemia

Induction 4–5 Weeks
1. Vincristine IV, weekly × 4 wk
2. Dexamethasone PO × 28 days for standard risk; prednisone PO × 28 days for high risk
3. L-Asparaginase *(E. coli):* IM 3 times/wk × 3 weeks; L-asparaginase (PEG): 1 dose
4. For high risk only: Daunomycin IV, weekly × 4 wk
5. Intrathecal cytosine arabinoside day 1, intrathecal methotrexate day 8

Consolidation
1. Intrathecal methotrexate, weekly × 4 wk
2. Cranial RT (high risk–slow responders: CNS disease at diagnosis)
3. Daily oral 6-MP
4. High-risk patients receive additional Cytoxan, cytosine arabinoside

Interim Maintenance*
1. Daily oral 6-mercaptopurine
2. Weekly oral methotrexate
3. Standard risk: vincristine once/month and 5-day, prednisone pulse once per month

Delayed Intensification*
1. Reinduction similar to induction, but dexamethasone replaces prednisone and adriamycin replaces daunomycin for high risk
2. Reconsolidation: ALL patients receive Cytoxan, cytosine arabinoside, and 6-thioguanine (replaces 6-mercaptopurine)

Maintenance*
1. Vincristine once per month
2. Dexamethasone (standard risk) or prednisone (high risk); pulses: 5 days/month
3. Daily oral 6-mercaptopurine
4. Weekly oral methotrexate

*Additional intrathecal methotrexate continues during these phases.

During induction, intrathecal instillation of some combination of methotrexate, cytosine arabinoside, and hydrocortisone is given to either eliminate existing CNS leukemia or prevent the development of CNS leukemia. In early studies of treatment for patients with childhood ALL who only received systemic therapy, approximately 25% of patients developed overt CNS leukemia within 6 months of diagnosis. Following successful remission induction, CNS therapy is intensified. For a short time (during consolidation), patients usually receive weekly intrathecal injections of methotrexate with or without cranial radiation. In the year 2000, only 10% of patients received cranial radiation for CNS prophylaxis. For high-risk patients, the use of intensive systemic chemotherapy in addition to the CNS-directed therapy during consolidation has resulted in significant improvement in overall outcome. Systemic chemotherapy during this phase often includes Cytoxan, cytosine arabinoside, and 6-mercaptopurine.

Most groups treating childhood ALL agree that some form of delayed intensification is required. In studies performed by the Children's Cancer Group, the delayed intensification phase is the most important element of treatment for patients with standard risk features. Delayed intensification tends to recapitulate the initial induction, except that dexamethasone is substituted for prednisone, adriamycin for daunomycin, and 6-thioguanine for 6-mercaptopurine.

Following delayed intensification, all patients receive at least 1–2 years of maintenance therapy. Maintenance therapy generally consists of a single monthly dose of vincristine, 5 days of oral prednisone, or daily oral 6-MP, and weekly oral dexamethasone. In certain protocols intrathecal chemotherapy is given every 3 months during maintenance. Relapse occurs most commonly in the bone marrow but also may occur in the CNS, testes, or other extramedullary sites. If relapse occurs while the patient is still receiving treatment, the prognosis is worse than if relapse occurs after discontinuation of therapy. Other additional remissions may be induced, but their duration is often short despite intensive therapy. Bone marrow transplant from a matched sibling donor or a matched unrelated donor is currently recommended for patients who have a bone marrow relapse while receiving initial chemotherapy. The treatment of acute nonlymphoblastic leukemia is quite different from that of ALL. In ALL, nonmyelosuppressive drugs such as vincristine, prednisone, and L-asparaginase are extremely active. This is not the case for AML. Repeated cycles of extremely intensive myelosuppressive chemotherapy are necessary to cure childhood AML. Induction therapy usually consists of cytosine arabinoside and an anthracycline, ± 6-thioguanine and etoposide. Induction seems to be most effective when two courses of drugs are given approximately 1 week apart, regardless of blood counts. Because of the poor outcome when standard chemotherapy is used, many centers recommend that all children with AML who have a matched sibling donor undergo bone marrow transplantation as soon as induction and consolidation therapy is completed. Most centers in the United States follow this strategy.

Complications. Certain major complications associated with the treatment of leukemia result from bone marrow suppression caused by chemotherapy. Patients may show bleeding manifestations and significant anemia that necessitates transfusion of platelets,

TABLE 15–10
Distribution of Childhood Non-Hodgkin Lymphoma by Histopathologic Type

Histologic Type	Marker	Incidence
Lymphoblastic		
	T cell (95%)	30%
	Precursor B (5%)	
Nonlymphoblastic		
Small noncleaved (Burkitt: non-Burkitt type)	Mature B-surface immunoglobulin	30%
Large cell	Mature B-surface immunoglobulin	20%
Anaplastic	Primarily T; occasionally null	15%
Other	Variable	5%

blood, or both. Low neutrophil counts predispose the patient to significant bacterial infection. Immunosuppression produced by chemotherapy can lead to the development of *Pneumocystis carinii* pneumonia. Bactrim prophylaxis can prevent this complication. Patients who have not previously had varicella are at risk for severe infection. Upon exposure, a nonimmune patient should receive zoster immune globulin. Long-term sequelae of therapy are now uncommon.

Lymphoma

Malignant lymphomas are the third most common tumors in childhood. There are two major types of lymphoma, Hodgkin disease (HD) (5.7 cases/million) and non-Hodgkin lymphoma (NHL) (7.4 cases/million).

Non-Hodgkin Lymphoma

Epidemiology. Non-Hodgkin lymphoma (NHL) occurs at least three times as frequently in boys as in girls. The peak incidence is between the ages of 7 and 11 years. Childhood NHL differs from adult NHL in a number of important features. Almost all cases of NHL in childhood are diffuse, highly malignant, and aggressive and show little differentiation. Originally, NHL was divided into two broad histologic groups, lymphoblastic and nonlymphoblastic (Table 15–10). The majority of nonlymphoblastic tumors have a mature B-cell immunophenotype characterized by the presence of surface immunoglobulin. Two major histologic variants, small noncleaved cell and large cell, make up the bulk of nonlymphoblastic NHL. Almost all lymphoblastic tumors are T-lineage. A distinct T-cell nonlymphoblastic NHL, the so-called anaplastic large-cell lymphoma, occurs in about 10% of children with NHL.

Distant, noncontiguous metastases are common in childhood NHL. Systemic chemotherapy therefore is mandatory and should be administered to all patients with NHL, even those with localized disease at diagnosis. NHL has been described in association with congenital or acquired immunodeficiency states following transplantation, chronic immune stimulation, autoimmune disease, and EBV-induced lymphoproliferation. Acquired immunodeficiency syndrome may be associated with B-cell NHL.

Clinical Manifestations. The abdomen, head, and neck are the most common sites for B-cell NHL, whereas the anterior mediastinum and peripheral nodes are the primary sites for T-cell lymphomas. Primary mediastinal, T-cell lymphoblastic lymphoma may produce airway or superior vena cava obstruction and pleural effusion. Diagnosis is established by results of a tissue biopsy or examination of pleural or peritoneal fluid. Systemic symptoms such as fever and weight loss may be present and are particularly prominent in patients with anaplastic large-cell lymphoma.

Treatment. T-cell lymphoblastic lymphoma and T-cell anaplastic large-cell lymphoma are generally treated with aggressive multidrug regimens similar to those used in ALL. For treatment purposes, B-cell NHL is divided into three groups. Patients with localized disease require minimal amounts of chemotherapy and have an outstanding outcome. Patients with disseminated B-cell NHL are divided into two groups based on the presence or absence of bone marrow and CNS involvement. The main drugs used in the treatment of mature B-cell NHL are Cytoxan, moderate- to high-dose methotrexate, cytosine arabinoside (Ara-C), adriamycin, ifosfamide, and VP-16. Radiation therapy is rarely used in patients with NHL because the disease is rarely localized and is highly chemotherapy sensitive.

Hodgkin Disease

Hodgkin disease (HD) in children is similar to that seen in adults. Hodgkin disease is seen most commonly in adolescents, and it is rare before 10 years of age. There is a 3:1 male predominance in early childhood Hodgkin disease. The sex ratio diminishes after puberty to the 1:4 ratio seen in adults. Hodgkin disease in childhood carries a very good prognosis. The etiology of Hodgkin disease is unknown, but indirect evidence has been uncovered suggesting an association with an infectious agent, possibly Epstein-Barr virus.

Clinical Manifestations. Painless, firm lymphadenopathy often confined to one or two lymph node areas (usually the supraclavicular and cervical nodes) is the most common clinical presentation of HD. Mediastinal lymphadenopathy producing cough or shortness of breath is another frequent initial presentation. High, spiking fever, drenching night sweats, and weight loss (>10%) are noted in 30% of children (B symptoms). Elevation of the erythrocyte sedimentation rate is a nonspecific finding but may correlate with prognosis. Cellular immunity, as determined by cutaneous antigen testing, occasionally reveals anergy.

Diagnosis and Staging. The pathologic hallmark of HD is the identification of Reed-Sternberg cells in tumor tissue. Histopathologic subtypes in childhood Hodgkin disease are similar to those in adults; 10–20% have lymphocyte predominant, 40–60% have nodular sclerosis, 20–40% have mixed cellularity, and <5% have lymphocyte depletion. As in adults, the lymphocyte predominant is the most favorable subtype and lymphocyte depletion the least favorable. Staging is according to the Ann Arbor system (Table 15–11). In the past, high-dose radiation therapy as the sole modality of treatment was used for early-stage Hodgkin disease in adults. Since radiation is a local treatment modality, staging laparotomy was often carried out to accurately assess the abdominal nodes, liver, and spleen. Since high-dose radiation is associated with unacceptable cosmetic and growth deformities in children, all children receive combination chemotherapy. Therefore, staging laparotomy is no longer used in children. In children, adequate staging information can generally be obtained from a CT scan of the neck, chest, abdomen, and pelvis and a gallium scan. For patients with stage III or IV disease and for patients with B symptoms, bone marrow aspiration and biopsy should be performed. Gallium is often concentrated in lymphomas. Since treated Hodgkin disease may leave a residual nonviable mass that is indistinguishable from residual Hodgkin disease on radiologic evaluation, gallium scanning is often done before and after chemotherapy. A mass that is initially gallium positive and becomes gallium negative is likely to represent scar or inactive disease. The generally accepted treatment for childhood Hodgkin disease is a combination of chemotherapy and low-dose involved field radiation (Table 15–12). With this treatment, the cure rate for childhood Hodgkin disease is over 90%. Chemotherapy usually consists of some combination of Cytoxan, vincristine, procarbazine, adriamycin, bleomycin, vinblastine, and etoposide. Steroids are also used in the treatment of Hodgkin disease. Many children and adolescents with Hodgkin disease can probably be safely treated with chemotherapy alone.

TABLE 15–11
Ann Arbor Staging Classification for Hodgkin Disease*

Stage I
Involvement of a single lymph node region (I), or a single extralymphatic organ or site (I_E)

Stage II
Involvement of two or more lymph node regions on the same side of the diaphragm (II), or localized involvement of an extralymphatic organ or site and of one or more lymph node regions on the same side of the diaphragm (II_E)

Stage III
Involvement of lymph node regions on both sides of the diaphragm (III), which may be accompanied by localized involvement of an extralymphatic organ or site (III_E), by involvement of the spleen (III_S), or both (III_{SE})

Stage IV
Diffuse or disseminated involvement of one or more extralymphatic organs or tissues, with or without associated lymph node enlargement

*Each stage is divided into "A" and "B" categories, in which "A" indicates no systemic symptoms and "B" indicates the presence of one or more of the following: (1) unexplained weight loss greater than 10% of body weight in preceding 6 months, (2) fever higher than 38° C, and (3) night sweats.
E, Extralymphatic; S, splenic involvement.

TABLE 15–12
Recommended Therapy for Children and Young Adults with Hodgkin Disease

Stage	Patient Features	Therapy
I, II (favorable)	No bulk disease; no hilar adenopathy	Four cycles of chemotherapy; low-dose radiotherapy to the involved areas
Other I, II, and all III	Bulk disease; hilar adenopathy; large mediastinal mass; unfavorable signs	Six cycles of hybrid chemotherapy; low-dose radiotherapy to the involved areas
IV		Six cycles of more aggressive chemotherapy; low-dose radiotherapy to the involved areas

Low-dose radiotherapy = 2000–2500 cGy.

Primary Central Nervous System Tumors

CNS tumors are the most common solid tumors in children and are second to leukemia in overall incidence. About 1200 new cases occur each year, and approximately 24 cases per million occur in children under the age of 15 years. Brain tumors in children differ from those in adults in that they are predominantly infratentorial tumors (posterior fossa) involving the cerebellum, midbrain, and brainstem (Table 15–13). Childhood brain tumors are differentiated further from those in adults in that they are usually low-grade astrocytomas or embryonic neoplasms (e.g., medulloblastoma, ependymoma, or germ cell tumor), whereas most CNS tumors in adults are malignant astrocytomas and metastatic carcinomas.

Clinical Manifestations. Brain tumors can cause symptoms by impingement on normal tissue, usually cranial nerves, or by an increase in intracranial pressure caused either by obstruction to cerebrospinal fluid flow or by a direct mass effect from the tumor (Table 15–14). Tumors that obstruct the flow of cerebrospinal fluid tend to become symptomatic quickly. Symptoms of CSF blockade are lethargy, headache, and vomiting (particularly in the morning upon awakening). Irritability, anorexia, poor school performance, or loss of developmental milestones may all be signs of slow-growing CNS

TABLE 15–13
Location, Incidence, and Prognosis of Central Nervous System Tumors in Children

Location	Incidence (%)	Five-Year Survival (%)
Infratentorial (Posterior Fossa)	55–60	
Astrocytoma (cerebellum)	20	90
Medulloblastoma	20	44–55
Glioma (brainstem)	15	High grade: 0–5; low grade: 30
Ependymoma	5	50–60
Supratentorial (Cerebral Hemispheres)	40–55	
Astrocytoma	15	10–50
Glioblastoma multiforme	10	0–5
Ependymoma	2.5	50–60
Choroid plexus papilloma	1.5	60–80
Midline		
Craniopharyngioma	6	70–90
Pineal (germinoma)	1	65–75
Optic nerve glioma	3	50–90

nosis of a CNS mass lesion should include arteriovenous malformation, aneurysm, brain abscess, parasitic infestation, granulomatous disease (e.g., tuberculosis or sarcoid), intracranial hemorrhage, pseudotumor cerebri, primary cerebral lymphoma, vasculitis, and rarely metastatic tumor.

Treatment. Once the diagnosis is established, high-dose dexamethasone is often administered to reduce tumor-associated edema. With improvements in neurodiagnosis, less surgical morbidity, and better chemotherapy programs, an aggressive approach to treatment of pediatric brain tumors has improved outcome. Surgical objectives are complete excision if possible and maximal debulking if a complete excision is not possible. In adults, radiation therapy has been the mainstay of the treatment of malignant CNS tumors. In children, radiation is often combined with chemotherapy given either before or after radiation. Primitive neuroectodermal tumors (including medulloblastoma) and germ cell tumors are sensitive to chemotherapy; high-grade gliomas are less sensitive to the effects of chemotherapy. Chemotherapy plays an especially important role, particularly in infants with brain tumors, in whom the effects of high-dose CNS radiation may be devastating.

Prognosis. The 5-year survival rate associated with all childhood CNS tumors is approximately 50%, resulting in large measure from the high curability of cerebellar astrocytomas and the increasing cure rate for patients with medulloblastoma.

Wilms Tumor

Wilms tumor is the most common renal malignant tumor of childhood, with a yearly incidence of 7.8 new cases per million children.

Epidemiology. The mean age at diagnosis is 3–3½ years of age, and no sex predilection is apparent. A hereditary form of Wilms tumor may be associated with a bilateral presentation and a young age at onset. A number of congenital anomalies frequently are identified in children with Wilms tumor, including sporadic aniridia, hemihypertrophy, and genitourinary abnormalities (e.g., hypospadias, cryptorchidism, horseshoe or fused kidneys, ureteral duplication, and polycystic kidneys). Wilms tumor with aniridia often is associated with a deletion of part of chromosome 11.

Clinical Manifestations. More than 80% of children with Wilms tumor have an abdominal mass that is usually discovered incidentally by the parents. Associated symptoms and laboratory abnormalities may be abdominal pain, fever, hypertension, and microscopic or gross hematuria. A CBC, urinalysis, and liver and renal function studies should be obtained. The first step in diagnosing a potential Wilms

tumors. In young children with open cranial sutures, an increase in head circumference may occur. Inability to abduct the eye as the result of a sixth cranial nerve palsy is a common sign of increased intracranial pressure. Seizures occur in 20–50% of patients with supratentorial tumors; focal weakness or sensory changes may also be seen. Optic pathway tumors lead to visual field defects. Cerebellar tumors are associated with ataxia and diminished coordination. Cranial nerve deficits other than sixth nerve palsy suggest involvement of the brainstem.

Diagnosis. A history and physical examination are fundamental for evaluation; this should involve a careful neurologic assessment, including visual fields and a funduscopic examination. If an intracranial lesion is suspected, an MRI is currently the examination of choice. Examination of cerebrospinal fluid by cytocentrifuge histology is essential to determine the presence of metastatic disease in primitive neuroectodermal tumors, germ cell tumors, and pineal region tumors. A lumbar puncture should not be undertaken before an MRI has been obtained. In addition to a primary brain tumor, differential diag-

TABLE 15–14
Manifestations and Treatment of Primary Central Nervous System Tumors

Tumor and Site	Manifestations	Treatment	Comments
Cerebellar astrocytoma	Onset between 5 and 8 yr of age; ↑ICP, ataxia, nystagmus, head tilt, intention tremor	Surgical excision plus adjuvant radiotherapy if a solid tumor; corticosteroids to ↓tumor edema	Symptoms present for 2–7 months; cystic tumors have favorable outcome
Medulloblastoma Cerebellar vermis and floor of fourth ventricle	Onset between 3 and 5 yr of age; ↑ICP, obstructive hydrocephalus, ataxia, cerebrospinal fluid metastasis, and spinal cord compression	Surgical excision and radiotherapy plus adjuvant chemotherapy,* corticosteroids to ↓tumor edema	Acute onset of symptoms; tumor is radiosensitive; cerebrospinal fluid checked for metastatic cells
Ependymoma Floor of fourth ventricle	↑ICP, obstructive hydrocephalus; rarely seeds spinal fluid	Surgical excision, radiotherapy, chemotherapy,* corticosteroids to ↓tumor edema	Onset intermediate between astrocytoma and medulloblastoma
Brainstem glioma	Onset between 5 and 7 yr of age; triad of multiple cranial nerve deficit (VII, IX, X, V, VI), pyramidal tract, and cerebellar signs; skip lesions common; ↑ICP is late	Excision impossible; radiotherapy is palliative; corticosteroids to ↓tumor edema; experimental chemotherapy*	Small size but critical location makes this tumor highly lethal
Pinealoma	Paralysis of upward gaze (Parinaud syndrome); lid retraction (Collier sign); hearing loss; precocious puberty; ↑ICP; may seed spinal fluid	Radiotherapy, chemotherapy; shunting of CSF	Germ cell line; germinoma, dermoid, teratoma, mixed lesions may calcify or secrete hCG or alpha-fetoprotein
Diencephalic glioma Hypothalamus	Onset between 2 and 5 mo of age; alert, euphoric, but emaciated appearance; emesis, optic atrophy, nystagmus	Radiotherapy	Patient may become obese after treatment

CSF, Cerebrospinal fluid; *hCG,* human chorionic gonadotropin; ↑ *ICP,* increased intracranial pressure: headache, vomiting (papilledema, III and VI nerve palsies, wide sutures); *TB,* tuberculosis.
*Chemotherapy may delay need for radiotherapy, thus avoiding treatment-related neurotoxicity. Chemotherapy includes alternating cycles of cyclophosphamide plus vincristine with cisplatin plus etoposide.

Continued

TABLE 15–14
Manifestations and Treatment of Primary Central Nervous System Tumors—cont'd

Tumor and Site	Manifestations	Treatment	Comments
Astrocytoma/ glioma			
Cerebral cortex	Onset between 5 and 10 yr of age; personality changes; headache, motor weakness, seizures; ↑ICP later	Location determines surgical resection or radiotherapy; anticonvulsant and corticosteroids; chemotherapy*	*Differential diagnosis:* Abscess, hydatid or porencephalic cyst; herpes simplex encephalitis, granuloma (TB, cryptococcus); arteriovenous malformation; hematoma; lymphoma
Optic glioma	Onset before 2 yr of age; poor visual acuity, exophthalmos, nystagmus; ↑ICP; optic atrophy, strabismus	Surgical resection or radiotherapy; chemotherapy*	Neurofibromatosis in 25% of patients
Craniopharyngioma			
Pituitary fossa	Onset between 7 and 12 yr of age; ↑ ICP, bitemporal hemianopia, sexual and growth retardation; growth hormone and gonadotropic deficiency	Begin cortisol replacement prior to surgery; total excision, adjuvant radiotherapy if extensive	Calcification above sella turcica; diabetes insipidus common postoperatively

CSF, Cerebrospinal fluid; *hCG,* human chorionic gonadotropin; ↑ *ICP,* increased intracranial pressure: headache, vomiting (papilledema, III and VI nerve palsies, wide sutures); *TB,* tuberculosis.
*Chemotherapy may delay need for radiotherapy, thus avoiding treatment-related neurotoxicity. Chemotherapy includes alternating cycles of cyclophosphamide plus vincristine with cisplatin plus etoposide.

tumor is abdominal ultrasound examination. An ultrasound examination can usually delineate an intrarenal mass from a mass in the adrenal gland or other surrounding structures. Evaluating the inferior vena cava is also crucial because tumor may extend from the kidney into the vena cava. A chest radiographic examination should be performed to look for pulmonary metastases. In most cases a CT scan of the chest, abdomen, and pelvis is also obtained.

Diagnosis. Differential diagnosis of Wilms tumor includes benign lesions such as hydronephrosis, polycystic disease of the kidney, other malignant tumors such as renal cell carcinoma, neuroblastoma, lymphoma, retroperitoneal rhabdomyosarcoma, certain benign renal tumors such as mesoblastic nephroma, and hemartoma. Prognostic factors are tumor stage and tumor histology. Anaplastic variants of Wilms tumor have a significantly worse outcome than the classic Wilms tumor. The 4-year relapse-free survival of patients with tumors of favorable histology is directly related to stage (Table 15–15). Cure rates for patients with localized Wilms tumor at di-

agnosis are above 85%, whereas patients with pulmonary metastases have event-free survivals of only approximately 70–80%.

Treatment. In centers in the United States, every attempt is made to obtain a complete resection before the initiation of chemotherapy, with or without radiation therapy. In European centers, however, preoperative chemotherapy is given in an effort to shrink the tumor and make definitive resection an easier process. In European centers, if a renal tumor has radiographic features of Wilms tumor, no biopsy is performed before initiation of chemotherapy. Patients with no metastatic lesions at the time of diagnosis receive vincristine and actinomycin D as preoperative therapy; patients with metastatic lesions (e.g., in the bone or lung) also receive adriamycin. The National Wilms Tumor Study chemotherapy for Wilms tumor with favorable histology includes vincristine and actinomycin D with or without adriamycin. In patients with stage III or IV disease the tumor bed or full abdomen, if necessary, is irradiated with a total dose of 1080 rads. Care must be taken to

TABLE 15–15
National Wilms Tumor Study Staging System*

Stage I

The tumor limited to the kidney and completely excised.

The surface of the renal capsule is intact; the tumor is not ruptured before or during removal.

No residual tumor is apparent beyond the margins of excision.

Stage II

The tumor extends beyond the kidney but is completely excised.

Regional extension of the tumor is present (i.e., penetration through the outer surface of the renal capsule into the perirenal soft tissues): vessels outside the kidney substance are infiltrated or contain tumor thrombus; the tumor may have been biopsied or local spillage of tumor confined to the flank has occurred; no residual tumor is apparent at or beyond the margins of excision.

Stage III

Residual nonhematogenous tumor confined to the abdomen is present.

Stage III—cont'd

Any of the following may occur:
- Lymph nodes on biopsy are found to be involved in the hilus, the periaortic chains, or beyond.
- Diffuse peritoneal contamination by the tumor has occurred, such as by spillage of tumor beyond the flank before or during surgery, or by tumor growth that has penetrated through the peritoneal surface.
- Implants are found on the peritoneal surfaces.
- The tumor extends beyond the surgical margins either microscopically or grossly.
- The tumor is not completely resectable because of local infiltration into vital structures.

Stage IV

Hematogenous metastases; deposits beyond stage III (e.g., lung, liver, bone, and brain)

Stage V

Bilateral renal involvement is seen at diagnosis.

An attempt should be made to stage each side according to the above criteria on the basis of extent of disease prior to biopsy.

*The clinical stage is decided by the surgeon in the operating room and is confirmed by the pathologist, who also evaluates the histology. It is done on the basis of gross and microscopic tumor distribution and is the same for tumors with favorable and with unfavorable histologic features. The patient is characterized, however, by a statement of both criteria (e.g., stage II, favorable histology, or stage II, unfavorable histology).

minimize radiation effects to the liver because radiation hepatotoxicity is potentiated by actinomycin D. Bilateral Wilms tumor is present in about 5% of children on initial presentation, whereas recurrent disease affects the opposite kidney in 4–5% of patients. Treatment for each patient with bilateral Wilms tumor should be individualized. Every effort should be made to retain as much functional nephrogenic tissue as possible.

Neuroblastoma

Neuroblastoma arises from primitive neural crest cells that form the adrenal medulla and the sympathetic nervous system.

Epidemiology. Neuroblastoma is the most common malignant tumor in infancy, with a median age of 20 months at onset. In childhood it ranks fourth in frequency after leukemia, lymphoma, and CNS tumors. Although neuroblastoma represents fewer than 8% of cases of childhood cancer, it is responsible for 15% of cancer deaths in children. The incidence of neuroblastoma is estimated to be 1 in 100,000 infants.

Clinical Manifestations. The most common presentation is an abdominal mass that is hard, smooth, and nontender. The mass is most often palpated in the flank. In the abdomen, 45% of tumors arise in the adrenal gland and 25% in the retroperitoneal sympathetic ganglia. Other common sites of origin are the pelvis, the posterior mediastinum, and the neck. Calcification within the tumor often is observed on plain films of the abdomen. The presentation must be differentiated from that of Wilms tumor, which also presents as an abdominal flank mass. Ultrasound examination is usually able to differentiate the two tumors.

Neuroblastoma may metastasize to multiple organs, including the liver, bone, bone marrow, and lymph nodes. In older children, fever and weight loss associated with a limp or back pain may be the presenting symptoms of neuroblastoma. Pulmonary involvement by neuroblastoma is uncommon. In infants, skin metastasis that manifests as "blueberry muffin" lesions may be seen. Vasoactive intestinal polypeptide secretion may produce watery diarrhea. Neuroblastoma is occasionally associated with opsoclonus and myoclonus.

Diagnosis. Diagnostic workup for neuroblastoma involves a CT scan of the chest, abdomen, and pelvis; a bone scan; bilateral bone marrow aspiration and biopsy; lumbar puncture; and a 24-hour urine collection for catecholamines. Most neuroblastomas secrete one or more catecholamines or their metabolic byproducts (vanillylmandelic acid or homovanillic acid). Neuroblastoma cells concentrate MIBG, a neurotransmitter precursor; thus MIBG scanning is a sensitive method for detecting neuroblastoma metastasis. More recently, octreotide scanning has also been used for patients with neuroblastoma. The international staging system for neuroblastoma is shown in Table 15–16. Appropri-

---

TABLE 15–16
International Neuroblastoma Staging System

Stage	Definition	Incidence (%)	Survival at 5 Years
1	Localized tumor with complete gross excision, with or without microscopic residual disease; representative ipsilateral lymph nodes negative for tumor microscopically (nodes attached to and removed with the primary tumor may be positive)	5	90% or greater
2A	Localized tumor with incomplete gross excision; representative ipsilateral nonadherent lymph nodes negative for tumor microscopically	10	70–80%
2B	Localized tumor with or without complete gross excision, with ipsilateral nonadherent lymph nodes positive for tumor. Enlarged contralateral lymph nodes must be negative microscopically		
3	Unresectable unilateral tumor infiltrating across the midline,* with or without regional lymph node involvement; or localized unilateral tumor with contralateral regional lymph node involvement; or midline tumor with bilateral extension by infiltration (resectable) or by lymph node involvement	25	40–70% (depending on completeness of surgical resection)
4	Any primary tumor with dissemination to distant lymph nodes; bone, bone marrow, liver, skin, and other organs (except as defined for stage 4S)	60	More than 60% if age at diagnosis is younger than 1 yr; 20% if age at diagnosis is older than 1 yr and under 2 yr; 10% if age at diagnosis is over 2 yr
4S	Localized primary tumor (as defined for stage 1, 2A, or 2B), with dissemination limited to skin, liver, and bone marrow† (limited to infants younger than 1 yr of age)	5	More than 80%

Modified from Brodeur GM et al: *J Clin Oncol* 11(8):1466–1477, 1993.
*The midline is defined as the vertebral column. Tumors originating on one side and crossing the midline must infiltrate to or beyond the opposite side of the vertebral column.
†Marrow involvement in stage 4S should be minimal (i.e., <10% of total nucleated cells identified as malignant on bone marrow biopsy or on marrow aspirate). More extensive marrow involvement would be considered to be stage 4. The MIBG scan (if performed) should be negative in the marrow.

ate evaluation of the biopsy specimen to provide important prognostic information is crucial. In addition to routine light microscopic examination, cytogenetic analysis and studies to detect N-*myc* amplification should be performed.

Prognosis. The age of the patient at presentation of the disease, the stage of the disease, the primary site, the presence or absence of metastasis, cytogenetics, DNA ploidy, amplification of the N-*myc* oncogene (poor prognosis), and histopathology all affect survival. In general, children with neuroblastoma can be divided into two large groups: those with favorable and those with unfavorable biology. Favorable biologic factors are tumor cell differentiation, no amplification of the N-*myc* oncogene, a triploid cytogenetic karyotype, and no loss of genetic material from the short arm of chromosome 1. Patients with favorable biology tend to be younger and often have localized disease. Patients younger than 1 year of age have a better prognosis than older patients, regardless of stage. This holds for patients with both favorable and unfavorable biology. Older patients with stage IV disease most commonly have unfavorable biology and a poor outcome with standard therapy.

Treatment. For patients with localized neuroblastoma, complete surgical excision is the initial treatment of choice. Children with favorable biology who undergo a gross total resection require no further therapy. In patients with advanced disease, combination chemotherapy is usually given after confirmation of the diagnosis. Delayed resection of the primary tumor is undertaken following a number of courses of chemotherapy. Radiation therapy is often given to the primary tumor bed and areas of metastatic disease. Until recently, the cure rate for older patients with stage IV disease has been very poor. In a recent study by the Children's Cancer Group, patients were randomly selected to receive either maintenance chemotherapy or high-dose chemotherapy with purged bone marrow rescue. Patients who attained a complete response to initial chemotherapy had significantly improved outcome if they received high-dose therapy with stem cell support. An additional finding of that study was that patients who received retinoic acid following either bone marrow transplant or maintenance chemotherapy had an improved outcome. The most common active agents are vincristine, cyclophosphamide, doxorubicin, cisplatin, and VP-16.

Soft Tissue Sarcomas

Rhabdomyosarcoma is the most common soft tissue sarcoma in children. Less common soft tissue sarcomas are fibrosarcoma, synovial sarcoma, malignant fibrous histiocytoma, alveolar soft-part sarcoma, epithelioid sarcoma, and extraosseous Ewing sarcoma. The incidence of rhabdomyosarcoma is about 4.5 cases per million, with a peak occurrence in children 2–6 years of age and a second peak in adolescence. Tumor arises primarily in skeletal muscle but may occur in any tissue derived from mesenchyme. The early peak is associated with tumors in the genitourinary region, head, and neck; the later peak is associated with tumors in the extremities, trunk, and male genitourinary tract. Tumors of the head and neck occur in the orbit, sinuses, nasopharynx, and soft tissues.

Clinical Manifestations. Clinical presentation of rhabdomyosarcoma varies, depending on the site of origin and subsequent mass effect. For example, swelling, proptosis, and limitation of extraocular motion may be seen with an orbital tumor; nasal mass, chronic otitis media, hemorrhage, ear discharge, obstruction, dysphagia, hearing abnormalities, and cranial nerve involvement may be noted with tumors in other head and neck sites. In the genitourinary tract, urethral or vaginal masses, paratesticular swelling, hematuria, and urinary frequency or retention may be noted. Trunk or extremity lesions tend to present as rapidly growing masses that may or may not be painful.

Diagnosis. Tissue biopsy is needed for definitive diagnosis. Two major histologic variants exist for rhabdomyosarcoma. Embryonal histology is most common in younger children with head and neck and genitourinary primary tumors. Alveolar histology occurs in older patients and is seen most commonly in trunk and extremity tumors. Alveolar rhabdomyosarcoma is often characterized by specific translocations: t(2;13) or t(1;13). Under the light microscope, rhabdomyosarcoma may appear as a small, round, blue cell tumor. In those cases immunohistochemical staining for muscle-specific proteins such as actin and myosin and other muscle-related proteins such as desmin and vimentin may help make the diagnosis. Metastatic workup for patients with rhabdomyosarcoma should involve a CT scan of the chest, abdomen, and pelvis, a bone scan, and bone marrow aspiration and biopsy. In patients with a parameningeal primary site (e.g., the middle ear, nasopharynx, or infratemporal fossa), a lumbar puncture is required.

Treatment. Treatment is currently based on a staging system that incorporates both the primary site and histology. The staging system also involves a local tumor group assessment based on the extent of initial surgery. In the intergroup rhabdomyosarcoma studies, the most common chemotherapy agents used are cyclophosphamide, vincristine, and actinomycin.

Most recently, topotecan and ifosfamide have been included in the treatment of rhabdomyosarcoma. Radiation is administered to all patients who have residual disease after initial surgery or who have had a biopsy only of the primary tumor. Patients with localized disease in favorable sites have an excellent prognosis when treated with vincristine and actinomycin D alone. Therapy for patients with metastatic disease at diagnosis remains inadequate.

MALIGNANT BONE TUMORS

The two most important malignant bone tumors in children are osteosarcoma and Ewing sarcoma.

Osteosarcoma

Osteosarcoma is a rare tumor. In children younger than 15 years old, only about 300 new cases occur each year in the United States. Males are affected 1½ times more than females.

Epidemiology and Etiology. Osteosarcoma most commonly affects adolescents, with the peak incidence occurring during the period of maximum growth velocity. The primary tumor most often is located at the epiphysis or metaphysis of anatomic sites that are associated with maximum growth velocity (e.g., distal femur, proximal tibia, or proximal humerus), but any bone may be involved. The cause is unknown; the correlation of the location of most tumors with a period of maximum bone growth suggests some relation to increased osteoblastic activity. Among patients with hereditary retinoblastoma, the incidence of osteosarcoma is increased 500 times; and deletions on the long arm of chromosome 13, which can occur in patients with retinoblastoma, have been found in some osteosarcomas. Osteosarcoma may arise in a previously radiated area.

Clinical Manifestations. Osteosarcoma generally presents with pain in a bony site. The pain may be associated with a palpable mass. X-ray examination of the affected region usually reveals a lytic lesion, often associated with calcification in the soft tissue surrounding the lesion.

Diagnosis. Needle biopsy is usually used to make the diagnosis of osteosarcoma. The presence of osteoid confirms the diagnosis of osteosarcoma. The extent of the primary tumor must be carefully delineated. MRI of the affected bone should be carried out at the time of diagnosis. Osteosarcoma tends to metastasize to bone and lung; therefore, a metastatic workup consists of a chest CT scan and a bone scan. Approximately 75–80% of patients with osteosarcoma have apparently localized disease at diagnosis. Before the availability of chemotherapy, patients with apparently localized

osteosarcoma of an extremity were treated with amputation alone. In approximately 80% of these patients, pulmonary metastases developed within 6 months of amputation. Therefore, osteosarcoma is characterized by a high incidence of micrometastatic disease at diagnosis. A number of biologic features of osteosarcoma, including p53 status, multiple–drug-resistance protein levels, and HER 2-NEU gene expression, have been looked at as potential prognostic factors.

Treatment. The current treatment of osteosarcoma involves preoperative combination chemotherapy followed by limb salvage or amputation and further postoperative chemotherapy. Agents effective against osteosarcoma are adriamycin, high-dose methotrexate, ifosfamide, and platinum drugs (cisplatin or carboplatin). After the completion of neoadjuvant chemotherapy, either limb salvage or amputation is performed. Patients whose tumor specimens show a high degree of necrosis related to the preoperative chemotherapy have an event-free survival rate greater than 80%. Patients who still have large amounts of viable tumor have a much worse prognosis. The outlook for patients who have metastatic osteosarcoma at diagnosis remains quite poor.

Ewing Sarcoma

Ewing sarcoma is a highly malignant, small, round, blue cell tumor most commonly found in bone. Ewing sarcoma is characterized by a specific chromosomal translocation, t(11;22). The incidence in white children is about 1.9 per million. Ewing sarcoma is quite rare in black children. The femur and pelvis are the most common sites, but lesions of the tibia, fibula, ribs, humerus, scapula, and clavicle also are encountered. The clinical manifestations are quite similar to those of osteosarcoma. An MRI of the primary lesion should be carried out to delineate the extent of the lesion and any associated soft tissue mass. Metastatic workup involves a bone scan, chest CT scan, and bone marrow aspiration or biopsy. The treatment for Ewing sarcoma is similar to that for osteosarcoma; preoperative chemotherapy is given, followed by local control measures and then further chemotherapy. Unlike osteosarcoma, Ewing sarcoma is radiation sensitive, although high doses of radiation are required to sterilize local lesions. Chemotherapy includes vincristine, cyclophosphamide, ifosfamide, VP-16, and doxorubicin. Actinomycin D, which was a mainstay in the therapy of Ewing sarcoma in earlier times, is used less frequently today. The cure rate for patients with localized Ewing sarcoma is approximately 60–70%. Patients who have lung metastasis at diagnosis have a cure rate of approximately 30–35%. All patients with metastases to other sites have a dismal outcome.

REFERENCES

Behrman RE, Kliegman RM, Jenson HB, editors: *Nelson textbook of pediatrics,* ed 16, Philadelphia, 2000, WB Saunders, Chapters 497–515.

Brodeur GM, Mans JM, Yamashiro DJ, et al: Biology and genetics of human neuroblastoma, *J Pediatr Hematol Oncol* 19(2):93–101, 1997.

Cokgor I, Friedman AH, Friedman HS: Gliomas, *Eur J Cancer* 34(12):1910–1915, 1998.

Deininger MWN, Goldman JM, Melo JV: The molecular biology of chronic myeloid leukemia, *Blood* 96(10):3343–3356, 2000.

Graf N, Tournade MF, DeKraker J: The role of preoperative chemotherapy in the management of Wilms tumor, *Urol Clin North Am* 27(3):443–454, 2000.

Grier HE: The Ewing's family of tumors, *Pediatr Clin North Am* 44(4):991–1004, 1997.

Keene DL, Hsu E, Ventureyra E: Brain tumors in childhood and adolescents, *Pediatr Neurol* 20(3):198–203, 1999.

Maris JM, Matthay KM: Molecular biology of neuroblastoma, *J Clin Oncol* 17(7):2264–2279, 1999.

Mason WP, Grovas A, Halpern S, et al: Intensive chemotherapy and bone marrow rescue for young children with newly diagnosed malignant brain tumors, *J Clin Oncol* 16(1):210–221, 1998.

Matthay KM, Villablanca JG, et al: Treatment of high risk neuroblastoma with intensive chemotherapy, radiotherapy, autologous bone marrow transplantation and B cis-retinoic acid, *N Engl J Med* 341(16):1165–1173, 1999.

Meyers PA, Gorlick R, Heller G, et al: Intensification of preoperative chemotherapy for osteogenic sarcoma: results of the Memorial Sloan Kettering (T12) protocol, *J Clin Oncol* 16(7):2452–2458, 1998.

Nachman JB, Sather TIN, Sensel MG, et al: Augmented post induction chemotherapy for children with high risk acute lymphoblastic leukemia and a slow response to initial therapy, *N Engl J Med* 338(23):1663–1671, 1998.

Packer RJ, Goldwein J, Nicholson SH, et al: Treatment of children with medulloblastoma with reduced dose craniospinal radiation therapy and adjuvant chemotherapy: a Children's Cancer Group study, *J Clin Oncol* 17(7):2127–2136, 1999.

Patte C: Non-Hodgkin's lymphoma, *Eur J Cancer* 34(3):359–362, 1998.

Pui CH, Evans WE: Acute lymphoblastic leukemia, *N Engl J Med* 339(9):605–615, 1998.

Ries LA, Smith MA, Gurney JG, et al: Cancer incidence and survival among children and adolescents: United States SEER Program 1975–1995, National Cancer Institute, SEER Program, NIH Publication No 99-4649, Bethesda, Md, 1999.

Ritter J: Acute myeloid leukemias—pediatric update, *Eur J Cancer* 34(6):862–872, 1998.

Rodman JH, Relling MV, Stewart CF, et al: Clinical pharmacokinetics and pharmacodynamics of anticancer drugs in children, *Semin Oncol* 20(1):18–29, 1993.

Ruymann FB, Grovas AC: Progress in diagnosis and treatment of rhabdomyosarcoma and related soft tissue sarcomas, *Cancer Invest* 18(3):223–241, 2000.

Sandlund JT, Downing JR, Crist WM: Non-Hodgkin's lymphoma in childhood, *N Engl J Med* 334(19):1238–1248, 1996.

Smith M, Arthur D, Camitta B, et al: Uniform approach to risk classification and treatment assignment for children with acute lymphoblastic leukemia, *J Clin Oncol* 14(1):18–24, 1996.

Stevens RF, Hann TM, Wheately K, et al: Marked improvements in outcome with chemotherapy alone in pediatric acute leukemia: results of the United Kingdom Medical Research Council's 10th AML trial. MRC Childhood Leukemia Working Party, *Br J Hematol* 101(1):130–140, 1998.

Wiener JS, Coppes MJ, Ritchey ML: Current concepts in the biology and management of Wilms tumor, *J Urol* 159(4):1316–1325, 1998.

CHAPTER 16

Nephrology: Fluids and Electrolytes

Aaron L. Friedman

Renal dysfunction is common in children. *Primary* dysfunction may be the result of diseases originating in the kidney or urinary tract (e.g., pyelonephritis, Wilms tumor, dysplasia, or minimal change nephrotic syndrome); *secondary* dysfunction may be the result of systemic illnesses that alter renal function, such as systemic lupus erythematosus (SLE), dehydration (e.g., acute tubular necrosis), heart failure (e.g., prerenal azotemia), hemolysis (e.g., hemoglobinuria), or nephrolithiasis (e.g., hyperparathyroidism). Renal involvement may be one manifestation of a systemic disorder (e.g., galactosemia or hemolytic-uremic syndrome), or the kidney may be the target organ for immune-mediated injury (poststreptococcal glomerulonephritis), but a limited number of manifestations of either primary or secondary renal disease exist (Table 16–1). Abnormalities of the many functions of the kidney appear predominantly as alterations in urine appearance or volume and disturbances of fluid and electrolyte or acid-base balance. Renal malformations and tumors (see Chapter 15) may be noted as flank or abdominal masses.

Because fetal urine production contributes to amniotic fluid volume, renal anomalies often are associated with reduced amniotic fluid volume (oligohydramnios) and less often with increased amniotic fluid volume (polyhydramnios). Renal and ureter anomalies are present in 3–4% of infants.

RENAL PHYSIOLOGY

The major functions of the kidney are to maintain body fluid and electrolyte homeostasis and to remove waste products of metabolism. This organ system has metabolic (gluconeogenesis) and endocrine functions (vitamin D activation, erythropoietin production) that also are important.

The major homeostatic functions of the kidney are carried out by the processes of glomerular ultrafiltration, tubular reabsorption, and tubular secretion. Glomerular ultrafiltration is the net result of opposing pressures acting within glomeruli, those pressures moving fluid across the glomerular capillary wall from blood to urinary space, and back pressure from glomerular filtrate in Bowman's space opposing this filtration.

Glomerular capillary hydrostatic pressure results from the systemic arterial pressure, which is modified by the afferent and efferent arteriolar tones. Because only minimal amounts of protein are filtered by the glomerulus, the oncotic pressure of the urinary space at the beginning of the proximal tubule generally is zero, and thus the pressure favoring filtration is essentially that of the capillary hydrostatic pressure. The hydrostatic pressure within the lumen of the urinary space of the early proximal tubule, plus the mean glomerular capillary oncotic pressure, opposes filtration. The hydrostatic pressure remains constant, but the oncotic pressure of the glomerular capillary progressively rises from the afferent to the efferent end as a result of the removal of fluid during filtration. Thus the pressures favoring filtration are maximal at the afferent end of the glomerulus and minimal at the efferent end. Alterations in systemic blood flow or in the internal regulation of glomerular pressures also alter the *glomerular filtration rate* (GFR). Obstruction of the renal tubules, ureter, or bladder may raise intratubular pressure and retard filtration. Changes in glomerular capillary protein concentration or in the permeability of the capillary wall also affect the glomerular filtration rate.

Glomerular filtration begins during the third month of gestation. Glomerulogenesis is completed at about 34 weeks of gestation, and subsequently the

TABLE 16–1
Common Manifestations of Renal Disease

Neonate	
Flank mass	Dysplasia, polycystic disease, hydronephrosis, tumor
Hematuria	Asphyxia, malformation, trauma, renal vein thrombosis
Anuria and oliguria	Agenesis, obstruction, asphyxia, vascular thrombosis

Child and Adolescent	
Cola-red colored urine	Hemoglobinuria (hemolysis); myoglobinuria (rhabdomyolysis); pigmenturia (porphyria, urate, beets, drugs); hematuria (glomerulonephritis, Henoch-Schönlein purpura, hypercalciuria)
Gross hematuria	Glomerulonephritis, benign hematuria, trauma, cystitis, tumor, nephrolithiasis
Edema	Nephrotic syndrome, nephritis, acute or chronic renal failure, cardiac or liver disease
Hypertension	Acute glomerulonephritis, acute or chronic renal failure, dysplasia, coarctation of the aorta, renal artery stenosis
Polyuria	Diabetes mellitus, central and nephrogenic diabetes insipidus, hypokalemia, hypercalcemia, psychogenic polydipsia, sickle cell anemia, polyuric renal failure, diuretic abuse
Oliguria	Dehydration, acute tubular necrosis, interstitial nephritis, acute glomerulonephritis, hemolytic-uremic syndrome
Urgency	Urinary tract infection, vaginitis, foreign body, hypercalciuria

glomerular filtration rate increases more rapidly than body size.

The GFR is measured most accurately by the infusion of a substance that is freely filtered by the glomerulus but is not metabolized, reabsorbed, or secreted, such as inulin. Clinically, creatinine is used to approximate GFR because it is excreted primarily through glomerular filtration and has little tubular reabsorption or secretion except in renal insufficiency. The GFR (measured using creatinine) is calculated as

$$GFR = UV/P \times 1.73/SA$$

where U = urine creatinine (mg/dL), V = volume collected over time (mL/min), P = serum creatinine (mg/dL), and SA = body surface area.

The GFR equation must be corrected for body surface area to achieve the standard nomenclature of mL/min/1.73 m^2. Creatinine clearance is therefore approximately 40 mL/min/1.73 m^2 in the full-term newborn. GFR increases during the first 2 years of life more rapidly than body size and achieves adult values/1.73 m^2 at this time (110–125 mL/min/ 1.73 m^2). Subsequently, GFR and body size increase proportionately, and thus GFR/1.73 m^2 remains stable throughout the remainder of childhood to adulthood (95–105 mL/min/1.73 m^2).

Plasma creatinine concentration alone is not an adequate measure of renal function. The "normal" lev-els of creatinine in most laboratories vary from 0.3–1.5 mg/dL, a range that encompasses individuals of all ages and sizes. The plasma creatinine concentration in a newborn equals the maternal value at delivery because of equilibration across the placenta. The neonate's own plasma creatinine level is achieved within 4–10 days of age in full-term infants.

Plasma creatinine depends on body mass, as well as on renal function; therefore, normal creatinine concentration is a gradually increasing absolute value throughout childhood. Classically, to determine the relationship between plasma creatinine and GFR in a particular child, the physician must measure creatinine clearance or another indicator of GFR. Because urine collections are somewhat difficult to obtain in the young child, another method is used to estimate the GFR; it has been demonstrated that plasma creatinine (P_{CR}), length in centimeters (L), and a constant of proportionality (k) reflect the relationship between urinary creatinine excretion and units of body size. The formula is

$$GFR \ (mL/min/1.73 \ m^2) = k \times L \ (cm)/P_{CR} \ (mg/dL)$$

The value for k is 0.33 in preterm infants, 0.45 in full-term infants, 0.55 in children and adolescent girls, and 0.7 in adolescent boys. This formula is useful only in infants and children whose body habitus is reasonably normal and whose renal function is stable.

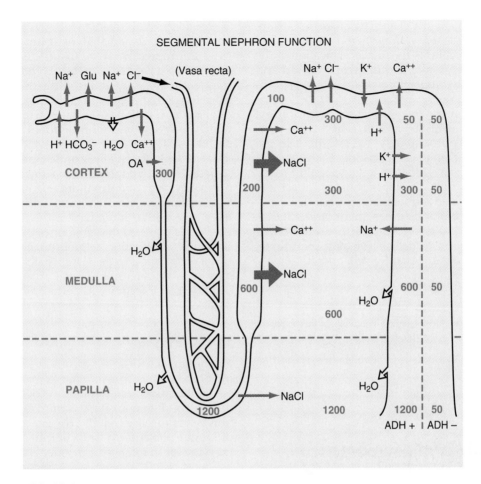

SEGMENTAL NEPHRON FUNCTION

FIG. 16–1

Major transport functions of each nephron segment, including representative osmolalities in vasa recta, interstitium, and tubule at different levels within the kidney. *ADH,* Antidiuretic hormone; *Glu,* glucose; *OA,* organic acid. (From Andreoli TE, Carpenter CCJ, Plum F, et al: *Cecil essentials of medicine,* Philadelphia, 1986, WB Saunders.)

FUNCTIONAL MORPHOLOGY

The *proximal tubule* is characterized by isosmotic reabsorption of the glomerular ultrafiltrate (Fig. 16–1). Normally, approximately two thirds of the glomerular ultrafiltrate is reabsorbed from the proximal tubule; a number of solutes, such as glucose and amino acids, are reabsorbed completely, and potassium is reabsorbed nearly completely. Most phosphate is reabsorbed from the proximal tubule, and calcium is absorbed in parallel with sodium reabsorption. The straight portion of the proximal tubule is responsible for secreting organic acids, including drugs such as penicillin.

The *loop of Henle* serves a major role, in that 25% of filtered sodium chloride is absorbed in this segment (Fig. 16–1). Differential permeabilities convert the isotonic fluid entering the loop of Henle from the proximal tubule into a hypotonic fluid delivered to the distal tubule. Preferential sodium chloride absorption (associated with active chloride transport) is the principal mechanism by which the countercurrent multiplier is activated and by which the medullary interstitial hypertonicity required for urinary concentration is accomplished. This principally occurs in the thick ascending limb. Salt and water movement across the thin limbs is driven primarily by osmotic gradients.

The *distal tubule* is made up of the *distal convoluted tubule,* which is water impermeable and continues to carry out the dilution of luminal fluid by way of active sodium chloride absorption, and the *collecting ducts,* which are the primary sites of *antidiuretic hormone* (ADH) activity. These distal segments are the sites of potassium and hydrogen ion secretion, which is responsible for the final acidification of the urine. The processes of sodium reabsorption and potassium and hydrogen ion secretion are all stimulated by aldosterone.

The maximum *urinary concentrating capacity* is less in the newborn (600–800 mOsm/L in the full-term newborn and approximately 400 mOsm/L in the preterm infant) than in children older than 1 year of age (>1200 mOsm/L). The neonate's ability to dilute the urine is fully developed, but the capacity to excrete a water load is quantitatively less. The newborn exhibits numerous other quantitative limitations, such as limits on the rate of excretion of sodium, potassium, hydrogen ion, and phosphate, but renal functions are qualitatively operative.

REFERENCES

Behrman RE, Kliegman RM, Jenson HB, editors: *Nelson's textbook of pediatrics*, ed 16, Philadelphia, 2000, WB Saunders, Chapters 516, 536.

Jones DP, Chesney RW: Development of tubular function, *Clin Perinatol* 19(1):33–57, 1992.

Robillard JE, Segar JL, Smith FG, et al: Regulation of sodium metabolism and extracellular fluid volume during development, *Clin Perinatol* 19(1):15–31, 1992.

CONGENITAL AND DEVELOPMENTAL ABNORMALITIES OF THE URINARY TRACT

Bilateral renal agenesis, which occurs in 1:4000 births, is the result of failure of development of or degeneration of the ureteric bud. Features associated with this condition are part of **Potter syndrome** (flat facies, clubfoot, and pulmonary hypoplasia), resulting from oligohydramnios and fetal compression by the uterus (see Chapter 19). Infants with bilateral renal agenesis usually die of respiratory insufficiency in the first week of life as a result of pulmonary hypoplasia, pneumothoraces, and pulmonary hypertension. *Unilateral renal agenesis* (1:1000 births) is associated with compensatory hypertrophy in the contralateral kidney and normal or minimally reduced renal function. Although this condition is compatible with normal renal function and normal life expectancy, an associated incidence of other abnormalities exists with unilateral renal agenesis, including abnormalities of the genital tract, skeletal system, and cardiovascular system. Unilateral renal agenesis also has been described as a component of the VACTERL* association, Turner syndrome, and Poland syndrome.

*VACTERL = Vertebral defects, imperforate anus, cardiac, tracheoesophageal fistula, renal dysplasia, limb abnormalities.

Renal hypoplasia refers to kidneys that are present but small in size and that, over time, predispose a child to progressive renal insufficiency because of their reduced nephron number. Hypoplastic kidneys frequently are scarred and difficult to distinguish from those that are chronically infected. Renal hypoplasia also may be associated with poor growth, which may become more evident in the second decade of life.

Renal dysplasia usually is unilateral and may be associated with hypoplasia. It is a developmental abnormality with abnormal organization and ductal differentiation. Most children with this disorder have obstructive anomalies of the urinary tract. It has been suggested that ureteric or urethral obstruction early in gestation is the primary factor leading to the dysplastic changes. Dysplastic (cystic) kidneys may with time resemble renal aplasia and lead to urinary tract infections, hypertension, or, less often, malignancy.

Cystic Dysplasias of the Kidney

Polycystic kidney disease is an inherited disease affecting both kidneys. The two major forms are an autosomal recessive type ("infantile" polycystic kidney disease) and an autosomal dominant type ("adult" polycystic disease [ADPKD]). The two conditions differ morphologically and clinically, although both may appear in infancy or in older children.

Autosomal Recessive Disease

The autosomal recessive type of polycystic kidney disease is characterized by marked enlargement of both kidneys with innumerable cysts throughout the cortex and medulla, which are dilated collecting ducts. Interstitial fibrosis and tubular atrophy may not be present at birth but progress with time, frequently to renal failure. Hepatic fibrosis is present and may lead to portal hypertension. Bile duct ectasia and biliary dysgenesis also occur. The kidneys of the newborn with the autosomal recessive form are spongy and markedly enlarged and maintain the usual renal configuration. Older children demonstrate less severe cyst formation but still show progressive renal fibrosis and tubular atrophy.

Although the *diagnosis* can be made in utero by ultrasonographic examination, many of the liveborn infants die in the neonatal period, often from respiratory distress resulting from pulmonary hypoplasia. Eighty percent of infants have clinical manifestations such as flank mass, hepatomegaly, pneumothorax, proteinuria, or hematuria.

Treatment is supportive, including the management of hypertension, renal failure, and poor nutrition. The *prognosis* is poor, in terms of both renal insufficiency and hepatic fibrosis. Ultimately, renal transplantation and treatment of hepatic fibrosis, including portosystemic shunts and liver transplantation, may be beneficial.

Autosomal Dominant

The autosomal dominant form of polycystic kidney disease (ADPKD) characteristically appears in the fourth or fifth decade of life but also presents in infancy or childhood. Infants have a clinical picture similar to that in autosomal recessive polycystic kidney disease, but older children may show a pattern similar to that of adults. Renal pathology shows glomerular and tubular cysts. Family history is usually positive. Hepatic cysts are present in this disease, and splenic and pancreatic cysts may also be seen. Cerebral aneurysms may be present and can be of clinical significance. The gene for ADPKD is on chromosome 6p21cen. The location or function of the ion pump may contribute to cyst formation.

Renal cysts are also observed in von Hippel-Lindau syndrome and tuberous sclerosis.

REFERENCES

Behrman RE, Kliegman RM, Jenson HB, editors: *Nelson's textbook of pediatrics*, ed 16, Philadelphia, 2000, WB Saunders, Chapter 529.

Kissane JM: Renal cysts in pediatric patients; a classification and overview, *Pediatr Nephrol* 4(1):69–77, 1990.

Woolf A, Winyard P: Unraveling the pathogenesis of cystic kidney disease, *Arch Dis Child* 72(2):103–105, 1995.

Vesicoureteral Reflux

Vesicoureteral reflux, the abnormal backflow of urine from the bladder to the ureter or kidney, usually results from a congenital incompetence of the vesicoureteral junction or, less often, from incompetence of the junction secondary to obstruction or infection. Reflux may be familial.

Pathophysiology. Reflux is potentially harmful because of the exposure of the kidney to *increased hydrodynamic pressure* during voiding. In addition, the incomplete emptying of the ureter and bladder on voiding predisposes the patient to **urinary tract infection** because in the presence of lower urinary tract infection, reflux allows bacteria to gain access easily to the pelvocalyceal system. **Reflux nephropathy** refers to the development and progression of *renal scarring*, often secondary to prolonged reflux, particularly if associated with infection or obstruction (bladder neck obstruction or posterior urethral valves). A significant number of children have end-stage renal disease as a result of reflux nephropathy, which also may be an important precursor to hypertension.

The normal vesicoureteral junction prevents reflux because of the oblique entry of the ureter into the bladder, the length of the ureteral tunnel traversing the bladder wall, and the 4–5:1 ratio of the length of this tunnel to the ureteral diameter. Primary reflux results from a short intramural tunnel ratio, as low as 1.5:1, and is characteristically associated with a lateral position of the ureteral orifice and an underdeveloped trigone. The shortened intramural tunnel decreases the efficiency of the valvular mechanism, allowing reflux to occur. Less often, duplications of the ureters that also exhibit ureteroceles may obstruct the upper collecting system. Reflux may be associated with ureteral diverticulum. Abnormalities of the neurogenic bladder associated with myelomeningocele are complicated by reflux in approximately one third to one half of affected children. Reflux also may be secondary to increased intravascular pressure when the bladder outlet is obstructed, to inflammation of the bladder (cystitis), or to surgical procedures performed on the bladder.

Clinical Manifestations. Reflux is characteristically discovered during radiologic evaluation following a urinary tract infection. Severe reflux may begin in utero and may be associated with neonatal renal insufficiency resulting from renal parenchymal loss. In neonates with urinary tract infection the incidence of reflux is high. Reflux may resolve with time.

Reflux and infection lead to the serious complication of renal scarring and may eventually result in renal insufficiency or failure. The younger the patient, the more likely reflux will be present; therefore, a *voiding cystourethrogram* (VCUG) should be performed in all infants and most children with a urinary tract infection. The *diagnosis* of previous renal scars can be made by nuclear medicine renal scan with radionuclides such as Tc-dimercaptosuccinic acid (DMSA). This scan defines the renal parenchyma and can diagnose acute pyelonephritis, chronic pyelonephritis, and scarring. The VCUG should be performed after the infection has been treated, but there is no need to wait days or weeks before performing the test. An international grading system has been used to describe reflux (Fig. 16–2). The incidence of scarring associated with the lowest grades of reflux is quite low (15%) but is very high with the higher grades of reflux (grade 4 or 5), in which scarring may occur in two thirds of the patients. Long-term follow-up suggests that reflux is likely to stop without surgical intervention in the low grades, specifically grades 1 and 2, but is far less likely to stop (in fewer than half of the patients) in grade 4 or 5.

Treatment. The finding of reflux indicates the need for long-term prophylactic antibiotic therapy that includes trimethoprim/sulfamethoxazole, sulfisoxazole, or nitrofurantoin. It has been recommended that a urine specimen be obtained for

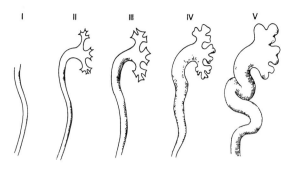

FIG. 16–2

International Classification of Vesicoureteral Reflux: Grade I, ureter only. Grade II, ureter, pelvis, and calyces. No dilation, normal calyceal fornices. Grade III, mild to moderate dilation or tortuosity of the ureter, and mild to moderate dilation of the renal pelvis; slight or no blunting of the fornices. Grade IV, moderate dilation or tortuosity of the ureter and moderate dilation of the renal pelvis and calyces. Complete obliteration of sharp angle of fornices but maintenance of the papillary impressions in the majority of calyces. Grade V, gross dilation and tortuosity of the ureter. Gross dilation of the renal pelvis and calyces. The papillary impressions are no longer visible in most of the calyces. Some authors consider grade IV or V with intrarenal reflux into the collecting ducts a high risk for scarring. (From Duckett JW, Bellinger MF: Cystographic grading of primary reflux as an indicator of treatment. In Johnston JH, editor: *Management of vesicoureteral reflux: international perspectives in urology,* vol 10, Baltimore, 1984, Williams & Wilkins.)

culture at regular (1–3-month) intervals until three consecutive cultures are negative; after that, the frequency can be further reduced. As noted earlier in grade 1 to grade 3 reflux, reflux generally disappears with time. More severe reflux is associated with significant ureteral dilation or upper tract changes on IVP, *renal ultrasound,* or radioisotope scan and often necessitates surgical intervention. In general, reflux of any grade found on *voiding cystourethrography* associated with a normal nephrosonogram or scan can be treated medically with long-term prophylactic antibiotics and serial urine cultures. However, if the IVP or renal scan reveals renal scarring and dilation or clubbing of the pelvocalyceal system, surgical intervention may be indicated at the outset. Surgical intervention is used commonly if reinfection occurs while the patient is receiving antibiotics. Surgical intervention clearly is needed if the reflux is associated with a ureterocele or other urinary tract obstruction. The presence of grade 4 to grade 5 reflux and the failure of time to resolve reflux over several years may be indications for medical or surgical treatment.

Complications of reflux nephropathy are hypertension and end-stage renal disease. The latter is pre-

dicted by proteinuria (>1 g/day) and is the result of the development of focal and segmental *glomerulosclerosis* and interstitial scarring.

Urinary Tract Obstruction

Obstruction of the urinary tract may occur at any anatomic level of the genitourinary system (Table 16–2). Severe obstruction early in gestation is thought to result in **renal dysplasia.** Ureteral obstruction later in fetal life or after birth results in dilation of the ureter and collecting system, often with alterations in renal parenchyma that may range from dilation to scarring and glomerular atrophy. The obstructed urinary tract is susceptible to infections, which may further worsen renal injury.

Clinical Manifestations. Obstructions may be silent but usually are discovered as a urinary tract infection or flank masses. In a newborn, bilateral abdominal masses frequently are hydronephrotic obstructed kidneys.

Diagnosis. *Renal ultrasound and voiding cystourethrography* are the standard tests for diagnosis of urinary tract obstruction. *Renal ultrasound* studies facilitate the identification of renal agenesis, renal hypoplasia, or cystic changes in the presence of obstruction, scarring, and dilation. The dilated upper urinary tract may or may not be obstructed. The radioisotope renogram, particularly used in conjunction with a diuretic agent, frequently allows differentiation of patients with a dilated urinary tract, which empties normally, from those with obstruction. Tc-DMSA scans are the most useful tests for evaluation of the presence of renal scars.

The urinary tract may be obstructed at multiple anatomic levels (Table 16–2). An obstruction of the ureteropelvic junction is the most common lesion in childhood. Such an obstruction may present as a palpable renal mass, urinary tract infection, hematuria (with or without trauma), or flank pain or may be discovered by routine fetal ultrasonographic examination. Twenty percent of ureteropelvic junction obstructions are bilateral.

Treatment. An obstructed ureteropelvic junction necessitates surgery. The success rate of pyeloplastics in relieving obstruction is high, although dilation may persist.

Obstructions of the ureter also may occur at the midureter or at the lower ureter in association with a ureterocele or with an ectopic ureteral orifice, which in turn is frequently associated with reflux. Ectopic ureters may drain a single collecting system or may drain the upper portion of a duplicated collecting system. Ectopic ureters frequently are obstructed; when this happens, prompt surgical intervention is required.

TABLE 16–2
Site and Etiology of Urinary Tract Obstruction

Site	Etiology
Infundibula	Congenital
	Calculi
	Infection
	Trauma
	Tumor
Pelvis	Congenital stenosis
	Infection
	Calculi
	Tumor
Ureteropelvic junction	Congenital stenosis*
	Calculi
	Tumor
	Trauma
Ureter	Obstructive megaureter*
	Ectopic ureter
	Ureterocele
	Valves
	Calculi*
	Primary renal tumor (Wilms tumor)
	Retroperitoneal tumor (lymphoma)
	Inflammatory bowel disease
	Retroperitoneal fibrosis
	Chronic granulomatous disease
Bladder	Neurogenic dysfunction*
	Tumor (rhabdomyosarcoma)
	Diverticula
	Ectopic ureter
Urethra	Posterior valves*
	Diverticula
	Strictures
	Atresia
	Ectopic ureter
	Foreign body
	Phimosis*
	Priapism

*Relatively common.

Prune-Belly Syndrome (Eagle-Barrett Syndrome)

The absence of or severe reduction in abdominal musculature associated with undescended testes and urinary tract abnormalities occurs in approximately 1:40,000 births. The characteristic dilation of the prostatic urethra without posterior urethral valves suggests severe but possibly transient urethral obstruction in fetal life. The reduced abdominal musculature may be the result of transient tense fetal ascites. Oligohydramnios and pulmonary hypoplasia may be present.

Urinary abnormalities include marked dilation of the ureters and calyceal system, a large bladder, and often a patent urachus. The kidneys may be dysplastic, and the testes are undescended in the abdomen. Anomalies of the bowel, heart, and musculoskeletal system may occur. The condition is rare in females. Usually no demonstrable obstruction of the urinary tract is present at birth.

Initial *treatment* consists of stabilization of the cardiopulmonary status and prevention of urinary tract infection. Renal ultrasound, measurement of renal function, radioisotope scan, and voiding cystourethrogram facilitate full assessment of the abnormalities. Therapy then is individualized to maintain renal function and prevent infection.

Posterior Urethral Valves

The posterior urethral valve is the most common cause of **bladder outlet obstruction** in males, present in 1:50,000 boys. The valves are sail-shaped membranes that arise from the verumontanum and attach to the contralateral wall of the urethra. In the presence of persistent valves the prostatic urethra becomes dilated, vesicoureteral reflux may be present, and a small bladder with hypertrophied walls develops. Renal dilation varies in degree, from mild hydronephrosis to severe hydronephrosis with dysplasia. Severe obstruction may be associated with oligohydramnios and subsequent lethal pulmonary hypoplasia. In the newborn period the male infant may exhibit a urinary tract infection, bilateral flank masses (hydronephrosis and hydroureter), a poor voiding stream, or little urinary output. Rupture of the renal pelvis produces **urinary ascites;** this is the most common cause of ascites in the newborn period. A child may come to medical attention later in infancy with a poor urinary stream, failure to thrive secondary to renal failure, urinary tract infection, or renal tubular acidosis. Infants with pulmonary hypoplasia often die early in infancy.

The *diagnosis* and extent of renal damage are established by ultrasonography and by voiding cystourethrography. In many cases the diagnosis is made before birth by fetal ultrasonography. Once the infant is stabilized, *treatment* consists of either preliminary decompression, valve ablation, or both, depending on the individual circumstances. Valve ablation is successful in most infants, and the serum creatinine level may return to normal by 1 year of age. Children having persistent elevated creatinine levels also may have associated renal dysplasia. Immediately after relief of the obstruction, a marked diuresis resulting from a defect in urine concentrating ability may be present. Careful follow-up to prevent urinary tract infection is essential.

REFERENCES

Behrman RE, Kliegman RM, Jenson HB, editors: *Nelson textbook of pediatrics,* ed 16, Philadelphia, 2000, WB Saunders, Chapters 545–548.

Jakobsson B, Söderlundhs S, Bert U: Diagnostic significance of ^{99m}Tc-dimercaptosuccinic acid (DMSA) scintigraphy in urinary tract infections, *Arch Dis Child* 67(11):1138–1142, 1992.

Schwartz GW, Brion LT, Spitzer A: The use of plasma creatinine concentration for estimating glomerular filtration rate in infants, children and adolescents, *Pediatr Clin North Am* 34(3): 571–590, 1987.

DISTURBANCES OF ELECTROLYTES, ACID-BASE BALANCE, AND FLUIDS

Because sodium is the principal extracellular cation, regulation of extracellular fluid parallels regulation of sodium balance. Intrarenal sodium conservation is regulated by the juxtaglomerular apparatus and the macula densa, which sense decreased effective renal blood flow and respond by releasing renin. Renin acts on angiotensinogen to produce angiotensin I. Angiotensin-converting enzyme then converts angiotensin I to angiotensin II, which stimulates the release of aldosterone. Aldosterone increases distal tubule sodium reabsorption. In conditions of severe sodium restriction, decreased intravascular volume (e.g., hemorrhage or sepsis), or decreased effective renal blood flow (e.g., heart failure) the urinary excretion of sodium approaches zero. In addition, baroreceptors in the atria, aortic arch, carotid bifurcations, and pulmonary vessels also sense volume depletion and signal the brain via cranial nerves IX and X. This signaling results in increased central nervous system (CNS) efferent sympathetic discharge, which regulates renal blood flow, vascular resistance, angiotensin II, and thus aldosterone release; the net result is sodium conservation.

The ADH system also senses volume changes. In conditions of hypovolemia, ADH, which increases renal reabsorption of water, is released. In normal day-to-day life this system functions to maintain osmolality within a narrow range because ADH secretion is stimulated during normovolemic states by high serum osmolality.

Atrial natriuretic peptide is synthesized in the cardiac atria and regulates sodium (and intravascular volume) by increasing the glomerular filtration rate and hydrostatic pressure, dilating afferent and constricting efferent arterioles. The hormone also blocks the tubular reabsorption of sodium and chloride.

Parenteral Fluid Therapy

Illnesses that lead to imbalances in fluids and electrolytes pose a greater risk to children than to adults. The younger the child is, the greater is the vulnerability to such disturbances because of the larger daily turnover of water relative to the total body water, the large extracellular fluid space, and in the neonate, the developmental limitations of renal function. The untoward effects of vomiting (reduced intake) and diarrhea (increased losses) appear much more rapidly in the infant than in the adult.

Fluid and electrolyte requirements and their provision are conveniently considered in terms of *maintenance, deficit,* and *supplemental therapy.* Therapeutic plans based on calculations of these needs must be modified constantly, based on a continuing clinical reassessment of the child's physical and mental status and the serial monitoring of levels of serum electrolytes, acid-base balance, blood urea nitrogen, and serum creatinine.

Maintenance Therapy

Ongoing, obligatory normal and abnormal losses of fluids and electrolytes from urine, sweat, feces, and lung must be replaced so that deficits do not occur. Disease states may modify the amount and type of such losses. Protein and calories also must be replaced when oral intake is restricted for a protracted time (see Chapter 2). Losses should be replaced orally, when possible, or intravenously.

Maintenance requirements of fluid and electrolytes are directly related to metabolic rate. An increased metabolic rate increases catabolism of metabolic fuels. This leads to increases in the rate of production of water of oxidation from carbohydrate, fat, and protein; in urinary excretion of solute and water; and in heat production, which increases water loss in insensible water loss, sweat, and respiratory gases. The turnover rates of electrolytes also are related closely to water loss and metabolic rate. Thus maintenance requirements for fluid and electrolytes can be calculated from a child's caloric expenditures.

Calculation of Normal Maintenance Requirements. A child's metabolic rate or caloric expenditure depends on age, body weight, degree of activity, temperature, and any pathologic state. Adjustments above basal caloric expenditures for activity are based on observation of the patient. The usual hospitalized patient burns calories at a rate 20–30% above basal caloric expenditures. Fever increases caloric expenditures by about 12%/1° C rise in temperature, and salicylism and hyperthyroidism increase caloric expenditures by 25–75%. Conversely, hypothermia results in similar decreases in caloric expenditure per incremental fall in temperature, and hypothyroidism results in a 10–25% decrease in basal metabolism.

Table 16–3 provides a simplified means of calculating expenditure for the average hospitalized child (nonneonate) engaged in the usual bed activity. Additional adjustments should be made for further activity, temperature, and disease states. The usual fluid and electrolyte losses that occur for each 100 kcal metabolized then also can be estimated. With this approach for replacing losses resulting from ongoing metabolism, 100 mL of fluid should be provided for every 100 kcal expended, and the solution should contain 35 mEq/L of sodium, 20 mEq/L of potassium, and 5% dextrose. This approach to providing maintenance requirements assumes that there is no kidney damage or disease state that would limit renal capacity to adjust urine flow rates and electrolyte excretion over wide ranges.

Modification of Maintenance Therapy as a Result of Disease. Maintenance requirements are decreased (30–45 mL/100 kcal of exogenous water is required to replace insensible water losses, such as sweat and water expired with breathing) in conditions of anuria or extreme oliguria or when excessive or inappropriate release of ADH occurs (i.e., meningitis, head trauma). Requirements for fluid and electrolytes are increased as a result of abnormal losses from gastrointestinal drainage, heat stress, adrenal insufficiency, diabetes mellitus, hyperventilation, loss of renal concentrating and diluting ability, diabetes insipidus, and burns. The amount and nature of the losses depend on the underlying disorder and the site of the loss.

TABLE 16–3
Calculation of Caloric Expenditure from Body Weight

Body Weight (kg)	Caloric Expenditure*
Up to 10	100 kcal/kg
11–20	1000 kcal + 50 kcal/kg for each kg above 10 kg
Above 20	1500 kcal + 20 kcal/kg for each kg above 30 kg

Modified from Behrman RE, editor: *Nelson textbook of pediatrics,* ed 14, Philadelphia, 1992, WB Saunders.
*1 kcal (kilocalorie) = 1000 calories.

Deficit Therapy

Deficits in body water and electrolytes occur from decreased intake and continuing normal losses, from increased losses with or without the usual intake, or from a combination of these events. Because deficits reflect ongoing physiologic readjustments, as well as direct losses, the amount of the deficits often is similar for a variety of precipitating conditions; therefore, they usually can be treated in a similar manner. Fluid and electrolyte treatment is related to a greater extent to the severity and type of deficit than to the underlying cause. The etiology also must be addressed specifically.

Severity. An acute loss of body weight greater than 1%/day reflects a loss of body fluid. The more rapidly a deficit develops, the less well it will be tolerated. Severe dehydration is frequently associated with shock, but even moderate deficits may cause circulatory instability if they develop over the course of a day (Table 16–4).

Pathophysiologic Types of Dehydration. Deficits from dehydration are classified as *isonatremic* (130–150 mEq serum Na^+/L), *hyponatremic* (hypotonic) (<130 mEq Na^+/L), or *hypernatremic* (hypertonic) (>150 mEq Na^+/L). Because plasma osmolality is reflected in sodium concentration, these forms usually are isotonic, hypotonic, and hypertonic, respectively. This may not be the case when another serum solute (such as glucose) is elevated, as occurs in diabetic ketoacidosis, which may result in hyponatremia and hypertonicity.

Isonatremic Dehydration. Approximately proportional fluid and electrolyte losses occur from the extracellular compartment, and because no resulting osmotic gradient across the cell walls takes place, intracellular fluid volume is not significantly changed.

Hypernatremic Dehydration. More water than sodium is lost from the extracellular space, or excess sodium is provided, increasing the osmolality of the extracellular fluid and causing water to move out of cells. This movement adds to the extracellular volume so that extracellular volume depletion is not as clinically severe as expected.

Hyponatremic Dehydration. Relatively more sodium than water is lost from the extracellular space, or excess water is provided. This leads to movement of water into cells, which further depletes the extracellular fluid, aggravating circulatory insufficiency.

Salt (sodium) poisoning or water intoxication may occur in the absence of dehydration and may produce hypernatremia and hyponatremia, respectively.

Clinical Assessment of Deficit. The patient history is the first critical step in the clinical assessment of the deficit. Table 16–5 indicates some of the important information that should be sought. For

TABLE 16–4
Assessment of Degree of Dehydration

	Mild	Moderate	Severe
Infant	5%	10%	15%
Adolescent	3%	6%	9%
Infants and young children	Thirsty; alert; restless	Thirsty; restless or lethargic but irritable or drowsy	Drowsy; limp, cold, sweaty, cyanotic extremities; may be comatose
Older children	Thirsty; alert; restless	Thirsty; alert (usually)	Usually conscious (but at reduced level), apprehensive; cold, sweaty, cyanotic extremities; wrinkled skin on fingers and toes; muscle cramps
Signs and Symptoms			
Tachycardia	Absent	Present	Present
Palpable pulses	Present	Present (weak)	Decreased
Blood pressure	Normal	Orthostatic hypotension	Hypotension
Cutaneous perfusion	Normal	Normal	Reduced and mottled
Skin turgor	Normal	Slight reduction	Reduced
Fontanel	Normal	Slightly depressed	Sunken
Mucous membrane	Moist	Dry	Very dry
Tears	Present	Present or absent	Absent
Respirations	Normal	Deep, may be rapid	Deep and rapid
Urine output	Normal	Oliguria	Anuria and severe oliguria

Modified from World Health Organization Guide.

TABLE 16–5
Historical Data for Evaluating Deficits

Weight change (preillness versus dehydrated weight)
Intake: quantity and composition of fluids and solids (including drugs) taken during illness
Output: quantity and pattern of output of urine; emesis; diarrhea; sweating; and drainage during illness
General medical status: respiratory function, cardiovascular status, renal function, central nervous system disease, and metabolic state (temperature) are especially relevant

Modified from Behrman RE, Kliegman RM, Jenson HB, editors: *Nelson textbook of pediatrics*, ed 16, Philadelphia, 2000, WB Saunders.

example, a history of fever and high-solute feedings in the presence of watery diarrhea favors hypernatremic dehydration. Physical examination may be complementary to the history and may be particularly helpful in characterizing the severity of dehydration (Table 16–6). Laboratory data may reflect hemoconcentration, although this may be masked by preexisting anemia or malnutrition. The level of blood urea nitrogen may be increased as a result of decreased blood flow and enhanced recycling of urea if the circulation is compromised, and creatinine levels usually are increased as a result of a decrease in glomerular filtration. Urine usually is concentrated and may transiently contain abnormal amounts of protein, casts, and cells. Serum electrolyte levels and acid-base data reflect specific deficits and their causes.

Supplemental Therapy

In certain disorders specific fluids and electrolytes may be needed in addition to those required to replace deficits and maintain homeostasis. For exam-

TABLE 16–6
Typical Patterns of Physical Signs in Moderate-Severe Dehydration

Sign	Isonatremic	Hyponatremic	Hyperna-tremic
Skin			
Color	Gray	Gray	Gray
Temperature	Cold	Cold	Cold
Turgor	Poor	Very poor	Fair
Feel	Dry	Clammy	Thick, doughy
Mucous membrane	Dry	Dry	Parched
Eyeball	Sunken and soft	Sunken and soft	Sunken
Fontanel	Sunken	Sunken	Sunken
State of consciousness	Lethargic	Very lethargic	Hyperirritable
Pulse	Rapid	Rapid	Moderately rapid
Blood pressure	Low	Very low	Moderately low

Modified from Behrman RE, Kliegman RM, Jenson HB, editors: *Nelson textbook of pediatrics,* ed 16, Philadelphia, 2000, WB Saunders.

TABLE 16–7
Oral Rehydration*

Status†	Mild Dehydration	Moderate Dehydration
Initial	50 mL/kg (over 4 hr)	100 mL/kg (over 6 hr)
Subsequent‡	100 mL/kg/24 hr	100 mL/kg/24 hr

*Amounts and rates should be increased or decreased based on evaluation of patient. Breast-feeding or plain water should be offered as needed.
†World Health Organization oral rehydration solution (ORS) is composed of 2 g glucose (CHO)/100 mL, 90 mEq Na^+/100 mL, 20 mEq K^+/100 mL, and 30 mEq HCO_3^-/100 mL. In the United States, commercially available oral rehydration solutions for the first 12 hours contain 2.0–2.5 g CHO/100 mL, 75 mEq Na^+/100 mL, 20 mEq K^+/100 mL, and 30 mEq HCO_3^-/100 mL. Solutions for subsequent use contain 2.0–2.5 g CHO/100 mL, 45–50 mEq Na^+/100 mL, 20 mEq K^+/100 mL, and 30 mEq HCO_3^-/100 mL.
‡Continue until diarrhea stops. Volume of ORS ingested should equal volume of stool losses. If losses cannot be measured, administer 10-15 mL ORS/kg/hr. Weigh child for best estimate of loss and repair.

ple, in pyloric stenosis sodium and potassium should be replaced as chloride salts because of gastric losses of hydrochloric acid, and burns may necessitate special replacement of the plasma lost by surface oozing and ultrafiltrate sequestrations around the burn site.

Principles of Therapy

Shock always must be treated as a medical emergency, with intravenous or (rarely) with intraosseous infusions (see Chapter 3). *Oral rehydration* may be appropriate in patients with mild to moderate dehydration (Table 16–7); this decision requires judgment about the etiology of the illness, the child's condition, and the capacity of the caregivers to provide adequate supervision of care.

Intravenous therapy should be provided for children when there is shock, severe dehydration, uncontrollable vomiting, diarrhea exceeding 10 mL/kg/hr, extreme fatigue, stupor, coma, severe gastric distention, or other serious complications. The goal of *initial therapy* is to treat or prevent shock through rapidly expanding the vascular volume by administering 10–30 mL/kg of an electrolyte solution such as isotonic saline (0.9%; Na^+ and Cl^+ both 155 mEq/L) or Ringer's lactate. This solution is given immediately, even before electrolyte values are known, because it is equally appropriate for isonatremic, hyponatremic, or hypernatremic dehydration and usually returns the serum sodium level toward normal. It is given as rapidly as possible for shock, or over 1–3 hours for less severely ill patients. Ordinarily, 20 mL/kg restores circulatory stability; if signs of shock persist, a second or third infusion of fluid (10–30 mL/kg) may be needed.

When the circulation is stabilized, *subsequent treatment* is directed at correcting the remaining water and sodium deficits and replacing ongoing abnormal and obligatory losses. Treatment usually is based on knowing the serum electrolyte concentrations. Unless hypokalemia is demonstrated or a condition known to be associated with severe potassium losses is present (e.g., pyloric stenosis, prolonged diarrhea, or diabetic acidosis), potassium losses are not replaced until urinary output is established.

Isonatremic Dehydration

In a patient with the isonatremic form of dehydration, sodium is lost from the extracellular space to the external environment and to the intracellular space, where it moves to compensate for intracellular potassium losses. To avoid subsequent overexpansion of the extracellular space after replacement of potassium as a result of sodium shift from the cells, one half of the deficit is replaced in the first 12-hour period, one quarter in the second, and one quarter in the third. In addition, the child should receive replacements for both ongoing normal losses (e.g., maintenance water, sodium, and potassium) and continuing abnormal losses during this 24-hour period.

Subsequently there should be 100% replacement of losses. Careful monitoring of weight is the best guide to successful fluid replacement. Serum electrolyte levels should be monitored. Potassium losses should be replaced slowly (over 36–48 hours) to avoid hyperkalemia. Potassium concentration in intravenous fluids should usually not exceed 40 mEq/L, at a rate not greater than 3 mEq/kg/24 hr, except under extraordinary circumstances.

Disturbances of Sodium Balance

Hyponatremia (Na⁺ ≤130 mEq/L)

Etiology and Pathophysiology. Reduced serum sodium content usually is associated with one of three mechanisms (Fig. 16–3). Because sodium is the main extracellular fluid cation, hyponatremia usually is associated with hypoosmolality. Occasionally, *pseudohyponatremia* is noted with isotonicity when plasma protein or triglyceride levels are elevated, with hyperosmolality when hypertonic infusions (e.g., mannitol or diatrizoate sodium) are given, or during hyperglycemia. For every 100 mg/dL increment of serum glucose, sodium levels decline by 1.6 mEq/L. *Hyperosmolar hyponatremia* is a result of osmotic fluid shifts from the intracellular space to the extracellular space; *isosmolar hyponatremia* is the result of an artifact of the laboratory analysis of sodium that measures the sodium content in serum drawn off after centrifugation, which contains both the plasma water and that component represented by excess lipid (hyperlipidemia) or protein (macroglobulinemia). Because sodium is present only in plasma (or serum) water and not in the lipid phase, measurements based on total volume (flame ionization) but not on plasma water yield pseudohyponatremia.

One frequent etiologic factor in true hyponatremia is the **syndrome of inappropriate ADH (SIADH) secretion**, which may be caused by a variety of disorders, including unregulated tumor production of ADH-like peptides, pulmonary disorders (e.g., pneumonia, positive end-expiratory pressure ventilation, asthma, cystic fibrosis, and pneumothorax), drugs (e.g., vincristine, opiates, carbamazepine, and cyclophosphamide), and direct irritation of the CNS (e.g., meningitis, encephalitis, hemorrhage, hypoxia, and trauma).

Hyposmolar hyponatremia accompanied by increased extracellular volume is also common in various edematous states, such as cardiac failure and cirrhosis. In these states water retention may be caused by a combination of reduced effective plasma volume, which is sensed by the aortic and carotid baroreceptors, and increased activity of the juxtaglomerular apparatus, signaling both ADH and renin secretion. The net result is both water and sodium retention and thus the formation of edema. Water retention in excess of sodium produces hyponatremia. This often is intensified when natriuretic (diuretic) agents are prescribed and the fluid intake is hyponatremic.

Hyponatremia without dehydration occurs in infants fed an inappropriately dilute formula because of errors in formula preparation or intentional formula dilution for the treatment of diarrhea or for reasons of financial difficulty. Hyponatremic dehydration may result during diarrhea when fluid replacement is more hypotonic than the diarrheal losses.

Clinical Manifestations. The symptoms of hyponatremia may include lethargy, apathy, disorientation, muscle cramps, anorexia, and agitation. The signs may include reduced mental status, decreased deep tendon reflexes, hypothermia, seizures, and pseudobulbar palsies. No clinical manifestations may be apparent. The more severe symptoms rarely occur unless the serum sodium level rapidly falls below 120 mEq/L if the serum sodium was in the normal range prior to the illness. Similar symptoms may occur associated with a rapid fall in the serum sodium level *into* the normal range if the serum sodium was elevated and dropped more than 15 or 20 mEq/L within 24 hours.

Treatment. The treatment depends on the mechanism of hyponatremia and on the presence or absence of serious clinical manifestations (Fig. 16–3). Acute-onset hyponatremia is more likely to be symptomatic than is chronic stable hyponatremia. Initial therapy should be calculated to raise the serum Na⁺ to 120 mEq/L rapidly, which usually stops seizures. Subsequent correction to 130 mEq Na⁺/L can be carried out over the next 24–36 hours. Rapid correction to levels greater than 130 mEq/L or more than 15 mEq/L/24 hr may be associated

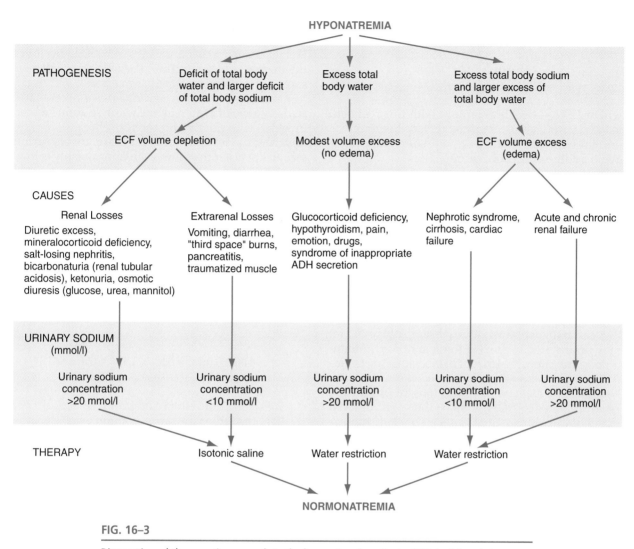

FIG. 16–3

Diagnostic and therapeutic approach to the hyponatremic patient. *ADH,* Antidiuretic hormone; *ECF,* extracellular fluid. (From Schrier RW, Berl T: Disorders of water metabolism. In Schrier RW, editor: *Renal and electrolyte disorders,* ed 2, Boston, 1980, Little, Brown.)

with severe adverse effects, such as central pontine myelinolysis. As a rule, the serum sodium level should not be raised or lowered more rapidly than 15 mEq/24 hr. Most patients with *acute SIADH* respond to fluid restriction, although sodium chloride (NaCl) infusion may be needed if hyponatremia is symptomatic.

Hyponatremic dehydration necessitates both sodium and fluid replacement in addition to the provision of supplements for ongoing losses and maintenance. Therapy is similar to that for isonatremic dehydration, except that when the sodium value to be infused is calculated, the extra loss of this ion

should be taken into account. This replacement usually should be spread over 36 hours. The sodium deficit in hyponatremic dehydration can be estimated by the following equation:

$$(\text{Desired Na}^+ - \text{Current Na}^+) \times 0.6 \times \text{Wt (kg)} = \text{mEq required}$$

Symptomatic hyponatremia may be treated with hypertonic (3%) saline (or normal saline) to raise the serum level to 120 mEq/L.

In situations of symptomatic hyponatremia without edema but with excess total body water, water diuresis (i.e., diuretics) may be helpful. The volume of diuresis needed to correct hyponatremia may be calculated by the following equation:

$$TBW = 0.6 \times wt \text{ (kg)}$$
$$\text{Excess water} = TBW - \text{Current } Na^+/\text{Desired } Na^+ \times TBW$$

where TBW = total body water. With this regimen, urine electrolytes also must be replaced with 3% or normal saline and sufficient potassium chloride to avoid additional electrolyte depletion.

Hypernatremia (Na⁺ ≥150 mEq/L)

Etiology and Pathophysiology. The serum sodium level is regulated by both ADH secretion and thirst. A high serum sodium level may be the result of water loss in excess of sodium loss (increased insensible water losses); insufficient ADH production (central diabetes insipidus) or reduced renal response to ADH (nephrogenic diabetes insipidus); poor response to thirst (hypodipsia); or salt poisoning, or less likely, excessive sodium retention (Fig. 16–4).

Central diabetes insipidus (absent ADH release) may be acquired (e.g., CNS trauma, tumor, autoimmunity, infection, hypoxia, or histiocytosis) or hereditary and sometimes with craniofacial anomalies. **Nephrogenic diabetes insipidus** (absent or reduced renal response to ADH) may be the result of renal pathology (e.g., interstitial nephritis or acute tubular necrosis), electrolyte disorders (e.g., hypercalcemia or hypokalemia), or drugs (e.g., lithium, demeclocycline, or amphotericin B) or may be hereditary. The hereditary illness appears in infants and is associated with polyuria, polydipsia, dehydration, fever, and growth and developmental retardation. It is most often an X-linked recessive disease and thus more often observed in males than in females. This defect is the result of mutations in the gene that encodes for the aquaporin-2 water channel.

Hypernatremic dehydration may occur in infants with a poor thirst mechanism or in breast-fed neonates of mothers whose milk supply is inadequate if these children have limited supplemental fluid intake. Failure to thrive, dehydration, hyperglycemia, hypocalcemia, acidosis, and prerenal azotemia are common associated findings. Infants with diarrhea and fever or those exposed to excessive environmental heat lose water in excess of sodium, placing them at risk for hypernatremia, especially if fluid replacement is hypertonic to losses.

Clinical Manifestations. The signs and symptoms relate to the primary disorder, dehydration. In hypernatremic dehydration, intravascular volume is conserved as a result of the hyperosmotic state, which results in a shift of water from the intracellular to the extracellular space. Therefore, the signs of dehydration are not as apparent as they are for an equivalent degree of isotonic dehydration. Based on skin turgor, tachycardia, and blood pressure, the severity of dehydration may be underestimated. Weight change remains the most reliable indicator of the degree of dehydration. Patients with salt poisoning may be in shock with seizures.

Treatment. *Hypernatremic dehydration* necessitates replacement of water in excess of sodium, which must be done slowly and carefully, because rapidly lowering the level of serum sodium lowers serum osmolality faster than intracellular osmolality is lowered, resulting in fluid crossing the cell membrane into the cell to reestablish osmotic equilibrium. This produces cellular swelling, which in the brain may lead to cerebral edema. Hemorrhage and thrombosis also may occur when the correction is too rapid, further contributing to the risk of seizures, coma, and death. Therefore, the serum sodium level should be lowered slowly toward normal at a rate of not more than 15 mEq/L/24 hr. The water deficit in hypernatremic dehydration can be estimated by using the following equation:

$$\text{Normal TBW} = 0.6 \times \text{Normal weight (kg)}$$
$$\text{Normal } Na^+/\text{Current } Na^+ \times TBW = \text{Current TBW}$$
$$\text{Deficit} = \text{Normal TBW} - \text{Current TBW}$$

The total fluid deficit should be corrected over 36–48 hours unless the serum sodium level is greater than 175 mEq/L. The most important aspects of treating hypernatremic dehydration are the initial management of shock, which reestablishes the circulation and renal blood flow, and then the slow replacement phase, which enables the now well-perfused kidneys to regulate water and sodium homeostasis. If the serum sodium level declines too quickly after treatment of shock, the rate of fluid replacement should be decreased.

Central **diabetes insipidus** necessitates ADH replacement. Nephrogenic diabetes insipidus will not respond to ADH and is treated with a low-salt and high-water diet. Thiazide diuretics may reduce urine output in children with nephrogenic diabetes insipidus by reducing intravascular volume, which may enhance proximal tubular salt and water reabsorption.

Disturbances of Potassium

Hypokalemia (K⁺ ≤3 mEq/L)

Etiology and Pathophysiology. Reduced serum potassium concentration may be the result of redistribution between the large intracellular potassium compartment and the smaller extracellular potassium space. Shifts of transcellular potassium from serum to cells are noted with acute alkalosis, insulin therapy, sympathomimetic agents, vitamin B_{12} therapy, and familial hypokalemic periodic paralysis.

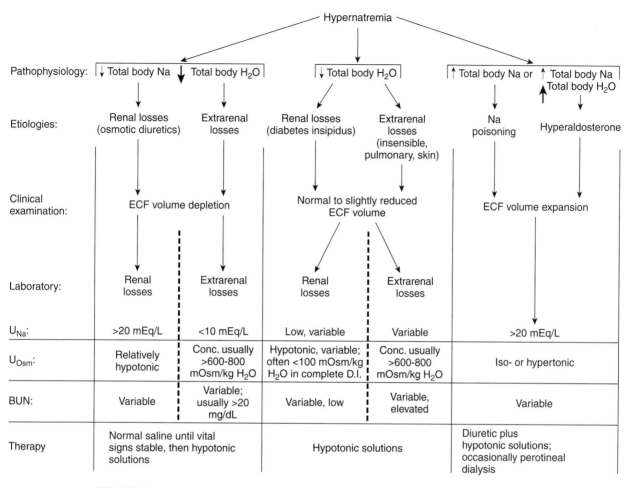

FIG. 16–4

Approach to hypernatremia. *BUN*, Blood urea nitrogen; *ECF*, extracellular fluid; U_{Na}, urinary sodium; U_{Osm}, urinary osmolality; ↓, less reduction; ⬇, more severe reduction. (From Norman M: In Fleisher G, Ludwig S, editors: *Textbook of pediatric emergency medicine*, Baltimore, 1983, Williams & Wilkins.)

Net renal loss of potassium is associated with the use of most diuretics, aminoglycosides, amphotericin B, platinum-containing cancer chemotherapy, excessive mineralocorticoid administration, renal disease such as renal tubular acidosis, and **Bartter syndrome.** Bartter syndrome is characterized by hypokalemic, hypochloremic metabolic alkalosis; hyperaldosteronism; hyperreninemia; increased urine chloride excretion; growth failure; normal blood pressure; hyperplasia of the juxtaglomerular apparatus; and increased urine prostaglandin E_2 excretion. It appears to be a defect in the Na-K-Cl cotransporter in the distal nephron.

Bartter syndrome presents in infancy as failure to thrive, salt craving, polyuria, muscle weakness, tetany, and constipation. *Gastrointestinal losses,* such as vomiting (which also results in renal potassium wasting secondary to alkalosis) and diarrhea in previously healthy children, frequently result in hypokalemia.

Gitelman syndrome is often confused with Bartter syndrome but is characterized by familial (autosomal recessive) hypokalemia and hypomagnesemia. Patients may be asymptomatic or may manifest transient weakness or tetany accompanied by emesis, fever, or abdominal pain.

Clinical Manifestations. The manifestations of hypokalemia are ileus, muscle weakness, nephrogenic diabetes insipidus, areflexic paralysis, and, especially with the use of digitalis, arrhythmias. The electrocardiogram in hypokalemia reveals ST segment depression, T-wave reduction, and the presence of a U wave. An approach to the evaluation of patients with hypokalemia is presented in Fig. 16–5.

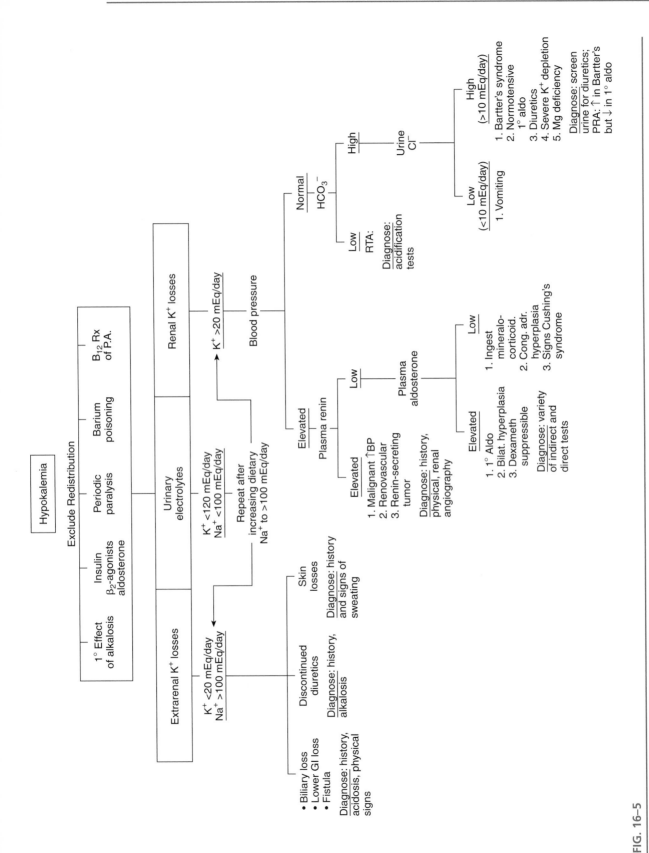

FIG. 16–5

Diagnostic approach to hypokalemia. *Aldo,* Aldosteronism; *BP,* blood pressure; *Cong. Adr,* congenital adrenal; *GI,* gastrointestinal; *PA,* pernicious anemia; *PRA,* plasma renin-angiotensin; *RTA,* renal tubular acidosis; *1°,* primary. (From Narins RG, Jones ER, Stom MC, et al: *Am J Med* 72:496, 1982.)

Treatment. The type of treatment selected depends on the underlying cause. Renal and gastrointestinal loss usually can be replaced by providing additional potassium chloride administered orally or intravenously. Bartter syndrome is treated with prostaglandin synthetase inhibitors (e.g., indomethacin or ibuprofen) together with potassium chloride and a potassium-sparing diuretic. Potassium losses should be replaced carefully to avoid hyperkalemia because potassium must pass through the extracellular space in order to replete the larger intracellular deficits. Gitelman syndrome responds to treatment with magnesium and does not usually necessitate potassium replacement.

Hyperkalemia (K⁺ ≥5.5 mEq/L)

An increased serum potassium level may be the result of transcellular shifts, increased potassium loss from cells, or decreased excretion (Table 16–8). The *clinical manifestations* of hyperkalemia are paresthesias, weakness, flaccid paralysis, and cardiac arrhythmias. The earliest electrocardiographic sign of hyperkalemia is peaked or tented T waves (K^+ 5.5–7.0 mEq/L). Higher levels (7.0–8.0 mEq/L) are associated with a prolonged PR interval, ST depression, and the initial widening of the QRS complex. The P wave may flatten as the potassium level increases. When the potassium level exceeds 8.0 mEq/L, the P wave may disappear, and the QRS complex widens and merges with the T wave, producing a sine wave pattern. Without treatment, asystole or ventricular fibrillation may occur. Hyponatremia, hypocalcemia, and acidosis intensify hyperkalemic cardiac effects.

The *treatment* of hyperkalemia involves measures to directly antagonize the membrane effects (e.g., calcium), redistribute potassium to the intracellular space (e.g., sodium bicarbonate, albuterol, and glucose with or without insulin), or remove potassium from the body. The administration of calcium gluconate, sodium bicarbonate, albuterol, and glucose are temporary measures that must be followed by procedures to remove potassium from the body. This can be accomplished by a forced diuresis or by the oral or rectal administration of a cation exchange resin (Kayexalate) that exchanges sodium for potassium and then binds potassium to be eliminated in stool. In situations of renal failure or when there is a need for rapid elimination, hemodialysis or peritoneal dialysis may be necessary.

Disturbances of Acid-Base Balance

Maintaining acid-base balance depends acutely on respiratory compensation (Table 16–9) and the tissue-buffering capacity of hemoglobin, albumin,

---

TABLE 16–8
Etiology of Hyperkalemia

Transcellular Shift
Acute acidosis, hyperkalemic familial periodic paralysis

Increased Endogenous Cell Release
Hemolysis, rhabdomyolysis, lysis of massive leukocytosis (leukemia)

Increased Exogenous Administration
Iatrogenic (intravenous route)

Decreased Excretion
Renal failure
Reduced renin-aldosterone production (Addison disease, adrenal genital syndrome, hypoaldosteronism, hyporeninemia)
Reduced tubular excretion (sickle cell anemia, systemic lupus erythematosus, obstructive uropathy, postrenal transplant)
Inhibition of tubular secretion by drugs (e.g., digitalis, spironolactone, amiloride, angiotensin-converting enzyme inhibitors)

---

bicarbonate, and bone. More chronic mechanisms involve increased renal excretion or reabsorption of bicarbonate through addition or subtraction of bicarbonate molecules to or from the buffering system. Pure acid-base disturbances are the result of alterations of only one of these functions, resulting in primary metabolic acidosis or alkalosis or primary respiratory acidosis or alkalosis. Rarely do compensating mechanisms completely correct a pure disorder, but they can provide significant improvement of pH. Mixed disturbances involve two or more primary disorders, such as occurs in a patient who has mixed respiratory-metabolic acidosis after a cardiopulmonary arrest.

Metabolic Alkalosis

A net gain of base or a net loss of acid produces a metabolic alkalosis (Table 16–10). However, unless there is a change in the usual renal mechanisms for reabsorbing bicarbonate or secreting hydrogen ion, the alkalosis will not persist. In situations of persistent extracellular volume depletion (especially with chloride loss), total body potassium depletion, persistent aldosterone secretion, or a combination of the above, increased proximal tubule reabsorption of bicarbonate develops and metabolic alkalosis becomes sustained. Most patients with metabolic alkalosis

TABLE 16–9
Characteristics of Primary Acid-Base Disturbances

Disorder	Etiology	Example	Compensation Mechanisms	Prediction of Pure Compensation
Metabolic				
Acidosis	$\downarrow HCO_3^-$	Hypoxia, drug ingestion, shock	$\downarrow Pco_2$ (acute) $\uparrow$Renal bicarbonate reabsorption (late)	1-mEq fall of HCO_3^- = 1–1.3 mm Hg fall of Pco_2
Alkalosis	$\uparrow HCO_3^-$ $\downarrow HCl$	$\uparrow$Bicarbonate/citrate, pyloric stenosis, gastric tube drainage losses	$\uparrow Pco_2$ (acute), renal bicarbonate excretion (late)	Pco_2 increases 6 mm Hg for 10-mEq increase of HCO_3^-
Respiratory				
Acidosis				
Acute (hr)	$\uparrow Pco_2$	Hypoventilation	$\uparrow HCO_3^-$ (renal)	HCO_3^- increases 1 mEq/L for each 10 mm Hg Pco_2
Chronic (days)	$\uparrow Pco_2$	BPD, cystic fibrosis	$\uparrow HCO_3^-$ (renal)	HCO_3^- increases 3–3.5 mEq/L for 10 mm Hg Pco_2
Alkalosis				
Acute (hr)	$\downarrow Pco_2$	Mechanical ventilation for $\uparrow$intracranial pressure, hysteria, hyperammonemia	$\downarrow HCO_3^-$ (renal)	HCO_3^- falls 2.5 mEq/L for 10 mm Hg of Pco_2
Chronic (days)	$\downarrow Pco_2$	Persistent mechanical ventilation	$\downarrow HCO_3^-$ (renal)	HCO_3^- falls 5 mEq/L for 10 mm Hg of Pco_2

Data from Narins R: In Maxwell M, Kleeman C, Narins R: *Clinical disorders of fluid and electrolyte metabolism,* ed 4, New York, 1987, McGraw-Hill; and DuBose T: *Med Clin North Am* 67:799, 1983.
BPD, Bronchopulmonary dysplasia.

have reduced total body potassium stores and hypokalemia, which results in increased hydrogen ion secretion by the distal tubule, maximizing bicarbonate reabsorption along the entire tubule and resulting in a *paradoxical aciduria.*

Clinical manifestations of metabolic alkalosis are mental confusion, tetany, poor cardiac output, enhanced digitalis toxicity, hypoventilation, and a shift of the hemoglobin oxygen curve to the left. The *treatment* of a metabolic alkalosis depends on the cause. Most cases caused by diuretics, vomiting, bicarbonate therapy, or nasogastric tube losses are "chloride responsive" and can be treated primarily with volume expansion and chloride replacement using normal saline and potassium chloride. Chloride repletion leads to enhanced renal bicarbonate excretion. "Chloride-unresponsive" patients may be hypertensive (e.g., in primary hyperaldosteronism or Cushing syndrome) or normotensive (in Bartter syndrome, magnesium deficiency, or severe hypokalemia) and require specific therapy for these disease states.

Metabolic Acidosis

The predominant causes of metabolic acidosis are a loss of bicarbonate (e.g., through diarrhea or urinary loss), endogenous production and retention of acids (e.g., inborn errors of metabolism or uremia), and exogenous administration of acid (e.g., salicylate or ethylene glycol). The **anion gap** can help differentiate bicarbonate loss from net acid gain as the *etiology* of acidosis (Table 16–11). In the presence of acidosis the undetermined anion above the normal anion gap range (10–14 mEq/L) is considered to be net acid gained. If the anion gap is normal, bicarbonate loss by the gastrointestinal system or kidney is the probable cause.

Lactic acidosis is a frequent cause of a net increase of endogenous acid production and is the result of multiple pathophysiologic mechanisms (Table 16–12).

The *clinical manifestations* of metabolic acidosis may be tachycardia, ventricular arrhythmias, reduced cardiac contractility, Kussmaul respiration, abdominal pain, increased serum uric acid, and hyperkalemia. The *treatment* of increased anion gap acidosis depends

TABLE 16–10
Etiology of Metabolic Alkalosis

Initiation	Maintenance	Maintenance Mechanism	Urine Chloride	Example
Loss of Acid				
GI tract	Volume contraction	↑Tubular HCO_3^- reabsorption	<10 mEq/L	Pyloric stenosis
	Decreased GFR	↑Fractional HCO_3^- reabsorption		Congenital chloride diarrhea
	Chloride depletion	↓GFR, ↓Cl^- causes ↑H^+ secretion; ↑renin		
Renal sodium delivery to tubule	K^+ depletion plus those for GI tract	↑Aldosterone, ↑H^+ secretion plus above	>20 mEq/L on diuretics, <10 mEq/L off therapy	Diuretics
Hyperreninemic states	As above	As above	>20 mEq/L	Bartter syndrome; primary hyperaldosteronism; licorice ingestion
High mineralocorticoid states				Renal artery stenosis
Gain of Base				
Alkalizing salts	Volume contraction	As above plus continued source	>20 mEq/L	Milk-alkali syndrome, citrate in blood products
	Continued base therapy, K^+ deficit	As above		
Posthypercapnic State	Volume contraction; decreased GFR; K^+ and Cl^- depletion	As above	<10 mEq/L	Slow correction of chronic respiratory acidosis

Data from Cogan M et al: *Med Clin North Am* 67:903, 1983; Sabatin S, Kurtzman N: In Maxwell M, Kleeman C, Narins R: *Clinical disorders of fluid and electrolyte metabolism,* ed 4, New York, 1987, McGraw-Hill.
GFR, Glomerular filtration rate; *GI,* gastrointestinal.

on the underlying disease and may involve insulin for diabetic ketoacidosis; dialysis for uremia; oxygen for carbon monoxide poisoning; removal of toxins (e.g., salicylate); and provision of sodium bicarbonate when acidosis is severe or not rapidly corrected by the above measures. The dose of bicarbonate (HCO_3^-) may be calculated by the following equation:

$$\text{Dose of bicarbonate} = (\text{Normal } HCO_3^- - \text{Current } HCO_3^-) \times 0.3 \times \text{Wt (kg)}$$

Overalkalinization should be avoided because it has detrimental effects, such as hypokalemia, reduced oxygen dissociation from hemoglobin, and further stimulation of lactate production. Partial correction of the acidosis is preferable while the under-

lying cause is being treated. Most children with diabetic ketoacidosis do not require bicarbonate because ketone body metabolism in the presence of insulin regenerates bicarbonate in the Krebs cycle. Intravenous bicarbonate in these patients may produce metabolic alkalosis and complicate recovery.

Renal Tubular Acidosis

Etiology and Classification. Renal tubular acidosis (RTA) is a condition characterized by hyperchloremic normal anion gap acidosis, which results from impaired renal acidification. Three distinctive types of renal tubular acidosis have been established:

- Type I: distal RTA
- Type II: proximal RTA

TABLE 16–11
Acidosis and the Anion Gap*

Increased Anion Gap Without Acidosis
Decreased calcium, magnesium, potassium, and other *cations*
Increased albumin, other *anions;* high-dose carbenicillin

Increased Anion Gap with Acidosis
Increased endogenous anions: lactate, sulfate, phosphate (uremia), ketones (diabetes), organic acids (inborn errors of metabolism)
Increased exogenous acids: salicylate, methanol, ethanol, paraldehyde

Normal Anion Gap with Acidosis
Bicarbonate losses; diarrhea, renal tubular acidosis, carbonic anhydrase inhibitor, ureterosigmoidostomy, dilutional acidosis, pancreatic fistula

Decreased Anion Gap Without Acidosis
Increased calcium, potassium, magnesium, bromide
Decreased albumin

Adapted from Oh W, Carroll H: *N Engl J Med* 297:814, 1977.
*Normal anion gap = $Na^+ (Cl^- + HCO_3^-)$ = 12 mEq/L.

TABLE 16–12
Etiology of Lactic Acidosis

Type A	
Tissue hypoxia	Shock, asphyxia, carbon monoxide toxicity
Type B	
Systemic disorders	Diabetes mellitus, renal failure, hepatic failure, malignancy, seizures, gut flora that produce D-lactate
Drugs	Biguanides, fructose, ethanol, salicylate, methanol, ethylene glycol
Inborn errors	Type I glycogen storage disease, pyruvate carboxylase deficiency, pyruvate dehydrogenase deficiency, mitochondrial myopathy, lactic acidemias, and other mitochondrial defects

■ Type IV: RTA associated with a **mineralocorticoid deficiency or decreased distal tubular responsiveness**

A type III was proposed but is most likely a variant of type I.

Proximal Renal Tubular Acidosis. The proximal form of RTA results from reduced proximal tubular reabsorption of bicarbonate, either as a result of a failure of hydrogen ion secretion proximally or as a result of deficient carbonic anhydrase activity. Normally, 85% of the filtered bicarbonate is reabsorbed in the proximal tubule. In proximal RTA, reabsorption is reduced. Distal tubular bicarbonate reabsorption cannot fully compensate for this load, and considerable filtered bicarbonate is excreted. The serum bicarbonate level falls until it reaches the new proximal tubule bicarbonate threshold, at which time bicarbonate wasting ceases. When the serum bicarbonate reaches this level (~15–16 mmol/L), bicarbonate reabsorption can be considered complete. The urine may become acidified because distal hydrogen ion secretion is normal. Severe hypokalemia is often an associated finding, resulting from extracellular volume contraction, leading to secondary hyperaldosteronism and distal tubule potassium loss.

Proximal RTA occurs as a primary disease, as a part of the **Fanconi syndrome,** and in a variety of other conditions (Table 16–13). Fanconi syndrome may be idiopathic or secondary to metabolic or toxic conditions, as noted in Table 16–13. In Fanconi syndrome a defect exists (sometimes reversible) in proximal tubular reabsorption of glucose, phosphate, potassium, and amino acids. This is associated with proximal RTA and a defect in vitamin D metabolism, leading to reduced levels of $1,25(OH)_2$ vitamin D.

Distal Renal Tubular Acidosis. The distal form of RTA results from an inability of the distal nephron to secrete hydrogen ion, preventing the reabsorption of the final 15% of bicarbonate (which reaches the distal tubule) and also the final acidification of the urine. In this condition the urinary pH cannot be reduced below 5.5–6.0, despite severe systemic acidosis. Hyperchloremia and hypokalemia accompany distal RTA. Distal RTA may be an isolated primary defect inherited as either an autosomal dominant or an autosomal recessive trait, or it may occur in association with a variety of disorders (Table 16–14). All forms of distal RTA may be complicated by nephrocalcinosis.

Mineralocorticoid Deficiency. Type IV RTA results from inadequate production of or reduced responsiveness to aldosterone. It is associated with *hyper*kalemic and hyperchloremic acidosis. This disorder may be primary or secondary to adrenal disease or parenchymal kidney damage, especially obstructive uropathy. *Hyporeninemic hypoaldosteronism* is another form of type IV RTA that also may result from renal disease associated with interstitial damage.

TABLE 16–13
Etiology of Proximal Renal Tubular Acidosis

Idiopathic or Primary
Sporadic
Fanconi syndrome

Secondary Metabolic Diseases
Cystinosis
Tyrosinemia
Galactosemia
Hereditary fructose intolerance
Type I glycogen storage disease
Lowe syndrome
Wilson disease
Osteopetrosis (carbonic anhydrase deficiency)

Drugs and Toxins
Heavy metals (lead, cadmium, mercury)
Outdated tetracycline
Carbonic anhydrase inhibitors
Vitamin D deficiency or altered metabolism

Miscellaneous
Hyperparathyroidism
Dysproteinemic states (monoclonal gammopathy)
Interstitial nephritis (renal transplant rejection, renal
    vein thrombosis)
Nephrotic syndrome
Prematurity
Pregnancy

TABLE 16–14
Etiology of Distal Renal Tubular Acidosis

Primary or Idiopathic
Sporadic
Familial

Secondary Inherited Diseases
Osteopetrosis
Sickle cell anemia
Wilson disease
Hypercalciuria

Hypercalciuria/Nephrocalcinosis
Hyperparathyroidism
Hypervitaminosis D
Hyperthyroidism
Medullary sponge kidney

Drugs and Toxins
Amphotericin B
Toluene
Amiloride
Lithium

Interstitial Renal Disease
Chronic pyelonephritis
Obstructive nephropathy
Renal transplantation rejection
Hyperoxaluria

Autoimmune and Hypergammaglobulinemic States
Systemic lupus erythematosus
Chronic active hepatitis
Cryoglobulinemia
Primary biliary cirrhosis
Sjögren syndrome
Thyroiditis
Pulmonary fibrosis

Clinical Manifestations. Children with RTA usually exhibit growth failure and acidosis. If Fanconi syndrome is present, rickets, polyuria, nausea, anorexia, and intermittent vomiting may also occur. Hypokalemia produces muscle weakness and polyuria. Patients with systemic acidosis and alkaline urine whose bicarbonate level is below 15 mEq/L most likely have distal RTA. In children with proximal RTA the urine becomes acidified when the bicarbonate threshold is attained. Primary RTA must be differentiated from secondary RTA because the latter requires specific therapy of the underlying disorder. For example, removal of galactose (in galactosemia) or fructose (in hereditary fructose intolerance) from the diet reverses these acquired forms of Fanconi syndrome.

Diagnosis. The diagnosis of RTA consists of determining the ability to secrete hydrogen ion (distal RTA) or the abnormal excretion of bicarbonate (proximal RTA). In a patient with a hyperchloremic metabolic acidosis, a measurement of the urine pH is essential. A urine pH less than 5.5 when the serum bicarbonate is below normal, and especially when the serum bicarbonate is 16 mEq or less, is very suggestive of proximal RTA. The provision of bicarbonate, either intravenously or in large doses orally, will increase the serum bicarbonate but will not increase it into the normal range; it will quickly raise the urine pH to >7.5. This means that the threshold for bicarbonate reabsorption has been exceeded despite a filtered load of bicarbonate that is below normal.

To diagnose distal RTA, a measurement of the *urine anion gap* (Na + K − Cl) is helpful. In normal patients under conditions of low serum bicarbonate levels, the gap will be negative because acidification of the urine leads to an increase in ammonium chloride excretion. Since the chloride is measured and the ammonium is not measured in the above equation, the anion gap will be negative. Normal individuals also have a low urine pH (<6). In patients with distal RTA, urinary acidification is not normal and ammonium chloride excretion is low. Therefore, the gap will be zero or positive. Affected patients will not have a urine pH <6.2. This test can be performed only when the serum bicarbonate level is low and the patient is not receiving bicarbonate therapy. The gold standard test for urinary acidification is an acid loading test, usually with the use of ammonium chloride. The finding of a further fall in serum bicarbonate without a decline in urine pH below 6.2 and without the development of a negative urine anion gap is proof of distal RTA.

Treatment. The goal of therapy is to correct the acidosis and achieve normal childhood growth. A sodium bicarbonate solution (1 mEq/mL) or tablet (8 mEq/tablet) or a sodium citrate–citric acid combination (e.g., Shohl solution; Bicitra) containing 1 mEq of Na citrate/mL of solution is administered. Alkali therapy plus potassium supplementation can be given in the form of Polycitra, which contains 1 mEq/mL of sodium citrate and 1 mEq/mL of potassium citrate. Patients with distal RTA require a smaller dose of alkalinizing agents, which is equal to endogenous acid production (1–2 mEq/kg/24 hr). However, because the urine cannot be acidified, nephrocalcinosis is common. Larger doses of alkali are required in proximal RTA to correct the acidosis because of the constant bicarbonate wasting resulting from the inability to reabsorb filtered bicarbonate. Proximal RTA, however, is more likely to resolve than is distal RTA. Type IV RTA most commonly results from obstructive uropathy and may resolve after the obstruction is corrected. Mineralocorticoid therapy may be needed for type IV RTA associated with aldosterone deficiency.

REFERENCES

Arnold WC, Kallen RJ: Fluid and electrolyte therapy, *Pediatr Clin North Am* 37(2):449–461, 1990.
Bartter F, Schwartz W: The syndrome of inappropriate secretion of antidiuretic hormone, *Am J Med* 42(5):790–806, 1967.
Battle DC, Hizon M, Cohen E, et al: The use of the urinary anion gap in the diagnosis of hyperchloremic metabolic acidosis, *N Engl J Med* 318(10):594–599, 1988.
Behrman RE, Kliegman RM, Jenson HB, editors: *Nelson textbook of pediatrics*, ed 16, Philadelphia, 2000, WB Saunders, Chapters 45–55, 537.
Caruana R, Buckalew V: The syndrome of distal (type 1) renal tubular acidosis, *Medicine* 67(2):84–99, 1988.
Gill JR Jr, Frolich JC, Bowden RE, et al: Bartter's syndrome: a disorder characterized by high urinary prostaglandins and a dependence of hyperreninemia on prostaglandin synthesis, *Am J Med* 61(1):43–51, 1976.
Narins R, editor: *Maxwell and Kleeman clinical disorders of fluid and electrolyte metabolism*, ed 5, New York, 1994, McGraw-Hill.
Oh M, Cavrol H: Anion gap, *N Engl J Med* 297(15):814–817, 1977.
Rodriguez-Soriano J: New insights into the pathogenesis of renal tubular acidosis—from functional to molecular studies, *Pediatr Nephrol* 14(12):1121–1136, 2000.
Rodriguez-Soriano J: Bartter and related syndromes: the puzzle is almost solved, *Pediatr Nephrol* 12(4):315–327, 1998.

RENAL DISEASES
Approach to the Child with Hematuria

When hematuria is a chief complaint, it generally is gross hematuria (seen with the naked eye), but microscopic hematuria may be the initial manifestation observed during routine urinalysis. Microscopic hematuria is defined as greater than three to five red blood cells per high-power field in freshly voided and centrifuged urine.

The child who exhibits gross hematuria needs prompt evaluation. The urinalysis should be repeated in the child who has the combination of microscopic hematuria, no proteinuria, normal blood pressure, and normal renal function. If the hematuria persists, further evaluation is appropriate. The first step in evaluating the child with hematuria is taking a careful history, performing a physical examination, and examining the urine. *The presence of red urine but a negative result on microscopic examination and negative dipstick reaction for blood* suggests that the red urine has been caused by a substance that has colored the urine, as might occur from the child's ingesting a medication such as acetophenetidin that has a metabolite that produces a dark wine-brown color; from a toxin such as benzene or carbon tetrachloride, both of which produce a red-brown color; from food dyes (beets); or from rifampin (orange-red color). The color also might be caused by the side effects of treatment, such as occurs after deferoxamine administration, or caused by poisoning with a heavy metal, such as lead, which produces a red-brown coloration of the urine. Urates are a common cause of an orange-red discoloration on the diaper of infants.

If the *urine test result is positive for blood but no red blood cells are seen* when the urine is promptly examined, the presence of free hemoglobin or myoglobin should be suspected. **Hemoglobinuria** may be present secondary to hemoglobin excretion from acute intravascular hemolysis (e.g., glucose-6-phosphate dehydrogenase deficiency or paroxysmal nocturnal hemoglobinuria) or from intravascular coagulation (e.g., sepsis or hemolytic-uremic syndrome [HUS]). It may be seen in freshwater drowning, mismatched blood transfusions, and other causes of hemolysis. Rhabdomyolysis and **myoglobinuria** (from a crush injury, burns, myositis, or asphyxia) also must be considered.

If *a significant number of red blood cells are present but no casts are observed*, bleeding beyond the glomerulus and renal tubules must be considered. However, it is important to remember that casts and red cells will hemolyze on standing, particularly in dilute urine; they also can be missed if the urine is not examined with reduced light and shortly after voiding.

Another mechanism for localizing hematuria to the glomerulus involves examining the morphology of the red blood cells. Carefully examining the urine by phase contrast microscopy frequently reveals altered red cell morphology in glomerular hematuria, whereas morphology characteristically is unaltered when nonglomerular causes are present. However, the absence of casts or the absence of alterations in red blood cell morphology by no means excludes a glomerular etiology.

The presence of red cells in the absence of casts is seen in some patients with hematuria associated with sickle cell trait or disease, in some children following marked exercise, and in patients after renal trauma. The presence of a coagulopathic condition (acute or inherited) may be associated with hematuria, although bleeding from the urinary tract in the absence of bleeding into other organ systems (e.g., skin or joints) is unusual. A family history of hematuria, renal failure, or deafness or the finding of hematuria on a urinalysis performed on siblings or parents suggests the possibility of a familial nephritis. Hypercalciuria is an important cause of isolated hematuria in children; 25–30% of children with isolated hematuria have calcium excretion rates greater than 4 mg/kg/24 hr or urinary calcium-to-creatinine ratios greater than 0.2:1.

Urolithiasis is one cause of painful hematuria. It may be seen in children who have idiopathic hypercalciuria, in children who have been immobilized for long periods, and in those with urinary tract malformations and recurrent infections. Idiopathic nephrolithiasis does occur with uric acid, calcium oxalate, and struvite, but it is uncommon. Urolithiasis also occurs in hyperparathyroidism, sarcoidosis, Lesch-Nyhan syndrome, diuretic use, cystic fibrosis, and inflammatory bowel disease. Nephrocalcinosis also may be seen in distal RTA, cystinuria, hyperoxaluria, the milk-alkali syndrome, and other uncommon conditions.

Abnormalities of the urinary tract must be considered in patients with hematuria. *Benign* (hemangioma, hamartoma) or *malignant* (Wilms-kidney, rhabdomyosarcoma-bladder) *tumors must be excluded in patients with hematuria.* Congenital obstruction, cystic disease, severe ureteral reflux, or an infiltrative process may be accompanied by hematuria. Nephrosonogram and (on occasion) IVP are important parts of the evaluation to rule out these possibilities. *Urinary tract infection* may present with hematuria, and a urine culture should be part of the initial evaluation of a child with hematuria. *Interstitial nephritis*, which may be drug induced or idiopathic, may present with hematuria, eosinophilia, and urinary eosinophils with or without casts.

The *differential diagnosis* of hematuria and its association with proteinuria and edema are noted in Table 16–15. The minimal screening evaluation for hematuria is described in Table 16–16.

TABLE 16–15
Differential Diagnosis of Proteinuria and Hematuria

Proteinuria	Hematuria	Edema	Etiology
Yes	No	No	Exercise, orthostatic (intermittent or fixed) fever, dehydration; benign; reflux nephropathy; focal segmental sclerosis; SLE
Yes	Yes	No or mild	Acute glomerulonephritis, IgA nephropathy (Berger disease), Henoch-Schönlein purpura, hemolytic-uremic syndrome, endocarditis, hereditary nephritis, interstitial nephritis, SLE, severe exercise
Yes	No	Yes	Minimal lesion (change) nephrotic syndrome; focal segmental sclerosis
Yes	Yes	Yes	Acute glomerulonephritis, atypical minimal lesion nephrotic syndrome, membranoproliferative (mesangiocapillary) glomerulonephritis, membranous nephropathy
No	Yes	No	Benign hematuria, IgA nephropathy, hereditary nephritis, sickle cell anemia, tumor, trauma, interstitial nephritis, nephrolithiasis, idiopathic hypercalciuria

IgA, Immunoglobulin A; *SLE,* systemic lupus erythematosus.

TABLE 16–16
Basic Workup of the Child with Hematuria

1. *History:* Present, past, family
2. *Physical examination:* Height, weight, blood pressure, optic fundi, presence or absence of abdominal mass, skin appearance, genitalia, edema, complete physical examination
3. *Laboratory:* Urinalysis; urine culture; complete blood count; smear; platelets; serum blood urea nitrogen; creatinine; calcium; streptozyme; serum complement (C3 as screen); quantitative urinary protein; calcium and creatinine; intravenous pyelogram, nephrosonogram, or both

---

If the urinalysis reveals the presence of *hematuria and casts,* one of a variety of glomerular diseases should be considered. Glomerular injury may be the result of immunologic injury (e.g., acute poststreptococcal glomerulonephritis), inherited disease (e.g., Alport syndrome), or vascular injury (e.g., acute tubular or cortical necrosis).

Microscopic Hematuria with Casts or Altered Red Cell Morphology but Little or No Proteinuria

Immunoglobulin A Nephropathy (Berger Disease). Microscopic hematuria or recurrent gross hematuria shortly after an upper respiratory infection (1–2 days) and not associated with the signs and symptoms of an acute nephritic syndrome (e.g., edema, hypertension, or renal insufficiency) suggests the possibility of immunoglobulin A (IgA) nephropathy or idiopathic hematuria (discussed in the following paragraph). The cause of IgA nephropathy disease is not known, but a consistent finding on renal biopsy is the presence of mesangial proliferation accompanied by mesangial deposits of IgA and variable deposition of IgG and IgM. The course generally is benign in children but may be associated with recurrent bouts of hematuria following or during respiratory infections. IgA nephropathy presents sporadically, with some reports of familial disease; is more common in males than in females; and is characteristically associated with normal renal function and normal serum levels of C3. Although the prognosis is good in children, progressive renal insufficiency and end-stage renal disease have been demonstrated to develop in about 25% of adults. No therapy currently is known that alters the course of the disease. Therapies that have been tried are glucocorticoids, immunosuppressive agents (e.g., cyclophosphamide, cyclosporine, and azathioprine), and fish oil.

Idiopathic Hematuria. Idiopathic hematuria may be familial or nonfamilial. *Benign familial hematuria* is a common nonprogressive, autosomal dominant disorder, demonstrating thinning of the glomerular basement membrane on electron microscopy; other family members (e.g., a parent or sibling) will also have hematuria, usually microscopic. Results of a renal biopsy in patients with the nonfamilial form may be normal or reveal only mild mesangial hypercellularity. Patients who have **Alport syndrome** often exhibit microscopic hematuria. This familial disorder is associated with progressive bilateral neurosensory deafness (high tones) and progressive renal failure during adolescence and young adulthood, particularly in males. Ocular findings include cataracts, keratoconus, and spherophakia. Electron microscopy of the renal biopsy reveals characteristic splitting and layering of the basement membrane of the glomerulus. The prognosis for patients with the nonfamilial or the non-Alport form of idiopathic familial hematuria is excellent, but long-term follow-up is required to exclude the progressive forms of familial hematuria.

Hematuria with Casts and Mild to Moderate Proteinuria

Children who have hematuria associated with casts and less than 1 g of proteinuria/m^2/24 hr usually have nephritis.

Acute Poststreptococcal Glomerulonephritis. Acute poststreptococcal glomerulonephritis (AGN) disorder is the prototype of the acute nephritic syndrome. AGN is associated with a sudden onset of gross hematuria in approximately two thirds of children, edema in three fourths, and hypertension in one half; it is also associated with variable degrees of renal insufficiency.

Etiology and Pathophysiology. AGN characteristically follows streptococcal pharyngitis or impetigo-pyoderma by 7–21 days. Only certain strains of group A beta-hemolytic streptococci are nephritogenic. Acute poststreptococcal glomerulonephritis is immunologically mediated by activation of the complement system, which initiates a glomerular proliferative and inflammatory response. Antigen-antibody complexes in the glomerular basement membrane induce complement activation. Edema is formed as a result of reduced GFR and hence decreased filtration plus enhanced distal Na^+ reabsorption. Plasma volume is elevated and plasma renin is suppressed.

Clinical Manifestations. Signs and symptoms may be delayed for 5 days to 3 weeks (10 days on average) after streptococcal infections. Children may have asymptomatic hematuria. Edema and tea- or cola-colored urine are the most common initial signs. Oliguria, edema, and hypertension may induce complications, such as heart failure and encephalopathy.

Diagnosis. The diagnosis is based on the typical findings of edema, hematuria, and hypertension.

Oliguria may occur, and pulmonary vascular congestion may be apparent on a chest roentgenogram. Encephalopathy or seizures may occur. In addition to hematuria, urinalysis reveals mild to moderate proteinuria, concentrated urine, and the presence of many casts, including coarse and fine granular and red cell casts. Previous streptococcal infection should be documented by the streptozyme test. Confirmation of activation of the complement system is determined by low C3 levels. Renal biopsy usually is not indicated in children with typical AGN; it reveals electron-dense deposits in the subepithelial space. The C3 returns to normal by 6–8 weeks. Renal failure, if present, usually resolves in 2–3 weeks, as do hypertension and gross hematuria.

Treatment. Specific therapy involves diuretics for hypertension, heart failure, pulmonary edema, and oliguria; and antihypertensive agents such as calcium channel blockers (e.g., nifedipine), angiotensin-converting enzyme inhibitors, or vasodilators (e.g., hydralazine) for hypertension. Proteinuria and edema characteristically decline fairly rapidly (in 5–10 days), but microscopic hematuria may persist for months or occasionally years, a circumstance that does not alter the generally excellent *prognosis* of this disease, from which greater than 95% of children recover completely.

The absence of evidence for a poststreptococcal glomerulonephritis does not exclude the diagnosis of *acute postinfectious glomerulonephritis,* because multiple etiologic factors (pneumococcus, *Staphylococcus,* and endocarditis-related pathogens) have been implicated. Hypocomplementemia persisting beyond 8 weeks of the illness, however, suggests the diagnosis of mesangiocapillary glomerulonephritis.

Mesangiocapillary (Membranoproliferative) Glomerulonephritis. Mesangiocapillary glomerulonephritis may present in a manner similar to that of acute poststreptococcal glomerulonephritis; characteristically, however, persistent hypocomplementemia is present. This disease frequently appears as a nephrotic syndrome that is present in fewer than 10% of patients with AGN (discussed under Nephrotic Syndrome in this chapter).

Hemolytic-Uremic Syndrome. HUS is characterized by a microangiopathic hemolytic anemia, renal cortical injury (sometimes progressing to renal cortical necrosis), and thrombocytopenia. HUS is a major cause of acute renal failure in children.

Etiology and Epidemiology. HUS may be sporadic, epidemic, and in some countries (e.g., Argentina) endemic. The disease typically occurs between the ages of 6 months and 4 years. Verotoxin has been implicated as one etiologic mechanism, especially if HUS follows *Escherichia coli* or *Shigella* enteritis. HUS following hemorrhagic colitis has been associated with a verotoxin-producing *Escherichia coli* O157:H7. Verotoxin is similar to Shiga toxin *(Shigella)* and binds to a specific receptor on endothelial cells, producing endothelial swelling. Familial disease may be the result of an alteration in the thromboxane-prostacyclin relationship, which favors endothelial platelet activation.

In most cases the primary event appears to be endothelial cell injury and subsequent localized clotting and platelet activation. Evidence for disseminated intravascular coagulation (DIC) rarely is present. Microangiopathic hemolytic anemia results from mechanical damage to red cells as they pass through the damaged vascular endothelium. Thrombocytopenia results from platelet adhesion.

Clinical Manifestations and Diagnosis. The onset of the syndrome usually appears as a gastroenteritis, most often with blood in the stool, followed in 7–10 days by weakness, lethargy, irritability, and oliguria. Physical examination reveals pallor, edema, petechiae, hepatosplenomegaly, and irritability. The diagnosis is supported by the presence of microangiopathic hemolytic anemia, thrombocytopenia, and acute renal failure. Seizures may indicate CNS involvement. A smear of peripheral red blood cells reveals schistocytes, helmet and burr cells, and fragmented erythrocytes. The reticulocyte count is elevated, and plasma haptoglobin levels are diminished. A Coombs test is negative. Leukocytosis is common. Urinalysis reveals microscopic hematuria, proteinuria, and casts. Other causes of microangiopathic hemolytic anemia should be excluded.

Treatment. The patient in acute renal failure requires immediate therapy. Many patients (30–50%) require early intervention with dialysis. Most children (>90%) survive the acute phase and recover normal renal function. Steroids, plasmapheresis, heparinization, and streptokinase are not helpful; platelet inhibitors, hyperimmune globulin, and plasma infusions have no proven benefit. Although careful medical management with early-onset dialysis frequently is associated with recovery, children nevertheless should be observed for the late development of hypertension, proteinuria, or chronic renal failure. Epidemic disease has the best *prognosis,* whereas familial cases, disease in older patients (older than 10 years of age) or in very young patients (younger than 8 months of age), HUS without diarrhea, and sporadic HUS have a poorer outcome.

Rapidly Progressive Glomerulonephritis. Rapidly progressive glomerulonephritis (RPGN) is a clinical syndrome of rapidly progressing nephritis accompanied by renal failure, the pathologic hallmark of which is epithelial cell proliferation and *crescent* formation. One histologic pattern is that of linear immunoglobulin and complement deposition (i.e., idiopathic, Goodpasture syndrome). The more common type is the appearance of immune complexes in a "lumpy" pattern in the basement membrane (in SLE, poststreptococcal AGN, polyarteritis, Henoch-Schönlein purpura, or mesangiocapillary or idiopathic glomerulonephritis). RPGN is more common in late childhood, when patients present with edema, gross hematuria, hypertension, and renal failure. Some children with rapidly progressive lupus nephritis respond to pulse prednisone or cyclophosphamide therapy, whereas other children (poststreptococcal glomerulonephritis) recover spontaneously. The prognosis for recovery of renal function is poor for the remaining types of RPGN. Fortunately, transplantation benefits most children who have end-stage renal disease associated with the "lumpy" immune complex pattern of RPGN. Transplantation is not as beneficial in conditions associated with antiglomerular basement membrane antibodies such as Goodpasture syndrome.

REFERENCES

Andreoli S: Chronic glomerulonephritis in childhood: membranoproliferative glomerulonephritis, Henoch-Schönlein purpura nephritis, and IgA nephropathy, *Pediatr Clin North Am* 42(6): 1487–1503, 1995.

Behrman RE, Kliegman RM, Jenson HB, editors: *Nelson textbook of pediatrics*, ed 16, Philadelphia, 2000, WB Saunders, Chapters 516–530.

Grimm PC, Ogborn MR: Hemolytic uremic syndrome: the most common cause of acute renal failure in childhood, *Pediatr Ann* 23(9):505–511, 1994.

Lieu TA, Grasmeder HM, Kaplan BS: An approach to the evaluation and treatment of microscopic hematuria, *Pediatr Clin North Am* 38:579, 1991.

Lim D, Walker D, Ellsworth P, et al: Treatment of pediatric urolithiasis between 1984 and 1994, *J Urol* 156(2 Pt 2):702–705, 1996.

Remuzzi G, Ruggenenti P: The hemolytic uremic syndrome, *Kidney Int* 48(1):2–19, 1995.

Siegler R, Pavia A, Cook J: Hemolytic uremic syndrome in adolescents, *Arch Pediatr Adolesc Med* 151(2):165–169, 1997.

Simekes A, Spitzer A: Poststreptococcal acute glomerulonephritis, *Pediatr Rev* 16(7):278–279, 1995.

Hematuria with Casts and Marked Proteinuria

Children who exhibit hematuria and marked proteinuria (greater than 1 g/m²/24 hr) may have a nephrotic syndrome (Table 16–15).

Approach to the Child with Proteinuria

(Table 16–17)
A small amount of protein is found in the urine of healthy children. The normal amount of urine protein is less than 4 mg/m²/hr or less than 100 mg/

TABLE 16–17
Evaluation of a Child with Proteinuria*

1. Complete history and physical examination
2. Confirmation of presence of proteinuria by repeat urinalysis
3. Twenty-four-hour urine collection to quantitate proteinuria; if quantitatively increased, proteinuria is present
4. Orthostatic test; if orthostatic test reveals fixed proteinuria, continue with tests listed in steps 5–7
5. Measurement of levels of serum BUN, creatinine (calculate creatinine clearance), total protein, albumin, cholesterol, and electrolytes
6. Measurement of streptozyme, C3, C4, ANA
7. Renal ultrasonography or intravenous pyelogram

---

*If steps 4–7 are abnormal, if there is a family history of renal disease, hematuria, hypertension, or edema, or if other manifestations of renal or systemic disease are present, biopsy may be needed.
ANA, Antinuclear antibody; *BUN,* blood urea nitrogen.

---

m²/24 hr. *Nephrotic proteinuria* is defined as greater than 40 mg/m²/hr or greater than 1 g/m²/24 hr. The intermediary amounts are abnormal but not within the nephrotic range. Qualitative proteinuria of 1+ or greater on at least two to three random urine specimens suggests proteinuria that should be confirmed quantitatively. A semiquantitative evaluation of proteinuria is possible with measurement of the urine protein-to-creatinine ratio on a single voided urine. The normal ratio generally is less than 0.2:1 when measured in the first morning specimen. The nephrotic urine protein-to-creatinine ratio is generally greater than 3.5:1.

Initially, it must be determined whether the proteinuria is transient or persistent. If it is persistent, the severity must be assessed (discussed later in this chapter under Glomerular Proteinuria). *Transient proteinuria* is seen after vigorous exercise and occasionally in children with fevers exceeding 38.5° C (101.3° F). The proteinuria usually is mild, transient, and reproducible.

Another type of transient proteinuria is *postural (orthostatic) proteinuria.* Patients excrete normal amounts of protein while recumbent but have significant, although moderate, proteinuria when in the upright position. Hematuria is absent and renal function, complement levels, and renal ultrasound or IVP are entirely normal. This transient proteinuria is best evaluated by collecting a timed urine specimen while the patient is recumbent (usually overnight), followed by a timed urine collection during a normally active day. The presence of significant, moderate proteinuria during the active period and a decrease in the proteinuria to normal or nearly normal levels during recumbency confirm the diagnosis of orthostatic proteinuria. It should be remembered that "fixed" proteinuria associated with renal disease also will have orthostatic accentuation during activity. Orthostatic proteinuria generally is thought to be benign. If proteinuria is *persistent* ("fixed"), renal disease should be considered (Table 16–15).

Tubular Proteinuria

In normal children, low-molecular-weight proteins are filtered and reabsorbed in the proximal tubule. Proximal tubular injury results in diminished reabsorptive ability (e.g., Fanconi syndrome) that produces mild to moderate proteinuria characteristically unassociated with edema.

Glomerular Proteinuria

Glomerular proteinuria is classified by its degree. Intermittent (mild) proteinuria (<0.5 g/m^2/day) is seen in pyelonephritis, renal cystic diseases, obstructive uropathies (congenital obstructions and reflux nephropathy), and mild glomerulonephritis. *Moderate proteinuria* (0.5–1 g/m^2/day) is seen in acute poststreptococcal glomerulonephritis, mild Henoch-Schönlein nephritis, severe pyelonephritis, chronic glomerulonephritis, and HUS. *Severe proteinuria* (>1 g/m^2/day) characteristically is associated with the nephrotic syndrome.

Nephrotic Syndrome

The nephrotic syndrome is an accumulation of symptoms and signs and is characterized by *proteinuria* (mainly albuminuria) greater than 1 g/m^2/24 hr, by *hypoproteinemia* (mainly albumin) with a total protein less than 5.5 g/dL and serum albumin less than 2.5 g/dL, by *hypercholesterolemia* (>250 mg/dL), and by *edema*. The primary disorder is an increase in glomerular permeability to proteins, most likely caused by a loss of the membrane sialoproteins, which in turn results in the loss of the negative charge on the basement membrane. This increase in glomerular permeability causes massive proteinuria accompanied by secondary hypoproteinemia. Plasma oncotic pressure is diminished, resulting in a shift of fluid from the vascular to the interstitial compartment and a contraction in plasma volume. Renal blood flow and GFR are not usually diminished, and in some instances GFR may be above normal. With profound hypoalbu-

minemia, GFR is diminished. In addition to hypoproteinemic reduction of plasma oncotic pressure, the formation of edema is enhanced by a reduction in effective blood volume and by an increase in tubular sodium chloride reabsorption produced by the activation of the renin-angiotensin-aldosterone system. Most serum lipids (including cholesterol and triglycerides) and levels of lipoprotein are elevated because hypoproteinemia stimulates hepatic lipoprotein synthesis; lipid metabolism is diminished.

Minimal Change Nephrotic Syndrome of Childhood

Minimal change nephrotic syndrome (MCNS) is the most common form of the nephrotic syndrome, seen in 80% of cases. The syndrome affects males more than females by 2:1 ratio. Typical nephrotic syndrome is defined as the absence of persistent hematuria, renal insufficiency, hypertension, and hypocomplementemia. Dependent pitting edema (pretibial, pedal, sacral, scrotal, labial, and periorbital) with weight gain or ascites is the most common presentation of nephrotic syndrome. Diarrhea (caused by intestinal edema) or respiratory distress (caused by pulmonary edema or pleural effusion) also may be present. Serum cholesterol usually is elevated and often markedly so (>400 mg/dL).

Of all childhood patients having MCNS, children 1–7 years old are likely to have steroid-responsive MCNS (87% of cases); therefore, corticosteroid therapy may be initiated without performing renal biopsy if the presentation is typical. Children 7–16 years of age still have a 50% chance of having MCNS on the basis of age alone, and if the children in this age group have a "typical" nephrotic syndrome, a trial of steroid therapy is indicated because prednisone responsiveness increases the chance of MCNS to 86%.

Management. If a child has the typical nephrotic syndrome, *treatment* consists of efforts to reduce edema and specific therapy with prednisone. The child who has a newly developed nephrotic syndrome usually requires hospitalization for diagnostic and therapeutic purposes.

The **edema** of the nephrotic syndrome is treated by restricting salt and water intake; by occasionally optimizing the excretion of these elements with the administration of diuretics; and, if the patient is refractory to diuretics alone, by increasing plasma volume. Sodium chloride intake should be restricted beyond a "no added salt" diet (<2 g Na per 24 hours). This salt restriction may be relaxed when the edema has resolved. At times, moderate fluid restriction is helpful. Diuretics may be required but should be given carefully because their overzealous use may further diminish plasma volume, resulting in hypotension and a fall in GFR.

Potassium supplementation may have to be provided if GFR is normal because considerable urine potassium can be lost as a result of a combination of secondary hyperaldosteronism and diuretic therapy. Hydrochlorothiazide often is effective in treating edema of the nephrotic syndrome unless the serum albumin is quite low or the GFR is impaired. If the GFR is normal, spironolactone may be added to minimize potassium losses. Furosemide generally is effective in inducing diuresis and natriuresis despite moderately decreased GFR and hypoalbuminemia. The administration of furosemide should be started with relatively small doses (1–2 mg/kg), and the patient should be monitored closely for volume depletion and electrolyte disturbances; occasionally even furosemide may be relatively ineffective in alleviating severe hypoalbuminemia in children. In these children, cautious volume expansion with salt-poor albumin (0.5 g/kg IV over 1–2 hours with furosemide 1–2 mg/kg) intravenously, infused during or immediately following albumin, usually results in diuresis. This therapy may be repeated once or twice, as needed. The infused albumin will be excreted rapidly (in 1–2 days) by patients with the nephrotic syndrome. Once adequate volume expansion has been achieved, further therapy with furosemide alone may suffice. Albumin should be given only in the presence of volume contraction, and the patient should be monitored closely for excessive volume expansion, which could lead to congestive cardiac failure.

Specific therapy is the administration of prednisone in a dosage of 2 mg/kg/day (60 mg/m²/24 hr) divided into two to four doses per day. Approximately 10% of patients respond (urine protein becoming negative or reduced to trace levels) by the end of 1 week, 70% by the end of 2 weeks, 85% by the end of 3 weeks, and 92% by the end of 4 weeks of therapy. The basics of therapy include continuing the dose until a negative or trace result is achieved on a urine protein dipstick for 4 consecutive days or for up to 4 weeks, whichever occurs first. At that point, the patient is switched to an every-other-day dosage at 60 mg/m². Prednisone should be given once on the dosage day for 2–4 weeks. Then a tapering schedule should be provided to have the patient discontinue receiving prednisone within another 4 weeks. Some evidence exists to suggest that a minimum of 2 weeks of daily prednisone therapy is preferred.

If a child does not respond to daily prednisone therapy, a renal biopsy is indicated because steroid resistance greatly increases the chance that the underlying pathology is other than MCNS. In these circumstances, the diagnosis most likely will be focal segmental glomerulosclerosis, mesangiocapillary (membranoproliferative) glomerulonephritis, or membranous nephropathy.

The treatment of each relapse of the nephrotic syndrome is similar to that given during the initial therapy. A relapse is defined either as persistent proteinuria for greater than 7 days in the absence of a respiratory infection or other intercurrent infection, or as the recurrence of edema. The definition is not simply the recurrence of proteinuria, because during an upper respiratory infection many children with the nephrotic syndrome have transient proteinuria that resolves spontaneously. Frequent relapses or steroid resistance may necessitate immunosuppressant therapy (e.g., with cyclophosphamide, chlorambucil, cyclosporine).

Complications. Infection is a major complication in children with the nephrotic syndrome (Table 16–18). Bacteremia and peritonitis may occur, particularly with *Streptococcus pneumoniae* or *E. coli*. A high index of suspicion and prompt evaluation are indicated in a febrile patient. Side effects of steroids are most common in initial nonresponders and frequently relapsing patients.

Focal Segmental Glomerulosclerosis

The presentation of focal segmental glomerulosclerosis (FSGS) may be identical to that of MCNS. In some cases, FSGS is thought to progress from MCNS, but in most circumstances it appears to be a separate entity. A circulating factor that increases glomerular permeability to albumin is found in some patients with FSGS. FSGS accounts for approximately 10% of children with the nephrotic syndrome. More than 80% of these patients are *steroid resistant*. Even those who initially respond frequently become steroid resistant subsequent to treatment. No clearly effective therapy for FSGS exists, although treatment with intravenous pulse methylprednisolone immunosuppressive agents

---

TABLE 16–18
Complications of Nephrotic Syndrome

Acute renal failure
Hypertension
Hypercoagulable state (renal vein thrombosis, pulmonary embolism)
Spontaneous bacterial peritonitis
Malnutrition
Exacerbation by immunization
Steroid-related toxicity
Immunosuppression-related toxicity

(cyclophosphamide, cyclosporine, and FK506) may produce remission in some patients and alleviate edema in others. Unfortunately, a considerable number of these patients progress to end-stage renal disease within 2–5 years. Children with FSGS who have progressed to end-stage renal disease and who have received kidney transplants also are more likely to have a recurrence in the transplanted kidney.

Membranous Nephropathy

Membranous nephropathy is an infrequent cause of the nephrotic syndrome in childhood. Approximately 1% of children with the nephrotic syndrome have this lesion. It is seen most commonly in adolescents and in children who have potentially curable systemic diseases such as hepatitis B, syphilis, malaria, and toxoplasmosis and as a result of drug therapy (e.g., with gold salts or penicillamine). These patients may exhibit the nephrotic syndrome or proteinuria only. Hematuria is common. The presence of proteinuria in a patient with one of the predisposing diseases is an indication for a renal biopsy.

Other Types of Nephrotic Syndrome

The nephrotic syndrome has been diagnosed in patients during therapy with penicillamine, gold, mercury compounds, and other drugs. It also has been described in association with several extrarenal neoplasms, such as lymphomas (particularly Hodgkin disease).

The **congenital nephrotic syndrome** appears in two forms during the first 6 months of life. The Finnish type is an autosomal recessive disorder most common in persons of Scandinavian descent. Prenatal diagnosis may be possible by detecting elevated levels of amniotic fluid alpha-fetoprotein; the placenta is enlarged. Proteinuria characteristically is present at birth, and the nephrotic syndrome becomes apparent within the first 3 months. Unfortunately, most of these children have died as a result of infection or renal failure by the age of 5 years. Renal transplantation may be of value. The other type of congenital nephrotic syndrome is a heterogeneous group of abnormalities, including diffuse mesangial sclerosis and conditions mostly associated with drugs or infections, such as syphilis and toxoplasmosis.

REFERENCES

Behrman RE, Kliegman RM, Jenson HB, editors: *Nelson textbook of pediatrics*, ed 16, Philadelphia, 2000, WB Saunders, Chapters 531–535.

Brodehl J: The treatment of minimal change nephrotic syndrome, *Eur J Pediatr* 150(6):380–387, 1991.

Cameron JS: Membranous nephropathy in childhood and its treatment, *Pediatr Nephrol* 4(2):193–198, 1990.

Habib R: Nephrotic syndrome in the first year of life, *Pediatr Nephrol* 7(4):347–353, 1993.

International Study of Kidney Diseases in Children: Minimal change nephrotic syndrome in children: deaths during the first 5–15 years of observation, *Pediatrics* 73(4):497–501, 1984.

McAdams A, Valentini R, Welch T: The nonspecificity of focal segmental glomerulosclerosis, *Medicine* 76(1):42–52, 1997.

Mendoza SA, Ture BM: Management of the difficult nephrotic patient, *Pediatr Clin North Am* 42(6):1459–1468, 1995.

Southwest Pediatric Nephrology Study Group: Focal segmental glomerulosclerosis in children with idiopathic nephrotic syndrome, *Kidney Int* 27(2):442–449, 1985.

ACUTE RENAL FAILURE

A significant decrease in GFR or in tubular function is designated as acute renal failure. This generally is associated with a GFR that is reduced sufficiently so that waste products (urea and phosphate) and water cannot be excreted and body fluid homeostasis is altered. Early recognition and management are critical.

Etiology and Pathophysiology. The major causes of acute renal insufficiency are listed in Table 16–19. *Prerenal renal failure* characteristically occurs when the circulating blood volume decreases, hypotension is present, or the effective blood volume decreases. Under these conditions, dehydration produced by vomiting, diarrhea, or a markedly increased insensible water loss can lead to hypovolemia. However, if the underlying cause of inadequate renal perfusion is reversed, renal function usually returns to normal. If the inadequate circulation persists, intrinsic renal damage supervenes.

Postrenal renal failure characteristically is obstructive in nature. Correcting or temporarily bypassing the obstruction will restore renal function unless renal parenchymal damage also has occurred. *Intrinsic renal failure* may be caused by vascular, immunologic, inflammatory, ischemic, or toxic injury to the kidney.

Acute Tubular Necrosis. Two principal mechanisms have been suggested to explain the renal failure exhibited in acute tubular necrosis. One hypothesis suggests that tubular injury caused by one of the conditions listed in Table 16–19 leads to decreased reabsorption of solutes and water. Thus delivery of salt and water to the distal nephron is increased, which stimulates the intrinsic renin-angiotensin system and tubuloglomerular feedback. The release of vasoactive substances produces increased cortical vascular resistance, which decreases cortical blood flow and produces further tubular injury. In addition, the release of vasoactive substances results in a diminished GFR, and, when severe, in acute renal failure. A second hypothesis suggests that tubular injury leads to tubular cell necrosis. Necrotic materials produce intratubular obstruction, raising intratubular resistance and thereby diminishing net

---

TABLE 16–19
Causes of Acute Renal Failure

Prerenal, Hypovolemic, Hypotension	**Postrenal (Obstruction)—cont'd**
Dehydration	Neurogenic bladder
Vomiting	Tumor lysis syndrome
Diarrhea	
Febrile illness	**Intrinsic**
Massive reduction in colloid oncotic pressure	Acute tubular necrosis
(protein-losing enteropathy, nephrotic syndrome)	Prolonged hypotension secondary to
Septic shock	Vomiting
Heart failure	Diarrhea
Hemorrhage	Shock
Burns	Nephrotoxins (drugs)
Peritonitis, ascites, cirrhosis	Glomerulonephritis
	Primary (poststreptococcal)
Postrenal (Obstruction)	Secondary (systemic lupus erythematosus and
Urethral obstruction	endocarditis)
Stricture	Interstitial nephritis
Posterior urethral valves	Primary
Diverticulum	Secondary
Phimosis	Drugs (allergic)
Ureteral obstruction	Toxins
Calculi	Vascular
Crystals (drugs or urate)	Renal vein thrombosis
Papillary necrosis	Arterial thromboemboli (umbilical artery catheter)
Clotted blood	Acute tubular necrosis
Tumor	Acute cortical necrosis
Ureterocele	Disseminated intravascular coagulation
Solitary renal unit with ureterovesical or ureteropelvic	Immune-mediated (scleroderma)
junction obstruction	Pigmenturia
Extrinsic tumor compressing bladder outlet	Hemoglobinuria
Extrinsic urinary tract tumors	Myoglobinuria

---

glomerular filtration and tubular flow, which results in acute renal failure. In addition, the cellular necrosis results in the loss of integrity of the renal tubule, with backleak of solute and fluid leading to reabsorption of most of the glomerular ultrafiltrate. Evidence exists for each of these theories, and it is probable that both play a role in the pathophysiology of acute renal failure.

Severe vascular compromise may lead to arterial or venous thrombosis or to *acute cortical necrosis.* Whereas acute tubular necrosis commonly is reversible, acute cortical necrosis leads to eventual scarring of the damaged glomeruli and permanent loss of renal function.

Diagnosis. History, physical examination, and laboratory data are helpful in evaluating the child with acute renal failure (Table 16–20).

The child with a *prerenal* cause of renal failure frequently has evidence of a precipitating illness associated with vomiting and diarrhea or an inadequate oral intake or has a history of one of the predisposing factors (Table 16–19). The physical examination may show signs of dehydration accompanied by decreased weight, decreased skin turgor, and perhaps tachycardia and hypotension. Mucous membranes of the mouth may be dry, and CNS signs of poor perfusion, such as irritability or lethargy, may be present. Urine volume characteristically is decreased.

Oliguric renal failure in adults is defined as less than 500 mL/day; oliguria in children is defined as less than 1–2 mL/kg/hr. *Nonoliguric renal failure* may occur and often is complicated by fluid and electrolyte disturbances, in addition to azotemia. Urinary osmolality is typically similar to serum osmolality. Measurement of urinary sodium usually reveals a sodium concentration between 20 and 40

TABLE 16–20
Laboratory Differential Diagnosis of Renal Insufficiency

	Prerenal		Renal		
	Child	**Neonate**	**Child**	**Neonate**	**Postrenal**
Urine Na$^+$ (mEq/L)	<20	<20–30	>40	>40	Variable, may be >40
FE$_{Na}$* (%)	<1	<2–5	>2	>2–5	Variable, may be >2
Urine osmolality (mOsm/L)	>500	>300–500	~300	~300	Variable, may be <300
RFI† (%)	<1	<2–5	>2	>2–5	Variable
Serum BUN-to-creatinine ratio	>20	≥10	~10	≥10	Variable, may be >20
Response to volume	Diuresis		No change		No change
Response to furosemide	Diuresis		No change		No change or diuresis
Urinalysis	Normal		RBCs, WBCs, casts, proteinuria		Variable to normal, possible crystals
Comments	Hx: diarrhea, vomiting, hemorrhage, diuretics Px: volume depletion		Hx: hypotension, anoxia, exposure to nephrotoxins Px: hypertension, edema		Hx: poor urine stream and output Px: flank mass, distended bladder

BUN, Blood urea nitrogen; *Hx,* history; *Px,* physical signs; *RBCs,* red blood cells; *WBCs,* white blood cells.
*FE$_{Na}$, Fractional excretion of sodium (%) = (urine sodium/plasma sodium urine creatinine ÷ plasma creatinine) × 100.
†*RFI,* Renal failure index = (urine sodium ÷ urine creatinine/plasma creatinine) × 100.

mEq/L, and the fractional excretion of sodium is usually greater than 1%. This is expressed as

$$\frac{U/p\,Na}{U/p\,creatinine} \times 100$$

Urinalysis reveals a specific gravity of 1.010–1.015 and frequently reveals nonspecific cellular elements.

Postrenal renal failure often is found in early infancy and is associated with an obstructive lesion. Physical findings of dehydration are absent. Urinary output may be decreased, normal, or increased. Urinary osmolality frequently is similar to that of plasma, urinary sodium concentration often is greater than 50 mEq/L, and fractional excretion of sodium is greater than 10%. Urinalysis reveals no sediment abnormalities. Renal ultrasonography, a voiding cystourethrogram, or a radionuclide scan is a useful test for assessing the possibility of postrenal failure.

The child with *intrinsic renal failure* may have a history compatible with one of the predisposing conditions. Physical examination may show signs of adequate, increased, or decreased fluid balance. Papilledema, hypertension, cardiac enlargement, or a gallop rhythm may be present, which would suggest vascular overload. Signs of systemic involvement resulting from underlying disease may be noted (e.g., in SLE, Henoch-Schönlein purpura, or HUS). Urine output characteristically is decreased. Urinary osmolality may be isotonic, hypotonic, or hypertonic. Urinary sodium concentration generally is increased, frequently to greater than 40 mEq/L, and the fractional excretion of sodium is greater than 1%. Urinalysis usually reveals red cell and granular casts. Usually, hematuria, proteinuria, and (sometimes) leukocyturia are exhibited. C3 complement may be depressed in acute poststreptococcal glomerulonephritis, SLE, or membranoproliferative (mesangiocapillary) glomerulonephritis. Evidence of an earlier infection may be present, which can be demonstrated by the presence of a positive streptozyme or hepatitis-B surface antigen. Anemia and thrombocytopenia may be present in conditions such as SLE or HUS. A chest roentgenogram may reveal evidence of pulmonary edema and cardiomegaly, suggesting vascular overload.

Treatment. Treatment depends on the cause of acute renal insufficiency, although certain modalities commonly are used for many children with acute renal failure. The first step is to develop a plan of comprehensive monitoring. The patient should be weighed at least at 12-hour intervals to determine fluid balance because acute weight changes reflect water loss or gain. Initial fluid and electrolyte therapy and a plan for frequent reevaluation should be established. Urine output and electrolyte composition should be determined frequently during the acute phase.

Reversible conditions that can be treated should be given prompt attention. Obstructions of the urinary tract should be corrected or bypassed. Infection and shock should be treated. Hypovolemia should be corrected promptly. Dopamine may improve renal blood flow in low doses and is effective in various states of poor cardiac output. In addition, dobutamine may improve renal perfusion by enhancing myocardial contractility. If the presence of severe, intrinsic renal failure is in question, a catheter may be placed into the bladder to assess whether urine is present and to remove the urine promptly. If acute renal failure is present, monitoring small volumes of urinary output present no advantage, because a urinary catheter may predispose to infection. Therefore, an indwelling catheter should not be maintained.

Fluid Requirements. The degree of dehydration should be estimated. If hypovolemia is apparent, intravascular volume should be expanded by intravenous administration of physiologic saline (0.9% sodium chloride); 20 mL/kg is given intravenously over 30–60 minutes. Once volume depletion has been corrected, an intravenous dose of furosemide (2 mg/kg) in the presence of anuria is reasonable. If urinary output is not increased, a second dose of furosemide may be given. If no response occurs, further infusion generally is not helpful and increases the risk of ototoxicity.

If the patient shows evidence of excessive weight gain or fluid overload, fluid intake should be reduced to insensible water loss, plus urinary and stool output, plus any fluid drainage (via nasogastric tube), minus a planned weight loss. Patients who have acute renal failure are catabolic and lose approximately 1% of body weight per day—in the form of tissue losses, not as fluid losses. When the patient maintains weight in the presence of acute renal failure, this generally indicates fluid retention. Diuretics can be attempted as initial therapy to mobilize retained fluids. However, with severe acute renal failure, the kidney may be unresponsive. Severe

fluid overload in the presence of marked oliguria or anuria is one indication for dialysis.

Hyperkalemia. Hyperkalemia is often seen in patients with acute renal failure resulting from the absence of potassium excretion and catabolism. Foods, fluids, and medications that contain high levels of potassium should be restricted until renal function is reestablished. Lead II of the electrocardiogram is useful for assessing cardiac changes caused by hyperkalemia (discussed earlier in the chapter under Disturbances of Electrolytes, Acid-Base Balance, and Fluids). The presence of hyperkalemia requires immediate attention. Severe hyperkalemia is an indication for dialysis.

Acidosis. Acidosis is common in renal failure as a consequence of catabolism and the inability of the failed kidney to secrete hydrogen ion. When the condition is severe, intravenous sodium bicarbonate should be administered as noted earlier, but should be given cautiously in order to avoid fluid overload, hypernatremia, and hypertension. Severe or unrelenting acidosis is an indication for dialysis.

Hypocalcemia. Hypocalcemia is seen commonly in acute renal failure in association with hyperphosphatemia. *Treatment* primarily involves efforts to lower the serum phosphorus level. Milk and other high-phosphorus foods should be severely restricted, and oral calcium carbonate should be given to bind phosphorus. Aluminum hydroxide gels previously used to treat hyperphosphatemia have been associated with aluminum intoxication (e.g., in dementia and rickets). If the patient shows evidence of tetany, an intravenous infusion of 10% calcium gluconate (0.5 mL/kg) may be given slowly.

Nutritional Needs. An adequate caloric intake must be maintained in patients with acute renal failure in order to minimize catabolism. At least 70% of the recommended daily allowance of calories and 0.5–1.0 g/kg/day of high-quality protein should be provided.

Dialysis. In children with renal insufficiency, dialysis is indicated in order to treat hyperkalemia unresponsive to medical therapy, acidosis unresponsive to medical therapy, hyperkalemia or acidosis in the presence of hypernatremia, fluid overload unresponsive to fluid restriction or to diuretics, or symptoms and signs of "uremia." The method used may be peritoneal dialysis, hemodialysis, or a modification of hemodialysis, such as hemofiltration or hemodiafiltration.

Complications. The most serious potential complications of acute renal failure are infections, vascular overload, and hyperkalemia. Other potential complications are uremic encephalopathy, seizures, pericardial effusion, hypertension, peptic ulceration, platelet dysfunction, and anemia. In addition, careful monitoring of blood levels of drugs excreted by the kidney and appropriate adjustment of either the total dose or the dosage interval are necessary to prevent complications or further renal injury (e.g., with acyclovir, aminoglycosides, penicillins, cephalosporins, vancomycin, ranitidine, or digoxin). The recovery phase of obstructive renal failure and acute tubular necrosis may be complicated by a polyuric phase associated with poor concentrating ability and hypokalemia, or hyperkalemia. The plan of management that minimizes the use of urinary catheters, avoids fluid overload and electrolyte excess, and effectively treats hyperkalemia generally is rewarded by the patient's recovery.

Prognosis. Recovery depends on the etiology of acute renal failure. Prerenal failure, postrenal failure, and intrinsic renal failure are reversible in most types of renal disease. In patients with acute tubular necrosis, the period of anuria/oliguria usually lasts 7–10 days and is followed by 2–7 days of polyuria. With good supportive care and steady monitoring, all patients should recover from acute tubular necrosis. Lack of improvement suggests acute cortical necrosis or some other cause. Renal failure associated with RPGN, renal vascular thrombosis, and cortical necrosis may not be reversible and may necessitate chronic dialysis and eventual renal transplantation.

REFERENCES

Behrman RE, Kliegman RM, Jenson HB, editors: *Nelson textbook of pediatrics,* ed 16, Philadelphia, 2000, WB Saunders, Chapters 542, 543.

Gaudio KM, Siegal NJ: Pathogenesis and treatment of acute renal failure, *Pediatr Clin North Am* 34(3):771–787, 1987.

Gouyon JR, Guignard JP: The management of acute renal failure in newborns, *Pediatr Nephrol* 14(10–11):1037–1044, 2000.

Thadhani R, Pascual M, Bonventre J: Acute renal failure, *N Engl J Med* 334(22):1448–1460, 1996.

CHRONIC RENAL FAILURE

Etiology. The cause of chronic renal failure in childhood is closely related to the age of the child at the time renal failure occurs. Between birth and 10 years of age, congenital and obstructive abnormalities are the most common causes. After age 10, acquired diseases such as focal segmental glomerulosclerosis, chronic glomerulonephritis, reflux nephropathy, HUS, and progressive hereditary disorders (e.g., Alport syndrome and cystic disease) are likely causes of chronic renal failure. In each category renal function progressively deteriorates and is accompanied by the contraction of the renal parenchyma with subsequent end-stage renal failure. The progression to end-stage renal failure is variable and depends on features such as hyperfiltration, ongoing immunologic injury, proteinuria, hypertension, secondary hyperparathyroidism, and infection.

Clinical Manifestations. Growth failure in children with chronic renal failure is prominent. The factors associated with growth retardation include undernutrition, osteodystrophy, hormonal abnormalities, medications (e.g., steroids), and acidosis. Increased calorie intake leads to a slight increase in growth, but considerably more calories are needed than are necessary to achieve comparable growth in children with normal renal function. Children with chronic renal failure also have progressive anemia, frequently are hypertensive, are at increased risk for infection or CNS disturbances, and demonstrate severe osteodystrophy.

Treatment. The management of children with chronic renal failure and their complex problems requires a team of pediatric nephrologists, clinical nursing specialists, nutritionists, social workers, psychiatrists, psychologists, recreational and occupational therapists, and various other professionals.

Diet. Children with chronic renal insufficiency have diminished growth velocity and progressive retardation of bone age before puberty. They should be provided with more than 80% of the recommended dietary allowance of calories. Infants often require greater than 125% of the recommended daily allowance to achieve moderate growth. Protein should be provided at a level of 1.5 g/kg/24 hr and should consist of high-biologic-value proteins. Milk and milk products must be restricted because of their high phosphate content. In infants a high-quality protein formula, such as PM60/40 (from Ross Laboratories), used in conjunction with calcium carbonate as a phosphate binder, may be indicated. Supplemental calcium usually is necessary because the child must avoid milk products. Children with renal insufficiency also need vitamin supplementation because they become deficient in water-soluble vitamins.

To keep the serum bicarbonate in the 19–20 mEq/L range, acidosis should be treated with appropriate doses of sodium bicarbonate or sodium citrate (Bicitra). Water balance usually is maintained reasonably well until dialysis is required; therefore, water restriction rarely is necessary. A "no added salt" diet provides adequate but not excessive sodium intake, although as a consequence of obstructive uropathies some children with renal insufficiency may be salt wasters, thus requiring increased salt intake. Patients with intrinsic renal disease usually have hypertension, for which salt restriction is needed. High-potassium foods should be avoided once renal failure is established. ACE inhibitors used to treat hypertension or proteinuria may result in hyperkalemia.

Renal Osteodystrophy. Renal osteodystrophy (most commonly, osteitis fibrosa) is a nearly constant accompaniment of chronic renal failure and is associated with hyperphosphatemia, high serum alkaline phosphatase activity, and secondary hyperparathyroidism. The initial therapy is to restrict phosphate in the diet, most commonly by restricting milk and milk products. In addition, calcium carbonate may be used to bind phosphate in the gastrointestinal tract. The phosphate level should be kept below the 5–6 mg/dL range to minimize secondary hyperparathyroidism while providing enough phosphate for new bone formation. Because milk restriction leads to inadequate calcium intake, a child should receive approximately 1 g of elemental calcium from all sources per day. Because that is not provided in the diet, calcium supplements should be given.

Chronic renal failure is associated with an inability of the kidney to convert 25-hydroxycholecalciferol to 1,25-dihydroxycholecalciferol. Therapy with either synthetic vitamin D (dihydrotachysterol) or 1,25-dihydroxycholecalciferol usually is necessary.

Anemia. Anemia is a common finding in chronic renal failure in children. Anemia results primarily from toxic depression of erythropoiesis by abnormal or retained metabolites and from a failure of the kidney to produce erythropoietin in response to anemia. Reduced serum iron and elevated iron-binding capacity are common but do not indicate iron deficiency because the anemia is normochromic and normocytic and the ferritin levels are normal or elevated. Transfusions are rarely needed if recombinant-produced erythropoietin is administered.

Growth. Therapy with recombinant-produced growth hormone is useful in children having chronic renal failure or receiving dialysis. Accelerated growth occurs with pharmacologic doses of human growth hormone. Growth hormone should be used when caloric intake, treatment of acidosis, and treatment to prevent renal osteodystrophy have been undertaken.

Treatment of End-Stage Renal Failure. The principal treatment of end-stage renal failure is *renal transplantation.* Cadaver donors and living related donors have been used extensively for renal transplantation. Children with progressive renal failure should be referred for evaluation to a center specializing in renal transplantation for children. Thoroughly evaluating the cause of chronic renal failure, listing potential donors, and beginning to prepare the family and child for dialysis and transplantation should begin before the threat of end-stage renal failure becomes immediate.

Dialysis is effective for sustaining the patient who is awaiting renal transplantation or in whom renal transplantation is not possible. The development of continuous ambulatory peritoneal dialysis (CAPD) and continuous cycling peritoneal dialysis (CCPD) has made chronic dialysis an effective and well-tolerated technique during the necessary time before transplantation. The principal complication of peritoneal dialysis is peritoneal infection, especially with *Staphylococcus (S. epidermidis* or *S. aureus).* For some the preferred mode of dialysis is hemodialysis. Because of improved techniques used in dialysis and immunosuppressive drugs used for transplantation (e.g., cyclosporine), the outlook for children with end-stage renal disease is encouraging. Patient and graft survival is highest in pediatric patients beyond infancy.

REFERENCES

Behrman RE, Kliegman RM, Jenson HB, editors: *Nelson textbook of pediatrics,* ed 16, Philadelphia, 2000, WB Saunders, Chapters 543, 544.

Bereket G, Fine RN: Pediatric renal transplantation, *Pediatr Clin North Am* 42(6):1603–1628, 1995.

Evans ED, Greenough LA, Ettenger RB: Principles of renal replacement therapy in children, *Pediatr Clin North Am* 42(2):1579–1602, 1995.

Fine R, Salusky I, Ettenger R: The therapeutic approach to the infant, children and adolescent with endstage renal disease, *Pediatr Clin North Am* 34(3):789–801, 1987.

Warady BA, Johns K: New hormones in the therapeutic arsenal of chronic renal failure: growth hormone and erythropoietin, *Pediatr Clin North Am* 42(6):1551–1577, 1995.

HYPERTENSION

Systolic and diastolic blood pressure values increase gradually between birth and 18 years of age. During this period and adulthood, most patients "track" in a constant percentile around the mean. The younger the hypertensive patient, the greater the chance the hypertension will be secondary to another disease rather than being essential hypertension.

Etiology. Hypertension in children may be the result of renal (Table 16–21), endocrine (Table 16–22), vascular (Table 16–23), and neurologic (Table 16–24) disorders and of miscellaneous disorders such as essential hypertension, drugs or foods (e.g., steroids or licorice), or prolonged immobilization.

Clinical Manifestations. The signs and symptoms of hypertension are heart failure, stroke, seizures, headache, coma, polyuria, oliguria, and blurred vision. However, many patients are asymptomatic, which emphasizes the importance of frequently obtaining a blood pressure reading from every infant and child. In young infants blood pressure may be measured with the Dynamap machine; in older patients standard sphygmomanometry and auscultation are sufficient. Additional physical findings are papilledema, abdominal bruits (renovascular), arm blood pressure greater than leg pressure (aortic coarctation), café-au-lait spots (neurofibromatosis), flank

TABLE 16–21
Renal Causes of Hypertension

Congenital Anomalies
Dysplastic kidney
Polycystic disease
Obstructive uropathy

Acquired Lesions
Wilms tumor
Acute glomerulonephritis
Hemolytic-uremic syndrome
Henoch-Schönlein purpura
Systemic lupus erythematosus
Familial nephritis (Alport syndrome)
Reflux nephropathy
Segmental hypoplasia (Ask-Upmark kidney)
Drugs, toxins (e.g., cyclosporine, steroids, lead)

TABLE 16–22
Endocrine Causes of Hypertension

Neuroblastoma
Pheochromocytoma
Adrenal genital syndrome (11-hydroxylase deficiency)
Cushing syndrome
Hyperparathyroidism-hypercalcemia
Hyperaldosteronism
Hyperthyroidism
Diabetic nephropathy
Liddle syndrome

TABLE 16–23
Vascular Causes of Hypertension

Coarctation of aorta
Postcoarctation repair
Renal artery embolism (neonate with umbilical artery catheter)
Renal vein thrombosis
Endocarditis
Renal artery stenosis
Fibromuscular dysplasia
Neurofibromatosis
Arteritis (Takayasu, periarteritis nodosa, or aortoarteritis)
Sarcoidosis
Essential hypertension (etiology uncertain)

TABLE 16–24
Neurologic Causes of Hypertension

Neurofibromatosis
Guillain-Barré syndrome
Subdural hemorrhage
Dysautonomia (Riley-Day syndrome)
Increased intracranial pressure (with bradycardia)
Poliomyelitis
Quadriplegia
Encephalitis
Stress, anxiety

Adapted from the chapter of John E. Lewy in the second edition.

masses (in hydronephrosis, renal dysplasia, neuroblastoma, and Wilms tumor), ataxia, opsoclonus (in neuroblastoma), tachycardia, flushing, diaphoresis (in pheochromocytoma), and truncal obesity, acne, striae, and buffalo hump (in Cushing syndrome).

Diagnosis. The diagnostic evaluation of patients with hypertension involves urinalysis; measurement of the levels of blood urea nitrogen, creatinine, electrolytes, and acid-base balance; a chest roentgenogram; and renal ultrasound. Clues from the history, physical examination, mode of presentation, initial laboratory data, and age should determine the next sequence of tests. A renal radionuclide scan and the determination of plasma hormone levels (e.g., catecholamines, thyroxine, cortisol, and renin) and urine hormone levels (vanillylmandelic acid, homovanillic acid, dopamine, and steroid hormones) are more specific and noninvasive methods. These should be undertaken if the history or physical examination suggests the possibility. Finally, renal arteriography and renal biopsy are invasive tests that may provide definitive diagnosis.

Treatment. Before treatment is initiated, it is important to determine whether the hypertension is persistent or intermittent; whether the measurements are accurate (using an appropriate size blood pressure cuff); and that the hypertension is not compensatory, as occurs with increased intracranial pressure or as a result of a coarctation of the aorta.

For mild hypertension, dietary manipulation (decreased salt intake), weight loss (for obese patients), and exercise should be considered. If drug therapy is desired, starting with a low dose of a diuretic such as thiazide might be considered. All diuretic therapy has the drawback of causing potassium loss in the urine, which may necessitate potassium supplementation. Other medications used as first-line therapy for mild to moderate hypertension are calcium channel blockers (nifedipine), angiotensin enzyme (ACE) inhibitors (captopril or enalapril), and beta blockers (propranolol, atenolol) or combined alpha and beta blockers (labetalol). The beta blockers are associated with the undesired side effects of lethargy and depression.

For severe hypertension, combined therapy (such as a diuretic and a calcium channel blocker, a diuretic and an ACE inhibitor, or perhaps all three options) might be appropriate. Renovascular hypertension, when amenable to treatment, can be managed with angioplasty or surgery on the involved vessel. Primary endocrine abnormalities or other primary diseases (e.g., coarctation of the aorta) require specific therapy. Hypertensive emergencies warrant intensive care and therapy with nifedipine, sodium nitroprusside, or labetalol.

Prognosis. The prognosis depends on the primary disorder. Essential hypertension, when present in adolescents and not associated with morbidity at presentation and untreated, contributes to the cardiovascular, CNS, and renal morbidity associated with hypertension in older patients.

REFERENCES

Behrman RE, Kliegman RM, Jenson HB, editors: *Nelson textbook of pediatrics*, ed 16, Philadelphia, 2000, WB Saunders, Chapter 451.

Harshfield GA, Alpert BS, Pullman DA, et al: Ambulatory blood pressure readings in children and adults, *Pediatrics* 94(2 Pt 1): 180–184, 1994.

Ingelfinger JR: Pediatric hypertension, *Curr Opinion Pediatr* 6(2): 198–206, 1994.

Sinaiko A: Hypertension in children, *N Engl J Med* 335(26):1968–1973, 1996.

Task Force on Blood Pressure Control in Children: Report of the Second Task Force on Blood Pressure Control in Children—1987, *Pediatrics* 79(1):1–25, 1987.

Tyagi S, Kaul U, Satsangi D, et al: Percutaneous transluminal angioplasty for renovascular hypertension in children: initial and long-term results, *Pediatrics* 99(1):44–49, 1997.

GENITAL DISORDERS
Anomalies of the Penis
Hypospadias

Hypospadias occurs in approximately 1:500 newborn infants. The urethral meatus is located below and proximal to its normal position, an abnormality resulting from a failure of the urethral folds to fuse completely over the urethral groove. The ventral foreskin also is lacking, and the dorsal portion gives the appearance of a hood.

Chordee is a term for a ventral curvature of the penile shaft. The meatus may be on the glans or at any point along the penis to the penile-scrotal junction. Rarely, the urethra opens onto the perineum. In this circumstance, the chordee is extreme, and the scrotum is bifid and sometimes extends to the dorsal base of the penis. Testes are undescended in 10% of boys with hypospadias, and inguinal hernias are common.

The *differential diagnosis* of severe hypospadias with undescended testes must include the various causes of ambiguous genitalia (e.g., congenital adrenal hyperplasia or masculinization of females). The frequency of other anomalies of the urinary tract in males with hypospadias is relatively low, except in those whose urethral opening is very close to the penile-scrotal junction.

Males with hypospadias should not be circumcised, because the foreskin often is necessary for later repair. The ideal age of repair remains controversial, although most pediatric urologists tend to operate before the patient is 18 months of age.

Phimosis

In 90% of uncircumcised male infants, the prepuce becomes retractable by the age of 3 years; after this age, the inability to retract the prepuce is termed phimosis. The condition may be congenital or a sequela to inflammation. Severe phimosis usually requires surgical enlargement of the opening or circumcision. Accumulation of smegma is not pathologic and does not require surgical treatment. *Paraphimosis* occurs when the prepuce is retracted behind the coronal sulcus and cannot be returned to its normal position, which usually is a result of venous stasis and edema and leads to severe pain. Occasionally, when the condition is discovered early, reduction of the foreskin is possible with lubrication. In some cases, circumcision is needed.

Disorders and Abnormalities of the Scrotum and Its Contents
Undescended Testes (Cryptorchidism)

Undescended testes are found in 0.7% of children after 1 year of age. The frequency is higher in full-term newborn infants (3.4%) than in older children. In cases discovered at birth, the percentage increases with prematurity (17% in infants with birth weights between 2000 and 2500 g and 100% in infants weighing less than 900 g). Although spontaneous testicular descent does not occur beyond the age of 1 year, failure to find one or both testes in the scrotum does not necessarily indicate undescended testicles.

Retractile testes, absent testes, and ectopic testes also may be the cause of cryptorchidism. The true undescended testis is found along the path of normal descent, usually with a patent processus vaginalis. The undescended testis commonly is associated with an *inguinal hernia*; it also is subject to *torsion*. A higher incidence of infertility in adulthood, a risk of development of tumor in the undescended testis, and untoward psychologic effects in adolescence and adulthood are associated with the condition. Cryptorchidism is bilateral in up to 30% of reported cases. Infertility is uniform in adults with untreated bilateral cryptorchidism. Because infertility also is common in adults with a history of unilateral undescended testicle, the contralateral descended testis may also be abnormal.

The undescended testis usually is histologically normal at birth, but atrophy and poor development are found by the end of the first year of life. Although cryptorchidism is still a subject of controversy, reports indicate that surgical correction at an early age results in a greater probability of fertility in adulthood. Stimulation with human chorionic gonadotropin (hCG) results in testosterone release from functioning testes. This helps in consideration of exploration for abdominal testes and often results in descent of retractile testes. The development of a malignant tumor in the cryptorchid testis has been reported to occur 20–44% of the time, usually in the third or fourth decade of life. The greatest risk seems to be in those who are untreated or who underwent surgical correction during or after puberty.

Indirect inguinal hernias accompany undescended testes and also are seen frequently with ectopic testes. Torsion, with or without infarction, may occur and probably is related to excessive mobility of these testes. *Orchidopexy* usually is undertaken in the second year of life. Most testes that are extraabdominal can be brought into the scrotum when the associated hernia is corrected. If the testis is not palpable, ultrasonography may determine its location. The closer the testis is to the internal inguinal ring, the better the chance of successful orchidopexy.

Retractile Testes

Retractile testes are normal testes that have retracted into the inguinal canal as a result of an exaggeration of the cremasteric reflex. The *diagnosis* of retractile testes is likely if testes are palpable in the newborn examination but not at a later examination. Retractile testes frequently can be identified and brought into the scrotum by palpation when the child is warm and relaxed, and they characteristically remain in the scrotum permanently with puberty. The retractile testis does not cause the complications commonly associated with a true undescended testis.

Torsion of the Testis

Torsion is an emergency that requires prompt diagnosis and treatment. It accounts for approximately 40% of cases of acute scrotal pain and swelling at all ages and is the major etiologic factor in patients younger than 6 years of age. It usually is caused by an abnormal fixation of the testis to the scrotum. If the tunica vaginalis covers both the testis and the epididymis, as well as the distal spermatic cord, the testis can rotate freely and torsion is facilitated. On examination, the swelling is apparent, tenderness is severe, and the cremasteric reflex is absent.

The *differential diagnosis* of torsion of the testes includes an incarcerated hernia and torsion of the testicular epididymal appendices. Torsion of the appendices is associated with point tenderness over the lesion and minimal swelling. In adolescence, the differential diagnosis of testicular torsion must also include **epididymitis.** Epididymitis is the most common cause of acute scrotal pain and swelling in older adolescents. The differential diagnosis frequently is helped by an antecedent history of sexual activity (e.g., infection with *Chlamydia* or gonococcus) or urinary tract infection (e.g., infection with *E. coli*). Testicular torsion must be considered as the principal diagnosis when severe acute testicular pain is present.

If radiologic studies are in doubt, prompt surgical exploration should be performed. If the testis is explored within 6 hours of torsion, the gonads will survive (in up to 90% of cases). The procedure is detorsion and fixation of the testis to the scrotum. The contralateral testis usually is fixed to the scrotum to prevent future torsion. If torsion of the appendices is found at the time of exploration, removal of the necrotic tissue is indicated.

REFERENCES

Behrman RE, Kliegman RM, Jenson HB, editors: *Nelson textbook of pediatrics*, ed 16, Philadelphia, 2000, WB Saunders, Chapters 552–554.

Berkowitz GS, Lapinski RH, Dolgun SE, et al: Prevalence and natural history of cryptorchidism, *Pediatrics* 92(1):44–49, 1993.

Davenport M: Problems with the penis and prepuce, *BMJ* 312 (7026):299–301, 1996.

Fallon B, Welton M, Hawtrey C: Congenital anomalies associated with cryptorchidism, *J Urol* 127(1):91–93, 1982.

John Radcliffe Hospital Cryptorchidism Study Group: Cryptorchidism: a prospective study of 7500 consecutive male births 1984–1988, *Arch Dis Child* 67(7):892–899, 1992.

URINARY TRACT INFECTION

Urinary tract infection (UTI) is the most common genitourinary disease of childhood.

Clinical Manifestations. The symptoms and signs of UTI vary markedly with age. *Neonates* commonly present with failure to thrive, feeding problems, diarrhea, vomiting, fever, and hyperbilirubinemia. The infant 1 month to 2 years of age with a UTI usually has non–urinary tract manifestations such as feeding problems, failure to thrive, diarrhea, and unexplained fever. This age group also presents with a UTI masquerading as gastrointestinal illness, such as "colic," irritability, and screaming periods. In the first month of life, a male preponderance is seen in patients with UTI. The sex ratio of UTI has a female preponderance from the second month of life to adulthood. The child 2–6 years of age may have gastrointestinal symptoms, but in this age group the classic signs of urinary tract infection, such as urgency, dysuria, frequency, and abdominal pain, begin to appear. The child 6–18 years of age most commonly has urgency, frequency, dysuria, and abdominal or flank pain. Urinary tract infections occur in 1–2% of school-age girls. In all children, *unexplained fevers* and sustained abdominal symptoms without explanation are indicators to examine the urine and obtain a urine specimen for culture.

Congenital genitourinary tract abnormalities predispose patients to UTI, and UTI should be suspected when unexplained fevers or other symptoms are found in a child with these problems.

Diagnosis. The diagnosis of a UTI is based on a *positive culture of bacteria* in the urine. The finding of any bacteria in urine obtained by bladder catheterization or by suprapubic bladder puncture indicates infection. A properly collected voided urine, promptly plated, that grows more than 100,000 colonies/mL of a single organism on quantitative bacterial culture has a 95% positive correlation with suprapubic aspiration. A count of less than 10^5 bacterial colonies on a voided specimen has diminished value. The presence of *leukocytes* in the urine suggests that infection may be present in the symptomatic child, but an inflammatory disease, such as acute poststreptococcal glomerulonephritis, is associated with leukocyturia. *Blood* in the urine may be present in a UTI, particularly in adolescent females, but the presence of blood or leukocytes in the urine is not diagnostic. The presence of numerous motile bacteria in a freshly voided and examined urine (uncentrifuged urine) specimen from symptomatic infants and children has a 94% correlation with a positive culture of a suprapubic aspiration. The presence of even scant bacteria has an 82% correlation with a positive suprapubic aspiration. A delay of 1–2 hours in the examination of a voided specimen frequently leads to bacterial multiplication and thus to a false impression of infection.

The most common cause of bacteriuria in the absence of a UTI is contamination of the urine by periurethral and anterior urethral flora. Colony counts will be low, however, if the urine is plated for culture promptly. In a few cases bacterial colony counts of less than 100,000 on a voided specimen occur when a UTI is present. This may happen in the well-hydrated child who is voiding frequently and has a dilute urine. It also may occur if the child has re-

ceived recent antimicrobial therapy or if bacterial inhibitors are present. Fewer than 10^5 bacterial colonies also may be seen when UTI is caused by fastidious organisms (e.g., as in tuberculosis).

Localization of a UTI is important because infection of the upper urinary tract is associated more frequently with anatomic abnormalities than is infection of the lower urinary tract. Unfortunately, the clinical presentation is of limited help in determining the site of infection in neonates, infants, and toddlers. Fever and abdominal pain can occur with either lower or upper UTI, although high fevers favor upper tract involvement. Direct methods of investigation, such as bladder washout specimens, usually are contraindicated because of their invasiveness. Indirect methods, including examining the urine for glitter cell and white cell casts (which, if present, indicate upper tract infection); finding evidence of an inability to maximally concentrate the urine; finding antibody-coated bacteria measured by immunofluorescence; beta$_2$-microglobulin excretion in 24-hour urine collections; and performing lactic dehydrogenase differential excretion all have been suggested, but these are of limited practical value in differentiating upper from lower UTIs. A high erythrocyte sedimentation rate (ESR), leukocytosis, and bacteremia are noted in pyelonephritis. Nephromegaly as seen with ultrasonography or renal scan suggests pyelonephritis more than other tests.

Predisposing Factors. The short urethra in girls predisposes them to UTI. Uncircumcised male infants are also at risk for UTI. The *E. coli* serotypes from bowel flora frequently are found in UTI. Furthermore, certain strains of bacteria have increased adherence to uroepithelial cells, which correlates with the presence of bacterial pili. A hydronephrotic kidney, vesicoureteral reflux, a poorly emptying bladder, congenital malformations, nephrolithiasis, and other factors leading to *urinary stasis* predispose the patient to a UTI. The specific role of vesicoureteral reflux in the pathogenesis of UTI is unclear. A high incidence of vesicoureteral reflux is reported in association with UTI, but its pathogenic significance remains unclear. However, the presence of vesicoureteral reflux and infection is a predisposing factor for chronic infection and renal scarring. Nonetheless, scarring may occur without reflux.

The most common bacteria isolated from symptomatic or asymptomatic children experiencing their first UTI, occurring at any age and in both boys and girls, is *E. coli*. Other organisms, such as *Klebsiella, Proteus,* enterococci, and *Staphylococcus saprophyticus,* appear more frequently in the presence of obstruction or abnormalities of the urinary tract.

Treatment. UTIs should be treated promptly. Neonates require 10–14 days of parenteral antibiotic therapy because a UTI is often associated with bacteremia. Older children with acute cystitis should receive at least a 5–7-day course of oral antibiotic therapy. The most common therapy is administration of amoxicillin or trimethoprim/sulfamethoxazole. In children with high fevers, white cell casts, or other symptoms or signs of *acute pyelonephritis,* the initial use of broad-spectrum parenteral antibiotics is indicated. In children with pyelonephritis who do not have toxic symptoms, treatment includes a parenteral antibiotic, such as ampicillin or a cephalosporin. Patients who exhibit evidence of toxicity (e.g., chills or a high fever) often are treated with ampicillin and gentamicin (or another aminoglycoside) or a third-generation cephalosporin alone. Once systemic toxicity has resolved and the patient is afebrile, oral therapy with an agent to which the cultured organism is sensitive should be administered to complete at least 14 days of therapy. The urine culture should be repeated 4–7 days after the therapy is discontinued because many relapses are asymptomatic. The UTI has a tendency to recur, even without predisposing factors. Some recommend that follow-up urine specimens should also be obtained for culture after recurrent cystitis or pyelonephritis, first at 1-month intervals and subsequently at 3-month intervals for at least 1 year.

Follow-Up Evaluation of the Urinary Tract. The decision as to whether to perform a workup after a UTI depends on the likelihood that complicating abnormalities are present. A history of treatment failure, the presence of unusual organisms, growth disturbances, suspicion of an anomaly or abscess, and frequent recurrences suggest a more complex problem. The indications for radiologic evaluation include the following:

- All children younger than 10 years of age
- A UTI in any male child

- A UTI in a female child older than 10 years of age who has signs or symptoms of pyelonephritis or who responds slowly to treatment
- Recurrent UTI in a prepubertal, non–sexually active female

The timing of evaluation is important. If the patient has toxic symptoms, responds slowly or poorly to therapy, or has a mass or bladder distention, prompt nephrosonography and ultrasound of the bladder are indicated. If the symptoms are those of lower UTI and response is rapid, it is best to wait until the patient is symptom free (VCUG). It is often useful to continue prophylactic therapy until the VCUG is completed. An experienced nephrosonographer can provide most of the important anatomic information by using renal ultrasound. However, small scars and slight calyceal dilations may be missed; therefore, it is sometimes suggested that in addition, a radionuclide study or IVP (discussed earlier in this chapter under Vesicoureteral Reflux) be performed. A voiding cystourethrogram is essential to assess reflux, bladder wall thickness, and bladder emptying.

REFERENCES

Behrman RE, Kliegman RM, Jenson HB, editors: *Nelson textbook of pediatrics,* ed 16, Philadelphia, 2000, WB Saunders, Chapters 546–551.

Benador D, Benador N, Slosman D, et al: Are young children at highest risk of renal sequelae after pyelonephritis? *Lancet* 349(9044):17–19, 1997.

Hellerstein S: Urinary tract infection: old and new concepts, *Pediatr Clin North Am* 42(6):1433–1457, 1995.

Strife C, Gelfand M: Renal cortical scintigraphy: effect on medical decision making in childhood urinary tract infection, *J Pediatr* 129(6):785–787, 1996.

CHAPTER 17

Endocrinology

Dennis M. Styne ▾ **Nicole S. Glaser**

The endocrine system regulates vital body functions by means of biochemical messengers (hormones). There is considerable overlap between the endocrine system and the nervous system; hormones can be regulated by nerve cells, and endocrine agents can also serve as neural messengers. Further, there is an intimate relationship between the endocrine system and the immune system. Hormones are classically defined as circulating messengers, with the location of their action at a distance from the specialized organ (gland) of origin of the secretion and production of the hormone. Consequently, signs and symptoms of an endocrine disorder may be related to the response of the peripheral tissue to a hormone excess or deficiency. Indeed, functioning endocrine tumors frequently produce profound physiologic changes that reveal the pathologic processes long before the appearance of signs and symptoms related to tumor mass. Hormone action also may be *paracrine* (acting on adjacent neighboring cells to the cell of origin of the hormone) or *autocrine* (acting on the cell of origin of the hormone itself); often, agents acting in these ways are called factors rather than hormones (Fig. 17–1). Hormones generally are regulated in a feedback loop so that the production of a hormone is controlled by its effect; for example, corticotropin-releasing factor (CRF) stimulates adrenocorticotropic hormone (ACTH) to produce cortisol, which in turn feeds back to suppress CRF and ACTH production so that an equilibrium is reached and levels of serum cortisol and ACTH remain in the normal range. The set point of the equilibrium may change with development; in prepuberty small amounts of sex steroids completely suppress gonadotropin secretion, but during pubertal development the sensitivity of this feedback loop decreases. Thus increased sex steroid production that causes the ensuing physical changes of puberty occurs before gonadotropin secretion is suppressed by these very sex steroids. A clinician

may determine the level of endocrine defect in the system by deduction after measuring the serum concentrations of hormones at various steps of the process.

Endocrine disorders generally manifest in one of four ways:

1. By excess hormone: in Cushing syndrome there is an excess of glucocorticoid present; if the excess is secondary to autonomous glucocorticoid secretion by a target organ (cortisol secretion by the adrenal gland), the trophic hormone ACTH will be suppressed.
2. By deficient hormone: in glucocorticoid deficiency, the level of cortisol is inadequate; if the

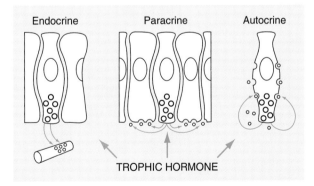

FIG. 17–1

Schematic representation of mechanisms of action of hormones and growth factors. Whereas traditional hormones are formed in endocrine glands and transported to distant sites of action through the bloodstream (endocrine mechanism), peptide growth factors may be produced locally by the target cells themselves (autocrine modality of action) or by neighboring cells (paracrine action). (From Wilson JD, Foster DW, editors: *Williams textbook of endocrinology*, ed 8, Philadelphia, 1992, WB Saunders.)

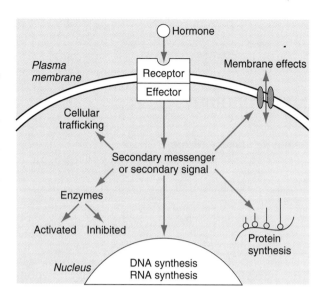

FIG. 17–2

A general model for the action of peptide hormones, catecholamines, and other membrane-active hormones. The hormone in the extracellular fluid interacts with the receptor at the cell membrane and activates an associated effector system, which leads to generation of an intracellular signal or second messenger that produces the final effects of the hormone. Abnormalities in the transmembrane domains of the receptors may cause disease (e.g., testotoxicosis). Abnormalities in the secondary messenger region may also cause disease (e.g., McCune-Albright syndrome). (From Wilson JD, Foster DW, editors: *Williams textbook of endocrinology,* ed 8, Philadelphia, 1992, WB Saunders.)

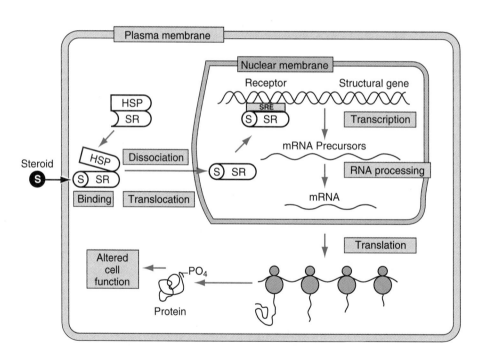

FIG. 17–3

Proposed mechanism of action of steroid hormones (e.g., glucocorticoids, estrogens, and progesterone) in activation of specific gene transcription. The steroid (S) diffuses across the plasma membrane and binds to a cytoplasmic receptor (SR). In the absence of steroid, the receptor resides in the cytoplasm as an inactive complex with heat shock protein (HSP). When the steroid binds to the receptor, the HSP dissociates from it. The steroid-receptor complex is translocated to the nucleus, where it binds to a chromatin receptor consisting of the steroid receptor response DNA element (SRE), thereby activating the transcription of specific genes involved in steroid hormone action. RNA transcripts are translated into proteins that mediate changes in cell function. Some models also suggest the presence of a membrane-associated glucocorticoid receptor. (Adapted from Chan L, O'Malley BW: *N Engl J Med* 294:1322, 1976.)

deficiency is at the target organ (the adrenal gland), the trophic hormone will be elevated (ACTH).
3. By an abnormal response of end organ to hormone; in pseudohypoparathyroidism there is resistance to parathyroid hormone.
4. By gland enlargement that may have effects as a result of size rather than function; with a large nonfunctioning pituitary adenoma, abnormal visual fields and other neurologic signs and symptoms will result even though no hormone is produced by the tumor.

Peptide hormones act through specific cell membrane receptors; when the hormone is attached to the receptor, the complex triggers various second messengers that cause the biologic effects (Fig. 17–2). Peptide hormone receptor number and avidity may be regulated by hormones; continuous rather than episodic exposure to gonadotropin-releasing hormone (GnRH) down-regulates GnRH receptor number, as well as receptor activity on pituitary gonadotropes. *Steroid hormones* exert their effects by attachment to intracellular receptors, and the hormone-receptor complex translocates to the nucleus, where it interacts with deoxyribonucleic acid (DNA) (hormone response elements upstream to the specific gene), causing appropriate effects (Fig. 17–3).

Because of the feedback loops, the interpretation of serum hormone levels must be related to their controlling factors; a given value of parathyroid hormone may be normal in a eucalcemic patient, but the same value may be inadequate in a hypocalcemic patient with partial hypoparathyroidism and this same value of parathyroid hormone may be excessive in a hypercalcemic patient who might have hyperparathyroidism.

HYPOTHALAMIC-PITUITARY AXIS

The *hypothalamus* controls many endocrine systems either directly or through the anterior pituitary gland; higher CNS centers, in turn, control the hypothalamus. Hypothalamic releasing or inhibiting factors travel down capillaries of the pituitary portal system to control the anterior pituitary gland, thereby regulating the hormones specific for the factor (Fig. 17–4). The pituitary hormones then enter the peripheral circulation and exert their effects on target glands, which, in turn, produce other hormones that feed back to suppress their controlling hypothalamic and pituitary hormones (e.g., insulin-like growth factor-1 [IGF1], cortisol, sex steroids, and thyroxine all feed back on the hypothalamic-pituitary system). Prolactin is the only pituitary hormone that is suppressed by a hypothalamic factor, prolactin inhibitory factor (dopamine). Thus hypothalamic de-

ficiency leads to a decrease in most pituitary hormone secretions but may lead to an increase in prolactin secretion. The hypothalamus is the location of vasopressin-secreting axons that either terminate in the posterior pituitary gland, and exert their effect via vasopressin secretion from this area, or terminate in the mediobasal hypothalamus, from which they can exert some effects on water balance, even in the absence of the posterior pituitary gland.

In childhood, *increased pituitary* secretion of various hormones as a result of an adenoma is rare, although cases of pituitary gigantism (growth hormone excess from a pituitary adenoma) do occur. Destructive lesions of the pituitary gland or hypothalamus are more common in childhood. A *craniopharyngioma*, a tumor of Rathke's pouch, may descend into the sella turcica, causing erosion of the bone and destruction of pituitary and hypothalamic tissue as it enlarges. Hypopituitarism in this case will be the result of lack of functioning pituitary or hypothalamic cells. Calcification of the tumor on plain radiographic examination of the CNS or on CT scan is frequent with a craniopharyngioma. Acquired hypopituitarism also may result from pituitary infections, from infiltration such as with Langerhans cell histiocytosis (histiocytosis X), lymphoma, and sarcoidosis, following radiation therapy or trauma to the CNS, and as a consequence autoimmunity to the pituitary gland.

Congenital hypopituitarism usually is caused by absence of hypothalamic releasing factors; thus the pituitary gland cannot release its hormone even though it has adequate supply, but the pituitary gland can be stimulated by exogenous hypothalamic-releasing factor administration. Congenital defects of pituitary secretion may also result from anatomic malformations of the hypothalamus, from pituitary hypoplasia or aplasia, or from more subtle defects of hormone secretion. Congenital defects associated with hypopituitarism range from **holoprosencephaly** (cyclopia, cebocephaly, orbital hypotelorism) to cleft palate (6% of cases of cleft palate are associated with GH deficiency). **Septooptic dysplasia** (optic nerve hypoplasia, absent septum pellucidum, or variations of both) may be associated with such significant visual impairment that pendular nystagmus (to and fro nystagmus caused by an inability to focus on a target) results. The MRI findings of congenital hypopituitarism may include an ectopic posterior pituitary gland "hot spot" and the appearance of a "pituitary stalk transection" and small pituitary gland.

Pituitary function testing is performed in some cases directly by measuring the specific pituitary hormone in the basal state and in some cases after stimulation. Indirect assessment of pituitary function can

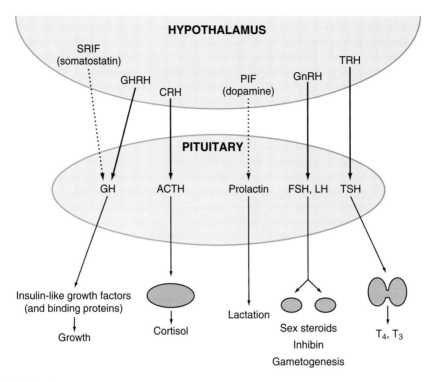

FIG. 17–4

Hormonal influences of the hypothalamus and pituitary gland. *Solid line* represents stimulatory influence; *dotted line* represents inhibitory influence. *SRIF,* Somatotropin release–inhibiting factor, somatostatin or SS; *GHRH,* growth hormone–releasing hormone or GRF; *CRH,* corticotropin-releasing hormone or CRF; *PIF,* prolactin inhibitory factor; *GnRH,* gonadotropin-releasing hormone or luteinizing hormone–releasing factor, LRF or LHRHoHormon; *TRH,* thyrotropin-releasing hormone or TRF; *GH,* growth hormone; *ACTH,* adrenocorticotropin; *FSH,* follicle-stimulating hormone; *LH,* luteinizing hormone; *TSH,* thyroid-stimulating hormone; T_4, thyroxine; T_3, triiodothyronine.

TABLE 17–1
Diagnostic Evaluation of Hypopituitarism

Manifestation	Cause	Tests*
Growth failure, hypothyroidism, or both	GH deficiency, TRH/TSH deficiency, or both	Provocative GH tests, free T_4, bone age, IGF1, IGF BP3
Hypoglycemia	GH deficiency, ACTH insufficiency, or both	Provocative GH tests, test of ACTH secretion, IGF1, IGF BP3
Micropenis, pubertal delay or arrest	Hypogonadotropic hypogonadism or GH deficiency	Sex steroids (E_2, testosterone), basal LH and FSH (analyzed by ultrasensitive assays) or after GnRH administration, provocative GH tests, IGF1, IGF BP3
Polyuria, polydipsia	ADH deficiency	Urine analysis (sp. gr.), serum electrolytes, urine and serum osmolality, water deprivation test

ADH, Antidiuretic hormone; E_2, estradiol; *FSH,* follicle-stimulating hormone; *GH,* growth hormone; *IGF1,* insulin-like growth factor; *IGF BP3,* insulin-like growth factor binding protein 3; *LH,* luteinizing hormone; *sp. gr.,* specific gravity; T_4, thyroxine; *TRH,* thyrotropin-releasing hormone; *TSH,* thyroid-stimulating hormone.
*Each patient with hypopituitarism should have a CNS MRI scan as part of evaluation to determine the etiology of the condition.

TABLE 17–2
Anterior Pituitary Hormone Function Testing

Random Hormone Measurements	Provocative Stimulation Test	Target Hormone Measurement
GH (useless as a random determination except in GH resistance or in pituitary gigantism)	Arginine (a weak stimulus) L-Dopa (useful clinically) Insulin-induced hypoglycemia (a dangerous but accurate test) Clonidine (useful clinically) GRH 12–24-hr integrated GH levels (of questionable utility)	IGF1, IGF BP3 (affected by malnutrition as well as GH deficiency)
ACTH (early AM sample useful only if in high normal range)	Cortisol after insulin-induced hypoglycemia (a dangerous test) 11-Desoxycortisol after metyrapone CRH ACTH stimulation test (may differentiate ACTH deficiency from primary adrenal insufficiency)	AM cortisol 24-Hr urinary free cortisol
TSH*	TRH	FT$_4$
LH, FSH*	GnRH (difficult to interpret in prepubertal subjects)	Testosterone Estradiol
Prolactin (elevated in hypothalamic disease and decreased in pituitary disease)	TRH	None

CRH, Corticotropin-releasing hormone; *FSH,* follicle-stimulating hormone; *FT$_4$,* free thyroxine; *GH,* growth hormone; *GRH,* growth hormone–releasing hormone; *IGF1,* insulin-like growth factor; *IGF BP3,* insulin-like growth factor binding protein 3; L-*dopa,* L-dihydroxyphenylalanine; *LH,* luteinizing hormone; *TRH,* thyrotropin-releasing hormone; *TSH,* thyroid-stimulating hormone.
*New supersensitive assays allow determination of abnormally low values found in hypopituitarism.

be obtained by measuring serum concentrations of the target gland hormones. (Table 17–1). Several tests of pituitary function are listed in Table 17–2.

GROWTH

Normal growth is the final common pathway of many factors, including endocrine, environmental, nutritional, and genetic influences (see Chapter 1). Maintenance of a normal linear growth pattern is good evidence of overall health and can be considered a "bioassay" for the condition of the whole child. The effects of certain hormones on growth and ultimate height are listed in Table 17–3. Just as various factors influence stature, stature itself influences psychologic, social, and, potentially, economic well-being. Parental concern about the psychosocial consequences of abnormal stature is a common factor that causes a family to seek medical attention.

Growth Hormone Physiology. Growth hormone secretion is stimulated by hypothalamic growth hormone–releasing factor (GRF, GHRH) and inhibited by growth hormone release inhibitory factor (somatostatin, SRIF, or SS), which interact with their individual receptors on the somatotrope in a noncompetitive manner. Growth hormone circulates with a growth hormone–binding protein (GHBP) that shares the same amino acid sequence as the extracellular domain of the membrane-bound growth hormone receptor; GHBP abundance reflects the abundance of growth hormone receptors. Growth hormone secretion causes production and secretion of insulin-like growth factor 1 and 2 (IGF1 and IGF2) in many tissues of the body, including the liver. IGF1 is most closely associated with postnatal growth, and serum concentrations of IGF1 follow serum concentration of GH. However, IGF1 production is also decreased in states of malnutrition in which,

TABLE 17–3
Hormonal Effects on Growth

Hormone	Bone Age	Growth Rate	Adult Height*
Androgen excess	Advanced	Increased	Diminished
Androgen deficiency	Normal or delayed	Normal or decreased	Increased slightly or normal
Thyroxine excess	Advanced	Increased	Normal or diminished
Thyroxine deficiency	Retarded	Decreased	Diminished
Growth hormone excess	Normal or advanced	Increased	Excessive
Growth hormone deficiency	Retarded	Decreased	Diminished
Cortisol excess	Retarded	Decreased	Diminished
Cortisol deficiency	Normal	Normal	Normal

Adapted from Underwood LE, Van Wyk JJ: Normal and aberrant growth. In Wilson JD, Foster DW, editors: *Textbook of endocrinology,* ed 8, Philadelphia, 1992, WB Saunders.
*Effect in most patients with treatment.

paradoxically, GH secretion is increased; in malnutrition the abundance of growth hormone receptors decreases and unlinks the relationship between rising growth hormone and rising IGF1 production. In obesity the opposite happens and GH secretion drops to low levels, but IGF1 concentrations remain normal. Growth hormone also stimulates the production of six different IGF binding proteins in the liver, kidney, and other tissues. Some IGF binding proteins are inhibitory, and some increase IGF activity. IGF BP3 is measurable in clinical assays and is itself growth-hormone dependent but less influenced by nutrition and age than is IGF1; measuring both IGF1 and IGF BP3 is useful in evaluating GH adequacy.

IGF1 acts primarily as a paracrine and autocrine agent, so the IGF1 measured in the peripheral circulation is far removed from the site of action and is an imperfect reflection of IGF1 physiology. IGF1 resembles proinsulin in structure, and the IGF1 receptor resembles the insulin receptor, so cross-reaction of one agent, if present in excess, can cause physiologic effects usually attributed to the other agent. Once IGF1 attaches to its membrane bound receptor, second messengers are stimulated to change the physiology of the cell and produce growth effects.

Measurement of Growth

Accurate measurements of height and weight should be plotted on the CDC growth charts for the timely diagnosis of growth disorders (see Chapter 1; the charts can be downloaded at www.cdc.gov/growth charts/). The correct measurement of an infant re-

quires one adult to hold the baby's head still and one other to extend the feet with the soles perpendicular to the lower legs. A caliper-like device such as an infantometer is used, or the movable plates on a baby scale are slid until one rests at the top of the baby's head and the other at the bottom of the baby's feet perpendicular to a ruler, so that the exact distance between the two plates can be determined. It is never accurate to measure a baby lying on a sheet of paper on the examining table by making a mark at the moving head and another at the moving feet and determining the distance between the two; if this technique is used, a true disorder of growth may be missed or a disorder of growth may be suspected in a normal child.

After 2 years of age, a child should be measured in the standing position. A decrease of roughly 1.25 cm in height measurement may occur when the child is measured in the standing position rather than in the lying position; many children who appear to be "not growing" are referred, when all that has changed is the position of the child at the time of measurement. Children measured in the standing position should be barefoot against a hard surface, where they can place the back with legs straight, bare feet together, and all aspects of the body pressed as far back as possible against the upright surface. Barrettes or hair buns must be removed. A Harpenden stadiometer or equivalent device is optimal for the measurement of stature, but the flexible bars that extend upward on some health scales are useless and may be misleading.

Measurement of arm span is essential when the diagnosis of Klinefelter syndrome, short-limbed dwarfism, or other dysmorphic conditions is considered. Arm span is measured as the distance between the tips of the fingers when the patient holds an outstretched arm horizontally while standing against a solid surface. The upper-to-lower segment ratio is the result of the division of the upper segment (determined by subtraction of the measurement from the symphysis pubis to the floor [known as the lower segment] from the total height) by the lower segment. This ratio changes with age. A normal term baby has an upper-to-lower ratio of 1.7:1, a 1-year-old has a ratio of 1.4:1, and a 10-year-old has a ratio of 1:1. Conditions of hypogonadism lead to greatly decreased upper-to-lower ratio in the adult, whereas hypothyroidism leads to a very high upper-to-lower ratio in the child.

Endocrine Factors Affecting Growth

Growth hormone (GH), somatotropin, is a 191–amino acid protein secreted by the pituitary gland under the control of GRF and SRIF (see Fig. 17–4). GH secretion is enhanced by alpha-adrenergic stimulation, hypoglycemia, starvation, exercise, early stages of sleep, and stress. GH secretion is inhibited by beta-adrenergic stimulation, hyperglycemia, and GH treatment itself. GH has direct effects (such as diabetogenic activity) and indirect effects (many aspects of growth) mediated by the IGFs. Serum concentrations of GH are low throughout the day except for occasional peaks within the 24-hour period. Thus, the determination of a random GH concentration is useless unless the sample is obtained during a brief episode of secretion. Inadequate secretion of GH is determined by a stimulation test to measure peak GH secretion (see Table 17–2). However, there is a high false-positive rate (on any day, about 10% of more normal children may not reach the normal peak GH following even two stimulatory tests and will falsely appear as growth hormone deficient). Thus indirect measurements of growth hormone secretion such as serum concentrations of IGF 1 and IGFBP3 are replacing GH stimulatory tests.

Most of the effects of GH on stature are the result of GH-stimulated production of IGFs. Serum IGF1 values are related to GH secretion, rising in GH excess and decreasing in GH deficiency. Since malnutrition lowers IGF1 levels even though it raises GH secretion, IGF1 is not an infallible reflection of GH secretion. IGF2 levels decrease in GH deficiency but do not rise above normal values in GH excess. IGF2 appears to have a prominent role in fetal growth.

The factors responsible for postnatal growth are not the same as those that mediate fetal growth. *Thyroid hormone* is essential for normal postnatal growth, although a thyroid hormone–deficient fetus will achieve a normal birth length; similarly, a GH-deficient fetus will have a normal birth length, although in IGF1 deficiency, resulting from growth hormone resistance (Laron dwarfism), fetuses are shorter than controls. Adequate thyroid hormone is necessary to allow the secretion of GH. Thus, hypothyroid patients may falsely appear to be GH deficient; with thyroid hormone repletion, growth hormone secretion normalizes. Gonadal steroids are important in the pubertal growth spurt. The effects of other hormones on growth are noted in Table 17–3.

Abnormalities of Growth
Short Stature of Nonendocrine Causes
(Tables 17–4 and 17–5)

Short stature is defined as subnormal height relative to other children of the same sex and age, taking family heights into consideration. The CDC growth charts use the 3rd percentile of the growth curve as the demarcation of the lower limit, but pathologic short stature is usually 3.5 standard deviations below the mean, which is far below the 3rd percentile; unfortunately, growth charts that demonstrate curves down to these low limits are rare (the Genentech company does have such charts available). *Growth failure,* however, denotes a slow growth rate irrespective of stature. Ultimately, a slow growth rate will lead to short stature, but a disease process will be caught sooner if the decreased growth rate is noted before the stature becomes short. Height velocity may be plotted on special charts. Plotted on a growth chart, growth failure appears as a curve that crosses percentiles and is associated with a height velocity below the 5th percentile of height velocity for age (Fig. 17–5). A corrected midparental height helps determine if the child is growing well for the family; it is calculated by finding the average height of the parents and adding 6.5 cm (2.5 inches) for a male patient or subtracting 6.5 cm from a female patient to correct for the average difference between adult height of males and females in the United States of 5 inches or 13 cm. To determine a range of normal height for the family under consideration, the corrected midparental height is bracketed by 2 standard deviations, which for the United States is approximately 4 inches. The range limited by 4 inches above and 4 inches below the corrected midparental height represents a range of expected adult height for the child or the target height. The presence of a height 3.5 standard deviations below the mean, a height velocity below the 5th percentile for age, or a height below the target height corrected for midparental height requires a diagnostic evaluation (Table 17–6).

Nutrition is the most important factor affecting

TABLE 17–4
Causes of Short Stature

Variations of Normal
Constitutional (delayed bone age)
Genetic (short familial heights)

Endocrine Disorders
GH deficiency
Congenital
   Isolated GH deficiency
   With other pituitary hormone deficiencies
   With midline defects
   Pituitary agenesis
   With gene deficiency
Acquired
   Hypothalamic/pituitary tumors
   Histiocytosis X (Langerhans cell histiocytosis)
   CNS infections and granulomas
   Head trauma (birth and later)
   Hypothalamic/pituitary radiation
   CNS vascular accidents
   Hydrocephalus
   Autoimmune
   Psychosocial dwarfism (functional GH deficiency)
   Amphetamine treatment for hyperactivity*
Laron dwarfism (increased GH and decreased IGF1)
Pygmies (normal GH and IGF2 but decreased IGF1)
Hypothyroidism
Glucocorticoid excess
   Endogenous
   Exogenous
Diabetes mellitus under poor control
Diabetes insipidus (untreated)
Hypophosphatemic vitamin D–resistant rickets
Virilizing congenital adrenal hyperplasia (tall child, short adult)
   P-450$_{c21}$, P-450$_{c11}$ deficiencies

Skeletal Dysplasias
Osteogenesis imperfecta
Osteochondroplasias

Lysosomal Storage Diseases
Mucopolysaccharidoses
Mucolipidoses

Syndromes of Short Stature
Turner syndrome (syndrome of gonadal dysgenesis)
Noonan syndrome (pseudo–Turner syndrome)
Autosomal trisomy 13, 18, 21
Prader-Willi syndrome
Laurence-Moon-Bardet-Biedl syndrome
Autosomal abnormalities
Dysmorphic syndromes (e.g., Russell-Silver, Cornelia de Lange)
Pseudohypoparathyroidism

Chronic Disease
Cardiac disorders
   Left-to-right shunt
   Congestive heart failure
Pulmonary disorders
   Cystic fibrosis
   Asthma
GI disorders
   Malabsorption (e.g., celiac disease)
   Disorders of swallowing
   Inflammatory bowel disease
Hepatic disorders
Hematologic disorders
   Sickle cell anemia
   Thalassemia
Renal disorders
   Renal tubular acidosis
   Chronic uremia
Immunologic disorders
   Connective tissue disease
   Juvenile rheumatoid arthritis
   Chronic infection
   AIDS
Hereditary fructose intolerance

Malnutrition
Kwashiorkor, marasmus
Iron deficiency
Zinc deficiency
Anorexia caused by chemotherapy of neoplasms

Modified from Styne DM: Growth disorder. In Fitzgerald PA, editor: *Handbook of clinical endocrinology*, Norwalk, Conn, 1986, Appleton & Lange.
AIDS, Acquired immunodeficiency syndrome; *CNS,* central nervous system; *GI,* gastrointestinal; *IGF,* insulin-like growth factor.
*Only if caloric intake severely diminished.

TABLE 17–5
Differential Diagnosis and Therapy of Short Stature

	Hypopituitarism GH Deficiency (Possibly with GnRH, CRH, or TRH Deficiency)	Constitutional Delay	Familial Short Stature	Deprivational Dwarfism	Turner Syndrome	Hypothyroidism	Chronic Disease
Family history positive	Rare	Frequent	Always	No	No	Variable	Variable
Gender	Both	Males more than females	Both	Both	Female	Both	Both
Facies	Immature or with midline defect (e.g., cleft palate or optic hypoplasias)	Immature	Normal	Normal	Turner facies or normal	Coarse (cretin if congenital)	Normal
Sexual development	Delayed	Delayed	Normal	May be delayed	Female prepubertal	Usually delayed, may be precocious if hypothyroidism is severe	Delayed
Bone age	Delayed	Delayed	Normal	Usually delayed; growth arrest lines present	Delayed	Delayed	Delayed
Dentition	Delayed	Normal; delay possible	Normal	Variable	Normal	Delayed	Normal or delayed
Hypoglycemia	Variable	No	No	No	No	No	No
Karyotype	Normal	Normal	Normal	Normal	45,X or partial deletion of X chromosome or mosaic	Normal	Normal

ACTH, Adrenocorticotropic hormone; *CRH,* corticotropin-releasing hormone; *GH,* growth hormone; *GnRH,* gonadotropin-releasing hormone; *T₄,* thyroxine; *TRH,* thyrotropin-releasing hormone.

Continued

TABLE 17–5
Differential Diagnosis and Therapy of Short Stature—cont'd

	Hypopituitarism GH Deficiency (Possibly with GnRH, CRH, or TRH Deficiency)	Constitutional Delay	Familial Short Stature	Deprivational Dwarfism	Turner Syndrome	Hypothyroidism	Chronic Disease
Free T$_4$	Low (if TRF-deficient) or normal	Normal	Normal	Normal or low	Normal: hypothyroidism may be acquired	Low	Normal
Stimulated GH	Low	Normal for bone age	Normal	Possibly low, or high if malnourished	Usually normal	Low	Usually normal
Insulin-like growth factor I	Low	Normal or low for chronologic age	Normal	Low	Normal	Low	Low or normal (depending on nutritional status)
Therapy	Replace deficiencies	Reassurance; sex steroids to initiate secondary sexual development in selected patients	None	Change or improve environment	Sex hormone replacement; GH; oxandrolone may be useful	T$_4$	Treat malnutrition, organ failure (e.g., dialysis, transplant, cardiotonic drugs, insulin)

ACTH, Adrenocorticotropic hormone; *CRH,* corticotropin-releasing hormone; *GH,* growth hormone; *GnRH,* gonadotropin-releasing hormone; *T$_4$,* thyroxine; *TRH,* thyrotropin-releasing hormone.

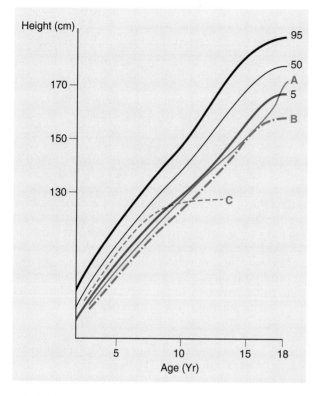

FIG. 17–5

Patterns of linear growth. Normal growth percentiles (5th, 50th, and 95th) are shown along with typical growth curves for constitutional delay of growth and adolescence (short stature with normal growth rate for bone age, delayed pubertal growth spurt, and eventual achievement of normal adult stature) *(A)*, familial short stature (short stature in childhood and as an adult with a normal growth rate) *(B)*, and acquired pathologic growth failure *(C)* (e.g., acquired untreated primary hypothyroidism). (See Chapter 1.)

TABLE 17–6
Growth Failure: Screening Test

Test	Rationale
CBC	*Anemia:* nutritional, chronic disease, malignancy *Leukocytosis:* inflammation, infection *Leukopenia:* bone marrow failure syndromes *Thrombocytopenia:* malignancy, infection
ESR, CRP	Inflammation of infection, inflammatory diseases, malignancy
Metabolic panel (electrolytes, liver enzymes, BUN)	Signs of acute or chronic hepatic, renal, adrenal dysfunction; hydration and acid-base status
Carotene, folate, and prothrombin time; celiac panel	Assess malabsorption; detect celiac disease
Urinalysis with pH	Signs of renal dysfunction, hydration, water and salt homeostasis; renal tubular acidosis
Karyotype	Determines Turner (XO) or other syndromes
Cranial imaging (MRI)	Assesses hypothalamic-pituitary tumors (craniopharyngioma, glioma, germinoma) or congenital midline defects
Bone age	Compare with height age, and evaluate height potential
IGF1, IGF BP3	Reflects growth hormone status or nutrition
Free thyroxine	Detects panhypopituitarism or isolated hypothyroidism
Prolactin	Elevated in hypothalamic dysfunction or destruction, suppressed in pituitary disease

BUN, Blood urea nitrogen; *CBC,* complete blood count; *CRP,* C-reactive protein; *ESR,* erythrocyte sedimentation rate; *IGF BP3,* insulin-like growth factor binding protein 3; *MRI,* magnetic resonance imaging.

growth on a worldwide basis (see Chapter 2). Failure to thrive may develop in the infant as a result of **maternal deprivation** (nutritional deficiency or aberrant psychosocial interaction) or as a result of organic illness (anorexia, nutrient losses through a form of malabsorption, or hypermetabolism caused by hyperthyroidism). Psychologic difficulties also can affect growth, as in **psychosocial or deprivation dwarfism,** in which the child develops functional temporary GH deficiency and poor growth as a result of psychologic abuse; when placed in a different, healthier psychosocial environment, growth hormone physiology normalizes and growth occurs.

The common condition known as **constitutional delay in growth and/or puberty** is a variation of normal growth, caused by a delayed tempo of physiologic development, and not a disease (Fig. 17–5 and Table 17–5). Usually, a family member has had delayed growth or puberty (e.g., a mother who had late onset of puberty or menarche or a father who started to shave late or grew in stature into his twenties) during childhood but achieved a near normal final height. The bone age is delayed more than two standard deviations from normal, but the growth rate remains appropriate for bone age. Constitutional delay usually leads to a delay in secondary sexual development. **Genetic** or **familial short stature** (Fig. 17–5 and Table 17–5) refers to a child born to a family with short parents who is expected to reach a lower than average height. Of course, if the parents were malnourished as children, grew up in a zone of war, or suffered famine, the heights of the parents are no longer predictive. The combination of constitutional growth delay and genetic short stature leads to more obvious short stature and brings the child to medical attention earlier and more frequently than a child who simply has one of the conditions. Although there are differences in height associated with ethnic differences, the most significant difference in stature between ethnic groups is the result of nutrition.

Recognizable physical syndromes of short stature often combine obesity and decreased height, whereas otherwise normal obese children are usually taller than average and have advanced skeletal development and physical maturation (Table 17–4). The **Prader-Willi syndrome** includes fetal and infantile hypotonia, small hands and feet (acromicria), postnatal acquired obesity and insatiable appetite, developmental delay, hypogonadism, almond-shaped eyes, and abnormalities of the SNRP portion of the 15th chromosome at 15q11-q13. Most cases have deletion of the paternal sequence, but about 20–25% have uniparental disomy, in which both chromosomes 15 derive from the mother; if both chromosomes 15 come from the father, Angelman syndrome develops. **Laurence-Moon-Bardet-Biedl syndrome** has retinitis pigmentosa, hypogonadism, and developmental delay with autosomal dominant inheritance pattern. However, Laurence-Moon syndrome is associated with spastic paraplegia, and Bardet-Biedl syndrome is associated with obesity and polydactyly. Pseudohypoparathyroidism leads to short stature and developmental delay with short fourth and fifth digits (Albright hereditary osteodystrophy phenotype), with resistance to PTH and resultant hypocalcemia and elevated levels of serum phosphorus.

Short Stature Caused by Growth Hormone Deficiency

(Tables 17–4 and 17–5)

Classic congenital or idiopathic GH deficiency occurs in about 1:4000 children. Idiopathic GH deficiency is a hypothalamic disease of inadequate GRF; the pituitary gland manufactures GH but does not secrete it. Less often, GH deficiency is caused by anatomic defects of the pituitary gland; or, in genetic forms, a portion of the GH gene is missing. Classic GH deficiency indicates virtually no secretion of GH, but intermediate forms of decreased GH secretion (partial GH deficiency or neurosecretory disorder)

occur. Acquired GH deficiency causing late-onset growth failure suggests a tumor.

Clinical Manifestations. Infants with congenital GH deficiency achieve a normal birth length and weight at term, but the growth rate slows after birth, and they become progressively shorter for age. They also tend to have an elevated weight for height and appear chubby and short. Careful measurements in the first year of life may suggest the diagnosis, but most patients do not receive the diagnosis until several years of age because of inaccurate height measurements and lack of suspicion. A patient with classic GH deficiency has the appearance of a cherub (a chubby, immature appearance), with a high-pitched voice resulting from an immature larynx. Unless severe hypoglycemia occurred or dysraphism (midline defects) of the head includes a CNS defect that affects mentation, the subject will have normal intellectual growth and age-appropriate speech. Male neonates with isolated GH deficiency with or without gonadotropin deficiency may have a **microphallus** (a stretched penile length of less than 2 cm). Severe fasting hypoglycemia leading to seizures in the newborn occurs because of decreased gluconeogenesis. Patients who lack adrenocorticotropic hormone (ACTH) in addition to GH may have more profound hypoglycemia because cortisol is another hormone that stimulates gluconeogenesis.

Growth hormone resistance is caused by abnormal number or function of GH receptors or to a postreceptor defect. Patients with the autosomal recessive Laron syndrome have a prominent forehead, blue sclera, delayed dentition and bone maturation, and low blood sugar. They have elevated serum GH concentrations, although serum IGF1 and IGF BP3 concentrations are low. The patients do not respond to the administration of growth hormone with an increase in growth or a rise in serum concentrations of IGF1 or IGF BP3. The characteristic decrease in the number of GH receptors is reflected in the decreased serum concentration of growth hormone–binding protein. Malnutrition or severe liver disease may cause acquired GH resistance because serum GH is elevated and IGF1 is decreased.

Diagnosis. If family or other medical history does not provide a likely diagnosis, screening tests should include a metabolic panel to evaluate kidney and liver function, a CBC to reflect nutrition, and a celiac panel and carotene and folate levels to rule out celiac disease and malabsorption. A urinalysis will aid in evaluation of renal function, and urinary pH and serum bicarbonate suggests whether renal tubular acidosis is present. In a girl without other explanation for short stature, a karyotype is obtained to rule out Turner syndrome.

After chronic disease or familial short stature is ruled out and routine laboratory testing is completed and normal (Table 17–6), two GH stimulatory tests are performed (Table 17–2). GH testing should be offered to a patient who is short (well below the 5th percentile and usually more than 3.5 standard deviations below the mean), who is growing poorly (below the 5th percentile growth rate or age), or who is below the target height when corrected for family heights.

Classic GH-deficient patients do not show an increase in serum GH levels after stimulation by various secretagogues, but some patients release GH in response to secretagogue testing but cannot spontaneously release GH during the day. Measuring serum IGF1 and its growth hormone–dependent binding protein (IGF BP3) is helpful but not infallible. Thus tests for growth hormone deficiency are imperfect, and in difficult cases an operational definition of GH deficiency might be that patients who require GH will grow significantly faster when administered a normal dose of GH than before treatment.

Treatment. GH deficiency is treated with biosynthetic recombinant DNA-derived GH; preparations differ as to form (powder that needs diluent versus premixed preparation), injection device (syringes, pen devices), and frequency of administration (daily, 6 times per week, or even every 2–4 weeks). Dosage is also titrated to the growth rate. Treatment with GH carries the risk of an increased incidence of slipped capital femoral epiphysis and pseudotumor cerebri. Human cadaver–derived pituitary GH is no longer used because of the risk of contamination with the neurodegenerative infectious Jakob-Creutzfeldt agent or prions.

Administration of GH to patients with normal GH responsiveness to secretagogues is controversial, but as noted above, diagnostic tests are imperfect; if the patient is growing very slowly without alternative explanation, growth hormone therapy is sometimes used. Indeed, GH is effective in increasing growth rate and final height in Turner syndrome and in chronic renal failure; growth hormone is also used for treatment of short stature and muscle weakness of Prader-Willi syndrome.

Psychologic support of children with severe short stature is important because they may become the object of ridicule by classmates. Although there is controversy, marital status, satisfaction with life, and vocational achievement may be decreased in children of short stature who are not given supportive measures.

Tall Stature

(Table 17–7)

Constitutional tall stature indicates an advancement of bone age and physical development leading to tall stature during childhood but an ultimate normal adult height. Moderate obesity may lead to this situation by

TABLE 17–7
Causes of Tall Stature

Variations of Normal
Constitutional
Genetic
Exogenous obesity

Endocrine Disorders
Pituitary gigantism
Sexual precocity
Thyrotoxicosis
Beckwith-Wiedemann syndrome

Nonendocrine Disorders
Marfan syndrome
Klinefelter syndrome
XYY syndrome
Cerebral gigantism (Sotos syndrome)
Homocystinuria
Weaver Smith syndrome

Modified from Styne DM: Growth disorder. In Fitzgerald PA, editor: *Handbook of clinical endocrinology,* Norwalk, Conn, 1986, Appleton & Lange.

advancing the bone age and leading to taller-than-average stature during the growing years but not necessary greater adult height. **Genetic tall stature** occurs in children of families who are tall; the child is tall during the growth period and in adulthood.

Therapy is not indicated for an otherwise normal child who is predicted to become "too" tall. In the past, high-dose estrogen administration was used to reduce final height in girls who are predicted to be more than 5 feet 10 inches by causing rapid pubertal progression, leading to early epiphyseal fusion. Boys were similarly treated with testosterone.

Cerebral gigantism or **Soto syndrome** manifests in infancy by increased growth rate, prominent forehead, sharp chin, high-arched palate, hypertelorism, and, frequently, developmental delay. By midchildhood, the growth rate normalizes.

Marfan syndrome combines tall stature usually with an increased arm span exceeding height, a decreased upper-to-lower segment ratio, long thin fingers (arachnodactyly) and toes, hyperextensibility of the joints, aortic dilation, mitral or other valve prolapse and regurgitation, and superior subluxations of the lens. Dural ectopia on MRI is suggested as an important diagnostic feature. The defective gene for fibrillin is at 15q21.1 in some reported cases. **Homocystinuria** may present with a pheno-type similar to that of Marfan syndrome but with the additional features of mental retardation and increased urinary secretion of homocysteine. The lens subluxation in this condition may be inferior.

Endocrine Etiology. **Pituitary gigantism** is caused by excess GH secretion.

Clinical Manifestations. If a GH-secreting adenoma occurs after puberty, a patient will have acromegaly, but if the adenoma occurs prior to epiphyseal fusion, the child will grow excessively. Height velocity is increased; coarse, leonine faces and acromegalic facial features may occur in teenagers with gigantism, as well as in adults with acromegaly. Organomegaly may be noted, and glucose intolerance or frank diabetes mellitus may result. Elevated fasting serum GH or IGF1 concentrations confirm the diagnosis. This is one the few situations in which a random GH sample can be diagnostic.

Diagnosis. If familial or constitutional tall stature or the noted syndromes are eliminated, serum GH and IGF1 are determined and MR imaging is performed to establish the diagnosis.

Treatment. Treatment of pituitary gigantism may include surgery (microadenomectomy) or medical therapy (somatostatin analog).

REFERENCES

Abernethy LJ: Imaging of the pituitary in children with growth disorders, *Eur J Radiol* 26(2):102–108, 1998.

Albertsson-Wikland K, Karlberg J: Postnatal growth of children born small for gestational age, *Acta Paediatr Suppl* 423:193–195, 1997.

Alpert BS: Tall stature, *Pediatr Rev* 19(9):303–305, 1998.

Guidelines for the use of growth hormone in children with short stature: a report by the Drug Therapeutics Committee of the Lawson Wilkins Pediatric Endocrine Society, *J Pediatr* 127(6): 857–867, 1995.

Parks J: Disorders of the hypothalamus and pituitary gland. In Behrman RE, Kliegman RM, Jenson HB, editors: *Nelson textbook of pediatrics*, ed 16, Philadelphia, 2000, WB Saunders.

Rosenbloom AL, Rosenfeld R, Guevano-Aguirre J: Growth hormone insensitivity, *Pediatr Clin North Am* 44(2):423–442, 1997.

Rosenfeld RG, Albertsson-Wikland K, Cassoria F, et al: Diagnostic controversy: the diagnosis of childhood growth hormone deficiency revisited, *J Clin Endocrinol Metab* 80(5):1532–1540, 1995.

Sklar CA: Growth and neuroendocrine dysfunction following therapy for childhood cancer, *Pediatr Clin North Am* 44(2):489–503, 1997.

Styne DM: Growth. In Greenspan FS, Gardner DG: *Basic and clinical endocrinology*, ed 6, New York, 2001, Lange Medical Books.

PUBERTY AND ITS DISORDERS

(See Chapters 1 and 7)

The staging of pubertal changes and the sequence of events are discussed in Chapter 7 (Figs. 7–1 to 7–4 and Tables 7–1 to 7–3).

Control of the onset of puberty involves adrenal maturation (*adrenarche,* the development of pubic and axillary hair) and hypothalamic-pituitary-gonadal maturation (genital development in boys and breast development in girls, gonadarche).

Hypothalamic gonadotropin–releasing hormone (GnRH) is produced by cells in the arcuate nucleus, is secreted from the median eminence of the hypothalamus into the pituitary portal system, and reaches the membrane receptors on the pituitary gonadotropes to cause the production and release of luteinizing hormone (LH) and follicle-stimulating hormone (FSH) into the circulation. In girls FSH stimulates the ovarian production of estrogen, and later in puberty causes the formation and support of corpus luteum. In boys LH stimulates the production of testosterone from the Leydig cells; later in puberty, FSH stimulates the development and support of the seminiferous tubules. In addition to their sex steroids, the gonads produce the protein inhibin. Both sex steroids and inhibin suppress the secretion of gonadotropins. It is the interplay of the products of the gonads and GnRH that modulates the serum concentrations of gonadotropins. GnRH is released in episodic pulses that vary during development and during the menstrual period. These pulses ensure that gonadotropins are released in a pulsatile manner, as well. With the onset of puberty, the amplitude of the pulses of gonadotropins increases, first at night and then throughout the day. Sex steroids are secreted in response, first during the night and then also throughout the day. This endocrine change of puberty may be demonstrated by obtaining frequent blood samples or by the administration of exogenous GnRH. This may be considered reactivation of the hypothalamic pituitary gonadal axis, which is quite active in the fetus and newborn but is suppressed in the childhood years until activity increases again at the onset of puberty.

Adrenarche occurs several years earlier than gonadarche and is heralded by increasing serum dehydroepiandrosterone (DHEA or DHEAS) values. Serum DHEA rises years before the appearance of its effects, such as the development of pubic or axillary hair. What controls adrenarche is not known , but it is not directed by gonadotropin secretion.

Delayed Puberty

(Table 17–8)

Puberty is delayed when there is no sign of pubertal development by age 13 years in girls and 14 years in boys living in the United States.

Constitutional Delay in Growth and Adolescence

(Table 17–5 and Abnormalities of Growth)

Patients who have a significantly delayed bone age (two standard deviations below the mean, which

---

TABLE 17–8
Classification of Delayed Puberty and Sexual Infantilism

Constitutional Delay in Growth and Puberty
Hypogonadotropic Hypogonadism
Central nervous system disorders
  Tumors (craniopharyngioma, germinoma, glioma)
  Congenital malformations
  Radiation therapy
  Other causes
Isolated gonadotropin deficiency
  Kallmann syndrome (anosmia-hyposmia)
  Other disorders
Idiopathic and genetic forms of multiple pituitary hormone deficiencies
Miscellaneous disorders
  Prader-Willi syndrome
  Laurence-Moon-Bardet-Biedl syndrome
  Functional gonadotropin deficiency
    Chronic systemic disease and malnutrition
    Hypothyroidism
    Cushing disease
    Diabetes mellitus
    Hyperprolactinemia
    Anorexia nervosa

Constitutional Delay in Growth and Puberty—cont'd
Hypogonadotropic Hypogonadism—cont'd
    Psychogenic amenorrhea
    Impaired puberty and delayed menarche in female athletes and ballet dancers (exercise amenorrhea)

Hypergonadotropic Hypogonadism
Klinefelter syndrome (syndrome of seminiferous tubular dysgenesis) and its variants
Other forms of primary testicular failure
Anorchia and cryptorchidism
Syndrome of gonadal dysgenesis and its variants (Turner syndrome)
Other forms of primary ovarian failure
XX and XY gonadal dysgenesis
  Familial and sporadic XX gonadal dysgenesis and its variants
  Familial and sporadic XY gonadal dysgenesis and its variants
Pseudo-Turner syndrome
Galactosemia

Modified from Grumbach MM, Styne DM: Puberty. In Wilson JD, Foster DW, editors: *Williams textbook of endocrinology*, ed 9, Philadelphia, 1998, WB Saunders.

---

is equal to a 1.5–2-year delay as a teenager) but who always have grown at the normal rate for their bone age and continue to do so may have delayed onset of their pubertal development as a variation of normal; this is often found in familial patterns. Spontaneous puberty usually begins in these patients by the time the bone age reaches 12 years of age in boys and 11 years in girls. Patients who have constitutional delay in puberty usually begin spontaneous pubertal development by 18 years of age. Other causes of delayed puberty as noted below must be eliminated before a diagnosis of constitutional delay in puberty is made.

Hypogonadotropic Hypogonadism

(Table 17–9; also Table 17–8)

Hypogonadotropic hypogonadism is a permanent condition that will not lead to spontaneous puberty. Patients with hypogonadotropic hypogonadism have eunuchoid proportions because their long bones grow for a longer than normal period, producing an upper-to-lower ratio below the lower limit of normal of 0.9 and an arm span wider than their height. If the patient has concurrent GH deficiency, stature will be exceptionally short.

Isolated Gonadotropin Deficiency. If there is an inability to release gonadotropins but no other pituitary abnormality, the patient has isolated gonadotropin deficiency (almost universally a result of absent GnRH). Patients grow normally until the time of the pubertal growth spurt, when they fail to experience accelerated growth.

Kallmann syndrome combines isolated gonadotropin deficiency with abnormal olfaction. There is genetic heterogeneity; some patients have a decreased sense of smell, others have abnormal reproduction, and some have both. This disorder is caused by mutations in the KAL gene at Xp 22.3 (X-chromosome) or other gene defects. The mutation causes the GnRH neurons to remain ineffectually located in the primitive nasal area rather than migrating to the correct location at the medial basal hypothalamus as occurs in the normal situation. Olfactory bulbs and olfactory sulci are often absent on magnetic resonance imaging (MRI) in affected patients.

TABLE 17–9
Differential Diagnostic Features of Delayed Puberty and Sexual Infantilism

	Stature	Plasma Gonadotropins	GnRH Test: LH Response	Plasma Gonadal Steroids	Plasma DHEAS	Karyotype	Olfaction
Constitutional Delay in Growth and Adolescence	Short for chronologic age, usually appropriate for bone age	Prepubertal, later pubertal	Prepubertal, later pubertal	Prepubertal, later normal	Low for chronologic age, appropriate for bone age	Normal	Normal
Hypogonadotropic Hypogonadism							
Isolated gonadotropin deficiency	Normal, absent pubertal growth spurt	Low	Prepubertal or no response	Low	Appropriate for chronologic age	Normal	Normal
Kallmann syndrome	Normal, absent pubertal growth spurt	Low	Prepubertal or no response	Low	Appropriate for chronologic age	Normal	Anosmia or hyposmia
Idiopathic multiple pituitary hormone deficiencies	Short stature and poor growth since early childhood	Low	Prepubertal or no response	Low	Usually low	Normal	Normal
Hypothalamo-pituitary tumors	Decrease in growth velocity of late onset	Low	Prepubertal or no response	Low	Normal or low for chronologic age	Normal	Normal
Primary Gonadal Failure							
Syndrome of gonadal dysgenesis and variants	Short stature since early childhood	High	Hyperresponse for age	Low	Normal for chronologic age	XO or variant	Normal
Klinefelter syndrome and variants	Normal to tall	High	Hyperresponse at puberty	Low or normal	Normal for chronologic age	XXY or variant	Normal
Familial XX or XY gonadal dysgenesis	Normal	High	Hyperresponse for age	Low	Normal for chronologic age	XX or XY	Normal

From Grumbach MM, Styne DM: Puberty. In Wilson JD, Foster DW, editors: *Williams textbook of endocrinology*, ed 9, Philadelphia, 1997, WB Saunders. *DHEAS*, Dehydroepiandrosterone sulfate; *GnRH*, gonadotropin-releasing hormone; *LH*, luteinizing hormone.

Abnormalities of the Central Nervous System. Central nervous system (CNS) tumors are an important cause of gonadotropin deficiency. Craniopharyngiomas have a peak incidence in the teenage years and may cause any type of anterior or posterior hormone deficiency. Craniopharyngiomas usually calcify, erode the sella turcica when they expand, and may impinge on the optic chiasm, leading to bitemporal hemianopsia and optic atrophy. Germinomas are noncalcifying hypothalamic or pineal tumors that frequently produce human chorionic gonadotropin (hCG), which may cause sexual precocity in boys who are of a prepubertal age (hCG stimulates the LH receptor because of the similarity of structure). Other tumors that may affect pubertal development include astrocytomas and gliomas.

Idiopathic Hypopituitarism. Congenital absence of various combinations of pituitary hormones may produce idiopathic hypopituitarism. Although this disorder may occur in family constellations following X-linked or autosomal recessive patterns, sporadic types of congenital idiopathic hypopituitarism are more common. Congenital hypopituitarism may manifest in a male with GH deficiency, with associated gonadotropin deficiency with a microphallus, or with hypoglycemia with seizures, especially if ACTH deficiency occurs as well.

Syndromes of Hypogonadotropic Hypogonadism. Weight loss resulting from voluntary dieting, malnutrition, or chronic disease will lead to decreased gonadotropin function when weight falls below 80% of ideal weight. **Anorexia nervosa** is characterized by striking weight loss and psychiatric disorders (see Chapters 2 and 3). Primary or secondary amenorrhea frequently is found in affected girls, and pubertal development is absent or minimal, depending on the level of weight loss and the age of onset. Regaining weight to the ideal level may not immediately reverse the condition. Increased physical activity, even without weight loss, can lead to decreased menstrual frequency and gonadotropin deficiency in **athletic amenorrhea;** when physical activity is interrupted, menstrual function may return. **Hypothyroidism** inhibits the onset of puberty and delays menstrual periods. Conversely, severe primary hypothyroidism may lead to precocious puberty (see below).

Hypergonadotropic Hypogonadism

Hypergonadotropic hypogonadism is characterized by elevated gonadotropin levels resulting from primary gonadal failure. This is a permanent condition.

Ovarian Failure. The Turner syndrome or the syndrome of gonadal dysgenesis is a common cause of ovarian failure and short stature. The karyotype is classically 45,XO, but other abnormalities of the X chromosome or mosaicism are possible. The incidence of Turner syndrome is 1:2000–5000 births (see Chapter 4). Patients with variants of Turner syndrome, other types of gonadal dysgenesis, and galactosemia, or those treated with radiation therapy or chemotherapy, also may have ovarian failure (Table 17–8). The features of a girl with Turner syndrome need not be classic, and the diagnosis must be considered in any girl who is short without a contributory history.

Testicular Failure. Klinefelter syndrome (seminiferous tubular dysgenesis) is the most common cause of testicular failure. The karyotype is 47,XXY, but variants with more X chromosomes are possible. The incidence is approximately 1:500–1000 in males. Testosterone levels may be close to normal, at least until midpuberty, because Leydig cell function may be spared; however, seminiferous tubular function characteristically is lost, causing infertility. The age of onset of puberty is usually normal, but secondary sexual changes may not progress because of inadequate Leydig cell function (see Chapter 4).

Primary Amenorrhea

Lack of menstruation in the presence of normal pubertal development might be the result of physiologic variation in which 5 years might pass before regular menstrual periods are established. When primary amenorrhea occurs, an anatomic defect may be responsible; the Rokitansky-Kuster-Hauser syndrome of congenital absence of the uterus occurs in 1:4000–5000 female births. Anatomic obstruction by imperforate hymen or vaginal septum also presents with normal secondary sexual development without menstruation. The complete syndrome of androgen insensitivity leads to normal feminization, no pubic or axillary hair, and primary amenorrhea, in this case resulting from absence of all mullerian structures, including ovaries. Undiagnosed Turner syndrome is another relatively common cause of amenorrhea, resulting from abnormal ovarian function. Secondary sexual development will also be absent or minimal.

Differential Diagnosis. Once it is determined that no secondary sexual development is present after the upper age limits of normal pubertal development, serum gonadotropin levels should be obtained to determine whether the patient has a hypogonadotropic (which may include constitutional delay in puberty since serum gonadotropin values are low) or hypergonadotropic hypogonadism (Table 17–9). Differentiation between constitutional delay in growth and hypogonadotropic hypogonadism is difficult if no family history for the former or no CNS or olfactory abnormalities for the latter are identified. Sometimes a period of observation for months or years is necessary before the diagnosis is confirmed by spontaneous pubertal development or lack of it.

Treatment. If a permanent condition is apparent, replacement with sex steroids is indicated. Girls are given low-dose ethinyl estradiol (e.g., 5–10 μg) or conjugated estrogens in low daily doses until breakthrough bleeding occurs, at which time cycling is started with a dose on the first 21 days of the month; on days 12–21 of the month, a progestational agent, such as medroxyprogesterone acetate (e.g., 5 mg), is added to mimic a normal menstrual period. In boys, testosterone enanthate or cypionate (e.g., 100 mg) is given IM once every 4 weeks. Oral agents are not used for fear of hepatic toxicity. This starting regimen is appropriate for patients with either hypo- or hypergonadotropic hypogonadism, and doses are gradually increased to adult levels. Those with apparent constitutional delay in puberty who have, by definition, passed the upper limits of normal onset of puberty may be given a 3-month course of low-dose, sex-appropriate gonadal steroids and then be observed to see if spontaneous puberty occurs. This course of therapy might be repeated once more without undue advancement of bone age. All patients with any form of delayed puberty are at risk for decreased bone density; adequate calcium intake is essential or this tendency might be magnified. Patients with hypogonadotropic hypogonadism may be able to achieve fertility by the administration of gonadotropin therapy or pulsatile hypothalamic-releasing hormone therapy administered by a programmable pump on an appropriate schedule; those with hypergonadotropic hypogonadism, by definition, have a primary gonadal problem and cannot achieve fertility.

Estrogen replacement for patients with Turner syndrome may be offered during the normal age of puberty in low doses to ensure feminization and to improve psychologic function, as well as to attempt to decrease the likelihood of osteoporosis. Growth hormone will increase the growth rate and final height of these patients. Patients with Turner syndrome have had successful pregnancies after in vitro fertilization with a donor ovum and endocrine support.

Sexual Precocity

(Tables 17–10 and 17–11)

Classification

Sexual precocity (precocious puberty) is classically defined as secondary sexual development occurring before the age of 9 years in boys or 8 years in girls. The lower limit of normal puberty may be 7 years in Caucasian girls and 6 years in African American girls.

The condition is **true precocious puberty** or **central precocious puberty,** if it emanates from premature reactivation of the hypothalamic-pituitary-gonadal axis (GnRH-dependent), or **incomplete precocious puberty,** if the hypothalamic-pituitary-gonadal axis is not involved in the process (GnRH-independent). Isosexual precocity is virilization in a boy and feminization in a girl, while contrasexual precocity is virilization in a girl and feminization in a boy. A boy may have incomplete isosexual precocious puberty as a result of autonomous production of testosterone or other androgens from the testes or adrenal glands or as a result of a tumor that produces hCG, stimulating the testes. A girl might have incomplete precocious puberty as a result of autonomous production of estrogens from the ovaries or adrenal glands.

Central (or Complete or True) Precocious Puberty (Constitutional or Familial Precocious Puberty). In **central precocious puberty** every endocrine (such as increased pulsatile gonadotropin secretion and increased response of luteinizing hormone [LH] to GnRH) and physical aspect of pubertal development is normal but occurs too early. Individuals who begin puberty only a few months early may have **constitutional** or **familial precocious puberty,** in which members of some families enter puberty before the lower age limits of normal; those who enter puberty much earlier have other forms of central precocious puberty. The clinical course of central precocious puberty may wax and wane. If no cause can be determined, the diagnosis is idiopathic precocious puberty; this condition occurs approximately nine times more often in girls than boys. Boys, on the other hand, have a higher incidence of CNS disorders, such as tumors and hamartomas, precipitating the precocious puberty. Thus, affected boys must always be suspected of harboring a tumor.

A CNS tumor or disease must be considered in all children with precocious puberty before the condition is diagnosed as idiopathic. **Hamartomas** of the tuber cinereum have a characteristic appearance on computed tomography (CT) or MRI, and biopsy is rarely required for diagnosis. The mass of GnRH neurons may act as an unrestrained ectopic hypothalamus that secretes GnRH and causes precocious puberty. These hamartomas are not true neoplasms because they do not grow. The resulting precocious puberty is quite responsive to medical therapy with GnRH agonists, and surgery is rarely indicated.

Other masses that cause precocious puberty are not so benign. **Optic or hypothalamic gliomas** (with or without neurofibromatosis), astrocytomas, and ependymomas may cause precocious puberty by exerting mass effects on those areas of the CNS that normally inhibit pubertal development. Although a tumor may cause precocious puberty, the radiation treatment of the tumor may precipitate growth hormone deficiency. Growth is greater than that found in age-matched controls but less than in GH replete patients with precocious puberty. Thus the growth hormone deficiency will not be as obvious as in growth hormone–deficient

---

TABLE 17–10
Classification of Sexual Precocity

True Precocious Puberty or Complete Isosexual Precocity
Idiopathic true precocious puberty
CNS tumors
  Hamartomas (ectopic GnRH pulse generator)
  Other tumors
Other CNS disorders
True precocious puberty after late treatment of congenital virilizing adrenal hyperplasia

Incomplete Isosexual Precocity (GnRH-Independent Sexual Precocity)
Males
  Chorionic gonadotropin-secreting tumors (hCG-dependent sexual precocity)
  CNS tumors (e.g., germinoma, chorioepithelioma, and teratoma)
  Tumors in locations outside the CNS (hepatoblastoma)
  LH-secreting pituitary adenoma
Increased androgen secretion by adrenal or testis
  Congenital adrenal hyperplasia (21-OH deficiency, 11-OH deficiency)
  Virilizing adrenal neoplasm
  Leydig cell adenoma
  Familial testotoxicosis (familial premature gonadotropin–independent Leydig cell and germ cell maturation)
Females
  Estrogen-secreting ovarian or adrenal neoplasms
  Ovarian cysts

Incomplete Isosexual Precocity (GnRH-Independent Sexual Precocity)—cont'd
Males and females
  McCune-Albright syndrome
  Primary hypothyroidism
  Peutz-Jeghers syndrome

Iatrogenic Sexual Precocity

Variations of Pubertal Development
Premature thelarche
Premature menarche
Premature adrenarche
Adolescent gynecomastia

Contrasexual Precocity
Feminization in males
  Adrenal neoplasm
  Increased extraglandular conversion of circulating steroids to estrogen
Virilization in females
  Congenital adrenal hyperplasia
  P-450$_{C21}$ deficiency
  P-450$_{C11}$ deficiency
  3β-ol deficiency
Virilizing adrenal neoplasms
Virilizing ovarian neoplasms (e.g., arrhenoblastomas)

From Grumbach MM, Styne DM: Puberty. In Wilson JD, Foster DW, editors: *Williams textbook of endocrinology*, ed 9, Philadelphia, 1998, WB Saunders.
CNS, Central nervous system; *GnRH*, gonadotropin-releasing hormone; *hCG*, human chorionic gonadotropin; *LH*, luteinizing hormone.

---

patients without precocious puberty. With GnRH treatment, the precocious puberty will be controlled and the growth rate will then decrease to that of a GH-deficient child. GH is, thus, additional therapy.

Almost any condition that affects the CNS, including hydrocephalus, meningitis, encephalitis, suprasellar cysts, head trauma, and irradiation, has been reported to precipitate central precocious puberty. Children with epilepsy and mental retardation also have an increased prevalence of precocious puberty.

Incomplete GnRH-Independent or Pseudoprecocious Puberty (Tables 17-10 and 17-11)

DISORDERS OF BOYS AND GIRLS. Because of a somatic mutation (which causes a mosaicism of affected cells but does not involve the germ cells) in the G-protein intracellular signaling system (specifically Gsα, which leads to unregulated constitutive activation of adenyl cyclase) several endocrine organs may autonomously function even in the absence of their stimulating trophic hormones, resulting in the **McCune-Albright syndrome.** Characteristically these patients have irregular café-au-lait spots in the so-called Coast of Maine form (caused by autonomous production of melanin), polyostotic fibrous dysplasia of the long bones (caused by autonomous activity of osteoblast progenitor cells), and precocious puberty (caused by GnRH-independent activation of testes or ovary). They also may have hyperthyroidism, hyperadrenalism, or acromegaly, all as a result of autonomous activity of the affected organs.

TABLE 17–11
Differential Diagnosis of Sexual Precocity

	Serum Gonadotropin Concentration*	LH Response to GnRH	Serum Sex Steroid Concentrations	Gonadal Size	Miscellaneous
True Precocious Puberty	Pubertal values	Pubertal	Pubertal values of testosterone or estradiol	Normal pubertal testicular enlargement or ovarian and uterine enlargement (by sonography)	MRI scan of brain to rule out CNS tumor or other abnormality; bone scan for McCune-Albright syndrome
Incomplete Sexual Precocity (Pituitary Gonadotropin–Independent)					
Males					
Chorionic gonadotropin–secreting tumor in males	High hCG (low LH)	Prepubertal (suppressed)	Pubertal values of testosterone	Slight to moderate uniform enlargement of testes	Hepatomegaly suggests hepatoblastoma; MRI scan of brain if chorionic gonadotropin–secreting CNS tumor suspected
Leydig cell tumor in males	Suppressed	Suppressed	Very high testosterone	Irregular asymmetric enlargement of testes	
Familial testotoxicosis	Suppressed	Suppressed	Pubertal values of testosterone	Testes symmetric and larger than 2.5 cm but smaller than expected for pubertal development; spermatogenesis may occur	Familial; probably sex-limited, autosomal dominant trait
Premature adrenarche	Prepubertal	Prepubertal	Prepubertal testosterone; DHEAS values appropriate for pubic hair stage 2	Testes prepubertal	Onset usually after 6 yr of age; more frequent in brain-injured children

Females

Granulosa cell tumor (follicular cysts may present similarly)	Suppressed	Suppressed	Very high estradiol	Ovarian enlargement on physical examination, MRI, CT, or sonography	Tumor often palpable on abdominal examination
Follicular cyst	Suppressed	Suppressed	Prepubertal to very high estradiol values	Ovarian enlargement on physical examination, MRI, CT, or sonography	Single or repetitive episodes; exclude McCune-Albright syndrome (e.g., perform skeletal survey and inspect skin)
Feminizing adrenal tumor	Suppressed	Suppressed	High estradiol and DHEAS values	Ovaries prepubertal	Unilateral adrenal mass
Premature thelarche	Prepubertal	Prepubertal	Prepubertal or early pubertal estradiol	Ovaries prepubertal	Onset usually before 3 yr of age
Premature adrenarche	Prepubertal	Prepubertal	Prepubertal estradiol; DHEAS values appropriate for pubic hair stage 2	Ovaries prepubertal	Onset usually after 6 yr of age; more frequent in brain-injured children

Modified from Grumbach MM, Styne DM: Puberty. In Wilson JD, Foster DW, editors: *Williams textbook of endocrinology*, ed 9, Philadelphia, 1997, WB Saunders. *CNS*, Central nervous system; *CT*, computed tomography; *DHEAS*, dehydroepiandrosterone sulfate; *GnRH*, gonadotropin-releasing factor; *hCG*, human chorionic gonadotropin; *LH*, luteinizing hormone; *MRI*, magnetic resonance imaging.
*In supersensitive assays.

Adrenal carcinomas usually secrete adrenal androgens such as DHEA; **adrenal adenomas** may virilize a child as a result of the production of androgen or may produce estrogen and feminize a child.

DISORDERS IN BOYS. Boys may have **familial premature Leydig and germ cell maturation** caused by an X-limited dominant defect producing constitutive activation of the LH receptor, which leads to continuous production and secretion of testosterone without requiring the presence of LH or hCG. An **hCG-secreting tumor** will stimulate LH receptors and increase testosterone secretion. Such tumors may be found in various places, including the pineal gland (dysgerminomas, which are radiosensitive) or the liver (hepatoblastoma, which may lead to death in just a few months after diagnosis).

DISORDERS IN GIRLS. Ovarian cysts may occur once or may be recurrent; high serum estrogen values may mimic ovarian tumors. **Congenital adrenal hyperplasia** is a cause of virilization in girls and is discussed in the following sections.

Evaluation of Sexual Precocity (Table 17-11). The first step in evaluating sexual precocity is to determine by physical examination whether effects characteristic of normal puberty are apparent (see Chapter 7) or whether only isolated estrogen or androgen effects are present in girls (e.g., the combination of pubic hair development and feminization in girls must indicate true precocious puberty, whereas the appearance of either might be the first sign of central precocious puberty or conversely might represent one of the causes of incomplete precocious puberty referred to previously). In boys it is important to note whether the testes are enlarged over 2.5 cm and whether the size is consistent with the degree of pubertal development, which suggests central (GnRH-dependent) precocious puberty. If the testes are not enlarged but virilization is progressing, the source of the androgens may be the adrenal glands or exogenous sources. If the testes are slightly enlarged but not consistent with the stage of pubertal development, ectopic production of hCG or familial Leydig and germ cell maturation may be the cause. Most of the enlargement of testes during puberty is the result of seminiferous tubule maturation. Therefore, if only Leydig cells are enlarged as in these conditions, the testes will make considerable testosterone but show only minimal enlargement.

Laboratory examinations include determination of sex steroid (testosterone estradiol, or DHEAS) and gonadotropin concentrations, usually in the GnRH-stimulated state. However, with modern ultrasensitive assays, basal determinations may suffice (Table 17–11). If values are in the normal pubertal range, central precocious puberty is likely, but discrepancies from the normal process suggest incomplete precocious puberty. Thyroid hormone determination is useful, since severe primary hypothyroidism can cause incomplete precocious puberty. If there is a suggestion of a CNS anomaly or a tumor (CNS, hepatic, adrenal, ovarian, or testicular), a CT or MRI scan of the appropriate location is indicated. The diagnosis of central precocious puberty mandates that an MRI of the CNS be performed.

Treatment (Table 17–12). Long-acting, superactive analogs of GnRH are the treatment of choice for central precocious puberty because they suppress gonadotropin secretion by down-regulating GnRH receptors in the pituitary gonadotropes. After a brief (2–3-day) increase in gonadotropin secretion, values drop and the pubertal process reverts to the prepubertal state. The early sexual development and increased height of the patient with precocious puberty mandate psychologic support or even counseling for children and families. Boys with GnRH-independent premature Leydig cell and germ cell maturation do not respond to GnRH analogs but require treatment with an inhibitor of testosterone synthesis (e.g., ketoconazole), an antiandrogen (e.g., spironolactone), or an aromatase inhibitor (e.g., testolactone). Patients with incomplete precocious puberty require removal of the hormone-secreting tumor, if possible. McCune-Albright syndrome is treated with testolactone and antiandrogens or antiestrogen such as tamoxifen. After successful therapy for the latter conditions, central precocious puberty may develop secondarily; GnRH agonist administration then becomes effective therapy.

Variations in Pubertal Development

Isolated Premature Thelarche (Premature Breast Development)

Benign premature thelarche is the isolated appearance of unilateral or bilateral breast tissue in girls, usually at ages 6 months to 3 years. There are no other signs of puberty and no evidence of excessive estrogen effect (e.g., vaginal bleeding, thickening of the vaginal secretions, increased height velocity, or bone age acceleration). Ingestion or dermal application of estrogen-containing compounds must be excluded as the etiology of the condition. Laboratory investigations are not usually necessary, but a pelvic ultrasound study may rarely be indicated to exclude ovarian pathology. Girls with this condition should be reevaluated at intervals of 6–12 months to ensure that apparent premature thelarche is not the beginning of isosexual precocious puberty. The prognosis is excellent; if no progression occurs, no treatment other than reassurance is necessary. There is no indication for a breast biopsy in a patient with established premature thelarche.

TABLE 17–12
Pharmacologic Therapy of Sexual Precocity

Disorder	Treatment	Action and Rationale
GnRH-dependent true or central precocious puberty	GnRH agonists	Desensitization of gonadotropes; blocks action of endogenous GnRH
GnRH-independent incomplete sexual precocity		
Girls		
Autonomous ovarian cysts	Medroxyprogesterone acetate	Inhibition of ovarian steroidogenesis; regression of cyst (inhibition of FSH release)
McCune-Albright syndrome	Medroxyprogesterone acetate*	Inhibition of ovarian steroidogenesis; regression of cyst (inhibition of FSH release)
	Testolactone* or fadrozole	Inhibition of P-450 aromatase; blocks estrogen synthesis
Boys		
Familial testotoxicosis	Ketoconazole*	Inhibition of $P-450_{c17}$ (mainly 17,20-lyase activity)
	Spironolactone* or flutamide *and* testolactone or fadrozole	Antiandrogen Inhibition of aromatase; blocks estrogen synthesis
	Medroxyprogesterone acetate*	Inhibition of testicular steroidogenesis

Modified from Grumbach MM, Kaplan SL: *Acta Paediatr Jpn* 30(Suppl):155, 1988.
FSH, Follicle-stimulating hormone; *GnRH,* gonadotropin-releasing hormone.
*If true precocious puberty develops, a GnRH agonist can be added.

Gynecomastia

In boys, the appearance of breast tissue is *gynecomastia,* which may occur to some degree in up to 45–75% of normal pubertal boys (see Chapter 7). Androgens are normally converted to estrogen by aromatization; in early puberty only modest amounts of androgens are produced and the estrogen effect can overwhelm the androgen effects at this stage. Later in pubertal development, the androgen production is so great that there is little effect from the estrogen produced by aromatization. Gynecomastia also accompanies Klinefelter syndrome as puberty progresses. Prepubertal gynecomastia suggests an unusual source of estrogen either from exogenous sources (oral or dermal estrogen administration is possible from contamination of food or ointments) or endogenous (from abnormal function of adrenal gland or ovary or from increased peripheral aromatization).

Isolated Premature Adrenarche (Pubarche)

The isolated appearance of pubic hair before the age of 6–7 years in girls or before the age of 9 years in boys is premature adrenarche and is relatively common. If the pubic hair is associated with any other feature of virilization (e.g., clitoral or penile enlargement or advanced bone age) or other signs (e.g., acne, rapid growth, or voice change), a detailed investigation for a pathologic cause of virilization is indicated because the cause might be life threatening. Measurements of serum testosterone, 17-hydroxyprogesterone (17-OHP), and dehydroepiandrosterone (DHEA) in basal and ACTH-stimulated states are indicated in heavily virilized patients. Excessive but glucocorticoid-suppressible 17-OHP or DHEA levels indicate an enzyme defect of congenital adrenal hyperplasia. Ultrasound studies may reveal a virilizing adrenal or ovarian tumor. Most patients with isolated pubic hair, however, do not have these abnormal signs of progressive virilization and simply have *premature* adrenarche or *(pubarche)* resulting from premature activation of DHEA secretion from the adrenal gland. Bone age may be slightly advanced and height slightly increased, but testosterone concentrations are normal. DHEA-S levels usually are high for prepuberty but are consistent with Tanner (Sexuality Maturity Rating) stages II and III (Figs. 7–1 and 7–4).

REFERENCES

Behrman RE, Kliegman RM, Jenson HB, editors: *Nelson textbook of pediatrics,* ed 16, Philadelphia, 2000, WB Saunders, Chapters 571–572.

Grumbach MM, Styne DM: Puberty. In Wilson JD, Foster DW, editors: *Williams textbook of endocrinology,* ed 9, Philadelphia, 1997, WB Saunders, pp 1509–1625.

Ringel M, Schwindinger W, Levine M: Clinical implications of genetic defects in G proteins, *Medicine* 75(4):171–184, 1996.

Rosenfeld RL: The ovary and female sexual maturation. In Sperling MA, editor: *Pediatric endocrinology*, Philadelphia, 1996, WB Saunders.

Styne DM: The testes: disorders of sexual differentiation and puberty. In Sperling MA, editor: *Pediatric endocrinology*, Philadelphia, 1996, WB Saunders.

Styne DM: Recent developments in disorders of puberty, *Pediatr Clin North Am* 44(2):505–529, 1997.

Styne DM: Puberty. In Greenspan FS, Gardner DG: *Basic and clinical endocrinology*, ed 6, New York, 2001, Lange Medical Books.

THYROID

Thyroid Physiology and Development

(Fig. 17–6)

Thyrotropin-releasing hormone (TRH), a tripeptide synthesized in the hypothalamus, stimulates the release of pituitary thyroid–stimulating hormone (TSH). Pituitary TSH is a glycoprotein that stimulates the synthesis and release of thyroid hormones by the thyroid gland. Plasma concentrations of TSH above the normal range indicate primary hypothyroidism, and those below the normal range indicate hypothalamic or pituitary deficiency or suppression of TSH secretion. Thyroid function develops in three stages:

1. Embryogenesis begins on the floor of the primitive oral cavity, and the gland descends to its definitive position in the anterior lower neck by the end of the first trimester. Thyroid glands that do not reach the normal location are ectopic but still may retain function (a lingual or sublingual site or even tissue found in a thyroglossal duct cyst may be the only functioning thyroid gland).
2. The hypothalamic-pituitary-thyroid axis becomes functional in the second trimester.
3. Peripheral metabolism of thyroid hormones matures in the third trimester.

Thyroxine (T_4), triiodothyronine (T_3), and TSH do not cross the placenta in significant amounts, so their concentration in fetal serum reflects fetal secretion and metabolism. However, antithyroid antibodies, thyroid-stimulating immunoglobulins (TSIs), iodides (including radioactive iodides), propylthiouracil, and methimazole do cross the placenta and affect fetal thyroid function. A baby born prematurely or intrauterine growth retarded (IUGR) may have an interruption of the normal maturational process and appear to have hypothyroidism by standard tests. It is controversial as to whether treatment is indicated in such situations.

The thyroid gland produces thyroid hormone in several steps. The thyroid gland (1) concentrates iodine and (2) attaches it (organifies it) to tyrosine molecules to produce either mono- or diiodotyrosine;

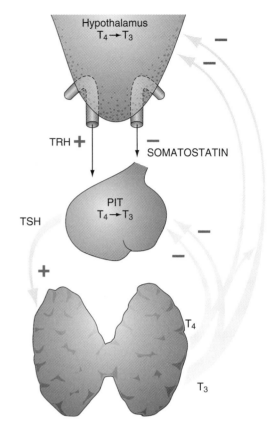

FIG. 17–6

Interrelationships of the hypothalamic-pituitary-thyroid axis. Thyroid-stimulating hormone (TSH) from the pituitary gland (PIT) stimulates the secretion of both thyroxine (T_4) and triiodothyronine (T_3) from the thyroid gland. These act at the pituitary gland level to control secretion of TSH by a negative feedback mechanism. In addition, T_4 is metabolized to the potent T_3 within the pituitary gland by a monoiodinase. Secretion of TSH is stimulated by thyrotropin-releasing hormone (TRH) from the hypothalamus and inhibited by somatostatin. Thyroid hormone acts at the hypothalamus to stimulate secretion of somatostatin (somatostatin acts as a negative signal to the pituitary secretion of TSH). (From Wilson JD, Foster DW, editors: *Williams textbook of endocrinology*, ed 8, Philadelphia, 1992, WB Saunders.)

with subsequent (3) coupling of two tyrosines, T_4 or T_3 is synthesized, representing the major thyroid hormones. The major fraction of circulating T_3 (~ two thirds) is derived from peripheral deiodination of T_4 to T_3, but some is produced by the thyroid gland itself. In Graves disease, a larger fraction originates in the thyroid gland. The conversion of T_4 to T_3 requires the removal of one iodine from the outer ring; removing an iodine from the inner ring results in reverse T_3 (rT_3), which has little biologic effect.

TABLE 17–13
Laboratory Test Results in Various Types of Thyroid Function Abnormalities in Children*

	Serum Total T_4	Free T_4	Serum TSH	Serum TBG
Primary hypothyroidism	↓	↓	↑	N
Hypothalamic (TRH) tertiary hypothyroidism	↓	↓	↓	N
Pituitary (TSH) secondary hypothyroidism	↓	↓	↓	N
TBG deficiency	↓	N	N	↓
TBG excess	↑	N	N	↑

N, Normal; ↓, decreased; ↑, increased; T_3, triiodothyronine; T_4, thyroxine; *TBG*, thyroid-binding globulin; *TRH*, thyroid-releasing hormone; *TSH*, thyroid-stimulating hormone.

Preferential conversion of T_4 to rT_3 rather than T_3 occurs in utero and in all forms of severe illness, including respiratory distress syndrome, fevers, anorexia, cachexia, and starvation. In contrast, conversion from T_4 to T_3 increases immediately after birth and throughout life. T_4 and T_3 are noncovalently bound to a specific serum carrier protein, thyroxine-binding globulin (TBG), and, to a lesser extent, to albumin. Only the small (<2%) fractions of T_4 and T_3 not bound to this or to other serum carriers, free T_4 (as it is converted to free T_3) and free T_3, are biologically active. Free T_3 exerts metabolic effects and negative feedback on TSH release.

At birth there are several dramatic changes in thyroid function. Serum TSH rises just after birth but soon reaches lower values considered normal for later life. T_4 secretion increases after birth, partially as a result of the peak in TSH and partially because of maturation of thyroid metabolism. T_4 rises to values so high as to be similar to hyperthyroidism in the adult during the first 2–4 days after birth. Serum thyroid hormone concentrations then decrease but only slowly reach values routinely found in adults. Free T_4 is the test of choice, since it eliminates the effects of variation in protein binding, which can be substantial.

A summary of laboratory test results in various types of thyroid abnormalities is illustrated in Table 17–13. Although thyroid scans rarely are indicated in pediatric thyroid disease, thyroid agenesis or ectopic thyroid tissue and hyperfunctioning "hot" nodules or nonfunctioning "cold" nodules may be detected by this test. A thyroid scan performed with short-lived ^{123}I will indicate the size, shape, and location of the thyroid gland as well as iodine concentrating ability. A solitary nodule is ominous, especially if it is solid and nonfunctional. An ultrasound study may determine whether it is cystic or solid. If solid, an ^{123}I scan will indicate its functional status. Solitary nodules are usually subject to excisional biopsies. Scans are rarely indicated in the diagnosis of Hashimoto thyroiditis or thyrotoxicosis.

Thyroid Disorders

Hypothyroidism

Hypothyroidism is diagnosed by a decreased serum-free T_4. This might be the result of thyroid disease (primary hypothyroidism) or of abnormalities of the pituitary gland (secondary) or the result of abnormality of the hypothalamus (tertiary). Hypothyroidism is divided into congenital or acquired disorders and may be associated with a goiter.

Congenital Hypothyroidism. Congenital hypothyroidism occurs in approximately 1:4000 live births and is usually caused by a dysgenetic (agenesis, aplasia, ectopia) malformation of the thyroid gland. Thyroid tissue usually is not palpable in these sporadic nongoitrous conditions. The free T_4 concentration is low and TSH levels are elevated, proving primary hypothyroidism. Routine neonatal screening programs to measure cord blood or heel stick TSH values are presently available in every state in the United States and in most countries. An immediate confirmatory serum sample should be obtained from any infant having a positive result on a screening test (low T_4, high TSH confirms the finding).

Congenital TBG deficiency occurs in about 1:10,000 live births and is associated with a low serum total T_4 concentration, a normal TSH and serum free T_4, and a euthyroid clinical status. Isolated secondary or tertiary hypothyroidism is rare, occurring in 1:100,000 live births; the free T_4 is normal to low in these conditions. When tertiary or secondary hypothyroidism is detected, assessment of other pituitary hormones and investigation of pituitary-hypothalamic anatomy via MRI are indicated.

Goitrous congenital hypothyroidism occurs in about 1 in 30,000 live births. The goiter reflects an inborn error of metabolism in the pathway of iodide incorporation or thyroid hormone biosynthesis or reflects the transplacental passage of antithyroid drugs given to the mother.

Clinical manifestations of congenital hypothyroidism in the immediate newborn period usually

TABLE 17–14
Causes of Hypothyroidism in Infancy and Childhood

Age	Manifestation	Cause
Newborn	No goiter	Thyroid gland dysgenesis or ectopic location
		Exposure to iodides
		TSH deficiency
		TRH deficiency
	Goiter	Inborn defect in hormone synthesis* or effect
		Maternal goitrogen ingestion, including propylthiouracil, methimazole, iodides
		Severe iodide deficiency (endemic)
Child	No goiter	Thyroid gland dysgenesis
		Cystinosis
		Hypothalamic-pituitary insufficiency
		Surgical after thyrotoxicosis or other thyroid surgery
	Goiter	Hashimoto thyroiditis: chronic lymphocytic thyroiditis
		Inborn defect in hormone synthesis or effect
		Goitrogenic drugs
		Infiltrative (sarcoid, lymphoma)

*Impaired iodide transport, defective thyroglobulin iodination, defective iodotyrosine dehalogenase, defective thyroglobulin, or its coupling to iodotyrosines.

are subtle but become more evident weeks or months after birth. Hence newborn screening is important to make an early diagnosis and initiate thyroid replacement therapy in the absence of definitive signs. However, findings at various stages after birth may include gestation greater than 42 weeks, birth weight greater than 4 kg, hypothermia, acrocyanosis, respiratory distress, large posterior fontanel, abdominal distention, lethargy and poor feeding, jaundice more than 3 days after birth, edema, umbilical hernia, mottled skin, constipation, large tongue, dry skin, and hoarse cry. Thyroid hormones are crucially important for maturation and differentiation of tissues such as bone (bone age is often delayed at birth because of intrauterine hypothyroidism) and brain (most thyroid-dependent brain maturation occurs in the 2–3 years after birth).

When *treatment* is initiated within 1 month or less after birth, the *prognosis* for normal intellectual development is excellent; screening programs usually offer therapy within 1–2 weeks of birth. If therapy is instituted after 6 months, when the signs of severe hypothyroidism (e.g., cretinism, a pejorative term not used when addressing families) are present, the likelihood of normal intellectual function is markedly decreased. Growth improves after thyroid replacement even in late diagnosed cases. The dose of thyroxine changes with age; 10–15 μg of T_4/kg is

used for a newborn, but about 3 μg/kg is used later in childhood. In neonatal hypothyroidism, the goal is to keep the serum free T_4 in the upper half of the range of normal but suppression of TSH is not necessary in all cases, as such suppression may lead to excessive doses of thyroxine.

Acquired Hypothyroidism. The *etiology* of acquired hypothyroidism is presented in Table 17–14, and the *clinical manifestations* are summarized in Table 17–15. The signs and symptoms may be subtle, and hypothyroidism should be suspected in any child who has a decline in growth velocity, especially if not associated with weight loss. The most common cause of acquired hypothyroidism in older children in the United States is lymphocytic autoimmune thyroiditis (Hashimoto thyroiditis). However, in many areas of the world, iodine deficiency is the etiology of endemic goiter (endemic cretinism). The failure of the thyroid gland may be heralded by a rise of TSH before T_4 levels fall. In contrast to untreated congenital hypothyroidism, acquired hypothyroidism is not a cause of permanent developmental delay.

Hashimoto Thyroiditis. Also known as autoimmune or *lymphocytic thyroiditis*, Hashimoto thyroiditis is a common cause of goiter and acquired thyroid disease in older children and adolescents. A family history of thyroid disease is present in 25–35% of patients, suggesting a genetic predisposition. The *etiol-*

TABLE 17–15
Symptoms and Signs of Hypothyroidism

Ectodermal	Poor growth
	Dull facies: thick lips, large tongue, depressed nasal bridge, periorbital edema
	Dry scaly skin
	Sparse brittle hair
	Diminished sweating
	Carotenemia
	Vitiligo
Circulatory	Sinus bradycardia/heart block
	Cold extremities
	Cold intolerance
	Pallor
	ECG changes: low-voltage QRS complex
Neuromuscular	Muscle weakness
	Hypotonia: constipation, potbelly
	Umbilical hernia
	Myxedema coma (CO_2 narcosis, hypothermia)
	Pseudohypertrophy of muscles
	Myalgia
	Physical and mental lethargy
	Developmental delay
	Delayed relaxation of reflexes
	Paresthesias (nerve entrapment: carpal tunnel syndrome)
	Cerebellar ataxia
Skeletal	Delayed bone age
	Epiphyseal dysgenesis, increased upper to lower segment ratio
Metabolic	Myxedema
	Serous effusions (pleural, pericardial, ascites)
	Hoarse voice (cry)
	Weight gain
	Menstrual irregularity
	Arthralgia
	Elevated CPK
	Macrocytosis (anemia)
	Hypercholesterolemia
	Hyperprolactinemia
	Precocious puberty in severe cases

CPK, Creatine phosphokinase; *ECG*, electrocardiogram.

ogy is an autoimmune process targeted against the thyroid gland with lymphocytic infiltration and lymphoid follicle and germinal center formation preceding fibrosis and atrophy.

Clinical manifestations include a firm, nontender euthyroid, hypothyroid or, rarely, hyperthyroid (hashitoxicosis) diffuse goiter with a pebble-like feeling; an insidious onset after 6 years of age (the incidence peaks in adolescence, with a female predominance); and sometimes a pea-sized "Delphian" lymph node above the thyroid isthmus. Associated autoimmune diseases include type 1 diabetes mellitus, adrenal insufficiency (Schmidt syndrome), and hypoparathyroidism. Type 1 autoimmune polyglandular disorder consists of hypoparathyroidism, Addison disease, mucocutaneous candidiasis, and often, hypothyroidism. Type 2 autoimmune polyglandular disorder consists of Addison disease, type 1 diabetes mellitus, and frequently autoimmune hypothyroidism. Trisomy 21 and Turner syndrome predispose to the development of autoimmune thyroiditis.

The *diagnosis* may be confirmed by serum antithyroid peroxidase (previously antimicrosomal) and antithyroglobulin antibodies. Neither biopsy nor thyroid scan is indicated in Hashimoto thyroiditis.

Treatment with thyroid hormone sufficient to suppress TSH to a normal level is indicated for hypothyroidism in Hashimoto thyroiditis. Patients without manifestation of hypothyroidism require periodic thyroid function testing (serum TSH and free T_4) every 6–12 months to detect the later development of hypothyroidism. Goiter with a normal TSH is not usually an indication for treatment.

Hyperthyroidism

Graves Disease. Most children with hyperthyroidism have Graves disease, the autonomous functioning of the thyroid caused by autoantibodies stimulating the thyroid gland (thyroid-stimulating immunoglobulins [TSIs]). The resulting excessive synthesis, release, and peripheral metabolism of thyroid hormones produce the clinical features. Hashimoto thyroiditis and thyrotoxicosis are on a continuum of autoimmune diseases, and there is overlap in their immunologic findings. Antimicrosomal and antithyroglobulin antibodies may be present in thyrotoxicosis, although the values are usually lower than found in Hashimoto thyroiditis. Exceptionally high titers of antibodies may indicate that the patient has the thyrotoxic phase of Hashimoto thyroiditis (hashitoxicosis caused by the release of preformed thyroid hormone), with the subsequent development of hypothyroidism. In Graves disease, serum T_4 and/or T_3 levels are elevated, whereas TSH is suppressed. Rare causes of hyperthyroidism include McCune-Albright syndrome, thyroid neoplasm, TSH hypersecretion, subacute thyroiditis, and iodine or thyroid hormone ingestion.

Clinical Manifestations. Graves disease presents as hyperthyroidism (Table 17–16). In children, Graves disease is about five times more common in females than in males, with a peak incidence in adolescence. Personality changes, mood instability, and poor school performance are common presenting problems. The tremor, anxiety, inability to concentrate, and weight loss may be insidious and confused with a psychologic disorder until thyroid function tests reveal the elevated serum free T_4 level. Serum T_4 may remain near normal while serum T_3 is selectively elevated (T_3 toxicosis). A firm, homogeneous goiter usually is present. Many patients complain of neck fullness and, in older subjects, a change in the size of their shirt collars. Thyroid gland enlargement is best visualized with the neck only slightly extended and with the examiner lateral to the patient; palpation of the thyroid gland is best performed

with the examiner's hands around the neck from the back. The patient swallows so the examiner can feel the size, consistency, nodularity, and motion of the gland. The thickness is estimated and the dimensions of each lobe are measured vertically and laterally. Auscultation may reveal a bruit over the gland.

Treatment. Three treatment choices are available: pharmacologic, surgical, and radioactive iodine.

Drugs. Medical therapy consists of propylthiouracil (PTU) to block thyroid hormone synthesis (5–7 mg/kg/24 hr PO in divided doses every 8 hours). Propranolol is started if symptoms are severe (2–3 mg/kg/24 hr orally) to control cardiac manifestations and is tapered as the PTU or methimazole takes effect. PTU usually is continued for 1–2 years

TABLE 17–16 Clinical Manifestations of Hyperthyroidism	
Increased catecholamine effects	Nervousness
	Palpitations
	Tachycardia
	Atrial arrhythmias
	Systolic hypertension
	Tremor
	Brisk reflexes
Hypermetabolism	Increased sweating
	Shiny, smooth skin
	Heat intolerance
	Fatigue
	Weight loss—increased appetite
	Increased bowel movement (hyperdefecation)
	Hyperkinesis
Myopathy	Weakness
	Periodic paralysis
	Cardiac failure—dyspnea
Miscellaneous	Proptosis, stare, exophthalmos, lid lag, ophthalmopathy
	Hair loss
	Inability to concentrate
	Personality change (emotional lability)
	Goiter
	Thyroid bruit
	Onycholysis
	Painful gland*
	Acute thyroid storm (hyperpyrexia, tachycardia, coma, high-output heart failure, shock)

* Unusual except in subacute thyroiditis with hyperthyroid phase.

because the remission rate is approximately 25% per year. In patients complying with the treatment regimen, the 2-year course of treatment can be repeated. PTU should suppress thyroid function to the point that thyroid hormone replacement is required and added to normalize serum free T_4. Complications of PTU are lupus-like syndrome, rash, granulocytopenia, and jaundice. These sometimes severe side effects are usually reversible after discontinuation of antithyroid therapy; failure to monitor and then discontinue PTU when complications arise may be fatal. Methimazole is an alternate agent to PTU and is given in approximately 10% of the dose of PTU. Iodine administration may suppress thyroid function, but it becomes ineffective in a few weeks. It is sometimes used as a preparation for surgery but never for long-term therapy.

Surgery. Surgical treatment consists of partial or complete thyroidectomy. Risks associated with thyroidectomy include the use of anesthesia and the possibility that the thyroid removal will be excessive, causing hypothyroidism, or that it will be inadequate, resulting in persistent hyperthyroidism. In addition, keloid formation, recurrent laryngeal nerve palsy, and hypoparathyroidism (transient postoperative or permanent) may occur. Thyroid storm caused by the release of large amounts of preformed hormone is a serious but rare complication. Even with optimal immediate postoperative results, patients may become hypothyroid within 10 years.

Radioiodine. Radioiodine (^{131}I) is slower in exerting therapeutic effects, may require repeated dosing, and may cause hypothyroidism. Although studies reveal no long-term consequences, concern remains about possible sequelae in children. Nonetheless, this method of treatment is entering the mainstream for adolescents as well as adults. Radioiodine given to a pregnant teenager will render the fetus hypothyroid and is, therefore, contraindicated.

Thyroid Storm. Thyroid storm (Table 17–16) is a rare medical emergency consisting of tachycardia and hyperthermia. *Treatment* includes reducing the hyperthermia with a cooling blanket and administering propranolol to control tachycardia. Iodine may be given to block thyroid hormone release. Cortisol may be indicated for relative adrenal insufficiency, and therapy for heart failure may include diuretics and digoxin.

Congenital Hyperthyroidism. This disorder results from transplacental passage of maternal TSIs. The *clinical* manifestations in the neonate may be masked for several days until the short-lived effects of transplacental maternal antithyroid medication wear off (assuming the mother was receiving such medication), at which time the effects of TSIs are observed. Irritability, tachycardia (often with signs of cardiac failure simulating "cardiomyopathy"), polycythemia, craniosynostosis, bone age advancement, poor feeding, and later failure to thrive are the clinical hallmarks. This condition may be anticipated if the mother is known to be thyrotoxic in pregnancy so that timely therapy can be offered. If the mother was cured of her hyperthyroidism before pregnancy by surgery or radioiodine treatment, which limits or curtails T_4 production but not the underlying immune disturbance producing TSIs, the infant may still be affected.

Treatment for the severely affected neonate includes oral propranolol at 2–3 mg/kg/24 hr in divided doses and propylthiouracil approximately 5 mg/kg/24 hr orally in three divided doses. Because the half-life of the immunoglobulin is several weeks, spontaneous resolution of neonatal thyrotoxicosis resulting from transplacental passage of TSIs usually occurs by 2–3 months of age. Observation without treatment is indicated in patients who are minimally affected.

Tumors of the Thyroid

Carcinoma of the thyroid is rare in children, but papillary and follicular carcinomas represent 90% of children's thyroid cancers. A history of therapeutic head or neck irradiation or radiation exposure from nuclear accidents predisposes a child to thyroid cancer. Carcinoma usually presents as a firm to hard, painless, nonfunctional solitary nodule and may spread to adjacent lymph nodes. Rapid growth, hoarseness (recurrent laryngeal nerve involvement), and lung metastasis may be present. If the nodule is solid on ultrasound, is "cold" on radioiodine scanning, and feels hard, the likelihood of a carcinoma is high. Excisional biopsy is usually performed, but fine-needle aspiration biopsy may also be diagnostic.

Treatment includes total thyroidectomy, selective regional node dissection, and radioablation with ^{131}I for residual or recurrent disease. The *prognosis* is usually good if the disease is diagnosed early.

Medullary carcinoma of the thyroid (MCT) may be asymptomatic except for a mass. *Diagnosis* is based on the presence of elevated calcitonin levels, either in the basal state or following pentagastrin stimulation, and histology. This tumor most often occurs with multiple endocrine neoplasia II (MEN), pheochromocytoma, or alone, possibly in a familial pattern. The presence of the RET oncogene is predictive of the development of MCT in some families. Therefore, screening the other members of the family is indicated after a proband is recognized.

REFERENCES

Behrman RE, Kliegman RM, Jenson HB, editors: *Nelson textbook of pediatrics,* ed 16, Philadelphia, 2000, WB Saunders, Chapters 573–579.

Dayan C, Daniel G: Chronic autoimmune thyroiditis, *N Engl J Med* 335(2):99–107, 1996.

Fisher DA: Hypothyroxinemia in premature infants: is thyroxine treatment necessary? *Thyroid* 9(7):715–720, 1999.

Fisher DA, Schoen EJ, La Franchi, et al: The hypothalamic-pituitary-thyroid negative feedback control axis in children with treated congenital hypothyroidism, *J Clin Endocrinol Metab* 85(8):2722–2735, 2000.

Foley TP: Disorders of the thyroid in children. In Sperling MA, editor: *Pediatric endocrinology*, Philadelphia, 1996, WB Saunders.

LaFranchi S: Disorders of the thyroid gland. In Behrman RE, Kliegman RM, Jenson HB, editors: *Nelson textbook of pediatrics*, ed 16, Philadelphia, 2000, WB Saunders.

Lazarus J: Hyperthyroidism, *Lancet* 349(9048):339–343, 1997.

Lindsay R, Toft A: Hypothyroidism, *Lancet* 349(9049):413–417, 1997.

DISORDERS OF SEXUAL DIFFERENTIATION

Normal Sexual Development

Gender is determined by a combination of karyotype (genotypic or chromosomal sex), which usually determines the morphology of internal organs and gonads (gonadal sex); the appearance of the external genitalia and the form of secondary sex characteristics (phenotypic sex); the self-perception of the individual (gender identity); and the perception of the individual by others (gender role). In most children these features blend and conform, but in some patients one or more features may not follow this sequence, leading to an intersex condition.

Ambiguous genitalia in a newborn must be considered an endocrine emergency. Insensitive handling of the situation may lead to a lifelong pattern of gender uncertainty in the patient and confusion in the parents. Complicating matters, the laboratory evaluations required may take days or weeks to be completed, thus delaying a sex assignment and naming of the infant.

Diagnosis and *treatment* of disorders of sex differentiation are best understood in terms of the embryology and hormonal control of normal sex differentiation. The internal and external genitalia are formed between the ninth and thirteenth week of gestation. Regardless of karyotype, a fetus is bipotential and has the capacity to develop a normal male or female phenotype. A female phenotype develops unless a specific "male" influence alters development. The male or female phenotype develops internally from bipotential gonads and ducts, and externally from bipotential anlage (Fig. 17–7). In the presence of a gene for the testes-determining factor identified as the SRY (sex reversing Y) gene, near the pseudoautosomal boundary on the Y chromosome, the primitive fetal gonad differentiates into a testis (Fig. 17–8). The testis secretes testosterone, which has direct effects (stimulation of development of the wolffian ducts) but also is locally converted to dihydrotestosterone (DHT) by the 5 α-reductase enzyme for other effects. DHT causes enlargement, rogation, and fusion of the labia majora into a scrotum; fusion of the ventral surface of the penis to enclose a penile urethra; and enlargement of the phallus with ultimate development of male external genitalia (Figs. 17–7 and 17–8). Testicular production and secretion of mullerian duct–inhibitory substance cause the regression and disappearance of the müllerian ducts and their derivatives, such as the oviducts and uterus. In the presence of testosterone, the wolffian ducts develop into the vas deferens, seminiferous tubules, and prostate.

In the absence of SRY, an ovary spontaneously develops from the bipotential, primitive gonad. In the absence of fetal testicular secretion of müllerian-inhibitory substance, a normal uterus, fallopian tubes, and posterior third of the vagina develop out of the müllerian ducts as the wolffian ducts degenerate. In the total absence of androgens, the external genitalia appear female. In the absence of adequate virilization because of abnormal development of the testes, biosynthetic defects of testosterone or DHT, or androgen receptor defects, any phenotype between normal female and male may develop; the result is a child having ambiguous genitalia. It is essential to note whether there is fusion of the posterior aspect of the vagina (which makes the vaginal opening small or even slit-like). This can occur only between 9–13 weeks of gestation and must occur if there is endogenous excessive production of androgen (as in congenital adrenal hyperplasia). If the vaginal opening is normal and there is no fusion, but the clitoris is enlarged without ventral fusion of the ventral urethra, the patient had later exposure to androgens. Further, a patient with a fully formed scrotum, even if small, and a normally formed but small penis, termed a microphallus, must have had normal exposure to and action of androgen during 9–13 weeks of gestation.

Abnormal Sexual Development

Virilization of the 46,XX Female (Female Pseudohermaphroditism)

Masculinization of the external genitalia of genotypic females (except for isolated enlargement of the clitoris, which can occur from later androgen exposure) is always caused by the presence of excessive androgens during the critical period of development (8–13 weeks gestation) (Table 17–17). The magnitude of the changes will reflect the quantity and duration of exposure to androgens. The degree of virilization can range from mild clitoral enlargement to the appearance of a "male" phallus with a penile urethra and

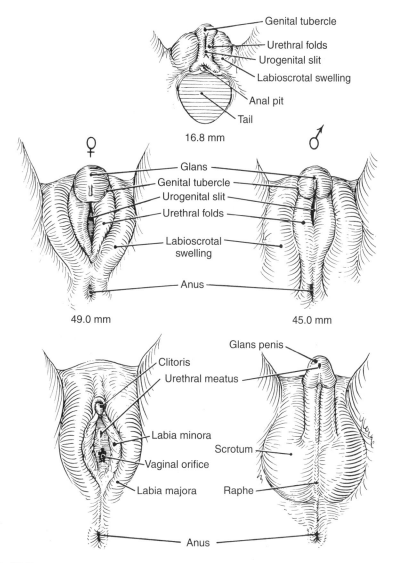

FIG. 17–7

Differentiation of male and female external genitalia as proceeding from a common embryonic anlage. Testosterone acts at 9–13 weeks of gestation to virilize the bipotential anlage. In the absence of testosterone action, the female phenotype develops. (From Grumbach MM, Conte FA: Disorders of sexual differentiation. In Wilson JD, Foster DW, editors: *Textbook of endocrinology,* ed 8, Philadelphia, 1990, WB Saunders. Adapted from Spaulding MH: *Contrib Embryol Carnegie Instit* 13:69–88, 1921.)

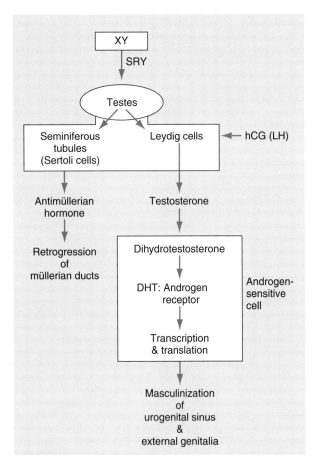

FIG. 17–8

A diagrammatic scheme of male sex determination and differentiation. *DHT*, Dihydrotestosterone; *SRY*, the gene for the testis-determining factor. (Modified from Wilson JD, Foster DW, editors: *Williams textbook of endocrinology*, ed 8, Philadelphia, WB Saunders, 1992.)

TABLE 17–17
Causes of Virilization in the Female

Condition	Additional Features
P-450$_{c21}$ deficiency	Salt loss in some
3β-Hydroxysteroid dehydrogenase deficiency	Salt loss
P-450$_{C11}$ deficiency	Salt retention/hypertension
Androgenic drug exposure (e.g., progestins)	Exposure between 9th and 12th wk gestation
Mixed gonadal dysgenesis or mosaic Turner syndrome	Karyotype = 46,XY/45,X
True hermaphrodite	Testicular and ovarian tissue present
Maternal virilizing adrenal or ovarian tumor	Rare, positive history

fused scrotum with raphe. Ambiguous genitalia in females is most commonly the result of an enzyme deficiency that impairs adrenal cortisol synthesis but does not affect androgen or precursor production. Congenital virilizing adrenal hyperplasia is the most common cause of ambiguous genitalia; ACTH stimulates hyperplasia of the adrenal cortex and excessive adrenal production of androgens (discussed in this chapter under Adrenal Gland).

Inadequate Masculinization of the 46,XY Male (Male Pseudohermaphroditism)

Underdevelopment of the male external genitalia occurs because of a relative deficiency of testosterone production or action (Table 17–18). The penis is small, with various degrees of hypospadias (penile or perineal) and associated chordee or ventral bind-

ing of the phallus; unilateral, but more often bilateral, cryptorchidism may be present. The testes should be carefully sought in the inguinal canal or labioscrotal folds by palpation or ultrasound. Very rarely, a palpable gonad in the inguinal canal or labioscrotal fold represents a herniated ovary or an ovotestis in a hermaphrodite. The latter patients have both ovarian and testicular tissue and usually an XX genotype, and ambiguous external genitalia. Production of testosterone by a gonad implies that testicular tissue is present and that at least some cells carry the SRY gene.

Testosterone production can be reduced by specific deficiencies of the enzymes needed for androgen biosynthesis or by dysplasia of the gonads. In the latter, if müllerian-inhibiting substance production also is reduced, a rudimentary uterus and fallopian tubes will be present. Enzyme defects in testosterone biosynthesis, which also block cortisol production, produce adrenal hyperplasia. Hypopituitarism with LH deficiency does not result in ambiguous genitalia because placental hCG in the fetal circulation stimulates fetal gonadal testosterone synthesis during the critical 9–13 weeks of gestation to allow development of a normal male phallus. Later in gestation, fetal LH is needed to stimulate the testes to produce adequate androgen to enlarge the fetal penis. Thus congenital gonadotropin deficiency may produce a normally formed but small penis (microphallus); this condition is often combined with deficiencies of GH and ACTH in neonatal hypopituitarism, causing neonatal hypo-

TABLE 17–18
Causes of Inadequate Masculinization in the Male

Condition	Additional Features
P-450$_{scc}$ (STAR) deficiency	Salt loss
3β-Hydroxysteroid dehydrogenase deficiency	Salt loss
P-450$_{c17}$ deficiency	Salt retention/hypokalemia/hypertension
Isolated P-450$_{c17}$ deficiency with 17,20-desmolase deficiency	Adrenal function normal
17β-Hydroxysteroid oxidoreductase deficiency	Adrenal function normal
Dysgenetic testes	Possible abnormal karyotype
Leydig cell hypoplasia	Rare
Complete androgen insensitivity or testicular feminization	Female external genitalia, absence of müllerian structures
Partial androgen insensitivity	As above with ambiguous external genitalia
5α-Reductase deficiency	Autosomal recessive, virilization at puberty

glycemia. Microphallus caused by this etiology will respond to testosterone treatment, resulting in an enlargement of the penis.

The complete form of androgen resistance or **testicular feminization syndrome** is the most dramatic example of androgen insensitivity. Absolute resistance of target tissues to the actions of the androgens in some patients occurs because the androgen receptor cannot bind DHT. In others, a postreceptor defect diminishes androgen action even though the number of androgen receptors is normal and they bind androgen normally. Affected patients have a 46,XY karyotype, normally formed testes (usually located in the inguinal canal or labia majora), and feminine-appearing external genitalia with a short vagina and no internal müllerian structures. At the time of puberty, testosterone concentrations rise to the normal male range. Because a portion of the testosterone is normally converted to estradiol in peripheral tissues and the estrogen cannot be opposed by the androgen, breast development ensues at the normal age of puberty without growth of pubic, facial, or axillary hair or, of course, the occurrence of menstruation. Gender identity and gender role are female.

5α-Reductase deficiency presents at birth with predominantly female phenotype or with ambiguous genitalia including perineoscrotal hypospadias. The defect is in 5α-reduction of testosterone to DHT. At puberty, spontaneous secondary sexual development occurs and the individual, raised as a girl until this age, in most cases converts to a male gender identity and male gender role. The interpretation of this change is controversial but is said by some to indicate that gender role, classically thought to be set by 2–4 years of age, can change much later in life. Others state that the child is recognized at birth as being different than a normal female and propose that the change in gender is less than complete from female to male.

Approach to the Infant with Genital Ambiguity

The major goal is a rapid identification of any life-threatening disorders (e.g., salt loss and shock caused by adrenal insufficiency). The decision of sex assignment is of great importance but is controversial because of the realization that prenatal androgen exposure (in an individual without complete androgen resistance) causes a tendency toward a male gender identity and male gender role. Although the classic approach to sex assignment has been based on the feasibility of genital reconstruction and potential fertility rather than on karyotype or gonadal histology, the effects of prenatal androgen must be considered. It may be inappropriate to raise a female infant who is severely virilized from virilizing congenital adrenal hyperplasia as a male; in most reported cases sex assignment and adult gender role remain female. If surgically corrected as a female, she will likely retain fertility because the internal organs are female. On the other hand, a 46,XY male with ambiguous genitalia and an extremely small phallus that will not increase in size with androgen therapy (partial androgen resistance) has classically been raised as a female because surgical construction of a fully functional phallus is very difficult. However, reported and anecdotal cases indicate that such patients frequently spontaneously revert to a male gender identity. Present management of ambiguous genitalia involves extensive open discussion with parents involving the biology of the infant and the likely prognosis. Treatment should be individualized and managed by an experienced pediatric endocrinologist.

Diagnosis. The first step toward diagnosis is to determine if the disorder represents virilization of a genetic female (androgen excess) or underdevelopment of a genetic male (androgen deficiency) (Fig. 17–8). Inguinal gonads that are evident on palpation usually are testes and indicate that incomplete development of a male phenotype has occurred; this pattern is not consistent, however, and ovaries and ovotestes may feel similar. Similarly, absence of female internal genitalia (detected by ultrasound) implies that müllerian-inhibiting substance was secreted by fetal testes. Karyotype determination, although helpful in diagnosis, is only one of many factors in deciding the sexual identity for purposes of rearing; the SRY gene may be found on chromosomes other than the Y chromosome and conversely, a Y chromosome may lack an SRY gene (it may have been translocated to an X chromosome, leading to the development of a 46,XX male).

Statistically, most virilized females have congenital adrenal hyperplasia, and 90% of those have 21-hydroxylase deficiency. The diagnosis is established by measuring the plasma concentration of 17-OHP (discussed in this chapter under Adrenal Gland), which typically is hundreds of times above the normal range. Other enzymatic defects also may be diagnosed by quantifying the circulating levels of the steroid that serves as the defective enzyme's substrate.

Accurate **diagnoses** are more difficult in underdeveloped males. When certain types of adrenal hyperplasia coexist with defects in androgen production of the testes, excessive ACTH secretion will elevate levels of specific adrenal steroid precursors substantially, allowing diagnosis. If the defect is restricted to testosterone biosynthesis, the measurement of testosterone and its precursors in the basal state and after stimulation by hCG may be required. Patients with normal levels of testosterone either have persistent androgen resistance (they will lack a response to exogenous testosterone) or have had an interruption of normal morphogenesis of the genitalia. Abnormalities of the sex chromosomes may be associated with dysgenetic gonads, which may be associated with persistence of müllerian structures.

Treatment. Treatment consists of replacing deficient hormones (e.g., cortisol in adrenal hyperplasia and testosterone to increase phallic size and facilitate puberty in a child with androgen biosynthetic defects who will be raised as male); surgical restoration to make the individual look more appropriate for the sex of rearing; and psychologic support of the whole family. Gonads and internal organs discordant for the sex of rearing are removed. Dysgenetic gonads should always be removed because gonadoblastomas or dysgerminomas may subsequently develop in the organ. Reconstructive surgery has usually been started by 2 years of age so that genital structure will reflect sex of rearing. This has itself become controversial; some advocate that the child should be involved in the decision about surgical reconstruction and sex of rearing, which would delay the decisions for years after birth.

REFERENCES

Behrman RE, Kliegman RM, Jenson HB, editors: *Nelson textbook of pediatrics,* ed 16, Philadelphia, 2000, WB Saunders, Chapters 592–598.

Griffin JE: Androgen resistance: the clinical and molecular spectrum, *N Engl J Med* 326(9):611–618, 1992.

Grumbach M, Conte F: Disorders of sexual differentiation. In Wilson J, Forest D, editors: *Williams textbook of endocrinology,* ed 8, Philadelphia, 1992, WB Saunders.

Styne DM: The testes: disorders of sexual differentiation and puberty. In Sperling MA, editor: *Pediatric endocrinology,* Philadelphia, 1996, WB Saunders.

Witchel SS, Lee PA: Ambiguous genitalia. In Sperling MA, editor: *Pediatric endocrinology,* Philadelphia, 1996, WB Saunders.

ADRENAL GLAND

The adrenal gland consists of an outer cortex, responsible for the synthesis of steroids, and an inner medulla derived from neuroectodermal tissue, which synthesizes catecholamines. The *adrenal cortex* consists of three zones: an outer glomerulosa whose end product is the mineralocorticoid aldosterone, which regulates sodium and potassium balance; a middle zone, the fasciculata, whose end product is cortisol; and an inner reticularis that synthesizes sex steroids. The general scheme of these synthetic steps is shown in Fig. 17–9.

The hypothalamic-pituitary-adrenal axis comprises a classic negative feedback system. Hypothalamic corticotropin-releasing hormone (CRH) stimulates the release of pituitary ACTH, derived by selective processing from pro-opiomelanocortin. ACTH governs the synthesis and release of cortisol and adrenal androgens. Primary adrenal insufficiency or cortisol deficiency from any defect in the adrenal gland results in an oversecretion of ACTH; cortisol deficiency also may occur from ACTH (secondary) or CRH (tertiary) deficiency, causing low serum ACTH concentrations as well as low cortisol. Endogenous (or exogenous) glucocorticoids feed back to inhibit ACTH and CRH secretion. The renin-angiotensin system, as well as potassium, regulates aldosterone secretion; ACTH has little effect on aldosterone production, except in excess, when it may increase aldosterone secretion.

Steroids that circulate in the free form (i.e., not bound to cortisol-binding protein [transcortin]) may cross the placenta from mother to fetus, but ACTH

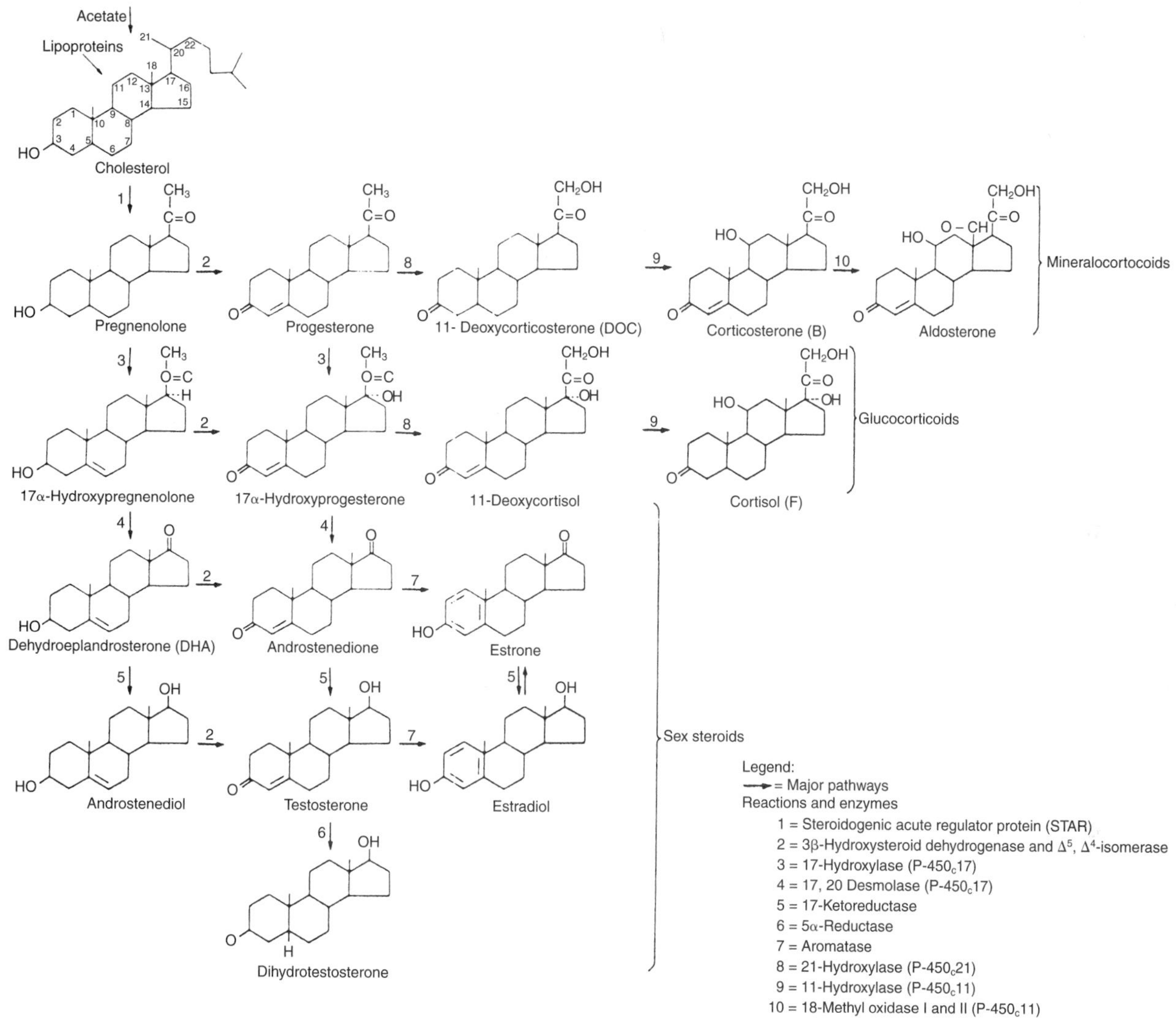

FIG. 17–9

Steroid hormone biosynthetic pathways. (From Styne DM: Sexual differentiation. In Fitzgerald PA, editor: *Handbook of clinical endocrinology*, Norwalk, Conn, 1986, Appleton & Lange.)

does not. The placenta plays an important role in steroid biosynthesis in utero, acting as a metabolic mediator between mother and child. Because the fetal CRH-ACTH-adrenal axis is operational in utero, deficiencies in cortisol synthesis lead to excessive ACTH secretion. If a virilizing adrenal enzyme defect is present, the fetal adrenal gland will secrete androgens, thus virilizing the fetus.

The normal variation of serum cortisol and ACTH levels leads to values that are high in early morning and lower at night. This normal diurnal variation may not be established until the end of the first to fourth year after birth.

Adrenal Insufficiency

The *clinical manifestations* of inadequate adrenal function result from the inadequate secretion or action of glucocorticoids, mineralocorticoids, or both (Table 17–19). In addition, in the case of enzyme defects that affect the gonad as well as the adrenal gland, overproduction or underproduction of potent androgens can occur, depending on the site of enzyme blockade (Fig. 17–9). Thus progressive virilization of the external genitalia may occur in females and males; incomplete virilization may occur in males. Ambiguity of the external genitalia is therefore a common manifestation of disordered

---

TABLE 17–19
Clinical Manifestations of Adrenal Insufficiency

Cortisol Deficiency	Aldosterone Deficiency—cont'd
Hypoglycemia	Salt craving
Inability to withstand stress	Acidosis
Vasomotor collapse	Failure to thrive
Hyperpigmentation (in primary adrenal insufficiency	Volume depletion
with excess of adrenocorticotropic hormone)	Hypotension
Apneic spells	Dehydration
Muscle weakness, fatigue	Shock
	Diarrhea
	Muscle weakness
Aldosterone Deficiency	
Hyponatremia	
Hyperkalemia	Androgen Excess or Deficiency (Caused by Adrenal
Vomiting	Enzyme Defect)
Urinary sodium wasting	Ambiguous genitalia in certain conditions

---

fetal adrenal enzyme function. Precise *diagnosis* is essential for the prescription of appropriate therapy, long-term outlook, and genetic counseling. Table 17–20 presents a diagnostic classification of adrenal insufficiency in infancy and childhood. In patients with enzyme defects, an elevation in the precursor steroid is present immediately proximal to the enzyme block, a deficiency of steroids is present subsequent to the block, and an excess of precursor is metabolized through remaining normal alternate enzyme pathways. These enzyme kinetics may be exploited in the diagnosis and treatment of congenital adrenal hyperplasia (Fig. 17–9).

The dominant clinical features of adrenal insufficiency in infancy are related to mineralocorticoid deficiency; these will develop only if there is impairment of mineralocorticoid secretion or action. Serum electrolyte measurement reveals hyponatremia and hyperkalemia usually developing by 5–7 days after birth but not, usually, immediately after birth. Vomiting, dehydration, and acidosis soon follow, as do shock and, if untreated, death. In females, ambiguous genitalia resulting from excessive androgen secretion may be caused by salt-losing congenital adrenal hyperplasia and, therefore, the ambiguous genitalia are a major clue to the presence of mineralocorticoid deficiency. All presentations of ambiguous genitalia should involve evaluation for mineralocorticoid deficiency. In males, the diagnosis of adrenal insufficiency may be overlooked or confused with pyloric stenosis. The most common form of congenital adrenal hyperplasia (CAH), 21-hydroxylase deficiency, does not cause abnormal genitalia in boys so there is no physical clue to salt loss as in girls. However, in pyloric stenosis, in contrast to salt-losing CAH, vomiting hydrochloric acid in stomach contents results in hypochloremia, serum potassium is normal or low, and alkalosis is present. This distinction may be lifesaving in preventing unnecessary investigations or inappropriate therapy.

In patients with congenital adrenal hypoplasia or adrenal hemorrhage, the secretion of all adrenal steroids will be low. In contrast, CAH leads to a diagnostic steroid pattern in blood and urine (Fig. 17–9). Deficiency of 21-hydroxylase is the most common form (95%) and serves as a paradigm for these disorders.

21-Hydroxylase Deficiency

The incidence of classical 21-hydroxylase deficiency is about 1:12,000 among various Caucasian populations. A higher incidence occurs in Yupic Eskimos, Yugoslavians, and Ashkenazi Jews. Nonclassical congenital adrenal hyperplasia may occur with an incidence of 1:50 in certain populations. Two genes on chromosome 6 code for 21-hydroxylase; if there is an affected proband, the genotype may be determined, permitting prenatal diagnosis in a subsequent pregnancy.

Deficient 21-hydroxylase activity (P-450$_{c21}$ deficiency) results in the decreased conversion of 17-OHP to 11-desoxycortisol and, in the salt-losing form, of progesterone to desoxycorticosterone, a mineralocorticoid proximal in the pathway to the production of aldosterone (Fig. 17–9). The obligatory decreased production of cortisol causes hypersecretion of ACTH, which, in turn, stimulates the synthesis of

TABLE 17–20
Causes of Adrenal Insufficiency in Infancy and Childhood

Congenital Adrenal Hypoplasia
Secondary to ACTH deficiency
Autosomal recessive
X-linked

Adrenal Hemorrhage, Necrosis, Thrombosis

Congenital Adrenal Hyperplasia
STAR deficiency
3β-Hydroxysteroid dehydrogenase deficiency
P-450$_{c21}$ (21-hydroxylase) deficiency
P-450$_{c11}$ (11β-hydroxylase) deficiency
P-450$_{c17}$ (17-hydroxylase) deficiency

Isolated Deficiency of Aldosterone Synthesis
P-450$_{c11}$ (18-hydroxylase) deficiency
P-450$_{c11}$ (18-hydroxysteroid dehydrogenase) deficiency

Pseudohypoaldosteronism—End-Organ
Unresponsiveness to Aldosterone

Congenital Adrenal Unresponsiveness to ACTH

Addison Disease
Autoimmune adrenal insufficiency*
Infections of the adrenal gland
  Tuberculosis
  Histoplasmosis
  Meningococcosis

Addison Disease—cont'd
Infiltration of the adrenal gland
  Sarcoidosis
  Hemochromatosis
  Amyloidosis
  Metastatic cancer, lymphoma
Adrenoleukodystrophy

Secondary—Pituitary-Hypothalamic
Craniopharyngioma
Histiocytosis
Empty sella syndrome
Pituitary irradiation
Sarcoidosis
Hypothalamic lesions
Postpartum pituitary necrosis
Head trauma

Drugs (Suppress Adrenal Steroidogenesis)
Acute withdrawal of steroid therapy given for more
  than 7–10 days
Metyrapone
Ketoconazole

ACTH, Adrenocorticotropic hormone.
*Isolated or as part of polyglandular syndrome type I (adrenal, hypoparathyroidism, mucocutaneous candidiasis) or type II (adrenal, thyroid, insulin-dependent diabetes).

steroids immediately proximal to the block and causes shunting of precursors to the androgen pathway, leading to the overproduction of testosterone. The latter results in many of the *clinical manifestations*. Virilization of the external genitalia of the female occurs in utero; the development of the ovaries, fallopian tubes, and uterus is unaffected. The degree of virilization in the external genitalia of the female is variable, ranging from mild clitoromegaly to complete fusion of labioscrotal folds, simulating a phallus (discussed in this chapter under Disorders of Sexual Differentiation). A male infant with this defect appears normal at birth, although penile enlargement may be apparent thereafter. The deficiency in aldosterone found in about 75% of patients causes salt wasting with shock and dehydration unless appropriate treatment is given.

Inadequately treated, P-450$_{c21}$ deficiency (assuming salt loss does not lead to serious complications) demonstrates postnatal virilization, causing excessive growth, early appearance of pubic hair, and progressive penile or clitoral enlargement. Although there is excessive linear growth initially, progressive advancement in the bone age is accompanied by early epiphyseal fusion, ultimately yielding short adult stature. Nonclassical P-450$_{c21}$ deficiency is noted years after birth, and affected subjects have milder manifestations without ambiguous genitalia, but they do have acne, hirsutism, and, in girls, irregular menstrual periods or amenorrhea. Late-onset

CAH in girls may be confused with ovarian hyperandrogenism polycystic ovarian disease.

Biochemical diagnostic studies demonstrate elevated levels of serum 17-OHP, the substrate for the defective P-450$_{c21}$ enzyme activity. In newborn infants with CAH the values are hundreds to thousands fold elevated, but in the nonclassical form, an ACTH stimulation test will be necessary to demonstrate an abnormally high response of 17 OHP. Serum cortisol and aldosterone levels (in salt losers) are low, whereas the level of testosterone is elevated, as it is derived from 17-OHP.

The **goals of** *treatment* are to achieve normal linear growth and bone age advancement. Chronic therapy consists of providing glucocorticoids at a dose of approximately 13–18 mg/m^2/24 hr of hydrocortisone or its equivalent. Mineralocorticoid therapy for salt losers consists of 9α-fludrocortisone (Florinef) at a dose of 0.1–0.2 mg/24 hr often with sodium chloride supplementation. Surgical correction of ambiguous external genitalia begins by 1 year of life to permit normal development of gender identity. The adequacy of glucocorticoid replacement therapy is often monitored by determining serum concentrations of adrenal metabolites, but the assessment of linear growth and skeletal age is the best reflection of appropriate therapy. To avoid adrenal insufficiency, threefold higher doses of glucocorticoids are given during stressful states, such as febrile illnesses and surgery, and subcutaneous glucocorticoid (Solu-Cortef) is used in severe emergencies. Mineralocorticoid therapy is monitored with serum sodium and potassium and plasma renin activity levels. Prenatal treatment with dexamethasone to suppress fetal ACTH-induced androgen production has been reported as successful in eliminating ambiguous genitalia in affected female fetuses, if begun at approximately the seventh week of gestation.

Other Enzyme Defects

The other enzyme defects are rare in contrast to 21-OH deficiency.

In **11-OH deficiency,** the next most common cause of CAH, virilization occurs with salt retention and hypokalemia, as a result of the buildup of desoxycorticosterone (Fig. 17–9), a potent mineralocorticoid. Hypertension develops as a result of excessive mineralocorticoid production.

A summary of the clinical and biochemical features of adrenal insufficiency in infancy is listed in Table 17–21.

Addison Disease

Addison disease is a rare acquired disorder of childhood, usually associated with autoimmune destruction of the adrenal cortex. It is a form of primary adrenal insufficiency, and there is absence of both glucocorticoid and mineralocorticoid. *Clinical manifestations* are hyperpigmentation, salt craving, postural hypotension, fasting hypoglycemia, and episodes of shock during severe illness. Baseline and ACTH-stimulated cortisol values are subnormal, thereby confirming the diagnosis; hyponatremia, hyperkalemia, and elevated plasma renin activity indicate mineralocorticoid deficiency. Associated autoimmune disorders include diabetes mellitus, thyroiditis, oophoritis, pernicious anemia and malabsorption, chronic hepatitis, vitiligo, alopecia, and mucocutaneous candidiasis (Table 17–20).

Replacement *treatment* with 13–18 mg/m^2/24 hr of hydrocortisone is indicated, with supplementation during stress at three times the normal maintenance dosage or the use of subcutaneous glucocorticoid (see above for CAH). The dose is titrated to allow a normal growth rate. Mineralocorticoid replacement with fludrocortisone is monitored by plasma renin activity and serum sodium and potassium determinations.

Cushing Syndrome

Classic *clinical manifestations* of Cushing syndrome in children include progressive central obesity, marked failure of longitudinal growth, hirsutism, weakness, a nuchal fat pad (buffalo hump), acne, striae, hypertension, and often hyperpigmentation (if ACTH is elevated). The etiology can be exogenous glucocorticoid administration or endogenous causes including adrenal adenoma, carcinoma, nodular adrenal hyperplasia, an ACTH-secreting pituitary microadenoma, resulting in bilateral adrenal hyperplasia (Cushing disease), or a very rare ACTH-secreting tumor. The high-dose dexamethasone suppression test (20 μg/kg orally every 6 hours for 48 hours) suppresses glucocorticoid secretion in Cushing disease but not in autonomous adrenal production of cortisol or in an ectopic ACTH-secreting tumor. Parenteral glucocorticoid therapy is necessary during and immediately after surgical treatment to remove the source of the excess glucocorticoids in order to avoid acute adrenal insufficiency.

Spontaneous Cushing syndrome is rare in childhood. Iatrogenic Cushing syndrome is far more common, produces similar clinical manifestations, and may be induced by the use of potent glucocorticoids for chronic inflammatory, neoplastic, and collagenvascular disorders and for suppression of the immune response. Depending on the potency of glucocorticoid used and its duration of use, both adrenal gland size and secretory ability and pituitary ACTH production and secretion are suppressed. Recovery of pituitary ACTH secretion precedes that of adrenal gland function. Hence, glucocorticoids should be

TABLE 17–21
Clinical and Biochemical Features in Newborn Adrenal Insufficiency

	Ambiguous Genitalia		Electrolyte Disturbance*	Serum					Urine		
	Virilized Female	Undervirilized Male		Cortisol	11-Deoxycortisol	17-OHP	DHEA	Aldosterone	17-OHCS	17-KS	Pregnanetriol
Hypoplasia	No	No	Severe	D	D	D	D	D	D	D	D
Hemorrhage	No	No	Moderate to severe	D	D	D	D	D	D	D	D
STAR deficiency	No	Yes	Severe	D	D	D	D	D	D	D	D
3β-HSD	Yes	Yes	Severe	D	D	D	I	D	D	I	D
P-450$_{c21}$ deficiency	Yes	No	Absent to severe	D	D	I	I	D	D	I	I
Aldosterone synthesis block	No	No	Severe	Nl	Nl	Nl	Nl	D	Nl	Nl	Nl
Pseudohypoaldosteronism	No	No	Severe	Nl	Nl	Nl	Nl	I	Nl	Nl	Nl
P-450$_{c11}$ deficiency	Yes	No	None	D	I	Nl or I	Nl	D	I	I	Nl–sl I
P-450$_{c17}$ deficiency	No	Yes	†	D	Nl–D	D	D	Nl–D	D	D	D
Unresponsiveness to ACTH	No	No	†	D	Nl–D	Nl–D	Nl–D	Nl–D	D	D	Nl–D

ACTH, Adrenocorticotropic hormone; *D,* decrease; *HSD,* hydroxysteroid dehydrogenase; *I,* increase; *Nl,* normal; *17-KS,* 17-ketosteroid; *17-OHCS,* 17-hydroxycorticosteroid.
*Usually manifested after 5 days of age.
†High normal Na$^+$ and low normal to low K$^+$.

withdrawn gradually over a number of weeks rather than cut abruptly when phasing out chronic treatment. During this tapering process, any emergency requires glucocorticoid therapy at triple the physiologic dose. The ability of the adrenal gland to respond to ACTH with a doubling of plasma cortisol to levels of at least 15–20 μg/dL indicates recovery of pituitary-adrenal function.

Treatment of Cushing syndrome is directed to the etiology. This may include excision of autonomous adrenal, pituitary, or ectopic ACTH-secreting tumors. Rarely, adrenalectomy or adrenal ablative agents (mitotane-*o,p'*-DDD) are needed to control the symptoms.

REFERENCES

Behrman RE, Kliegman RM, Jenson HB, editors: *Nelson textbook of pediatrics,* ed 16, Philadelphia, 2000, WB Saunders, Chapters 584–591.

Miller WL: Pathophysiology, genetics and treatment of hyperandrogenism, *Pediatr Clin North Am* 44(2):375–395, 1997.

Oelkers W: Adrenal insufficiency, *N Engl J Med* 335(16):1206–1212, 1996.

Saenger P: New developments in side-chain cleavage enzyme deficiency and StAR protein, *Pediatr Clin North Am* 44(2):397–421, 1997.

Speiser PW, New MI: Prenatal diagnosis and treatment of congenital adrenal hyperplasia, *J Pediatr Endocrinol* 7(3):183–191, 1994.

BONE AND MINERAL ENDOCRINOLOGY
Parathyroid Hormone and Vitamin D

(See Chapter 2)

Calcium and phosphate are regulated mainly by diet and three hormones: parathyroid hormone (PTH), vitamin D, and calcitonin. These hormones maintain plasma ionized calcium levels in the normal range. PTH is secreted in response to a decrease in serum ionized calcium level. It attaches to its membrane receptor and then acts via adenylate cyclase to mobilize calcium from bone into the serum and to enhance fractional reabsorption of calcium by the kidney while inducing phosphate excretion, all of which help to raise the serum calcium concentration and decrease serum phosphate. Lack of PTH effect is heralded by low serum Ca in the presence or elevated PO_4 for age. Because PTH increases renal 1-α-hydroxylase activity, it also acts indirectly to elevate serum calcium concentration by stimulating the production of 1,25-dihydroxyvitamin D from 25-hydroxyvitamin D. Calcitonin increases the deposition of Ca into bone; in normal states the effect is subtle, but calcitonin may be used to suppress extremely elevated serum Ca values.

1,25-Dihydroxyvitamin D enhances calcium absorption from the gastrointestinal tract, resulting in increased serum calcium levels and increased bone mineralization. Vitamin D derived from exposure of the skin to ultraviolet rays (usually via the sun) or ingestion must be sequentially modified first to 25-hydroxyvitamin D in the liver and then 1α-hydroxylated to the metabolically active form (1,25-dihydroxyvitamin D) in the kidney. The serum concentration of 25-hydroxyvitamin D is a better reflection of vitamin D sufficiency than the measurement of 1,25-hydroxyvitamin D.

Hypocalcemia

The *clinical manifestations* of hypocalcemia (ionized calcium <4.5 mg/dL; total calcium <8.5 mg/dL if serum protein is normal) result from increased neuromuscular irritability and include muscle cramps, carpopedal spasm (tetany), weakness, paresthesia, laryngospasm, or seizure-like activity (patient is often awake and aware during these episodes in contrast to many episodes of epilepsy). Latent tetany can be detected by the *Chvostek sign* (facial spasms are produced by lightly tapping over the facial nerve just in front of the ear) or by the *Trousseau sign* (carpal spasms are demonstrated when arterial blood flow to the hand is occluded for 3–5 min with a blood pressure cuff inflated to 15 mm Hg above systolic blood pressure). Total serum calcium concentration is usually measured, even though a determination of serum ionized calcium (~half the total Ca in normal circumstances), the biologically active form, is preferable. Albumin is the major reservoir of protein-bound calcium. Therefore, disorders that alter plasma pH or serum albumin concentration must be considered when circulating calcium concentrations are being evaluated. The fraction of ionized calcium is inversely related to plasma pH; *alkalosis* can precipitate hypocalcemia by lowering ionized calcium without changing total serum calcium. Alkalosis may result from hyperpnea caused by anxiety or from hyperventilation related to physical exertion. Hypoproteinemia may lead to a false suggestion of hypocalcemia, as the serum total calcium level is low even though the ionized Ca^{++} remains normal. Therefore, it is best to measure serum ionized calcium if hypocalcemia or hypercalcemia is suspected.

Primary hypoparathyroidism causes hypocalcemia but does not cause rickets. The etiology of primary hypoparathyroidism may be as follows:

1. Congenital malformation (e.g., the DiGeorge syndrome) resulting from developmental abnormalities of the third and fourth brachial arches, leading to hypoparathyroidism and mandibular hypoplasia, hypertelorism, short philtrum, low-set and malformed ears, and malformations of the heart and great vessels such as ventricular and

atrial septal defects, right aortic arch, interrupted aortic arch, and truncus arteriosus (see Chapters 8 and 13)

2. Surgical procedures such as thyroidectomy or parathyroidectomy, in which parathyroid tissue is removed either deliberately or as a complication of surgery for another goal

3. Autoimmunity, which may destroy the parathyroid gland

Pseudohypoparathyroidism may occur in one of three forms:

1. Type Ia: an abnormality of the Gsα-protein linking the PTH receptor to adenyl cyclase; biologically active PTH is secreted in great quantities but exerts no effect, since there is no way for PTH to stimulate its receptor

2. Type Ib: normal Gsα with other abnormalities in the production of adenyl cyclase

3. Type II: normal production of adenyl cyclase but a distal defect eliminates the effects of PTH

Pseudohypoparathyroidism is an autosomal dominant condition that may present at birth or later. Other *clinical manifestations* of pseudohypoparathyroidism associated with **Albright hereditary osteodystrophy** (AHO) include short stature, stocky body habitus, round facies, short fourth and fifth metacarpals, calcification of the basal ganglia, subcutaneous calcification, and often developmental delay. AHO may be inherited separately from pseudohypoparathyroidism, so that a patient may have a normal appearance with hypocalcemia or may have the AHO phenotype with normal serum Ca, PO$_4$, PTH, and response to PTH (pseudopseudohypoparathyroidism).

During the first 3 days after birth, serum calcium concentrations normally decline in response to withdrawal of the maternal calcium supply via the placenta. Sluggish PTH response in the neonate may result in a transient hypocalcemia. Hypocalcemia caused by attenuated PTH release is found in infants of mothers with hyperparathyroidism and hypercalcemia; the latter suppresses fetal PTH release, thereby causing **transient hypoparathyroidism** in the neonatal period.

Normal serum magnesium concentrations also are required for normal parathyroid gland function and action. Thus **hypomagnesemia** may cause a secondary hypoparathyroidism that will respond poorly to therapies other than magnesium replacement.

Neonatal tetany resulting from excessive phosphate consumption classically occurs in the 1-week-old to 1-month-old infant who is fed cow's milk. The resultant hyperphosphatemia drives down the serum calcium level, causing symptomatic hypocalcemia (see Chapter 6). Cow's milk contains more calcium than human milk but also has more phosphorus. Excessive phosphate retention, as occurs in patients with renal failure, also produces hypocalcemia.

The **etiology of hypocalcemia** usually can be discerned by combining features of the clinical presentation with determinations of serum ionized calcium, phosphate, alkaline phosphatase, PTH (preferably at a time when the calcium is low), magnesium, and albumin. X-rays of the long bones and hands and knees are important if the problem occurs after the neonatal period. If the PTH concentration is not elevated appropriately relevant to a low serum Ca, hypoparathyroidism (transient, primary, or caused by hypomagnesemia) is present. Vitamin D stores can be estimated by measuring serum 25-hydroxyvitamin D and renal function assessed by a serum creatinine measurement or determination of creatinine clearance (Table 17–22).

Treatment of severe tetany or seizures resulting from hypocalcemia consists of intravenous calcium gluconate (1–2 mL/kg of 10% solution) given slowly over 10 minutes while cardiac status is monitored by EKG for bradycardia, which can be fatal. Chronic treatment of hypoparathyroidism involves administering vitamin D, preferably in the form of 1,25-dihydroxyvitamin D, and calcium. Therapy is adjusted to keep the serum calcium in the lower half of

TABLE 17–22
Important Physiologic Changes in Bone and Mineral Diseases

Condition	Calcium	Phosphate	Parathyroid Hormone	25(OH)D
Primary hypoparathyroidism	↓	↑	↓	Nl
Pseudohypoparathyroidism	↓	↑	↑	Nl
Vitamin D deficiency	Nl(↓)	↓	↑	↓
Familial hypophosphatemic rickets	Nl	↓	Nl (sl↑)	Nl
Hyperparathyroidism	↑	↓	↑	Nl
Immobilization	↑	↑	↓	Nl

Nl, Normal; *sl*, slight; ↑, high; ↓, low; *25(OH)D*, 25-hydroxyvitamin D.

the normal range to avoid episodes of hypercalcemia that might produce nephrocalcinosis and pancreatitis.

Rickets

(See Chapter 2)

Rickets is defined as decreased or defective bone mineralization in growing children; **osteomalacia** is the same condition in adults. The proportion of osteoid (the organic portion of the bone) is excessive. As a result, the bone becomes soft, and the metaphyses of the long bones widen. Poor linear growth, bowing of the legs on weight bearing (often painful), thickening at the wrists and knees, and prominence of the costochondral junctions (rachitic rosary) of the rib cage occur. At this stage, the x-ray findings are diagnostic.

In **nutritional vitamin D deficiency,** calcium is not adequately absorbed from the intestine (see Chapter 2). Poor vitamin D intake (food fads or poor maternal diet, both affecting breast milk vitamin D) or avoidance of sunlight also may contribute to the development of rickets. Fat malabsorption resulting from hepatobiliary disease (biliary atresia, neonatal hepatitis) or other causes also may produce vitamin D deficiency because vitamin D is a fat-soluble vitamin. Defects in vitamin D metabolism by the kidney (renal failure, autosomal recessive deficiency of 1α-hydroxylation, **vitamin D–dependent rickets)** or liver (defect in 25-hydroxylation) also can cause rickets. Very-low-birth-weight infants have an increased incidence of rickets of prematurity (see Chapter 6).

In **familial hypophosphatemic rickets,** the major defect in mineral metabolism is failure of the kidney to resorb filtered phosphate adequately so that serum phosphate decreases and urinary phosphate is high. The *diagnosis* of this X-linked disease usually is made within the first few years of life and typically is more severe in males. This may be the most common cause of rickets in the United States.

The *etiology* of rickets usually can be determined by assessment of the mineral and vitamin D (25-hydroxyvitamin D <8 ng/mL suggests nutritional vitamin D deficiency) status as outlined for the different disorders (Table 17–22). Further testing of mineral balance or measurement of other vitamin D metabolites may be required in more difficult cases.

Several chemical forms of vitamin D can be used for *treatment* of the different rachitic conditions, but their potencies vary widely and required dosages depend on the condition being treated (see Chapters 2 and 16). Rickets is usually treated with 1,25-hydroxyvitamin D and supplemental calcium. In hypophosphatemic rickets, phosphate supplementation (not calcium) must accompany vitamin D therapy, which is given to suppress secondary hyperparathyroidism. Adequate therapy restores normal skeletal growth and produces resolution of the roentgenographic signs of rickets. Nutritional rickets is treated with vitamin D in one large dose or multiple smaller replacement doses. Surgery may be required to straighten legs in long-standing untreated patients.

Hypercalcemia

Hypercalcemia is rare in children. Symptoms include mental disturbances, anorexia, constipation, lethargy, vomiting, weakness, and polyuria. With time, uncontrolled chronic hypercalcemia usually will produce pancreatitis or nephrolithiasis, renal insufficiency, or both. There are many causes of hypercalcemia, including hyperparathyroidism, immobilization (body casts), hypervitaminosis D (food faddism or incorrectly prepared commercial formula), fat necrosis, maternal hypoparathyroidism with subsequent fetal hypocalcemia stimulating fetal PTH production, autosomal dominant–familial hypocalciuric hypercalcemia, Williams syndrome, and malignancy. MEN type I combines hyperparathyroidism with pituitary adenomas. MEN type II is associated with medullary carcinoma of the thyroid, parathyroid adenomas, and pheochromocytoma; the hyperparathyroidism initially arises to combat hypocalcemia caused by calcitonin secretion and then becomes autonomous.

REFERENCES

Behrman, RE, Kliegman RM, Jenson HB, editors: *Nelson textbook of pediatrics,* ed 16, Philadelphia, 2000, WB Saunders, Chapters 580–583.

Carpenter TO: New perspectives on the biology and treatment of X-linked hypophosphatemic rickets, *Pediatr Clin North Am* 44(2):443–446, 1997.

Feinmesser R, Lubin E, Segal K, et al: Carcinoma of the thyroid in children: a review, *J Pediatr Endocrinol Metab* 10(6):561–568, 1997.

Glorieux FH: Rickets, the continuing challenge, *N Engl J Med* 325(26):1875–1877, 1991.

Guise TA, Mundy GR: Clinical review 69: evaluation of hypocalcemia in children and adults, *J Clin Endocrinol Metab* 80(5):1473–1478, 1995.

Lteif AN, Zimmerman D: Bisphosphonates for treatment of childhood hypercalcemia, *Pediatrics* 102(4 Pt 1):990–993, 1998.

Mimouni FB, Root AW: Disorders of calcium metabolism in the newborn. In Sperling MA: *Pediatric endocrinology,* Philadelphia, 2000, WB Saunders.

DIABETES MELLITUS

Diabetes mellitus is characterized by hyperglycemia and glycosuria and occurs as a common end point of many disease processes (Table 17–23). The most common type occurring in childhood is **type I diabetes mellitus (DM1),** which is caused by autoimmune destruction of the pancreas. Patients with DM1 have severe and usually permanent insulin deficiency and require insulin for survival and prevention of life-threatening episodes of ketoacidosis. **Type 2 diabetes mellitus** (DM2) is less common in children. Individuals with DM2 are not dependent on insulin for survival, but they may require insulin to achieve adequate glycemic control. DM2 most commonly results from insulin resistance, with inability of the pancreas to maintain adequate compensatory hyperinsulinemia. Less common subtypes of DM2 result from genetic defects of the insulin receptor or inherited abnormalities in sensing of ambient glucose concentration by pancreatic beta cells (Table 17–23).

Definition

A *diagnosis* of diabetes mellitus can be made if a fasting serum glucose concentration is greater than 126 mg/dL or a 2-hour postprandial serum glucose concentration is greater than 200 mg/dL on two separate occasions. A patient is considered *glucose intolerant* if fasting serum glucose concentrations are greater than 110 mg/dL but less than 126 mg/dL and if 2-hour postprandial values are greater than 140 mg/dL but less than 200 mg/dL. Sporadic **hyperglycemia** occurs in children, usually in the setting of an intercurrent illness. When the hyperglycemic episode is clearly related to an illness or other physiologic stress, the probability that this represents incipient diabetes is small (<5%). Sporadic hyperglycemia occurring without a clear precipitating physiologic stress, however, is of more concern, as diabetes eventually develops in at least 30%.

Insulin-Dependent (Type 1) Diabetes Mellitus

Epidemiology. DM1 is the most common pediatric endocrine disorder, affecting approximately 1 in 300–500 children under 18 years of age. Different ethnic populations vary in their susceptibility to diabetes. The annual incidence in children ranges from a high of 30:100,000 among Scandinavian populations to a low of 1:100,000 in Japan. In the United States, the annual incidence is approximately 15:100,000. The prevalence of DM1 in the United States is highest among Caucasian Americans and is lower among African Americans and Hispanic Americans.

TABLE 17–23
Classification of Diabetes Mellitus in Children and Adolescents

Type	Comment
Type 1 (Insulin-Dependent)	
Transient neonatal	Presents immediately after birth; lasts 1–3 mo
Permanent neonatal	Other pancreatic defects possible
Classic type I	Glycosuria, ketonuria, hyperglycemia, islet cell antibody to glutamic acid decarboxylase positive; definite genetic component
Type 2 (Non-Insulin-Dependent)	
Secondary	Cystic fibrosis, hemochromatosis, drugs (e.g., L-asparaginase)
Adult type (classic)	Associated with obesity, insulin resistance; definite genetic component
Maturity onset diabetes of youth (MODY)	Autosomal dominant, onset before 25 years of age; not associated with obesity or autoimmunity; single gene mutations include: hepatocytic nuclear factors 1-beta, 1-alpha, 4-alpha; glucokinase; insulin promoter factor 1
Mitochondrial diabetes	Associated with deafness and other neurologic defects, maternal transmission—mtDNA point mutations
Other	
Gestational diabetes	Abnormal glucose tolerance only during pregnancy, which reverts to normal post partum; increased risk for later onset of diabetes

GCK, Glucokinase; *MODY,* maturity-onset diabetes of youth; *mtDNA,* mitochondrial deoxyribonucleic acid; *TCF,* transcription factor.

Genetic determinants play a role in the suscepti-bility to DM1, although the mode of inheritance is complex and likely multigenic. Siblings or offspring of patients with diabetes have a risk of 3–6% for de-velopment of diabetes; an identical twin has a 30–50% risk. Genetic factors do not fully account for suscepti-bility to DM1; environmental factors also play a role.

The association of DM1 susceptibility with the human leukocyte antigen (HLA) region on chromo-some 6 is the strongest determinant of susceptibility, accounting for approximately 40% of the familial in-heritance of DM1. Specific HLA alleles (HLA DR3 and DR4) have been determined to increase the risk of developing DM1, whereas other specific HLA al-leles have been found to exert a protective effect. More than 90% of children with DM1 possess HLA DR3, DR4 alleles, or both. The insulin gene region V on chromosome 11 has also been linked to DM1 sus-ceptibility, and there is some evidence for associa-tion of at least 18 other loci with DM1.

Etiology. In addition to the presence of diabetes susceptibility genes, an environmental insult must occur to trigger autoimmune destruction of the islet cells. The nature of this environmental insult, how-ever, is unknown. Scandinavian studies have sug-gested an increased incidence of DM1 in children ex-posed to cow's milk before 2 years of age. These studies lead to theories that cross-reactivity of anti-bodies to bovine serum albumin (BSA) with islet cell antigens might be involved. Viral infectious agents have possibly been implicated, including coxsackie

B virus, cytomegalovirus (CMV), mumps, and rubella. Potential mechanisms for viral initiation of the autoimmune response include direct beta cell damage through viral infection, antibody cross-reac-tivity, and polyclonal activation of B lymphocytes.

Antibodies to islet cell antigens can be demon-strated in the sera of susceptible individuals months to years before the onset of beta cell dysfunction and most likely indicate an ongoing destructive process (Fig. 17–10). A number of different antibodies to beta cell antigens can be detected, including islet cell an-tibodies (ICA), insulin autoantibodies (IAA), and an-tibodies to glutamic acid decarboxylase (GAD). Studies of family members of patients with DM1 have shown that the risk for diabetes increases with the number of antibodies detected in the serum. In individuals with only one detectable antibody, the risk is only 10–15%; in individuals with three or more antibodies, the risk is 55–90%.

Once initiated, the autoimmune destructive pro-cess is thought to continue until 80–90% of the beta cell mass has been destroyed. At that point, the re-maining beta cell mass is insufficient to maintain glycemic control and clinical manifestations of dia-betes result (Fig. 17–10).

Clinical Manifestations. When insulin secretory ca-pacity becomes inadequate to support peripheral glucose uptake and to suppress hepatic glucose pro-duction, hyperglycemia results. The initial manifes-tation of insulin deficiency is postprandial hyper-glycemia. Fasting hyperglycemia then develops.

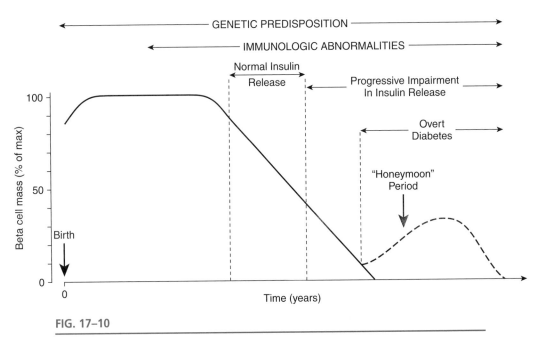

FIG. 17–10

Schematic representation of the autoimmune evolution of diabetes in genetically predisposed individuals.

Ketogenesis is a sign of severe insulin deficiency. Lack of suppression of gluconeogenesis, glycogenolysis, and fatty acid oxidation contributes to the hyperglycemia and results in the generation of ketone bodies (acetoacetate and beta-hydroxybutyrate) and acetone. Protein stores in muscle and fat stores in adipose tissue are broken down to provide substrates for gluconeogenesis and fatty acid oxidation.

Glycosuria occurs when the serum glucose concentration exceeds the renal threshold for glucose reabsorption (at approximately 180 mg/dL). Glycosuria causes an osmotic diuresis (including obligate loss of sodium, potassium, and water), leading to dehydration. Polydipsia occurs as the patient attempts to compensate for the excess fluid losses. Weight loss results from the persistent catabolic state, as well as the loss of ingested calories through glycosuria and ketonuria. The classic presentation of DM1 includes polyuria, polydipsia, polyphagia, and weight loss.

Diabetic Ketoacidosis. If the clinical features of DM1 are not detected early, diabetic ketoacidosis (DKA) can occur. DKA can also occur in patients with known diabetes if insulin injections are omitted or during periods of intercurrent illness when insulin requirements are increased as a result of elevated concentrations of the counterregulatory hormones, glucagon, cortisol, and catecholamines. In the setting of hyperglycemia, DKA can be considered to be present if (1) the arterial pH is less than 7.25, (2) the serum bicarbonate level is less than 15 mEq/L, and (3) ketones are detected in serum or urine.

Pathophysiology. In the absence of adequate insulin secretion, persistent partial hepatic oxidation of fatty acids to ketone bodies occurs. An excess of these organic acids results in a metabolic acidosis with an elevated anion gap. Lactic acidosis can also contribute when severe dehydration results in decreased tissue perfusion. Hyperglycemia causes an osmotic diuresis that is initially compensated for by increased fluid intake. As the hyperglycemia and diuresis worsen, most patients are unable to maintain the large fluid intake required and dehydration occurs. Vomiting as a result of intestinal ileus and increased insensible losses caused by tachypnea worsen the state of dehydration. Electrolyte abnormalities occur secondary to loss of electrolytes in the urine and transmembrane alterations resulting from acidosis. As hydrogen ions accumulate as a result of ketoacidosis, exchange of hydrogen ions for intracellular potassium occurs. Serum concentrations of potassium rise initially, then decrease as excess serum potassium is cleared by the kidney. Depending on the duration of ketoacidosis, serum potassium concentrations at diagnosis may be increased, normal, or decreased, but intracellular potassium concentrations are depleted. Phosphate depletion can also occur as a result of the increased renal phosphate excretion required for elimination of excess hydrogen ions. Sodium depletion is also common in DKA, resulting from renal losses of sodium caused by osmotic diuresis and vomiting (Fig. 17–11).

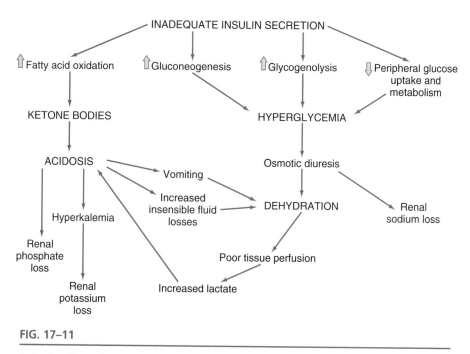

FIG. 17–11

Pathophysiology of diabetic ketoacidosis.

Presentation. Patients with DKA present initially with a history of polyuria, polydipsia, and nausea and vomiting. Abdominal pain occurs frequently and can mimic an acute abdomen. The presence of polyuria, despite a state of clinical dehydration, is indicative of osmotic diuresis and differentiates patients with DKA from those with gastroenteritis or other gastrointestinal disorders. Respiratory compensation for acidosis results in tachypnea with deep (Kussmaul) respirations. The "fruity" odor of acetone can frequently be detected on the patient's breath. The abdomen may be distended secondary to paralytic ileus. An altered mental status can occur, ranging from disorientation to coma. Signs of dehydration may be minimal because increased serum osmolality results in preservation of intravascular volume.

Laboratory studies reveal hyperglycemia, with serum glucose concentrations ranging from 200 mg/dL to greater than 1000 mg/dL. Arterial pH is less than 7.25, and the serum bicarbonate concentration is less than 15 mEq/L. Serum sodium concentrations may be elevated, normal, or low, depending on the balance of sodium and free water losses. The measured serum sodium concentration, however, is artificially depressed because of hyperglycemia. A "corrected" sodium concentration can be calculated according to the following formula:

Corrected sodium concentration = Measured sodium concentration + [1.6 × (Serum glucose concentration − 150)/100]

Hyperlipidemia can also contribute to the decrease in measured serum sodium. Potassium concentrations may be elevated, normal, or low, depending on the duration of DKA. The level of blood urea nitrogen (BUN) can be elevated with prerenal azotemia secondary to dehydration. The white blood cell count is usually elevated and can be left-shifted in the absence of infection. Fever, however, is unusual and should prompt a search for infectious sources that may have triggered the episode of DKA.

Treatment. Therapy for patients with DKA involves careful replacement of fluid deficits, correction of acidosis and hyperglycemia via insulin administration, correction of electrolyte imbalances, and monitoring for complications of treatment. The optimal approach to management of DKA is controversial, since the cause of the most serious complication—cerebral edema—is unknown. Therapeutic strategies must strike a balance between adequate correction of fluid losses to avoid complications of severe dehydration and avoidance of rapid shifts in osmolality and fluid balance.

Dehydration. The patient presenting in DKA can be assumed to be approximately 10% dehydrated. If a recent weight measurement is available, the precise extent of dehydration can be calculated. An initial intravenous fluid bolus of a glucose-free isotonic solution (normal saline, lactated Ringer's) at 10–20 mL/kg should be given to restore intravascular volume and renal perfusion. The remaining fluid deficit after the initial bolus should be added to maintenance fluid requirements, and the total should be replaced slowly over 36–48 hours. Ongoing losses resulting from osmotic diuresis usually do not need to be replaced unless urine output is very large or signs of poor perfusion are present. Osmotic diuresis is usually minimal when the serum glucose concentration falls below 300 mg/dL. To avoid rapid shifts in serum osmolality, 0.9% NaCl can be used as the replacement fluid for the initial 4–6 hours, followed by 0.45% NaCl.

Hyperglycemia. Insulin should be administered intravenously at a dose of 0.1 U/kg/hr. An initial bolus of 0.1 U/kg of regular insulin is sometimes given; use of a bolus is controversial. Proponents of this approach suggest that maximal insulin binding to receptors may occur more rapidly. Opponents argue that use of an insulin bolus may contribute to a rapid decrease in serum glucose, resulting in potentially harmful shifts in serum osmolality.

Optimally, serum glucose concentrations should decrease at a rate no faster than 100 mg/dL/hr. When serum glucose concentrations fall below 250–300 mg/dL, glucose should be added to the intravenous fluids. If serum glucose concentrations fall below 200 mg/dL before correction of acidosis, the glucose concentration of the intravenous fluids should be increased, but the insulin infusion should not be decreased.

Acidosis. Insulin therapy promotes metabolism of ketone bodies, and this process alone is usually sufficient to correct acidosis. Bicarbonate therapy should be avoided unless severe acidosis (pH <7.0) results in hemodynamic instability or symptomatic hyperkalemia is present. Potential adverse effects of bicarbonate administration include paradoxic increases in CNS acidosis caused by increased diffusion of carbon dioxide across the blood-brain barrier, potential tissue hypoxia caused by shifts in the oxyhemoglobin dissociation curve, abrupt osmotic changes, and increased risk of development of cerebral edema.

As acidosis is corrected, urine ketone concentrations may appear to rise. This occurs because beta-hydroxybutyrate, which is not detected in urine ketone assays, is converted to acetoacetate with treatment. Urine ketone concentration, therefore, is not a useful index of the adequacy of therapy.

Electrolyte Imbalances. Regardless of the serum potassium concentration at presentation, total body potassium depletion is very likely. Potassium concentrations can decrease rapidly as insulin therapy improves the acidotic state and potassium is exchanged for intracellular hydrogen ions. Once adequate urine output is demonstrated, potassium should be added to the intravenous fluids. Potassium replacement should be given as 50% potassium chloride and 50% potassium phosphate at a concentration of 20–40 mEq/L. This combination provides phosphate for replacement of deficits and avoids excess phosphate administration, which may precipitate hypocalcemia.

Monitoring. A flow sheet should be used to monitor fluid balance and laboratory measurements. Initial laboratory measurements should include serum glucose, sodium, potassium, chloride, bicarbonate, BUN, creatinine, calcium, phosphate, and magnesium concentrations as well as arterial or venous pH and a urinalysis. Serum glucose measurement should be repeated every hour during therapy and electrolyte concentrations every 2–3 hours. Calcium, phosphate, and magnesium concentrations should be measured initially and every 4–6 hours during therapy. Neurologic and mental status should be assessed at frequent intervals, and complaints of headache or deterioration of mental status should prompt rapid evaluation for possible cerebral edema.

Complications. Clinically apparent cerebral edema occurs in 1–5% of cases of DKA. Cerebral edema is the most serious complication of DKA, with a mortality rate of 20–80%. The pathogenesis of this complication is incompletely understood. Subclinical cerebral edema is common in patients with DKA, but the factors that exacerbate this process leading to symptomatic brain swelling and possible cerebral herniation are not clearly defined. Cerebral edema typically occurs 6–10 hours after therapy for DKA is begun, often following a period of apparent clinical improvement. Factors that have been found to correlate with increased risk for cerebral edema include:
- Higher initial BUN concentration
- Lower initial Pco_2
- Failure of the serum sodium concentration to rise as glucose concentration falls during treatment
- Treatment with bicarbonate

Signs of advanced cerebral edema include obtundation, papilledema, pupillary dilation or inequality, hypertension, bradycardia. and apnea. *Treatment* involves the use of intravenous mannitol, endotracheal intubation, and hyperventilation.

Other complications of DKA are intracranial thrombosis or infarction, acute tubular necrosis with acute renal failure caused by severe dehydration, pancreatitis, arrhythmias caused by electrolyte abnormalities, pulmonary edema, and bowel ischemia.

Peripheral edema occurs commonly 24–48 hours after therapy is initiated and may be related to residual elevations in antidiuretic hormone (ADH) and aldosterone.

Transition to Outpatient Management. Once the acidosis has been corrected and the patient can tolerate oral feedings, the intravenous insulin infusion can be discontinued and a regimen of subcutaneous insulin injections initiated. Typical starting doses are approximately 0.5 U/kg/24 hr for prepubertal patients and approximately 0.7 U/kg/24 hr for adolescents; two thirds of the total daily insulin dose should be given as intermediate-acting insulin (NPH or Lente), and one third should be given as short-acting (regular) insulin. The dose should be divided into two daily injections, with two thirds given in the morning, 30 minutes before breakfast, and one third given in the evening, 30 minutes before dinner (Fig. 17–12). The first subcutaneous insulin dose should be given 30–45 minutes before discontinuation of the intravenous insulin infusion. Further adjustment of the insulin dose should be made over the following 2–3 days.

Another alternative for making the transition to subcutaneous insulin is to begin by giving injections of regular insulin before each meal and NPH at bedtime. This regimen can then be converted to a twice-daily regimen of NPH and regular insulin after the patient is able to tolerate a full diet and serum glucose concentrations stabilize.

Serum glucose concentrations should be assessed before each meal, at bedtime, and at 2–3 AM to provide information for adjustment of the regimen.

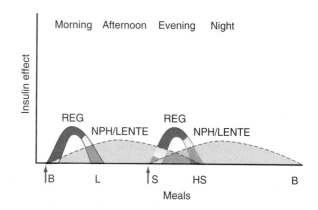

FIG. 17–12

Representative profile of insulin effect using a twice-daily injection regimen that combines an intermediate-acting insulin (NPH or Lente) with regular (short-acting) insulin. (From Schade DS, Santiago JV, Sykler JS: *Intensive insulin therapy,* New York, 1983, Excerpta Medica.)

Patients and their families should begin learning the principles of diabetes care as soon as possible. Demonstration of ability to administer insulin injections and test glucose concentrations using a glucometer is necessary prior to discharge, as is knowledge of hypoglycemia management and meal planning.

Honeymoon Period. In patients with new onset of DM1, often the beta cell mass has not been completely destroyed by the autoimmune process. With insulin treatment, the remaining functional beta cells recover from the state of exhaustion and are again able to produce insulin. When this occurs, insulin requirements decrease and there is a period of stable blood glucose control, often with nearly normal glucose concentrations. This phase of the disease, known as the honeymoon period, usually continues for a few months, but can last up to 2 years.

Outpatient DM1 Management. Long-term management of DM1 in children requires a comprehensive approach, with attention to medical, nutritional, and psychosocial issues. Therapeutic strategies should be flexible, with the individual needs of each patient taken into account. Optimal care involves a team of diabetes professionals including a physician, a diabetes nurse educator, a dietitian, and a social worker.

Goals. The Diabetes Control and Complications Trial (DCCT) established that intensive insulin therapy, with the goal of maintaining blood glucose concentrations as close to normal as possible, can delay the onset and slow the progression of complications of diabetes, including retinopathy, nephropathy, and neuropathy. In this trial, intensive insulin therapy also resulted in a two- to threefold increase in severe hypoglycemia. One should give careful consideration to the balance of these two features when planning the treatment goals for children with DM1. Although the risk for diabetic complications increases with duration of diabetes, the rate of increase in risk may be slower in the prepubertal years than in adolescence and adulthood. Thus the gains from achieving tight control of blood glucose concentrations in childhood appear somewhat less than in adulthood. Furthermore, the adverse effects of hypoglycemia in young children may be significant because the immature CNS may be more susceptible to damage during episodes of glycopenia.

The goals of therapy will therefore differ, depending on the age of the patient. For children under 5 years of age, an appropriate goal is maintenance of blood glucose concentrations between 100 and 200 mg/dL. For school-age children, 80–180 mg/dL is a reasonable target range. For adolescents, the goal is 70–150 mg/dL. Goals of therapy should also take into account other individual characteristics, such as a past history of severe hypoglycemia and the abilities of the patient and family.

Insulin Regimens. A number of different types of insulin differ in duration of action and time to peak effect (Table 17–24). These insulins can be used in various combinations, depending on the needs and goals of the individual patient. The most commonly used regimen in school-aged children involves two subcutaneous injections per day of intermediate-acting insulin (NPH or Lente) and short-acting insulin (regular) (Fig. 17–12). This regimen is preferred because it does not require the patient to give an insulin injection at midday, during school hours. Patients using this regimen must adhere to a relatively rigid meal schedule, however, and this can be difficult to coordinate with variations in daily activities. Other regimens use multiple injections of short-acting insulin given before meals in combination with a long-acting basal insulin (such as Ultralente or Glargine) or with an intermediate-acting insulin given at bedtime. These regimens provide more flexibility but require the patient to administer many injections per day and thus are more suitable for adolescents than young children. Pumps that provide a continuous subcutaneous infusion of short-acting insulin are also available and have been used by children and adolescents who are highly motivated to achieve tight control.

Two insulin analogs are available in which altered amino acid positioning results in more or less rapid absorption. Lispro is a synthetic human insulin analog in which the amino acids at positions 28 and 29 (lysine and proline) are reversed. This alteration in

TABLE 17–24
Insulin Preparations

Type of Insulin	Onset	Peak Action	Duration
Very Short-Acting			
Lispro	15–30 min	30–90 min	2–4 hr
Short-Acting			
Regular	30 min–1 hr	2–4 hr	6–10 hr
Intermediate-Acting			
NPH			
Lente	1–4 hr	4–12 hr	12–24 hr
Long-Acting			
Protamine zinc	4–6 hr	8–20 hr	24–30 hr
Ultralente			
Glargine	1–2 hr	No peak	24–30 hr

the insulin structure results in rapid absorption and onset of action (Table 17–24). Lispro insulin can be substituted for short-acting insulins and may be particularly useful in patients who have problems with postprandial hypoglycemia. Because of the short duration of action, Lispro must be used in combination with an intermediate-acting or long-acting insulin. Glargine is a new insulin analog in which the amino acid glycine is substituted for asparagine in the A-chain of insulin and two arginine molecules are added to the C-terminus of the B-chain. These alterations result in increased solubility at acidic pH and decreased solubility at physiologic pH.

When insulin Glargine is injected subcutaneously, it precipitates and is thus absorbed very slowly. In clinical studies, Glargine has been demonstrated to have a duration of action >24 hours and to have essentially no peak of activity.

Total daily insulin doses differ, depending on the age and pubertal stage of the patient and the duration of diabetes. Newly diagnosed patients in the honeymoon period may require as little as 0.2–0.4 U/kg/24 hr. Prepubertal patients with a duration of diabetes greater than 1–2 years typically require 0.5–1.0 U/kg/24 hr. During midadolescence, when elevated GH concentrations produce relative insulin resistance, insulin requirements increase by 40–50% and doses of 1–2 U/kg/24 hr are typical.

Nutrition. Balancing the daily meal plan with the dosages of insulin is critical for maintaining serum glucose concentrations within the target range and avoiding hypoglycemia. The content and schedule of meals will vary according to the type of insulin regimen used; however, it is recommended that carbohydrates contribute 50–65% of the total calories, protein 12–20%, and fat less than 30%. Saturated fat should contribute less than 10% of the total caloric intake, and cholesterol intake should be less than 300 mg/24 hr. High fiber content is recommended. It should be emphasized that these recommendations describe a healthy diet for anyone, regardless of the presence of diabetes. Participation of the entire family is critical to ensure compliance.

Children using a combination of intermediate-acting and short-acting insulins given twice a day need to maintain a relatively strict meal schedule so that peaks of carbohydrate absorption correspond with peaks in insulin action. A typical meal schedule for a patient using this type of regimen involves three meals and three snacks daily. The total carbohydrate content of the meals and snacks should be kept constant. Patients using multiple injection regimens or the insulin pump can maintain a more flexible meal schedule with regard to the timing of meals and the carbohydrate content. These patients give an injection of insulin before each meal, with the total dose calculated according to the carbohydrate content of the meal. Further adjustments in the dose can be made based on the measured serum glucose concentration and plans for exercise during the day.

Monitoring. Routine monitoring of children with IDDM involves daily blood glucose determinations, assessment of long-term glycemic control, screening for complications of diabetes, and evaluation for other disorders that can occur with increased frequency in patients with IDDM.

Blood Glucose Testing. Blood glucose should be routinely monitored (with rapid, portable glucose meters) before each meal and at bedtime. Hypoglycemia during the night or excessive variability in the morning glucose concentrations should prompt additional testing at 2 or 3 AM to ensure that there is no hypoglycemia leading to the Somogyi effect or rebound hyperglycemia, at the morning (prebreakfast) sample. During periods of intercurrent illness or when blood glucose concentrations are greater than 300 mg/dL, urine ketones should also be tested.

Long-Term Glycemic Control. Measurements of glycohemoglobin or hemoglobin A_{1c} reflect the average blood glucose concentration over the preceding 3 months and provide a means for assessing long-term glycemic control. Glycohemoglobin or hemoglobin A_{1c} should be measured four times a year and the results used for counseling of patients. Table 17–25 summarizes the correlation between hemoglobin A_{1c} or glycohemoglobin and daily blood glucose measurements. Measurements of glycohemoglobin or hemoglobin A_{1c} are inaccurate in patients with hemoglobinopathies. Glycosylated albumin or fructosamine can be used in these cases.

TABLE 17–25
Biochemical Indices of Glycemic Control

Poor Control
HgbA$_{1c}$ >10.0%
Average blood glucose >240 mg/dL

Average Control
HgbA$_{1c}$ >8.0–10.0%
Average blood glucose 180–240 mg/dL

Intensive Control
HgbA$_{1c}$ 6.0–8.0%
Average blood glucose 120–180 mg/dL

HgbA$_{1c}$, Hemoglobin A$_{1c}$.

Complications. Patients with DM1 of greater than 3–5 years' duration should receive an annual ophthalmologic examination for retinopathy. Urine should be collected annually for assessment of microalbuminuria; if present, microalbuminuria is suggestive of early renal dysfunction and indicates a high risk of progression to nephropathy. *Treatment* with angiotensin-converting enzyme (ACE) inhibitors may halt the progression of microalbuminuria. In children with DM1, annual cholesterol measurements and periodic assessment of blood pressure are recommended. Early detection of hypertension and hypercholesterolemia with appropriate intervention can help to limit future risk of coronary disease.

Other Disorders. Diseases with an autoimmune basis are more prevalent in children with diabetes than in the general population. Chronic lymphocytic thyroiditis is particularly common and can result in hypothyroidism. Because symptoms can be subtle, thyroid function tests should be performed annually. Other disorders that occur with increased frequency in children with DM1 include celiac disease, immunoglobulin A (IgA) deficiency, and peptic ulcer disease.

Special Problems

Hypoglycemia. Iatrogenic hypoglycemia occurs commonly in patients with DM1. Patients using conventional insulin therapy have an average of one episode per week of symptomatic hypoglycemia, and those on intensive regimens have an average of two episodes per week. Severe episodes of hypoglycemia, resulting in seizures or coma or requiring assistance from another person, occur in 10–25% of these patients per year. Approximately 4% of deaths in patients with DM1 can be attributed to hypoglycemia, usually as a result of nonintentional trauma.

Hypoglycemia in patients with DM1 results from a relative excess of insulin in relation to the serum glucose concentration. This excess can be caused by alterations in the dose, timing, or absorption of insulin, alterations in carbohydrate intake, or changes in insulin sensitivity resulting from exercise. Defective counterregulatory responses also contribute to hypoglycemia. Abnormal glucagon responses to falling serum glucose concentrations develop within the first few years of the disease, and abnormalities in epinephrine release occur after a somewhat longer duration.

Lack of awareness of hypoglycemia occurs in approximately 25% of patients with diabetes. Recent episodes of hypoglycemia may play a role in the pathophysiology of hypoglycemia unawareness; following an episode of hypoglycemia, autonomic responses to subsequent episodes are reduced. A return of symptoms of hypoglycemia can be demonstrated in these patients after 2–3 weeks of strict avoidance of hypoglycemic episodes.

Symptoms of hypoglycemia include those resulting from neuroglycopenia (e.g., headache, visual changes, confusion, irritability, or seizures) and those resulting from the catecholamine response (e.g., tremors, tachycardia, diaphoresis, or anxiety; also discussed in this chapter under Hypoglycemia). Mild episodes can be treated with administration of rapidly absorbed oral glucose (glucose gel or tablets, fruit juices, and nondiet or non–artificially sweetened sodas). More severe episodes that result in seizures or loss of consciousness at home should be treated with glucagon injections. Intravenous glucose should be given in hospital settings.

Early-Morning Hyperglycemia. A variety of situations can lead to early-morning hyperglycemia. The most frequent assumption is that the evening dose of intermediate-acting insulin is inadequate, but this is not always the case. Hypoglycemia that occurs during the night can result in increased secretion of counterregulatory hormones and rebound hyperglycemia, a situation known as the *Somogyi phenomenon.* Patients experiencing nighttime hypoglycemia also may experience headache on awakening, diaphoresis, and nightmares.

In some children the evening intermediate-acting insulin is given early and the dose wanes by the early morning, resulting in a rise in glucose concentrations. Increased secretion of GH during the early morning hours can also contribute to morning hyperglycemia, particularly during midadolescence. This situation is known as the *dawn phenomenon.* Testing of blood glucose concentrations at 2 or 3 AM can distinguish between these possibilities. Depending on the results, the evening intermediate-acting insulin dose may need to be changed or given at bedtime.

Prognosis. Long-term complications of DM1 include retinopathy, nephropathy, neuropathy, and macrovascular disease. Evidence of tissue damage caused by hyperglycemia is rare in patients with a duration of diabetes of less than 5–10 years, and clinically apparent disease rarely occurs before a duration of 10–15 years. Therefore, pediatricians encounter these complications infrequently. The eventual morbidity and mortality attributable to these disorders, however, are substantial. Some degree of diabetic retinopathy eventually occurs in nearly 100% of patients with DM1 and is the cause of approximately 5000 new cases of blindness in the United States yearly. Nephropathy eventually occurs in 30–40% and accounts for approximately 30% of all new adult cases of end-stage renal disease. Neuropathy occurs in 30–40% of postpubertal patients with DM1 and leads to sensory, motor, or autonomic deficits. Macrovascular disease results in an increased risk of myocardial infarction and stroke among individuals with diabetes.

The DCCT convincingly demonstrated that intensive control of diabetes, employing frequent blood glucose testing and multiple daily injections of insulin or an insulin pump, can substantially reduce the development or progression of diabetic complications. Intensive management resulted in a 76% reduction of risk for retinopathy, a 39% reduction in microalbuminuria, and a 60% reduction in clinical neuropathy. For pubertal and adult patients, these benefits of intensive therapy likely outweigh the increase in risk for hypoglycemia. For younger patients, in whom the risks for hypoglycemia are greater and the benefits of tight glucose control may be lower, a somewhat less intensive regimen may be appropriate.

Research efforts have focused on prevention of diabetes in patients known to be at risk. In first-degree relatives of patients with DM1, the future risk for development of DM1 can be determined on the basis of measurements of antibodies to beta cell antigens and insulin responses to stimulation. A preliminary study demonstrated that administration of small doses of subcutaneous insulin to individuals at high risk for development of DM1 may delay or prevent onset of diabetes.

Non-Insulin-Dependent (Type 2) Diabetes Mellitus (DM2)

Epidemiology. DM2 was thought to be uncommon in childhood; however, the prevalence of this disorder in children is increasing, perhaps as a reflection of the increased prevalence of childhood obesity. DM2 is currently thought to account for approximately 8–15% of cases of diabetes in childhood. The prevalence is highest among children of ethnic groups with a high prevalence of DM2 among adults, including Native Americans, Hispanic Americans, and African Americans. Obesity and a family history of DM2 are risk factors.

Pathophysiology. DM2 can occur as the result of various pathophysiologic processes; however, the most common form results from peripheral insulin resistance with failure of the pancreas to maintain compensatory hyperinsulinemia (Table 17–23). The precise defects underlying the insulin-resistant state and the eventual pancreatic beta cell failure are complex and poorly understood. Other subtypes of DM2 can also occur in children. Maturity-onset diabetes of youth (MODY) comprises a group of dominantly inherited forms of relatively mild diabetes. Insulin resistance does not occur in these patients; instead, the primary abnormality is an insufficient insulin secretory response to glycemic stimulation (Table 17–23). DM2 in childhood can also result from rare inherited defects in mitochondrial genes. Other rare subtypes of DM2 are syndromes of severe insulin resistance caused by mutations in the insulin receptor gene and diabetes resulting from the secretion of abnormal forms of insulin.

Differential Diagnosis. Differentiating DM2 from DM1 in children can be challenging. The possibility of DM2 should be entertained in patients who are obese, have a strong family history of DM2, have a finding of acanthosis nigricans (increased pigmentation of skin in flexural areas) on physical examination (a dermatologic manifestation of hyperinsulinism), or have absence of antibodies to beta cell antigens at the time of diagnosis of diabetes. Although ketoacidosis occurs far more commonly in DM1, it can also occur in patients with DM2 under conditions of physiologic stress and thus cannot be used as an absolute differentiating factor. The diagnosis of DM2 can be confirmed by evaluation of insulin or C-peptide responses to stimulation with oral carbohydrate.

REFERENCES

Behrman RE, Kliegman RM, Jenson HB, editors: *Nelson textbook of pediatrics,* ed 16, Philadelphia, 2000, WB Saunders, Chapter 599.

Diabetes Control and Complications Trial Research Group: The effect of intensive treatment of diabetes on the development and progression of long-term complications in insulin-dependent diabetes mellitus, *N Engl J Med* 329(2):977–986, 1993.

Diabetes Control and Complications Trial Research Group: Effect of intensive diabetes treatment on the development and progression of long-term complications in adolescents with insulin-dependent diabetes mellitus, *J Pediatr* 125(2):177–188, 1994.

Fagot-Campagna A, Pettitt DJ, Engelgau MM, et al: Type 2 diabetes among North American children and adolescents: an epidemiologic review and a public health perspective, *J Pediatr* 36(5):664–672, 2000.

Glaser NS: Non-insulin dependent diabetes mellitus in childhood and adolescence, *Pediatr Clin North Am* 44(2):307–337, 1997.

Krane E: Diabetic ketoacidosis: biochemistry, physiology, treatment, prevention, *Pediatr Clin North Am* 34(4):935–960, 1987.

Owerbach D, Gabbay KH: The search for IDDM susceptibility genes: the next generation, *Diabetes* 45(5):544–551, 1996.

Rosenbloom AL, Schatz DA, Krischer JP, et al: Therapeutic controversy: prevention and treatment of diabetes in children, *J Clin Endocrinol Metab* 85(2):494–522, 2000.

Sperling MA: The etiology of insulin-dependent diabetes mellitus, *Pediatr Clin North Am* 44(2):269–284, 1997.

Verge CF, Gianani R, Kawasaki F, et al: Prediction of type 1 diabetes in first-degree relatives using a combination of insulin, GAD, and ICA512bdc/IA-2 autoantibodies, *Diabetes* 45(7):926–933, 1996.

HYPOGLYCEMIA

Hypoglycemia in infancy and childhood can result from a large variety of hormonal and metabolic defects (Table 17–26). Hypoglycemia occurs most frequently in the early neonatal period, often as a result of inadequate energy stores to meet the disproportionately large metabolic needs of premature or small-for-gestational-age newborns. Hypoglycemia in the first few days of life in an otherwise normal newborn, however, is less frequent and warrants concern (see Chapter 6). After the initial 2–3 days of life, hypoglycemia is far less common and is more frequently the result of endocrine or metabolic disorders.

Definition

Beyond the early neonatal period, serum glucose concentrations less than 45 mg/dL are considered to be abnormal and necessitate treatment. Serum glucose concentrations less than 55 mg/dL can occasionally occur in normal individuals, especially with prolonged fasting, but should be considered suspect, particularly if there are concurrent symptoms of hypoglycemia (Table 17–27). The *diagnosis* of hypoglycemia should be made on the basis of a low serum glucose concentration, symptoms compatible with hypoglycemia, and resolution of the symptoms after administration of glucose.

TABLE 17–26
Classification of Hypoglycemia in Infants and Children

Abnormalities in the Hormonal Signal Indicating Hypoglycemia
Counterregulatory Hormone Deficiency
Panhypopituitarism
Isolated growth hormone deficiency
ACTH deficiency
Addison disease
Glucagon deficiency
Epinephrine deficiency
Hyperinsulinism
Infant of a diabetic mother
Infant with erythroblastosis fetalis
Persistent hyperinsulinemic hypoglycemias of infancy
Beta cell adenoma (insulinoma)
Beckwith-Wiedemann syndrome
Anti-insulin receptor antibodies

Inadequate Substrate
Prematurity/small-for-gestational-age infant
Ketotic hypoglycemia
Maple syrup urine disease

Disorders of Metabolic Response Pathways
Glycogenolysis
Glucose-6-phosphatase deficiency
Amylo-1,6-glucosidase deficiency
Liver phosphorylase deficiency
Glycogen synthase deficiency
Gluconeogenesis
Fructose-1,6-diphosphatase deficiency
Pyruvate carboxylase deficiency
Phosphoenolpyruvate carboxykinase deficiency

Fatty Acid Oxidation
Long-, medium-, or short-chain fatty acid acyl-CoA dehydrogenase deficiency
Carnitine deficiency (primary or secondary)
Carnitine palmitoyltransferase deficiency
Other
Enzymatic defects
    Galactosemia
    Hereditary fructose intolerance
    Propionicacidemia
    Methylmalonic acidemia
    Tyrosinosis
    Glutaric aciduria
Global hepatic dysfunction
Reye syndrome
Hepatitis
Heart failure
Sepsis-shock
Carcinoma/sarcoma (IGF-2 secretion)
Malnutrition-starvation
Hyperviscosity syndrome

Drugs/Intoxications
Oral hypoglycemic agents
Insulin
Alcohol
Salicylates
Propranolol
Valproic acid
Pentamidine
Ackee fruit (unripe)
Quinine
Trimethoprim/sulfamethoxazole (with renal failure)

IGF, Insulin-like growth factor.

Clinical Manifestations. The symptoms and signs of hypoglycemia result from both direct depression of the CNS owing to lack of energy substrate and the counterregulatory response to low glucose via catecholamine secretion (Table 17–27). The manifestations in infants differ when compared with those in older children. Symptoms and signs of hypoglycemia in infants are relatively nonspecific and include jitteriness, feeding difficulties, pallor, hypotonia, hypothermia, episodes of apnea and bradycardia, and seizures. In older children, symptoms and signs include confusion, irritability, headaches, visual changes, tremors, pallor, sweating, tachycardia, weakness, seizures, and coma.

Failure to recognize and treat hypoglycemia can result in serious long-term morbidity, including mental retardation and nonhypoglycemic seizures. Younger infants and patients with more severe or prolonged hypoglycemia are at greatest risk for adverse outcomes.

Pathophysiology. Normal regulation of serum glucose concentrations requires appropriate interaction of a number of hormonal signals and metabolic pathways. An overview of these pathways is presented in Fig. 17–13. The components required for glycemic regulation fall into three basic categories:
1. The hormonal signal indicating hypoglycemia
2. Energy stores adequate to supply substrates for the metabolic pathways
3. Functioning metabolic-enzymatic pathways for glucose and ketone body generation
4. Defects in any of these categories can result in hypoglycemia

The Hormonal Signal

In a normal individual, a fall in serum glucose concentrations will lead to suppression of insulin secretion and increased secretion of the counterregulatory hormones (growth hormone, cortisol, glucagon, and epinephrine). This hormonal signal promotes the release of amino acids (particularly alanine) from muscle to fuel gluconeogenesis and the release of triglyceride from adipose tissue stores to provide free fatty acids (FFAs) for hepatic ketogenesis. Both FFAs and

---

TABLE 17–27
Symptoms and Signs of Hypoglycemia

Features Associated with Epinephrine Release*	Features Associated with Cerebral Glucopenia
Perspiration	Headache
Palpitation (tachycardia)	Mental confusion
Pallor	Somnolence
Paresthesia	Dysarthria
Trembling	Personality changes
Anxiety	Inability to concentrate
Weakness	Staring
Nausea	Hunger
Vomiting	Convulsions
	Ataxia
	Coma
	Diplopia
	Stroke

*These features may be blunted if the patient is receiving beta-blocking agents.

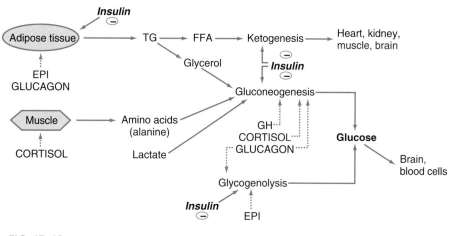

FIG. 17–13

Regulation of serum glucose. – represents inhibitions. *EPI*, Epinephrine; *FFA*, free fatty acid; *GH*, growth hormone; *TG*, triglyceride.

ketones serve as alternate fuels. It also stimulates the breakdown of hepatic glycogen and promotes gluconeogenesis. Failure of any of the components of this hormonal signal can lead to hypoglycemia.

Hyperinsulinemia. Failure of suppression of insulin secretion in response to low serum glucose concentrations can occur in infants but is uncommon beyond the neonatal period. In neonates this situation arises most frequently in infants of diabetic mothers who have been exposed to high concentrations of glucose in utero resulting in fetal islet cell hyperplasia. The hyperinsulinemic state is transient, usually lasting hours to days (see Chapter 6).

Hyperinsulinism that persists beyond a few days of age can result from a condition previously referred to as "nesidioblastosis" but more appropriately called **persistent hyperinsulinemic hypoglycemia of the newborn (PHHN).** In these infants hyperplasia of the islet cells develops in the absence of excess stimulation by maternal diabetes. Some patients with PHHN have genetic abnormalities of the sulfonylurea receptor or other genetic defects that alter the function of the ATP-sensitive potassium channel that regulates insulin secretion. Hyperinsulinism can also occur in the **Beckwith-Wiedemann syndrome,** a condition characterized by macrosomia, macroglossia, omphalocele, visceromegaly, and earlobe creases.

Regardless of the cause, infants with hyperinsulinism are characteristically large for gestational age. Hypoglycemia is severe and frequently occurs within 1–3 hours of a feeding. Glucose requirements are large, often two to three times the normal basal glucose requirement of 4–8 mg/kg/min. The *diagnosis* of hyperinsulinism is confirmed by the detection of serum insulin concentrations above 5 µU/mL during an episode of hypoglycemia. The absence of serum and urine ketones at the time of hypoglycemia is an important diagnostic feature, distinguishing hyperinsulinism from defects in counterregulatory hormone secretion.

Treatment initially involves the infusion of intravenous glucose at high rates and of diazoxide to suppress insulin secretion. If this therapy is unsuccessful, long-acting somatostatin analogs can be tried. Often, medical therapy for PHHN is unsuccessful and subtotal (90%) pancreatectomy is required to prevent long-term neurologic sequelae of hypoglycemia.

In children hyperinsulinemia is rare and usually results from an islet cell adenoma. Children with this condition characteristically have a voracious appetite, obesity, and accelerated linear growth. As in infants, *diagnosis* requires demonstration of insulin concentrations >5 µU/mL during an episode of hypoglycemia. A CT or MRI scan of the pancreas should be attempted, but visualization of an adenoma is usually difficult. Surgical removal of the adenoma is curative.

Factitious Hyperinsulinemia. In rare cases, insulin is administered to a child as a form of child abuse or **Munchausen syndrome by proxy.** This *diagnosis* should be suspected if extremely high insulin concentrations are detected (>100 µU/mL). C-peptide concentrations are low or undetectable, which confirms that the insulin was from an exogenous source.

Defects in Counterregulatory Hormones. Abnormalities in the secretion of counterregulatory hormones that produce hypoglycemia usually involve GH, cortisol, or both. Deficiencies in glucagon and epinephrine secretion have been described but are rare. GH and cortisol deficiency occur as a result of hypopituitarism. Hypopituitarism results rarely from congenital hypoplasia or aplasia of the pituitary, or more commonly from deficiency of hypothalamic releasing factors. Clues to this diagnosis in infants include the presence of hypoglycemia in association with midline facial or neurologic defects (such as cleft lip and palate or absence of the corpus callosum); pendular nystagmus (indicating possible abnormalities in the development of the optic nerves and visual impairment, which can occur in septooptic dysplasia); and the presence of microphallus and cryptorchidism in males (indicating abnormalities in gonadotropin secretion). Jaundice and hepatomegaly can also occur, simulating neonatal hepatitis. Despite the presence of GH deficiency, these infants are usually of normal size at birth. Older children with hypopituitarism, however, usually have short stature and a subnormal growth velocity.

Deficient cortisol secretion can also occur in primary adrenal insufficiency resulting from a variety of causes. In infants, primary adrenal insufficiency often results from congenital adrenal hyperplasia, most frequently as a result of 21-hydroxylase deficiency (discussed earlier in the chapter under Disorders of Sexual Differentiation). In older children, primary adrenal insufficiency is most frequently seen in **Addison disease,** but it can also occur in adrenoleukodystrophy and other disorders (discussed earlier under Adrenal Gland). Addison disease should be suspected if there is hyperpigmentation of the skin, a history of salt cravings, hyponatremia, and hyperkalemia.

Confirmation of GH or cortisol deficiency as the cause of hypoglycemia requires the detection of low serum GH and cortisol concentrations during an episode of hypoglycemia or after other stimulatory testing. In contrast to hyperinsulinism, serum and urine ketones are positive at the time of hypoglycemia and FFAs are elevated. Treatment involves supplementation of the deficient hormones in physiologic doses.

Energy Stores

Sufficient energy stores in the form of glycogen, adipose tissue, and muscle are necessary to respond appropriately to hypoglycemia. Deficiencies in these stores are a common cause of hypoglycemia in neonates who are small for gestational age or premature (see Chapter 6). Beyond the early neonatal period, energy stores are usually sufficient to meet the metabolic requirements except in malnourished children Release of substrate from energy stores, however, is thought to be abnormal in one common form of childhood hypoglycemia, ketotic hypoglycemia.

Ketotic Hypoglycemia. This disorder is usually seen in children between 18 months and 5 years of age. It is the most common cause of new-onset hypoglycemia in children over 2 years of age. Typically, these patients have symptoms of hypoglycemia after a period of prolonged fasting, often in the setting of an intercurrent illness. Children with this disorder are often thin and small and may have a history of being small for gestational age. Defective mobilization of alanine from muscle to fuel gluconeogenesis is thought to be the cause. Because there are no specific diagnostic tests for this disorder, ketotic hypoglycemia is a *diagnosis of exclusion*.

Treatment involves avoidance of fasting and frequent feedings of a high-protein, high-carbohydrate diet. Patients may require hospitalization for intravenous glucose infusion if they cannot maintain adequate oral intake during a period of illness. The disorder usually resolves spontaneously by 7–8 years of age.

Maple Syrup Urine Disease. Maple syrup urine disease is a defect in branched chain amino acid catabolism and results in inadequate release of alanine from muscle. Affected patients may have hypoglycemia along with vomiting, lethargy, seizures, hyperammonemia, and metabolic acidosis. The urine has a characteristic maple syrup odor. Measurement of serum amino acids is required to make the diagnosis.

Metabolic Response Pathways

Maintenance of normal serum glucose concentrations in the fasting state requires both glucose production via glycogenolysis and gluconeogenesis and the production of alternative energy sources (e.g., free fatty acids and ketones) via lipolysis and fatty acid oxidation.

Glycogenolysis. Glycogen storage diseases present in a variety of subtypes that differ in severity (see Chapter 5). Among the subtypes that result in hypoglycemia, the most severe form is glucose-6-phosphatase deficiency. This subtype is characterized by severe hypoglycemia, massive hepatomegaly, growth retardation, and lactic acidosis. In contrast, deficiencies in the glycogen phosphorylase enzymes may cause isolated hepatomegaly with or without hypoglycemia.

The *diagnosis* of glycogen storage disease is suggested by a finding of hepatomegaly without splenomegaly. Ketosis occurs with hypoglycemic episodes. Confirmation of the diagnosis requires specific biochemical studies of leukocytes or liver biopsy specimens.

Treatment involves frequent high-carbohydrate feedings during the day and continuous feedings at night via nasogastric tube. Feedings of uncooked cornstarch during bedtime are sufficient to maintain serum glucose concentrations in some patients.

Gluconeogenesis. Defects in gluconeogenesis are uncommon and include fructose-1,6-diphosphatase deficiency and phosphoenolpyruvate carboxykinase deficiency. Affected patients exhibit fasting hypoglycemia, hepatomegaly caused by fatty infiltration, lactic acidosis, and hyperuricemia. Ketosis occurs, and FFA and alanine concentrations are high.

Treatment involves frequent high-carbohydrate, low-protein feedings.

Fatty Acid Oxidation. These disorders of ketogenesis include the fatty acid acyl-coenzyme A (CoA) dehydrogenase deficiencies; long-chain, medium-chain, and short-chain acyl-CoA dehydrogenase deficiency, and hereditary carnitine deficiency. Of these disorders, medium-chain acyl-CoA dehydrogenase deficiency (MCAD) is the most common. MCAD occurs in 1 in 9000–15,000 live births. Patients often are well in infancy and can have the first episode of hypoglycemia at 2 years of age or older. Episodes of hypoglycemia usually occur with prolonged fasting or during episodes of intercurrent illness.

Mild hepatomegaly may be present along with mild hyperammonemia, hyperuricemia, and mild elevations in hepatic transaminases. Ketone concentrations are low or undetected. The *diagnosis* is confirmed by the finding of elevated concentrations of dicarboxylic acids in the urine. *Treatment* involves avoidance of fasting.

Other Metabolic Disorders. A number of metabolic disorders in addition to those just described can lead to hypoglycemia. These include galactosemia, hereditary fructose intolerance, and a number of disorders of organic acid metabolism (Table 17–26). Hypoglycemia in these disorders is usually a reflection of global hepatic dysfunction secondary to the buildup of hepatotoxic intermediates. Many of these disorders present with low concentrations of ketone bodies because ketogenesis is also affected. The finding of non–glucose-reducing substances in the urine suggests a diagnosis of galactosemia or hereditary fructose intolerance. Occurrence of symptoms following ingestion of fructose or sucrose suggests hereditary fructose intolerance. *Treatment* requires dietary restriction of the specific offending substances.

Medications and Intoxication

Hypoglycemia can occur as an adverse effect of a number of medications, including insulin, oral hypoglycemic agents, and propranolol, and as a result of salicylate intoxication. Valproate toxicity can cause a disorder similar to that seen in the fatty acid oxidation defects. Ethanol ingestion can also cause hypoglycemia, especially in younger children, because the metabolism of ethanol results in the depletion of cofactors necessary for gluconeogenesis.

Reactive Hypoglycemia

The term "reactive hypoglycemia" has been used to describe hypoglycemia occurring 2–3 hours after a meal. This condition can occur in patients who have the *dumping syndrome* as a consequence of gastric surgery. Rapid gastric emptying results in a rapid rise of serum glucose and excess stimulation of insulin secretion. Rarely, transient reactive hypoglycemia can occur in patients who later have IDDM. Delayed insulin secretion in response to elevations in serum glucose concentrations is thought to be responsible for this phenomenon. Except for the patients just described, true reactive hypoglycemia is rare.

Diagnosis. Because the list of causes of hypoglycemia is long and complex, establishing the *etiology* in a particular patient can be difficult. Frequently, it is not possible to make an accurate diagnosis without obtaining a *critical sample* of blood and urine at the time of the hypoglycemic episode. In a child with unexplained hypoglycemia, a serum sample should be obtained before treatment for the measurement of glucose and insulin, GH, cortisol, FFAs, and β-hydroxybutyrate. Measurement of serum lactate levels should also be considered. A urine specimen should be obtained for measuring ketones and reducing substances. The results of this initial testing can establish whether endocrine causes are responsible and, if not, provide initial information regarding which types of metabolic disorders are most likely. Whenever possible, additional samples of blood and urine should be frozen for further analysis if necessary.

Emergency Management. Acute care of the patient with hypoglycemia consists of rapid administration of intravenous glucose (2 mL/kg of 10% dextrose in water is usually sufficient). Following the initial bolus of glucose, an infusion of intravenous glucose should be established to provide approximately one and one half times the normal hepatic glucose production rate (8–12 mg/kg/mm in infants, 6–8 mg/kg/mm in children). Higher infusion rates may be needed for hyperinsulinemic states. This allows for suppression of the catabolic state and prevents further decompensation in patients with certain metabolic disorders. If adrenal insufficiency is suspected, stress doses of glucocorticoids should be administered.

REFERENCES

Behrman RE, Kliegman RM, Jenson HB, editors: *Nelson textbook of pediatrics,* ed 16, Philadelphia, 2000, WB Saunders, Chapter 88.

Cornblath M, Ichord R: Hypoglycemia in the neonate, *Semin Perinatol* 24(2):136–149, 2000.

Dunne MJ, Kane C, Sheperd RM, et al: Familial persistent hyperinsulinemic hypoglycemia of infancy and mutations in the sulfonylurea receptor, *N Engl J Med* 336(10):703–706, 1997.

Haymond MW, Sunehag A: Controlling the sugar bowl: regulation of glucose homeostasis in children, *Endocrinol Metab Clin North Am* 28(4):663–694, 1999.

Service F: Hypoglycemic disorders, *N Engl J Med* 332(17):1144–1152, 1995.

Sperling MA, Menon RK: Hyperinsulinemic hypoglycemia of infancy: recent insights into ATP-sensitive potassium channels, sulfonylurea receptors, molecular mechanisms, and treatment, *Endocrinol Metab Clin North Am* 28(4):695–708, 1999.

Stanley CA, Hale DE: Genetic disorders of mitochondrial fatty acid oxidation, *Curr Opin Pediatr* 6(4):476–481, 1994.

CHAPTER 18

Neurology

Ira Bergman ▼ Michael J. Painter

Neurologic disorders include diseases of the central nervous system (CNS), peripheral nervous system, muscle, and special senses. These diseases may involve a single anatomic or functional part of the nervous system or may be widespread throughout the entire nervous system. The nervous system may be the primary site of the disease process or may be secondarily affected by diseases whose primary pathology is in other organs and tissues. The pathogenesis of neurologic disorders includes congenital anomalies, inborn errors of metabolism, infection, intoxication, neoplasm, vascular occlusion, trauma, anoxia, nutritional deficiency, autoimmunity, and cellular degeneration.

The primary symptoms of neurologic disease are headache; dizziness; visual or hearing loss; impairment of swallowing or respiration; weakness; numbness or paresthesias; difficulty walking or talking; incontinence; deterioration of thinking, coordination, or memory; change in personality; or seizures. These symptoms may be congenital or acquired, acute or chronic, progressive or static, and reversible or irreversible.

DEVELOPMENT OF THE CENTRAL NERVOUS SYSTEM

The precursor of the nervous system is the neural plate of the embryonic ectoderm, which develops at 18 days of gestation. The neural plate gives rise to the neural tube, which forms the brain and spinal cord, and the neural crest cells, which form the peripheral nervous system, meninges, melanocytes, and adrenal medulla.

The neural tube begins to form on the twenty-second day of gestation. The rostral end forms the brain, and the caudal region forms the spinal cord. The lumen of the neural tube forms the ventricles of the brain and the central canal of the spinal cord.

Congenital Anomalies of the Nervous System

Defective closure of the caudal neural tube at the end of the fourth week of gestation results in anomalies of the lumbar and sacral vertebrae or spinal cord called *spina bifida*. These anomalies range in severity from clinically insignificant defects of the L5 or S1 vertebral arches to major malformations of the thoracic spinal cord that lies uncovered by skin or bone on the baby's back. The latter severe defect, called a myelocele, results in total paralysis and loss of sensation in the legs and incontinence of bowel and bladder. In addition, affected children usually have an associated anomaly of the brainstem, called an Arnold-Chiari malformation, that results in hydrocephalus and weakness of face and swallowing. In a meningocele the spinal canal and cystic meninges are exposed on the back, but the underlying spinal cord is anatomically and functionally intact. In spina bifida occulta, the skin of the back is apparently intact, but defects of the underlying bone or spinal canal are present. These defects include tethering of the spinal cord to a thick filum terminale, lipoma or dermoid cyst, or a tiny epithelial tract extending from the skin surface to the meninges. A small dimple or tuft of hair may be present over the affected vertebra. Patients with spina bifida occulta may have difficulties controlling their bowel or bladder, weakness and numbness in the feet, and recurrent ulcerations in the areas of numbness. Bladder dysfunction may result in repeated episodes of urinary tract infections, reflux nephropathy, and renal insufficiency. An epithelial tract may predispose to recurrent episodes of meningitis. The spina bifida malformation can be prevented in a significant number of cases by folate administration to the pregnant mother. Because the defect occurs so early in gestation, all women of childbearing age are advised to take 0.4 mg of oral folate every day.

Meningomyelocele

Neonates with meningomyelocele must undergo operative closure of their open spinal defects and treatment of hydrocephalus by placement of a ventriculoperitoneal shunt. Toddlers and children with lower spinal cord dysfunction require physical therapy and bracing of the lower extremities and intermittent bladder catheterization. Children with meningomyelocele who do not have associated brain anomalies are likely to have normal intelligence. Meningomyelocele in the fetus is suggested by an elevated alpha-fetoprotein in the mother's blood and confirmed by ultrasound examination and high concentrations of alpha-fetoprotein and acetylcholinesterase in the amniotic fluid.

Diastematomyelia

In diastematomyelia, a bone spicule or fibrous band divides the spinal cord into two longitudinal sections. An associated lipoma that infiltrates the cord and tethers it to the vertebrae may be present. Symptoms include weakness and numbness of the feet and urinary incontinence. Reflexes in the feet are diminished or absent. Surgical treatment to free the cord prevents further neurologic deterioration and may improve preexisting symptoms.

Cranial Defects

Defective closure of the rostral neural tube produces anencephaly or encephalocele. Neonates with anencephaly have a rudimentary brainstem or midbrain but no cortex or cranium. This is a rapidly fatal condition. Patients with encephalocele usually have a skull defect and exposure of meninges alone or meninges and brain. Occasionally the defect can produce protrusion of frontal lobe into the nose without a noticeable skull or skin defect. The recurrence risk in subsequent pregnancies for either cranial or spinal neural tube defects is 10%. Within a family, an anencephalic birth may be followed by the birth of a second child affected with a lumbar-sacral meningomyelocele. The inheritance of neural tube defects is polygenic.

Macrocephaly and Microcephaly

Macrocephaly may be the result of *macrocrania*, increased skull thickness; *hydrocephalus*, enlargement of the ventricles; or *megalencephaly*, enlargement of the brain. Macrocrania may be caused by diseases of bone metabolism or hypertrophy of the bone marrow resulting from hemolytic anemia. Megalencephaly may be the result of an embryologic disorder causing abnormal proliferation of brain tissue, such as neurofibromatosis, tuberous sclerosis, Sotos syndrome, Riley-Smith syndrome, and hemimegalencephaly, or of accumulation of abnormal metabolic substances as seen in Alexander, Canavan, and Tay-Sachs diseases, and the mucopolysaccharidoses.

Rarely, small head, microcephaly, is the result of premature closure of one or more skull sutures called *craniosynostosis*, but this diagnosis is readily made by the abnormal shape of the skull. In most circumstances, microcephaly reflects micrencephaly, a small brain. Brain growth is rapid during the perinatal period, and any insult (e.g., infectious, metabolic, toxic, or vascular disorder) sustained during this period or early infancy is likely to impair brain growth and result in microcephaly. *Microcephaly vera* is an autosomal recessive genetic disorder producing severe hypoplasia of the frontal regions of the brain and skull. These children are severely mentally retarded. A myriad of syndromes and metabolic disorders are associated with microcephaly, some of which are hereditary (Table 18–1). As a rule, macrocephaly and microcephaly raise a concern about cognitive ability, but head circumference alone should never be used to establish a prognosis for intellectual development.

REFERENCES

Behrman RE, Kliegman RM, Jenson HB, editors: *Nelson textbook of pediatrics*, ed 16, Philadelphia, 1996, WB Saunders, Chapter 601.

McComb JG: Spinal and cranial neural tube defects, *Semin Pediatr Neurol* 4(3):156–166, 1997.

MRC Vitamin Study Research Group: Prevention of neural tube defects: results of the Medical Research Council vitamin study, *Lancet* 338(8760):131–137, 1991.

Volpe J: *Neurology of the newborn*, ed 4, Philadelphia, 2001, WB Saunders.

NEUROLOGIC EVALUATION

Examining children is challenging because often the children are not ready to follow directions, and because they sometimes actively resist the examination. The process and interpretation of the examination vary with chronologic age. The examination of the newborn is unique, whereas examination of the older child is similar to that of the adult.

An important clue to the disease process is provided by the evolution of symptoms. Symptom evolution is defined as static, progressive, intermittent, or salutatory. Neurologic abnormalities that are observed in the first few months of life and do not change in character over time are static. They are probably caused by congenital abnormalities of brain or brain injury sustained during the prenatal or neonatal period. Steadily progressive disorders suggest degenerative disease or neoplasm. Symptoms that are *intermittent* and *brief* suggest epileptic or migraine syndromes. *Salutatory* disorders, characterized by bursts of symptoms followed by partial recovery, are seen with demyelinating and vascular diseases.

Findings on the general examination often are clues to diagnosis. Abnormalities of hair, skin, teeth, and nails are frequent accompaniments of congeni-

TABLE 18–1
Microcephaly

Etiology	Comment
Recognized Chromosomal Disorders	
Trisomy 13	Cleft lip, midface defects
Trisomy 18	Weak cry, early death
5P-	Cri-du-chat syndrome
Genetic Disorders	
Microcephaly vera	
Microcephaly with lissencephaly, schizencephaly, pachygyria, micropolygyria, and agenesis of the corpus callosum	Autosomal recessive
Sex-linked microcephaly	Sex-linked recessive, autosomal dominant
Microcephaly with normal intelligence and minor malformations	
Microcephaly with Syndromes	
Angelman syndrome	Characteristic mental retardation, ataxia, seizures
Prader-Willi syndrome	Hypotonia, cryptorchidism, obesity
Smith-Lemli-Opitz syndrome	Cryptorchidism, hypospadias, vomiting, seizures
Cornelia de Lange syndrome	Anteverted nostrils, low birth weight, carp mouth, micromelia, synophrys
Seckel dwarf syndrome	Bony defects, joint dislocations
Cockayne syndrome	Retinal degeneration, cataracts, brain calcifications
Rubinstein-Taybi syndrome	Broad thumbs and toes, narrow nose, maxillary hypoplasia
Hallermann-Streiff syndrome	Microphthalmia, small nose
Infections (Congenital)	
Rubella	
Cytomegalovirus (CMV)	
Toxoplasmosis	
Syphilis	
Toxic	
Radiation of the fetus	
Fetal alcohol syndrome	
Phenylketonuria (PKU)	
Hypoxic-ischemic or other severe brain injury	
Intrauterine or neonatal	

tal brain disorders because all of these tissues arise for the embryonic *ectoderm*. Café-au-lait spots are flat, light brown areas of skin more than 0.5 cm in size that are numerous in neurofibromatosis. Adenoma sebaceum is fibrovascular lesions that look like acne on the nose and malar face regions and is commonly seen in older children and adults with tuberous sclerosis. The *head circumference* is measured in its largest occipitofrontal diameter and plotted against appropriate standard growth curves (see Chapter 1, Figs. 1–4 and 1–10). A measurement three standard deviations above the mean defines macrocephaly, and three standard deviations below the mean defines microcephaly. Measurements plotted over time may show an accelerating pattern, indicating hydrocephalus, or a decelerating pattern, indicating brain injury.

During infancy, the anterior fontanel is slightly depressed and pulsatile when the infant is placed in the sitting position. When the fontanel is tense or bulging, increased intracranial pressure is suspected. An unusual shape of the head may indicate premature closure of one or more of the sutures (craniosynostosis). Abnormal shape, location, and condition of the ears are found in a number of genetic syndromes. An examination of the eyes should include a search for epicanthal folds, coloboma, conjunctival telangiectasias, or cataracts. Examining the optic fundus with a direct ophthalmoscope helps assess the status of the optic discs and macula. A complete examination of the retina requires dilating the pupil and using an indirect ophthalmoscope. Examining the hands and feet reveals the presence of abnormal creases, polydactyly, or syndactyly (see Chapter 19). An examination of the neck and spine should include searching for *midline defects,* which may be obvious, such as spina bifida with myelomeningocele, or subtle, such as cutaneous dimples, small openings or sinus tracts, or tufts of hair or subcutaneous lipomas. Kyphosis and scoliosis may result from abnormalities of the central or peripheral nervous systems.

Neonatal Examination

Because the cortex and subcortical white matter of the neonate are immature, the neurologic examination of the neonate is used mainly to assess the function of the basal ganglia and more caudal structures. The results of the examination should be used cautiously in predicting developmental outcome.

Reflexes

A number of primitive reflexes present at birth (Table 18–2) assess the functional integrity of the brainstem and basal ganglia. As a group, they are symmetric and disappear at 4–6 months of age, indicating the normal maturation of descending inhibitory cerebral influences. The *Landau* and *parachute* reflexes become apparent after the newborn period, indicating proper maturation of appropriate brain structures. The *grasp* and *rooting* reflexes are inhibited by maturation of frontal lobe structures and

TABLE 18–2
CNS Reflexes of Infancy

Reflex	Description	Age of Appearance	Age of Disappearance	Origin in Central Nervous System
Moro	Sudden head extension causes extension followed by flexion of the arms and legs	Birth	4–6 mo	Brainstem vestibular nuclei
Grasp	Placing a finger in palm results in flexing of the infant's fingers, accompanied by flexion at elbow and shoulder	Birth	4–6 mo	Brainstem vestibular nuclei
Rooting	Tactile stimulus about the mouth results in the infant's mouth pursuing the stimulus	Birth	4–6 mo	Brainstem trigeminal system
Trunk incurvation	Stroking the skin along the edge of the vertebrae produces curvature of the spine with the apex opposite to the direction of the stroke	Birth	9–6 mo	Spinal cord
Placing	Infant places foot on examining surface when dorsum of foot is brought into contact with the edge of the surface	Birth	4–6 mo	Cerebral cortex
Crossed extension	One leg held firmly in extension and the dorsum and sole of the foot stimulated results in a sequence of flexion, extension, and adduction, followed by toe fanning of the opposite leg	Birth	4–6 mo	Spinal cord
Tonic neck	With the infant supine, turning of the head results in ipsilateral extension of the arm and leg in a "fencing" posture	Birth	4–6 mo	Brainstem vestibular nuclei
Parachute	With the infant sitting, tilting to either side results in extension of the ipsilateral arm in a protective fashion	6–8 mo	Never	Brainstem vestibular nuclei
Landau	With the infant held about the waist and suspended, extension of the neck produces extension of the arms and legs	6–8 mo	15 mo–2 yr	Brainstem

may reappear later in life with frontal lobe lesions. Asymmetry of the primitive reflexes often indicates focal brain or peripheral nerve lesions.

Posture

Posture is defined as the position that the infant naturally assumes when placed supine. An infant at 28 weeks of gestation demonstrates total extension, whereas at 32 weeks a slight increase in tone of the lower extremities is noted. At 34 weeks, the lower extremities are flexed and the upper extremities are extended. At term, the infant flexes both lower and upper extremities. *Recoil* is defined as a liveliness with which an arm or leg springs back to its original position after passive stretching and release. Recoil is essentially absent in the small premature infant but is brisk at term.

Movement and Tone

Spontaneous movements of the small premature infant are slow and writhing, whereas those of the term infant are more rapid. The popliteal angle, heel-to-ear maneuver, scarf maneuver, and head control are used in assessing muscle tone and estimating gestational age (see Chapter 6 and Fig. 6–6).

NEUROLOGIC EXAMINATION AT ALL AGES

Cranial Nerve Evaluation

The evaluation of cranial nerve function depends on the stage of maturation of the child's brain and on the ability of the child to cooperate. Lesions of the neuromuscular apparatus, including the anterior horn cell, peripheral nerves, neuromuscular junction, and muscle, are called lower motor neuron lesions, whereas lesions of tracts that originate above the brainstem and synapse on the anterior horn cells are called upper motor neuron lesions.

Cranial Nerve I

The sense of smell can be assessed in verbal, cooperative children at the age of 2–3 years. Aromatic substances such as perfumes and ground coffee should be used, not volatile substances (such as ammonia) that irritate the nasal mucosa and do not test smell. Anosmia may be congenital or the result of head trauma, cribriform plate fractures, meningitis, diseases of the nose, or brain tumors.

Cranial Nerve II

Full-term newborns in the quiet awake state will follow a human face, light in a dark room, or a large, brightly colored optico-kinetic strip. Visual acuity has been estimated to be 20/150 in the newborn and 20/20 at 6 months of age. Standard visual charts that display pictures instead of letters can be used to assess visual acuity in toddlers, and peripheral vision can be tested by surreptitiously bringing objects into the visual field from behind. Lesions of the anterior visual pathways, including the retina, optic nerves, chiasm, and tract, are expressed by a reduced pupillary reaction to light. Unilateral lesions are readily identified by the "swinging flashlight test." The light is shone in the normal eye, and both pupils constrict. When the light is moved to the abnormal eye, both pupils dilate. This is called an afferent pupillary defect. Lesions of the posterior visual pathway, including the lateral geniculate, optic radiations, and occipital cortex, are expressed by loss of visual fields and normal pupillary light reactions.

Cranial Nerves III, IV, and VI

Extraocular movements may be assessed by observation of spontaneous, pursuit, and saccadic eye movements. Pursuit movements are slow and occur when the eyes are following an object. Saccadic movements are rapid and occur when the eyes move from fixation on one object to fixation on a different object. Pursuit and saccadic eye movements are controlled by different CNS mechanisms. Rotating the head or spinning the infant can help assessment of oculocephalic vestibular reflexes. The oculocephalic reflex is said to be uninhibited when turning of the head in one direction elicits an immediate movement of the eyes in the opposite direction. This response is normal in the newborn. However, in a child or adult an uninhibited response indicates that the cortex is not functioning properly to inhibit the brainstem. A normal response is the occurrence of multiple, random saccadic eye movements as the head is turned. The oculocephalic response is said to be incomplete when the eyes do not move fully and conjugately in response to head turning. An incomplete response indicates dysfunction of the brainstem.

Cranial nerve III (oculomotor nerve) innervates the pupil, levator palpebrae superioris, medial, superior, and inferior recti, and the inferior oblique muscles. Cranial nerve IV (trochlear nerve) innervates the superior oblique muscle, and cranial nerve VI (abducens nerve) innervates the lateral rectus muscle. Abnormalities of these cranial nerves, which control eye movement, may cause diplopia. Diseases may affect these cranial nerves within the brainstem, in the subarachnoid space, in the cavernous sinus, or in the globe. Because cranial nerve VI has a long intracranial route within the subarachnoid space, failure of abduction of one or both eyes is a frequent nonspecific sign of increased intracranial pressure.

The pupillary light reaction is present by 30 weeks of gestation. Lesions of the third cranial nerve produce a dilated, mydriatic pupil, whereas lesions of the facial sympathetic fibers produce a constricted, meiotic pupil. Third nerve lesions may be associated with incomplete eye movements, and sympathetic lesions may produce a Horner syndrome with meiosis, ptosis, and unilateral facial anhidrosis. Drugs given systemically or instilled in the conjunctiva may affect pupil size. Anticholinergic and sympathomimetic drugs dilate the pupil, and cholinergic, narcotic, and sedative drugs constrict the pupil.

Cranial Nerve V

In newborns and small infants, the muscles of mastication can be observed as the infant sucks and swallows. The masseter muscles may be directly palpated. In later childhood, as cooperation improves, pterygoid function may be assessed by voluntary jaw deviation. The left pterygoid muscle moves the jaw to the right. The *corneal reflex* can be tested (cranial nerves V and VII) at any age. Facial sensation of light touch and pain can be determined with cotton gauze and pinprick.

Cranial Nerve VII

In newborns and small infants, the examiner can assess the facial muscles by observing the face at rest, with crying and with blinking. A common harmless anomaly in infants is unilateral absence of the depressor anguli oris muscle that produces an asymmetry of the face when the child cries. The lower lip on the involved side does not pull down. Cooperative children can be asked to smile, blow out their cheeks, blink forcibly, and furrow their foreheads. Weakness of all muscles of the face, including the forehead, eye, and mouth, indicates a lesion of the facial nerve. Weakness of the lower face and mouth with sparing of the forehead and eye closure indicates a unilateral lesion of the brain because the upper face receives cortical innervation from both hemispheres. The most common cause of facial nerve palsy is a transient inflammation called Bell's palsy. Commonly, taste in the anterior two thirds of the tongue is affected, as is the stapedial nerve, causing sounds to seem loud on the involved side. However, tearing is normal because the inflammation occurs distal to the geniculate ganglion.

Cranial Nerve VIII

Symptoms of lesions of cranial nerve VIII include deafness, tinnitus, and vertigo. Neonates who are alert will blink in response to a bell, and 4-month-old infants will turn their head and eyes to localize a sound stimulus. Hearing can be tested in the verbal child by whispering a word in one ear while covering or masking the opposite ear. Hearing loss can be conductive because of a lesion of the middle ear or sensorineural because of a lesion of the cochlea or auditory nerve. Tuning fork testing at 512 Hz can distinguish these two types. In *Rinne testing*, a tuning fork is placed alternately with the tines next to the pinna and with the stem on the mastoid process. Air conduction should sound louder and last longer than bone conduction. If bone conduction produces a better quality sound than air conduction, middle ear disease is likely. In Weber testing, the stem of the tuning fork is placed on the middle of the forehead. The sound should be equal in the two ears. If the sound is heard better in one ear, the problem is either a sensorineural loss in the opposite ear or a conductive loss in the ipsilateral ear. A conductive loss produces less air masking in the involved ear and an apparent improved bone conduction to that ear.

Lesions of the vestibular component of cranial nerve VIII produce symptoms of vertigo, nausea, vomiting, diaphoresis, and nystagmus. The *differential diagnosis* of vertigo is noted in Table 18–3. Nystagmus is an involuntary beating eye movement with a rapid phase in one direction and a slow phase in the opposite direction. By convention, the direction of the nystagmus is defined by the fast phase

---

TABLE 18–3
Differential Diagnosis of Vertigo*

Peripheral Causes
Benign positional vertigo
Acute vestibulopathy (labyrinthitis)
Ménière syndrome
Toxic labyrinthopathy
Motion sickness

Central Causes
Multiple sclerosis
Cerebrovascular disease
Cerebellopontine tumors (acoustic neuroma)
Migraine

---

*Peripheral vertigo has no other auditory (except Ménière syndrome) or neurologic deficits. Often, an intense sense of severe spinning with nausea, vomiting, a positive Romberg test, past pointing, and rotatory or horizontal nystagmus is present. Vertical nystagmus is often the result of brainstem lesions.

and may be horizontal, vertical, or rotatory. Lesions of the eighth cranial nerve commonly occur in the cerebellopontine angle but may also occur within the brainstem or within the petrous bone.

Cranial Nerves IX and X

The gag reflex is brisk at all ages except in the very immature neonate. An absent gag suggests a lower motor neuron lesion of either the brainstem, cranial nerves IX or X, neuromuscular junction, or pharyngeal muscles. Uvula deviation toward one side suggests palsy of cranial nerves IX or X on the opposite side. Weak, breathy, or nasal speech, weak sucking, drooling and inability to handle secretions, and gagging and nasal regurgitation of food are additional symptoms of cranial nerve X dysfunction.

Cranial Nerve XI

Observing the infant's posture and spontaneous activity assesses the functions of the trapezius and sternocleidomastoid muscles. Head tilt and drooping of the shoulder are suggestive of lesions involving cranial nerve XI. In later childhood, strength in these muscles can be tested directly and individually.

Cranial Nerve XII

Atrophy and fasciculation of the tongue, usually indicating a lesion of the anterior horn cells, can be observed at any age and are most reliably assessed when the infant is asleep. By 1 year of age, having the child follow a lollipop with the tongue can assess specific tongue movements. The tongue deviates toward the weak side in unilateral lesions.

Motor Examination

Strength

Strength in infants is assessed by observation. Arm and leg movements should be symmetric, and the limbs should easily be lifted off the bed. Symmetry of movements is seen best when the infant is held supine, with one hand supporting the buttocks and one the shoulders. Strength in toddlers is assessed by functional abilities. The child should be able to reach high above his or her head, wheelbarrow walk, run, hop, easily go up and down stairs, and arise from the ground. Cooperative children can undergo individual muscle strength testing. The primary symptom of lower motor neuron disease is weakness, whereas the primary symptom of upper motor neuron disease is stiffness. When the corticospinal pathway is interrupted, the affected limb can still move, but movements are coarse, slow, and stiff. Extrapyramidal motor pathway lesions may produce similar symptoms or may produce movement disorders such as tremor,

chorea, or athetosis. Muscle fasciculations indicate denervation from disease of the anterior horn cell or peripheral nerve.

Tone

In infants, two types of tone are assessed. Passive tone is the resistance to stretch felt as the limb is flexed and extended by the examiner. Lower motor lesions produce decreased passive tone, and chronic upper motor lesions produce increased passive tone. Active tone is the posture that an infant adopts when he or she is placed in a particular position. When the hands are grasped and the infant is pulled from supine to sitting, the infant's arms should pull on the examiner's fingers, and the head should not lag behind the shoulders. When the child is held upright with the examiner's hands in the infant's axillae, the infant's shoulders should be exerting downward force on the examiner's hands, and the infant's legs should be extended and pushing down on the examining table. When the child is held carefully above the table in prone or supine suspension, the child should have no difficulty raising the limbs and head above the plane of the body. Active tone is decreased with lesions of both the upper and lower motor neuron. In upper motor lesions, the infant demonstrates abnormal postures, such as standing on tiptoes instead of flatfooted and the hands constantly fisted with the thumb within the fist. In extrapyramidal disease, an increase in resistance is present throughout passive movement of a joint (*rigidity*). In pyramidal disease, increased resistance to passive movement that is velocity dependent and that suddenly gives way at a critical point (*clasped knife response*) is noted. Observation, palpation, and comparison to contralateral extremities assess muscle bulk. Excessive muscle bulk is seen in myotonia congenita and pseudohypertrophic muscular dystrophy.

Coordination

Observation and functional analysis help assess coordination in infants and toddlers. Intention tremor is the major symptom of cerebellar dysfunction. With cooperative children, having the children do repetitive finger or foot tapping can test rapid alternating movements. Both cerebellar and corticospinal tract dysfunction produce slow, rapidly alternating movements; the finger or foot tapping test alone cannot distinguish between the two.

Gait

Locomotion is assessed in infants by observation of creeping, crawling, and cruising. The toddler gait is normally wide based and somewhat unsteady. The base narrows with age, so that by the sixth year a child is able to tandem walk. At that time, the child should be able to walk high on the toes and heels. Cerebellar dysfunction results in a broad-based, unsteady gait accompanied by difficulty in executing turns. Corticospinal tract dysfunction produces a stiff, scissoring gait, with the child walking on the toes. Arm swing is decreased and the arm is held flexed across the body. Extrapyramidal dysfunction produces a slow, shuffling gait with dystonic postures. There may also be choreoathetotic movements. Lower motor neuron disease results in either a waddling gait if the proximal muscles are weak or a steppage gait if the distal muscles are weak. Each of these abnormal gaits is readily recognized in its pure form, but analysis of gait, like analysis of speech, is frequently extremely difficult and indeed frustrating because these are complex patterns with inputs from every part of the nervous system.

Reflexes

Myotactic reflexes at the triceps, biceps, brachioradialis, knee, and ankle are elicited by sudden tendon stretch and can be obtained at any age. These reflexes are decreased in lower motor neuron disease and increased with the development of clonus in chronic upper motor neuron disease. The Babinski response with upward movement of the great toe and flaring of the toes upon noxious stimulation of the side of the foot is a sign of corticospinal tract dysfunction. It is not helpful in the neonate because the normal response at this age may be either extensor or flexor. The plantar response is consistently flexor after 2 years of age.

Developmental reflexes of the neonate are described in Table 18–2.

Involuntary Movements

Involuntary movements are discussed under Movement Disorders.

Sensory Examination

The sensory examination of the newborn and infant is limited to observing the response to light touch or gentle sterile pinprick. Stimulation of the limb should produce a facial grimace. Movement of only the limb may be produced by a spinal reflex. In a cooperative child, the senses of pain, touch, temperature, vibration, and joint position can be individually tested. The cortical areas of sensation must be intact to identify by touch an object placed in the hand (stereognosis) or a number written in the hand (graphesthesia) or to distinguish between two sharp objects applied simultaneously and closely on the skin (two-point discrimination).

Mental Status Evaluation

The assessment of mental status is a critical aspect of the examination. *Alertness* is assessed in the newborn and small infant by observing spontaneous activities, feeding behavior, and the ability of the infant to visually fix and follow the movement of objects. The infant's response to tactile, visual, and auditory stimuli is noted. Does the infant localize sound, follow objects visually, and verbalize to noxious stimuli? In circumstances of altered consciousness, the response to painful stimuli is noted. Does the infant simply withdraw from pain, or is vigorous withdrawal accompanied by vocalization? Toddlers are expected to play at a level appropriate for their age, and older children can be tested for orientation to time, place, person, and purpose. (See the *Glasgow Coma Scale* under Disorders of Consciousness.)

Language function is both expressive (involving speech and the use of gestures such as pointing or shaking the head) and receptive (understanding speech or gesture). Abnormalities of language resulting from disorders of the cerebral hemispheres are referred to as *aphasias.* Anterior, expressive, or Broca aphasia is characterized by sparse, nonfluent language. Posterior, receptive, or Wernicke aphasia is characterized by an inability to understand language. Speech is fluent but nonsensical. Global aphasia refers to impaired expressive and receptive language.

The use of a Denver Developmental Standard Screening Test is an efficient means of relating the child's behavior to appropriate age norms (see Chapter 1). In addition to expressive and receptive language function, older children can be tested for reading, writing, numerical skills, general fund of knowledge, abstract reasoning, judgment, humor, and memory.

Special Diagnostic Procedures
Cerebrospinal Fluid Analysis

Analysis of cerebrospinal fluid (CSF) is essential when CNS infection is suspected and can provide important clues to various other diagnoses as outlined in Table 18–4. Differentiating a hemorrhagic CSF caused by a traumatic lumbar puncture (LP) from a true subarachnoid hemorrhage may be difficult. In most cases of traumatic LP, the fluid clears significantly over time. In addition, usually the person performing the LP has a good sense of whether the tap was traumatic or atraumatic. LP should be avoided in patients with clinical evidence of raised intracranial pressure for fear of causing cerebral herniation. Warning signs are papilledema or depression of consciousness with focal neurologic deficits. CT may indicate critical compression by demonstrating effacement of the cisterns around the midbrain.

TABLE 18-4
Analysis of CSF

	>1 Month Old	<1 Week Old
Normal CSF		
Cell count	$<5/mm^3$	$<10\text{-}40/mm^3$
Protein	<40 mg/dL	$<65\text{-}150/dL$
Sugar	$>\frac{2}{3}$ blood sugar or >60 mg/dL	$>\frac{2}{3}$ blood sugar or >40 mg/dL

↑ Polymorphonuclear WBCs, ↓ sugar
Bacterial infection
Parasitic infection
Leak of dermoid contents

↑ Lymphocytes, ↓ sugar
Mycobacterial infection
Fungal infection
Carcinomatous meningitis
Sarcoidosis

↑ Lymphocytes, normal sugar
Viral infection
Parainfectious disease
Parameningeal infection
Vasculitis
Lead intoxication

↑↑ CSF protein
Infection
Venous thrombosis
Hypertension
Spinal block (Freund syndrome)
Guillain-Barré syndrome

Mild CSF pleocytosis
Tumor
Infarction
Multiple sclerosis
Subacute bacterial endocarditis

Bloody CSF
Subarachnoid hemorrhage
Subdural hemorrhage
Intraparenchymal hemorrhage
   Trauma
   Vascular malformation
   Coagulopathy

Electroencephalography

The electroencephalograph (EEG) records electrical activity generated by the cerebral cortex. EEG rhythms mature throughout childhood. The EEG of the premature infant is discontinuous and accompanied by a predominance of slower frequencies (2–4 Hz) until 36 weeks of gestation, when the waking portion of the record is continuous. Sleep remains characterized by a discontinuous pattern (trace alternans). In later childhood, the occipital portion of the EEG is characterized by 8–12 Hz activity (alpha), whereas faster rhythms (13–30 Hz) (beta) are seen anteriorly. Theta rhythms (4–7 Hz) are intermixed. Fixed slow-wave foci (1–3 Hz) delta rhythms suggest an underlying structural abnormality. When delta activity is seen diffusely, increased intracranial pressure or other encephalopathy is suspected. Spikes, polyspikes, and spike-and-wave abnormalities indicate an underlying seizure tendency.

Evoked Responses

Evoked responses are computer-analyzed CNS responses to afferent stimuli. The stimulus (a click for auditory testing, a flash or pattern stimulus for visual testing, and a vibratory stimulus for somatosensory testing) is applied, and the CNS response is monitored over the scalp. Repetitive stimuli are computer averaged, and a response pattern is obtained. Abnormalities of the components of the response pattern can be localized to specific areas of the CNS. Somatosensory responses are of value in assessing peripheral nerve, spinal cord, and cerebral hemispheric function, whereas visual and auditory responses are of value in assessing hearing, central auditory function, and abnormalities of visual acuity and the visual pathways. Auditory evoked responses also are known as brainstem-evoked responses because they assess auditory pathways at the level of the brainstem. Evoked responses are of particular value in small infants and patients with altered consciousness.

Electromyography

Electromyography (EMG) is used primarily to assess abnormalities of the neuromuscular apparatus, including anterior horn cells, peripheral nerves, neuromuscular junctions, and muscles. Normal muscle is electrically silent at rest, and the presence of spontaneous discharge of motor *fibers* (fibrillations) or *groups of muscle fibers* (fasciculation) is indicative of denervation. Denervation indicates dysfunction of anterior horn cells or peripheral nerve. Abnormal responses in the muscle to repetitive nerve stimulation are seen with diseases of the neuromuscular junction such as myasthenia gravis and botulism. The amplitude and duration of the muscle compound action potential are decreased in primary diseases of muscle. Nerve conduction velocities are slowed in neuropathies.

Neuroradiology

Imaging the brain and spinal cord is accomplished using CT, myelography, cerebral angiography, and magnetic resonance imaging (MRI). Ultrasonography is a bedside procedure that can visualize the brain and ventricles of infants with open fontanels.

REFERENCES

Behrman RE, Kliegman RM, Jenson HB, editors: *Nelson textbook of pediatrics*, ed 16, Philadelphia, 2000, WB Saunders, Chapters 541, 542, 552, 555.
Jones KL: *Smith's recognizable patterns of human malformation*, ed 5, Philadelphia, 1997, WB Saunders.

DISORDERS OF CONSCIOUSNESS

Consciousness is a process by which a person is aware of self and environment. Coma is defined as being unresponsive to stimuli. Coma differs from sleep, in that the person in a coma cannot be aroused. Arousal is impaired by small lesions involving the reticular activating system (RAS), extensive bilateral cerebral lesions, or unilateral cerebral lesions that distort the upper brainstem (i.e., herniation syndromes). The RAS is a network of neurons located in the core of the brainstem extending from the mid pons through the midbrain and hypothalamus to the thalamus. The RAS projects widely to the cerebral cortex and serves a general arousing function.

Depression of consciousness may be acute, chronic, transitory, or recurring.

Acute Disorders of Consciousness

(See Chapter 3)

Approach. Acute changes in consciousness vary in degree from mild lethargy and confusion to deep coma. The *differential diagnosis* of altered consciousness is presented in Table 18–5. An initial approach to the comatose patient is discussed in Chapter 3. In childhood, the most common causes of coma are infections, hypoxia-ischemia (after cardiac arrest or drowning), intoxication, head trauma, and the ictal or postictal state.

Metabolic derangement may necessitate adjustments of certain blood chemistries (e.g., glucose, calcium, sodium, bicarbonate, blood urea nitrogen [BUN], and ammonia) by intravenous infusions or dialysis. Toxic ingestion may necessitate gastric lavage, charcoal administration, forced diuresis, dialysis, or specific antidotes (see Chapter 3). Infections are treated with antibiotics or antiviral agents (see Chapter 10). Structural brain lesions may necessitate surgical excision or medical treatment of raised intracranial pressure (see Chapter 3).

Clinical Manifestations. A detailed history and physical examination usually provide sufficient clues to

TABLE 18–5
Diagnostic Approach to Coma

Cause	Diagnostic Approach
Metabolic Derangements	Na^+, K^+, Cl^-, CO_2, BUN, creatinine, AST, ALT, PT, PTT, blood gas, ammonia, lead level, pyruvate, lactate, urinalysis, and urine amino and organic acids
Hypoglycemia	
Hyponatremia or its correction	
Hypernatremia or its correction	
Hyperosmolarity or its correction	
Hypercapnia	
Uremia	
Hyperammonemia	
Hepatic failure	
Reye syndrome	
Urea cycle enzyme deficiency	
Fatty acid/acyl-coenzyme A dehydrogenase deficiency	
Methylmalonicaciduria	
Propionicaciduria	
Idiopathic of prematurity	
Mitochondrial diseases	
Diabetes mellitus—ketoacidosis or hypoglycemia	
Lead intoxication	
Causes with CSF Abnormalities	CSF analysis, CT, MRI, angiogram
See Table 18-4	
Causes with CT or MRI Abnormalities	CT, MRI
Infarction	
Global (anoxia)	
Multifocal	
Unilateral, large	
Focal midbrain, hypothalamus, or thalamus	
TTP-HUS	
Mass lesion	
Tumor	
Hemorrhage	
Hydrocephalus	
Abscess	
Inflammatory mass	
Cyst	
Postinfectious demyelination	
Cerebral edema	
Trauma	
Hypoxia-ischemia	
Rapid correction of hyperosmolarity (hyperglycemia, hypernatremia)	
Infectious-postinfectious	
Toxins—lead	
Causes with Normal CT and CSF	Blood and urine analyses for toxic substances, EEG
Drug intoxication or withdrawal	
Epilepsy	
Concussion	
Migraine	
Hypoxic-ischemic injury	

ALT, Alanine aminotransferase (formerly SGPT); *AST,* aspartate aminotransferase (formerly SGOT); *BUN,* blood urea nitrogen; *CSF,* cerebrospinal fluid; *CT,* computed tomography; *EEG,* electroencephalogram; *HUS,* hemolytic-uremic syndrome; *MRI,* magnetic resonance imaging; *PT,* prothrombin time; *PTT,* partial thromboplastin time; *TTP,* thrombotic thrombocytopenic purpura.

differentiate among the three major diagnostic categories producing coma: metabolic or toxic, infectious, and structural. Fever, petechiae, chills, and sweats suggest infection. Pain on neck flexion, photophobia, and pain on movement of the eyes are symptoms of meningeal irritation. Symptoms of abdominal pain, diarrhea, sore throat, conjunctivitis, cough, or rash point to viral encephalitis or a parainfectious syndrome. Neck motion should be avoided in patients with suspected trauma or drowning until the cervical spine films rule out vertebral fracture or subluxation. Headache and severe vomiting can be caused by raised intracranial pressure. A very abrupt loss of consciousness suggests a stroke. Stupor progressing to deep, unarousable "sleep" over hours suggests drug intoxication. A chronic gradual fading of alertness over weeks suggests a growing intracranial mass. Chronic medical conditions or their treatment (e.g., diabetes mellitus, insulin administration, and leukemia), head trauma, use of "street drugs," social and emotional difficulties, exposure to sick animals, or travel to areas with known endemic diseases (e.g., Rocky Mountain spotted fever, Lyme disease) all provide specific clues.

Neurologic examination begins with observation. Breathing patterns, posture, and spontaneous actions often provide important clues to the depth, localization, and etiology of the depressed consciousness. Important recognizable respiratory patterns include *Cheyne-Stokes respiration,* central neurogenic hyperventilation, and gasping respiration. In Cheyne-Stokes respiration, a period of hyperventilation with a crescendo-decrescendo pattern alternates with a shorter period of apnea. Cerebral, thalamic, or hypothalamic modulation of respiration has been lost, but brainstem control is intact. This pattern also can be observed in patients with heart failure or primary respiratory disease. Midbrain disease yields *central neurogenic hyperventilation,* which consists of sustained rapid deep breathing. Gasping respirations are irregularly irregular. They indicate dysfunction of the low brainstem–medulla and usually are followed by terminal apnea.

Body posture can indicate the degree of depression of consciousness. Mild depression is manifested by a comfortable "sleeping" posture, with limbs slightly flexed, body tilted to one side, and eyes fully closed. Frequent readjustments of position, yawns, and sighs are observed. Patients who lie in a flat, extended, unvarying position with eyes half-open exhibit deep coma. An asymmetric posture suggests motor dysfunction of one side.

Observation reveals focal and generalized seizures, tremors, myoclonus, asterixis, choreoathetosis, dystonia, and ballismus. Focal seizures imply focal brain disease but also may be noted in children with meningitis or hypoglycemia. Generalized tremors, myoclonus, and asterixis are seen with

metabolic-toxic diseases. Choreoathetosis, dystonia, and ballismus imply basal ganglia dysfunction.

Hallucinations can involve any sensory modality. Typically, olfactory and gustatory hallucinations indicate structural brain disease; visual and tactile hallucinations indicate metabolic-toxic disease; and auditory hallucinations indicate psychiatric illness.

Formal assessment of the degree of unconsciousness is performed using the *Glasgow Coma Scale* (Table 18–6). Unresponsive patients are stimulated with noise, light touch, and pain. The various stages of depression of consciousness are defined in Table 18–7.

TABLE 18–6
Glasgow Coma Scale

Response	Score
Best Motor Response	
Nil (flaccid)	1
Extensor response	2
Abnormal flexion	3
Withdrawal	4
Localization of pain	5
Obeys commands	6
Best Verbal Response	
Nil	1
Incomprehensible sounds	2
Inappropriate words	3
Confused conversation	4
Oriented, fluent speech	5
Best Eye Opening Response	
Nil	1
To pain	2
To speech	3
Spontaneous	4

TABLE 18–7
Stages of Depressed Consciousness

Stage	Manifestations
Lethargy-irritability	Sleepy, poor attention, fully arousable
Confusion	Poor orientation
Delirium	Agitated confusion, hallucinations, autonomic abnormalities (e.g., excess sweating, tachycardia, hypertension)
Obtundation	Arousable only to severe stimuli
Stupor	Unarousable, localizes pain
Coma	Unarousable, does not localize pain

The detailed neurologic examination of the comatose patient focuses on the eyes and patterns of motor movement and tone. Eye movements are observed and then elicited with the *doll's head maneuver* (oculocephalic response) and cold caloric stimulation (oculovestibular response) (Fig. 18–1). The comatose patient may have no spontaneous eye movements, or the eyes may spontaneously rove slowly side to side. Doll's head movement should not be performed until it is clear that the cervical spine has not sustained a fracture or subluxation. People who are awake always can move their eyes whenever and wherever they wish by either saccadic or pursuit eye movements. Cold water placed in the external ear of a conscious person elicits nystagmus to the opposite side and extreme vertigo. Cold water placed in the ear of a comatose patient elicits tonic eye deviation to the same side. The oculocephalic response to head turning elicits uninhibited eye movements in the comatose patient if the brainstem is intact and incomplete eye movements if the brainstem is injured. With uninhibited eye movements, the eyes move opposite to the direction of head movement at exactly the same pace, as if they were freely floating "ball bearings" within the orbits. With complete loss of oculomotor function, the eyes remain in the center of the orbit, as if they are "painted on," regardless of any stimulation.

Certain characteristic postures and tone can define the level or locus of neurologic disability. *Decorticate posturing* consists of rigid extension of the legs and feet, flexion and supination of the arms, and fisting of the hands. It occurs when the midbrain and red nucleus control body posture without inhibition by diencephalon, basal ganglia, and cortical structures. *Decerebrate posturing* consists of rigid extension of legs, arms, trunk, and head with hyperpronation of lower arms. It indicates pontine and vestibular nucleus control of posture without inhibition from more rostral structures. These postures may be exhibited unilaterally or bilaterally, indicating equal or unequal dysfunction of the two sides of the brain. Sometimes, stereotyped rigid postures are exhibited that do not fall easily into the category of decerebrate or decorticate positions. These postures also indicate lack of cerebral and diencephalic control of upper brainstem motor reflexes.

Metabolic causes of acute coma are suggested by spontaneous fluctuations in the level of consciousness; tremors, myoclonus, and asterixis; visual and tactile hallucinations; and deep coma with preservation of pupillary light reflexes. Acute metabolic or toxic disorders usually produce a hypotonic limp state, but hypertonia, rigidity, and decorticate and decerebrate posturing sometimes are observed in coma caused by hypoglycemia, hepatic encephalopathy, and short-acting barbiturates. Focal abnormalities, including hemiparesis, cortical blindness, choreoathetosis, and ataxia, suggest *structural brain disease.*

Intracranial Pressure Evaluation. Papilledema or cranial nerve III palsies in patients with depressed consciousness are strong evidence of elevated intracranial pressure (ICP), which is a medical emergency. More commonly, progressive loss of consciousness accompanied by a characteristic progression of motor, oculomotor, pupillary, and respiratory signs, as detailed in Table 18–8, warns of incipient transtentorial herniation. Uncal herniation is another sign of severe increased ICP with early unilateral third nerve palsy and contralateral hemiparesis. Medical therapy must be instituted and emergency cranial CT performed. The initial study is done without contrast material so that blood and calcifications are easily identified. Contrast material can then be administered to identify inflammatory and neoplastic lesions. Some metabolic derangements give rise to severe elevations of ICP without producing recognizable CT abnormalities. These derangements include hepatic encephalopathy, Reye syndrome, hyponatremia, lead encephalopathy, trauma, treatment of diabetic ketoacidosis, and global or multifocal hypoxic-ischemic injury. Lumbar puncture increases the risk of transtentorial herniation in patients with raised ICP and should be avoided.

Differential Diagnosis. See Table 18–5.

Toxic or Metabolic Abnormalities. Metabolic imbalances associated with depression of consciousness are most severe when the metabolic derangement has developed acutely and rapidly. The neurologic deficits associated with uremia and hypercapnia without hypoxia usually are fully reversible. The other metabolic disorders, however, may produce permanent neurologic disability if they are not treated at an early stage. Pathologic examination of brain tissue has revealed neuronal loss in the presence of hypoglycemia; vascular damage and parenchymal hemorrhages with hypernatremia; cerebral edema with hyponatremia, hepatic failure, Reye syndrome, and lead encephalopathy; and astrocytosis with hepatic failure. Focal deficits are uncommon in metabolic encephalopathy. The presence of asterixis signals hepatic or uremic encephalopathy or hypercapnia. Reye syndrome produces an easily recognizable clinical picture consisting of pernicious vomiting, lethargy, belligerence, hyperventilation, and large pupils.

Systemic acidosis and alkalosis do not significantly depress consciousness but are characteristic features of a number of diseases that produce encephalopathy. Consciousness often is reduced in patients with diabetic ketoacidosis, but the severity of unresponsiveness correlates with the degree of hyperosmolarity, not with the degree of acidosis.

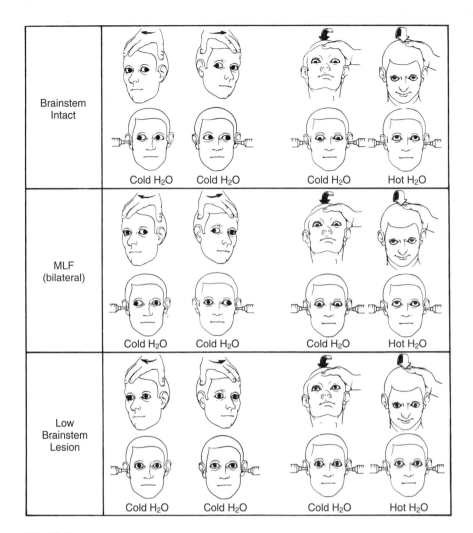

FIG. 18–1

Ocular reflexes in unconscious patients. *Top,* Oculocephalic *(above)* and oculovestibular *(below)* reflexes in an unconscious patient whose brainstem ocular pathways are intact. Horizontal eye movements are illustrated on the left and vertical eye movements on the right. Lateral conjugate eye movements (upper left) to head turning are full and opposite in direction to the movement of the face. A stronger stimulus to lateral deviation is achieved by irrigating cold water against the tympanic membrane. There is tonic conjugate deviation of both eyes toward the stimulus; the eyes usually remain tonically deviated for 1 minute or more before slowly returning to the midline. Because the patient is unconscious, there is no nystagmus. Extension of the neck in a patient with an intact brainstem produces conjugate deviation of the eyes in the downward direction, and flexion of the neck produces deviation of the eyes upward. Bilateral cold water against the tympanic membrane likewise produces conjugate downward deviation of the eyes, whereas hot water (no warmer than 44° C [111.2° F]) causes conjugate upward deviation of the eyes. *Middle,* Effects of bilateral medial longitudinal fasciculus (MLF) lesions on oculocephalic and oculovestibular reflexes. The left portion illustrates that oculocephalic and oculovestibular stimulation deviates the appropriate eye laterally and brings the eye, which normally would deviate medially, only to the midline, because the medial longitudinal fasciculus, with its connections between the abducens and oculomotor nuclei, is interrupted. Vertical eye movements often remain intact. *Bottom,* Effects of a low brainstem lesion. On the left, neither oculovestibular nor oculocephalic movements cause lateral deviation of the eyes because the pathways are interrupted between the vestibular nucleus and the abducens area. Likewise, in the right portion, neither oculovestibular nor oculocephalic stimulation causes vertical deviation of the eyes. On rare occasions, particularly with low lateral brainstem lesions, oculocephalic responses may be intact even when oculovestibular reflexes are abolished. (From Plum F, Posner J: *The diagnosis of stupor and coma,* ed 3, Philadelphia, 1980, FA Davis.)

TABLE 18–8
Progression of Stages and Anatomic Levels of Transtentorial Central Herniation

Signs	Thalamus →	Midbrain →	Medulla*
Consciousness	Confusion; stupor	Coma	Coma
Respirations	Sighs; Cheyne-Stokes type	Central neurogenic hyperventilation	Gasping; absent
Pupils	Small, reactive	3–5 mm, fixed	Unreactive
Extraocular movements	Roving; uninhibited	Incomplete, dysconjugate	Absent
Motor response	Spastic; decorticate	Decerebrate	Flaccid

*Uncal herniation with unilateral oculomotor nerve palsy and/or hemiplegia is another sign of severe increased intracranial pressure.

Proper treatment results in rapid return of full consciousness (see Chapter 17). In rare instances, patients with diabetes lapse into stupor hours after treatment is begun because of the development of brain swelling and central herniation; mortality is high. Medical therapy to reduce cerebral swelling may be quite effective if instituted when consciousness first wanes (see Chapter 3).

The *common drugs* and *toxins* that cause stupor and coma and their effects on pupillary size are listed in Table 18–9. Amphetamines, cocaine, psychedelics, anticholinergics, and withdrawal from alcohol or barbiturates can produce delirium. The clinical profile of depressant drug overdose consists initially of lethargy, ataxia, dysarthria, and nystagmus. This is followed by coma in a flaccid state, with diminished stretch reflexes, incomplete extraocular muscle responses, and small, reactive pupils.

Cerebrospinal Fluid Abnormalities. Red blood cells in the cerebrospinal fluid CSF indicate primary subarachnoid hemorrhage or parenchymal hemorrhage that has ruptured into the CSF. The former usually is caused by rupture of a saccular "berry" aneurysm of one of the major cerebral arteries in the circle of Willis. These aneurysms are presumed to result from localized developmental defects in the arterial walls. Rupture is rare in childhood. The usual *clinical manifestations* are the sudden onset of intense headache followed by collapse and loss of consciousness. Focal neurologic deficits are variable, but nuchal rigidity almost invariably is present. Retinal or subhyloid hemorrhages are common. Treatment should take place in an intensive care unit (ICU) and consists of bed rest, sedation, and therapy to eliminate vascular spasm until surgical or endovascular elimination of the aneurysm is feasible.

Spontaneous parenchymal hemorrhages in children are usually caused by arteriovenous malformations (AVMs). These are developmental anomalies

---

TABLE 18–9
Effect of Coma-Producing Toxins on Pupillary Size

Pupils Small
Narcotics (except meperidine)
Sedatives
    Barbiturates
    Alcohol
Major tranquilizers
Phenothiazines
Cholinergic agonists
    Organophosphate insecticides
    Nicotine
    Certain plants and mushrooms

Pupils Large
Anticholinergics
    Antihistamines
    Tricyclic antidepressants
    Phenothiazines
Glutethimide

Pupils Normal
Salicylates
Acetaminophen

---

consisting of tangled or dilated vessels that form a communication between the arterial and venous systems. The entire complex may enlarge slowly with age. Clinical presentation most commonly occurs between 10 and 40 years of age with intraparenchymal and subarachnoid hemorrhages, seizures, headaches, or slowly progressive neurologic deficits. The rare AVM that produces a very enlarged "vein of Galen aneurysm" can cause heart failure in infancy as a result of large-volume blood flow through the shunt. In early childhood these AVMs also can cause hydrocephalus as a result of compression of the aqueduct by the enlarged vein of Galen. A loud cranial bruit, if present, suggests an AVM.

Treatment of AVMs consists of surgical removal of the entire lesion, if possible. Intravascular resins or embolization with particulate matter also has been used to halt flow.

Other causes of parenchymal hemorrhages are cerebral trauma, disorders of hemostasis, hypertension, tumors, or hemorrhagic infarctions.

White blood cells in the CSF usually denote infectious meningitis or meningoencephalitis but also may be associated with subacute bacterial endocarditis, vasculitis, carcinomatous meningitis, or a parainfectious syndrome.

Parainfectious syndromes (e.g., disseminated encephalomyelitis) closely resemble episodes of viral meningoencephalitis but are the consequence of acute multifocal, immunologically mediated demyelination rather than of direct viral invasion of the brain. Fever, stiff neck, depression of consciousness, and focal neurologic deficits occur a few days after a benign systemic viral syndrome. The course is variable, but most children recover without sequelae within a few days to weeks. Systemic viral infection appears to trigger the syndrome by an unknown mechanism. These syndromes were first described following measles, mumps, rubella, and chickenpox and after vaccination against smallpox and rabies.

CT Abnormalities. Cerebral CT of a child with an acute disorder of consciousness may disclose either a space-occupying or a destructive lesion. To depress consciousness, unilateral cerebral lesions must directly compress and distort the diencephalon and brainstem, increase intracranial pressure by their bulk and associated edema, or block CSF pathways and produce hydrocephalus with increased ICP. Focal midbrain and diencephalic lesions that impair the RAS also can depress consciousness. Space-occupying lesions include tumors, abscesses, hemorrhages, cysts, and inflammatory masses.

Destructive lesions include infarcts and demyelinating plaques. When visible by CT, both appear as low-density areas, but the latter are confined to the white matter. Cerebral infarctions can impair consciousness when the lesions are global, multifocal, located in the midbrain, or unilateral and large. The latter create brain swelling and elevations of ICP, which then depress consciousness.

The major diseases that produce demyelinating plaques are multiple sclerosis and the parainfectious syndromes. The former is a chronic condition that occasionally presents in an acute disseminated man-

ner to produce coma. Parainfectious syndromes, in contrast, usually occur acutely and frequently give rise to multifocal lesions that impair consciousness. Cerebral MRI produces the best image of small infarctions and small demyelinating plaques. Almost all cerebral lesions, except calcifications and acute hemorrhages, are visualized better on MRI than CT. CT remains the preferred imaging technique in emergency situations because it can be performed very rapidly and accurately identifies acute hemorrhages and large space-occupying lesions, as well as edema and shifts of the midline.

Hypoxic-Ischemic Injury (see Chapter 6). Deprivation of oxygen to the brain, caused by either deficient oxygen in the blood (hypoxemia) or deficient delivery of blood to the brain (ischemia), impairs consciousness (Table 18–10). Severe ischemia produces loss of consciousness within seconds and permanent brain damage within a few minutes. Sometimes progressive deterioration in functioning takes place for several hours after a severe hypoxic-ischemic insult. Some irreversibly damaged cells may continue to function for a brief period and then die. Release of metabolites from dead and dying cells may initiate a chemical cascade, leading to loss

---

TABLE 18–10
Causes of Hypoxia and Ischemia

Hypoxia
Po₂ Decreased
Pulmonary disease
Cardiac disease; right-to-left shunt
Hypoventilation
  Exogenous (e.g., drowning, choking, suffocation)
  Neuromuscular disease
  Central respiratory drive decreased
Po₂ Normal; Decreased O₂ Content
Severe anemia
Carbon monoxide poisoning
Methemoglobinemia

Ischemia
Cardiac disease (decreased cardiac output)
Myocardial infarction
Arrhythmia
Valvular disease
Pericarditis
Pulmonary embolism
Hypotension, shock
Hanging, strangulation
Extensive cerebrovascular disease

of membrane stability in adjacent cells, intracellular influx of calcium ions, and cell death. In addition, the development of circulatory failure from anoxic cardiac injury, disseminated intravascular coagulation (DIC), or cerebral edema may compound the initial injury.

Rarely, patients undergo delayed *postanoxic encephalopathy.* An initial hypoxic-ischemic event causes stupor or coma. The patients awaken in 24–48 hours, but several days to weeks later they become irritable, apathetic, and confused. Then a spastic quadriplegia accompanied by pseudobulbar palsy develops. Pathologic and radiologic studies reveal severe bilateral leukoencephalopathy. The pathogenesis is unknown. Patients may die, recover completely, or remain in a spastic state.

The *prognosis* of cerebral hypoxic-ischemic injury is extremely variable in children. In general, short duration of coma (hours to 1–2 days) and presence of intact brainstem function on admission to the hospital imply a good prognosis. The most common permanent neurologic sequelae are spasticity, ataxia, choreoathetosis, parkinsonian syndrome, intention or action myoclonus, memory loss, visual agnosia, and impairments of learning and attention. Improvement can occur for several months to 1 year following the insult. *Treatment* involves physical therapy, occupational therapy, rehabilitative services, and education.

Occult Etiology. Some causes of coma remain unclear after the entire diagnostic workup is completed. The most common occult causes are drug or toxin exposure, cranial trauma, seizures, hypoxic-ischemic injury, migraine, and viral encephalitis. Sometimes a diagnosis is verified only as the natural history of the illness unfolds and the results of repeated examinations and testing are known.

Prognosis. The outcome of coma relates to many variables, including the etiology (intoxication carries a good prognosis, hypoxia carries a bad prognosis), the duration of coma, the age (children have a better outcome than adults), and the Glasgow Coma Scale on admission. Complete recovery from traumatic coma of several days' duration is possible in children. However, some survivors of severe coma are left in a persistent vegetative state or with severe neuropsychiatric disability.

Brain Death. Death of the whole brain (cortex and brainstem) generally is accepted as death of the person. Brain death means irreversible cessation of all functions. Table 18–11 lists the usual guidelines. In addition, total absence of cerebral blood flow on four-vessel intracranial angiography or nuclide brain scanning is definitive confirmation of brain death. Application of the criteria of brain death can be very difficult, particularly in newborns.

Transient Recurrent Depression of Consciousness

Seizures, migraine, cardiac arrhythmia, or hypoglycemia can cause episodic depression of consciousness with full recovery.

Consciousness can be impaired during seizures or in the postictal state. Nonconvulsive status epilepticus that is either generalized or partial complex can directly impair consciousness. Some patients may have a prolonged postictal state following an unrecognized seizure.

Basilar artery migraine attacks last hours and may consist of confusion accompanied by agitation, ataxia, cortical blindness, vertigo, or cranial nerve palsies. Headache may precede or follow the neurologic signs. Ischemia of the tissues supplied by the basilar artery also can produce amnesia and, infrequently, total loss of consciousness.

Cardiac arrhythmia or an obstructive cardiomyopathy (e.g., septal hypertrophy, left atrial myxoma, or critical aortic stenosis) can cause recurrent episodes of syncope. Children with unexplained syncope require a complete cardiac examination.

Hypoglycemia can give rise to recurrent episodes of lethargy, confusion, seizures, or coma. Anxiety, excess sweating, tremulousness, and hunger often herald attacks. A typical spell usually can be aborted by feeding the child orange juice or other sugar-containing solutions.

Several metabolic disorders cause recurrent bouts of hyperammonemia (Table 18–5). Symptoms include

---

TABLE 18–11
Guidelines for Determination of Brain Death*

No spontaneous movements, communication, or interaction with the environment

No supraspinal response to externally applied stimuli (pain, touch, light, sound)

Absence of brainstem reflexes (including pupillary light, oculocephalic, oculovestibular, corneal, oropharyngeal-gag, and tracheal-cough)

Apnea

Electrocerebral silence on electroencephalogram

---

*All of the criteria listed should be present on multiple examinations at least 6–24 hours after the onset of coma and apnea. There must be documented absence of drug intoxication (including sedatives and neuromuscular blocking agents), hypothermia, and cardiovascular shock. A cause of coma sufficient to account for the loss of brain function should be established.

nausea, vomiting, lethargy, confusion, ataxia, hyperventilation, and coma. Unlike episodes of hypoglycemia, which evolve over minutes, these spells worsen over hours. High-protein dietary intake or systemic viral infections often precipitate them. Early intravenous therapy is required to prevent permanent brain damage or death.

REFERENCES

Behrman RE, Kliegman RM, Jenson HB, editors: *Nelson textbook of pediatrics*, ed 16, Philadelphia, 1996, WB Saunders, Chapters 549–551.
Hossmann KA: The hypoxic brain: insights from ischemia research, *Adv Exp Med Biol* 474:155, 1999.
Plum F, Posner JB: *The diagnosis of stupor and coma*, Philadelphia, 1980, FA Davis.
Task Force for the Determination of Brain Death in Children: Guidelines for the determination of brain death in children, *Ann Neurol* 21:616, 1987.

CRANIOCEREBRAL TRAUMA

Children with head trauma may have depression of consciousness and neurologic deficits or may be alert without neurologic deficits. The former necessitates neurosurgical management, and the latter necessitates neurologic observation. Most serious trauma results from motor vehicle accidents, sports, recreation-related injuries, and violence.

Patients with Neurologic Deficits

Patients with neurologic deficits may have awakened following the injury (lucid interval) and then relapsed into coma or may have remained abnormal from the time of injury. Some patients are stable; others progressively deteriorate and require immediate neurosurgical care. These patients should all be managed in a skilled trauma center. The circulation must be supported, bleeding controlled, and all systemic problems identified. Proper intravenous fluids must be administered, the neck carefully immobilized in a neutral position, and the cerebral lesions managed immediately. A baseline neurologic evaluation should be followed by intubation, ventilation if indicated, and pharmacologic paralysis or sedation. If the patient is consciousness and the neurologic deficits are stable, other life-threatening problems (e.g., an acute abdomen) may take precedence over immediate neurosurgical evaluation or treatment. Skull and cervical spine roentgenograms and cranial CT are obtained as soon as possible. Syndromes of posttraumatic hemorrhage are summarized in Table 18–12.

TABLE 18–12
Syndromes of Posttraumatic Intracranial Hemorrhage

Syndrome	Clinical and Radiologic Characteristics	Treatment
Epidural	Onset over minutes to hours Uncal herniation with third nerve palsy and contralateral hemiparesis Lens-shaped extracerebral hemorrhage compressing brain	Surgical evacuation or observation Prognosis good
Acute subdural	Onset over hours Uncal herniation Focal neurologic deficits Crescentic extracranial hemorrhage compressing brain	Surgical evacuation Prognosis guarded
Chronic subdural	Onset over weeks to months Anemia, macrocephaly Seizures, vomiting Crescentic, low-density mass on CT	Subdural taps or subdural shunt as necessary Prognosis good
Intraparenchymal	Depressed consciousness Focal neurologic deficits Additional multiple contusions	Supportive care Prognosis guarded
Subarachnoid	Stiff neck Late hydrocephalus	Supportive care Prognosis variable
Contusion	Focal neurologic deficits Brain swelling with transtentorial herniation CT: multifocal low-density areas with punctate hemorrhages	Medical treatment of elevated intracranial pressure Prognosis guarded

CT, Computed tomography.

If surgery is not required, the child should be managed in an intensive care unit (see Chapter 3). If the child's neurologic condition worsens or the child already is comatose, ICP monitoring may be indicated.

Children with cerebral contusion who survive the acute cerebral swelling may improve rapidly or slowly or remain vegetative. Those who show daily improvement starting within days of the injury usually will recover completely. Maximal recovery may take weeks, months, or even a year in some patients. Caution must be used in providing families with a prognosis. Coma lasting for weeks following head trauma still is compatible with an ultimately good outcome, although the risk of late sequelae is increased. Patients who remain in a vegetative state for months following head injury are unlikely to improve.

Awake, Alert Children Without Neurologic Deficits Who Have Headaches, Sleepiness, or Vomiting

Most children in this category recover fully and uneventfully. A few of these patients experience early or late complications that must be recognized and treated.

Concussion

Concussion is a brief period of unconsciousness, lasting seconds or minutes, that occurs immediately after head trauma. Amnesia often follows concussion. *Retrograde amnesia* is the inability to remember events immediately before the trauma and may extend backward in time for minutes, hours, days, or weeks. Usually, retrograde memory gradually is regained and permanent amnesia lasts only for the few minutes immediately prior to the blow. *Antegrade amnesia* is the inability to form new memories and becomes manifest by the patient incessantly repeating the same questions shortly after they have been answered (e.g., "Where am I?" "Why am I here?"). This state often persists for hours. The period of amnesia, both retrograde and antegrade, usually correlates with the severity of the trauma.

The pathophysiology of concussion is thought to be a shearing lesion of white matter as the brain is shaken within the cranium, resulting in a temporary failure of axon conduction. If loss of consciousness is maintained for longer than an hour or if recovery of consciousness is slow and accompanied by focal neurologic deficits, the pathophysiology is likely to include contusion and laceration, which may lead to focal or generalized *brain swelling*.

Repeated concussions, especially within a short time frame such as days or weeks, are thought to carry a significant risk of permanent brain injury. A commonly used guideline is that children who sustain a sports-related concussion can resume participation 4 weeks after the injury if they have been asymptomatic at rest and with exertion for 2 weeks. Many neurologists will prohibit a child from playing a sport in which they have sustained two or three concussions.

Hemorrhage

See Table 18–12.

Malignant Posttraumatic Cerebral Swelling

Occasionally, epidural hemorrhage, other intracranial hemorrhage, or a rapid life-threatening increase in ICP develops unexpectedly in children who appear stable for hours following head trauma. *Diagnosis* and *treatment* proceed as detailed in Table 18–12.

Syncope

Some patients faint a few minutes after head trauma or on awakening from their initial concussion. These patients complain of "dizzy" lightheadedness and loss of vision and slowly slump to the ground in a sleeplike state. Spontaneous arousal to full orientation occurs within a couple of minutes. Presumably, the psychic trauma produces a vagal discharge resulting in bradycardia and hypotension. *Treatment* consists of keeping the patient lying down until he or she is fully aroused, well perfused, and reassured that all is well.

Transient Neurologic Disturbance

Transient neurologic disturbances sometimes develop in a few minutes after minor or severe head trauma and last for minutes to hours before clearing. The most common symptoms are cortical blindness and a confusional state, but hemiparesis, ataxia, or any other neurologic deficit may appear. These symptoms may represent migraine precipitated by trauma in susceptible children.

Posttraumatic Seizures

Posttraumatic seizures are discussed in the following section under Seizure Disorders.

Drowsiness, Headache, and Vomiting

Drowsiness, headache, and vomiting are common following head trauma and are not by themselves of concern if consciousness is preserved and results of the neurologic examination are normal. Children are especially susceptible to severe sleepiness following head trauma but should be easily arousable to alert wakefulness. If these symptoms persist unabated for more than 1–2 days, CT or MRI is indicated.

Skull Fractures

Skull fractures may be linear, diastatic (spreading the suture), depressed (an edge displaced inferiorly), or compound (bone fragments breaking the skin surface).

Linear and diastatic fractures necessitate no treatment but indicate severe trauma capable of producing an underlying hematoma.

Small depressed fractures have the same significance as linear fractures, but if the depression is more than 0.5–1 cm, surgical elevation of bone fragments and repair of associated dural tears are recommended.

Compound fractures or penetrating injuries necessitate surgical débridement but not prophylactic antibiotic therapy. Tetanus prophylaxis must be ensured. The risk of local brain contusion and early seizures is high.

Clinical *manifestations* of skull fracture include localized bogginess and pain; subcutaneous bleeding over the mastoid process (*Battle sign)* or around the orbit (*raccoon eyes);* blood behind the tympanic membrane (*hemotympanum);* or CSF leak from the nose (*rhinorrhea)* or ear (*otorrhea).*

Rarely, following linear skull fractures, a soft, pulsatile scalp mass is palpable within a few weeks to months. Radiographically, the fracture edges are separated by a soft tissue mass that consists of fibrotic and accumulated brain and meningeal tissue and perhaps a leptomeningeal cyst. The recommended *treatment* involves surgical excision of abnormal tissue and dural repair.

Cerebrospinal Fluid Leak

CSF leak occurs when a skull fracture tears adjacent dura, creating communications between the subarachnoid space and the nose, paranasal sinuses, mastoid air cells, or middle or external ear. Clear fluid that leaks from the nose or ear following head trauma is presumed to be CSF. The presence of air within the subdural, subarachnoid, or ventricular space also indicates a dural tear and open communication between the nose or paranasal sinuses and brain. In most cases, the dura heals spontaneously when the patient's head is kept elevated. If the leak persists or recurs or if meningitis supervenes, the fracture site is identified and the dura is surgically repaired.

Cranial Nerve Palsies

Palsies following laceration or contusion resulting from skull fracture may be transitory or permanent. Longitudinal fractures of the petrous bone produce conductive hearing loss and facial palsy, which begin hours after the injury and usually resolve spontaneously. Transverse petrous fractures produce sensorineural hearing loss and immediate facial palsy, with a poor prognosis for spontaneous recovery. Disruption of the ossicular chain is a cause of hearing loss and necessitates surgery. Permanent loss of olfaction after a head injury is the result of a vibra-

tional rupture of the thin olfactory nerves within the cribriform plate. Disruption of cranial nerves III, IV, or VI produces ophthalmoplegia, diplopia, and head tilt.

Cervical Spine Injuries

Cervical spine injuries should be suspected in any unconscious child, especially if bruises are present on the back. In conscious children, findings of neck or back pain, burning or stabbing pains radiating to the arms, paraplegia, quadriplegia, or asymmetric motor or sensory responses of arms or legs are indications of spinal cord injury. Cervical spine injury (displaced or fractured vertebra) also may result in complete transection of the cord with spinal shock, loss of sensation, and flaccid paralysis. A contused cord (without vertebral abnormality) may be exhibited in a similar manner. Any patient with a clinical or radiologic abnormality of the spine requires immediate spine and cardiopulmonary stabilization and neurosurgical consultation. High-dose (30 mg/kg bolus, then 5.4 mg/kg/hr for 23 hours) intravenous methylprednisolone is indicated in cases of spinal cord trauma and improves the ultimate degree of recovery of function.

Subdural Fluid

The presence of subdural fluid can be the result of either active accumulation of fluid or atrophy of adjacent brain tissue. The former process usually begins with a subdural hemorrhage. Vascular membranes arising from dura surround the hemorrhage. Leakage of proteinaceous exudate or small hemorrhages from these membranes may enlarge the subdural collection. Symptoms consist of slowly evolving focal neurologic deficits, focal seizures, or evidence of raised ICP. Treatment may require repeated subdural taps or a subdural-peritoneal shunt.

Post–Head Trauma Syndrome

Some children complain of headache, dizziness, forgetfulness, inability to concentrate, slowing of response time, mood swings, irritability, and other subtle aberrations of cerebral function for days or weeks following an uncomplicated concussion. These deficits almost always resolve spontaneously. Children may require brief periods of special schooling, home tutoring, and reassurance. Persistent severe headaches often respond to prophylactic therapy with propranolol, 1 mg/kg/24 hr.

Management. Children who have been unconscious from a head injury or who have amnesia after a blow to the head should be examined in an emergency room. High-risk patients include those with persistent depressed level of consciousness, focal neurologic signs, decreasing level of consciousness, penetrating skull injury, or depressed skull fractures. These patients warrant care in a skilled trauma center and CT or MRI examination.

The period of observation should increase with the severity of the injury, and there should be no hesitation to admit children without neurologic deficits to the hospital for observation. If the child appears well after several hours and is discharged home, parents should be instructed to call their physician for any change in alertness, orientation, or neurologic functioning. An increase in headache or vomiting is cause for concern.

Prognosis. Children suffering from concussion without subsequent neurologic deficits do well. Late sequelae are rare. Children with moderate contusions usually make good recoveries even when neurologic signs persist for weeks. Long-term sequelae may include poor memory and slowing of motor skills or a generalized decrease in cognitive skills, behavioral alterations, and attention deficits. Language function, especially in the young child, frequently makes a good recovery. Rehabilitation consists of physical therapy, behavior management, and appropriate education. *Poor prognostic features* include a Glasgow Coma Scale score of 3–4 on admission without improvement in 24 hours, absent pupillary light reflexes, and persistent extensor plantar reflexes. Extracranial trauma also contributes to the morbidity of these patients (e.g., adult respiratory distress syndrome, sepsis, and emboli).

REFERENCES

Behrman RE, Kliegman RM, Jenson HB, editors: *Nelson textbook of pediatrics,* ed 16, Philadelphia, 2000, WB Saunders, Chapters 64, 692.

Chiles B, Cooper P: Acute spinal injury, *N Engl J Med* 334(8): 514–520, 1996.

Duhaime AC, Alario AJ, Lewander WJ, et al: Head injury in very young children: mechanisms, injury types, and ophthalmologic findings in 100 hospitalized patients younger than 2 years of age, *Pediatrics* 90(2 Pt 1):179–185, 1992.

Lieh-Lai MW, Theodorou AA, Sarnaik AP, et al: Limitations of the Glasgow Coma Scale in predicting outcome in children with traumatic brain injury, *J Pediatr* 120(2 Pt 1):195–199, 1992.

White RJ, Likavec MJ: The diagnosis and initial management of head injury, *N Engl J Med* 327(21):1507–1511, 1992.

INCREASED INTRACRANIAL PRESSURE

Pathophysiology and Etiology. Increased intracranial pressure (ICP) is both a symptom of serious intracranial pathology and a cause of irreversible neurologic injury. The skull is a rigid container enclosing a fixed volume, which includes the brain, cerebrospinal fluid, and blood. Normally, the brain accounts for 80–85% of the volume, CSF 10–15%, and blood 5–10%. As intracranial volume and ICP rise, the same increments in volume cause larger and larger increases in ICP in a rapidly worsening vicious cycle. The brain can accommodate raised ICP initially by expelling CSF and blood from the intracranial compartment into the spinal subarachnoid space. When the limits of this accommodation are reached, the brain itself begins to shift in response to the continuing elevation of ICP. The intracranial space is divided into compartments by dural extensions that are called the falx and the tentorium. Brain shifts are called herniations and may occur under the falx, through the tentorial notch or into the foramen magnum. Supratentorial masses will produce transtentorial herniation; infratentorial masses will produce foramen magnum herniation, and unilateral frontal masses will produce transfalcial herniation. Transtentorial herniation is more likely to occur with a unilateral hemispheric lesion than with diffuse supratentorial brain swelling. Transtentorial and foramen magnum herniations are immediately life threatening and indicate critically raised ICP (Table 18–13). Herniations produce infarction of vital thalamic and brainstem structures by interference with their arterial and venous blood supply and distortion of their structures. Lumbar puncture is contraindicated in the presence of increased ICP because leak of CSF through a puncture wound in the lumbar thecal sac promotes brain shifts and herniations.

The causes of increased intracranial pressure (ICP) are listed in Table 18–14 and can be broadly categorized as follows: (1) mass lesion, (2) hydrocephalus, (3) brain swelling.

Symptoms and Signs. The symptoms and signs of raised ICP include headache, vomiting, lethargy, irritability, sixth nerve palsy, strabismus, diplopia, and papilledema. Infants who have an open fontanel will usually not develop papilledema or abducens palsy. Specific signs of raised ICP in infants consist of a bulging fontanel, suture diastasis, distended scalp veins, a persistent downward deviation ("sunsetting") of the eyes, and rapid growth of head circumference. Specific signs of raised ICP in the infratentorial compartment (posterior fossa) include stiff neck and head tilt.

Focal neurologic deficits will reflect the site of the lesion that is producing the increased ICP and may include hemiparesis from supratentorial lesions and ataxia from infratentorial lesions.

The major specific sign of *critically increased ICP* is dilation and poor reactivity of one or both pupils. Cushing triad is a late sign of critically increased ICP and consists of elevated blood pressure, decreased pulse, and irregular respirations.

TABLE 18–13
Herniation Syndromes

Location	Description	Clinical Findings
Transtentorial		
Central	Caudal displacement of cerebral hemispheres, resulting in downward displacement of diencephalon and midbrain	Altered mental status Cheyne-Stokes to central neurogenic hyperventilation Decorticate to decerebrate posturing Loss of oculovestibular reflexes Death
Uncal	Temporal lobe displacement into the tentorial opening Third nerve, posterior cerebral artery, and midbrain compression	Unilateral pupillary dilation followed by oculomotor paralysis with or without ptosis Hemiplegia Death
Cerebellar		
Downward	Cerebellar tonsils displaced through the foramen magnum Compression of medulla, posterior inferior cerebellar artery	Neck stiffness Respiratory, cardiac arrest Lower cranial nerve dysfunction Death
Upward	Cerebellar tissue displaced through tentorial opening Compression of midbrain and superior cerebellar arteries	Paralysis of upgaze Pupillary dilation Central hyperventilation Death
Transfalcial		
Cingulate	Unilateral cerebral lesions result in displacement of the cingulate gyrus beneath the falx cerebri, compromising the cingulate gyrus and the callosal and pericallosal arteries	Cingulate gyrus necrosis and ischemia lead to edema and central transtentorial herniation

Diagnosis. The cause of increased ICP is determined by brain imaging with either CT or MRI. CT is usually preferred because of its ready availability, speed of imaging, and clear delineation of acute hemorrhage. Mass lesions, hydrocephalus, and trauma are easily diagnosed. Diffuse brain swelling produced by hypoxic-ischemic injury, meningitis, encephalitis, metabolic abnormalities, or toxins is more difficult to recognize. The best evidence of severely increased ICP on CT scan consists of effacement of the dorsal perimesencephalic cisterns.

Conditions with Focal Lesions on CT Scan

Brain Abscess. Brain abscesses or any mass lesion may produce increased ICP not only by virtue of large size but also by blockage of CSF, blockage of venous outflow, or production of cerebral edema. This vasogenic edema is produced by leakage of plasma proteins and fluid through a damaged blood-brain barrier at the level of the endothelial cell. Brain abscesses usually present as mass lesions, producing focal neurologic signs and increased ICP. Symptoms of infection, including fever, malaise, anorexia, and stiff neck, may also be present or may be absent. Edema is usually severe and extensive in the surrounding white matter. The diagnosis of brain abscess is suspected in children with chronic cardiac or pulmonary disease that may embolize infected material to their brains. Lumbar puncture is particularly contraindicated in children with suspected brain abscess because the risks of transtentorial herniation are high as a result of the extensive unilateral white matter edema.

Hydrocephalus. Hydrocephalus usually produces a slowly evolving syndrome of increased ICP extending over weeks or months. Pressure is exerted by both enlarging ventricles and interstitial edema

---

TABLE 18–14
Causes of Increased Intracranial Pressure

Focal Lesion Revealed on CT	Diffuse Swelling Revealed on CT; Mental Status Abnormal—cont'd
Hydrocephalus	Fulminant hepatic encephalopathy
Infarction	Pulmonary insufficiency with hypercarbia
Mass lesion	Lead intoxication
Hemorrhage	
Tumor	**No Focal Lesion Revealed on CT; Mental Status**
Abscess	**Normal (Pseudotumor Cerebri Syndrome)**
Cyst	Intracranial venous sinus thrombosis
Inflammatory mass	Drugs
	Vitamin A; retinoic acid
Diffuse Swelling Revealed on CT; Mental Status	Tetracycline; nalidixic acid
Abnormal	Endocrinologic disturbance
Hypoxic-ischemic injury	Withdrawal of chronic steroid administration
Trauma	Addison disease
Infection	Hypoparathyroidism
Meningitis	Obesity in women with menstrual irregularities
Encephalitis	Iron-deficiency anemia
Hypertension	Catch-up growth in infants with malnutrition (e.g., cystic fibrosis)
Metabolic derangement or toxin	High-altitude brain edema
Hyponatremia	Idiopathic pseudotumor cerebri
Diabetic ketoacidosis	
Dialysis disequilibrium syndrome	
Reye syndrome	

in the periventricular white matter created by transudation of CSF through the ependymal barrier. CSF is an ultrafiltrate of plasma continuously produced by the choroid plexus of the lateral, third, and fourth ventricles. The normal volume of CSF is approximately 50 mL in neonates and 150 mL in adults. CSF normally flows from the lateral ventricles through the intraventricular foramen of Monro to the third ventricle. From the third ventricle, it passes through the cerebral aqueduct to the fourth ventricle. CSF exits the fourth ventricle from the single midline foramen of Magendie and the two lateral foramina of Luschka. Subarachnoid flow occurs superiorly to the cisterns of the brain and inferiorly to the spinal subarachnoid space. Absorption of CSF is accomplished predominantly by the arachnoid villi, which are microtubular invaginations into the large dural sinuses and are most concentrated along the superior sagittal sinus.

The *etiology* of hydrocephalus is obstruction of CSF flow anywhere along its course (Table 18-15). Obstructive or internal hydrocephalus is caused by a block before CSF reaches the subarachnoid space. Impairment of CSF flow within the subarachnoid space or impairment of absorption is known by the misnomer communicating hydrocephalus (actually extraventricular obstructive hydrocephalus) or external hydrocephalus. Hydrocephalus caused by overproduction of CSF without true obstruction is seen in choroid plexus papillomas, which account for 2–4% of childhood intracranial tumors and manifest in early infancy.

Ventricular distention and increased intracranial pressure cause the clinical manifestations of hydrocephalus. Dilation of the lateral ventricles results in stretching of the corticopontocerebellar and corticospinal pathways, which sweep around the lateral margins of these ventricles to reach the cerebral peduncles. This stretching results in ataxia and spasticity that initially are most marked in the lower extremities because the leg fibers are closest to the ventricles. Distention of the third ventricle may compress the hypothalamic regions and result in endocrine dysfunction. The optic nerves, chiasm, and tracts also are in proximity to the anterior third ventricle, and visual dysfunction results when these structures are compressed. Dilation of the cerebral aqueduct compresses the surrounding periaqueductal

TABLE 18–15
Causes of Hydrocephalus

Obstruction Region	Clinical Characteristics	Etiology
Intraventricular foramina	Acutely or slowly evolving, unilateral ventricular dilation; can be exhibited at any age	Congenital, parasellar mass, intraventricular tumors
Aqueduct of Sylvius (cerebral aqueduct)	May be exhibited in utero or in adults; usually noted in infancy; slowly evolves	Neurofibromatosis, intrauterine toxoplasmosis, postmumps meningoencephalitis; periaqueductal mass lesions: tumors, vein of Galen malformations; congenital dysplasia; hereditary, sex-linked
Impaired flow from the fourth ventricle		
Dandy-Walker malformation	Enlarged occipital shelf; slowly evolving; marked transillumination of the posterior fossa; usually is exhibited in infancy but may be delayed until adult life	Referred to as atresia of the foramina of Luschka and Magendie but actually due to agenesis of the cerebellar vermis, resulting in cystic dilation of the fourth ventricle and aqueductal compression
Arnold-Chiari malformation	May or may not be associated with myelomeningocele; may be exhibited in later life with cranial nerve dysfunction, with or without hydrocephalus	Congenital malformation resulting in a small posterior fossa, caudal displacement of the fourth ventricle and cerebellum, and distortion of the brainstem
Congenital bone lesions of the cranial base	Slowly evolving hydrocephalus, stiff neck; lower cranial nerve dysfunction	Achondroplasia, rickets, basilar impression; these lesions compress the posterior fossa, preventing CSF flow and distorting the brainstem
Extraventricular obstruction (communicating)	Acutely or slowly evolving; is exhibited at any age	Congenital, due to hypoplasia of the arachnoid villi; following infection or hemorrhage due to destruction of arachnoid villi or subarachnoid fibrosis, causing obstruction to CSF flow (following superior sagittal sinus occlusion, preventing absorption of CSF)

CSF, Cerebrospinal fluid.

vertical gaze center, causing paresis of upward gaze. Manifestations of increased ICP may evolve slowly when obstruction to CSF flow is not complete and there is time for transependymal absorption of CSF into the veins of the white matter, or rapidly when obstruction is abrupt and complete (as in subarachnoid hemorrhage) and compensation cannot occur.

The *treatment* of hydrocephalus is both medical and surgical. Following subarachnoid hemorrhage or meningitis, the flow or absorption of CSF may be transiently impaired. In this circumstance, the use of agents such as acetazolamide, which transiently decreases CSF production, may be of benefit. Surgical management consists of removing the obstructive lesion (tumor, cyst, or AVM) or placing a shunt. A shunt consists of polyethylene tubing extending usually from a lateral ventricle to the peritoneal cavity. Shunts carry the hazards of infection (e.g., with *Staphylococcus epidermidis* or *Corynebacterium)* or sudden occlusion with signs and symptoms of acute hydrocephalus.

Conditions with No Focal Lesion on CT Scan: Mental Status Abnormal

Diffuse brain swelling in an acutely ill child usually results from hypoxic-ischemic injury, trauma, infection, metabolic derangement, or toxic ingestion, as listed in Table 18–14. Hypoxic-ischemic injury produces cytotoxic edema, which consists of swelling of neurons, glia, and endothelial cells because of damage to the cellular metabolic machinery.

Meningitis. Bacterial meningitis may produce increased ICP by blockage of CSF pathways, toxic cerebral edema, increase in cerebral blood flow, or multifocal cerebral infarctions. Most children with bacterial meningitis can safely undergo lumbar puncture because the brain swelling is diffuse and evenly distributed throughout the brain and spinal CSF compartments. However, a small number of patients with meningitis demonstrate transtentorial herniation within a few hours of a spinal tap. Focal neurologic signs, poorly reactive pupils, or a tense fontanel is a contraindication to lumbar puncture in the infant or child with suspected bacterial meningitis. Children with bacterial meningitis and depression of consciousness should be examined frequently within the first 12 hours following a lumbar puncture. If the pupils dilate or other evidence of increased ICP becomes evident, immediate treatment must be undertaken and may be life saving.

Conditions with No Focal Lesion on CT Scan: Mental Status Normal

Pseudotumor Cerebri Syndrome. Pseudotumor cerebri is a benign cause of increased ICP that is associated with diffuse brain swelling. Critical herniations do not occur. The patients do not appear critically ill and exhibit headache, diplopia, abducens palsy, and papilledema. Brain imaging studies are usually normal. This syndrome has been associated with the ingestion of certain drugs, endocrine disturbances, and intracranial venous sinus thrombosis. Most commonly however, this condition is idiopathic and affects children who are otherwise perfectly well. Usually, idiopathic intracranial hypertension will resolve spontaneously over several weeks or months. Treatment with acetazolamide, several lumbar punctures, or a short course of corticosteroids is sufficient. Rarely, chronic papilledema from persistent pseudotumor cerebri produces visual impairment, and more aggressive management is required.

Treatment. The treatment of increased ICP includes rigorous support of the vital signs, as well as the following specific interventions. Mannitol is used acutely to produce an osmotic shift of fluid from the brain to the plasma. Corticosteroids reduce vasogenic cerebral edema over several hours. Acetazolamide and furosemide transiently decrease CSF production. Intubation and hyperventilation produce cerebral vasoconstriction, leading to decreased cerebral blood volume. A ventricular catheter is used to remove CSF and to continuously monitor the intracranial pressure. Pentobarbital-induced coma reduces pressure by severely suppressing cerebral metabolism and cerebral blood flow.

All treatments for increased ICP are temporary measures intended to prevent critical herniations until the underlying disease process either is treated or resolves spontaneously. Timely intervention can reverse the vicious cycle of cerebral herniation, and a complete neurologic recovery is possible even after clear signs of transtentorial or foramen magnum herniation have begun. Once these signs are completed, however, with bilaterally dilated, unreactive pupils, absent eye movements, and flaccid quadriplegia, recovery is no longer possible.

REFERENCES

Behrman RE, Kliegman RM, Jenson HB, editors: *Nelson textbook of pediatrics,* ed 16, Philadelphia, 1996, WB Saunders, Chapters 62–64, 72, 607, 610, 612, 692.

Miller D: Intracranial pressure monitoring, *Arch Neurol* 42(12): 1191–1193, 1986.

Packer RJ: Brain tumors in children, *Arch Neurol* 56(4):421–425, 1999.

HEADACHE AND MIGRAINE

The evaluation of children with *headache* is straightforward. If the neurologic examination reveals any abnormalities, cranial CT or MRI is obtained. If neurologic and general physical examinations are negative, the likely diagnoses are either migraine or tension headaches.

Any space-occupying lesion within the cranium can cause headache, either by pressure on adjacent pain-sensitive structures or by obstruction of CSF circulation and the production of hydrocephalus. Lesions within the posterior fossa usually produce occipital pain, whereas supratentorial lesions produce frontal, temporal, or vertex pain. Hydrocephalus usually causes early morning frontal headache that may awaken the child, and often is associated with vomiting with or without nausea. Aneurysms almost always present as an acute subarachnoid hemorrhage and are characterized by severe headache, change in consciousness, and stiff neck. Pseudotumor cerebri presents with severe daily headaches and with signs of increased ICP.

Hypertension, trauma, lumbar puncture, fever, various drugs, and infection also may cause acute headache. Headache is a common symptom in patients with meningitis, encephalitis, sinusitis, pharyngitis, and systemic viral illnesses and may be associated with a variety of disorders involving the eyes, ears, nose, teeth, and neck.

Many patients with headache visit a doctor only for reassurance that there is no serious underlying disease, and thereafter are content to treat the headache symptomatically. An unremarkable history and physical examination are sufficient to provide this reassurance. Sometimes the neurologic examination yields equivocal findings or the history is so compelling for serious intracranial pathology that CT or MRI is required despite a normal examination. Worrisome headaches are those that are most severe on awakening, that awaken the patient in the middle of the night, that are severely exacerbated by coughing or bending, that are acute without a previous history of headache, that are present daily and getting progressively more severe in a crescendo pattern, and that are accompanied by vomiting with or without nausea.

Migraine and *tension headache*s are the most common causes of recurrent headaches in both children and adults (Table 18–16). The pathogenesis of migraine is unknown, but there is paroxysmal hyperexcitability of the sensory pathways of the fifth cranial nerve, followed by release of inflammatory mediators. There may be a phase of intracerebral arterial constriction followed by a phase of extracranial, and sometimes intracranial, arterial dilation. Migraine frequently begins in childhood. Infants and toddlers who are unable to verbalize the source of their discomfort may exhibit spells of irritability, sleepiness, pallor, and vomiting. Young children with migraine frequently lack many of the typical features. Periodic headaches in children accompanied by nausea or vomiting and relieved by rest are likely to be migraine. Sometimes even the periodic nature of the headache is not appreciated because the children will have frequent mild to moderate headaches between major attacks of severe headaches. The name "common migraine" sometimes is attached to these moderate atypical headaches.

The most characteristic symptom of migraine is a visual aura that immediately precedes the headache and persists for 15–20 minutes. The visual aura consists of spots, flashes, or lines of light that flicker in one visual field. Migraine auras may also consist of brief episodes of unilateral or perioral numbness, unilateral weakness, or vertigo. Sometimes patients with migraine have episodes of neurologic deficits that persist for hours and then resolve completely. These episodes are called "complicated migraine" and typically consist of hemiparesis, monocular blindness, ophthalmoplegia, or confusion. The *diagnosis* is frequently uncertain during the first attack, and brain imaging may be required.

Treatment of migraine includes prophylactic medications taken daily to reduce the frequency and severity of attacks and symptomatic medications taken during attacks to reduce their intensity and duration (Table 18–17). The first step in migraine prophylaxis is to identify precipitating agents and eliminate as many as possible. Prophylactic medications are used when headaches are occurring frequently and interfering with activities of daily life.

TABLE 18–16
Features of Classic Migraine and Tension Headaches

Migraine
Aura
   Flashes of light
   Wavy or zigzag lines
   Enlarging scotoma surrounded by luminous changes
   Unilateral numbness
   Duration of 10–30 min
Unilateral (hemicrania)
Throbbing
Nausea/vomiting
Photophobia, audiophobia
Relief by rest
Periodic attacks (lasting hours)*
Precipitating factors
   Psychologic stresses
   Lack of food or sleep
   Menses
   Exertion
   Foods or drugs
      Monosodium glutamate
      Cheeses
      Chocolate
      Oral contraceptive pills
Exacerbated by head movement
Family history

Tension Headache
Daily with work or school
Present all day with worsening in afternoon
Moderate band-like or boring pain
Multiple somatic complaints (e.g., shortness of breath, abdominal pain, dizziness)

---

*Migraines may last as long as 72 hours but usually are less than 24 hours.

Symptomatic therapy requires early administration of analgesic and sedative medications, immediate rest, and sleep in a quiet, dark room. Unfortunately, administration of oral medication often is impossible because of severe nausea and vomiting. Triptans are serotonin receptor agonists that may abort migraine attacks within 15–20 minutes following oral, nasal, or subcutaneous administration. They may produce serious cardiovascular side effects in patients with coronary artery disease.

Tension headaches can be acute and related to environmental stresses or can be chronic and a symp-

TABLE 18–17
Treatment for Migraine

Nonmedical
  Eliminate precipitating factors
  Reassurance
  Biofeedback
  Psychotherapy
Analgesics
  Aspirin
  Acetaminophen
  Nonsteroidal antiinflammatory drugs (NSAIDs)
    (e.g., naproxen)
Minor tranquilizers
  Barbiturates
  Benzodiazepine
  Chloral hydrate
  Antihistamines
Antiemetics
  Metoclopramide
  Promethazine
Ergot alkaloids
Combinations of symptomatic medicines
Triptans (serotonin agonists)
Prophylactic agents
  Tricyclic antidepressants (amitriptyline, nortripty-
    line, desipramine)
  Serotonin reuptake inhibitors (fluoxetine)
  Beta-adrenergic blocker (propranolol)
  Calcium channel blocker (verapamil)
  Valproic acid
  Cyproheptadine
  Methysergide

TABLE 18–18
Paroxysmal Disorders of Childhood

Seizure disorders
Migraine
Transient ischemic attack
Breath-holding spells
Night terrors
Hypoglycemia
Narcolepsy, cataplexy
Paroxysmal torticollis
Paroxysmal vertigo (benign)
Paroxysmal dystonia or choreoathetosis
Shudder attacks
Pseudoseizures

tom of underlying psychiatric illness, such as anxiety neurosis, hysterical neurosis, or depression. These *tension headaches* have a different clinical profile than that of migraine (Table 18–16). *Treatment* consists of psychologic support or counseling, biofeedback, mild analgesics, mild tranquilizers, antidepressants, or psychiatric intervention.

REFERENCES

Annequin D, Tourniaire B, Massiou H: Migraine and headache in childhood and adolescence, *Pediatr Clin North Am* 47(3):617–631, 2000.
Behrman RE, Kliegman RM, Jenson HB: *Nelson textbook of pediatrics*, ed 16, Philadelphia, 2000, WB Saunders, Chapter 604.
Davies NP, Hanna MG: Neurological channelopathies: diagnosis and therapy in the new millennium, *Ann Med* 31(6):406–420, 1999.
Ptacek LJ: Ion channel diseases: episodic disorders of the nervous system, *Semin Neurol* 19(4):363–369, 1999.

PAROXYSMAL DISORDERS

Paroxysmal disorders of the nervous system are characterized by the abrupt onset of a clinical episode that tends to be stereotyped and repetitive, lasts seconds to minutes (rarely hours), and ends abruptly. Depending on the etiology of the episode, there may be a warning before or a state of altered awareness afterward, but the child usually recovers quickly. The differential diagnosis of transient paroxysmal disorders in childhood includes seizures, migraine, transient ischemic attack, syncope, vertigo, hypoglycemia, breathholding spells, tics, and conversion reactions. The EEG is most useful in distinguishing seizure from nonepileptic paroxysmal disorders. However, on occasion normal children have epileptiform EEG patterns, and children with seizures may have normal interictal EEGs. Simultaneous video and EEG monitoring of the patient during a spell may be necessary to make a clear diagnosis. The *differential diagnosis* of paroxysmal disorders is listed in Table 18–18.

Seizure Disorders
Classification

A classification of individual seizures and some of the more frequently seen epileptic syndromes is presented in Table 18–19. The clinical seizure classification describes individual events, whereas epileptic syndromes consider age of onset, etiology, and association of seizure types. Etiology of seizures is presented in Table 18–20.

Generalized Tonic, Clonic, and Tonic-Clonic Seizures. Tonic, clonic, and tonic-clonic seizures are the most common childhood type. They may occur alone or be associated with other seizure types. Typically,

TABLE 18–19
Classification of Epileptic Seizures and Some Epileptic Syndromes

Clinical Seizures
Partial Seizures
Simple partial (consciousness not impaired)
   Motor signs
   Special sensory (visual, auditory, olfactory, gustatory,
      vertiginous, or somatosensory)
   Autonomic
   Psychic (déjà vu, fear, and others)
Complex partial (consciousness impaired)
   Impaired consciousness at onset
   Development of impaired consciousness
Generalized Seizures
Absence
   Typical
   Atypical

Generalized Seizures—cont'd
Tonic-clonic
Atonic
Myoclonic
Tonic
Clonic
Unclassified
Neonatal

Epileptic Syndrome
Benign focal epilepsy
Juvenile myoclonic epilepsy
West syndrome
Lennox-Gastaut syndrome
Acquired epileptic aphasia
Benign neonatal convulsions

TABLE 18–20
Etiology of Seizures

Perinatal Conditions
Cerebral malformation
Intrauterine infection
Hypoxic-ischemic*
Trauma
Hemorrhage*

Infections
Encephalitis*
Meningitis*
Brain abscess

Metabolic Conditions
Hypoglycemia*
Hypocalcemia
Hypomagnesemia
Hyponatremia
Hypernatremia
Storage diseases
Reye syndrome
Degenerative disorders
Porphyria
Pyridoxine dependency (deficiency)

Poisoning
Lead
Cocaine

Poisoning—cont'd
Drugs (see Chapter 3)
Drug withdrawal

Neurocutaneous Syndromes
Tuberous sclerosis
Neurofibromatosis
Sturge-Weber syndrome
Klippel-Trenaunay-Weber syndrome
Linear sebaceous nevus
Incontinentia pigmenti

Systemic Disorders
Vasculitis (CNS or systemic)
SLE
Hypertensive encephalopathy
Renal failure
Hepatic encephalopathy

Other
Trauma*
Tumor
Febrile*
Idiopathic*
Familial

CNS, Central nervous system; *SLE,* systemic lupus erythematosus.
*Common.

the attack begins abruptly but occasionally is preceded by a series of myoclonic jerks. Consciousness and control of posture are lost, followed by tonic stiffening and upward deviation of the eyes. Pooling of secretions, pupillary dilation, diaphoresis, hypertension, and piloerection are common. Clonic jerks follow the tonic phase, and then the child is briefly tonic again. Thereafter, the child remains flaccid, and urinary incontinence may occur. As the child awakens, irritability and headache are common. During an attack, the EEG demonstrates repetitive synchronous bursts of spike activity followed by periodic paroxysmal discharges. Brief seizures of any type are not believed to produce brain damage directly. However, generalized tonic-clonic activity lasting longer than 30 minutes is defined as *status epilepticus* and may lead to brain damage

It is important to distinguish primary generalized tonic and clonic seizures from *partial seizures* with secondary generalized spread. Most children with exclusively primary generalized tonic-clonic seizures have genetic epilepsy, whereas partial seizures are frequently associated with focal brain lesions. The presence of an aura indicates a focal origin of the attack. Young children often are unaware of an aura or focal onset of their seizure, and caretakers frequently witness only the generalized aspects of the event.

Treatment is outlined in Table 18–21.

Febrile Seizures. Seizures with fever may be caused by infection of the nervous system, epilepsy triggered by fever, or *simple febrile convulsions.* The latter represent a common genetic predisposition to seizures in infancy that is precipitated by a rapid rise in body temperature. They occur in 2–4% of children between ages 6 months and 7 years, with half occurring between ages 1 and 2 years. Uncomplicated febrile seizures are generalized seizures lasting less than 15 minutes that occur only once in a 24-hour period. If focal, prolonged, or multiple, the seizure is referred to as a *complex febrile seizure.*

The prognosis of children with febrile seizures is excellent. Intellectual achievements are normal. Many children will have further febrile seizures, but the development of epilepsy, afebrile seizures, is rare. Febrile seizures will recur in 50% of children who have their first febrile seizure at less than 1 year of age and in 28% of those with onset after 1 year of age. About 10% of children with febrile seizures have three or more recurrences. The risk of multiple recurrences is greater in infants with onset in the first year. Children with complex febrile seizures have only an 8% risk of having further complicated febrile seizures. The risk of epilepsy in most children with febrile seizures is no greater than the general population and is 1%. Factors that increase the risk for the development of epilepsy include abnormal neurologic examination or development, family history of epilepsy, and complex febrile seizures. The probability of developing epilepsy is 2% if one risk factor is present and 10% if two or three risk factors are present.

Because febrile seizures are brief and the outcome is benign, most children who have them require no treatment. Rectal diazepam can be administered during a seizure to abort a prolonged event. Daily administration of phenobarbital or valproic acid prevents febrile seizures, but serious potential side effects limit their use. Valproic acid can rarely cause fatal hepatic necrosis, and this complication is more common in young children under two years of age. Phenobarbital causes serious behavioral disturbances in about one third of children. Phenobarbital is ineffective when given at the onset of a febrile illness because a therapeutic level cannot be achieved rapidly enough.

Benign Neonatal Convulsions. Benign neonatal convulsions are an autosomal dominant genetic disorder localized to *chromosome 20.* This seizure syndrome is characterized by generalized clonic seizures occurring toward the end of the first week of life. Response to *treatment* is variable, but the outlook generally is favorable.

Status Epilepticus. Status epilepticus is a seizure of sufficient duration or frequency to create a fixed epileptic condition. The duration of seizure activity necessary to reach status epilepticus varies, but after 20–30 min of convulsive status, reductions in cortical partial pressure of oxygen occur in experimental animals, indicating a risk of irreversible brain injury. About 25% of children exhibiting status epilepticus have an acute brain injury, such as purulent or aseptic meningitis, encephalitis, electrolyte disorder, or acute anoxia. Twenty percent are children with a history of brain injury or congenital malformation. In 50% of the cases of status epilepticus, there is no definable etiology, but in 50% of this group, status is associated with fever. Sudden cessation of anticonvulsant medication is another frequent cause. Overall, the mortality rate of status epilepticus is less than 10%.

The first priority of *treatment* is to ensure an adequate airway and to assess the cardiovascular status (see Chapter 3). The child's mouth and throat should be cleared, the oral pharynx suctioned, and a plastic oral airway placed. Oxygen is administered. If there is any doubt concerning the adequacy of the airway, the child should be intubated. If violent muscle activity impairs ventilation, muscle paralysis should be instituted. The child should be examined for focal neurologic signs and evidence of meningeal irritation. A history is obtained with specific reference to

TABLE 18–21
Treatment of Seizure Disorders*

Seizure Type	Drugs†	Therapeutic Serum Levels (μg/mL)	Drug Complications
Tonic-clonic	Carbamazepine	8–12	Drowsiness, agranulocytosis, dizziness, hyponatremia; aplastic anemia
	or		
	Phenytoin	10–20	Gingival hyperplasia, hirsutism, nystagmus, pseudolymphoma; Stevens-Johnson syndrome, SLE, rickets
	or		
	Phenobarbital	15–40	Sedation, reduced cognition; Stevens-Johnson syndrome; hyperactivity
	or		
	Valproate	50–100	Drowsiness, pancreatitis, fatal liver failure (Reye-like syndrome) if under 2 yr old
	or		
	Topiramate	2–20	Cognitive, neuropsychiatric, kidney, staring, paresthesias
Partial	Carbamazepine		
	or		
	Phenytoin		
	or		
	Valproate‡		
Absence	Ethosuximide	40–100	Nausea, lethargy, hiccups, SLE, Stevens-Johnson syndrome; blood dyscrasia
	or		
	Valproate		
	Clonazepam as alternative	0.013–0.072	Ataxia, lethargy, blood dyscrasia, depression, salivation
Atonic, myoclonic	Valproate	2–20	Toxic epidermal necrolysis; Stevens-Johnson syndrome
	or		
	Lamotrigine		
	Clonazepam as alternative		
Infantile spasms	ACTH		Immunosuppression, hypertension, infection
	or		
	Corticosteroids		Adrenal suppression, cataracts, osteoporosis, hypertension, immunosuppression, infection
	Clonazepam, valproate, vigabatrin as alternatives		

Modified from *Med Lett* 28:91, 1986.
*Surgical approaches to seizures have been successful in children with recurrent, difficult to treat seizures or children with serious drug reactions. Surgery ablates the epileptiform focus or prevents generalization. Surgery is most beneficial in mesial temporal lobe epilepsy. Vagal pacing may be an alternative.
†See Appendix I for dosages.
‡Gabapentin is also effective for complex partial seizures with secondary generalizations. Levels need not be monitored.
ACTH, Adrenocorticotropic hormone; *SLE*, systemic lupus erythematosus.

previous seizures and anticonvulsant treatment. An intravenous infusion should be started, and laboratory evaluation be undertaken as detailed in the following sections.

The International Symposium on Status Epilepticus recommends the simultaneous administration of diazepam, 0.2–0.4 mg/kg (up to 10 mg) given intravenously at a rate of 1 mg/min, and phenytoin, 20 mg/kg (up to 1.0–1.5 g) at a rate of 1 mg/kg/min. Diazepam distributes rapidly to the brain but has a short duration of action, whereas phenytoin distributes more slowly but has a longer duration. Alternative agents include lorazepam (0.1–0.15 mg/kg intravenously) or, if seizures do not stop, a continuous infusion of intravenous diazepam. If diazepam and phenytoin are ineffective, a loading dose of 10 mg/kg of phenobarbital is given, which may be repeated in 10 minutes. If this approach is ineffective, preparations for general anesthesia are undertaken. While anesthesia is being awaited, continuously infused diazepam or pentobarbital is recommended. Once status epilepticus stops, maintenance therapy is initiated with the appropriate anticonvulsant.

Absence Seizures. Approximately 6–20% of epileptic children have typical absence seizures. The clinical hallmark of absence seizures is a brief loss of environmental awareness accompanied by eye fluttering or simple automatisms such as head bobbing and lip smacking. Seizures usually begin between 4 and 6 years of age. There is a 75% concordance rate in monozygotic twins, which suggests a genetic etiology. Neurologic examination and brain imaging are normal. The characteristic EEG patterns consist of synchronous 3-Hz spike-and-wave activity with frontal accentuation. The clinical seizure invariably is accompanied by the electrical discharge, and both are provoked by hyperventilation or flashing light stimulation. Approximately 40–50% of children with absence seizures have associated generalized seizures; 60% occur before and 40% after the onset of absence seizures.

Differentiating absence from partial complex seizures can be difficult. Both seizure types are characterized by stoppage of activity, staring, and alteration of consciousness and may include automatisms. The automatisms of partial complex seizures are usually more complicated than those seen in absence seizures and may involve repetitive swallowing, picking of the hands, or walking in nonpurposeful circles. Partial complex seizures often are followed by postictal confusion, whereas absence seizures are not. Absence seizures are provoked by hyperventilation and usually last a few seconds, whereas partial complex seizures occur spontaneously and usually last several minutes. Children may have dozens of absence seizures per day, whereas they rarely have more than one or two partial complex seizures in a day. *Treatment* is outlined in Table 18–21.

Myoclonic, Tonic, Atonic, and Atypical Absence Seizures. Myoclonic, tonic, atonic, and atypical absence seizures make up 10–15% of childhood epilepsies. They are frequently associated with underlying structural brain disease and are difficult to treat and classify. They often occur in combination with each other and with generalized tonic-clonic seizures.

Atypical Absence Seizures. Atypical absence seizures manifest as episodes of impaired consciousness with automatisms, autonomic phenomena, and motor manifestations, such as eye opening, eye deviation, and body stiffening. The EEG shows slow spike and wave activity at 2–3 Hz.

Myoclonus. Myoclonus is a lightning-like jerk of part of the body. The phenomenon is epileptic if the EEG shows epileptiform discharges during the jerk and nonepileptic if it does not. Nonepileptic myoclonus may originate in the basal ganglia, brainstem, or spinal cord and may be benign, as in sleep myoclonus, or indicative of serious pathology. Myoclonic epilepsy is usually associated with multiple seizure types. The underlying illness producing myoclonic epilepsy may be developmental and static or progressive and associated with neurologic deterioration (e.g., neuronal ceroid lipofuscinosis, Lafora body, and Unverricht-Lundborg disease).

Myoclonic absence refers to the body jerks that commonly accompany absence seizures and atypical absence seizures. Bilateral massive epileptic myoclonus is symmetric and varies in intensity. The peak age of occurrence is within the first year (37%), and status epilepticus is the first ictal manifestation in 77% of patients.

Juvenile Myoclonic Epilepsy. Juvenile myoclonic epilepsy (Janz) occurs in adolescence and is an autosomal dominant disorder with variable penetrance. The genetic abnormality is localized on chromosome 6. Myoclonus, predominantly in the morning, with or without generalized clonic and absence seizures characterizes the disorder. Seizures usually resolve promptly with therapy with valproic acid, but therapy must be maintained for life.

Astatic-Akinetic or Atonic Seizures. These usually have their onset between 1 and 3 years of age. The seizures last 1–4 seconds and are characterized by a loss of body tone, with falling to the ground, dropping of the head, or pitching forward or backward. A tonic component usually is associated. These seizures frequently result in repetitive head injury if the child is not protected with a hockey or football helmet. They are most frequent on awakening and on falling to sleep. Fifty or more daily seizures are usual. Children with astatic-akinetic seizures usually have mental retardation and underlying brain abnormalities. Tuberous sclerosis is a frequent cause.

Infantile Spasms. Infantile spasms (West syndrome) are characterized by a brief contraction of the neck, trunk, and arm muscles, followed by a phase of sustained muscle contraction lasting from 2–10 seconds. The initial phase consists of flexion and extension in various combinations such that the head may be thrown either backward or forward. The arms and legs may be either flexed or extended. As with most seizures, spasms occur most frequently when the child is awakening from sleep or going to sleep. Each jerk is followed by a brief period of relaxation and is then repeated multiple times in clusters of unpredictable and variable duration. Many clusters occur each day. The EEG during the waking state, hypsarrhythmia, is dramatically abnormal, consisting of high-voltage slow waves, spikes, and polyspikes accompanied by background disorganization. Commonly, burst suppression patterns are seen during sleep. The peak age of onset is 3–8 months, and 86% of infants experience the onset of seizures before the age of 1 year. In circumstances in which flexion of the thighs and crying are prominent, this syndrome often is mistaken for colic.

This seizure type carries a poor prognosis. The etiology is not determined in 40% of children. This cryptogenic group has a better response to therapy than the group with a clear etiology, and about 40% will have a good intellectual outcome. Etiology will be determined in 60%; this symptomatic group responds poorly to anticonvulsant therapy and has a very poor intellectual prognosis. Tuberous sclerosis is the most common recognized cause. The *etiology* of infantile spasms is outlined in Table 18–22.

Treatment of infantile spasms includes adrenocorticotropic hormone (ACTH), oral corticosteroids, benzodiazepines, and valproic acid. The Food and Drug Administration (FDA) does not yet approve vigabatrin, a promising drug available in Europe and Canada, because it can cause visual field deficits. Irritability, swelling, hypertension, glycosuria, and severe infections are complications to be anticipated with steroid therapy.

Lennox-Gastaut Syndrome. Lennox-Gastaut syndrome is an epileptic syndrome with variable age of onset, but most children have the syndrome before the age of 5 years. Multiple seizure types, including atonic-astatic, partial, atypical absence, and generalized tonic, clonic, or tonic-clonic varieties, characterize the disorder. Many children have underlying brain injury or malformations. These seizures usually respond poorly to *treatment*, but some patients have a good response to valproic acid.

Partial Seizures. Partial seizures constitute 40–60% of the classifiable epilepsies of childhood. Simple partial seizures arise from a specific anatomic focus, and clinical symptomatology may include motor, sensory, psychic, or autonomic abnormalities. Location and direction of spread of the seizure focus determine clinical symptomatology. Complex partial seizures are similar, but in addition, consciousness is impaired. When partial seizures spread to involve the whole brain and produce a generalized tonic-clonic seizure, they are said to show secondary generalization. Focal brain lesions cause many partial epilepsies, but some are genetic epilepsies.

Partial seizures that manifest only with psychic or autonomic symptoms can be difficult to recognize. Uncinate seizures arising from the medial temporal

| TABLE 18–22 |
| Etiologies of Infantile Spasms |

Metabolic
Phenylketonuria
Biotinidase deficiency
Maple syrup urine disease
Isovalericacidemia
Ornithine accumulation
Nonketotic hyperglycinemia
Pyridoxine dependency
Hypoglycemia
Lipidosis

Developmental Malformations
Polymicrogyria
Lissencephaly
Schizencephaly
Down syndrome and other chromosomal disorders
Aicardi syndrome
Organoid nevus syndrome

Neurocutaneous Syndromes
Tuberous sclerosis
Sturge-Weber syndrome

Congenital Infections
Toxoplasmosis
Cytomegalovirus
Syphilis

Encephalopathies
Postasphyxia
Posttraumatic
Posthemorrhagic
Postinfectious
Postimmunization (pertussis)

lobe manifest with an olfactory hallucination of an extremely unpleasant odor. Gelastic seizures originating from hypothalamic tumors are spells of uncontrolled laughter. Lip smacking seizures arise from the anterior temporal lobe and episodes of macropsia, micropsia, altered depth perception, and vertigo from the posterior temporal lobe. Limbic temporal lobe discharges result in dream-like states (déjà vu and bizarre psychic abnormalities). Episodic autonomic phenomena such as fever, tachycardia, shivering, and increased gastrointestinal motility may rarely be seizures of temporal lobe origin.

Treatment is outlined in Table 18–21.

Benign Focal Epilepsy. Also known as rolandic epilepsy, benign focal epilepsy usually begins between the ages of 5 and 10 years. The incidence may be as high as 21:100,000, comprising 16% of all afebrile seizures in children below the age of 15 years. The seizures usually are focal motor with generalized spread. In approximately half of the children, seizures occur only during sleep or on awakening. Symptoms commonly include abnormal movement or sensation around the face and mouth. Speech and swallowing are impaired. A family history of similar seizures is found in 13% of patients. The disorder is called benign because the seizures usually respond promptly to anticonvulsant therapy, because intellectual outcome and brain imaging are normal, and because epilepsy resolves after puberty.

Acquired Epileptic Aphasia. Acquired epileptic aphasia (Landau-Kleffner syndrome) is characterized by the onset in early childhood of a cortical auditory deficit and language disability. The patients develop partial and generalized seizures, and the EEG is highly epileptiform in sleep. It is unclear whether frequent temporal lobe seizures cause the language disability or whether unknown and perhaps inflammatory temporal lobe pathology is responsible for both the seizures and language loss.

Rasmussen encephalitis is a chronic, progressive focal inflammation of the brain of unknown origin. Both an autoimmune origin and a focal viral encephalitis have been postulated. The usual age of onset is 6–10 years. The disease begins with focal, persistent motor seizure activity including epilepsia partialis continua. Over months, the children develop hemiplegia and cognitive deterioration. EEG shows focal spikes and slow wave activity. Brain imaging studies are initially normal and then show atrophy in the involved area. Hemispherectomy has been the only successful therapy as measured by seizure eradication and prevention of cognitive deterioration, but permanent hemiparesis is an inevitable consequence.

Pseudoseizures. Children with hysteria or malingering occasionally may have seizures, and children with seizure disorders may consciously or subconsciously exhibit activity that simulates their own seizures. Pseudoseizures differ clinically from epileptic seizures in that tremulousness or thrashing rather than true tonic-clonic activity is noted. Verbalization and pelvic thrusting are more commonly seen in pseudoseizures, and pseudoseizures are more likely to be initiated or terminated by suggestion. An EEG performed during pseudoseizure activity does not demonstrate typical epileptiform patterns.

Laboratory Evaluation of Seizures

A complete laboratory evaluation of a child with the new onset of seizures includes a CBC; measurement of blood chemistries, including glucose, calcium, sodium, potassium, chloride, bicarbonate, urea nitrogen, creatinine, magnesium, and phosphorus; blood or urine toxicology screening; analysis of CSF; and EEG and brain imaging. Neonates may also require testing of blood ammonia and inborn errors of metabolism; CSF glycine, lactate and herpes simplex PCR; urine and stool culture of viruses, especially CMV and enterovirus; and a clinical trial of pyridoxine. Analysis of CSF is not necessary if the patient is afebrile and has no neurologic signs and if the history does not suggest a meningeal infection. MRI is far superior to CT in demonstrating brain pathology, but in the acute ER setting CT may be desirable because it can be performed very rapidly and demonstrates acute intracranial hemorrhage more clearly than MRI. Children with simple febrile seizures who have completely recovered may require little or no laboratory evaluation. MRI is unlikely to be abnormal in patients with primary generalized epilepsies, such as typical absence and myoclonic epilepsy of Janz, but will reveal lesions in about 25% of other patients even when the examination and EEG do not show focal features. Lesions may be progressive, such as malignant and benign tumors, AVM, and neuroepithelial and dermoid cysts, or static, such as malformations, old strokes, gliosis, and focal atrophy. Identification of some static lesions, such as cortical dysplasia, hamartoma, and mesial temporal sclerosis, may allow consideration of surgical correction of medically refractory epilepsy.

Principles of Seizure Therapy

Treatment is not necessary for most benign febrile seizures. Absence seizures, infantile spasms, atypical absence seizures, and astatic-akinetic seizures are universally recurrent at the time of diagnosis, and therapy is indicated. The overall risk of recurrence for children whose first seizure is generalized tonic-clonic is approximately 50%, and it seems reasonable to wait for recurrence before therapy is instituted.

When treatment is initiated, the goal is to achieve optimal function. Medication risks should be weighed against the risk of seizure type. Initially, a single agent should be chosen, because this reduces cost, improves compliance, and avoids toxicity. Approximately 50% of children obtain satisfactory seizure control with one drug. A second agent is considered only after therapeutic anticonvulsant levels are obtained with the first drug. Anticonvulsant levels are helpful in adjusting medication but should be interpreted in light of the patient's clinical state. Because of phenobarbital's long half-life, phenobarbital plasma levels can be determined anytime throughout the day. Levels of carbamazepine and phenytoin may vary significantly between peak and trough as a result of their shorter half-lives. When hepatic and renal disease is present, drug binding is likely to be altered, and free and bound anticonvulsant determinations can be helpful. Hazardous physical activities are best avoided, and many advise against direct contact sports such as football. Children with epilepsy have a greater risk of submersion accidents, but the risk can be minimized by maintaining anticonvulsant drug levels in the therapeutic range and appropriate supervision.

The duration of anticonvulsant therapy varies by seizure type. Children with generalized tonic, clonic, and tonic-clonic seizures, absence seizures, and certain partial seizures may not require therapy for more than 2–4 years. The risk of recurrence is higher when partial seizures occur. Children with myoclonic seizures, progressive myoclonic epilepsy, atypical absence seizures, and the Lennox-Gastaut syndrome require treatment for life. As a rule, children who are neurologically abnormal, have seizures that were initially difficult to control, and have persistently epileptiform EEGs are at highest risk for recurrence when therapy is discontinued.

REFERENCES

Baumann RJ, Duffner PK: Treatment of children with simple febrile seizures: the AAP practice parameter, *Pediatr Neurol* 23(1):11–17, 2000.
Behrman RE, Kliegman RM, Jenson HB, editors: *Nelson textbook of pediatrics*, ed 16, Philadelphia, 2000, WB Saunders, Chapter 602, 603.
Camfield PR, Camfield CS: Advances in the diagnosis and management of pediatric seizure disorders in the twentieth century, *J Pediatr* 136(6):847–849, 2000.
Camfield PR, Camfield CS: Treatment of children with "ordinary" epilepsy, *Epileptic Disorders* 2(1):45–51, 2000.
Holmes GL: Use of EEG in childhood epilepsy, *Int Pediatr* 7:223, 1992.
Morton LD, Pellock JM: Overview of childhood epilepsy and epileptic syndromes and advances in therapy, *Curr Pharm Design* 6:879, 2000.
Shields WD: Catastrophic epilepsy in childhood, *Epilepsia* 41(Suppl 2):S2–S6, 2000.
Shinnar S, Berg A, Moshe S, et al: The risk of seizure recurrence after a first unprovoked afebrile seizure in childhood: an extended follow-up, *Pediatrics* 98(2 Pt 1):216–225, 1996.
Wyllie E: Surgical treatment of epilepsy in pediatric patients, *Can J Neurol Sci* 27(2):106–110, 2000.

ACUTE ATAXIA

Ataxia is an abnormality of coordination resulting in an impairment of direction, rate, and strength of voluntary movement. The usual symptoms are a broad-based unsteady gait and tremor. Tremor worsens with intentional movement of the limbs and is called dysmetria. Classically these symptoms stem from disorders of the cerebellum and cerebellar pathways, including the cerebellar peduncles in the brainstem, spinocerebellar tract in the spinal cord, and thalamic nuclei. Peripheral nerve lesions causing loss of proprioception and bilateral frontal lobe lesions can lead to similar symptoms.

The most common causes of acute ataxia in childhood are postinfectious acute cerebellar ataxia and drug intoxications. Some causes, such as tumors in the posterior fossa, hydrocephalus, multiple sclerosis, strokes, and hemorrhages, are easily identified by asymmetric clinical findings, associated noncerebellar neurologic signs, and abnormalities on CT or MRI of the brain. Other causes, such as the paraneoplastic opsoclonus-myoclonus syndrome associated with neuroblastoma, mild inborn errors of metabolism, labyrinthine dysfunction, head trauma, epilepsy, postictal state, migraine, and Guillain-Barré and Miller Fisher syndromes, are difficult to prove or require special tests for their identification.

Postinfectious Acute Cerebellar Ataxia

Postinfectious acute cerebellar ataxia may follow chickenpox, infectious mononucleosis, or a mild respiratory or gastrointestinal viral illness by about a week. It begins abruptly, causing staggering and frequent failing, and can progress to difficulty with standing and sitting. Truncal ataxia may be the only symptom or may be accompanied by dysmetria of the arms, dysarthria, nystagmus, vomiting, irritability, and lethargy. Symptoms usually peak within 2 days, then stabilize and resolve over 1–2 weeks. Recovery is usually complete.

CSF examination sometimes demonstrates a mild lymphocytic pleocytosis or mild elevation of protein content. Brain imaging is usually normal. The pathogenesis of the syndrome is uncertain and may represent either a direct viral infection of the cerebellum or an autoimmune response directed to the cerebellar white matter and precipitated by the preceding viral infection. No specific therapy is available.

Drug Intoxication

Overdosage with any sedative-hypnotic agent can produce ataxia and lethargy, but ataxia without lethargy usually results from intoxication with alcohol, phenytoin, or carbamazepine. It is important to ask whether anyone in the household or a house that the child visits (such as a grandparent) is taking anticonvulsant or antipsychotic medications. Treatment is supportive, and the toxic agent is removed.

Tumors and Paraneoplastic Opsoclonus-Myoclonus Syndrome

Posterior fossa tumors, primarily involving the cerebellum or the brainstem, produce ataxia that may be acute or gradual in onset. Once begun, the symptoms worsen progressively. The common tumors are medulloblastoma, ependymoma, cerebellar astrocytoma, and brainstem glioma. The ataxia and dysmetria may result from the primary cerebellar lesion or from obstruction of the CSF pathways and hydrocephalus. Hydrocephalus causes ataxia by pressure on the corticopontocerebellar pathways as they sweep over the lateral ventricles. Rarely, a neuroblastoma located in the adrenal medulla or anywhere along the paraspinal sympathetic chain in the thorax or abdomen is associated with degeneration of Purkinje cells and the development of severe ataxia, dysmetria, irritability, myoclonus, and opsoclonus. The myoclonic movements are irregular, lightning-like movements of a limb or the head. Opsoclonus is a very rapid, multidirectional, conjugate movement of the eyes that suddenly dart in random directions. The presence of this sign in infants and toddlers should prompt a vigorous search for an occult neuroblastoma, including urine testing of the adrenergic metabolites VMA and HVA, chest x-ray examination, abdominal ultrasound, and MRI with contrast of the entire sympathetic chain. These tumors tend to be localized and curable by surgical resection, unlike neuroblastoma without opsoclonus. The current hypothesis is that an immunologic reaction directed toward the tumor is misdirected to also attack Purkinje cells and other neuronal elements. Treatment with corticosteroids often relieves the acute neurologic symptoms, but 64% of children are left with persistent cerebellar deficits and 36% with intellectual deficits.

Inborn Errors of Metabolism

Several inborn errors of metabolism can present with intermittent episodes of ataxia, as well as somnolence. These include Hartnup disorder, branched chain ketoaciduria (maple syrup urine disease), multiple carboxylase deficiency (biotinidase deficiency), disorders of the urea cycle, and abnormalities of pyruvate metabolism.

Labyrinthine Dysfunction

Difficulty walking with a severe staggering gait is one manifestation of labyrinthine dysfunction, but the diagnosis is usually clarified by the associated symptoms of a severe sense of spinning dizziness, nausea and vomiting, and the associated signs of pallor, sweating, and nystagmus.

PSYCHOMOTOR RETARDATION

See Chapter 1.

Nonprogressive Psychomotor Retardation

In many children with severe mental retardation, the history and general physical examination are unremarkable. No focal neurologic deficits are present, and laboratory evaluation is unrevealing. Most chil-

dren with this idiopathic condition probably have microscopic aberrations of CNS development involving the structure of neurons or neuronal organelles, aggregation of neurons, myelinization of white matter, synapse formation, or interneuronal connections. *Treatment* includes infant stimulation and educational programs, but no treatment program can increase inherent learning capacity.

Congenital Malformations of the Brain

Most brain malformations can be produced by a variety of injuries occurring during a vulnerable period of gestation. These precipitating factors include chromosomal, genetic, and metabolic abnormalities (see Chapters 4 and 5); infections (cytomegalovirus, TORCH*; see Chapters 6 and 10); and exposure to irradiation, certain drugs, and maternal illness during pregnancy.

In all types of congenital hydrocephalus, the degree of ventricular enlargement correlates roughly with outcome, but examples of neonates with severe hydrocephalus who receive ventriculoperitoneal shunts and then have normal development are well known. Children with congenital hydrocephalus often have associated defects in the closure of the neural tube.

Hydranencephaly is a condition in which the brain presumably develops normally but then is destroyed by an intrauterine, probably vascular, insult. The result is a virtual absence of the cerebrum with an intact skull. The thalamus, brainstem, and some occipital cortex are present. The child may have a normal outward appearance but does not achieve developmental milestones.

Holoprosencephaly represents varying degrees of failure of the primary cerebral vesicle to divide and expand laterally and often is associated with midline facial defects (e.g., hypotelorism, cleft lip, and cleft palate). This anomaly may occur in an isolated fashion or be associated with a chromosomal or genetic disorder. The *prognosis* for infants with severe holoprosencephaly is uniformly poor.

A number of malformations detailed in the following sections result from the failure of normal migration of neurons from the germinal matrix zone around the ventricle to the cortical surface at 1–5 months of gestation. Often, multiple malformations exist in the same patient. Neurologic development with all of these anomalies is variable and depends on the type and extent of the malformations.

Schizencephaly is characterized by symmetric bilateral clefts within the cerebral hemispheres that extend from the cortical surface to the ventricular cavity. *Clinical manifestations* include severe mental and

---

*TORCH = *t*oxoplasmosis, *o*ther (syphilis, hepatitis, zoster), *r*ubella, *c*ytomegalovirus, and *h*erpes simplex.

motor retardation. Some children have unilateral schizencephaly manifested by hemiparesis and mild mental impairment.

Lissencephaly indicates smooth brain with absence of sulcation. The normal six-layered cortex does not develop, and affected children have seizures and profound developmental retardation. This anomaly most commonly is part of a genetic or chromosomal disorder.

In macrogyria the gyri are few in number and too broad, whereas in polymicrogyria the gyri are too many and too small. Sometimes macrogyria and polymicrogyria affect an entire hemisphere, producing enlargement of that hemisphere and a clinical syndrome of severe, medically intractable seizures that begin in early infancy. Hemispherectomy is required to stop the seizures. Gray matter heterotopias are abnormal islands within the central white matter of neurons that have never completed the migratory process.

Agenesis of the corpus callosum may be partial or complete and may occur in an isolated fashion or in association with other anomalies of cellular migration.

Dandy-Walker malformation is diagnosed on the basis of the classic triad: complete or partial agenesis of the vermis, cystic dilatation of the fourth ventricle, and enlarged posterior fossa. There may be associated hydrocephalus, absence of the corpus callosum, and neuronal migration abnormalities. Intelligence may be normal or impaired, depending on the degree of associated cerebral neuronal defects.

Megalencephaly, or large brain, is diagnosed by finding a large head with radiographically normal-appearing intracranial contents. Most often this is a familial trait of no clinical significance. Sometimes it is associated with disorders of neuronal migration and a clinical syndrome of developmental retardation. Neurofibromatosis and Soto syndrome (cerebral gigantism) are two genetic syndromes associated with megalencephaly and sometimes with mental retardation. Megalencephaly is also a feature of a number of metabolic diseases that produce a progressive, degenerative encephalopathy.

Microcephaly usually is produced by failure of normal brain growth. Any injury to the brain, intrauterine or postnatal, can retard subsequent brain growth. Autosomal recessive genetic illnesses resulting in microcephaly and mental retardation have been described. Brain malformations often are associated with microcephaly. In general, children with head circumferences more than three standard deviations below the mean, regardless of the cause, exhibit retarded intellect.

Congenital disorders producing chronic, nonprogressive ataxia are described in Table 18–23.

TABLE 18–23
Congenital Causes of Chronic Ataxia

Disorder	Age of Presentation	Clinical Manifestations	Mechanism of Ataxia, Diagnoses, and Treatment
Cerebellar hypoplasia	Early infancy (occasionally delayed)	Developmental delay, hypotonia, athetosis, chorea, delayed walking, ataxic gait	Absent cerebellar granular cells; CT shows small cerebellum
Vermal aplasia: Dandy-Walker malformation	Early infancy	Macrocephaly, enlarged occipital region; ataxia	Hydrocephalus and cystic dilation of the fourth ventricle; treatment is by shunting of hydrocephalus and/or the posterior fossa cyst
Joubert syndrome	Early infancy	Neonatal episodic hyperpnea and apnea; hypotonia, nystagmus	MRI and CT demonstrate agenesis of the superior cerebellar vermis
Arnold-Chiari malformation	Variable	Headache, neck pain, lower cranial nerve dysfunction, nystagmus, ataxia; this variety does not have associated myelomeningocele	MRI and CT demonstrate a caudal fourth ventricle; distortion of the brainstem; treatment is by posterior fossa decompression
Hydrocephalus	Variable	Macrocephaly, vomiting, ataxia	CT and MRI demonstrate enlarged lateral ventricles; in aqueductal stenosis, the third ventricle is particularly large, whereas the fourth ventricle is normal or small

CT, Computed tomography; *MRI*, magnetic resonance imaging.

Chromosomal Disorders

Chromosomal abnormalities such as trisomy 21 are associated with mental retardation (see Chapter 4). The most common form of familial mental retardation, affecting 1 in 1250 males, is the fragile X syndrome. Expansion of a trinucleotide repeat, CGG, and abnormal methylation of a CpG island of the FMR-1 gene at chromosome position Xq27.3 cause it. The features are varying degrees of mental retardation, autistic behavior, large ears, macroorchidism, and an elongated, narrow face. Females may be affected, but usually not as severely as males.

Two other syndromes associated with mental retardation are caused by deletions of the same region of the long arm of chromosome 15. Angelman syndrome is caused by the loss of the maternal allele and is manifested by severe mental retardation, severe seizures, tremulousness, a characteristic facies, and a happy external demeanor. Prader-Willi syndrome is caused by the loss of the paternal allele and is manifested by severe hypotonia and feeding difficulties in the neonatal period, cryptorchidism, small hands and feet, mild mental retardation, and almond-shaped eyes. The difference in phenotype, depending on loss of the maternal or paternal allele, supports the genetic phenomenon of *imprinting* (see Chapter 4).

Progressive Mental Retardation

A complete laboratory evaluation is listed in Table 18–24. Degenerative hereditary and metabolic diseases usually are symmetric in their manifestations and slowly progressive over weeks, months, and years. However, some acquired diseases can simulate this clinical picture and must be excluded because they are more likely to be treatable than the degenerative conditions.

Acquired Illnesses Mimicking Degenerative Diseases

Some children with epilepsy have seizures so frequently that they are continuously in either an ictal or postictal state and appear stuporous. A treatment program employing high doses of multiple anticonvulsants may compound this problem. The children's decline in alertness arouses suspicion of a progressive illness, but readjustment of medications and amelioration of the seizure disorder return the children to previous levels of functioning.

Chronic drug overdose with sedatives, tranquilizers, anticholinergics, and anticonvulsants can bring about progressive mental confusion, lethargy, and ataxia. Lead poisoning may cause chronic learning difficulties or may present acutely with irritability, listlessness, anorexia, and pallor, progressing to

---

TABLE 18–24
Laboratory Evaluation for Degenerative Neurologic Metabolic Diseases

Blood
CBC (leukocyte vacuolations)
Blood gas determination
Ammonia
Na^+, K^+, Cl^-, CO_2 (anion gap), CPK, uric acid, fasting blood glucose, cholesterol, triglycerides
Lactate, pyruvate
Amino acids
Very-long-chain fatty acids
Acyl-carnitine
Biotinidase level

Lysosomal Enzymes
WBCs
Serum fibroblasts

DNA Probes
Many disorders

Urine
Ketones
Screen for inborn errors
Organic acids
24-Hour amino acids
24-Hour mucopolysaccharides
Carnitine: free, esterified, total
Sialyloligosaccharides

Imaging
Skull
Vertebrae
Long bones
CNS, MRI

Biopsy
Skin
Bone marrow
Conjunctiva
Rectum
Muscle
Nerve

CBC, Complete blood count; *CNS*, central nervous system; *CPK*, creatine phosphokinase; *DNA*, deoxyribonucleic acid; *MRI*, magnetic resonance imaging; *WBCs*, white blood cells.

fulminant encephalopathy. Vitamin deficiency of thiamine, niacin, B_{12}, and E can produce encephalopathy, as well as peripheral neuropathy and ataxia. Both congenital and acquired hypothyroidism impair intelligence and retard movement. Congenital hypothyroidism produces irreversible damage if it is not treated immediately after birth. Structural brain diseases, such as hydrocephalus and slowly growing tumors, also may mimic dementia.

Certain indolent brain infections such as rubeola (measles), rubella (German measles), syphilis, prion disease, and some fungi cause mental and neurologic deterioration over months and years. Congenital HIV infection causes both failure of normal developmental and regression of acquired skills.

Severe psychosocial deprivation in infancy can give rise to apathy and failure to attain developmental milestones. Depression in older children can lead to blunting of affect, social withdrawal, and poor school performance that raise the question of encephalopathy and dementia.

Hereditary and Metabolic Degenerative Diseases

Degenerative diseases may affect white matter, gray matter, or focal regions of the brain. Many of the white and gray matter degenerative illnesses result from enzymatic disorders within subcellular organelles, including lysosomes, mitochondria, and peroxisomes. Disorders of lysosomal enzymes typically impair metabolism of brain sphingolipids and gangliosides. These enzyme deficiencies have classic patterns of expression with specific names such as Niemann-Pick disease, Gaucher disease, and Tay-Sachs disease, but the same apparent deficiencies can produce unusual clinical syndromes that differ greatly from the classic patterns. The age of onset, rate of progression, and even the neurologic signs may be entirely different. For this reason, any patient with a degenerative neurologic condition of unknown cause should have leukocytes or skin fibroblasts harvested for measurement of a standard battery of lysosomal, peroxisomal, and mitochondrial enzymes (see Chapter 5).

Degenerative Diseases with Focal Manifestations. Ataxia indicates disease of the cerebellum or spinocerebellar pathways. Abnormalities of extraocular movement or respiration indicate disease of the brainstem. Choreoathetosis or dystonia indicates disease of the motor basal ganglia. Paraplegia indicates disease of the spinal cord. Hereditary-degenerative diseases causing ataxia are described in Table 18–25.

Friedreich ataxia is a relentlessly progressive, autosomal recessive disorder that becomes manifest in the early teenage years with ataxia, dysmetria, dysarthria, pes cavus, hammer toes, diminished proprioception and vibration, diminished or absent reflexes, upgoing toes, kyphoscoliosis, nystagmus, and a hypertrophic cardiomyopathy. It is caused by a homozygous GAA expansion of 120–1700 trinucleotide repeats of the first intron of the frataxin gene on chromosome 9. The GAA repeats are unstable on transmission. The size of the GAA expansion determines the frequency of cardiomyopathy and loss of reflexes in the upper limbs.

Lesch-Nyhan syndrome is a sex-linked recessive disorder caused by deficiency of hypoxanthineguanine phosphoribosyltransferase, leading to the formation of excess uric acid. Infants appear normal until late in the first year of life, when they exhibit psychomotor retardation, choreoathetosis, spasticity, and severe self-mutilation. These patients never achieve ambulation. Gouty arthritis and renal calculi with renal failure also occur. The hyperuricemia and renal complications are treated with allopurinol, a xanthine oxidase inhibitor, but no effective treatment for the neurologic disease is available.

Wilson disease is a treatable degenerative condition that exhibits signs of both cerebellar and basal ganglia dysfunction. It is an autosomal recessively inherited inborn error of copper metabolism. Serum copper and ceruloplasmin levels are low, and abnormal copper deposition is found in the liver, producing cirrhosis; in the peripheral cornea, producing a characteristic green-brown (Kayser-Fleischer) ring; and in the CNS, producing neuronal degeneration and protoplasmic astrocytosis. Neurologic symptoms characteristically begin in the early teenage years with dysarthria, dysphasia, drooling, fixed smile, tremor, dystonia, and emotional lability. MRI always shows abnormalities of the basal ganglia. *Treatment* is with a copper-chelating agent, such as oral penicillamine.

Ataxia-telangiectasia (AT) is an autosomal recessive genetic disorder of DNA repair that produces a neurologic disorder, immunologic deficiency, lymphoid malignancy, and gonadal dysgenesis. The neurologic symptoms manifest between 1 and 2 years of age with progressive ataxia, dystonia, chorea, swallowing difficulty, poor facial movements, and severe abnormalities of saccadic and pursuit eye movements. Most characteristically, the patients develop oculomotor apraxia, a disorder in which the child focuses by making quick darting head movements in order to compensate for the inability to generate saccadic eye movements. There is presently no therapy for the disease or the neurologic symptoms and the patients are in wheelchairs in childhood. Intellect is preserved. The external hallmark of the disease, conjunctival telangiectasia, does not manifest until about 5 years of age. Telangiectasia also develops on the ear, malar face, neck, elbow, knee, hands, and

TABLE 18–25
Hereditary Causes of Ataxia

Disorder	Usual Age of Onset	Hereditary Pattern	Clinical Characteristics	Etiology and Treatment
Friedreich ataxia	2–16 yr	Recessive	Ataxia, scoliosis, pes cavus, posterior column sensory loss, areflexia, cardiomyopathy	Chromosome 9 trinucleotide repeat expansion; supportive
Machado-Joseph disease	12–15 yr	Dominant	Cerebellar, pyramidal, extrapyramidal degeneration; anterior horn cell disease; Portuguese ancestry	Chromosome 14 trinucleotide repeat expansion; supportive
Vitamin E deficiency	2–16 yr	Recessive	Resembles Friedreich ataxia	Vitamin E
Spinocerebellar ataxia 1	6–60 yr	Dominant	Nystagmus, dysarthria, hyperreflexia, ataxia	CAG trinucleotide repeat expansion; supportive
Spinocerebellar ataxia 2	2–65 yr	Dominant	Resembles spinocerebellar ataxia 1 but also oculomotor paresis	Chromosome 12; CAG–trinucleotide repeat expansion; supportive
Ataxia-telangiectasia	Early infancy (1–2 yr)	Recessive	Ataxia, oculomotor apraxia, sinopulmonary infections, telangiectasia of conjunctiva and skin	B- and T-cell dysfunction; cellular immunity is impaired; supportive
Metachromatic leukodystrophy	1–2 yr	Recessive	Ataxia, spasticity, optic atrophy, dementia	Aryl-sulfatase deficiency; supportive
Refsum disease	4–7 yr	Recessive	Ataxia, neuropathy, retinitis pigmentosa, ichthyosis	Phytanic acid hydroxylase deficiency; phytol-free diet
Leigh disease	Infancy to adolescence	Recessive	Ataxia, lactic acidosis, hypotonia, abnormalities of respiration	Some have disorders of pyruvate metabolism; supportive
Wilson disease	Infancy to adulthood	Recessive	Hepatic disease, tremor, dystonic athetosis, chorea	Copper transport disorder; penicillamine
Abetalipoproteinemia	5–15 yr	Recessive	Ataxia, dysmetria, fat malabsorption, acanthocytosis, retinitis pigmentosa, sensory loss	Low-fat diet, vitamin E and A supplementation
Juvenile gangliosidosis	3–5 yr	Recessive GM₁ or GM₂ forms	Ataxia, spasticity, rigidity, dementia	None available
Ramsay Hunt syndrome	7–10 yr	Sporadic	Ataxia, tremor, myoclonus, dementia	Supportive
Marinesco-Sjögren syndrome	Infancy to 5 yr	Recessive	Cataracts, ataxia, growth failure, mental retardation	Supportive

MLD, Metachromatic leukodystrophy.

feet. In addition, prematurely gray hair and atrophic skin develop in patients. Recurrent sinopulmonary infections are a problem in some patients from infancy. Thirty percent of patients die of lymphoid cancers. Laboratory clues to the diagnosis include elevation of blood alpha-fetoprotein levels and depression of blood IgA and circulating T-cell levels. Patients with IgA deficiency are at risk of anaphylaxis following blood transfusion that includes IgA.

Many of the pathophysiologic aspects of this disease are exceptionally well understood. The ATM gene is a large gene on 11q22-23. Most mutations are unique; most patients are compound heterozygotes; and most mutations are nonsense. It is therefore impractical to find the mutation by base pair analysis, but in 80% of cases a genetic diagnosis can be made by failure to detect the ATM protein on Western blot. The protein is a DNA-binding protein kinase related to other kinases involved in cell cycle progression and cellular response to DNA damage. The basic pathologic defect is an inability to properly respond to homologous double-stranded DNA breaks by either DNA repair or induction of apoptosis. These DNA breaks occur normally during meiosis and V(D)J recombination in formation of antigen receptors. They can also occur as a toxic response to UV irradiation and alkylating agents. Mature T cells are sparse because accurate recombination is required to form T-cell receptors and the presence of receptors is necessary for T-cell maturation. IgA is deficient because the constant region for IgA is most distant from the V region on the immunoglobulin gene complex and most likely to be affected by abnormal recombination. Gonadal dysgenesis occurs because meiotic chromosomes must undergo homologous recombination to form gametes. The dermatologic manifestations result from improperly repaired UV injury. Lymphoid malignancies result from improper repair of V(D)J breaks with translocation of the T-cell receptor promoter to a chromosomal position that stimulates an oncogene. The neurologic symptoms are most difficult to explain. It is possible that neurons are unable to effectively repair DNA damage from normal oxidative stress.

Subacute necrotizing encephalomyelopathy, or Leigh disease, is a neuropathologically defined degenerative inherited CNS disease primarily involving the periaqueductal region of the brainstem, caudate, and putamen. Symptoms usually begin before 2 years of age and consist of hypotonia, feeding difficulties, respiratory irregularity, weakness of extraocular movements, and ataxia. Blood and CSF lactate and pyruvate levels are elevated. Different disorders of mitochondrial function can produce this clinical syndrome. Decreased pyruvate carboxylase or pyruvate dehydrogenase activity, biotinidase deficiency, and

cytochrome *c* oxidase deficiency have been identified as causative in some cases. Vitamin therapies have been attempted but with little success except in children with biotinidase deficiency.

Degenerative Diseases of the White Matter. The prominent signs of diseases affecting primarily white matter are spasticity, ataxia, optic atrophy, and peripheral neuropathy. Seizures and dementia are late manifestations. In general, life expectancy ranges from months to a few years. Metachromatic leukodystrophy is an autosomal recessive lipidosis caused by deficiency of the enzyme aryl-sulfatase. Demyelination of the central and peripheral nervous systems occurs, and children present between 1 and 2 years of age, with stiffening and ataxia of gait, spasticity, optic atrophy, intellectual deterioration, absent reflexes, upgoing toes, raised CSF protein, and slowing of motor nerve conduction velocities.

Krabbe disease (globoid cell leukodystrophy) presents a similar clinical picture that begins at 6 months of age and includes irritability, macrocephaly, hyperacusis, and seizures. The same combination of upper and lower motor neuron signs is noted as a result of demyelination of both the central and peripheral nervous systems. Krabbe disease is also an autosomal recessive lipidosis and is caused by a deficiency of the enzyme galactocerebrosidase.

Adrenoleukodystrophy is a sex-linked, recessively inherited disorder associated with progressive central demyelination and adrenal cortical insufficiency. It is caused by an impaired capacity of a subcellular organelle, the peroxisome, to degrade saturated unbranched very-long-chain fatty acids, particularly hexacosanoate (C26:0). The diagnosis is established by finding an elevated hexacosanoate level in plasma lipids and typical abnormalities of neuroimaging. The most common presentation is in boys of early school years who develop subtle behavior changes and intellectual deterioration, followed by cortical visual and auditory deficits and stiff gait. Later, spastic quadriparesis, coma, and seizures supervene. Symptomatic adrenocortical insufficiency with fatigue, vomiting, and hypotension develops in 20–40% of patients, usually at the same time as the neurologic illness. The disease can also present with slowly progressive paraplegia in young men and is then called adreno-myelo-leukodystrophy.

Degenerative Diseases of the Gray Matter with Visceromegaly (See Chapter 5). The prominent signs of gray matter encephalopathy are dementia and seizures. To aid diagnosis, these diseases are divided into those with and without hepatosplenomegaly. All the illnesses discussed next are genetic disorders. All are autosomal recessive traits except for Hunter syndrome, which is a sex-linked recessive trait, Rett syndrome, which is a sex-linked dominant trait, and the mitochondrial encephalopathies, in which the disease may be transmitted through either nuclear or mitochondrial DNA defects.

In the *mucopolysaccharidoses*, degradation of mucopolysaccharides (MPSs) is defective because of the absence of a variety of lysosomal hydrolases. MPSs are important matrix constituents of connective tissue, skin cartilage, bone, and cornea. In these diseases, they accumulate within lysosomes and abnormally large amounts are excreted in the urine. The clinical manifestations of these disorders are dwarfism, kyphoscoliosis, coarse facies, hepatosplenomegaly, cardiovascular abnormalities, and corneal clouding. Neurologic involvement is seen in MPS types 1H (Hurler syndrome), II (Hunter syndrome), III (Sanfilippo syndrome), and VII. Children with Hurler syndrome, the most severe of these illnesses, appear normal during the first 6 months of life and then develop the characteristic skeletal and neurologic features. Mental deficiency, spasticity, deafness, and optic atrophy are progressive. Hydrocephalus frequently occurs because of obstruction to CSF flow by thickened leptomeninges.

Mucolipidosis II (I-cell disease), *mucolipidosis III*, GM_1 *gangliosidosis, fucosidosis,* and *mannosidosis* resemble Hurler syndrome clinically but do not exhibit excess excretion of MPS and involve different disorders in lysosomal hydrolases. The diagnosis is confirmed by analysis of enzymes in white blood cells, serum, and skin fibroblasts.

Classic *Niemann-Pick disease* is caused by a deficiency of the enzyme sphingomyelinase. Sphingomyelin accumulates in foam cells of the reticuloendothelial system of the liver, spleen, lungs, and bone marrow; it also distends neurons of the brain. Intellectual retardation and regression, myoclonic seizures, hypotonia, hepatosplenomegaly, jaundice, and, sometimes, retinal cherry-red spots are noted within the first year of life. The diagnosis is confirmed by finding foam cells in the bone marrow and sphingomyelinase deficiency in leukocytes and skin fibroblasts.

Although the most common form of *Gaucher disease* is an indolent illness of adults, there is a rapidly fatal infantile form featuring severe neurologic involvement caused by deficiency of the enzyme glucocerebrosidase. Glucoceramide accumulates in the liver, spleen, and bone marrow. The characteristic neurologic signs are neck retraction, extraocular movement palsies, trismus, difficulty swallowing, apathy, and spasticity. Gaucher cells are found in bone marrow, and the level of serum acid phosphatase is increased.

Degenerative Disease of the Gray Matter Without Visceromegaly. *Tay-Sachs disease* occurs most commonly in Jewish children of Eastern European background. The disease is confined to the CNS. It is caused by deficiency of hexosaminidase A and the accumulation of GM_2 ganglioside in cerebral gray matter and cerebellum. Infants are normal until 6 months of age, when they develop listlessness, irritability, hyperacusis, intellectual retardation, and a retinal cherry-red spot. The ganglion cells of the retina and macula are distended with ganglioside and appear as a large area of white surrounding a small red fovea that is not covered by ganglion cells. Within months, blindness, convulsions, spasticity, and opisthotonos develop.

Rett syndrome is a common neurodegenerative disorder affecting only females, with onset at about 1 year of age. It is characterized by the loss of purposeful hand movements and communication skills; social withdrawal; gait apraxia; stereotypic repetitive hand movements that resemble washing, wringing, or clapping of the hands; and acquired microcephaly. The illness then plateaus for many years before seizures, spasticity, and kyphoscoliosis develop. The etiology is a mutation on an X-chromosome gene coding for a transcription factor called methyl-CpG-binding protein 2 (MeCP2). The exact phenotype is influenced by whether the mutation is missense or truncating and on the pattern of X-chromosome inactivation in the individual patient.

Neuronal ceroid lipofuscinosis represents a family of genetic diseases characterized histologically by the accumulation in lysosomes of autofluorescent hydrophobic material, consisting of hydrophobic proteins and esterified dolichol lipopigments. The clinical features are dementia, retinal degeneration, and severe myoclonic epilepsy. Visceral symptoms, despite the presence of the storage process, are absent. The disease may present at any age. Pathogenesis at the molecular level is now being elucidated. The original infantile form of NCL (NCL1) is now defined as palmityl protein thioesterase deficiency (gene at the 1p32 locus), the late infantile form (NCL2) as pepstatin resistant proteinase deficiency (gene at the 11p15.5 locus), and the original juvenile form (NCL3) as a defect in a gene (locus 16p11.2-12.3) whose product, the NCL3 protein, still lacks functional characterization.

Mitochondrial diseases can produce the Leigh phenotype described above but can also produce an incredibly diverse set of neurologic, myopathic, and visceral symptoms. Moreover, this group of diseases is probably the most common cause of neurodegenerative disorders. CNS symptoms include failure of development or dementia, severe myoclonic epilepsy, ataxia, ophthalmoplegia, optic atrophy, deafness, and stroke-like episodes. Myopathic symptoms include hypotonia and weakness. Nonneurologic symptoms are short stature, diabetes mellitus, hypertrophic cardiomyopathy, and renal tubular acidosis. The etiology may be defects of mitochondrial DNA or nuclear DNA that codes for mitochondrial proteins. Laboratory clues to the diagnosis are elevations of blood and CSF lactate and pyruvate. When myopathy is present, blood creatine phosphokinase may be elevated, EMG shows a myopathic pattern, and skeletal muscle biopsy reveals ragged red fibers representing proliferating abnormal mitochondrial elements. Specific genetic diagnoses are often difficult to identify because clinical features are pleotropic within individual defects and overlap between different defects and also because analysis of mitochondrial protein function is technically very demanding. Specific syndromes include MELAS (*mitochondrial myopathy, encephalopathy, lactic acidosis, and stroke-like episodes*), MERRF (*myoclonus, epilepsy, and ragged red fibers*), which includes dementia, hearing loss, optic nerve atrophy, ataxia, and loss of deep sensation, and NARP (*neuropathy, ataxia, and retinitis pigmentosa*).

Many degenerative encephalopathies defy diagnosis despite extensive laboratory analysis. The diagnosis of leukodystrophy usually can be made confidently on the basis of extensive cerebral white matter changes on CT or MRI. The diagnosis of hereditary or metabolic gray matter encephalopathy when histologic and biochemical studies are normal is much less secure. Acquired lesions (infectious, inflammatory, vascular, or toxic) are difficult to exclude completely. Brain biopsy is not likely to be helpful unless specific lesions are demonstrated on neuroimaging.

REFERENCES

Amir RE, Van den Veyver IB, Schultz R, et al: Influence of mutation type and X chromosome inactivation on Rett syndrome phenotypes, *Ann Neurol* 47(5):670–679, 2000.

Behrman RE, Kliegman RM, Jenson HB, editors: *Nelson textbook of pediatrics*, ed 16, Philadelphia, 1996, WB Saunders, Chapters 601, 605, 607, 608.

Gressens P: Mechanisms of cerebral dysgenesis, *Curr Opin Pediatr* 10(6):556–560, 1998.

Nowaczyk MJ, Whelan DT, Heshka TW, et al: Smith Lemli-Opitz syndrome: a treatable inherited error of metabolism causing mental retardation, *CMAJ* 161(2):165–170, 1999.

Opitz J: Mental retardation: biologic aspects of concern to pediatricians, *Pediatr Rev* 2:41, 1980.

WEAKNESS

Neuroanatomy

Voluntary movement is directed by a conscious "will," using a large number of subconscious motor mechanisms. Maintenance of proper tone and coordination of agonist, antagonist, synergistic, and fixating muscle groups involve motor nuclei of the spinal cord, cerebellum, brainstem, thalamus, basal ganglia, and motor cortex of the cerebrum.

The corticospinal tract and its neurons that subserve voluntary motor activity are known as the *upper motor neuron*. The *lower motor neuron* includes the anterior horn cells in addition to their motor roots and peripheral motor nerves, the neuromuscular junctions, and the muscles. Destruction of the upper motor neuron causes loss of voluntary control but not total loss of movement. Motor nuclei of the basal ganglia, thalamus, and brainstem have their own tracts that innervate anterior horn cells and produce simple or complex stereotyped patterns of movement. Destruction of the spinal cord leaves intact simple, stereotyped reflex movements coordinated by local spinal reflexes below the level of the lesion. Destruction of the lower motor neuron leads to total absence of movement because it is the final common pathway producing muscle activity.

Weakness caused by disease of the lower motor unit is different in quality from weakness produced by central, corticospinal tract lesions. The latter often is not so much an inability to move the limb as a loss of dexterous movements. The corticospinal tract permits fine motor activity, and its function is best tested by asking the patient to perform rapid alternating movements of the distal extremities. Mild dysfunction produces slowed, stiff motions. More severe dysfunction produces stiff, abnormal postures that do not respond to voluntary command. Characteristically, the posture in corticospinal tract disease consists of the forearm being flexed at the elbow and wrist and adducted close to the chest, with the leg extended and adducted. Disease of the lower motor unit produces progressive loss of strength with hypotonia and no abnormality of posture. Function is best tested by measuring the strength of individual muscle groups or, in the young child, by observing the ability to perform tasks requiring particular muscle groups (e.g., walk up or down stairs, arise from the ground, walk on toes or heels, raise the hands above the head, and squeeze a ball). Table 18–26 characterizes the findings in weakness of upper and lower motor neuron type.

Disease of the Upper Motor Neuron

Stroke is an important and often preventable cause of damage to the corticospinal tract. Tumors, trauma, infections, demyelinating syndromes, and metabolic and degenerative diseases also injure the corticospinal tract.

Stroke in Childhood

Obstruction of blood flow may occur in arteries or veins and may be caused by local thrombosis or

TABLE 18–26
Corticospinal (Upper) and Neuromuscular (Lower) Loss of Motor Function

Clinical Sign	Neuromuscular	Corticospinal
Posture	Flaccid	Arm flexed, leg extended
Tone	Decreased	Increased
Reflexes	Decreased	Increased
Babinski reflex	Absent	Present
Atrophy	Possible	Absent
Fasciculations	Possible	Absent

TABLE 18–27
Causes of Stroke in Childhood

Cardiac or other embolic source
Infectious vasculitis
  Bacterial meningitis
  Chickenpox
Vessel wall pathology
  Arterial dissection
    Traumatic
    Spontaneous
  Moya-Moya
  Vasculitis
Atlantoaxial dislocation
Carcinomatous meningitis
Fibromuscular dysplasia
Atheroclerosis
Amphetamine-cocaine abuse
Coagulopathies
  Sickle cell disease
  Disseminated intravascular pathology
  Hemolytic-uremic syndrome
  Antiphospholipid antibodies
  Pregnancy/oral contraceptive pills
  Malignancy
  L-Asparaginase
  Nephrotic syndrome
  Liver disease
  Genetic procoagulopathy
    Factor V Leiden deficiency
    Protein C deficiency
    Protein S deficiency
    Antithrombin III deficiency
    Homocystinuria
Neonatal
  Emboli from dead twin
  Emboli from involuting umbilical vessels
  Polycythemia

embolization from distant sites. Cerebral embolization characteristically occurs without warning, produces its full deficit within seconds, and may be associated with focal seizures, headache, and hemorrhagic infarction. The most common sources of cerebral emboli are the heart and the carotid artery in the neck. Cerebral thrombosis may be preceded by transient ischemic attacks that resolve completely. The deficits themselves evolve over hours in a stepwise or stuttering progression. The sudden emergence of neurologic deficits implies cerebrovascular disease, and the site of occlusion is suggested by the neurologic deficits. An evolving stroke is distinguished from an attack of neurologic migraine by abnormal findings on diffusion-weighted MRI.

A wide diversity of causes produces stroke in childhood (Table 18–27). The most common causes are congenital heart disease, sickle cell anemia (SS), and meningitis. If clinical assessment does not reveal the cause of the stroke, a complete laboratory investigation should be promptly undertaken. There is no treatment to repair the neurologic lesion after it has occurred, whereas prevention of stroke in children is often possible if the etiology is known.

Heart disease and its complications may give rise to thromboses in cerebral arteries or veins or to emboli in cerebral arteries. Cerebral venous and arterial thromboses occur in 1–2% of infants with unrepaired cyanotic congenital heart disease and probably are related to local congestion of blood flow. Predisposing factors include acute episodes of severe cyanosis, febrile illnesses, dehydration, polycythemia, hyperventilation, and iron-deficiency anemia. Sources of emboli include mural thrombi from dilated poorly contracting cardiac chambers, bacterial endocarditis, nonbacterial endocarditis, valvular disease, atrial myxoma, cardiac catheterization, and cardiac surgery. Septic emboli producing cerebral infarcts occur in 10–20% of patients who develop bacterial endocarditis.

Often, a thorough evaluation of the child with a stroke does not reveal the etiology. Angiography may disclose the site of vascular occlusion, but the pathogenetic mechanism remains unknown. This condition has been labeled as acute hemiplegia of childhood.

A similar problem in defining etiology pertains to children with congenital hemiplegia. Affected infants typically present at 6–9 months of age with decreased use of one side of the body. CT reveals an area of encephalomalacia in the contralateral cerebral hemisphere. The details of the child's intrauterine, labor, delivery, and postnatal history often are unremarkable. Some neonates manifest focal seizures. The timing of the injury is unknown.

Completed strokes do not benefit from medical treatment. Strokes in evolution, transient ischemic attacks, or ongoing cerebral embolization may be treated with anticoagulants (e.g., intravenous heparin, subcutaneous low-molecular-weight heparin and oral warfarin [Coumadin]), platelet antiaggregants (aspirin and dipyridamole), thrombolysis via arterial or venous catheters, or surgery to enlarge stenosed channels, excise sources of emboli, or provide alternative sources of intracerebral blood flow.

Disease of the Lower Motor Neuron

Each motor neuron (anterior horn cell) in the spinal cord and brainstem gives rise to a single myelinated axon that extends to muscle. After numerous branching, each axon twig terminates in a synapse with a single muscle fiber. The presynaptic axon terminal releases acetylcholine, which traverses the synaptic cleft, binds to receptors on the muscle membrane, initiates muscle contraction, and is inactivated by acetylcholinesterase. The lower motor unit consists of all of these components.

Neuromuscular disease is illness of any component of the motor unit. The distribution of muscle weakness can point toward specific diseases (Table 18–28). Diseases affecting each component of the motor unit are listed in Table 18–29 and briefly summarized below.

Disease of the Spinal Cord

Acute spinal cord disease may produce a flaccid, areflexic paralysis that simulates neuromuscular disease. A child who demonstrates an acute or subacute flaccid paraparesis is most likely to have either an acute cord syndrome or the Guillain-Barré syndrome. The acute cord syndrome may be the result of transverse myelitis, a cord tumor, infarction, demyelination, or trauma. The hallmarks of spinal cord disease are a sensory level, a motor level, disturbance of bowel and bladder function, and local spinal pain or tenderness. Transverse myelitis is treated with high-dose steroids; trauma and tumor necessitate immediate neurosurgical management.

Diseases of the Anterior Horn Cell

Werdnig-Hoffmann Disease or Spinal Muscular Atrophy. Progressive degeneration of anterior horn cells is the sole manifestation of this genetic illness, which may begin in intrauterine life or anytime thereafter and may progress at a rapid or slow pace. In general, the earlier in life that the process starts,

TABLE 18–28
"Topography" of Neuromuscular Diseases

Proximal Muscle Weakness
Dystrophy
Duchenne
Limb-girdle
Dermatomyositis; polymyositis
Kugelberg-Welander disease (late-onset spinal muscular atrophy)

Distal Limb Weakness
Polyneuropathy (Guillain-Barré syndrome, others)
HMSN I
HMSN II
Myotonic dystrophy
Distal myopathy

Ophthalmoplegia and Limb Weakness
Myasthenia gravis
Botulism
Myotonic dystrophy
Congenital structural myopathy
Miller Fisher variant of Guillain-Barré syndrome

Facial and Bulbar Weakness
Myasthenia gravis
Botulism
Polio
Miller Fisher variant of Guillain-Barré syndrome
Myotonic dystrophy
Congenital structural myopathy
Facioscapulohumeral dystrophy

HMSN, Hereditary motor sensor neuropathy.

the more rapid the progression. Infants who already are affected at birth or who become weak within the first several months of life usually progress to flaccid quadriplegia with bulbar palsy, respiratory failure, and death within the first year of life. This early fulminant form of the illness is called Werdnig-Hoffmann disease. A mild form of the illness, Kugelberg-Welander syndrome, begins in late childhood with proximal weakness of the legs and progresses slowly over decades. Between these extremes the illness may be unpredictable. It may begin between 6 months and 6 years of age and may progress rapidly or slowly, or may progress rapidly initially and then seemingly plateau. SMA is one of the most frequent autosomal recessive diseases, with

TABLE 18–29
Diseases of the Lower Motor Unit in Infants and Children

Anterior Horn Cell	**Neuromuscular Junction—cont'd**
Spinal muscular atrophy*	Congenital*
Poliomyelitis (natural or vaccine)	Botulism*
Enteroviruses	Aminoglycosides
Peripheral Nerve	**Muscle**
Guillain-Barré syndrome	Dystrophy
Tick paralysis	Duchenne
Hereditary*	Becker
Vitamin E, B_{12}, and B_1 deficiencies	Limb-girdle
Toxins	Facioscapulohumeral
Lead, thallium, arsenic, mercury	Myotonic*
Hexane	Congenital*
Acrylamide	Myositis (viral, polymyositis)
Organophosphates	Congenital structural myopathy
Diphtheria	Central core
Collagen-vascular disease	Nemaline rod
Porphyria	Centronuclear
Paraneoplastic	Congenital fiber type of disproportion
Drugs	Congenital muscular dystrophy
Amitriptyline	Miscellaneous types
Dapsone	
Hydralazine	**Metabolic, Endocrine, and Mineral**
Isoniazid	Glycogen storage disease II (Pompe disease)
Nitrofurantoin	Carnitine metabolism abnormalities
Vincristine	Mitochondrial abnormalities
	Thyroid excess or deficiency
Neuromuscular Junction	Cortisol excess or deficiency
Myasthenia gravis	Hyperparathyroidism; calcium excess
Acquired	Potassium excess or deficiency (periodic paralysis)
Neonatal transitory*	

*Infants.

a carrier frequency of 1 in 50. All types of SMA are caused by mutations in the survival motor neuron gene (SMN1). There are two almost identical copies, SMN1 and SMN2, present on chromosome 5q13. Only homozygous absence of SMN1 is responsible for SMA, whereas homozygous absence of SMN2, found in about 5% of controls, has no clinical phenotype. However, the number of SMN2 copies modulates the SMA phenotype.

The *clinical manifestations* usually are similar in all affected siblings within a single family. Infants exhibit progressive proximal weakness, decreased spontaneous movement, and floppiness. Atrophy may be marked. Head control is lost. With time, the legs stop moving altogether, and the children play only with toys placed in their hands. The range of facial expression diminishes, and drooling and gurgling increase. The eyes remain bright, open, mobile, and engaging. Weakness is flaccid, with early loss of reflexes. Fasciculations sometimes can be seen in the tongue and are best identified when the child is asleep. The infants have normal mental, social, and language skills and sensation. Breathing becomes rapid, shallow, and predominantly abdominal. In the very weak child, respiratory infections lead to atelectasis, pulmonary infection, and death. The level of creatine phosphokinase may be mildly elevated. The electromyogram (EMG) shows fasciculations, fibrillations, positive sharp waves, and high-amplitude, long-duration motor units.

No *treatment* for the condition exists. Symptomatic therapy is directed toward minimizing contractures, preventing scoliosis, aiding oxygenation, preventing aspiration, and maximizing social, language, and intellectual skills. Respiratory infections are managed early and aggressively with pulmonary toilet, chest physical therapy, oxygen, and antibiotics. The use or nonuse of artificial ventilation must be individualized for each patient in each stage of the illness.

Poliomyelitis. See Chapter 10.

Peripheral Neuropathy

The principal peripheral nerve diseases in childhood are (1) Guillain-Barré syndrome, (2) hereditary motor sensory neuropathy (Charcot-Marie-Tooth disease), and (3) tick paralysis. Peripheral neuropathy produced by diabetes mellitus, alcoholism, chronic renal failure, amyloid, exposure to industrial or metal toxins, vasculitis (often as mononeuritis multiplex), or the remote effects of neoplasm is a common cause of weakness and sensory loss in adults but is rare in infants and children.

Guillain-Barré Syndrome. Guillain-Barré syndrome is an idiopathic peripheral neuropathy that often occurs after a respiratory or gastrointestinal infection. Infection with *Campylobacter jejuni* is associated with a severe form of the illness. The characteristic symptoms are areflexia, flaccidity, and relatively symmetric weakness beginning in the legs and ascending to involve the arms, trunk, throat, and face. Progression can occur rapidly, in hours or days, or more indolently, over weeks.

Typically, the child complains of numbness or paresthesia in the hands and feet and then experiences a heavy weak feeling in the legs, followed by inability to walk. The examination often demonstrates complete absence of reflexes even when strength is good. Objective signs of sensory loss usually are minor compared with the dramatic weakness. Meningeal signs frequently are noted. Progression to bulbar and respiratory insufficiency may occur rapidly, and close monitoring of respiratory function is necessary. Neuropathy is distinguished from a spinal cord syndrome by normal bowel and bladder function, loss of arm reflexes, absence of a sensory level, and lack of spinal tenderness. Dysfunction of autonomic nerves can lead to hypertension, hypotension, orthostatic hypotension, tachycardia, and other arrhythmias, urinary retention or incontinence, stool retention, or episodes of abnormal sweating, flushing, or peripheral vasoconstriction. A cranial nerve variant of GBS called the Miller Fisher syndrome manifests with ataxia, partial ophthalmoplegia, and areflexia.

Porphyria and tick paralysis may simulate Guillain-Barré syndrome. Other causes of peripheral neuropathy include vasculitis, heredity, nutritional deficiency (vitamins B_1, B_{12}, and E), endocrine disorders, infections (e.g., diphtheria or Lyme disease), and toxins (e.g., organophosphate or lead).

CSF in GBS often is normal in the first week of the illness and then shows elevated protein levels without pleocytosis. Nerve conduction velocity and EMG also may be normal early in the disease but then show delay in motor nerve conduction velocity and decreased amplitude and temporal dispersion of the evoked compound motor action potential.

This illness resolves spontaneously, and 75% of patients recover normal function within 1–12 months. Twenty percent of patients are left with mild to moderate residual weakness in the feet and lower legs. The mortality rate is 5%, and death is caused by autonomic dysfunction (hypertension-hypotension, tachycardia-bradycardia, and sudden death), respiratory failure, or complications of mechanical ventilation, cardiovascular collapse, or pulmonary embolism.

Children with moderate or severe weakness or rapidly progressive weakness should receive *treatment* in a pediatric intensive care unit. Endotracheal intubation should be performed electively in patients who exhibit early signs of hypoventilation, accumulation of bronchial secretions, or obtunded pharyngeal or laryngeal reflexes. Prior to mechanical ventilation, respiratory sufficiency is monitored by frequent spirometric studies, including vital capacity and maximum inspiratory force. Therapy is symptomatic and rehabilitative and directed at hypertension, hypotension, and cardiac arrhythmia; pulmonary embolism; nutrition, fluids, and electrolytes; pain; skin, cornea, and joints; bowel and bladder; infection; psychologic support; and communication. Controlled studies have not supported the efficacy of ACTH or steroids but suggest that plasma exchange and intravenous immunoglobulin (IVIG) may be beneficial in rapidly progressive disease. Most patients are initially treated with IVIG (total dose 2 g/kg given over 4–5 days).

Hereditary Motor Sensory Neuropathy (Charcot-Marie-Tooth Disease). Hereditary motor and sensory neuropathy (HMSN), commonly called Charcot-Marie-Tooth (CMT) disease, is a chronic, genetic polyneuropathy characterized by weakness and wasting of distal limb muscles. Most often, complaints begin in the preschool years with *pes cavus deformity of feet* and weakness of the ankles with frequent tripping. Examination shows high-arched feet, bilateral weakness of foot dorsiflexors, and normal sensation despite occasional complaints of paresthesia. Progression is slow, extending over years and decades. Eventually, patients develop weakness and atrophy of the entire lower legs and hands and mild to moderate sensory loss in the hands and feet. Some patients never have more than a mild deformity of the feet, loss of ankle reflexes, and electrophysiologic abnormalities, whereas others in the same family may be confined to a wheelchair and have difficulties performing everyday tasks with their hands.

HMSN type I is a demyelinating illness with severely decreased nerve conduction velocity and hypertrophic changes on nerve biopsy. The most common form (CMT 1A) is due to a *duplication* of DNA at 17p11.2–12, a region containing the peripheral myelin protein (PMP 22) gene. A *deletion* in this region gives rise to a much milder condition, called hereditary neuropathy, with liability to pressure palsies. An X-linked form of CMT is caused by mutations of the gap junction protein, connexin 32. HMSN type II is a neuronal form with normal or mildly decreased nerve conduction velocity and no hypertrophic changes. Both type I HMSN and type II HMSN are inherited as autosomal dominant traits with variable expressivity.

Specific *treatment* is not available, but braces such as those that maintain the feet in dorsiflexion can improve function measurably. Early surgery is contraindicated because progression of the disease destabilizes even a good repair.

Neuromuscular Junction

Acquired Myasthenia Gravis. Classic myasthenia gravis may begin in the teenage years with the acute onset of ptosis, diplopia, ophthalmoplegia, and weakness of extremities, neck, face, and jaw. *Clinical manifestations* are least prominent on awakening in the morning and worsen as the day progresses or with exercise. In some children, the disease never advances beyond ophthalmoplegia and ptosis; in others, however, a progressive and potentially life-threatening illness develops that involves all musculature, including that of respiration and swallowing.

Edrophonium chloride (Tensilon) intravenously transiently improves strength and decreases fatigability. Anti–acetylcholine receptor antibodies usually can be detected in the serum, and EMG reveals a decremental response to repetitive nerve stimulation at 1–3 Hz.

Treatment includes an acetylcholine esterase inhibitor, such as pyridostigmine (Mestinon), thymectomy, prednisone, plasmapheresis, and immunosuppressive agents. When respiration is compromised, immediate intubation and admission to an intensive care unit are indicated.

Neonatal Transitory Myasthenia Gravis. In 10–20% of neonates born to mothers with myasthenia gravis, a transitory myasthenic syndrome develops that persists for 1–10 weeks (the mean is 3 weeks). Almost all infants born to mothers with myasthenia demonstrate anti–acetylcholine receptor antibody, and neither antibody titer nor extent of disease in the mother predicts which neonates will display clinical disease. Symptoms and signs include ptosis, ophthalmoplegia, weak facial movements, poor sucking and feeding, hypotonia, and variable extremity weakness.

The *diagnosis* is made by demonstrating clinical improvement lasting approximately 45 minutes following intramuscular (IM) administration of neostigmine methylsulfate, 0.1 mg. *Treatment* with oral pyridostigmine (Mestinon) or neostigmine 30 minutes before feeding is continued until spontaneous resolution occurs.

Muscle Disease
Duchenne Dystrophy

Muscular dystrophy is a common sex-linked recessive trait appearing in 20–30:100,000 boys. Boys exhibit the trait at about 3 years of age with inability to run properly or keep up athletically with their peers. Some have an antecedent history of mild slowness in attaining motor milestones such as walking and climbing stairs. Examination shows calf hypertrophy and mild to moderate proximal leg weakness exhibited by a hyperlordotic and waddling gait and inability to arise from the ground easily. The child typically arises from sitting by using his arms to climb up his legs and body, the *Gower sign*. Weakness progresses such that arm weakness is evident by 6 years of age, and most boys are confined to a wheelchair by 12 years of age. By 16 years, little mobility of arms remains and respiratory difficulties increase. Death is caused by pneumonia or congestive heart failure resulting from myocardial involvement.

Serum creatine phosphokinase levels are always markedly elevated. Muscle biopsy shows muscle fiber degeneration and regeneration accompanied by increased intrafascicular connective tissue. This disease results from absence of a large protein called dystrophin that is associated with the muscle fiber plasma membrane. Becker muscular dystrophy arises from an abnormality in the same gene locus that results in the presence of dystrophin that is abnormal in either amount or molecular structure. It has the same clinical symptoms as Duchenne dystrophy, but onset is later and progression is slower. Prenatal *diagnosis* of both diseases is possible by genetic testing. Approximately one third of cases represent new mutations.

Treatment is supportive, with physical therapy, bracing, proper wheelchairs, and prevention of scoliosis. A multidisciplinary approach is recommended.

Limb-Girdle Dystrophy

Limb-girdle dystrophy is usually an autosomal recessive disease presenting with proximal leg and arm weakness. The *clinical manifestations* are similar to those of Duchenne dystrophy but are seen in an older child or teenager and progress slowly over years. By midadult life, most patients are wheelchair bound and incapacitated. The genetic defect may lie with one of the many muscle proteins that make up the muscle fiber plasma membrane cytoskeleton complex.

Facioscapulohumeral Dystrophy

Facioscapulohumaral dystrophy is usually an autosomal dominant disease presenting in teenagers with facial and proximal arm weakness. The child has mild ptosis, a decrease in facial expression, inability to pucker the lips or whistle, neck weakness, difficulty in fully elevating the arms, scapular winging, and thinness of upper arm musculature. Progression is slow, and most patients retain excellent functional capabilities for decades. Genetic diagnosis is possible by finding a characteristic 4q35 deletion.

Myotonic Dystrophy

Myotonic dystrophy is exhibited either at birth, with severe generalized weakness, or in adolescence, with slowly progressive facial and distal extremity weakness and myotonia. The adolescent type is the classic illness and is associated with cardiac arrhythmias, cataracts, male pattern baldness, and infertility in males (hypogonadism). The facial appearance is characteristic, with hollowing of muscles around temples, jaw, and neck; ptosis; facial weakness; and drooping of the lower lip. The voice is nasal and mildly dysarthric.

Some mothers with myotonic dystrophy give birth to children with the disease who are immobile and hypotonic, with expressionless faces, tented upper lips, ptosis, absence of sucking and Moro reflexes, and poor swallowing and respiration. Often, weakness and atony of uterine smooth muscle during labor lead to associated hypoxic-ischemic encephalopathy and its sequelae. The presence of congenital contractures, clubfoot, or a history of poor fetal movements indicates intrauterine neuromuscular disease.

Myotonic dystrophy is an autosomal dominant genetic disease caused by progressive expansion of a triplet repeat, GCT, on chromosome 19q13.2–13.3 in a gene designated myotonin protein kinase (MP-PK) (see Chapter 4).

Congenital Structural Myopathies

Congenital structural myopathies are a group of congenital, often genetic, either nonprogressive or slowly progressive myopathies characterized by abnormal appearance of the muscle biopsy (see Table 18–29). The *etiology* is uncertain.

The typical *clinical manifestations* consist of a hypotonic infant with moderately diffuse weakness involving limbs and face, often accompanied by congenitally dislocated hips, high-arched palate, clubfoot, and contractures at hips, knees, ankles, or elbows secondary to intrauterine weakness. The attainment of motor milestones is moderately to severely delayed, and the illness is either static or slowly progressive. Progressive kyphoscoliosis represents a significant problem in some children. Reflexes are diminished, creatine phosphokinase levels may be mildly elevated, EMG shows a nonspecific myopathic pattern or is normal, and muscle biopsy demonstrates characteristic changes for each entity.

Juvenile Dermatomyositis

Juvenile dermatomyositis (DM) is the most common chronic idiopathic inflammatory myopathy in childhood. The clinical features include progressive proximal muscle weakness; erythematous rash around the eyes (heliotrope), knuckles (Gottron rash), and on the extensor surfaces of the knees, elbows, and toes; and subcutaneous calcinosis. Other organs such as the intestines may be involved in the inflammatory process. The pathogenesis includes a complement-dependent humoral attack on an unidentified vascular endothelial cell antigen leading to a distinctive microangiopathy in skin, muscle, and other affected organs. Myositis-specific autoantibodies may be identified in the serum. Diagnostic testing includes measurement of serum creatine phosphokinase (CPK) levels, an electromyogram (EMG), and MRI of muscle and muscle biopsy. Therapy for 2 years with corticosteroids often cures the disease in children.

Metabolic Myopathies

Glycogen storage disease type II (Pompe disease) and muscle carnitine deficiency are discussed in Chapter 5.

Mitochondrial myopathies are characterized by muscle biopsy specimens that display ragged red fibers, representing collections of abnormal mitochondria. Hypotonia, ophthalmoplegia, and progressive weakness are the typical symptoms. The mitochondrial disease is systemic, but the symptoms may involve various combinations of muscle, brain, and visceral organs as discussed above.

Endocrine myopathies including hyperthyroidism, hypothyroidism, hyperparathyroidism, and Cushing syndrome are associated with proximal muscle weakness (see Chapter 17). *Hypokalemia* and *hyperkalemia* produce weakness and loss of tendon jerks.

Laboratory Evaluation

Laboratory evaluation is required in patients who have a neuromuscular disease and in whom a careful history and physical examination have not revealed a specific diagnosis (Table 18–30). When planning a laboratory evaluation, it is important to keep in mind that EMG and nerve conduction velocity testing are moderately painful and that muscle biopsy usually requires general anesthesia.

Patients with Duchenne muscular dystrophy, central core myopathy, and other myopathies are susceptible to the life-threatening syndrome of **malignant hyperthermia.** This may occur during administration of anesthesia consisting of succinylcholine or of potent inhalation agents such as halothane. Often, a family history of unexplained death during operations is noted. The symptoms of myopathy may be subtle such as mild ptosis, facial muscle wasting, kyphoscoliosis, foot deformity, dislocated hips, hypermobile hips, dislocated patella, and other musculoskeletal anomalies. Malignant hyperpyrexia can also occur in children without muscle disease as an autosomal dominant genetic disorder. *Diagnosis* of the condition in the patient and family with idiopathic malignant hyperthermia is possible with genetic testing or the in vitro muscle

contraction test. Excessive tonic contracture on exposure to halothane and caffeine in vitro indicates susceptibility. Malignant hyperpyrexia is manifested as a rapid rise of body temperature and Pco_2, muscle rigidity, cyanosis, hypotension, arrhythmias, and convulsions. *Treatment* with intravenous dantrolene, sodium bicarbonate, and cooling is helpful.

Sequelae

The major *complications* of neuromuscular illness are the development of contractures, scoliosis, and pneumonia. *Prevention* and *treatment* of contractures with active range of motion exercises and bracing are important because contractures can be painful or inhibit function even when strength is adequate. Surgery to release contractures or to realign tendons is most helpful in nonprogressive or in very slowly progressive conditions. Kyphoscoliosis produces loss of function, disfigurement, and when severe, life-threatening decrease of ventilatory reserve. Vigorous prophylaxis and treatment are achieved by maintaining ambulation for as long as possible, a properly fitted wheelchair, bracing, and surgery. Pneumonia in the weak patient may produce heavy secretions that are difficult to clear, progressive atelectasis, and respiratory failure. Anticipatory treatment with antibiotics, hospitalization, chest physical therapy, oxygen, and ventilatory support helps in most cases.

Neonatal and Infantile Hypotonia

Neonatal and infantile hypotonia poses certain distinctive diagnostic dilemmas. First, some neuromuscular diseases are characteristic of this age. Second, the distinction between neuromuscular paralysis and cerebral depression is much more difficult in neonates than in older children who, when awake and aware, can communicate. Finally, in some infants a unique syndrome of hypotonia, "floppiness," and hypomotility develops, accompanied by only a small loss of observable strength. This syndrome carries a *differential diagnosis* quite different from that of the definitely weak infant (Table 18–31).

Neonatal Immobility

The first step in evaluating an infant who does not move spontaneously or in response to stimulation is to determine whether *awareness* is intact. If the child is bright-eyed, able to follow, and tries to smile but is unable to move, cortical activity is intact. If the face and eyes are immobile and the eyelids are ptotic, the problem is more difficult. Certain clinical questions may help assess the mental status of the poorly mobile infant. Does the infant respond promptly in some way to a flashlight, bell, or nasal cotton stimulation?

TABLE 18–30
Evaluation of Neuromuscular Disease

Examine parents and obtain complete history
Complete blood count, differential, ESR, electrolytes, BUN, creatinine, glucose, Ca^{2+}, PO_4^- alkaline phosphatase, Mg^{2+}, bilirubin, blood gases, CPK, lactate, pyruvate
Chest roentgenogram, ECG
Stool: botulism culture and toxin, *Campylobacter* culture
Cerebral spinal fluid (protein, cells)
Tensilon test, neostigmine test
EMG-NCV
Muscle biopsy
MRI of spinal cord

BUN, Blood urea nitrogen; *CPK,* creatine phosphokinase; *ECG,* electrocardiogram; *EMG,* electromyogram; *ESR,* erythrocyte sedimentation rate; *MRI,* magnetic resonance imaging; *NCV,* nerve conduction velocity.

TABLE 18–31
Approach to Differential Diagnosis of the Floppy Infant

Weakness	No Weakness
Awareness Intact	*Acute systemic illness*
Neuromuscular disease	*Mental retardation*
Spinal cord disease	Specific syndromes
Trauma	Down syndrome
Tumor	Cerebrohepatorenal (Zellweger peroxisomal
Vascular compromise	disorder)
Malformation	Oculocerebrorenal (Lowe syndrome)
Spina bifida	Kinky hair disease (Menkes syndrome–copper
Syringomyelia	metabolism disorder)
Cerebral Depression (Flaccid Encephalopathy)	Neonatal adrenal leukodystrophy
Severe brain illness	*Prader-Willi syndrome*
Structural	*Connective tissue disorder*
Infectious	Ehlers-Danlos syndrome
Metabolic (e.g., anoxia)	Marfan syndrome
Intoxication through mother	Congenital laxity of ligaments
Magnesium sulfate	*Nutritional-metabolic disease*
Barbiturates	Rickets
Narcotics	Renal tubular acidosis
Benzodiazepines	Celiac disease
General anesthesia	Biliary atresia
Metabolic abnormality	Congenital heart disease
Hypoglycemia	*Benign congenital hypotonia*
Kernicterus	

Do the eyes follow if the lids are lifted? Are reflexes increased as in cerebral disease, or are they absent? If clinical examination does not settle the question, an EEG will be helpful; cerebral disease sufficient to suppress all movement produces severe slowing of the EEG. If the EEG is normal or near normal and the infant is immobile, a disease of the neuromuscular unit or spinal cord is present.

If the cause of the child's immobility is depression of consciousness, the *differential diagnosis* is quite broad (Table 18–5). The most common causes of neonatal immobility are severe hypoxic-ischemic encephalopathy (HIE), metabolic encephalopathy, and intoxication. Severe HIE can result acutely in a flaccid, areflexic infant with complete ptosis, ophthalmoplegia, absent corneal and gag reflexes, and pupillary reactions that may be absent or preserved. Intoxication can be direct from sedative medications the child receives or indirect from medicines given to the mother. Mothers who receive drugs during labor that are cerebral depressants, such as magnesium sulfate, barbiturates, narcotics, benzodiazepines, and inhalation anesthetics, can give birth to children who are transiently floppy, apneic, and unresponsive. Rarely, neuromuscular weakness develops in infants treated with an aminoglycoside for suspected sepsis whose mothers received magnesium sulfate, because both these drugs inhibit acetylcholine release at the neuromuscular junction. Infants with severe hypoglycemia or hyperbilirubinemia that produces kernicterus can exhibit a flaccid encephalopathy. Seizures frequently accompany HIE and metabolic encephalopathies but are unusual with drug intoxication.

Hypotonia Without Major Weakness

Some infants who appear to move well when supine in their cribs clearly are "floppy" when handled or moved. When placed on their backs, most of these children are bright-eyed, have expressive faces, and can lift their arms and legs without apparent difficulty. When they are lifted, however, their heads flop, they "slip through" at the shoulders, do not stand upright on their legs, and form an "inverted U" in prone suspension. When placed prone as neonates, they may lie flat instead of having their arms tucked underneath them and their rumps up in the air. Passive tone is decreased, but reflexes are normal. This clinical picture may be associated with significant cerebral disease or may be a benign phenomenon that is outgrown.

Prader-Willi syndrome presents with severe neonatal hypotonia, severe feeding problems leading to failure to thrive, small hands and feet, and in the male, small penis, small testicles, and cryptorchidism. Paradoxically, severe hyperphagia and obesity develop in early childhood. Approximately 60–70% of affected individuals have an interstitial deletion of paternal chromosome 15q11q13. Many other syndromes also present with severe neonatal floppiness and mental dullness (Table 18–31).

Children who have a connective tissue disorder, such as Ehlers-Danlos syndrome, Marfan syndrome, or familial laxity of the ligaments, may exhibit marked passive hypotonia, "double jointedness," and increased skin elasticity. They have normal strength and cognition and achieve motor and mental milestones normally. They have peculiar postures of their feet or an unusual gait when examined by an orthopedist.

Finally, there are children who have benign congenital hypotonia. Typically, they exhibit the condition at 9–12 months, with delayed motor skills. They are unable to sit, creep, or crawl but have good verbal, social, and manipulative skills and an intelligent appearance. Strength appears normal, and the children can briskly kick arms and legs and bring their toes to their mouths. However, the children display head lag, slip-through in ventral suspension, and floppiness of passive tone. Parents may remember that the infant has seemed floppy from birth. This *diagnosis* represents a miscellaneous category of unknown causes. Some children may have mild congenital myopathies, and others may have mild cerebellar immaturity or dysfunction, but extensive laboratory investigation is unrevealing and not warranted. A complete physical examination, CBC, electrolytes, bicarbonate, BUN, creatinine, calcium, CPK, bilirubin, ALT, AST, and urinalysis are necessary and sufficient to exclude occult disease of the bone marrow, heart, liver, or kidneys. Most of these children catch up to their peers and appear normal by 3 years of age. Often, other family members have exhibited a similar developmental pattern.

REFERENCES

Andersson PB, Rando TA: Neuromuscular disorders of childhood, *Curr Opin Pediatr* 11:497, 1999.

Behrman RE, Kliegman RM, Jenson HB, editors: *Nelson textbook of pediatrics*, ed 16, Philadelphia, 1996, WB Saunders, Chapters 614–622.

Duggan D, Gorospe J, Fanin M, et al: Mutations in the sarcoglycan genes in patients with myopathy, *N Engl J Med* 336(9):618–624, 1997.

Evans O, Vedanarayqnan V: Guillain-Barré syndrome, *Pediatr Rev* 18(1):10–16, 1997.

Ouvrier R: Correlation between the histopathologic, genotypic, and phenotypic features of hereditary peripheral neuropathies in childhood, *J Child Neurol* 11(2):133–136, 1996.

Plasma Exchange Sandiglobulin Guillain-Barré Syndrome Trial Group: Randomized trial of plasma exchange, intravenous immunoglobulin, and combined treatments in Guillain-Barré syndrome, *Lancet* 349(9047):225–230, 1997.

Rivkin MJ, Volpe JJ: Strokes in children, *Pediatr Rev* 17(8):265–278, 1996.

Sebire G, Hollenberg H, Meyer L, et al: High dose methylprednisolone in severe acute transverse myelitis, *Arch Dis Child* 76(2):167–168, 1997.

Shanske S, DiMauro S: Diagnosis of the mitochondrial encephalomyopathies, *Curr Opin Rheumatol* 9(6):496–503, 1997

Tsao CY, Mendell JR: The childhood muscular dystrophies: making order out of chaos, *Semin Neurol* 19(1):9–23, 1999.

NEUROCUTANEOUS DISORDERS

The skin, teeth, hair, nails, and brain are derived embryologically from *ectoderm*, and abnormalities of these surface structures may indicate abnormal brain development. The term *phakomatosis* means "mother spots" or "birthmarks" and refers to tuberous sclerosis and neurofibromatosis. Not all of the so-called neurocutaneous disorders, however, have characteristic cutaneous lesions, and not all are of ectodermal origin. Von Hippel-Lindau disease does not have characteristic cutaneous lesions, and both von Hippel-Lindau disease and Sturge-Weber disease are of mesenchymal rather than ectodermal origin. More than 40 conditions are referred to as neurocutaneous syndrome, but neurofibromatosis, tuberous sclerosis, Sturge-Weber disease, von Hippel-Lindau disease, and ataxia-telangiectasia are the major disorders.

Neurofibromatosis

Neurofibromatosis refers to two distinct genetic diseases. Neurofibromatosis 1 (NF1), also known as von Recklinghausen disease, is a common autosomal-dominant disorder with an incidence of approximately 1 in 3,000. It is caused by mutations of the NF1 gene, which is located at chromosome 17q11.2 and codes for neurofibromin. Spontaneous new mutations occur in 30–50% of cases. Somatic mosaicism, in which an abnormality in one copy of the NF1 gene is present in some cells but not others, indicating a postzygotic mutation, has been identified and called segmental NF. The cardinal features of the disorder are café-au-lait spots, axillary freckling, cutaneous neurofibromas, and iris hamartomas (Lisch nodules). Common complications are learning disability, scoliosis, macrocephaly, headache, and optic gliomas. Other complications such as sphenoid wing dysplasia, cortical thinning of the long bones with pseudarthrosis, peripheral nerve malignancy, pheochromocytoma, renovascular hypertension, and epilepsy are individually rare. Hyperintense lesions on T2-weighted MRI scans in the basal ganglia, internal capsule, thalamus, cerebellum, and brainstem are common and distinctive for the disease. They are benign and disappear in adulthood. NF1 is a tumor suppressor gene, and neurofibromin is a major negative regulator of a key signal transduction pathway in cells, the Ras pathway, which transmits mitogenic signals to the nucleus. Loss of neurofibromin leads to increased levels of activated Ras (bound to GTP), and thus increased downstream mitogenic signaling. The average life expectancy of patients with NF1 is probably reduced by 10–15 years, and malignancy is the most common cause of death. Genetic and psychologic counseling are important components of care for this chronic disorder.

Café-au-lait spots are present in more than 90% of patients who have NF1. They typically appear in the first few years of life and increase in number and size over time. The presence of six or more spots larger than 5 mm suggests the diagnosis. *Lisch nodules* also increase in frequency with age and are present in more than 90% of adults who have NF1. Approximately 25% of children exhibit these iris nodules.

Neurofibromas are composed of various combinations of Schwann cells, fibroblasts, mast cells, and vascular elements. Dermal neurofibromas are nearly universal and consist of discrete, small, soft lesions that lie within the dermis and epidermis and move passively with the skin. They rarely cause any symptoms. Plexiform neurofibromas are large, occasionally nodular, subcutaneous lesions that lie along the major peripheral nerve trunks. They often cause symptoms including pain, weakness, and invasion of adjacent viscera or spinal cord. Sarcomatous degeneration occurs. Surgical treatment is attempted, but results are often unsatisfactory. Other tumors that occur in NF1 are optic nerve gliomas, astrocytomas of brain and spinal cord, and malignant peripheral nerve tumors.

NF2 is an incurable disease that predisposes patients to multiple intracranial and spinal tumors, including bilateral vestibular schwannomas, schwannomas of other cranial and spinal nerves, meningiomas, and gliomas. Peripheral nerve tumors, including schwannomas and neurofibromas, are uncommon. The average life span is less than 40 years. Posterior capsular or cortical cataracts are common, but Lisch nodules, café-au-lait spots, and axillary freckling are not features of the disease. NF2 is an autosomal-dominant disorder with an incidence of 1 in 33,000. Half the cases have no family history. The NF2 is a tumor suppressor gene on chromosome 22 that codes for a protein called merlin. Merlin is similar to a family of proteins that serve as linkers between integral membrane proteins and the cy-

toskeleton and are involved in Rho-mediated signal transduction.

Tuberous Sclerosis

Tuberous sclerosis (TS) is an autosomal dominant genetic disorder characterized by hamartomas in many organs, especially the brain, eye, skin, kidneys, and heart. The incidence is 1:10,000 births. Two thirds of cases are sporadic and are thought to represent new mutations. Germline mosaicism is uncommon but explains how parents who apparently do not have the disease can have multiple children with TS. Mutations affecting either of the presumed tumor-suppressor genes TSC1 (chromosome 9) or TSC2 (chromosome 16) cause TS. Both appear to function as tumor suppressors because in accordance with the Knudsen "two-hit" hypothesis, somatic loss or intragenic mutation of the corresponding wild-type allele is seen in the associated hamartomas. Among sporadic TS cases, mutations in TSC2 are more frequent and often accompanied by more severe neurologic deficits. The TSC1 and TSC2 genes encode distinct proteins, hamartin and tuberin, respectively, that are widely expressed in the brain and may interact as part of a cascade pathway that modulates cellular differentiation, tumor suppression, and intracellular signaling. Tuberin has a GTPase-activating protein-related domain that may contribute to a role in cell cycle passage and intracellular vesicular trafficking.

The classic clinical features are facial angiofibromas, formerly referred to as adenoma sebaceum; mental retardation (MR); and severe epilepsy. Less than 50% of patients with TS exhibit all three features. Other major signs are ungual fibromas, retinal hamartomas, hypopigmented macules, shagreen patches, renal angiomyolipoma, cardiac rhabdomyoma, brain tubers, and brain subependymal nodules and astrocytomas. Facial angiofibromas do not develop until 2–5 years of age, but hypomelanotic macules, called ash-leaf spots, are present in infancy and best detected with a Wood's lamp under ultraviolet light. *Shagreen patches* are elevated, rough plaques of skin with a predilection for the lumbar and gluteal regions that develop in late childhood or early adolescence. Cardiac rhabdomyomas are largest during prenatal life and in infancy and are rarely symptomatic. Occasionally they may cause arrhythmias or cardiac outflow obstruction. Renal angiomyolipomas may undergo malignant transformation and are the most common cause of death in adults with TS. Tubers in the cerebral cortex are areas of cerebral dysplasia that in combination with other microscopic areas of abnormal development are responsible for the symptoms of MR and epilepsy. Sub-ependymal nodules (SENs) are hamartomas that may mutate into a growth phase and become subependymal giant-cell astrocytomas. These obstruct CSF outflow and cause hydrocephalus. These brain lesions can be detected directly by MRI and indirectly by CT, which demonstrates periventricular calcifications within the SEN, especially around the foramen of Monro.

TS is one of the most common causes of infantile spasms. These children often develop intractable epilepsy, with myoclonic, atonic, partial and grand mal seizures, as well as MR, autism, and hyperactivity.

Sturge-Weber Syndrome

The Sturge-Weber syndrome (SWS) is characterized by angiomas of the leptomeninges overlying the cerebral cortex in association with an ipsilateral facial port-wine nevus that, at the least, covers part of the forehead and upper eyelid but may have a much more extensive, and even a bilateral, distribution. This nevus flammeus is an ectasia of superficial venules, not a hemangioma, because it has no endothelial proliferation. Ocular defects of SWS include glaucoma and hemangiomas of the choroid, conjunctiva, and episclera. Glaucoma is present in 30–50% of patients and may be progressive. SWS is sporadic and not genetic.

The most common associated neurologic abnormality is the presence of seizures. Seizures develop because of ischemic injury to the brain underlying the meningeal angiomas. Angiomas are most commonly located in the posterior parietal, posterior temporal, and anterior occipital lobes. These angiomas consist of thin-walled veins within the pia mater and produce venous engorgement and presumably stasis within the involved areas. Positron emission tomography has demonstrated hypoperfusion and hypometabolism in these areas. In some children with SWS, progressive ischemia of the underlying brain develops, resulting in hemiparesis, hemianopia, intractable focal seizures, and dementia. Calcium becomes detectable in the gyri of the brain underlying the angioma, and, as the intervening sulci are spared, the radiologic picture of "tram track" or "railroad track" calcifications is seen in about 60% of cases. Many children with SWS are intellectually normal, and seizures are well controlled with standard anticonvulsants. Hemispherectomy has been proposed for infants whose seizures begin early in life and are difficult to control. Intellectual and even motor outcome appears improved, but the surgical risks of the procedure are considerable.

Laser surgery is the most promising therapeutic option for cosmetic management of the facial nevus flammeus. Expert ophthalmologic management of glaucoma and choroidal hemangiomas is required.

REFERENCES

Behrman RE, Kliegman RM, Jenson HB, editors: *Nelson textbook of pediatrics*, ed 16, Philadelphia, 2000, WB Saunders, Chapter 605.
Crino PB, Henske EP: New developments in the neurobiology of the tuberous sclerosis complex, *Neurology* 53(7):1384–1390, 1999.
Kihiczak NI, Schwartz RA, Jozwiak S, et al: Sturge-Weber syndrome, *Cutis* 65(3):133–136, 2000.
Ruggieri M: The different forms of neurofibromatosis, *Childs Nerv Syst* 15(6–7):295–308, 1999.

MOVEMENT DISORDERS

Movement disorders are the result of abnormalities of the extrapyramidal system, which is composed of the basal ganglia and its connections. Disorders of movement may be *bradykinetic,* slowness of movement; *hypokinetic,* paucity of movement; or *hyperkinetic,* excessive involuntary movements. Bradykinesia and hypokinesia describe the agonizingly slow gait, halting speech patterns, apparent inactivity, and paucity of facial expression seen in children with extrapyramidal disorders. The hyperkinetic disorders are associated with many disease states and as a group are activated by stress and fatigue but disappear in sleep. *Segmental myoclonic* abnormalities refer to activity in isolated muscle groups (e.g., the palatal myoclonus) that does not disappear in sleep.

Chorea

Chorea is a hyperkinetic, rapid, unsustained, irregular, purposeless, nonpatterned movement. Muscle tone is decreased. Choreiform movement abnormalities may be congenital, familial, metabolic, vascular, toxic, infectious, or neoplastic in origin. The movements may occur alone or as part of a more extensive neurologic disorder (e.g., Sydenham chorea, Huntington chorea, cerebral palsy, Wilson disease, or reactions to toxins and drugs). Fidgety behavior, inability to sit still, clumsiness, dysarthria, and an awkward gait may occur. The exact site of dysfunction within the extrapyramidal system is unknown.

Athetosis

Athetosis is a hyperkinetic, slow, coarse, writhing movement that is more pronounced in distal muscles. Muscle tone is increased. Athetosis frequently is seen in combination with chorea (choreoathetosis) and usually is present in conjunction with other neurologic signs. It may be seen in virtually all the disorders mentioned for chorea, but the most prominent cause is encephalopathy. Athetosis is a prominent feature of Hallervorden-Spatz disease, Wilson disease, and Pelizaeus-Merzbacher dystrophy.

Dystonia

Dystonia is a hyperkinetic, sustained, slow, twisting motion (torsion spasm) that may progress to a fixed posture and can be activated by repetitive movement (i.e., action dystonia). It usually begins in the legs when appendicular muscles are involved and in the neck or trunk when axial muscles are involved. Dystonia is a movement disorder with many causes and associated neurologic signs. *Tardive dyskinesia* usually is associated with antipsychotic drug use; darting tongue movements, incessant flexion and extension of the distal muscles, standing and marching in place, and a perception of restlessness are common.

Tremor

Tremor is a hyperkinetic, rhythmic, oscillatory movement caused by simultaneous contractions of antagonistic muscles. The amplitude and frequency are regular. In children, tremor is usually of physiologic, familial, or cerebellar origin but may be seen in association with other disease processes (e.g., thyrotoxicosis, hypoglycemia, or Wilson disease) or drugs (e.g., bronchodilators, amphetamines, or tricyclic antidepressants).

Myoclonus

Myoclonus is a hyperkinetic, brief flexion contraction of a muscle group, resulting in a sudden jerk. Myoclonus may be epileptic or nonepileptic. Nonepileptic myoclonus is distinguished from tremor in that it is a simple contraction of an agonist muscle, whereas tremor is a simultaneous contraction of agonist and antagonist muscles. Myoclonus is seen as a manifestation of various epilepsies and of infectious, toxic, and metabolic encephalopathies.

Tic

Tic movements are similar to myoclonus but are much more stereotyped and involve the face, shoulder, and arm. Motor tics in association with vocal tics are characteristic of Tourette syndrome.

Tourette syndrome consists of a chronic tic disorder that begins in early childhood. The severity and form of the tics vary over months and years; vocal tics are common. The tics vary from simple twitches and grunts to complex stereotyped movement patterns. Obsessive-compulsive disorder and attention-deficit/hyperactivity syndrome may also be present in some children. The prevalence is at least 5:10,000, with a male-to-female ratio of 4:1. The pathophysiology underlying the tics is unknown, but a family history of tics is elicited in more than 50% of cases. Imaging of the brain is always normal and does not have to be performed. Many children with Tourette syndrome are comfortable with their tics and require no therapy, whereas others benefit from psychologic support and pharmacologic therapy with neuroleptics.

REFERENCES

Behrman RE, Kliegman RM, Jenson HB, editors: *Nelson textbook of pediatrics*, ed 16, Philadelphia, 2000, WB Saunders, Chapter 606.
Janavs JL, Aminoff MJ: Dystonia and chorea in acquired systemic disorders, *J Neurol Neurosurg Psychiatry* 65(4):436–445, 1998.
Robertson MM: Tourette syndrome, associated conditions and the complexities of treatment, *Brain* 123(Pt 3):425–462, 2000.

CHAPTER 19

Common Orthopaedic Problems of Children

George H. Thompson

GENERAL CONSIDERATIONS

Multiple congenital and acquired mechanisms may produce orthopaedic problems specific to childhood; other pathologic mechanisms are common to all age groups (Table 19–1). Most pediatric orthopaedic problems involve the spine and lower extremities, especially the hips and feet. Upper extremity abnormalities, other than trauma, occur less frequently. In addition to the challenge of identifying pathologic processes and choosing nonoperative versus operative management, the necessity of clearly discerning ongoing physiologic, developmental, or maturational changes from abnormal events confronts the pediatrician. What may be physiologic at one age may be pathologic at another.

IN UTERO POSITIONING

The in utero position produces joint and muscle contractures and affects torsional and angular alignment of long bones, especially of the lower extremities (Fig. 19–1). All normal full-term newborns have 20–30-degree hip and knee flexion contractures. These decrease to neutral by 4–6 months of age. The newborn hip externally rotates in extension 80–90 degrees and has limited internal rotation of 0–10 degrees. The normal newborn foot also may reflect the in utero position. Most commonly, in utero the feet are in the tucked-under position, which can be observed after birth. On inspection the forefoot appears adducted or deviated inwardly with respect to the hindfoot; the heel may be inverted; and the foot tends to be in equinus or pointed down at the ankle. If the foot can be positioned so that the lateral border is straight, the heel slightly everted, and the foot dorsiflexed to above a right angle, the clinical diagnosis of normal in utero positioning is validated.

The face may be distorted by in utero positioning, whereas the spine and upper extremities are less af-

fected. The effects of normal in utero position are physiologic in origin but produce parental concern. The child may be 3–4 years of age before the intrauterine effects completely resolve.

DEVELOPMENTAL MILESTONES AND NEUROLOGIC MATURATION

Neurologic maturation, marked by the achievement of motor milestones at the regular intervals, is important for normal musculoskeletal development (see Chapter 1). A trophic relationship exists between skeletal form and gross motor development. Normal neurologic development must be included in the definition of a normal musculoskeletal system. Any process that produces a neurologic abnormality may secondarily cause an aberration of musculoskeletal growth. Any disorder that primarily affects skeletal muscle may produce abnormalities of skeletal growth and development. Normal muscle function is necessary for normal skeletal growth.

GAIT

Disturbances of gait, including *limp,* are common manifestations of pediatric orthopaedic disorders (Tables 19–2 and 19–3). Understanding the normal development aspects of gait is helpful in distinguishing maturational from pathologic processes. Normal gait (walking on level ground) is composed of a stance phase and a swing phase. The gait cycle is the interval between stance phases on the same limb. The stance phase (60% of gait) is performed when the foot, which bears weight, contacts the ground; it begins with the heel strike and ends with the toe-off. In the swing phase (40%), the foot is off the ground. The early child's or toddler's (12–18 months) gait is quite hesitant and inconsistent. The gait is broad based and characterized by rapid cadence, short

TABLE 19–1
Mechanisms of Common Pediatric Orthopaedic Problems

Category	Mechanism	Example
Congenital		
Malformation	Teratogenesis prior to 12th wk of gestation	Spina bifida
Disruption	Amniotic band constriction	Extremity amputation
	Fetal varicella infection	Limb scar/atrophy
Deformation	Leg compression	Developmental dysplasia of the hip (DDH)
	Neck compression	Torticollis
Dysplasia	Abnormal cell growth or metabolism	Osteogenesis imperfecta
		Skeletal dysplasias
Acquired		
Infection	Pyogenic-hematogenous spread	Septic arthritis, osteomyelitis
Inflammation	Antigen-antibody reaction	Systemic lupus erythematosus
	Immune mediated	Juvenile rheumatoid arthritis
Trauma	Mechanical forces, overuse	Child abuse, sports injuries, unintentional injury, fractures, dislocations, tendonitis
Tumor	Primary bone tumor	Osteosarcoma
	Metastasis to bone from other site	Neuroblastoma
	Bone marrow tumor	Leukemia, lymphoma

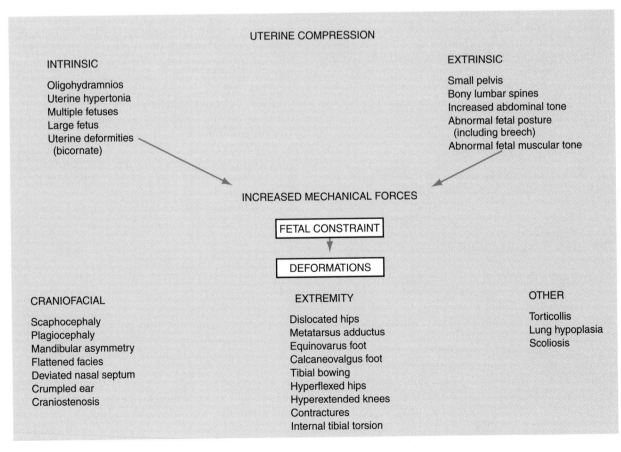

FIG. 19–1

Deformation abnormalities resulting from uterine compression.

TABLE 19–2
Differential Diagnosis of Gait Disturbances (Limping)

Early Walker (1–3 Years Old)
Painful Limp
Septic arthritis and osteomyelitis
Transient monoarticular synovitis
Occult trauma ("toddler's fracture")
Intervertebral discitis
Painless Limp
Developmental dysplasia of the hip (DDH)
Neuromuscular disorder
Cerebral palsy
Lower extremity length inequality

Child (3–10 Years of Age)
Painful Limp
Septic arthritis and osteomyelitis
Transient monoarticular synovitis
Trauma
Rheumatologic disorders
    Juvenile rheumatoid arthritis (JRA)
    Intervertebral discitis
Legg-Calvé-Perthes disease (LCPD)

Painless Limp
Developmental dysplasia of the hip (DDH)
Legg-Calvé-Perthes disease (LCPD)
Lower extremity length inequality
Neuromuscular disorder
    Cerebral palsy
    Muscular dystrophy (Duchenne)

Adolescent (11 Years of Age to Maturity)
Painful Limp
Septic arthritis and osteomyelitis
Trauma
Rheumatologic disorder
Slipped capital femoral epiphysis (SCFE): acute; unstable
Painless Limp
Slipped capital femoral epiphysis (SCFE): chronic; stable
Developmental dysplasia of the hip (DDH): acetabular dysplasia
Lower extremity length inequality
Neuromuscular disorder

TABLE 19–3
Mechanisms of Gait Disturbances and Extremity Pain

Mechanical
Trauma, fracture, sprain
Sports injury; overuse injury
Child abuse
Developmental dysplasia of the hip (DDH)

Osseous
Legg-Calvés-Perthes disease (LCPD)
Slipped capital femoral epiphysis (SCFE)
Osteomyelitis
Discitis
Osteoid osteoma

Articular
Septic arthritis
Toxic synovitis
Rheumatic disease (JRA, SLE)
Hemophilia

Neurologic
Guillain-Barré syndrome (other peripheral neuropathies)
Intoxication
Cerebellar ataxia

Neurologic—cont'd
Brain tumor
Lesion occupying spinal cord space
Myopathy
Hemiplegia
Sympathetic reflex dystrophy

Hematologic
Sickle cell pain crisis
Leukemia
Metastatic tumor
Bone tumor
Langerhans cell histiocytosis

Other
Kawasaki disease
Conversion reaction
Gaucher disease
Scurvy
Rickets
Psoas abscess

DDH, Developmental dysplasia of the hip; *JRA*, juvenile rheumatoid arthritis; *SLE*, systemic lupus erythematosus.

steps, flatfoot initial ground contact, and nonaccompaniment by the reciprocal arm swing. A 2-year-old has increased velocity and step length and a diminished cadence. Normal adult gait is achieved by 3–7 years of age.

Limping is either painless or painful (Table 19–2). A painful limp is characterized by acute onset and usually is caused by trauma, infection (septic arthritis and osteomyelitis), or acquired disorders (Table 19–3). Stance phase and stride length are shortened in an attempt to decrease standing on the involved limb. Trunk shift to the opposite side also decreases stress and maintains balance. This is referred to as an **antalgic gait.** A painless limp is characterized by normal stance phase but a persistent trunk sway. This type of gait is called a **Trendelenburg gait.**

Painless limping (Table 19–2) may be associated with neuromuscular disorders producing muscle weakness about the hip, especially in the gluteus medius muscle, the major hip abductor. This muscle stabilizes the pelvis during stance phase and prevents a pelvic drop to the opposite side. Trauma or weakness of this muscle or inflammatory hip disorders are the most common causes of limping. Disorders that have bilateral involvement produce a **waddling gait.**

Knee pathology, usually from trauma, can produce a limp by limiting knee flexion and causing the child to circumduct the leg and elevate the pelvis during swing phase. It also produces a shortened stance phase. Poor dorsiflexion of the foot resulting from weakness (peroneal nerve injury or peripheral neuropathy) or trauma causes increased knee flexion for toe clearance during the swing phase, resulting in a **drop-foot gait.**

Toe-walking, which is common in early walkers, may be the result of habit, leg length discrepancy, underlying neuromuscular disorder (cerebral palsy), or a congenital contracture of the gastrocnemius and soleus muscles (Achilles tendon or heel cord).

GROWTH AND DEVELOPMENT

During the growing years, the ends of long bone contain a much greater proportion of cartilage than after maturity (Fig. 19–2). The high cartilage content (articular and physeal) leads to a unique vulnerability from trauma and metaphyseal infections. The infections may involve the metaphysis, joint space, or both.

Special anatomic features within the child's skeletal system stimulate and support the various kinds of skeletal growth that continuously occur in the immature skeletal (Fig. 19–3). The epiphyseal growth plate, also called the *physis*, provides for longitudinal growth of the bones. Articular cartilage provides for enlargement of the bone ends and also for growth of

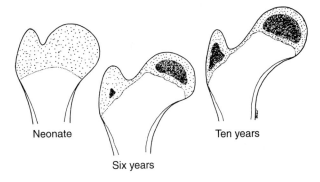

FIG. 19–2

Lightly stippled areas represent cartilage composition, whereas heavily darkened areas are zones of ossification. (From Tachjidan MO: *Congenital dislocation of the hip,* New York, 1982, Churchill Livingstone.)

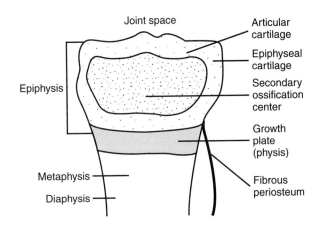

FIG. 19–3

Schematic of long bone structure. The shaft, or *diaphysis,* is distal to the *metaphysis,* which is the closest extension of endochondral bone. The epiphyseal growth plate *(physis)* is the avascular cartilage between the articular surface and the metaphyseal bone. The growth plate is the region of longitudinal bone growth. The contribution to eventual bone length varies: 80% for the proximal humerus, 20% for the distal humerus, 75% for the distal radius, 80% for the distal ulna, 70% for the distal femur, 57% for the proximal tibia, and 60% for the proximal fibula. When growth is complete, the epiphyseal growth plate is ossified or closed. The cartilaginous epiphyseal plate is supported by internal interdigitation with the metaphyseal bone and externally by the insertion of the fibrous periosteum. (Modified from Shapiro F: *N Engl J Med* 317:1702, 1987.)

some of the small bones largely covered by articular cartilage, such as the carpals and tarsals. The perichondrium and the periosteum provide appositional growth or circumferential growth of the cartilage and skeletal structures, respectively. Trauma, infection, nutritional deficiency (rickets), regional soft tissue

TABLE 19–4
Glossary of Orthopaedic Terminology

Abduction	Movement away from the midline
Adduction	Movement toward and possibly across the midline
Anteversion	Increased angulation of the femoral head and neck with respect to the knee in the frontal plane
Apophysis	Bone growth center that is not a growth plate and that has a strong muscle insertion (e.g., greater trochanter of femur)
Arthroplasty	Surgical reconstruction of a joint
Arthrotomy	Surgical incision into a joint
Calcaneus	Dorsiflexion of hindfoot
Cavovarus	High longitudinal or medial arch of foot with plantar-flexed supinated forefoot and hindfoot varus
Cavus	High longitudinal arch of the foot (usually plantar-flexed forefoot)
Dislocation	Complete loss of contact between two joint surfaces
Equinus	Plantar flexion of the forefoot, hindfoot, or entire foot
Extension	Means to straighten, and is the reverse of flexion
External rotation	External rotation, away from the midline
Flexion	Means to bend
Internal rotation	Inward rotation, toward the midline
Osteotomy	Surgical division of a bone
Subluxation	Incomplete loss of contact between two joint surfaces
Valgum	Angulation of a bone or joint in which the apex is toward the midline; genu valgum or knock-knee
Varum	Angulation of a bone or joint away from the midline; genu varum or bowleg

processes, inborn errors of metabolism (e.g., mucopolysaccharidosis, mucolipidosis, Gaucher disease, and disorders of collagen or cartilage synthesis), and other metabolic processes (e.g., oxalosis, renal tubular acidosis, uremia, and endocrine excess or deficiencies) may affect each of these processes, producing a distinct aberration in the particular growth function.

ORTHOPAEDIC TERMINOLOGY

The terminology used in orthopaedics to describe position, motion, and function can be confusing. Some common orthopaedic terms are presented in Table 19–4.

REFERENCES

Behrman RE, Kliegman RM, Jenson HB, editors: *Nelson textbook of pediatrics*, ed 16, Philadelphia, 2000, WB Saunders, Chapters 678–679.
Myers MT, Thompson GH: Imaging the child with a limp, *Pediatr Clin North Am* 44(3):657–658, 1997.
Sutherland DH, Olsten R, Cooper L, et al: The development of mature gait, *J Bone Joint Surg Am* 62(3):336–353, 1980.
Thompson GH: Gait disturbances. In Kliegman RM, editor: *Practical strategies in pediatric diagnosis and therapy*, Philadelphia, 1996, WB Saunders.

THE HIP

The hip is a ball (femoral head) and socket (acetabulum) joint that provides the skeleton with structural balance and stability. The femoral head and acetabulum have a trophic relationship and are interdependent for normal growth and development (Fig. 19–4). When this trophic relationship is interrupted, abnormal hip development follows. Muscle balance and activity related to appropriate gross motor development are essential to normal development of the hip. The blood supply to the capital femoral epiphysis (CFE) or femoral head is unique because the CFE and femoral neck lie intracapsularly, but the blood supply from the retinacular vessels is extraosseous, lying on the surface of the femoral neck and entering the epiphysis peripherally. The blood supply to the femoral head is vulnerable to damage from septic arthritis, trauma, and other vascular insults. *Avascular necrosis* or *osteonecrosis*, either as an idiopathic process or secondary to other disorders, is common in children.

Developmental Dysplasia of the Hip

Developmental dysplasia of the hip represents abnormal development or dislocation of the hip; at

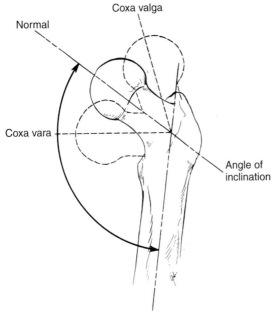

FIG. 19–4

Coxa vara and coxa valga. The neck-shaft angle is measured on an anteroposterior roentgenogram. This angle is formed by a line drawn through the femoral shaft center and one bisecting the head and neck. Normally, the value of this angle decreases with age. A reasonably accurate neck-shaft angle measurement may be made on an anteroposterior pelvic roentgenogram by placing the patient's hips in maximum internal rotation. Otherwise, because of the illusion caused by anteversion or external rotation on a one-plane roentgenogram, the measured neck-shaft angle value may be considerably larger than the true value. Internal femur rotation has a negligible effect on the neck-shaft angle. (From Chung SMK: *Hip disorders in infants and children*, Philadelphia, 1981, Lea & Febiger.)

birth, the hips usually are not dislocated but rather "dislocatable." Dislocations tend to occur after delivery. Because dislocations are not truly congenital in origin, the term developmental dysplasia of the hip (DDH) is more appropriate than congenital dysplasia or dislocation of the hip (CDH). DDH is classified into two major groups: *typical*, in a neurologically normal infant, and *teratologic*, when an underlying neuromuscular disorder (myelodysplasia or arthrogryposis multiplex congenita) or syndrome complex is present. The teratologic type of dislocation occurs in utero. Typical DDH is the most common form.

Etiology. The causes of DDH are multifactorial. *Physiologic* factors are a positive family history (in

20% of cases), generalized ligamentous laxity, maternal estrogen and other hormones associated with pelvic ligament relaxation, and female predominance (9:1). *Mechanical* factors are primigravida, breech presentation, oligohydramnios, and postnatal positioning. The positive family history and the generalized ligamentous laxity are related factors. Maternal estrogens and other hormones associated with pelvic relaxation also result in further, although temporary, relaxation of the newborn hip joint.

Approximately 60% of children with typical DDH are first-born, and 30–50% are in a breech position. In this presentation the fetal pelvis is positioned in the maternal pelvis, which results in extreme hip flexion and limitation of hip motion. Increased hip flexion results in stretching of the already lax capsule and ligamentum teres. It also produces posterior uncoverage of the femoral head. This position, as well as decreased hip motion, alters the normal trophic relationship of the hip, resulting in abnormal development of the cartilaginous acetabulum.

The sex ratio of infants with DDH who are breech is 2:1 female to male. This decline substantiates the importance of the mechanical factors of the breech position in the development of DDH. Congenital muscular torticollis (in 14–20% of cases) and metatarsus adductus (1–10%) are also associated with DDH. The presence of either of these two conditions necessitates a careful examination of the hips.

Postnatal factors also are important. Maintaining the hips in the position of adduction and extension is a major factor leading to dislocation. Placing the extremities in this position puts the unstable hip under pressure as a result of the normally present hip flexion and abduction contractures. As a consequence, the femoral head can be displaced from the acetabulum over several days, weeks, or perhaps months.

Clinical Manifestations. Particular test results and other physical findings are common in infants with DDH.

The *Barlow test* is the most important maneuver in examination of the newborn hip. This is a provocative test that attempts to dislocate an unstable hip. The examiner stabilizes the infant's pelvis with one hand and then flexes and adducts the opposite hip and applies a posterior force (Fig. 19–5). If the hip is dislocatable, this is usually readily felt. After release of the posterior pressure, the hip will usually relocate spontaneously. It has been estimated that 1:100 newborns has clinically unstable hips (subluxation or dislocation), but only 1:800–1000 infants develops a persistent dislocation.

The *Ortolani test* is a maneuver to reduce a recently dislocated hip. The result is most likely to be

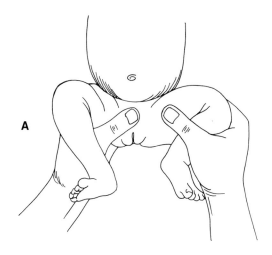

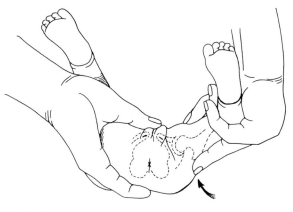

FIG. 19–6

Ortolani (reduction) test. With the infant relaxed and content on a firm surface, the hips and knees are flexed to 90 degrees. The hips are examined one at a time. The examiner grasps the infant's thigh with the middle finger over the greater trochanter, and lifts the thigh to bring the femoral head from its dislocated posterior position to opposite the acetabulum. Simultaneously, the thigh is gently abducted, reducing the femoral head into the acetabulum. In a positive finding, the examiner senses reduction by a palpable, nearly audible "clunk."

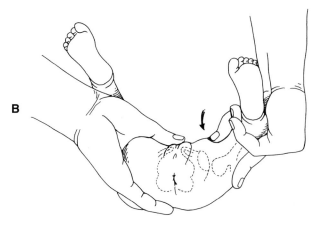

FIG. 19–5

Barlow (dislocation) test. Reverse of Ortolani test. If the femoral head is in the acetabulum at the time of examination, the Barlow test is performed to discover any hip instability. **A,** The infant's thigh is grasped as shown and adducted with gentle downward pressure. **B,** Dislocation is palpable as the femoral head slips out of the acetabulum. Diagnosis is confirmed with the Ortolani test.

positive in infants 1–2 months of age, because adequate time must have passed for the true dislocation to have occurred. In this test, the infant's thigh is flexed and abducted and the femoral head is lifted anteriorly toward the acetabulum (Fig. 19–6). If reduction is possible, the relocation will be felt as a "clunk," not as a "click." After 2 months of age, manual reduction of a dislocated hip is not usually possible because of the development of soft tissue contractures.

Limitation of hip abduction is indicative of soft tissue contractures and may indicate DDH (Fig. 19–7). Conversely, hip abduction contractures may indicate dysplasia of the contralateral hip.

An *asymmetric number of thigh skin folds* and apparent shortening of an extremity (uneven knee levels) when the supine infant's feet are placed together on the examining table with the hips and knees flexed (positive Galeazzi sign) is suggestive of DDH because these findings indicate proximal displacement of the femoral head. In older or walking children, complaints of limping, waddling (bilateral DDH), increased lumbar lordosis (swayback), toe-walking, and in-toeing may be associated with an unrecognized DDH.

A common concern regarding an unstable hip is the presence of a hip "click." This click is usually not pathologic and is secondary to breaking the surface tension across the hip joint, snapping of gluteal tendons, patellofemoral motion, or femorotibial (knee) rotation.

Roentgenographic Evaluation. Ultrasonography is used for initial evaluation and to follow the results of conservative treatment in newborns and infants (<3 months) with DDH. Hip stability and acetabular development can usually be assessed accurately. Unfortunately, this is expensive and requires considerable experience to perform accurately.

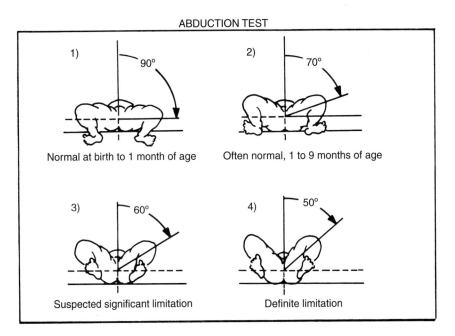

ABDUCTION TEST

1) 90°
Normal at birth to 1 month of age

2) 70°
Often normal, 1 to 9 months of age

3) 60°
Suspected significant limitation

4) 50°
Definite limitation

FIG. 19–7

Hip abduction test. Place the infant supine, flex the hips 90 degrees, and fully abduct. While the normal abduction range is quite broad, one can suspect hip disease in any patient who lacks more than 35–45 degrees of abduction. (From Chung SMK: *Hip disorders in infants and children,* Philadelphia, 1981, Lea & Febiger.)

Roentgenographic evaluation is useful in older infants (>3 months) and includes an anteroposterior (AP) and Lauenstein (frog) position lateral roentgenograms of the pelvis. The ossific nucleus does not appear until 4–6 months of age and may be further delayed in infants with DDH. Line measurements usually are made to determine the relationship of the femoral head to the acetabulum. Arthrography, computed tomography (CT), and MRI may be beneficial in select or difficult cases.

Treatment. The treatment of DDH is individualized and depends on the child's age at diagnosis. The goal is a concentric and stable reduction that results in normal growth and development of the hip.

When an unstable hip is recognized at birth, maintenance of the hip in the position of flexion and abduction ("human" position) for 1–2 months usually is sufficient. This position maintains reduction of the femoral head and allows for tightening of the ligamentous structures, as well as for stimulation of normal growth and development of the acetabulum. Usually, double or triple diapers are sufficient in neonates. Treatment usually is continued until clinical stability of the hip is seen and the radiographic or

ultrasonography measurements are within normal limits. Between 1 and 6 months of age, the Pavlik harness is indicated. It places the hips in the human position by flexing the hips more than 90 degrees (preferably 100–110 degrees) and providing gentle abduction. This redirects the femoral head toward the acetabulum. Usually, spontaneous relocation of the femoral head occurs within 3–4 weeks. The Pavlik harness is approximately 95% successful in dysplastic or subluxated hips and 80% in true dislocations.

If a reduction does not occur, a surgical closed reduction is attempted. This consists of preliminary skin traction for 1–3 weeks to stretch the soft tissue contractures, percutaneous adductor tenotomy, closed reduction, and application of a hip spica cast in the "human" position. In the older infant (6–18 months), surgical closed reduction is the major method of treatment. If the hip shows significant residual instability at the time of closed reduction, an open reduction may be indicated. Beyond 18 months of age, the dysplastic changes are so advanced that open reduction followed by pelvic or femoral osteotomy, or both, is usually necessary.

Complications. The most important and severe complication of DDH is iatrogenic avascular necrosis (osteonecrosis) of the capital femoral head (CFE). Reduction of the femoral head under pressure produces cartilaginous compression, which can lead to occlusion of the intraarticular, extraosseous epiphyseal vessels and produce partial or total CFE infarction. Revascularization follows, but abnormal growth and development may occur, especially if the physis is severely damaged. The hip is most vulnerable to this complication before the development of the ossific nucleus (4–6 months).

Redislocation and subluxation of the femoral head and residual acetabular dysplasia are other common complications.

Septic Arthritis and Osteomyelitis

See Chapter 10.

Transient Monoarticular Synovitis

Transient synovitis of the hip is a common cause of limping in young children and is characterized by acute onset of pain, limp, and mild restriction of hip motion, especially abduction and internal rotation. This is a diagnosis of exclusion because septic arthritis or osteomyelitis of the hip must be excluded.

Etiology. The etiology of transient synovitis remains uncertain. Possible causes have included active or recent viral infection and hypersensitivity. Approximately 70% of involved children have a nonspecific viral upper respiratory infection 7–14 days before the onset of hip symptoms.

Diagnosis. Biopsy specimens from the hip joints of patients with transient synovitis have demonstrated synovial hypertrophy secondary to nonspecific inflammatory reaction. Hip joint aspirations, if necessary, will be negative, although a small effusion is common. The differential diagnosis includes septic arthritis, juvenile rheumatoid arthritis, fractures, psoas abscess, leukemia and other malignancies, osteonecrosis, and other disorders that are listed in Tables 19–2 and 19–3.

Clinical Manifestations. The mean age of onset is 6 years; most patients are 3–8 years of age. The male-to-female ratio is 2:1. The acute onset of pain is felt in the groin, anterior thigh, or knee. It must be remembered that any child with nontraumatic anterior thigh or knee pain must be evaluated carefully for hip pathology because this is the site of referred pain. Patients usually are ambulatory, and the hip is not usually held in the flexed, abducted, and externally rotated position typical of bacterial infection unless a significant effusion is present. Children are usually afebrile, and the white blood cell count and erythrocyte sedimentation rate (ESR) are normal or slightly elevated. Patients at high risk for septic arthritis usually have temperature >38.5° C, an ESR >20, leukocytosis, severe pain, tenderness to palpation, spasm, and refusal to walk.

Roentgenographic Evaluation. AP and frog lateral roentgenograms of the pelvis are usually normal. Ultrasound examination of the hip may be useful in demonstrating the hip joint effusion. Aspiration of fluid may improve symptoms and improve local blood flow. Bone scans may help differentiate a septic process.

Treatment. Bed rest and non–weight bearing until the pain resolves, followed by limited activities (for 1–2 weeks) are the treatments of choice. This sometimes is difficult because children want to return to normal activities when their symptoms resolve. If the child returns to normal activities too early, exacerbation of symptoms can occur. Nonsteroidal antiinflammatory agents (NSAIDs) are helpful. Lack of improvement necessitates further evaluation for more serious disorders.

Legg-Calvé-Perthes Disease

Legg-Calvé-Perthes disease (LCPD) is idiopathic avascular necrosis (osteonecrosis) of the CFE and the associated complications in a growing child. This disorder is caused by an interruption of the CFE blood supply. It is more common in males (4–5:1) and is bilateral in approximately 20% of patients. Children with LCPD have delayed bone ages, disproportionate growth, and mild short stature.

Clinical Manifestations. The clinical onset occurs between the ages of 2 and 12 years, with a mean age of 7 years. Mild or intermittent pain in the anterior thigh and a limp may each be present. The classic presentation is a "painless" limp. The pertinent early physical findings include antalgic gait; muscle spasm and mild restriction of motion, especially abduction and internal rotation; proximal thigh atrophy; and mild shortness of stature.

Roentgenographic Evaluation. Roentgenographic assessment is necessary to determine the extent of CFE involvement, follow disease progression, assess sphericity of the femoral head, the possibility of CFE collapse and extrusion, and the response to treatment. AP and frog lateral pelvic roentgenograms usually are adequate, but occasionally additional procedures such as arthrography, bone scans, and MRI may be useful. Bone scans and MRI are helpful in recognizing early LCPD but are of limited value in assessing the extent of CFE involvement or following the disease progression.

Prognosis. The short-term prognosis concerns femoral head deformity at the completion of the healing stage. The long-term prognosis involves the potential for osteoarthritis of the hip in adulthood.

The prognostic factors for the development of late degenerative arthritis include femoral head deformity and age at clinical onset. Older children with significant residual femoral head deformity are at risk for development of degenerative arthritis. The incidence is essentially 100% in children who are 10 years of age or older at onset. This rate is in contrast to a negligible risk in children 5 years or younger and a 38% risk when onset occurs between 6 and 9 years of age. Additional prognostic features are femoral head containment, hip range of motion, and premature CFE closure.

Treatment. LCPD is a local, self-healing disorder. Prevention of femoral head deformity and secondary osteoarthritis is the only justification for treatment. There are four basic treatment goals:

- Elimination of hip irritability
- Restoration and maintenance of a good range of hip motion
- Prevention of CFE collapse, extrusion, or subluxation
- Attainment of a spherical femoral head at healing

Treatment uses the concept of containment; the femoral head is contained within the acetabulum so that the latter acts as a mold for the reossifying CFE. Containment is indicated for children 6 years of age (perhaps 5 years in females) or older in whom more than one half the CFE is involved. This is accomplished by nonsurgical containment using abduction casts and orthoses or by surgical containment with proximal femoral varus osteotomy, with or without derotation, and pelvic osteotomies to redirect the acetabulum and thereby contain the femoral head in the position of weight bearing. The long-term results of surgical containment treatment are 85–90% satisfactory (round or oval femoral head).

Slipped Capital Femoral Epiphysis

Slippage of the capital femoral epiphysis (SCFE) is the most common adolescent hip disorder.

Etiology. The etiology of SCFE is unknown. An endocrine basis has been suggested because SCFE frequently occurs in adolescents who either are obese and have delayed skeletal maturation or are tall and thin, following a recent growth spurt. In obese children a low level of sex hormones has been postulated; in tall, thin children an overabundance of growth hormone is implicated. It is known that both sex hormones and growth hormones alter the rate of proliferation of the cartilage cells in the physis and the rate of skeletal growth. SCFE also can occur as a complication of an underlying endocrine disorder, such as hypothyroidism, pituitary disorders, pseudohypoparathyroidism, and treatment with recombinant growth hormone. When a SCFE occurs before puberty, a hormonal abnormality or systemic disorder should be suspected. Nonetheless, the histopathology of SCFE indicates mechanical factors as the ultimate cause of slippage. Obesity produces high shear forces across the weakened and obliquely oriented growth plate.

Roentgenographic Evaluation. AP and frog lateral roentgenograms of the pelvis are used for assessment of the hips. The earliest sign of SCFE is widening of the physis without slippage. This is considered a preslip condition. As slippage occurs, the CFE stays in the acetabulum, and the femoral neck rotates anteriorly and occasionally superiorly, resulting in a varus, retroverted femoral head and neck (Fig. 19–8). The degree of slippage between the CFE and the femoral neck can be classified into mild (0–33%), moderate (34–50%), and severe (>50%) by roentgenographic measurements. Slippage resulting in a valgus deformity is rare except

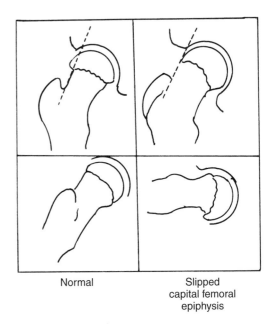

Normal

Slipped capital femoral epiphysis

FIG. 19–8

Klein's line extends along the lateral femur neck and normally passes through a small part of the lateral femoral head. In slipped capital femoral epiphysis (SCFE), the line will not pass through the head or may just touch its lateral margin. A frog-leg lateral, rather than an anteroposterior, projection gives the clearest view of SCFE. (From Chung SMK: *Hip disorders in infants and children*, Philadelphia, 1981, Lea & Febiger.)

in metabolic disorders, such as renal osteodystrophy and Marfan syndrome, and as a sequela to irradiation therapy.

Classification. SCFE is classified as stable or unstable depending on the continuity between the CFE and femoral neck.

Stable SCFE. Continuity and stability are seen between the CFE and femoral neck. The deformity occurs as a slow slippage through the physis. Initially the physis will be wide; this is a preslip condition. The patient may have mild discomfort, but the physical findings are usually normal. Preslips frequently are seen in the opposite hip of an adolescent with a previous SCFE. As slippage occurs, symptoms will increase. This now represents a chronic SCFE, the most common type. The patient usually has a history of symptoms lasting several months. However, because of continuity between the femoral neck and CFE, the symptoms are not severe and the child is able to walk, albeit with a mildly antalgic, externally rotated gait.

Unstable SCFE. In unstable SCFE, the continuity between the CFE and femoral neck is disrupted, producing instability and acute symptoms. Usually, antecedent symptoms are absent or mild, such as pain and limp for less than 3 weeks. Slippage occurs suddenly, with or without significant trauma; the pain is so severe that the child usually is unable to stand or bear weight.

An unstable SCFE can also occur on an existing chronic or stable SCFE. Affected adolescents have had previous symptoms (pain, limp, out-toed gait) for several months. Trauma, usually mild, is a potential underlying factor that results in the sudden slippage.

Clinical Manifestations. The physical findings in SCFE depend on the degree of slippage and stability of the CFE. In an unstable SCFE the physical examination is limited by pain with any attempted hip motion. In stable, chronic SCFE the patient has an antalgic gait, and the affected extremity is externally rotated. Hip range of motion will demonstrate a lack of internal rotation and increased external rotation. As the hip is flexed, it will become progressively externally rotated. Limitation of flexion and abduction also may be present as a result of a varus deformity of the proximal femur. Adolescents, especially those who are obese, with nontraumatic knee pain (referred pain) should be evaluated carefully for SCFE.

Treatment. The goals of treatment for SCFE are prevention of further slippage and minimization of complications. These are accomplished by epiphysiodesis of the CFE. The technique selected depends on CFE stability and the severity of the slippage. The current methods include in situ internal fixation with pins or screws (single or multiple); open bone graft epiphysiodesis; closed bone graft epiphysiodesis; osteotomies of the femoral neck or subtrochanteric regions to realign the proximal femur; and hip spica cast immobilization.

Complications. The two serious complications in SCFE are avascular necrosis and chondrolysis. Avascular necrosis occurs as a result of injury to the retinacular vessels. This can be caused by forced manipulation of an unstable slip, compression from intracapsular hematoma, or direct injury during surgery. Partial forms of avascular necrosis also may occur following internal fixation as a result of disruption of the intraepiphyseal blood vessels. Chondrolysis occurs when there is destruction of the articular cartilage of the hip joint. The etiologic mechanism of this complication is unclear but has been demonstrated to be associated with more severe slips, black race, pins or screws protruding out of the femoral head, and female gender.

REFERENCES

Beach R: Minimally invasive approach to management of irritable hip in children, *Lancet* 355(9211):1202–1203, 2000.

Behrman RE, Kliegman RM, Jenson HB, editors: *Nelson textbook of pediatrics,* ed 16, Philadelphia, 2000, WB Saunders, Chapter 684.

Committee on Quality Improvement, Subcommittee on Developmental Dysplasia of the Hip: Clinical practice guidelines: early detection of developmental dysplasia of the hip. American Academy of Pediatrics, *Pediatrics* 105(4 Pt 1):896–905, 2000.

Guille JT, Pizzutillo PD, MacEwen GD: Developmental dysplasia of the hip from birth to six months, *J Am Acad Orthop Surg* 8(4):232–242, 2000.

Kocher MS, Zurakowski D, Kasser JR: Differentiating between septic arthritis and transient synovitis of the hip in children: an evidence-based clinical prediction algorithm, *J Bone Joint Surg Am* 81(12):1662–1670, 1999.

Reynolds RA: Diagnosis and treatment of slipped capital femoral epiphysis, *Curr Opin Pediatr* 11(1):80–83, 1999.

Roy DR: Current concepts in Legg-Calvé-Perthes disease, *Pediatr Ann* 28(12):748–752, 1999.

THE LOWER EXTREMITIES

Torsional (in-toeing and out-toeing) and angular (physiologic bowlegs and knock-knees) variations of the lower extremities are common reasons parents seek medical attention for a child. Most of these complaints do not necessitate active treatment because they are physiologic and will resolve with normal growth. It is important to understand the natural history to reassure a concerned family.

Angular Variations

Reasons for angular deformities can be either physiologic (variations) or pathologic (deformities). Physiologic torsional and angular variations, fortunately,

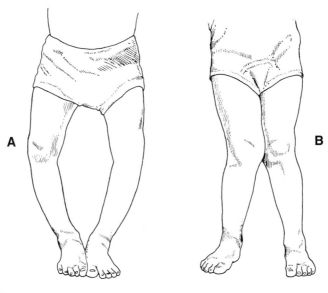

FIG. 19–9

A, Bowleg deformity. Bowlegs are referred to as varus angulation (genu varum) because the knees are tilted away from the midline of the body. **B,** Knock-knee or valgus deformity of the knees. The knee is tilted toward the midline. (From Scoles P: *Pediatric orthopedics in clinical practice,* ed 2, Chicago, 1988, Year Book Medical Publishers.)

are the most common. These occur predominantly in the tibia. The femur is less commonly involved.

Physiologic Bowlegs (Genu Varum)

The lower extremities of newborns and infants (younger than 1 year of age) commonly have mild to moderate bowing and internal rotation (Fig. 19–9). This is caused by in utero positioning, in which the hips are flexed, abducted, and externally rotated; the knees flexed and lower legs internally rotated; and the feet in slight equinus, supination, and contact with the posterolateral aspect of the opposite thigh. This position produces hip flexion, abduction, and external rotation contractures; knee flexion contractures and internal tibial torsion; and mild supination of the feet. The bowed appearance is actually a torsional combination from the external rotation of the hip (tight posterior capsule) and the internal tibial torsion. With the onset of standing and independent walking, the bowing spontaneously corrects over a period of 6–12 months. Significant improvement does not occur during the first year of life. The typical infant has 15 degrees of genu varum or bowleg configuration. This decreases to approximately 10 degrees by 1 year of age. By 2 years of age, the majority of children have straight or neutrally aligned lower extremities. *Treatment* may be indicated for children 2–3 years or older

in whom there has been no documented improvement with growth, but this is rarely necessary.

Physiologic Knock-Knees (Genu Valgum)

As the spontaneous correction of physiologic bowlegs continues, there is typically an overcorrection, of variable degree, into mild genu valgum or knock-knee (Fig. 19–9). This physiologic angular variation commonly is seen between 3 and 4 years of age but resolves spontaneously between 5 and 8 years. As with physiologic bowlegs, *treatment* rarely is indicated.

Torsional Variations

The common causes of in-toeing and out-toeing are delineated in Table 19–5.

In-Toeing

Internal Femoral Torsion or Anteversion. Internal femoral torsion or anteversion is the most common cause of in-toeing in children 2 years of age or older. It occurs more commonly in females than males (2:1). Most children with this condition have generalized ligamentous laxity. The *etiology* of femoral torsion is controversial; it may be congenital (persistent infantile femoral anteversion) or acquired secondary to abnormal sitting habits.

| **TABLE 19–5** |
| **Common Causes of In-Toeing and Out-Toeing** |

In-Toeing
Internal femoral torsion or anteversion
Internal tibial torsion
Metatarsus adductus
Talipes equinovarus (clubfoot)

Out-Toeing
External femoral torsion
External tibial torsion
Calcaneovalgus feet
Hypermobile pes planus (flatfoot)

Clinical Manifestations. The primary clinical feature of internal femoral torsion is an in-toed gait. While watching the undressed child walk, the examiner notes the entire lower leg to be internally rotated. The hip has 80–90 degrees of internal rotation in the extended position; as a result, external rotation is limited to 0–10 degrees. Generalized ligamentous laxity, resulting in elbow and finger hyperextension, knee recurvatum, and hypermobile flatfeet (pes planus), is present. These children sit almost exclusively in the "television" or "W" position. This position may allow the lower leg to act as a lever, thereby producing the torsional change in the "biologically plastic" femur. Although this condition is also called *femoral anteversion,* which implies an abnormality of the proximal femur, it is actually a torsional abnormality throughout the femoral shaft that results in a change in the normal alignment between the hip and knee.

Roentgenographic Evaluation. Roentgenographic evaluation for internal femoral torsion is not routinely necessary. Clinical measurements usually are quite accurate. CT of the hip and knee can be used to precisely measure the degree of torsion roentgenographically, but is usually not necessary.

Treatment. Management consists primarily of observation. It was incorrectly believed that internal femoral torsion was associated with bunions, back pain, degenerative osteoarthritis of the hip and knee, and difficulty with athletic ability. Correction of abnormal sitting habits usually allows this torsional variation to resolve with normal growth and development. However, it can take 1–3 years for complete correction to occur. Children over 10 years of age and young adolescents may not have enough remaining musculoskeletal growth for spontaneous correction to occur. After these children have been followed up for 1–2 years without improvement and

if there is significant cosmetic or functional disability, surgical correction may be beneficial.

Internal Tibial Torsion. Internal or medial tibial torsion is the most common cause of in-toeing in children younger than 2 years of age and is the result of normal in utero positioning. This condition may be associated with metatarsus adductus. It also is the major component of physiologic bowlegs.

Clinical Manifestations. The degree of tibial torsion can be measured by the supine or prone thigh-foot angle. In both tests, the child's knee is flexed to 90 degrees to neutralize the normal tibiofemoral rotation, and the foot is placed in a neutral or simulated weight-bearing position. The long axis of the foot is compared to the long axis of the thigh (prone test) or tibia (supine test). An inwardly rotated foot is assigned a negative value and represents internal tibial torsion. The measurements must be recorded on each visit to document improvement. Roentgenographic measurements usually are of no value in assessment of internal tibial torsion.

Treatment. Internal tibial torsion is a physiologic condition, and spontaneous resolution with normal growth and development can be anticipated. If there has been no documented improvement by 2 years of age, a nighttime orthosis such as a Denis Browne splint may be considered. There are no prospective studies documenting the efficacy of an orthosis. Rarely, persistent internal tibial torsion in an older child or adolescent may necessitate surgical derotation.

Out-Toeing

External tibial torsion is common and usually associated with a calcaneovalgus foot (discussed later in this chapter under The Foot). Both are the result of a variation in normal in utero position. When these two conditions are combined with the normally externally rotated hip (tight posterior hip capsule), a very externally rotated or out-toed appearance is the result. Fortunately, external tibial torsion is physiologic and undergoes spontaneous resolution with normal growth similar to internal tibial torsion.

Pathologic Genu Varum
Tibia Vara (Blount Disease)

Idiopathic tibia vara, or Blount disease, is the most common pathologic disorder producing a progressive genu varum deformity. It is characterized by abnormal growth of the medial aspect of the proximal tibial epiphysis, resulting in a progressive varus angulation below the knee. Tibia vara can occur at any age in a growing child. It is classified according to the age at clinical onset: infantile (1–3 years), juvenile (4–10 years), and adolescent (11 years or older). The infantile group is the most common; the juvenile and adolescent forms are typically combined as late-onset tibia vara, which occurs much less frequently.

Etiology. Although the exact cause of tibia vara remains unknown, it appears to be secondary to growth suppression from increased compressive forces across the medial aspect of the knee.

Clinical Manifestations. The characteristics of infantile tibia vara include predominance of black race, female gender, marked obesity, approximately 80% bilateral involvement, a prominent medial metaphyseal beak, internal tibial torsion, and lower extremity length inequality. Characteristics of the juvenile and adolescent (late-onset) form are black race, predominance of males, marked obesity, approximately 50% bilateral involvement, slow, progressive genu varum deformity, pain rather than deformity as the primary initial complaint, no palpable proximal medial metaphyseal beak, minimal internal tibial torsion, mild medial collateral ligament laxity, and mild lower extremity length inequality.

The differences between the three tibia vara groups appear to be related primarily to the age at clinical onset, the amount of remaining growth, and the magnitude of the medial compression forces on the involved side. Thus the infantile-onset group has the potential for the greatest deformity and the adolescent-onset group has the least.

Roentgenographic Evaluation. Standing AP and lateral roentgenograms of the lower extremities are necessary to assess pathologic genu varum deformities. Roentgenographically, fragmentation with a protuberant step deformity and beaking of the proximal medial tibial metaphysis are considered the major features of infantile tibia vara. The changes of the proximal medial tibia are less conspicuous in the late-onset forms and are characterized by wedging of the medial portion of the epiphysis, a mild posteromedial articular depression, a serpiginous cephalad curved physis of variable width, and mild or no fragmentation or beaking of the proximal medial metaphysis.

The major deformity that must be differentiated from infantile tibia vara is the physiologic genu varum deformity. It is difficult to differentiate roentgenographically between these two disorders in children younger than 2 years of age.

Treatment. Once the roentgenographic findings confirm the diagnosis, treatment should begin immediately. Orthotic management may be considered for children 3 years of age or younger with a mild deformity. Approximately 50% of children with this criterion may achieve adequate correction using orthoses. Conservative management in the late-onset forms of tibia vara is contraindicated. The children are too large, compliance is poor, and the remaining growth too small to allow for adequate correction.

The indications for surgical treatment in infantile tibia vara include 4 years of age or older, failure of orthotic management, and moderate to severe deformity. Proximal tibial valgus osteotomy with associated fibular diaphyseal osteotomy is the procedure of choice.

Lower Extremity Length Discrepancies

Length discrepancies in the femur, tibia, or both are common problems. The *differential diagnosis* is extensive; some of the common causes are in Table 19–6.

Normal Growth and Development

Approximately 65% of the growth of the entire lower extremity comes from the distal femoral (38%) and proximal tibial (27%) physeal plates. Thus growth disturbances about the knee can have the most adverse effect on lower extremity length, depending on the amount of remaining growth.

Methods of Limb Length Measurement

Clinical Measurements. Clinical measurements are less accurate than the roentgenographic tech-

---

TABLE 19–6
Common Causes of Lower Extremity Length Inequality

Congenital
Proximal femoral focal deficiency
Coxa vara
Hemiatrophy and hemihypertrophy (anisomelia)

Developmental
Developmental dislocation of the hip (DDH)
Legg-Calvé-Perthes disease (LCPD)

Neuromuscular
Polio
Cerebral palsy (hemiplegia)

Infectious
Pyogenic osteomyelitis with physeal damage

Trauma
Physeal injury with premature closure
Overgrowth
Malunion (shortening)

Tumor
Physeal destruction
Radiation-induced physeal injury
Overgrowth

niques. A common clinical measurement is from the anterior superior iliac spine to the medial malleolus. This minimizes measurement error secondary to pelvic obliquity. The most accurate clinical method for measuring limb length involves leveling the pelvis. Blocks of various thickness may be placed beneath the foot on the involved side until the iliac crests are level. The height of the blocks indicates the amount of discrepancy.

Roentgenographic Measurements. Roentgenographic evaluations are the most accurate method of assessment of leg length. The *teleoroentgenogram* is a single exposure of both lower extremities. Its primary indication is for young children, usually under 5 years of age. A small amount of magnification error is present, but this type of measurement has the advantage of showing angular deformities.

The *orthoroentgenogram* consists of three separate, slightly overlapping exposures of the hips, knees, and ankles on a long cassette. Bone length is measured directly on the roentgenogram. Less magnification is present, and angular deformities are demonstrated. It has the disadvantage of being bulky and difficult to handle.

The *scanogram* is the most accurate method and consists of three narrow exposures of the hips, knees, and ankles on a standard cassette with a roentgenographic ruler next to the extremity. Minimal magnification is present, and accurate measurements can be made. However, angular deformities cannot be visualized fully, which may lead to errors in interpretation. Currently, *CT scanogram* techniques are being used with the best accuracy.

The measured discrepancy is followed with the Moseley and Green-Anderson graphs. An AP roentgenogram of the left hand and wrist for bone age determination is necessary to assess maturation.

Treatment. Issues in management include etiology of the discrepancy, skeletal age, ultimate discrepancy, anticipated adult height, neuromuscular status of the extremities, joint involvement, and psychologic aspects of the child and parents. Discrepancies of greater than 2 cm at maturity usually necessitate treatment. Equalization can be achieved by nonsurgical and surgical methods. The nonsurgical methods include orthotic and prosthetic devices; surgical methods include shortening of the longer extremity, lengthening of the shorter extremity, or a combination of both. Discrepancies of 2–5 cm are treated by epiphysiodesis (surgical physeal closure) of the affected side and discrepancies greater than 5 cm by lengthening.

REFERENCES

Behrman RE, Kliegman RM, Jenson HB, editors: *Nelson textbook of pediatrics,* ed 16, Philadelphia, 2000, WB Saunders, Chapters 681, 682.

Heath CH, Staheli LT: Normal limits of knee angles in white children: genu varum and genu valgum, *J Pediatr Orthop* 13(12): 259–262, 1993.

Staheli LT: Instructional Course Lecture: rotational problems in children, *J Bone Joint Surg* 75A:939, 1993.

Thompson GH: Angular deformities of the lower extremities in children. In Chapman MN, editor: *Operative orthopaedics,* ed 2, Philadelphia, 1993, JB Lippincott.

Yun AG, Severino R, Reinker K: Attempted limb lengthenings beyond twenty percent of the initial bone length: results and complications, *J Pediatr Orthop* 20(2):151–159, 2000.

THE KNEE

The knee joint is unique because the movement of the tibiofemoral articulation is constrained only by soft tissues rather than by the usual geometric fit between the ends of articulating bone (Fig. 19–10). Paramount among these constraints are the medial and lateral collateral ligaments, the anterior and posterior cruciate ligaments, and the medial and lateral menisci. Weight is transmitted by load path that includes both the points of articular cartilage and the menisci. A second clinically important area, the patellofemoral joint, is part of the knee and a common site of problems, especially in adolescents.

Accumulation of fluid *(effusion)* in the knee is common during childhood and adolescence. When fluid accumulates rapidly after an injury, blood is usually in the joint *(hemarthrosis);* this may indicate an occult fracture or an injury to one of the ligaments or menisci. If there has been repeated trauma, an accumulation of synovial fluid may indicate a chronic

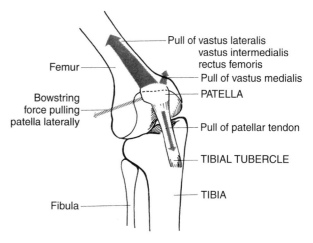

FIG. 19–10

Diagram of the knee extensor mechanism. The major force exerted by the quadriceps muscle tends to pull the patella laterally out of the intercondylar sulcus. The vastus medialis muscle pulls medially to keep the patella centralized. (From Smith JB: *Pediatr Clin North Am* 33:1443, 1986.)

internal derangement, usually a tear of a meniscus. Unexplained accumulation of fluid may occur with arthritis (septic, viral, postinfectious, Lyme, juvenile rheumatoid arthritis, or systemic lupus erythematosus), in association with ligamentous laxity (hypermobile joint syndrome), and with overactivity. In addition to the evaluation of other systemic manifestations and the clinical history (e.g., fever, hemophilia, rash, or trauma), an analysis of an aspiration of fluid from the joint generally is indicated and expedites precise diagnosis (see Chapter 10).

Discoid Lateral Meniscus

Each meniscus is semilunar in shape, but occasionally the lateral meniscus persists as a solid disc, an entity referred to as *discoid lateral meniscus*. A normal meniscus is attached about its periphery and glides anteriorly and posteriorly with knee motion, but a discoid meniscus is less mobile and may become torn. Occasionally there is no peripheral attachment about its posterolateral aspect. During knee flexion, the entire discoid meniscus may suddenly displace anteriorly to produce a loud audible "click" or "clunk." Most commonly, the patient comes to clinical attention during late childhood and early adolescence (11–15 years of age). AP roentgenograms may show widening of the lateral aspect of the knee joint. Arthroscopy, arthrography, and MRI are diagnostic.

Treatment in most cases involves excision of tears and reshaping of the meniscus arthroscopically. Peripheral reattachment is performed when possible.

Popliteal Cyst

A popliteal cyst ("Baker cyst") is commonly seen during the middle childhood years (Fig. 19–11). The cause is distention of the gastrocnemius and semimembranosus bursa along the posteromedial aspect of the knee by synovial fluid from the tendon sheaths. In childhood the cysts usually are benign and resolve with time, even though several years may be required. Knee roentgenograms are normal; the *diagnosis* is confirmed by ultrasound or aspiration. *Treatment* should be directed at reassurance because surgery is rarely indicated.

Osteochondritis Dissecans

Osteochondritis dissecans commonly involves the knee and occurs when an area of bone adjacent to the articular cartilage becomes avascular and separates from the underlying bone. In the older child or young adolescent this condition usually affects the lateral portion of the medial femoral condyle. AP,

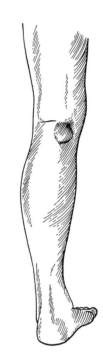

FIG. 19–11

Diagram of popliteal cyst location: posterior and medial aspect of knee, usually inferior to knee crease. (From Ferguson A: *Orthopedic surgery in infancy and childhood*, ed 5, Baltimore, 1981, Williams & Wilkins.)

lateral, and "tunnel" roentgenograms of the knee are diagnostic and are used to follow the course of the disease. In the young patient the overlying articular cartilage usually remains intact, and the area of avascular necrosis revascularizes and heals spontaneously. With increasing age, the risk increases for fracture of the articular cartilage and separation of the bony fragment. MRI is helpful in determining the integrity of the articular cartilage. In the young adolescent, the physician must decide whether to follow the lesion expectantly or to attempt to stimulate healing surgically. Once cartilage fracture takes place, surgical treatment is necessary; this may consist of arthroscopic excision, drilling of the lesion to promote revascularization and healing, and possible internal fixation.

Osgood-Schlatter Disease

The portion of the patellar ligament inserted into the tibial tubercle, an extension of the proximal tibial epiphysis, is vulnerable to microfracture during late childhood and early adolescence. This condition, Osgood-Schlatter disease, is more common in males.

The natural history is usually benign, with activity-related pain persisting for 12–24 months. Physical examination demonstrates swelling and prominence of the tibia tubercle and exquisite local tenderness. Roentgenograms are necessary to rule out other lesions. Frequently, bony enlargement of the tibial tubercle will be a consequence of the healing response. Rest, restriction of activities, and occasionally a knee immobilizer may be necessary, combined with an isometric exercise program. Antiinflammatory medications may also be beneficial.

Patellofemoral Disorders

The patellofemoral joint depends on a subtle balance among restraining ligaments, muscle forces, alignment, and articular anatomy for normal function (Fig. 19–10). On its deep surface, the patella has a V-bottom shape; it moves through a matching groove in the distal femur called the *trochlea.* The force of the muscle pulling through the quadriceps tendon and the patellar ligament does not act in a straight line because the patellar ligament inclines in a slightly lateral direction with respect to the line of the quadriceps tendon. This lateral movement, coupled with the movement of the restraining ligaments, tends to move the patella in a lateral direction. The vastus medialis muscle functions to counteract the laterally acting forces. An abnormality of any one or a group of these factors makes the patellofemoral joint function abnormally; the usual clinical manifestation is knee pain.

Idiopathic anterior knee pain is common in adolescents. This condition was once called **chondromalacia patellae,** but this term was incorrect because the joint surfaces of the patella are normal. Abnormal mechanics and variables associated with puberty are possible etiologic factors. The condition is easily assessed by directly palpating the extended knee and also by compressing the patellofemoral joint. To elicit the latter sign, the physician merely exerts manual pressure over the patella with the knee extended. Crepitus may be elicited. Roentgenograms are rarely helpful. Running and climbing stairs elicit pain when the knee is flexed. The pain usually is perceived maximally as the knee comes to within 15–20 degrees of full extension. Although it may be reasonable to treat recent or mild cases empirically with antiinflammatory medication and an exercise program aimed at developing strength and bulk in the vastus medialis muscle, persistent or refractory cases should be referred to an orthopaedist. Patellofemoral pain is particularly prevalent among young athletes (participating in running, basketball, and soccer) and in adolescent women.

Recurrent *patellar subluxation* and *dislocation* resulting from similar muscle imbalance also can occur in late childhood and early adolescence. Several other predisposing factors are known, including generalized ligamentous laxity, internal femoral torsion, genu valgum, and lateral femoral condyle hypoplasia. Acute traumatic dislocations can occur in a normal knee.

Initial *treatment* is nonoperative, with a vigorous physical therapy program to strengthen predominantly the quadriceps muscles. If this fails, surgical correction is necessary.

REFERENCES

Behrman RE, Kliegman RM, Jenson HB, editors: *Nelson textbook of pediatrics,* ed 16, Philadelphia, 2000, WB Saunders, Chapter 683.

Davids JR: Pediatric knee: clinical assessment and common disorders, *Pediatr Clin North Am* 43(5):1067–1090, 1996.

Roach JW: Knee disorders and injuries in adolescents, *Adolesc Med* 9(3):589–597, 1998.

Sales deGauzy J, Mansat C, Darodes PH, et al: Natural course of osteochondritis dissecans in children, *J Pediatr Orthop B* 8(1):26–28, 1999.

Stanitski CL: Instructional course lecture: anterior knee pain syndromes in the adolescent, *J Bone Joint Surg* 75A:1407, 1993.

VanRhijn LW, Jansen EJ, Prujis HE: Long-term follow-up of conservatively treated popliteal cysts in children, *J Pediatr Orthop B* 9(1):62–64, 2000.

THE FOOT

In the newborn and nonambulatory infant, the difference between posturing and deformity must be remembered. Posturing is the habitual position in which the infant holds the foot; passive range of motion is normal. Deformity produces an appearance similar to posturing, but the motion is restricted. Most pediatric foot disorders are painless. However, foot pain does occur, especially in older children. The *differential diagnosis* of foot pain in children is presented in Table 19–7.

Metatarsus Adductus

Congenital metatarsus adductus is a common problem of infants and young children. It also is known as *metatarsus varus* if the forefoot is both supinated and adducted. The condition occurs equally in males and females and is bilateral in 50% of patients. Metatarsus adductus has hereditary tendencies and is more common in firstborn than in later children because of the molding effect from the smaller primigravida uterus and abdominal wall. Approximately 10% of children with metatarsus adductus have DDH; careful examination of the hips is necessary.

Clinical Manifestations. The forefoot is adducted and occasionally supinated. The hindfoot and midfoot are normal. The lateral border of the foot is convex and the base of the fifth metatarsal appears prominent.

TABLE 19–7
Differential Diagnosis of Foot Pain by Age

0–6 Years of Age	6–12 Years of Age	12–20 Years of Age
Poor-fitting shoes	Poor-fitting shoes	Poor-fitting shoes
Foreign body	Sever disease	Stress fracture
Fracture	JRA	Foreign body
Osteomyelitis	Foreign body	Ingrown toenail
Juvenile rheumatoid arthritis (JRA)	Accessory tarsal navicular	Metatarsalgia
Leukemia	Tarsal coalition	Plantar fasciitis
Puncture wound	Ewing sarcoma	Osteochondritis dissecans
Dactylitis	Hypermobile flatfoot	Avascular necrosis of metatarsal (Freiberg infarction) or navicular bone (Köhler disease)
	Trauma (fractures; sprains)	Sever disease
	Puncture wound	Achilles tendinitis
		Trauma (fractures; sprains)
		Plantar warts
		Tarsal coalition
		Accessory ossicles (navicular, os trigonum)

The medial border of the foot is concave. The interval between the first and second toes is usually increased, with the great toe being held in a greater varus position. Ankle dorsiflexion and plantar flexion are normal. Forefoot flexibility can vary from flexible to rigid. To perform an assessment, the examiner stabilizes the hindfoot and midfoot in a neutral position and applies pressure over the first metatarsal head. In the walking child with an uncorrected metatarsus adductus deformity, an in-toed gait is noted. Abnormal shoe wear is also commonly seen.

Roentgenographic Evaluation. Routine roentgenograms of the foot usually are not necessary for metatarsus adductus, because they will not demonstrate mobility. AP weight-bearing roentgenograms demonstrate adduction of the metatarsals at the tarsometatarsal articulation and an increased intermetatarsal angle between the first and second metatarsals.

Treatment. The feet may be classified into three groups, depending on forefoot flexibility.

Type I deformities concern flexible feet that can actively and passively achieve the overcorrected (abducted) position. Voluntary correction can be elicited by stroking the lateral border of the foot to stimulate the peroneal musculature. Usually, no treatment is needed.

Type II deformities concern feet that can be corrected to the neutral position, both passively and actively. These feet may benefit from a trial of corrective shoes, such as straight- or reversed-last shoes. These shoes are worn full time (22 hr/day), and the child is reevaluated in 4–6 weeks. If the condition has improved, treatment can be continued. If no improvement occurs, serial plaster casts are necessary.

Type III deformities are rigid and cannot be corrected. These feet are treated with serial casts that are changed at intervals of 1–2 weeks. Usually, complete correction can be obtained in 4–6 weeks, depending on the child's age and the severity of deformity. The best results are obtained when casting is initiated before the child is 8 months of age.

For metatarsus adductus deformities persisting or presenting after 4 years of age, surgical intervention is usually required. Children 4–6 years of age with a fixed deformity usually are considered for soft tissue release. Older children usually do not benefit from the soft tissue release and require metatarsal osteotomies.

Calcaneovalgus Feet

The calcaneovalgus foot is a relatively common finding in the newborn and appears to be secondary to in utero positioning. This condition is manifested by a hyperdorsiflexed foot with forefoot abduction and heel valgus and usually is associated with external tibial torsion. These variations usually are unilateral but may be bilateral. In utero the plantar surface of the foot was against the wall of the uterus, forcing it into a hyperdorsiflexed, abducted, and externally rotated position. When calcaneovalgus feet and external tibial torsion are combined with the normal newborn external rotation of the hip (tight posterior capsule), an excessively externally rotated lower extremity is the result.

Clinical Manifestations. The infant typically has an externally rotated extremity. The dorsum of the foot can be brought into contact with the anterior aspect of the tibia, and the forefoot will have an abducted appearance.

The most common condition that must be distinguished from the calcaneovalgus foot is a congenital vertical talus. The differentiation usually can be made clinically because a vertical talus is a rigid deformity.

Roentgenographic Evaluation. Simulated weight-bearing AP and lateral roentgenograms of the feet may be necessary to differentiate between the calcaneovalgus foot and a congenital vertical talus. In a calcaneovalgus foot the roentgenograms either are normal or show a slight increase in hindfoot valgus. In congenital vertical talus, the hindfoot is in equinus and the midfoot dorsally displaced (**rocker-bottom deformity**).

Treatment. The typical calcaneovalgus foot requires no treatment. The hyperdorsiflexion of the foot resolves during the first 3–6 months of life. The external tibial torsion, however, persists and follows the same natural history as internal tibial torsion. Spontaneous improvement does not occur until the child begins to pull to stand and walk independently. Most involved infants will have normally aligned feet and lower extremities by 2 years of age.

Talipes Equinovarus (Clubfoot)

A clubfoot is a deformity of not only the foot but also the entire lower leg. Clubfoot can be congenital, teratologic, or positional. The congenital clubfoot is usually an isolated abnormality, whereas the teratologic form is associated with a neuromuscular disorder such as spina bifida, arthrogryposis multiplex congenita, or a syndrome complex. Positional clubfoot is a normal foot that has been held in a deformed position in utero.

Etiology. The cause of a congenital clubfoot is unknown. Inheritance may be multifactorial, with a major influence possibly from a single autosomal dominant gene. Biopsy studies of the extrinsic muscles of the calf have suggested a nonprogressive neuromuscular etiology.

Clinical Manifestations. The congenital clubfoot, which constitutes 75% of cases, is characterized by the absence of other congenital abnormalities, variable rigidity of the foot, mild calf atrophy, and mild hypoplasia of the tibia, fibula, and bones of the foot. It occurs more commonly in males (2:1) and is bilateral in 50% of cases. The probability of random occurrence is approximately 0.1%, but within involved families the probability is approximately 3% for subsequent siblings and 20–30% for offspring of involved parents.

Examination of the infant clubfoot demonstrates hindfoot equinus, hindfoot varus, forefoot adduction, and variable rigidity. All are secondary to the medial dislocation of the talonavicular joint. In the older child the calf and foot atrophy is more obvious than in the infant, regardless of how well corrected or functional the foot. These findings are the result of the neuromuscular etiology of clubfoot.

Roentgenographic Evaluation. AP and lateral standing or simulated weight-bearing and a maximum dorsiflexion lateral roentgenograms are used in the assessment of clubfoot (Fig. 19–12). Useful measurements in assessing clubfoot are the AP talocalcaneal angle, the lateral talocalcaneal angle, and the talocalcaneal overlap. The navicular, which is the primary site of deformity, does not ossify until 3 years of age in the female and 4 years of age in the male. Thus line measurements are necessary to determine the position of the unossified navicular.

Treatment

Conservative Management. Conservative methods of treatment are taping and the use of malleable splints and serial plaster casts. Taping and malleable splints are particularly useful in premature infants until they attain an appropriate size for casting. Serial plaster casts are the major method of treatment. Failure to achieve clinical and roentgenographic correction by 3 months of age is an indication for surgical treatment. Further attempts at conservative management may lead to articular damage and a midfoot breech (rocker-bottom deformity).

Surgical Management. The most common method of initial surgical treatment is a complete soft tissue release that simultaneously corrects all components of the clubfoot deformity. Satisfactory long-term results can be expected in 75–90% of these cases. Unsatisfactory results require additional treatment and usually are secondary to extrinsic muscle imbalance (neuromuscular etiology) rather than incomplete correction.

Hypermobile Pes Planus (Flexible Flatfeet)

Hypermobile or pronated feet are common sources of parental concern. The affected child is usually asymptomatic and has no limitations of activities. Flexible flatfeet are common in neonates and toddlers as a result of associated ligamentous laxity and fat in the area of the medial longitudinal arch; significant improvement is noted by 6 years of age. In the older child flexible flatfeet usually are secondary to generalized ligamentous laxity.

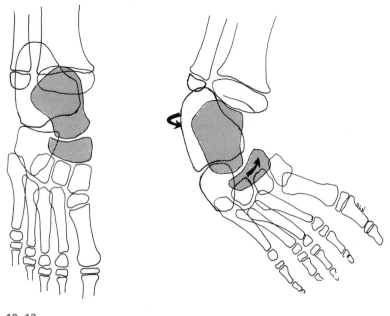

FIG. 19–12

Diagram of anteroposterior roentgenogram of a normal foot and talipes equinovarus. (From Tachdjian MO: *Pediatric orthopedics*, Philadelphia, 1972, WB Saunders.)

Clinical Manifestations. In the non–weight-bearing position in the older child with a flexible flatfoot, the normal medial longitudinal arch is present; in the weight-bearing position the foot becomes pronated, with varying degrees of pes planus and heel valgus. Subtalar motion is normal or slightly increased. Loss of subtalar motion may indicate a rigid flatfoot. Common causes of **rigid flatfeet** include a tight Achilles tendon (heel cord), tarsal coalitions, and neuromuscular abnormalities (e.g., with cerebral palsy). Rigid flatfeet also may be a familial trait.

Roentgenographic Evaluation. Roentgenograms of asymptomatic flexible flatfeet usually are not indicated.

Treatment. The treatment of flexible flatfeet is conservative; the diagnosis is not possible until after 6 years of age. Treatment is indicated only for persistent symptoms not attributable to other causes or abnormal shoe wear. Feet that are symptomatic with vigorous physical activities usually respond readily to the use of a commercially available medial longitudinal arch support.

Peroneal Spastic Flatfoot (Tarsal Coalition)

Peroneal spastic flatfoot is a common disorder. It is characterized by a painful, rigid valgus deformity of the midfoot and hindfoot (flatfoot) and peroneal (lateral calf) muscle spasm, without true spasticity. Peroneal spastic flatfoot usually is synonymous with tarsal coalition, a congenital fusion or (more likely) failure of segmentation between two or more tarsal bones. However, any condition that alters the normal gliding and rotary motion of the subtalar joint may produce the appearance of a peroneal spastic flatfoot. Thus congenital malformations, arthritis or inflammatory disorders, infection, neoplasms, and trauma are potential, although uncommon, causes.

The most common tarsal coalitions occur at the middle talocalcaneal (subtalar) facet and between the calcaneus and navicular bones (calcaneonavicular coalition). Coalitions can be fibrous, cartilaginous, or osseous. Tarsal coalitions are bilateral in approximately 50% of affected children.

Clinical Manifestations. The onset of symptoms usually occurs during the second decade of life. Although mild limitation of subtalar motion and a valgus deformity are present beginning in early childhood, the onset of symptoms varies with the age at which the fibrous or cartilaginous bar begins to ossify and further decrease motion. The talonavicular coalitions ossify between 3 and 5 years; the calcaneonavicular coalitions, between 8 and 12 years; and the medial facet talocalcaneal coalitions, between 12 and 16 years of age. The pain typically is felt laterally in the hindfoot and radiates proximally along the lateral malleolus and distal fibula (peroneal muscle spasm). Symp-

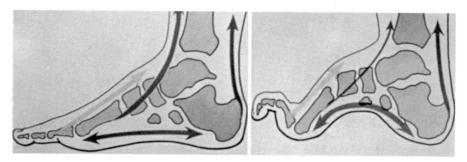

FIG. 19–13

The normal muscular balance of the foot is demonstrated on the left. A right triangle of muscle forces is generated by the gastrocnemius-soleus muscle group posteriorly, the plantar muscles inferiorly, and the tibialis anterior muscle. Weakness, as demonstrated in the diagram on the right, causes imbalance in the foot with resultant pes cavus. (Redrawn from Chuinard E, Baskin M: *J Bone Joint Surg* 55A:351, 1973.)

toms frequently are aggravated by sports or by walking on uneven ground. The foot is pronated in both the weight-bearing and the non–weight-bearing positions. Subtalar or midtarsal joint motion is diminished or absent, and attempts at motion produce pain. Frequent ankle "sprains" may occur.

Roentgenographic Evaluation. The diagnosis of tarsal coalition is confirmed roentgenographically by AP, lateral weight-bearing, and oblique roentgenograms of the foot. Beaking of the anterior aspect of the talus on the lateral view suggests a tarsal coalition. Axial views through the posterior and middle talocalcaneal joints can be useful in the diagnosis of the middle facet talocalcaneal coalition. CT is the procedure of choice in the evaluation of tarsal coalitions, especially those involving the middle facet.

Treatment. The treatment of symptomatic tarsal coalition varies according to the type of coalition, the age of the patient, the extent of the coalition, the presence or absence of degenerative osteoarthritis, and the degree of disability. Nonoperative treatment consists of cast immobilization, shoe inserts, or orthotics. When this fails, excision of the coalition and soft tissue interposition to prevent hematoma formation and reossification of the coalition are quite effective in relieving pain, improving subtalar motion, and allowing resumption of normal activities.

Cavus Feet

Cavovarus foot, an exaggerated medial longitudinal arch associated with a varus alignment of the hindfoot, often appears during the middle childhood years (Fig. 19–13). Both idiopathic and neuromuscular types may be seen; in either instance cavovarus is usually a progressive deformity leading to considerable compromise of foot function. In hypermobile

pes planus the foot rotates externally; in high arch or cavovarus posture, however, the foot rotates internally. The cavovarus foot also tends to be rigid. Aggressive treatment is warranted and usually involves reconstructive surgery. Special shoes and shoe modifications are not helpful but sometimes may be warranted for symptomatic treatment. Because a neuromuscular etiologic mechanism is possible whenever such a deformity of the foot exists, careful assessment of the patient's neurologic function is mandatory. Spinal cord pathology, poliomyelitis, and peripheral neuropathy (Charcot-Marie-Tooth disease) must always be considered.

Congenital Vertical Talus

Congenital vertical talus is an uncommon foot deformity producing a rigid, rocker-bottom shape to the foot. The talus is vertically oriented, with dorsal displacement of the navicular bone. Hindfoot equinovalgus, a convex plantar surface, midfoot and forefoot dorsiflexion and abduction, and rigidity are present. Most affected children have an underlying syndrome, such as spina bifida, arthrogryposis multiplex, or a congenital or chromosomal abnormality (e.g., trisomy 18). The diagnosis is confirmed roentgenographically with AP and lateral weight-bearing or simulated weight-bearing views. A maximum plantar flexion lateral roentgenogram demonstrates the inability to align the forefoot and midfoot with the hindfoot.

Treatment. Treatment is similar to that for a congenital clubfoot. Serial manipulations and casts are attempted in infancy but are only occasionally successful. Most children need surgical intervention with an extensive soft tissue release. The navicular must be reduced onto the head of the talus.

Occasionally, transfer of the tibialis anterior tendon to the neck of the talus is necessary to support the talus and prevent recurrence.

Osteochondroses

Both the tarsal navicular (in Kohler disease) and the head of the second metatarsal (in Frieberg disease) may undergo idiopathic avascular necrosis. These conditions are relatively uncommon, and both produce pain in the affected site on activity or weight bearing. The pathologic process involves infarction and subsequent revascularization, resorption, and reformation of the affected bone. Symptomatic treatment based on the severity of the child's complaints is appropriate.

As the child enters the adolescent growth spurt, the insertion of major muscle groups to bone is vulnerable to microfracture through the fibrocartilage, resulting in inflammatory and healing responses. The usual site of microfracture in the foot is at the attachment of the triceps surae to the os calcis, producing **Sever disease.** Symptoms wax and wane, depending on the level of activity, until skeletal maturity is achieved. The usual residual manifestation, if any, is some bony enlargement at the tendon insertion site when the cartilage, which proliferated as part of the healing response, undergoes its normal maturation to become bone. *Treatment* is symptomatic and includes the use of antiinflammatory agents, rest, icing, and elevation.

The major cause of adolescent heel pain is a tight Achilles tendon (heel cord) caused by rapid growth. A stretching exercise program is usually effective in relieving symptoms. Enthesitis secondary to juvenile rheumatoid arthritis must also be considered.

Adolescent Bunions

Bunions, or hallux valgus deformities, are common in adolescents. Typically, the family has a positive history of the condition. The deformity is usually bilateral and occurs predominantly in females. Most commonly, a congenital malalignment of the first metatarsal (metatarsus primus varus) is present. The hallux valgus deformity, enlargement of the medial aspect of the first metatarsal head, and symptoms usually begin in early adolescence.

Roentgenograms of the feet are necessary to assess the deformity; the AP and lateral weight-bearing views are selected.

Treatment is directed toward relief of symptoms. Initially this consists of appropriately fitting shoes with a wide toe-box and, occasionally, orthotics if there is associated pes planus. If this measure fails,

---

TABLE 19–8
Syndromes Associated with Polydactyly
Ellis–van Creveld syndrome
Rubinstein-Taybi syndrome
Carpenter syndrome
Meckel-Gruber syndrome
Polysyndactyly
Trisomy 13
Orofaciodigital syndrome

---

surgical realignment is necessary. Surgery is quite effective in relieving symptoms, although it usually does not restore the appearance of the foot to normal.

Toe Deformities

Curly toes is the most common lesser toe deformity of childhood. Flexion is present at the proximal interphalangeal joint with lateral rotation. The fourth and fifth toes are most commonly involved. The deformity is caused by tightness of the flexor digitorum longus and brevis tendons. Observation is recommended for infants and young children, because 25–50% of cases resolve spontaneously. Deformities persisting after 3–4 years of age are treated by open tenotomies of the flexor tendons.

Extra toes **(polydactyly)** usually are recognized at birth, and it is appropriate to decide on a management strategy at that time. When the extra toe is attached to the foot by only a tag of skin and soft tissue, as commonly occurs adjacent to the fifth toe, simple amputation or ligation through the stalk is effective. When the abnormality involves the great toe or the middle toes or when there is some rudiment of cartilage or bone connecting it with the foot proper, delayed surgical treatment targeted at the specific abnormality is indicated. Malformation syndromes may be associated with polydactyly (Table 19–8).

Fusing of the toes **(syndactyly)** is more common than polydactyly and is usually a benign cosmetic problem that does not warrant treatment. Syndromes also may be associated with syndactyly (Table 19–9).

Puncture Wounds

Puncture wounds of the foot are common and generally trivial. For most of these injuries, cleaning the wound, ensuring prophylaxis for tetanus infection, and administering broad-spectrum oral antibiotic

TABLE 19–9
Syndromes Associated with Syndactyly

Apert syndrome
Carpenter syndrome
de Lange syndrome
Holt-Oram syndrome
Orofaciodigital syndrome
Polysyndactyly
Fetal hydantoin syndrome
Laurence-Moon-Biedl syndrome
Fanconi pancytopenia
Trisomy 21
Trisomy 13
Trisomy 18

TABLE 19–10
Classification of Spinal Deformities

Scoliosis
Idiopathic
Infantile
Juvenile
Adolescent
Congenital
Failure of formation
   Wedge vertebrae
   Hemivertebrae
Failure of segmentation
   Unilateral bar
   Bilateral bar
Mixed
Neuromuscular
Neuropathic diseases
Upper motor neuron
   Cerebral palsy
   Spinocerebellar degeneration
      Friedreich ataxia
      Charcot-Marie-Tooth disease
   Syringomyelia
   Spinal cord tumor
   Spinal cord trauma
Lower motor neuron
   Myelodysplasia
   Poliomyelitis
   Spinal muscular atrophy
Myopathic diseases
   Duchenne muscular dystrophy
   Arthrogryposis
   Other muscular dystrophies
Syndromes
Neurofibromatosis
Marfan syndrome
Compensatory
Leg length inequality

Kyphosis
Postural roundback
Scheuermann disease
Congenital kyphosis

Adapted from the Terminology Committee of the Scoliosis Research Society, 1975.

prophylaxis are all that is needed. When infection occurs despite these measures, *Pseudomonas aeruginosa* and *Staphylococcus aureus* are the offending organisms in most cases of osteomyelitis or osteochondritis, supposedly because these organisms normally colonize the skin surface of the foot as a result of the moist environment in an athletic shoe.

Treatment of these infections involves débriding the wound to remove necrotic tissue, which invariably is present, and administering parenteral antibiotics, initially with methicillin and gentamicin. Subsequent antibiotic treatment should be based on culture and sensitivity studies. After surgery, parenteral antimicrobial therapy is required for 10–14 days.

REFERENCES

Behrman RE, Kliegman RM, Jenson HB, editors: *Nelson textbook of pediatrics*, ed 16, Philadelphia, 2000, WB Saunders, Chapter 680.

Blakemore LC, Cooperman DR, Thompson GH: The rigid flatfoot: tarsal coalition, *Foot Ankle Clin* 3:609, 1998.

Drennan JC: Instructional course lecture: congenital vertical talus, *J Bone Joint Surg* 77A:1916, 1995.

Farsetti P, Weinstein SL, Ponseti IV: The long-term functional and radiographic outcomes of untreated and non-operatively treated metatarsus adductus, *J Bone Joint Surg* 76A:257–265, 1994.

Laughlin TJ, Armstrong DJ, Caporusso J, et al: Soft-tissue and bone infections from puncture wounds in children, *West J Med* 166:126–128, 1997.

Mosca VS: Flexible flatfoot and skewfoot, *J Bone Joint Surg* 77A: 1937, 1995.

Sullivan JA: Pediatric flatfoot, *J Am Acad Orthop Surg* 7:44–53, 1999.

Thompson GH: Bunions and deformities of the toes in children and adolescents, *J Bone Joint Surg* 77A:1924, 1995.

SPINE

A simplified classification of the common spinal abnormalities is presented in Table 19–10.

Clinical Examination

A complete physical examination is necessary for any child or adolescent with a spinal deformity because the deformity may indicate an underlying disease. The back is examined with the patient in the standing position, and viewed from behind (Fig. 19–14). The levelness of the pelvis is assessed first. Lower extremity length inequality results in pelvic obliquity and can produce the appearance of *scoliosis*, termed compensatory scoliosis. When the pelvis is level or has been leveled with wood blocks placed under the foot, the spine is examined for symmetry. The back is observed for areas of deformity, spinal curvature, cutaneous lesions (e.g., hemangioma or hair tuft), and areas of tenderness.

After the spine is examined for levelness, the patient is asked to bend forward with the hands directed between the feet (Adams forward bend test). A tangential view of the spine while standing behind (thoracic area) and in front (lumbar area) allows the observer to determine the symmetry of the back. The presence of a hump is the hallmark of a scoliotic deformity. The corresponding area opposite the hump typically is depressed. The reason for these "humps and valleys" is *spinal rotation*. Scoliosis represents a rotational malalignment of one vertebra on another. This results in rib elevation when the curve is in the thoracic area and paravertebral muscle elevation when the curve is in the lumbar region. When the trunk is viewed from the side with the patient still in the forward flexed position, the degree of roundback can be ascertained. A sharp, abrupt forward angulation in the midline thoracic or thoracolumbar region is indicative of a *kyphotic deformity*.

In a patient with scoliosis other areas of the body also must be examined, including the skin (hairy patches, nevi, and lipomas are suggestive of *spinal dysraphism* and café-au-lait spots for neurofibromatosis), the extremities (for skeletal dysplasia), the heart (checking for murmurs indicative of Marfan syndrome), and the neurologic system, to determine whether the scoliosis is truly idiopathic or possibly secondary to an underlying neuromuscular disorder or producing neurologic complications.

Roentgenographic Evaluation. Initial roentgenograms of the spine include a posteroanterior (PA) and lateral standing roentgenogram of the entire spine. This allows assessment for scoliosis, kyphosis, lordosis, congenital malformations, and, if the iliac crests are visible, the skeletal maturity of the patient. The degree of curvature is measured from the most tilted or end vertebra of the curve superiorly and inferiorly using the *Cobb method* (Fig. 19–15).

Scoliosis

Alterations in normal spinal alignment that occur in the AP or frontal plane are termed scoliosis. Most scoliotic deformities are idiopathic (i.e., of unknown causation). Others, however, can be congenital, secondary to an underlying neuromuscular disorder, or compensatory from a lower extremity length inequality.

Idiopathic Scoliosis

Idiopathic scoliosis is the most common form of scoliosis. It occurs in healthy, neurologically normal children, and its etiology is unknown. The incidence is only slightly higher in females, but the condition is more likely to progress and necessitate treatment in females. Hereditary tendencies are associated with the condition; approximately 20% of patients have other family members with the same condition.

Idiopathic scoliosis is classified into three age groups: infantile (birth to 3 years), juvenile (4–10 years), and adolescent (11 years and older). *Idiopathic adolescent scoliosis* (found in 80% of cases) is the most common cause of spinal deformity. The right thoracic curve is the most common pattern. *Infantile* scoliosis is quite rare in the United States but is common in England. *Juvenile* scoliosis is not common, but many children with the diagnosis of adolescent scoliosis actually had the juvenile-onset type but the diagnosis was not made until later.

Clinical Manifestations. Idiopathic scoliosis is usually a painless disorder. Any child with scoliosis and back pain requires a careful neurologic examination. Left thoracic curves and back pain are associated with an increased incidence of intraspinal pathology, such as a syrinx or tumor. These children should be evaluated by MRI of the spine.

Treatment. Treatment of idiopathic scoliosis is based on the maturation of the patient and whether the curve is progressive or nonprogressive. No treatment is necessary for nonprogressive deformities. The possibility for progression varies with several factors: sex, age, curve location, and curve magnitude. The risk for progression is much higher for females (5:1). The younger the child, the higher the risk for progression. The treatment of progressive idiopathic adolescent scoliosis involves observation, an orthosis, or surgery; exercises alone are ineffective. Typically, curves less than 25 degrees are observed. Progressive curves between 25 and 45 degrees in a skeletally immature patient are managed by an orthosis. Curves greater than 45 degrees generally necessitate surgery.

Congenital Scoliosis

Abnormalities of vertebral formation during the first trimester lead to structural deformities of the

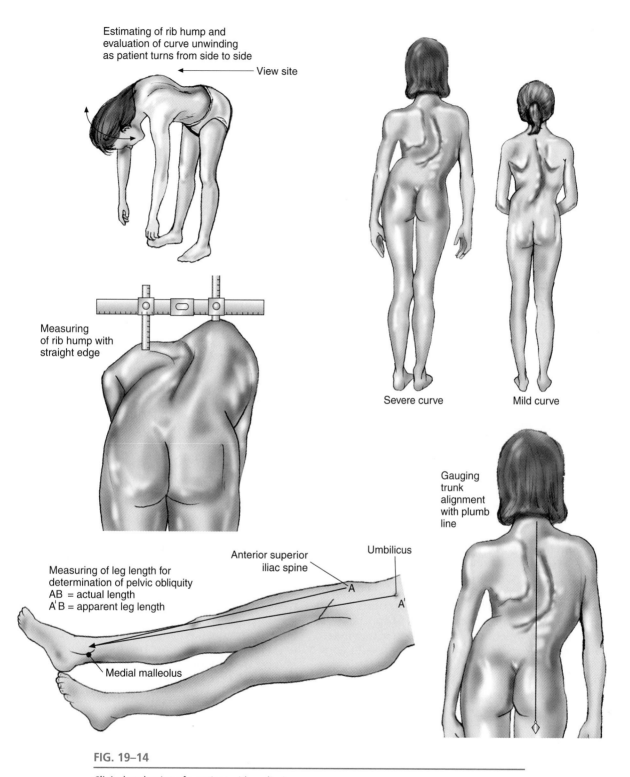

Estimating of rib hump and
evaluation of curve unwinding
as patient turns from side to side

View site

Measuring
of rib hump with
straight edge

Severe curve

Mild curve

Gauging
trunk
alignment
with plumb
line

Measuring of leg length for
determination of pelvic obliquity
AB = actual length
A'B = apparent leg length

Anterior superior
iliac spine

Umbilicus

A

A'

Medial malleolus

FIG. 19–14

Clinical evaluation of a patient with scoliosis.

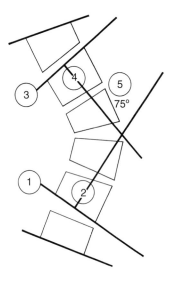

FIG. 19–15

Scoliosis; measurement of a curve by the Cobb (roentgenographic) method. *1,* Bottom vertebra: lowest one whose bottom tilts to concavity of curve. *2,* Erect perpendicular from bottom of bottom vertebra. *3,* Top vertebra: highest one whose top tilts to concavity of curve. *4,* Drop perpendicular from top of top vertebra. *5,* Measure intersecting angle. This is the accepted method of measurement of a curve according to the Scoliosis Research Society. Curves of 0–20 degrees are mild, 20–40 degrees are moderate, and above 40 degrees are severe. (From Ferguson A: *Orthopedic surgery in infancy and childhood,* ed 5, Baltimore, 1981, Williams & Wilkins.)

spine that are evident at birth or in early childhood. Congenital scoliosis can be classified as (1) partial or complete failure of vertebral formation (wedge vertebrae or hemivertebrae), (2) partial or complete failure of segmentation (unsegmented bars), or (3) mixed (Fig. 19–16). The condition may occur as a single anomaly or in combination with other bone, neural, or soft tissue abnormalities of the axial or appendicular skeleton. Congenital genitourinary malformations occur in 20% of children with congenital scoliosis. Unilateral renal agenesis is the most common abnormality, but 6% of affected children may have a silent, obstructive uropathy. Overall, 30–34% have extravertebral anomalies or syndromes such as VATER syndrome, or Klippel-Feil syndrome.

Renal ultrasonography is performed in all patients to assess for possible genitourinary problems. Congenital heart disease may be found in 10–15% of patients. Spinal dysraphism occurs in approximately 20% of patients with congenital scoliosis. This includes tethered spinal cord, intradural lipomas, syringomyelia, diplomyelia, and diastematomyelia.

These abnormalities frequently are associated with cutaneous lesions of the back (e.g., hairy patches, skin dimples, and hemangiomas) and abnormalities of the feet and lower extremities (e.g., cavus feet, calf atrophy, asymmetric foot size, and neurologic changes). MRI of the spine is the procedure of choice for evaluation of possible spinal dysraphism.

The risk of progression of spinal deformity in a child with congenital scoliosis is variable, depending on the growth potential of the malformed vertebra. Defects such as a block vertebra have little growth potential, whereas unilateral unsegmented bars typically produce progressive deformities. Seventy-five percent of involved patients demonstrate some progression that continues until skeletal growth stops; approximately 50% require treatment. Rapid progression can be expected during periods of rapid growth, before 2 years and after 10 years of age. Thoracolumbar curves and multiple hemivertebras are associated with rapid progression, whereas nonsegmented hemivertebra is the least likely to progress.

Early *diagnosis* and prompt *treatment* of progressive curves are essential elements in the care of congenital spinal deformity. Orthotic treatment is of limited value because these curves tend to be rigid. A spinal fusion without instrumentation is the most common procedure. If severe, the scoliosis may produce deformity, pulmonary restriction (cor pulmonale), and neurologic compression.

Neuromuscular Scoliosis

Progressive spinal deformity is a common and potentially serious abnormality associated with many neuromuscular disorders, such as cerebral palsy, Duchenne muscular dystrophy, spinal muscular atrophy, and spina bifida. Progression is usually continuous once scoliosis begins. The magnitude of the deformity depends on the severity and pattern of weakness, whether the disease process is progressive, and the amount of remaining musculoskeletal growth. In nonambulatory patients, the curves tend to be long and sweeping, produce pelvic obliquity, involve the cervical spine, and alter pulmonary function, producing restrictive lung disease. As these curves progress, sitting balance can be lost and the affected individuals must use their arms to support an upright position. Spinal alignment must be part of the routine examination of a child with a neuromuscular disorder. Ambulatory patients have a much lower incidence of spinal deformity than nonambulatory or more severely involved patients. The standing or sitting forward bending test can be used to assess the symmetry of spinal alignment.

Any asymmetry is an indication for *roentgenographic evaluation,* which should include a PA and

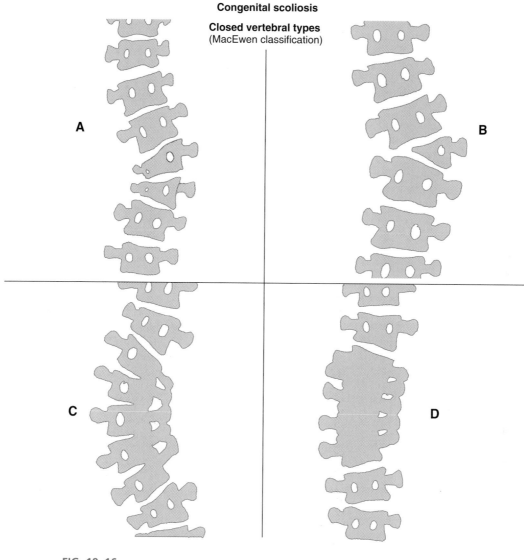

Congenital scoliosis

Closed vertebral types
(MacEwen classification)

FIG. 19–16

Types of closed vertebral and extravertebral spinal anomalies that result in congenital scoliosis. **A,** Partial unilateral failure of formation (wedge vertebrae). **B,** Complete unilateral failure of formation (hemivertebra). **C,** Unilateral failure of segmentation (congenital bar). **D,** Bilateral failure of segmentation (block vertebra).

lateral standing or AP and lateral sitting view of the entire spine. If the child or adolescent cannot sit unsupported, a supine AP radiograph may be necessary.

The goal of *treatment* is to prevent progression and loss of function. Nonambulatory patients usu-ally are more comfortable, are more independent, and have better respiratory function when they are able to sit erect without external support. Orthotic management or bracing is not usually effective; surgery is necessary in most cases. The current in-strumentation systems are sufficiently strong and distribute the corrective forces such that postoperative immobilization is usually not necessary.

Compensatory Scoliosis

Adolescents with lower extremity length inequality may have a positive screening examination for scoliosis. With a pelvic obliquity, the patient's spine curves in the same direction as the obliquity. The magnitude of the lower extremity length discrepancy can be measured radiographically by a scanogram of the lower extremities. Distinguishing between a structural and a compensatory spinal deformity is important.

Kyphosis

The term kyphosis refers to a roundback deformity or to an increased angulation in the thoracic or thoracolumbar spine in the sagittal plane. Roundback deformities can be postural, structural **(Scheuermann kyphosis)**, or congenital in origin.

Postural Roundback

Postural kyphosis is secondary to bad posture and is a common concern of parents. Postural kyphosis is voluntarily corrected in both the standing and prone positions. Radiographically, no vertebral abnormalities are present. There may be some increase in the normal kyphosis of the thoracic region, but a supine hyperextension film will show complete correction. The child is responsible for correcting posture. Active *treatment* is not indicated.

Scheuermann Disease

Scheuermann disease is common and second only to idiopathic scoliosis as a cause of pediatric spinal deformity. It occurs equally among male and female adolescents. Its *etiology* is unknown; hereditary factors are present, but with no definite pattern of inheritance. The differentiation between postural kyphosis and Scheuermann disease is determined by clinical and roentgenographic evaluation.

Clinical Manifestations. A patient with Scheuermann disease cannot correct the kyphosis in either the standing or the prone, hyperextended position. When viewed from the side in the forward flexed position, patients with Scheuermann disease usually show an abrupt angulation in the mid to lower thoracic region (Fig. 19–17). A patient with a postural roundback shows a smooth, symmetric contour. In both conditions the normal lumbar lordosis is increased when the patient stands erect. Approximately 50% of patients with Scheuermann disease have apical back pain, especially with thoracolumbar kyphosis.

The classic roentgenographic findings of Scheuer-

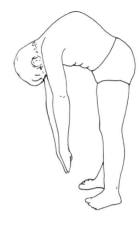

FIG. 19–17

Note the sharp break in the contour in the child with kyphosis. (From Behrman RE, editor: *Nelson textbook of pediatrics*, ed 14, Philadelphia, 1992, WB Saunders.)

mann kyphosis include narrowing of disc space; loss of the normal anterior height of the involved vertebra, producing wedging of 5 degrees or more in three or more vertebrae; irregularities of the end plates; and Schmorl nodes.

Treatment. Treatment of Scheuermann kyphosis is similar to that for scoliosis and is dependent on the maturation age of the patient, the degree of deformity, and the presence or absence of pain in the apical region. Nonoperative treatment consists of a corrective plaster cast followed by an orthosis. Permanent correction of the kyphotic deformity can be achieved with nonoperative management. Surgical treatment in Scheuermann disease rarely is necessary and is indicated for those patients who have completed growth, who have a severe deformity, or who have chronic, intractable pain.

Congenital Kyphosis

Congenital kyphosis includes congenital failure of the formation of all or part of the vertebral body, but with preservation of the posterior elements; failure of anterior segmentation of the spine (anterior unsegmented bar); or both. The more severe deformities usually are recognized at birth and rapidly progress thereafter. The less obvious deformities may not appear until years later. Once the progression begins, it does not cease until the end of growth. The most important factor regarding congenital kyphosis is that a progressive deformity in the thoracic spine can result in *paraplegia*. This usually is associated with the failure of vertebral body formation.

Treatment, when necessary, is operative. Orthotic management is ineffective.

Spondylolysis and Spondylolisthesis

Spondylolysis is a defect in the pars interarticularis without forward slippage of the involved vertebra on the one below. *Spondylolisthesis* refers to the forward slippage or displacement of the involved vertebra. The lesions are not present at birth but occur in 5% of children by 6 years of age. Children involved in certain sports, such as gymnastics, have an even higher incidence of spondylolysis. This has been attributed to repetitive hyperextension stresses resulting in a fatigue fracture of the pars interarticularis.

Spondylolisthesis is classified according to the degree of slippage of one vertebra on the other: grade 1, less than 25%; grade 2, 25–50%; grade 3, 50–75%; grade 4, 75–100%; and grade 5, complete displacement. The most common location of spondylolisthesis is the fifth lumbar vertebra on the sacrum (first sacral vertebra).

Clinical Manifestations. Physical examination for spondylolysis or spondylolisthesis is similar to that for any disorder of the spine. A palpable "step-off" at the lumbosacral area and a vertically oriented sacrum indicate severe spondylolisthesis. A neurologic examination must be performed because nerve root involvement can occur, especially with severe displacement.

Roentgenographic Evaluation. Roentgenographic evaluation should include standing PA and lateral views of the entire spine, with an oblique radiograph of the lumbar spine. MRI may be required in patients with neurologic findings.

Treatment. Children and adolescents with asymptomatic spondylolysis require periodic evaluation during growth to assess for possible slippage; treatment rarely is required. Painful spondylolysis may benefit from orthotic management. If this does not relieve pain, surgical intervention with an in situ posterior spinal fusion may be required.

Adolescents with spondylolisthesis may require treatment, which depends on age, type of defect, degree of the slippage, and associated malalignment in the involved area.

- *Grade 1:* Usually, no treatment is required unless there is chronic pain. Conservative management may be tried initially; if this fails, surgical intervention may be necessary.
- *Grade 2:* Usually, a spinal fusion is required because of the high risk for further progression.
- *Grade 3* and *grade 4:* Usually, fusion is required to prevent further deformity.

Disc Space Infection

A disc space infection may be regarded as an infection of the disc without producing an acute osteomyelitis of the vertebral body. The most common organism is *S. aureus*. The infection can occur at any age. The disc space may at times be sterile. Children may have back pain, but they also may have abdominal or pelvic pain, irritability, and refusal to walk.

Clinical Manifestations. The child typically maintains the spine in a straight, stiff, or splinted position and refuses to flex the lumbar spine. The normal lumbar lordosis is reversed, and there may be paravertebral muscle spasms. However, in comparison with other forms of osteomyelitis, there are inconsistent systemic symptoms, such as fever and an elevated white blood cell count. The ESR typically is elevated.

Roentgenographic Evaluation. The roentgenographic features will vary according to the interval between the onset of symptoms and delay in diagnosis. AP, lateral, and oblique radiographs of the lumbar spine or thoracic spine, depending on the location of symptoms, usually are necessary to make the diagnosis. Typically, the disc space is narrowed, with irregularity of the adjacent vertebral body end plates. In very early cases, bone scan or (more often) MRI studies may be helpful because they may be positive before routine roentgenographic changes are present; MRI can be used to differentiate discitis from the distinct, more serious condition of vertebral osteomyelitis.

Treatment. The treatment of disc space infection usually is antibiotic therapy. Blood cultures may be helpful in establishing a precise organism. Aspiration needle biopsy of the disc space is reserved for children who do not respond to initial treatment with antistaphylococcal antibiotics. Immobilization of the spine may be used on a symptomatic basis. In most children, however, symptoms rapidly resolve with intravenous antibiotics. Intravenous antibiotics are continued for 1–2 weeks and followed by oral antibiotics for an additional 4 weeks.

Torticollis

The literal definition of torticollis is twisted neck, but the traditional definition is shortening of one sternocleidomastoid muscle. Shortening and secondary contractures can be a primary abnormality of the sternocleidomastoid muscle (muscular torticollis) or secondary to central nervous system or upper cervical spine abnormalities.

Infants and young children with muscular torticollis have the ear pulled down toward the clavicle on the ipsilateral side. The face looks upward toward the contralateral side. Early in infancy, a "tumor" or thickening is palpated in the lower to mid portion of the sternocleidomastoid muscle. This represents swelling or fibrosis of the central portion of the muscle and often is a precursor of the subsequent contracture. Skull and facial asymmetry or plagiocephaly may be present in congenital cases.

Etiology. In infants, in utero malposition, birth trauma, sternocleidomastoid muscle compartment syndrome, and heredity have been implicated as etiologic factors. In acquired torticollis in children, central nervous system mass lesions, abnormalities of the cervical spine, and local head and neck infections are more likely. Psychiatric causes may occur during adolescence.

Diagnosis. A thorough neurologic examination should be performed and AP and lateral radiographs of the cervical spine obtained. A CT scan or MRI of the head and neck is necessary for any patient with persistent neck pain or with neurologic signs and symptoms.

Treatment. Treatment goals include ruling out an underlying disorder, increasing range of motion of the neck, and correcting the cosmetic deformity. Some infants with muscular torticollis may respond to nonoperative measures, which include range of motion exercises of the head and neck and stretching of the restrictive muscles several times daily. General indications for nonoperative management include age younger than 1 year, positive response to stretching exercise over several weeks, and no underlying cervical spine abnormalities or central nervous system findings.

Principles of surgical management of patients with muscular torticollis include identifying and releasing all restricting bands involving the sternocleidomastoid muscle and other neck structures, moving the head through a full range of motion before completion of the surgery, and resuming physical therapy within 2 weeks of operation to prevent recurrent contracture.

BACK PAIN IN CHILDREN

Back pain in children is unusual and should be viewed with concern. In contrast to adults, in whom back pain frequently is mechanical or psychologic in origin, back pain in children is usually the result of organic causes, especially in the preadolescent. Back pain lasting more than a few days requires careful investigation. Approximately 85% of children with back pain of more than 2 months have a specific lesion: 33% posttraumatic (occult fracture, spondylolysis), 33% developmental (kyphosis, scoliosis), and 18% infection or tumor. In the remaining 15% the diagnosis will be undetermined.

Clinical Manifestations. The history should include the onset and duration of symptoms; antecedent factors; general health; family history; location, character, and radiation of pain; and neurologic symptoms such as muscle weakness, sensory changes, and bowel or bladder dysfunction. Physical examination should include a complete musculoskeletal and neurologic evaluation. Spinal alignment, mobility, muscle spasm, and areas of tenderness should be evaluated and recorded. Muscle strength, sensory assessment (such as pain and light touch), deep tendon reflexes, and pathologic reflexes (such as the Babinski sign) are tested. The danger signs in childhood back pain are persistent or increasing pain; systemic symptoms such as fever, malaise, or weight loss; neurologic findings; bowel or bladder dysfunction; young age, especially under 4 years (suspect tumor); and painful left thoracic spinal curvatures.

Roentgenographic Evaluation. The first diagnostic procedure is PA and lateral standing films of the entire spine with right and left oblique views of the involved area. Other roentgenograms may be necessary, depending on the location of the pain and the differential diagnoses. These include bone scans, CT scan, and MRI. MRI is especially useful when intraspinal pathology is suspected.

Laboratory Evaluation. Laboratory studies such as CBC, ESR, and tests for the juvenile forms of arthritis (juvenile rheumatoid arthritis and ankylosing spondylitis) may be necessary.

Differential Diagnosis. The differential diagnosis in pediatric back pain is extensive (Table 19–11).

Treatment. The treatment of back pain is based on the specific diagnosis. If no definite diagnosis is established, an initial trial of physical therapy is recommended.

REFERENCES

Behrman RE, Kliegman RM, Jenson HB, editors: *Nelson textbook of pediatrics*, ed 16, Philadelphia, 2000, WB Saunders, Chapter 685.

Cheng JC, Tang SP, Chen TMK, et al: The clinical presentation and outcome of treatment of congenital muscular torticollis in infants: a study of 1,086 cases, *J Pediatr Surg* 35:1091–1096, 2000.

Fernandez M, Carrol CL, Baker CJ: Discitis and vertebral osteomyelitis in children: an 18-year review, *Pediatrics* 105:1299–1304, 2000.

Herman MJ, Pizzutillo PD: Cervical spine disorders in children, *Orthop Clin North Am* 30:457–466, 1999.

Little DG, Song KM, Katz D, et al: Relationship of peak growth velocity to other maturation indicators in idiopathic scoliosis in girls, *J Bone Joint Surg* 82A:685–693, 2000.

Lonstein JE: Spondylolisthesis in children: course, natural history and management, *Spine* 24:2640–2648, 1999.

Lowe TG: Scheuermann's disease, *Orthop Clin North Am* 30:475–487, 1999.

McCarthy RE: Management of neuromuscular scoliosis, *Orthop Clin North Am* 30:435–449, 1999.

McMaster MJ, Singh H: The natural history of congenital scoliosis and kyphoscoliosis: a study of one hundred and twelve patients, *J Bone Joint Surg* 81A:1367–1383, 1999.

Prahinski JR, Polly DW, McHale, KA, et al: Occult intraspinal anomalies in congenital scoliosis. *J Pediatr Orthop* 20:59–63, 2000.

Roach JW: Adolescent idiopathic scoliosis, *Orthop Clin North Am* 30:353–365, 1999.

Scoles PV: Back pain in children and adolescents. In Kliegman RM et al, editors: *Practical strategies in pediatric diagnosis and therapy*, Philadelphia, 1996, WB Saunders.

TABLE 19–11
Differential Diagnosis of Back Pain

Inflammatory Diseases
Discitis (common before 6 years of age)
Vertebral osteomyelitis (pyogenic or tuberculous)
Spinal epidural abscess
Pyelonephritis
Pancreatitis

Rheumatologic Diseases
Pauciarticular juvenile rheumatoid arthritis
Reiter syndrome
Juvenile ankylosing spondylitis
Psoriatic arthritis

Developmental Diseases
Spondylolysis
Spondylolisthesis
Scheuermann syndrome
Scoliosis (especially left thoracic)

Mechanical Trauma and Abnormalities
Hip and pelvic anomalies
Herniated disc
Overuse syndromes (common with athletic training
  and in gymnasts and dancers)
Vertebral stress fractures
Compression fracture (steroids, sickle cell anemia)
Upper cervical spine instability

Neoplastic Diseases
Primary vertebral bone tumors (osteogenic sarcoma)
Metastatic tumor (neuroblastoma)
Primary spinal tumor (neuroblastoma, astrocytoma)
Malignancy of bone marrow (ALL, lymphoma)
Benign tumors (eosinophilic granuloma, osteoid
  osteoma)

Other
After lumbar puncture
Conversion reaction
Juvenile osteoporosis

ALL, Acute lymphocytic leukemia.

THE SHOULDER

The shoulder joint has minimal geometric stability because of the relatively small glenoid fossa that articulates with a proportionately large hemispheric humeral head. A large range of motion is gained at the expense of intrinsic stability; consequently, the musculature about the shoulder, particularly the muscles of the rotator cuff, must function with normal glenohumeral contact. Scapulothoracic movement greatly expands the range of motion possible at the shoulder area; the scapula, just as is the case with the glenohumeral joint, requires strong coordinated musculature to function with stability.

Sprengel Deformity

Failure of the scapula to descend to its normal location is Sprengel deformity, which occurs with varying degrees of severity. The scapula is located abnormally high with respect to the child's neck and thorax. Webbing of the neck or skin of the neck and a low posterior hairline may be associated findings. In the severe form, a bone (omovertebral) may connect the scapula with the lower cervical spine and virtually no scapulothoracic movement may be possible; often, associated muscle anomalies are present that further limit strength and stability of the shoulder girdle. In the mild form, the scapula is slightly high riding, with less than normal motion. Association with congenital cervical vertebral anomalies, particularly the **Klippel-Feil anomaly,** occurs and suggests the possibility of significant problems in other organ systems. The best outcome in severe Sprengel deformities is achieved in early childhood by surgically repositioning and occasionally partially resecting the scapula. This improves cosmesis and motion, especially shoulder abduction.

Brachial Plexus (Obstetric) Palsy

See Chapter 6.

Dislocation of the Shoulder

Dislocation of the shoulder is uncommon in childhood but becomes more frequent in adolescence. The younger the individual at the time of the initial dislocation, the more likely that recurrent dislocation will develop. The chances of redislocation are so high that many orthopaedic surgeons now favor early reconstruction rather than instituting conservative treatment and awaiting further dislocations.

Epiphysiolysis of the Proximal Humeral Epiphysis

The youngster who engages regularly in a throwing sport is at risk for traumatic epiphysiolysis of the proximal humeral physis. This disorder is a fatigue separation through the physis; it heals with rest and avoidance of repetitive throwing. Pain about the shoulder is the usual presenting complaint.

Overuse Syndromes

Overuse syndromes, inflammatory responses in tendons and bursae subjected to repetitive mild trauma, are uncommon in childhood but may be seen in the adolescent. Subacromial **bursitis**, for example, occurs in tennis players and swimmers. Bicipital **tendinitis** is uncommon in the young but may produce a sensation of something snapping in the shoulder or shoulder pain when the bicipital groove is shallow and the tendon can subluxate from it. In these types of inflammatory responses, direct tenderness over the involved anatomic structure is diagnostic.

REFERENCES

Behrman RE, Kliegman RM, Jenson HB, editors: *Nelson textbook of pediatrics*, ed 16, Philadelphia, 2000, WB Saunders, Chapter 687.

Cho TJ, Choi IH, Chung CY, et al: Sprengel deformity: morphometric analysis using 3D-CT and its clinical relevance, *J Bone Joint Surg* 82B:711–718, 2000.

Epps HR, Salter RB: Orthopaedic conditions of the cervical spine and shoulder, *Pediatr Clin North Am* 43:919–931, 1996.

Kawan M, Sinclair J, Letts M: Recurrent posterior shoulder dislocation in children: the results of surgical treatment, *J Pediatr Orthop* 17:533–538, 1997.

THE ELBOW

The elbow joint consists of three articulations: the ulna and the humerus, the radius and the humerus, and the proximal radius and the ulna. Collectively, they provide for a hinge-type joint that allows for a palm-up (supination) and a palm-down (pronation) positioning of the wrist and hand. The elbow has great geometric stability, and the musculature moving the joint primarily motor flexion and extension at the elbow joint, but there are smaller muscles that primarily serve to rotate the radius about its long axis.

Nursemaid's Elbow

The radial head is not as bulbous in the infant as in older children. During infancy, the annular ligament that passes around its base can partially slip off the head with traction across the elbow. When the ligament slips, the entity is known as nursemaid's elbow, or subluxation of the annular ligament (Fig. 19–18). The subluxation is initiated by a jerk on the extended elbow when a child falls with the hand being held or when a child is forcefully lifted by the hand. When the subluxation occurs, the hand typically is held in a palm-down position, and the child may refuse to use the hand or may cry when the elbow is moved. Moving the hand to a palm-up position with pressure over the radial head usually reduces the ligament subluxation and restores full normal use of the extremity. The parents should be educated about the mechanism of injury and should be encouraged to avoid picking the child up by holding the hand or forearm. Once subluxation has occurred, there is a propensity for subsequent episodes. Generally, the problem resolves with maturation.

Panner Disease

Panner disease is an osteochondrosis that involves the ossific nucleus of the capitellum, the lateral portion of the distal humeral epiphysis. It is most common in adolescents, especially those involved in throwing activities. They complain of pain and may

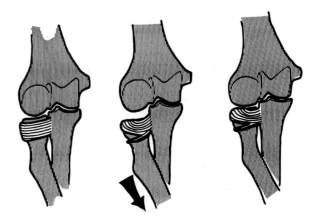

FIG. 19–18

The pathology of pulled elbow. The annular ligament is torn when the arm is pulled. The radial head moves distally and, when traction is discontinued, the ligament is carried into the joint. (From Rang M: *Children's fractures*, ed 2, Philadelphia, 1983, JB Lippincott.)

have crepitation and loss of motion. AP, lateral, and oblique roentgenograms, CT, or MRI may be helpful. In the absence of a loose osteocartilaginous body, *treatment* is conservative; if such a body is present, surgery is indicated.

Throwing Injuries

The elbow is especially vulnerable to throwing injuries in the skeletally immature child. The most common pathology results from abnormal compressive forces acting across the radial side of the joint. In addition to Panner disease, the radial head may become asymmetric compared with the opposite side or may be fragmented. Some irregularity in shape of the cartilaginous radial head is present. Additionally, there may be irregularity of the capitellum. Rarely, small pieces of bone and cartilage (loose bodies) from the capitellum or radial head become entrapped in the joint. Before the problem becomes established or severe, the child complains of an aching pain about the elbow, which generally is worse after throwing than during the time spent at the throwing activity. On physical examination, an early loss of supination (the palm-up position of the hand) can be detected. Children in whom these lesions develop generally have a high emotional investment in their particular sport, most commonly baseball, and nonparticipation is a difficult option for them to accept. Avoidance of pitching until the elbow is normal on physical examination with follow-up roentgenogram is the best solution. Often, switching the baseball player to another position allows the child to avoid pitching. Behind such highly motivated youngsters is usually an overzealous parent or coach in need of appropriate counseling.

REFERENCES

Behrman RE, Kliegman RM, Jenson HB, editors: *Nelson textbook of pediatrics*, ed 16, Philadelphia, 2000, WB Saunders, Chapter 687.

DeSilva MF, Williams JS, Fadale PD, et al: Pediatric throwing injuries about the elbow, *Am J Orthop* 27:90, 1998.

THE WRIST AND HAND

Multiple small joints, a delicately balanced intrinsic muscle system, a powerful extrinsic muscle system, dense sensory innervation, and specialized skin combined to make the hand a highly mobile, sensitive, and delicate yet powerful anatomic part.

The extrinsic muscles, those whose muscle origin is in the forearm and that motor the hand via tendons that pass to it, provide great power, whereas the intrinsic muscles, those that are located in the hand itself, modulate the effects of the powerful extrinsic musculature and provide for delicate coordinated movement. Asking the patient to open the hand, extending and spreading the fingers and

thumb, and, subsequently, clenching the hand to a fist, yields much insight because these maneuvers require coordinated function of both the intrinsic and extrinsic musculature, as well as full range of motion in the small joints of the hand. After this maneuver, having the individual squeeze the examiner's fingers gives further information about the strength of the hand.

FINGER ABNORMALITIES

Extra digits **(polydactyly)** occur as both simple and complex varieties (Table 19–8). Those skin tags and digit remnants typically seen near the metacarpophalangeal joint of the small finger or of the thumb that do not have palpable bone in their base or possess voluntary movement may be excised while the child is still in the nursery. Varieties of polydactyly more complex than this should be referred for amputation.

Syndactyly also occurs in both simple and complex patterns (Table 19–9). There always is concern about the sharing of common important structures between the digits and about the tethering effect of the syndactyly on the growth of the affected digits. Referral for delineation of the specific pathology and development of a treatment strategy are indicated when the condition is recognized.

Isolated thickening in the flexor pollicis longus tendon may produce a **trigger thumb.** As the nodule enlarges, it may snap or trigger as it passes through the first pulley that prevents bowstringing of the tendon. Ultimately, it may not pass through at all, producing a flexion deformity at the interphalangeal joint. The nodule is usually palpable at the level of the metacarpophalangeal joint on the volar surface. These children should be referred because many need surgery, release of the first pulley, to correct the triggering or the contracture.

Ganglion

A synovial fluid–filled cyst about the wrist, a *ganglion*, is common in childhood. The usual site is the dorsum of the wrist near the radiocarpal joint, and a secondary site is over the volar radial aspect of the wrist. The essential pathology is a defect in one of the joint capsules; with wrist use, synovial fluid is pumped into the soft tissue, where it becomes walled off by reactive fibrous tissue. Often, in the skeletally immature child, the process is benign and tends to disappear with the passage of time. In the event that a ganglion is sufficiently large to cause pain or interfere with normal tendon function, aspiration and injection of the cyst are sometimes helpful; in refractory cases, surgical excision of the cyst accompanied by removal of the tract that extends into the joint is curative.

REFERENCES

Behrman RE, Kliegman RM, Jenson HB, editors: *Nelson textbook of pediatrics,* ed 16, Philadelphia, 2000, WB Saunders, Chapter 687.

Dunsmuir RH, Sherlock DA: The outcome of treatment of trigger thumb in children, *J Bone Joint Surg* 82B:736–738, 2000.

Netscher DT: Congenital hand problems: terminology, etiology, and management, *Clin Plast Surg* 25:537–552, 1998.

Watson S: The principles of management of congenital anomalies of the upper limb, *Arch Dis Child* 83:10–17, 2000.

MUSCULOSKELETAL TRAUMA

Fractures in children have been estimated to account for 10–15% of all childhood injuries. Children are not small adults; their skeletal systems have anatomic, biomechanical, and physiologic differences from those of adults. These result in different fracture patterns, including epiphyseal injuries, problems of diagnosis, and variation in management techniques.

The anatomic differences in the pediatric skeleton include the presence of preosseous cartilage, physes, and thicker, stronger periosteum that produces callus more rapidly and in greater amounts. Biomechanically, the pediatric skeletal system can absorb more energy before deformation and fracture than adult bone can. This has been attributed to lower ash content and the greater porosity of young bone. As maturation occurs, the porosity decreases and the cortical bone becomes thicker and stronger. The thick periosteum of a child is a major determinant in whether a fracture becomes displaced. The thick periosteum also can act as an impediment to closed reduction because of the hinging phenomenon. Conversely, it can help stabilize a fracture following reduction.

Unusual Features
Fracture Remodeling

Remodeling occurs by a combination of periosteal resorption and new bone formation. Thus, anatomic alignment in certain pediatric fractures is not always necessary. The major factors affecting fracture remodeling are the child's age, the proximity of the fracture to a joint, and the relationship of the fracture to the plane of joint motion. The amount of remaining musculoskeletal growth provides the basis for remodeling; the younger the child, the greater the remodeling potential. Certain physes also have a relatively greater growth potential than others. Fractures adjacent to a physis undergo the greatest amount of remodeling, provided that the residual deformity is in the plane of motion of that joint. Fracture remodeling is not effective in displaced intraarticular fractures, diaphyseal fractures, malrotation, and fracture displacement or deformity not in the plane of joint motion. The amount of remodeling will be significantly diminished as a child approaches skeletal maturity.

Overgrowth

Overgrowth, especially in long bones such as the femur, is the result of the increased blood flow associated with fracture healing. Femoral fractures in children under 10 years of age frequently overgrow 1–3 cm. This accounts for the concept of *bayonet apposition* to compensate for the overgrowth that may occur over the next 1–2 years. After 10 years of age, overgrowth is less of a problem and end-on alignment is recommended.

Progressive Deformity

Injuries to a physis can result in complete or partial closure. As a consequence, angular deformity, shortening, or both can occur. The magnitude depends on the bone involved and the amount of remaining growth. Growth arrest most commonly occurs in the distal femur, distal tibia, and proximal tibia.

Healing Rate

Fractures heal more quickly in children than in adults. This effect is due to their growth potential and thicker, more metabolically active periosteum. As the older child and adolescent mature, the rate of healing slows and approaches that of an adult.

Pediatric Fracture Patterns
Nonepiphyseal Fractures

Complete. Complete fractures occur when both sides of the bone are fractured. This is the most common fracture type. These fractures may be classified as spiral, transverse, oblique, or comminuted, depending on the direction of the fracture line.

Buckle or Torus Fracture. Compression of bone produces a buckle or torus fracture. These fractures typically occur in the metaphyseal areas in young children, especially the distal radius. They are inherently stable and usually heal in 2–3 weeks with simple immobilization.

Greenstick. When a bone is angulated beyond the limits of plastic deformation, a greenstick fracture may occur. This represents bone failure on the tension side and compression or bend deformity on the opposite side. The energy has been insufficient to result in a complete fracture.

Bowing or Bend Fractures. Traumatic bowing or bend deformities are due to plastic deformation of bone. The bone was angulated beyond its limit of plastic deformation but did not fracture. Thus no fracture line is visible roentgenographically.

Epiphyseal Fractures

Fractures involving the physes are common and comprise 15–20% of all children's fractures. There is a male-to-female ratio of 2:1, and the upper extremity is involved twice as frequently as the lower. The peak incidence in males is 13–14 years and in females 11–12 years. The distal radius is the most common site, followed by the distal tibia.

Ligaments frequently insert into epiphyses. As a consequence, traumatic forces supplied to an extremity may be transmitted to the physis. The strength of the physes is enhanced by their shape and perichondrial ring. However, the physis still is not as strong biomechanically as the metaphyseal or diaphyseal bone. The physis is most resistant to traction and least resistant to torsional or angular forces.

Classification. Salter and Harris have classified epiphyseal injuries into five groups (Fig. 19–19):
- *Type I,* epiphyseal separation through the physis
- *Type II,* fracture through a portion of the physis but exiting across the metaphysis
- *Type III,* fracture through the physis but exiting across the epiphysis into the joint
- *Type IV,* a fracture line extending across the metaphysis, physis, and epiphysis
- *Type V,* a crush injury to the physis

This classification allows generalized prognostic information regarding the risk for premature physeal closure and the indications for treatment. A *type VI* injury (injury to the perichondral ring that often results in a peripheral bony bridge and rapid angular deformities) has also been suggested.

Treatment. Types I and II fractures usually can be managed by closed reduction techniques and do not require perfect alignment. A major exception is type II fractures of the distal femur. Fractures in this location carry a poor prognosis unless almost anatomic alignment is obtained by either closed or open methods. Types III and IV epiphyseal fractures require anatomic alignment because of displacement of the physis and the articular surfaces. Type

V fractures usually are recognized in retrospect and invariably result in premature growth plate closure.

Management of Pediatric Fractures

Closed Treatment

Most pediatric fractures can be managed by closed methods.

Operative Treatment

Certain pediatric fractures have been demonstrated to have better prognosis if the fractures are reduced, by either open or closed techniques, and then internally fixed. Approximately 3-4% of pediatric fractures require internal fixation. The common indications for internal fixations in children and adolescents with open physes include:
- Displaced epiphyseal fractures
- Displaced intraarticular fractures
- Unstable fractures
- Fractures in the multiply injured child
- Open fractures

In children the goals of surgery and type of internal fixation device used are different. The goals of surgery are not rigid internal fixation but, rather, attainment and maintenance of anatomic alignment. Thus, simple fixation with the use of Steinmann pins, Kirschner wires, and small cortical screws is indicated. Fractures subsequently are protected with external immobilization, usually a plaster cast, until satisfactory healing has occurred. All internal fixation devices are removed following fracture healing to prevent incorporation into the callus formation and bone and to prevent physeal damage if a physis has been transgressed by a smooth wire or pin.

External fixation also has been quite successful for certain pediatric fractures. The major indications

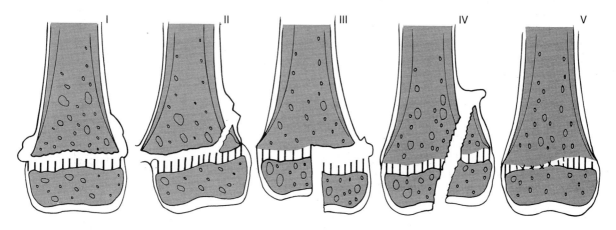

FIG. 19–19

The types of growth plate injury as classified by Salter and Harris. (From Salter RB, Harris WR: *J Bone Joint Surg* 45A:587, 1963.)

have been pelvic and open extremity fractures, especially those with extensive soft tissue loss, burns, or vascular and nerve repairs.

SPECIAL PROBLEMS

Neurovascular Injuries

The most common sites of neural or vascular injuries are the distal humerus, in which supracondylar fractures occur, and the knee, in which dislocations and physeal fractures or dislocations occur. Careful neurovascular examination is necessary for all fractures and should be documented in the patient's medical record.

Compartment Syndromes

Hemorrhage and soft tissue swelling within tight fascial compartments may result in muscle ischemia and neurovascular compromise unless decompressed surgically. This condition is called compartment syndrome. The forearm and lower leg are the major sites, and these syndromes tend to occur following supracondylar fractures at the distal humerus and tibial shaft fractures. The common findings are tense compartments, severe pain, decreased sensation in the nerves that transverse the involved compartment, and pain with passive stretch (fingers or toes) of involved muscles. In addition, once an injured extremity is placed in a cast, it is possible that a cast-induced compartment syndrome may develop. It is the responsibility of the treating physician to ensure that parents understand the signs of ischemia and appreciate that it is an emergency. The parents must contact the physician or return to the hospital immediately.

Toddler's Fracture

An oblique fracture of the distal one third of the tibia without a fibula fracture can occur with minimal trauma in children 1–3 years of age and occasionally up to 6 years of age. Limping or inability to bear weight is a common complaint. These fractures may not be visible roentgenographically, but occasionally oblique roentgenograms may be helpful. A physical examination may show minimal soft tissue swelling, pain, and slight warmth.

Child Abuse

Fractures attributable to child abuse constitute a special issue that constantly must be considered in trauma assessment of the infant and younger child, especially those 3 years of age or less (see Chapter 1). Multiple fractures that are visible roentgenographically at different stages of healing are a classic sign. If a child has been shaken, frequently areas adjacent to the epiphysis on the metaphyseal side will fracture, producing the appearance of metaphyseal "corner" fractures.

Long bone fractures, especially spiral fractures of the humeral, tibial, or femoral shaft, suggest that someone has forcefully twisted the extremity. When there is any suspicion of abuse, the child should be admitted to the hospital for full assessment. Roentgenograms of a specific area are appropriate, but a bone scan may be more helpful in identifying other fractures, old and new. A thorough physical examination focusing on soft tissues, the skeletal system, and the cranium, along with a careful examination of the retina for hemorrhage or detachment, is important.

REFERENCES

Behrman RE, Kliegman RM, Jenson HB, editors: *Nelson textbook of pediatrics,* ed 16, Philadelphia, 2000, WB Saunders, Chapter 689.

Green NE, Swiontkowski MF: *Skeletal trauma in children,* ed 2, vol 3, Philadelphia, 1998, WB Saunders.

King J, Kiefendorf D, Apthorp J, et al: Analysis of 429 fractures in 189 battered children, *J Pediatr Orthop* 8:585–589, 1988.

Metabolic Bone Disease

Metabolic bone disease may occur from disorders that primarily affect bone, cartilage, and collagen or that indirectly affect bone mineralization. Primary bone disorders often occur in the fetus or young infant, such as the skeletal dysplasia-like syndromes (e.g., achondroplasia, Kneist syndrome, and osteogenesis imperfecta).

Patients with metabolic disorders that produce indirect effects may appear normal at birth, and signs of bone disease may develop later. The signs of bone disease may occur after or concomitant with the manifestations produced by the underlying metabolic disorder (e.g., homocystinuria, Marfan syndrome, Gaucher disease, or renal rickets). The *treatment* of primary disorders of bone is limited, and therapy of inborn errors of metabolism must be tailored to the specific disease (see Chapter 5).

REFERENCES

Engelbert RHH, Uiterwaal CSPM, Gulmans VAM, et al: Osteogenesis imperfecta in childhood: prognosis for walking, *J Pediatr* 137:397–402, 2000.

Shaw NJ, Boivin CM, Crabtree NJ: Intravenous pamidronate in juvenile osteoporosis, *Arch Dis Child* 83:143–145, 2000.

Bone Tumors and Cystic Lesions

Benign bone tumors and cystic lesions are common in childhood. Some represent fibrous dysplasia and others are benign tumors, whereas subacute osteomyelitis **(Brodie abscess)** and eosinophilic granuloma represent lesions unrelated to abnormal osseous or cartilage growth (Table 19–12). Many

TABLE 19–12
Benign Bone Tumors and Cysts

Disease	Characteristics	Roentgenography	Treatment	Prognosis
Osteochondroma (osteocartilaginous exostosis)	Common; distal metaphysis of femur, proximal humerus, proximal tibia; painless, hard, nontender mass	Bony outgrowth, sessile or pedunculated	Excision, if symptomatic	Excellent; malignant transformation rare
Multiple hereditary exostoses	Osteochondroma of long bones; bone growth disturbances	As above	As above	Recurrences
Osteoid osteoma	Pain relieved by aspirin; femur and tibia; predominantly found in boys	Dense sclerosis surrounds small radiolucent nidus, less than 1 cm	As above	Excellent
Osteoblastoma (giant osteoid osteoma)	As above, but more destructive	Osteolytic component; size greater than 1 cm	As above	Excellent
Enchondroma	Tubular bones of hands and feet; pathologic fractures, swollen bone; Ollier disease if multiple lesions are present	Radiolucent diaphyseal or metaphyseal lesion; may calcify	Excision or curettage	Excellent; malignant transformation rare
Nonossifying fibroma	Silent; rare pathologic fracture; late childhood, adolescence	Incidental roentgenographic finding; thin sclerotic border, radiolucent lesion	None or curettage with fractures	Excellent; heals spontaneously
Eosinophilic granuloma	Age 5–10 yr; skull, jaw, long bones; pathologic fracture; pain	Small, radiolucent without reactive bone; punched out lytic lesion	Biopsy, excision rare; irradiation	Excellent; may heal spontaneously
Brodie abscess	Insidious local pain; limp; suspected as malignancy	Circumscribed metaphyseal osteomyelitis; lytic lesions with sclerotic rim	Biopsy; antibiotics	Excellent
Unicameral bone cyst (simple bone cyst)	Metaphysis of long bone (femur, humerus); pain, pathologic fracture	Cyst in medullary canal, expands cortex; fluid-filled unilocular or multilocular cavity	Curettage; steroid injection into lesion	Excellent; some heal spontaneously
Aneurysmal bone cyst	As above; contains blood, fibrous tissue	Expands beyond metaphyseal cartilage	Curettage, bone graft	Excellent

of these lesions produce pain, pathologic fractures, or limp; others may be incidental findings on roentgenographic examination. The *prognosis* usually is excellent. *Treatment* is summarized in Table 19–12. Malignant bone tumors are discussed in Chapter 15.

REFERENCES

Behrman RE, Kliegman RM, Jenson HB, editors: *Nelson textbook of pediatrics,* ed 16, Philadelphia, 2000, WB Saunders, Chapters 507, 514, 706–713.

Gitelis S, Wilkins R, Conrad EU III: Benign bone tumors, *J Bone Joint Surg* 77A:1756, 1995.

CHAPTER 20

Pediatric Dermatology

David M. Allen ▼ Beth A. Drolet

BASIC DERMATOLOGIC DIAGNOSIS

The history is an essential component in evaluating a patient with a skin lesion (Table 20–1). Onset, cutaneous symptoms, and associated systemic signs or symptoms are important. Unlike other organ systems, the skin is readily available for self-diagnosis and self-treatment. Patients make diagnostic assumptions and institute therapy before seeking medical opinion. Many over-the-counter remedies are available, which may dramatically alter the appearance of a rash. Obtaining an accurate description of the original lesion improves diagnostic accuracy. Patients do not consider a topical antibiotic or anti-itch medication "treatment"; thus a severe contact dermatitis to neomycin may be missed if the patient does not admit to applying a topical antibiotic.

Dermatologists have integrated a descriptive nomenclature of skin lesions to assist with diagnosis. This nomenclature is divided into primary and secondary lesions (Tables 20–2, 20–3, and 20–4). Using these terms helps not only with generating a differential diagnosis, but also with communication between providers.

A careful examination of the skin requires both a visual and a tactile assessment. Examination of the skin must be performed systematically. The body parts must be separated into segments. Mucous membranes, hair, nails, and teeth, all of ectodermal origin, may also be involved in cutaneous disorders and should be assessed. Determination of the primary or secondary nature of the lesion is the cornerstone of dermatologic diagnosis. The primary lesion is defined as the lesion that arises de novo and is most characteristic of the disease process (Figs. 20–1, 20–2, 20–3, and 20–4). A primary lesion is not necessarily the first lesion the patient notices; two different types of primary lesions may be present. In most cases, secondary lesions are the residue, or result, of the effects of the primary lesion and rarely may be seen in the absence of a primary lesion.

The color, texture, configuration, and distribution of the lesion should be recorded. Detailed evaluation of color is important because even subtle variation may imply quite different diagnoses. When evaluating color, the physician must take into consideration the background pigmentation of the patient. For example, in deeply pigmented patients redness is masked, and subsequent assessment of the severity of the eruption may be greatly diminished. A detailed observation of configuration (Table 20–5) and distribution is also helpful. A localized or grouped eruption may suggest a cutaneous infection, whereas widespread and symmetric involvement of extensor surfaces may suggest a primary skin disorder such as psoriasis.

BIRTHMARKS

"Birthmark" is a term that describes congenital anomalies of the skin. It should not be used as a definitive diagnosis because congenital skin lesions vary greatly in their appearance and prognosis (Table 20–6).

Hemangiomas and Vascular Formations

Vascular lesions can be divided into two major categories: hemangiomas and vascular malformations. Hemangiomas are benign "tumors" (cell proliferation) of the vascular endothelium characterized by proliferative and involutional phases. Malformations are developmental defects derived from the capillary, venous, arterial, or lymphatic vessels. These lesions remain relatively static; growth is commensurate with growth of the child. Differentiating between these two entities is important because they have different prognoses and clinical implications.

TABLE 20–1
Evaluation of Patient with a Skin Lesion

Demographic Data
What are the age, gender, and race of the patient?

Morphology (Primary and Secondary Lesion)
What did the lesion or rash look like when it was first noted?
How has it changed?
Is what we are seeing today typical (e.g., a good day or bad day)?
Has the lesion blistered, bled, or drained?

Chronologic Course of the Eruption or Lesion
When did you first notice the lesion or eruption?
How long does an individual lesion last?
Do the lesions or eruptions appear in crops?
If transient, is the eruption seasonal?
Is the eruption worse at one particular time of the day?

Distribution
Where did the eruption begin?
How did it spread?
Is there a pattern to the spreading?
Does it occur on the face?
Does it occur on the palms or soles?
Any changes in hair, nails, or teeth?

Symptoms
Does the lesion or eruption itch?
Is the lesion or eruption painful?
Have there been any associated fevers?
Are there any symptoms of temperature instability?
What appears to trigger the lesion or eruption?
What appears to help alleviate symptoms?
Review of related systems?

Treatment and Skin Care
Have any prescription creams, ointments, or gels been applied?
Have any prescription or over-the-counter medications been given orally (e.g., prednisone, antibiotics, antihistamines, or antifungals)?
What over-the-counter creams, ointments, gels, lotions, or powders have been applied (e.g., topical antibiotics, steroids, antihistamines, antifungals, or emollients)?

Medical History
Has the patient had any prior skin disorders?
Does the patient have a history of chronic or recurrent infections (cutaneous, otitis, sinusitis pneumonia)
Does the patient have a history of atopy (e.g., asthma, environmental, food, or seasonal allergies)?
Does the patient have a history of drug allergies?

Family History
Does the family have a history of skin disease?
Does the family have a history of skin cancer?
Does the family have a history of atopy (asthma, seasonal allergies, drug allergies, or atopic dermatitis)?

Social History
Who lives with the patient?
Who are the caregivers?
Does the patient go to day care?
Has the patient had any contacts with similar eruptions or lesions?

Is the Patient Sexually Active?

TABLE 20–2
Terminology of Primary Lesions

Macule	Flat, well-circumscribed lesion with color up to 1 cm in size
Patch	Similar to a macule, but large (>1 cm)
Papule	Circumscribed, elevated, solid lesion <1 cm in diameter
Nodule	An elevated, solid lesion with depth up to 2 cm
Tumor	A large circumscribed lesion with depth >2 cm
Plaque	An elevated lesion >2 cm in size
Pustule	A papule that contains purulent exudate, <1 cm
Vesicle	Circumscribed, elevated, fluid filled, <1 cm diameter
Bulla	Fluid-filled lesion >1 cm
Wheal	Rounded or flat-topped edematous plaque that is transient; varies greatly in size

TABLE 20–3
Terminology of Secondary Lesions

Scale	Results from abnormal keratinization
	May be fine, or sheet-like
Crust	Dried collection of serum and cellular debris
Erosion	Caused by loss of the epidermis
	Moist, shallow lesion
Ulcer	Circumscribed, depressed, focal loss of entire epidermis into dermis
	Heals with scarring
Atrophy	A shallow depression
	Results from thinning of epidermis or dermis
Scar	Thickened, firm, and discolored collection of connective tissue
	The result of dermal damage
	Initially pink, and lightens with time
Sclerosis	Circumscribed or diffuse hardening of skin, usually forms in a plaque
Lichenification	Accentuated skin lines/markings
	Results from thickening of the epidermis
Excoriation	Superficial erosion, linear, caused by scratching
Fissures	Linear breaks within the skin surface
	Usually painful

TABLE 20–4
Special Terms in Dermatology

Telangiectasia	Dilated superficial blood vessels
Petechiae	Small, circumscribed macule resulting from extravasated blood
Purpura	Large, circumscribed patch or plaque of extravasated blood (ecchymosis/bruise); does not blanch with applied pressure
Milia	Superficial, white, small epidermal keratin cyst
Cyst	A papule or nodule with an epidermal lining composed of fluid or solid material
Comedone	A plugged hair follicle (whitehead/blackhead)

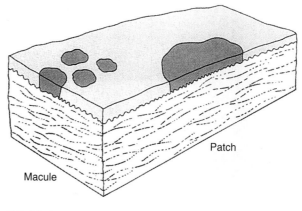

FIG. 20–1

Primary lesions. Flat, nonpalpable. (From Swartz MH: *Textbook of physical diagnosis: history and examination,* Philadelphia, 1989, WB Saunders.)

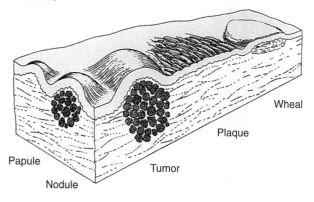

FIG. 20–2

Primary lesions. Palpable, elevated, solid masses. (From Swartz MH: *Textbook of physical diagnosis: history and examination,* Philadelphia, 1989, WB Saunders.)

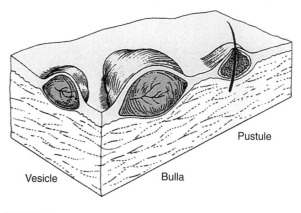

FIG. 20–3

Primary lesions. Palpable, elevated, fluid-filled masses. (From Swartz MH: *Textbook of physical diagnosis: history and examination,* Philadelphia, 1989, WB Saunders.)

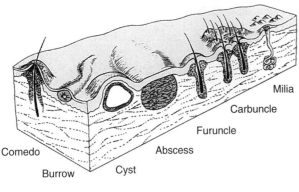

FIG. 20–4

Special primary lesions. (From Swartz MH: *Textbook of physical diagnosis: history and examination*, Philadelphia, 1989, WB Saunders.)

TABLE 20–5
Configuration of Lesions

Linear	Lesions arranged in straight lines that may imply external insult or could imply developmental anomaly occurring along embryonic lines (lines of Blaschko)
Nummular	Round, coin-sized and -shaped
Annular	Circular or ring-like with central clearing: Polycyclic/serpiginous variations and confluence of annular lesions
Iris/targetoid	Ring-like with central dark redness giving a characteristic "bull's-eye" appearance
Grouped	Clustered
Reticular	Lacy or net-like
Dermatomal	Following dermatomal distribution
Zosteriform	Following dermatomal distribution

Hemangiomas

Hemangiomas are the most common soft tissue tumors of infancy, occurring in approximately 5–10% of 1-year-old infants. True hemangiomas are characterized by a growth phase, marked by endothelial proliferation and hypercellularity, and by an involutional phase. Hemangiomas are heterogeneous, their appearance dictated by the depth and location in the skin, as well as by the stage of evolution. In the newborn, hemangiomas may originate as a pale white macule with thread-like telangiectasia. When the tumor proliferates, it assumes its most recognizable

form, a bright red, slightly elevated, noncompressible plaque. Hemangiomas that lie deeper in the skin are soft, warm masses with a slightly bluish discoloration. Frequently, hemangiomas have both a superficial and a deep component. They range from a few millimeters to several centimeters in diameter and are usually solitary; up to 20% involve multiple lesions. Hemangiomas occur predominantly in females (3:1) and have an increased incidence in premature infants. Approximately 55% are present at birth; the remainder develop in the first weeks of life. Superficial hemangiomas have reached their maximal size by 6–8 months, but deep hemangiomas may grow for 12–14 months. They then undergo slow, spontaneous resolution, which takes 3–10 years.

Despite the benign nature of most cutaneous hemangiomas, a small number cause functional compromise or permanent disfigurement. Ulceration, the most frequent complication, can be painful and has a risk of infection, hemorrhage, and scarring.

The **Kasabach-Merritt phenomenon,** a complication of a rapidly enlarging vascular lesion, is characterized by hemolytic anemia, thrombocytopenia, and coagulopathy. These massive tumors are usually a deep red-blue color, are firm, grow rapidly, have no sex predilection, and tend to proliferate for a longer period (2–5 years). Most patients with Kasabach-Merritt phenomenon do not have typical hemangiomas but have other proliferative vascular tumors, usually kaposiform hemangioendotheliomas or tufted angiomas. The Kasabach-Merritt phenomenon necessitates aggressive (often multimodality) treatment and carries a significant mortality rate.

Periorbital hemangiomas pose considerable risk to vision (i.e., amblyopia) and should be carefully monitored. Hemangiomas involving the ear may decrease auditory conduction, which ultimately may cause speech delay. Multiple cutaneous **(diffuse hemangiomatosis)** and large facial hemangiomas may be associated with visceral hemangiomas. **Subglottic hemangiomas** are manifested as hoarseness and stridor; progression to respiratory failure may be rapid. Approximately 50% of affected infants have associated cutaneous hemangiomas; therefore, "noisy breathing" in an infant with a cutaneous hemangioma involving the chin, lips, mandibular region, and neck warrants direct visualization of the airway. Symptomatic airway hemangiomas develop in over 50% of infants with extensive facial hemangiomas in the "beard" distribution.

Extensive cervicofacial hemangiomas may be associated with multiple anomalies, including *p*osterior fossa malformations, *h*emangiomas, *a*rterial anomalies, *c*oarctation of aorta and cardiac defects, and *e*ye abnormalities **(PHACES syndrome).** This syndrome has a marked female predominance (9:1)

TABLE 20–6
Common Birthmarks

Color/Lesion	Birthmark	Location	Other
Brown/macule or patch	Café-au-lait macule	Variable, trunk	Associated with neurofibromatosis
Brown (<20 cm)/ plaque (see text)	Congenital melanocytic nevus	Scalp, trunk	Possible increased risk of melanoma
Brown (>20 cm)/ plaque (see text)	Giant melanocytic nevus	Trunk most common	3–7% risk of melanoma, neuro-cutaneous melanosis
Brown-flesh colored/ plaque	Epidermal nevus	Variable, trunk and neck	
Red/patch	Port-wine stain	Variable, face most common	Associated with Sturge-Weber syndrome
Red/papule or plaque	Hemangioma	Variable, head and neck most common	Facial lesions (beard distribu-tion) associated with airway lesions
Red-purple/plaque	Lymphatic malformation	Variable, trunk, proximal leg	Often have a vesicular appearance
Gray-blue/patch	Mongolian spot (dermal melanosis), nevus of Ito	Buttocks, lower trunk	Usually resolve spontaneously
Gray-blue/patch	Nevus of Ota	Forehead and eyelids	Ocular pigmentation
Gray-blue/patch	Nevus of Ito	Posterior shoulder	
Blue/nodule	Dermoid cyst	Scalp, face, neck	May connect to CNS if midline
Blue-purple/nodule	Cephalhematoma	Scalp	
Blue-purple/plaque	Venous malformation	Variable	Enlarge slowly over time
Yellow-orange/plaque	Nevus sebaceus	Scalp, face, neck	Basal cell carcinoma may arise within lesion
Yellow-orange/nodule	Congenital juvenile xanthogranuloma	Trunk	
Yellow-brown/papule or nodule	Mastocytoma	Variable	May become urticarial or blister
Hypertrichosis/plaque	Congenital melanocytic nevus	Scalp, trunk	
Hypertrichosis/tumor	Plexiform neurofibroma	Trunk most common	Associated with neurofibromatosis
Hypertrichosis/plaque	Smooth muscle hamartoma	Trunk	
White/patch	Nevus anemicus	Variable	
White/patch	Nevus depigmentosus	Variable	

and is thought to represent a developmental field defect that occurs during the eighth to tenth week of gestation. Strokes are common. **Lumbosacral hemangiomas** suggest an occult spinal dysraphism with or without anorectal and urogenital anomalies. Imaging of the spine is indicated in all patients with midline cutaneous hemangiomas in the lumbosacral area.

Most hemangiomas do not necessitate medical intervention and will involute spontaneously; however, if complications arise and treatment is warranted, oral systemic corticosteroids are the mainstay of therapy.

Pyogenic Granuloma

A pyogenic granuloma is not congenital but is an acquired, benign vascular tumor. These lesions are most commonly seen in toddlers and young children. They occur on the face in the periocular region and on the oral mucosa, hands, fingers, proximal upper extremity, and the shoulders. Initially they appear to be inconsequential, pink-red papules that often appear after minor trauma. The lesions grow slowly over a period of months to produce a bright red, vascular, often-pedunculated papule measuring 2–10 mm. The lesions often have the appearance of granulation tissue and are very friable. When traumatized, these lesions may bleed profusely, often requiring emergent medical attention. Pulsed-dye laser therapy or surgical excision provides the most definitive treatment option.

Vascular Malformations

Vascular malformations are congenital abnormalities that are composed of anomalous capillaries, veins, lymphatics, or any combination of the three.

Transient Macular Stains (Salmon Patches)

Transient macular stains (salmon patches) are present in up to 70% of normal newborns. They are usually found on the nape of the neck, the eyelids, and the glabella. Most of the facial lesions fade by 1 year of age, but those on the neck are more persistent. Surveys of adult populations confirm the persistence of the nuchal lesions in approximately 25% of the population.

Port-Wine Stain

Port-wine stains (nevus flammeus) are malformations of the superficial capillaries of the skin. These lesions are present at birth and should be considered permanent developmental defects. Port-wine stain lesions may be only a few millimeters in diameter or may cover extensive areas, occasionally involving up to half the body surface. They do not proliferate after birth; any apparent increase in size is caused by growth of the child. A port-wine stain may be localized to any body surface, but facial lesions are the most common. Port-wine stains are pink-red, sharply demarcated macules and patches in infancy. With time they darken to a purple or "port wine" color and may develop a pebbly or slightly thickened surface.

The most successful treatment modality in use is the pulsed-dye laser, which is usually quite effective in fading these lesions. Treatment is more effective if undertaken in infancy.

Most port-wine stains occur as isolated defects and do not indicate systemic malformations. Rarely, they may suggest ocular defects or specific neurocutaneous syndromes. Children with facial port-wine stains involving skin innervated by the V1 branch of the trigeminal nerve should have a thorough ophthalmologic and neuroimaging evaluation in infancy, because these children are at risk for Sturge-Weber syndrome. **Sturge-Weber syndrome** (encephalofacial angiomatosis) consists of a facial port-wine stain, usually in the cutaneous distribution of the first branch of the trigeminal nerve; a leptomeningeal angiomatosis; mental retardation; seizures; hemiparesis contralateral to the facial lesions; and ipsilateral intracortical calcification. Ocular manifestations are frequent and include buphthalmos, glaucoma, angioma of the choroid, hemianoptic defects, and optic atrophy. Roentgenograms of the skull of the older child show pathognomonic "tramline," double-contoured calcifications in the cerebral cortex on the same side as the port-wine stain. Computed tomography (CT) scan may detect the calcifications in the younger child before they are apparent on roentgenograms; magnetic resonance imaging (MRI) has replaced the CT scan as the diagnostic modality of choice. The prognosis depends on the extent of cerebral involvement, rapidity of progression, and response to treatment. Anticonvulsant therapy and neurosurgical procedures have been of value in some patients.

Klippel-Trénaunay syndrome is characterized by a cutaneous vascular malformation (usually a port-wine stain), venous varicosities, and overgrowth of the bony structures and soft tissues of the involved part. Complications are severe edema, phlebitis, thrombosis, ulceration of the affected area, and vascular malformations involving the viscera. Port-wine stains also occur with moderate frequency in **Beckwith-Wiedemann syndrome** (macroglossia, omphalocele, macrosomia, hyperinsulinemic hypoglycemia, and cytomegaly of the fetal adrenal gland), **Roberts syndrome,** and **Cobb syndrome** (cutaneomeningospinal angiomatosis).

Venous and Lymphatic Malformations

Venous malformations present as soft, blue, compressible plaques and nodules that may occur on any skin surface. They appear at birth and enlarge slowly with time secondary to engorgement of the anomalous vessels. Venous malformations may be quite small and of minimal concern, or very large lesions that can be severely disfiguring and may be complicated by thrombosis, infection, and edema of surrounding tissue.

Lymphatic malformations (lymphangiomas) are composed of dilated lymph channels that are lined by normal lymphatic endothelium. They may be superficial or deep and often is are associated with anomalies of the regional lymphatic vessels.

The term *lymphangioma circumscriptum* is used to describe the most common type of lymphatic malformation, which may be present at birth or appear in early childhood. Areas of predilection are the oral mucosa, the proximal limbs, and the joint flexures. These lesions consist of clustered red to purple, gelatinous papules measuring 2–5 mm in size.

Cystic hygroma is a benign, congenital, multilocular mass of anomalous cystic lymph vessels. It is usually found in the neck region. Surgical excision or sclerotherapy is the available treatment option for venous and lymphatic malformations. The tumors tend to increase in size and should be treated by surgical excision.

Epidermal Nevi

Epidermal nevi are a group of lesions that are found in the neonatal period. Most consist of an overgrowth of keratinocytes that often have an identifiable differentiation toward one of the cutaneous appendages. They vary considerably in their size, clinical appearance, histologic characteristics, and evolution, depending on their topographic location. Lesions occurring in sites normally rich in sebaceous glands (e.g., the scalp) may look like sebaceous nevi, whereas others, found in areas where the epidermis is thick (e.g., the elbow) look primarily warty in nature.

The most common type of epidermal nevus in the newborn infant is the nevus sebaceus, a hairless, papillomatous, yellow or pink, slightly elevated plaque on the scalp, forehead, or face. These lesions have a characteristic shape, often being oval or lancet shaped. Because a significant incidence of basal cell epitheliomas occurs in these lesions after puberty, they should be removed surgically.

REFERENCES

Behrman RE, Kliegman RM, Jenson HB, editors: *Nelson textbook of pediatrics*, ed 16, Philadelphia, 2000, WB Saunders, Chapters 650, 651, 653.

Drolet BA, Esterly NB, Frieden IJ: Hemangiomas of children, *N Engl J Med* 341(3):173–181, 1999.

Enjolras O, Mulliken J. Vascular tumors and vascular malformations, new issues, *Adv Dermatol* 13:375–423, 1998.

Enjolras O, Riche MC, Merland JI: Facial port-wine stains and Sturge-Weber syndrome, *Pediatrics* 76(1):48–51, 1985.

PIGMENTED LESIONS AS BIRTHMARKS
Dermal Melanosis (Mongolian Spot)

The most frequently encountered pigmented lesion is the mongolian spot, which occurs in 70–96% of black, Oriental, and Native American infants and in approximately 5% of white infants. Although most of these lesions are found in the lumbosacral area, they also occur at other sites. The lesion is macular and gray-blue, lacks a sharp border, and may cover an area 10 cm or larger. Most lesions gradually disappear during the first few years of life; aberrant lesions in unusual sites are more likely to persist.

Café-au-Lait Macules

Café-au-lait spots are pigmented macules that may be present in the newborn infant but tend to develop during childhood. They range in color from very light brown to a chocolate brown. Classically, café-au-lait macules are associated with neurofibromatosis. As many as five café-au-lait macules are found in 1.8% of newborns and 25–40% of normal children, and have no significance. Children with multiple café-au-lait macules should be evaluated carefully for additional stigmata of neurofibromatosis type 1. Six or more lesions (>0.5 cm in length) are suggestive of the diagnosis, especially when accompanied by "freckling" in the flexures. The axillary and inguinal freckles actually represent tiny café-au-lait macules. Café-au-lait spots are usually the first cutaneous lesions to appear in a patient with neurofibromatosis, but additional genetic and clinical investigations may be needed to establish a diagnosis (Table 20–7).

The pigmented patches of McCune-Albright syndrome (polyostotic bone dysplasia, café-au-lait spots, and multiple endocrine disorders) are also referred to as café-au-lait macules; however, they are usually unilateral, elongated, and large (>10 cm) and often have a ragged, irregular border (see Chapter 17).

Congenital Melanocytic Nevi

Approximately 1–2% of newborn infants have melanocytic nevi. Small lesions (as opposed to giant pigmented nevi) are flat or slightly elevated plaques, often with an oval or lancet configuration. Most lesions are dark brown; scalp lesions may be red-brown at birth. The pigmentation within an individual lesion is often variegated or speckled with an accentuated epidermal surface ridge pattern. Textural changes, deeper pigmentation, and elevation help to differentiate these lesions from café-au-lait macules. Thick, dark, coarse hair is frequently associated with congenital melanocytic nevi. These lesions vary in site, size, and number but are most often solitary. Histologically they are characterized by the presence of nevus cells in the dermis; most have nevus cells extending into the deeper dermis. These lesions pose a slightly increased risk for the development of malignant melanoma, mostly during

TABLE 20–7
NIH Consensus Criteria for Neurofibromatosis Type 1
• Definitive diagnosis requires at least two criteria
• Six or more café-au-lait macules >0.5 cm (children) or >1.5 cm (adults)
• Two or more neurofibromas or one plexiform neurofibroma
• Axillary or inguinal freckling
• Optic glioma
• Two or more Lisch nodules of the iris
• Distinctive bone changes
• First-degree relative with neurofibromatosis type 1

adult life. For this reason many dermatologists advise removal of these lesions before or near the time of puberty. Should the family elect to observe rather than excise the nevus, periodic evaluation of the lesion for surface changes and associated symptoms should be performed. Excisional biopsy is indicated in instances in which malignant change is suspected.

Congenital Giant Melanocytic Nevi

Giant congenital nevi are nevi that will be approximately 20 cm in adulthood (smaller in the newborn, approximately 5–12 cm) and are one of the most dramatic birth defects. These nevi may occupy 15–35% of the body surface, most commonly involving the trunk or head and neck region. The pigmentation often is variegated from light brown to black. The affected skin may be smooth, nodular, or leathery. Prominent, dark hypertrichosis is often present. Numerous smaller (1–5 cm) light-brown patches (satellite nevi) are diffusely distributed. Malignant melanoma develops in the nevus in approximately 2–10% of affected patients over a lifetime.

Neurocutaneous melanosis is rarely associated with giant congenital melanocytic nevi in an axial distribution; affected patients have hydrocephalus, seizures, and death from an intracranial melanoma in early childhood. Because of the significant incidence of malignant degeneration, the hideous deformity, and the intense pruritus that may accompany these lesions, staged surgical excision is usually attempted. The use of tissue expansion techniques has greatly improved the capability for surgical removal of large lesions.

Peutz-Jeghers Syndrome

The cutaneous lesions of the Peutz-Jeghers syndrome may be present at birth or develop soon thereafter. They consist of brown to blue-black macules (darker than freckles) that develop around the nose and mouth. The lips and oral mucosa are often involved, as are the hands, fingertips, and toes. Macular hyperpigmentation is the only visible sign of this autosomal dominant disorder until adolescence. In adolescence intussusception, bleeding, and subsequent anemia begin to develop; this is evidence of coexisting small bowel polyposis.

Postinflammatory Hyperpigmentation

Hyperpigmentation may be secondary to any inflammatory process in the skin and thus has many causes, including primary irritant dermatitis, infections, panniculitis, and hereditary diseases such as epidermolysis bullosa. The hyperpigmentation may result from enhanced melanosome production, larger melanin deposits in basal cells, greater numbers of keratinocytes, an increase in the thickness of the stratum corneum, or deposits of melanin in dermal melanophages.

Acquired Nevi

Acquired melanocytic nevi or "moles" are common skin lesions. Melanocytic nevi may occur at any age; however, the lesions appear to develop most rapidly in prepubertal children and teenagers. Melanocytic nevi are well delineated, round to oval brown papules. Lesions are most numerous on the face, chest, and upper torso. Family history, skin type, and sun exposure are considered major etiologic factors. Irregular pigmentation, rapid growth, bleeding, and a change in configuration or borders are worrisome signs of malignant degeneration. Surgical excision and histologic examination are indicated in moles that are changing rapidly or have such features.

Malignant melanoma is rare in childhood; however, there is an alarming increase in incidence in adolescence. Education of parents and children regarding sun exposure, sun protection, and observation of changes in moles that are suggestive of malignancy is important.

Blue nevi are rare, oval, dome-shaped, blue or deep black papules or tumors 1–3 cm in size found on the upper half of the body. They grow slowly and have little tendency to become malignant but may be difficult to differentiate clinically from vascular tumors or atypical melanocytic nevi. If the diagnosis is in question, excisional biopsy is diagnostic and curative.

REFERENCES

Behrman RE, Kliegman RM, Jenson HB, editors: *Nelson textbook of pediatrics,* ed 16, Philadelphia, 2000, WB Saunders, Chapter 657.
Chamlin SL, Williams ML: Moles and melanoma, *Curr Opin Pediatr* 10(4):398–404, 1998.
DeDavid M, Orlow S, Provost N, et al: A study of large congenital nevi and associated malignant melanoma: review of cases in the New York University registry and the world literature, *J Am Acad Dermatol* 36(3 Pt 1):409–416, 1997.
Korf BR: Diagnostic outcome of children with café au lait spots, *Pediatrics* 90(6):924–927, 1992.

VESICOBULLOUS DISEASES

In diagnosing and treating vesicobullous diseases, important historical facts are the distribution of the initial blistering, age of onset, family history, exacerbating factors, and associated symptoms. In addition to identifying the size and distribution of the primary lesions, physical examination should note the presence or absence of mucosal lesions, with particular attention paid to mucosal surfaces (the eyes and oropharynx). Signs of scarring and the presence of secondary infection must also be sought.

Accurate and timely diagnosis is essential because there are many distinct causes of cutaneous blistering. Disease severity can range from well-localized lesions of bullous impetigo to the intensely inflammatory urticarial bullae of bullous pemphigoid and the widespread, life-threatening desquamation seen in toxic epidermolytic necrolysis (Table 20–8).

The depth of separation in the skin dictates the clinical appearance of the blister (Fig. 20–5). Bullous diseases may result from loss of adhesion very superficial in the skin (subcorneal), within the epidermis (intraepidermal), or at the junction of the epidermis and dermis (subepidermal). Blisters residing beneath the stratum corneum and within the epidermis tend to be flaccid and are easily ruptured. Often no blisters are present, and all that may be appreciated are eroded areas with crust and desquamated skin. Patients with widespread intraepidermal blistering may also display the **Nikolsky sign,** which is elicited when there is an absence of cohesion between the keratinocytes of the superficial epidermis so that the separated layers are easily made to slip laterally

---

TABLE 20–8
Vesiculobullous Eruptions

Entity	Clinical Clues
Hereditary	
Epidermolysis bullosa (AR, AD)	Bullae at birth in more severe forms
	Localized or widespread
	Dystrophic nails in some forms
	Bullae induced by trauma, friction; may occur spontaneously
	Mucosal involvement in severe forms
Incontinentia pigmenti (X-linked recessive)	Crops of blisters at birth or early infancy
	Often linear
	May have coexistent streaky hyperpigmentation
	Eosinophilia
	Associated CNS, dental, ocular, cardiac, skeletal abnormalities
	Females affected; males may have Klinefelter syndrome
Porphyria cutanea tarda (AD or acquired)	On dorsal hands, other sun-exposed skin
	Heal with milia formation
	Increased fragility of skin
	Hypertrichosis
Epidermolytic hyperkeratosis (bullous congenital ichthyosiform erythroderma) (AR)	Verruciform scales in flexural surfaces
	Bullae within first week of life
	Hyperkeratosis after third month
	Collodion membrane at birth in some cases
Autoimmune	
Linear IgA disease (chronic bullous disease of childhood)	Onset usually before 6 yr of age
	Sites of predilection: perioral, periocular, lower abdomen, buttocks, anogenital region
	Annular or rosette configuration of tense blisters—"cluster of jewels"
	Mucous membranes commonly involved
	Spontaneous remission
	DIF shows linear deposits of IgA at DEJ

From Nopper AJ, Rabinowotz RG: Rashes and skin lesions. In Kliegman RM, editor: *Practical strategies in pediatric diagnosis and therapy,* Philadelphia, 1996, WB Saunders.
AD, Autosomal dominant; *AR,* autosomal recessive; *CNS,* central nervous system; *DEJ,* dermoepidermal junction; *DIF,* direct immunofluorescence; *Ig,* immunoglobulin; *KOH,* potassium hydroxide.

Continued

TABLE 20–8
Vesiculobullous Eruptions—cont'd

Entity	Clinical Clues
Autoimmune—cont'd	
Bullous pemphigoid	Large, tense subepidermal bullae
	Lower abdomen, thighs, face, flexural areas
	Oral lesions common
	DIF shows linear deposits of C3 and IgG at DEJ
Pemphigus vulgaris	Flaccid bullae, persistent erosions
	Seborrheic distribution
	Mucosal involvement very common, usually the initial manifestation
	Positive Nikolsky sign
	DIF with intercellular (desmosomal) deposits of IgG, C3
Pemphigus foliaceus	Small flaccid bullae or shallow erosions with scaling, crusting
	Back, scalp, face, upper chest, abdomen
	Oral lesions uncommon
	May resemble a generalized exfoliative dermatitis
	DIF shows intercellular deposition of IgG, C3 in superficial epidermis
Dermatitis herpetiformis	Intensely pruritic
	Associated with gluten-sensitive enteropathy
	Extensor surfaces: elbows, knees, buttocks, shoulders, neck
	Hemorrhagic lesions on palms and soles
	DIF shows granular deposition of IgA in dermal papillae
Infectious	
Bacterial	
Staphylococcal scalded skin syndrome (SSSS)	Generalized, tender erythema
	Positive Nikolsky sign
	Occasionally associated with underlying infection such as osteomyelitis, septic arthritis, pneumonia
	Desquamation, moist erosions observed
	More common in children younger than 5 years of age
Bullous impetigo	Localized benign SSSS
Viral	
Herpes simplex virus	Grouped vesicles on erythematous base
	May be recurrent in same site—lips, eyes, cheeks, hands
	Reactivated by fever, sunlight, trauma, stress
	Positive Tzanck smear, herpes culture
Varicella	Crops of vesicles on erythematous base—"dewdrops on rose petal"
	Highly contagious
	May see multiple stages of lesions simultaneously
	Associated with fever
	Positive Tzanck smear, varicella-zoster culture

From Nopper AJ, Rabinowotz RG: Rashes and skin lesions. In Kliegman RM, editor: *Practical strategies in pediatric diagnosis and therapy*, Philadelphia, 1996, WB Saunders.
AD, Autosomal dominant; *AR*, autosomal recessive; *CNS*, central nervous system; *DEJ*, dermoepidermal junction; *DIF*, direct immunofluorescence; *Ig*, immunoglobulin; *KOH*, potassium hydroxide.

TABLE 20–8
Vesiculobullous Eruptions—cont'd

Entity	Clinical Clues
Viral—cont'd	
Herpes zoster	Grouped vesicles on erythematous base limited to one or several adjacent dermatomes
	Usually unilateral
	Burning, pruritus
	Positive Tzanck smear; varicella-zoster culture
	Thoracic dermatomes most commonly involved in children
Hand-foot-mouth syndrome (coxsackievirus)	Prodrome of fever, anorexia, sore throat
	Oval blisters in acral distribution, usually few in number
	Shallow oval oral lesions on erythematous base
	Highly infectious
	Peak incidence in late summer and in fall
Fungal	
Tinea corporis	Annular scaly plaques, usually with central clearing
	Pustule formation common
	Positive KOH, fungal culture
Tinea pedis	Vesicles and erosions on instep
	Interdigital fissuring
	Positive KOH, fungal culture
Scabies	Burrow formation
	Interdigital web spaces, genitalia, ankles, lower abdomen, wrist
	Intensely pruritic
	Very contagious
	Positive scabies preparation
Hypersensitivity	
Erythema multiforme major (Stevens-Johnson syndrome)	Prodrome of fever, headache, malaise, sore throat, cough, vomiting, diarrhea
	Involvement of two mucosal surfaces, usually see hemorrhagic crusts on lips
	Target lesions progress from central vesiculation to extensive epidermal necrosis; may have sheets of denuded skin
	Associated with infections and drugs
Toxic epidermal necrolysis	Possible extension of erythema multiforme major involving more than 30% of body surface
	Severe exfoliative dermatitis
	Older children and adults
	Frequently related to drugs (e.g., sulfonamides, anticonvulsants)
	Positive Nikolsky sign
Extrinsic	
Contact dermatitis	Irritant or allergic
	Distribution dependent on the irritant or allergen
	Distribution helpful in establishing diagnosis
Insect bites	Occur occasionally following flea or mosquito bites
	May be hemorrhagic bullae
	Often in linear or irregular clusters
	Very pruritic

AD, Autosomal dominant; *AR,* autosomal recessive; *CNS,* central nervous system; *DEJ,* dermoepidermal junction; *DIF,* direct immunofluorescence; *Ig,* immunoglobulin; *KOH,* potassium hydroxide.

Continued

TABLE 20–8
Vesiculobullous Eruptions—cont'd

Entity	Clinical Clues
Extrinsic—cont'd	
Burns	Irregular shapes and configurations
	May be suggestive of abuse
	Vary from first to third degree, bullae with second and third degree
Friction	Usually on acral surfaces
	May be related to footwear
	Often activity related
Miscellaneous	
Urticaria pigmentosa	Positive Darier sign
	Coexistent pigmented lesions
	Usually presents during infancy
	Dermatographism commonly seen
Miliaria crystallina	Clean, 1–2-mm superficial vesicles occurring in crops, rupture spontaneously
	Intertriginous areas, especially neck and axillae

From Nopper AJ, Rabinowotz RG: Rashes and skin lesions. In Kliegman RM, editor: *Practical strategies in pediatric diagnosis and therapy,* Philadelphia, 1996, WB Saunders.

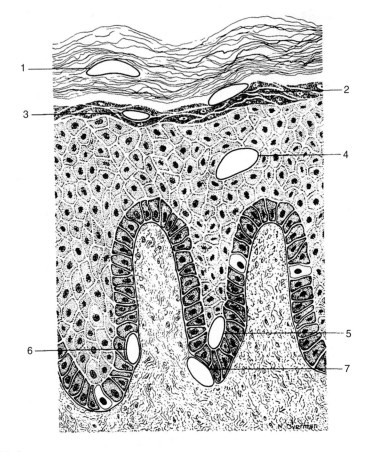

FIG. 20–5

Blister cleavage sites in the skin. *1,* Intracorneal. *2,* Subcorneal. *3,* Granular layer. *4,* Intraepidermal. *5,* Suprabasal. *6,* Junctional (between the basal cell membrane and basement membrane). *7,* Subepidermal. (From Nopper AJ, Rabinowotz RG: Rashes and skin lesions. In Kliegman RM, editor: *Practical strategies in pediatric diagnosis and therapy,* Philadelphia, 1996, WB Saunders.)

with minimal pressure. In the absence of external trauma and secondary infection, blistering diseases that result in skin separation above the basement membrane zone (BMZ) heal without scarring. In contrast, bullous disorders characterized by a plane of separation below the BMZ heal with scarring, whereas diseases characterized by a pathogenic split within the BMZ heal with variable scarring. Disorders resulting in a plane of separation within or below the BMZ demonstrate tense blisters.

The desmosomes, hemidesmosomes, and anchoring fibrils facilitate cell-to-cell adhesion. Genetic abnormalities or immune destruction of these structures leads to blistering. Desmosomes anchor adjacent keratinocytes to each other and function as intradermal adhesion plaques. Loss of the integrity of desmoglein 1 or 3 proteins results in defective desmosomal plaques and intraepidermal blister formation. Hemidesmosomes are vital in epidermal adhesion to the underlying dermis. Type XVII collagen (also known as BP180 or bullous pemphigoid antigen 2) and $\alpha_6\beta_4$ integrin are key molecules found within the hemidesmosomal plaque. Compromise of these proteins leads to defective hemidesmosome integrity and subsequent skin separation within the BMZ. Anchoring fibrils, made of type VII collagen, anchor the hemidesmosome to the underlying superficial dermis, thus providing epidermal attachment. Defects in type VII collagen have been shown to result in scarring forms of blistering diseases. Compromise of any of the above components can occur through genetic disorders or via antibody.

Autoimmune Bullous Disorders

Circulating autoantibodies recognize and attack otherwise normal "self" antigens. The clinical manifestations correlate with the location and disruption of the function of the antigens. Disruption of any of the molecules that maintain skin integrity leads to blister formation. Confirming a clinical suspicion of autoimmune bullous disease requires a skin biopsy and immunofluorescence to determine the specific component targeted. Management, course, and prognosis depend on the specific diagnosis.

Linear IgA Bullous Dermatosis and Chronic Bullous Disease of Childhood

The childhood form of linear IgA bullous dermatosis, known as chronic bullous disease of childhood (CBDC), is an acquired, self-limited, rare, immune-mediated disorder characterized by subepidermal blisters and a circulating IgA anti-BMZ antibody that targets a portion of type XVII collagen found in the hemidesmosome. There are oval or sausage-shaped, tense blisters 1–2 cm in diameter preferentially developing on the trunk, buttocks, genitals, and thighs. They are classically clustered in an annular rosette, often referred to as a "crown of jewels." Blistering may also occur on the scalp and perioral area. There is significant erythema at the base of the bullae and intense pruritus that causes the patient to rupture the bullae, leaving extensive erosions and ulcerations. Because the plane of skin separation occurs below the epidermis, the Nikolsky sign is negative. Intraoral and mucosal lesions are uncommon. Direct immunofluorescence performed on a biopsy of perilesional skin reveals a linear deposition of IgA distributed along the BMZ. The average age of onset is 5 years, with most cases remitting within 8–10 years. There is a slight female predominance. Vancomycin has been implicated in precipitating isolated cases of linear IgA disease.

Treatment is usually successful with either dapsone or sulfapyridine. Occasionally, symptomatic control can be maintained with topical steroids alone, but systemic corticosteroids are usually required. Untreated, the disease runs a chronic, relapsing course that usually resolves in the early teen years.

Dermatitis Herpetiformis

Dermatitis herpetiformis (DH) is a chronic, intensely pruritic, episodic eruption that occurs symmetrically on the extensor surfaces. Lesions occur in crops and are usually small (2–7 mm), excoriated vesicles. Rarely, lesions may be bullous, papular, or urticarial. Classically the vesicles are preceded by hours of intense pruritus. Sites of predilection include the elbows, knees, buttocks, sacrum, scapula, scalp, and face. Mucosal involvement is uncommon. Although no specific antigen has been implicated, IgA deposits are found in the skin of affected patients.

Gluten, a protein found in rye, wheat, and barley, plays a role in the pathogenesis of DH. Atrophy of jejunal villi and inflammation of the small bowel occur, with subsequent enteropathy. If the diet is high in gluten, an enteropathy identical to that of celiac disease develops in patients with DH. However, the majority of these patients do not exhibit gastrointestinal manifestations (see Chapter 11).

DH disease affects adults 20–60 years old but can occur in children as young as 10 years of age. The disease has a slight male predilection. DH patients have a higher risk of thyroid disorders, non-Hodgkin lymphoma, and small bowel lymphoma. Dapsone and sulfapyridine are the drugs of choice for treatment of DH. The need for systemic therapy can be reduced drastically by a gluten-free diet. A team approach involving the patient's family, dermatologist, pediatrician, gastroenterologist, and a skillful dietitian is helpful.

Pemphigus Vulgaris

Pemphigus is a rare autoimmune disease caused by circulating autoantibodies to desmoglein 1 and 3, desmosomal proteins involved in the intercellular adhesion of epithelial cells, resulting in intraepidermal separation and blister formation. The disease is rare in children, occurring more often in children older than 10 years of age. Round, flaccid bullae 1–4 cm in size develop on normal skin and mucous membranes. The blisters rupture easily; often only the resultant erosion and crust are present on examination. Because of the intraepidermal separation, the Nikolsky sign is present. Pemphigus vulgaris tends to heal very slowly with hyperpigmented macules and patches. Frequently these children will present with intraoral ulceration, pain, and weight loss. They often receive a misdiagnosis of recurrent aphthous ulcers or Stevens-Johnson syndrome. In many, oral lesions are the only presenting sign of pemphigus vulgaris. Stomatitis may be severe and extensive, extending into the esophagus (esophagitis dissecans superficialis) and larynx. Severe pain and dysphagia are major causes of morbidity and may necessitate use of narcotic analgesics. Diagnosis is made by clinical impression and skin biopsy for direct immunofluorescence to detect intercellular autoantibodies.

Pemphigus vulgaris is considered a serious disease. The prognosis in children is relatively good with appropriate treatment. In most children the severity of their disease is such that they require long-term corticosteroid administration. Oral prednisone 60–100 mg/day, or IV methylprednisolone 1 g/day × 5 days should be used initially in adolescent-size patients. Because of the effects of long-term corticosteroid therapy, steroid-sparing agents such as azathioprine, cyclosporine, methotrexate, cyclophosphamide, and mycophenolate may be instituted.

The differential diagnosis includes aphthous stomatitis, herpes stomatitis, herpangina, inflammatory bowel disease, and cicatricial pemphigoid.

Bullous Pemphigoid

Bullous pemphigoid (BP) is a severe inflammatory, blistering disease with circulating autoantibodies targeting type XVII collagen (BP180). It rarely occurs in young children. It is characterized by large, tense bullae that have a predilection for the intertriginous areas and flexural aspects of the arms. In children most cases begin with blistering distributed over the hands and feet; facial involvement is common. Oral involvement varies from 10–30%, but involvement of other mucosal surfaces is uncommon. Often, intensely pruritic urticarial plaques associated with outbreaks are present; occasionally, targetoid lesions may be seen. Young girls may initially exhibit vulvar involvement, which is misdiagnosed as child abuse.

The disease is chronic, with a frequently relapsing course. In adults BP tends to last 6–7 years. In children it is usually less severe, with a duration of less than 1 year. The majority of cases in children last less than 6 months. The prognosis is excellent in children, with most patients having a lasting remission.

Treatment usually requires systemic corticosteroids and oral antihistamines for pruritus.

Epidermolysis Bullosa

Epidermolysis bullosa (EB) is a group of rare, inherited, blistering disorders characterized by blister formation caused by minor trauma. These diseases are the result of genetic defects in dermal-epidermal adhesion molecules, which anchor the basal keratinocytes to the underlying papillary dermis. Over 20 subtypes of EB have been divided into three major forms (simplex, junctional, and dystrophic), based on the level of skin separation, the pattern of inheritance, and the presence of scarring. Internal involvement may occur and may be life threatening. Because blister formation is caused by defective adhesion components and is not antibody mediated, inflammation is not a factor in EB.

Epidermolysis Bullosa Simplex

Six subtypes of epidermolysis bullosa simplex (EBS) have been described; all but one has autosomal dominant inheritance. A rare form associated with muscular dystrophy is an autosomal recessive disorder. EBS is caused by defective keratin filaments, which result in fracturing of the keratinocytes in the epidermis, and subsequent blistering with minor trauma. Because the plane of skin separation is above the basement membrane zone, lesions heal without scarring. The presentation and clinical course of each subtype vary. In general, blistering begins at birth from passage through the birth canal. In the neonate blistering and large erosions primarily affect the feet, hands, neck, and lower legs. As the child begins to crawl and walk, blister formation is predominantly seen on the knees, feet, buttocks, elbows, and hands. The severity of each phenotype varies greatly.

Junctional Epidermolysis Bullosa

Junctional epidermolysis bullosa (JEB) is an autosomal recessive mechanobullous disorder with subepidermal blistering occurring within the dermal-epidermal junction. Several key molecules of the hemidesmosomes are defective or absent in JEB, which results in blister formation on minor trauma. Hemidesmosomal plaques function as glue that cements the epidermis to the underlying dermis. Several subtypes of JEB have been described, encompassing a spectrum from life-threatening disease to relatively minor involvement. Herlitz-JEB is the most severe variant of all EB and is associated with a 50–80% mortality in the first 2 years of life. Affected infants have massive erosions that heal very slowly, often forming thick granulation tissue. These infants are prone to infection, electrolyte imbalance, temperature instability, and high metabolic demands. Herlitz-JEB is associated with numerous systemic complications, including growth retardation, ocular problems, respiratory distress, and several gastrointestinal diseases. One subset of JEB is associated with pyloric atresia.

The prognosis of JEB depends on the specific subtype. With the exception of the early mortality of Herlitz-JEB, affected individuals generally have a normal life span but have significant morbidity resulting from their skin fragility. JEB usually heals without scarring, but the disease may leave an atrophic appearance.

Dystrophic Epidermolysis Bullosa

In dystrophic epidermolysis bullosa (DEB), blister formation occurs below the dermal-epidermal junction in the superficial papillary dermis. It is inherited in both autosomal dominant and recessive patterns, with the dominant variant being mild and the recessive form more severe. In recessive dystrophic-EB, widespread blistering begins at birth and results in contractures with marked scarring. Fusion of the digits with encasement of the fingers and toes and subsequent autoamputation leads to the classic "mitten deformities" of recessive dystrophic-EB. Systemic involvement may be severe, with gastrointestinal complications being the most common. Oral mucosal involvement leads to severe dysphagia; esophageal stenosis occurs from recurrent scarring. During infancy and early childhood, septicemia, pneumonia, and secondary cutaneous infections may arise. Urethral lesions may induce urinary retention, urethral stenosis, and occasionally hydronephrosis. Patients with recessive dystrophic-EB are also at increased risk for the development of nonmelanoma skin cancers. As a rule, nail changes are seen in all forms of DEB.

Management

The management of all forms of EB is symptomatic and palliative, consisting of good wound care, prevention of trauma, and treatment of infection. Intact bullae should be drained because this increases comfort and prevents extension of the blister when it is compressed.

Erythema Multiforme, Stevens-Johnson Syndrome, and Toxic Epidermal Necrolysis

Erythema multiforme minor (EM), Stevens-Johnson syndrome (SJS, or EM major), and toxic epidermal necrolysis (TEN) are acute hypersensitivity reactions characterized by cutaneous and mucosal necrosis. These disorders may represent a continuum. The clinical spectrum ranges from the well-localized lesions of EM to the serious and life-threatening extensive desquamation of TEN. These syndromes represent a T-cell–mediated hypersensitivity reaction to a number of etiologic agents; infectious organisms and drugs are the most common. Infectious agents are more closely associated with eruptions of EM minor and SJS, whereas drugs are implicated with the more severe reactions of TEN.

Erythema Multiforme Minor

Erythema multiforme minor is a common, self-limiting, acute hypersensitivity syndrome characterized by the abrupt onset of 1–3 cm, oval or round, deep red, well-demarcated, flat macules with a dusky gray or bullous center. Some of the lesions have a wheal-like appearance; unlike urticaria, these are fixed and represent epidermal cell necrosis rather than the transient tissue edema of urticaria. The classic "target lesion" consists of three concentric rings; the outermost is red, the intermediate is white, and the center is a dusky red or blue. If blistering occurs, it is mild and involves <10% of the body surface area. Mucous membrane involvement tends to be minimal and affects no more than one mucosal surface. Cutaneous lesions are symmetric and involve the upper extremities, with the dorsal hands, palms, and extensor surfaces most commonly involved.

EM minor is less severe than Stevens-Johnson syndrome and accounts for nearly 80% of EM cases. The majority of EM cases in children are precipitated by herpes simplex virus infection and may recur with each episode of herpes infection. A positive clinical history of herpes labialis is obtained in 50% of cases. Herpes simplex virus DNA is detected in 80% of children with EM, suggesting that it is the primary cause of EM minor in children. Symptomatic treatment is usually sufficient. Oral antihistamines help suppress the pruritus, stinging, and burning. The use of systemic steroids is controversial and usually not indicated. Children with recurrent lesions associated with documented herpes simplex virus infections may be candidates for pro-phylactic oral acyclovir. The prognosis is excellent, with most lesions lasting no more than 2 weeks. Healing occurs without scarring.

Stevens-Johnson Syndrome (Erythema Multiforme Major)

Stevens-Johnson syndrome is a severe, life-threatening, blistering hypersensitivity reaction. It is usually preceded by a febrile respiratory illness 1–14 days before the onset of cutaneous lesions. Involvement of at least two mucous membrane surfaces is requisite for diagnosis and is a distinguishing characteristic from EM minor. Children have extreme irritability, anorexia, and fever. The upper and lower lips are swollen and bright red with erosions and hemorrhagic crusts. Erosions of the tongue, buccal mucosa, and gingival margin may be seen. The eyelids are usually swollen. Early in the disease process there is bilateral conjunctival injection; however, this usually progresses to conjunctival erosions. There may be erosions of the vaginal or perianal mucosa. Urogenital, esophageal, and tracheal surfaces may be involved in the most severe cases. The extent of skin involvement is variable. There may only be mucosal lesions, or a combination of mucosal and skin lesions. Red macules and target-like lesions appear suddenly and tend to coalesce into large patches, with a predominant distribution over the face and trunk. Skin lesions evolve rapidly into frank bullae and areas of necrosis. The extent of epidermal detachment is 10–20% of the body surface area.

Drugs and *Mycoplasma pneumoniae* infections are the most common causes of SJS in children. HSV appears to have no role in the pathogenesis of SJS. Other precipitating factors are other viral infections, bacteria, syphilis, and deep fungal infections. The most common drugs implicated are nonsteroidal antiinflammatory drugs (NSAIDs), followed by sulfonamides, anticonvulsants, penicillins, and tetracycline derivatives.

SJS disease occurs in children 2–18 years of age and appears to be more common in younger patients than erythema multiforme. The diagnosis of SJS is clinical; there are no diagnostic tests. Confusion with potentially toxin-mediated diseases (e.g., Kawasaki disease, scarlet fever, toxic shock syndrome, and staphylococcal scalded skin syndrome) and rheumatologic disorders (e.g., Behçet disease) may occur. Patients with Kawasaki disease have conjunctival injection and hyperemia of the mucous membranes. Necrosis of the mucosal surfaces does not occur; therefore, blistering, erosions, and severe crusting are not observed. The mucosal changes of staphylococcal scalded skin syndrome are minor, and frank erosions are not present. The blistering of the skin is superficial and involves larger areas of the face and intertriginous regions. Rheumatologic disorders can usually be excluded by their chronic, less abrupt course.

SJS is a serious illness with a 5–15% mortality rate. Discontinuation of the offending agent, pain management, and supportive care are the mainstays of therapy. Children often require prolonged hospitalization. They have severe intraoral pain, resulting in very poor oral intake. Parenteral or nasogastric feeding should be instituted early, because this may accelerate the healing process. Careful fluid management and monitoring of electrolytes are essential. Skin cultures for potential infections should be performed and appropriate parenteral antibiotics given if warranted. Systemic steroids have not been demonstrated to be beneficial; they may actually increase morbidity and mortality.

The most common serious long-term sequelae of SJS involve ocular complications. Keratitis, corneal ulcerations, uveitis, severe conjunctivitis, and panophthalmitis may occur, leading to partial or complete blindness. An ophthalmology consultation with close follow-up is essential.

Toxic Epidermal Necrolysis

Toxic epidermal necrolysis (TEN) is a severe, life-threatening condition characterized by extensive skin necrosis equivalent to a second-degree burn. It is distinguished from EM minor and SJS by larger body surface area involvement (>30%) and massive, sheet-like denudation of skin. Typically >50% body surface area is affected. Individual lesions overlap with those of erythema multiforme but are more abrupt in occurrence and evolution. An upper respiratory prodrome may have been present 1–3 days before skin manifestations. Toxic epidermal necrolysis presents with high fever, severe irritability, and the abrupt onset of diffuse, deep red or dusky discoloration of the skin. The children have exquisite pain of their skin and appear to have a toxic condition. The dusky redness rapidly progresses into sheet-like peeling of the entire epidermis, leaving deep erosions. Mucous membrane involvement is usually less than that of SJS; significant overlap can occur.

Drugs (e.g., NSAIDs, particularly ibuprofen and Naprosyn) are the most common precipitating factors. Sulfonamides, anticonvulsants, penicillins, and tetracyclines have also been reported to cause TEN. Infectious organisms are not associated with the development of TEN. TEN is a severe disease with a mortality of 30–50%. Supportive care with aggressive fluid and electrolyte management, wound care, and pain control results in decreased morbidity and mortality. Superinfection and respiratory failure are the major causes of death. Severely affected children may benefit from the wound-care expertise of a burn unit. The use of systemic corticosteroids is controversial and is thought to increase the risk of infection and decrease wound healing. Intravenous gamma globulin and cyclosporine have been used with some encouraging results; controlled studies are not currently available.

Mastocytosis

Mast cell disease is a rare cutaneous disease of childhood and can result in a solitary mast cell tumor, a disseminated maculopapular eruption (urticaria pigmentosa), a bullous eruption, or a diffuse infiltration of the skin. The diagnosis can be made by demonstration of excessive numbers of mast cells on skin biopsy. A solitary mast cell tumor (mastocytoma) is the most common form and may be present at birth or develop in the first year of life.

Mastocytomas are ovoid, light tan to pink papules measuring 0.4–6 cm in size. The lesions are conspicuous by their tendency to urticate (form wheals) when rubbed; rarely in the newborn, they develop overlying blisters. Solitary lesions involute spontaneously within months to years.

Urticaria pigmentosa manifests as numerous, pink-brown, 1–2-cm oval macules. The lesions are usually located centrally and often develop later in infancy. Systemic manifestations of histamine release, such as flushing attacks, diarrhea, or generalized pruritus, may rarely be observed in patients with urticaria pigmentosa. The disseminated form may be complicated by mast cell infiltrates in internal organs. Treatment is usually not necessary, but in symptomatic patients distressing cutaneous symptoms such as dermatographism and pruritus may be helped with oral antihistamines.

Zinc Deficiency (Acrodermatitis Enteropathica)

Zinc deficiency occurs in the genetic disorder **acrodermatitis enteropathica** and as an acquired condition attributable to inadequate zinc intake. Acrodermatitis enteropathica, a rare disorder, is inherited as an autosomal recessive trait. It is characterized by acute vesicobullous, eczematous, and psoriasiform eruptions around the hands, feet, eyes, mouth, and genitals of infants. The disease is often misdiagnosed as refractory atopic dermatitis. The onset may be as early as the third week of life, but more frequently it occurs later in infancy after weaning from breast milk. Failure to thrive, hair loss, ocular changes, marked irritability, and paronychial lesions are additional features. Chronic, severe, and intractable diarrhea is the most serious manifestation. The disease is caused by a defect in zinc absorption or trans-

port; very low plasma zinc levels have been documented in untreated patients. A similar clinical picture may be seen rarely in preterm, breast-fed infants. It is theorized that their mother's milk is deficient inzinc and that preterm infants are at increased risk because their zinc stores may not be fully developed. Supplemental oral zinc sulfate is the treatment of choice and induces dramatic remissions of the disease.

REFERENCES

Amos B, Deng JS, Flynn K, et al: Bullous pemphigoid in infancy: case report and literature review, *Pediatr Dermatol* 15(2):108–111, 1998.

Assier H, Bastuji-Garin S, Revuz J, et al: Erythema multiforme with mucous membrane involvement and Stevens-Johnson syndrome are clinically different disorders with distinct causes, *Arch Dermatol* 131(5):539–543, 1995.

Behrman RE, Kliegman RM, Jenson HB, editors: *Nelson textbook of pediatrics*, ed 16, Philadelphia, 2000, WB Saunders, Chapter 660.

Diaz LA, Giudice GJ: End of the century overview of skin blisters, *Arch Dermatol* 136(1):106–112, 2000.

Esterly NB, Furey NL, Kirschner BS, et al: Chronic bullous dermatosis of childhood, *Arch Dermatol* 113(1):42–46, 1997.

Fine JD, Eady RA, Bauer EA, et al: Revised classification system for inherited epidermolysis bullosa: report of the second International Consensus Meeting on Diagnosis and Classification of epidermolysis bullosa, *J Am Acad Dermatol* 42(6):1051–1066, 2000.

Robinson ND, Hashimoto T, Amagai M: The new pemphigus variants, *J Am Acad Dermatol* 40(5 Pt 1):649–671, 1999.

Roujeau JC, Kelly JP, Naldi L, et al: Medication use and the risk of Stevens-Johnson syndrome or toxic epidermal necrolysis, *N Engl J Med* 333(24):1600–1607, 1995.

Roujeau JC: Stevens-Johnson syndrome and toxic epidermal necrolysis are severity variants of the same disease, which differs from erythema multiforme, *J Dermatol* 24(11):726–729, 1997.

DISORDERS OF THE EPIDERMIS
Atopic Dermatitis

See Chapter 8.

Contact Dermatitis

Inflammation in the top layers of the skin caused by direct contact with a substance is divided into two subtypes: contact irritant dermatitis and contact allergic dermatitis.

Primary contact irritant dermatitis is common and observed after the skin surface is exposed to an irritating chemical or undergoes repeated exposure to a substance that dries the skin. The eruption is characterized by ill-defined red patches and plaques with secondary scales. The eruption is localized to skin surfaces that are exposed to the irritant. For example, irritant diaper dermatitis is distributed in the perianal region and on the buttocks, areas repeatedly exposed to urine and feces. Contact irritant dermatitis is frequently observed on the dorsal surface of the hands in patients who repeatedly wash their hands with an irritating soap.

Allergic contact dermatitis is a form of cell-mediated immunity. This reaction can be divided into two phases, the sensitization phase and the elicitation phase. The antigens involved in allergic contact dermatitis are called haptens. These haptens can readily penetrate the epidermis and then are bound by the antigen-presenting cells (Langerhans cells) of the epidermis. The hapten is presented to T lymphocytes, and an immune cascade follows.

Contact allergic dermatitis is usually an acute and severe reaction limited to exposure sites. The initial lesions are bright red, pruritic patches, often in linear or sharply marginated, bizarre configurations. Within the patches are clear vesicles and bullae with a serosanguineous drainage. Signs and symptoms of the disease may be delayed for 7–14 days after exposure if the patient has not been previously sensitized. Upon reexposure, symptoms begin within hours and are usually more severe. The eruption may persist for weeks. Distribution of the dermatitis and a detailed exposure history are the most useful diagnostic tools. Involvement of the lower legs and distal arms suggests exposure to plants of the *Rhus* species (poison ivy or poison oak). Dermatitis of the ears (earrings), wrist (bracelet or watch), or periumbilical region (buckle of jeans or pants) suggests a metal allergy to nickel. Distribution on the dorsal surface of the feet is highly indicative of a shoe allergy, usually to dyes, rubber, or leather. Topical antibiotics (e.g., neomycin) and fragrances (e.g., soap, perfumes, and cosmetics) are frequent causes of allergic contact dermatitis.

Topical steroids are effective in treatment of allergic and irritant contact dermatitis. High potency steroids may be necessary for severe reactions of allergic contact dermatitis. Oral antihistamines or oral steroids may be required to control itching. Every effort should be made to identify the trigger because reexposure often leads to more severe reactions.

Psoriasis

Psoriasis is a common papulosquamous condition notable for well-demarcated, erythematous, scaling papules and plaques. Psoriasis occurs at all ages, including infancy; 30% of cases have an onset during childhood. The disease is characterized by a chronic and relapsing course, although spontaneous remissions can occur. Infections, stress, trauma, and medications are known to cause disease exacerbations. The disease also tends to worsen during the fall and winter, probably secondary to decreased humidity within the environment.

Various subtypes of psoriasis exist. The most common variety is plaque-type (psoriasis vulgaris), which can be localized or generalized. The lesions consist of round, well-demarcated, red plaques measuring 1–7 cm. The so-called micaceous scale is distinctive in its thick, silvery appearance, with pinpoint bleeding points (Auspitz sign) revealed upon removal of the scales. The lesions of psoriasis have a distinctive distribution, involving the extensor aspect of the elbows and knees, posterior occipital scalp, periumbilical region, lumbosacral region, and intergluteal cleft. Children often have facial lesions involving the upper inner aspect of the eyelids. Nail plate involvement is common and includes pitting, onycholysis, subungual hyperkeratosis, and "oil staining" (reddish brown subungual macular discoloration).

Guttate (drop-like) psoriasis is seen exclusively in children and young adults. Numerous 0.5–2 cm, oval or lancet-shaped, scaling, red papules and small plaques distributed over the upper torso and proximal extremities typify this form of psoriasis. Many physicians attribute the onset of guttate psoriasis to prior streptococcal infections. The possibility of concurrent streptococcal infection (including perianal streptococcal cellulitis) should be investigated in cases of new onset and flares of guttate psoriasis.

Inverse psoriasis describes the presence of marginated, bright red, macerated, scaling patches and plaques in the axillary and inguinal regions. This can be differentiated from seborrheic dermatitis, candidiasis, and noninfectious intertrigo by the well-delineated nature of the patches and plaques. The typical psoriatic scale is not seen in this variant.

Erythrodermic and pustular forms of psoriasis are severe and potentially fatal, generalized forms of psoriasis that are uncommon in children. Acute onset of generalized erythema with subsequent exfoliative scaling typifies erythrodermic psoriasis, whereas spreading, bright red plaques with the sudden onset of fine, 2–3-mm sterile pustules at the periphery of the lesions characterizes pustular psoriasis. Patients can have fever, leukocytosis, temperature instability, electrolyte and fluid abnormalities, and rarely high-output cardiac failure. The treatment of psoriasis with oral systemic corticosteroids can induce pustular psoriasis and should be avoided.

The cornerstone of topical therapy is corticosteroids. Because of the risk of atrophy, striae, and telangiectases, especially when potent fluorinated corticosteroid preparations are chronically administered, the goal is to use the least potent corticosteroid. Topical calcipotriene (vitamin D analog) is a useful adjuvant to topical steroids. Guttate psoriasis is generally quite difficult to treat with topical agents, and phototherapy is usually instituted in affected patients. Generalized erythrodermic psoriasis and pustular psoriasis may necessitate systemic intervention or Goeckerman therapy involving UVB irradiation and tar.

Seborrheic Dermatitis

Seborrheic dermatitis is an inflammatory skin disease and is common in all ages. In infancy, "cradle cap" describes the thick, waxy, yellow-white scaling of the scalp. Extension to forehead and postauricular areas is common. Diaper and intertriginous areas can have sharply demarcated erythematous patches with yellowish, "greasy," or waxy-appearing scale. Significant erythema may be present, particularly if the eruption spreads onto the face and torso. Significant postinflammatory hypopigmentation may occur after the inflammation has faded. The eruption is usually asymptomatic, which helps to differentiate it from infantile atopic dermatitis. In adolescence involvement of the scalp, eyebrows, nasal bridge, and nasolabial folds is more typical. Seborrheic dermatitis is responsive to low-potency steroids. Treatment for 3–5 days is usually adequate. Cradle cap is self-limited and resolves during the first year of life. In all ages, shampooing with zinc pyrithione (Head and Shoulders, SHS Zinc), selenium sulfide 1–2.5%, salicylic acid (TSal), or ketoconazole (Nizoral) can treat scalp scale.

Lichen Planus

Lichen planus is an uncommon dermatosis in childhood, with children accounting for less than 5% of cases. The primary lesion is a pruritic, flat-topped, polygonal, and violaceous papule, which most often arises on the flexor wrists, knees, feet, anterior shins, and shaft of the penis. Close inspection of the surface of the papule reveals a fine, whitish reticulation or streaking (Wickham striae). Mucous membranes are involved in 50% of cases, with lacy, white plaques on the buccal mucosa and infrequently on the palate, lips, and tongue. The oral and genital lesions may become erosive and extremely painful. Nail involvement may occur; characteristic findings are nail plate ridging, dystrophy, subungual hyperkeratosis, or pterygia. Variants of lichen planus are bullous, annular, linear, and hypertrophic lichen planus.

Typically, lichen planus is a chronic disorder, lasting an average of about 12–15 months, and may be cyclic, recurring 7–8 years later. More chronic cases can persist for years, with episodes of remissions and exacerbations. The underlying etiol-

ogy of lichen planus is unknown; rarely, systemic medications have been associated with lichen planus–like eruptions. Treatment includes the use of systemic antihistamines (e.g., hydroxyzine or diphenhydramine) for pruritus and the use of corticosteroids (topical, intralesional, and systemic).

Pityriasis Rosea

Pityriasis rosea is a benign, self-limited eruption occurring at any age, with peak incidence during adolescence. A solitary 2–5-cm, pink, round patch that often has a hint of central clearing, the so-called herald patch, is the first manifestation of the eruption. This herald patch is typically found on the breast, lower torso, or proximal thigh and is often misdiagnosed as fungal or eczematous in origin. One to 2 weeks later, multiple 0.5–2.0-cm, oval-to-oblong, red or tan ("fawn"-colored) macules with fine, branlike scale erupt on the torso and proximal extremities in a characteristic arrangement parallel to skin tension lines ("Christmas tree" pattern). Papular and papulovesicular variants may be seen in infants and young children. Rarely, the eruption may have an inverse distribution involving the axillae and groin. Usually the condition is asymptomatic, but mild prodromal symptoms may be present with the appearance of the herald patch; pruritus can be present in 25%. The eruption lasts 4–14 weeks, with gradual resolution. Residual hyperpigmentation or hypopigmentation can take additional months to clear. Currently there is no known etiology, although several factors suggest a viral infection (with human herpesvirus 7). There are seasonal clustering (in fall and spring), rare involvement of multiple family members, reports of prodrome, and the tendency for lifelong immunity (although rare reports of recurrent episodes exist). The differential diagnosis includes secondary syphilis, drug eruption, and another viral exanthem. Treatment is unnecessary. Pruritus can be managed with oral antihistamines, phototherapy, and low-potency topical corticosteroids.

Uncommon Papulosquamous Disorders

Gianotti-Crosti syndrome (papular acrodermatitis of childhood) was related to hepatitis B infection in Europe and Asia. In the United States, it has been associated with other infectious agents and may represent the cutaneous manifestation of a host response to multiple viral infections. The peak incidence occurs between the ages of 1–6 years. The eruption begins with the acute onset of multiple, tiny (1–2 mm), lichenoid, flesh-colored to red papules, which can coalesce to form plaques. Many of the papules look vesicular; they are very firm to palpation. The eruption involves the face, buttocks, and the ventral surface of the distal extremities, with relative sparing of the torso. The children are generally well, but pruritus may be severe. The condition is self-limited, with gradual resolution in 2–8 weeks. This eruption is usually preceded by an upper respiratory infection and may be associated with generalized lymphadenopathy and hepatosplenomegaly. Laboratory testing reveals normal complete blood counts and erythrocyte sedimentation rate; liver function tests can be elevated. Treatment involves supportive care with bland emollients and oral antihistamines if itching is severe.

PLEVA (pityriasis lichenoides et varioliformis acuta) and **PLC (pityriasis lichenoides chronica)** represent acute and chronic forms of a papulosquamous disorder of unknown etiology. Generalized crops of reddish brown macules progress to crusted papulovesicles with central necrosis. The condition has a benign course and resolves in weeks to months without significant scar formation. These eruptions may be pruritic; postinflammatory hyperpigmentation is common. Symptomatic care with oral antihistamines (e.g., diphenhydramine and hydroxyzine) and medium-potency topical corticosteroids (e.g., triamcinolone 0.1% in equal volume with Eucerin) is usually quite beneficial. Oral erythromycin (30 mg/kg/day, divided tid) has been reported to shorten the course of the eruption. Phototherapy (natural sunlight or UVB) can also ameliorate symptoms, analogous to what is usually observed in pityriasis rosea.

DISORDERS OF THE DERMIS
Granuloma Annulare

Granuloma annulare is a benign, common cutaneous disorder of childhood. Granuloma annulare may occur at any age but is most often seen in patients 6–10 years of age. The lesions are red to brown in color and annular or circinate in configuration. They are distributed on the dorsal aspect of the feet and the hands and on the extensor surface of the elbows and knees. Rarely, lesions may be distributed more widely. The lesions of granuloma annulare are asymptomatic and are often misdiagnosed as tinea corporis. The distribution, color, and lack of scaling can help to differentiate this disorder from a tinea infection. A palisading granulomatous infiltrate is seen on histologic examination. The lesions will spontaneously resolve without scarring over a period of years; thus treatment is not usually recommended.

Juvenile Xanthogranuloma

Juvenile xanthogranuloma is a benign, self-healing infiltrate of lipid-laden macrophages in the upper dermis. Twenty percent of lesions are present at birth, with 90% of lesions present by 1 year of age. The lesions of juvenile xanthogranuloma are red-yellow papules that measure 3–20 mm in size; they may be solitary or multiple. Rarely, congenital lesions will be larger (5–10 cm) and tend to have central ulceration. The plaques are round to oval in shape and frequently have overlying telangiectasia. They may occur anywhere but are most frequently seen on the scalp, face, and neck. They may be multiple and rarely may involve internal organs such as the liver, spleen, and lung. Juvenile xanthogranulomas may also involve the eye; complications include glaucoma and hyphema. The cutaneous lesions are asymptomatic and resolve spontaneously over a period of 3–6 years. No treatment is necessary.

Morphea

The term scleroderma is used to describe thickening and tightening of the skin from increased dermal fibrosis. Systemic scleroderma with internal involvement as described in adults is quite rare during childhood. Morphea is the term used for localized thickening of the skin without internal involvement; this disease is almost exclusively seen in children and carries a very different prognosis from scleroderma. Morphea most commonly affects children of school age and is quite rare in infants.

Several subtypes of morphea are known, and the clinical appearance may be quite variable. The diagnosis is often made only after histologic confirmation. Linear morphea is the most common variant and occurs in late childhood and adolescence. The lesions of linear morphea are most often solitary and affect the limbs. Early in the disease process there is red-violaceous discoloration of the skin, often associated with itching or burning. As the process progresses, the skin becomes firm and bound down, qualities that can be appreciated only by firm palpation of the skin. The purple discoloration is replaced by a white, shiny texture, and finally with brown hyperpigmentation often speckled with hypopigmentation. When fully evolved, the lesions of morphea are often lancet or linear in shape and may traverse an entire limb. Contractures may occur, resulting in significant morbidity. Morphea "en plaque" refers to a less common variant that tends to affect older children. Here the lesions are round to oval in shape, often multiple, and occur on the trunk. "En coup de sabre" (stripe of the tiger) is the term used to describe a devastating, rare variant that occurs exclusively on one side of the face. The lesions often begin on the forehead and extend down onto the nose and cheek. Here the disease process involves not only the skin, but also the underlying musculature and bone, resulting in severe facial hemiatrophy.

The pathogenesis of morphea is not fully understood. Most subtypes of childhood morphea are self-limited and resolve with minimal cutaneous changes. A notable exception to this is the coup de sabre deformity, which almost uniformly results in significant disfigurement. Potent topical steroids have been used with minimal success, but appear to be of some benefit if instituted early. Systemic immunosuppressive therapy may be used for the most severe cases.

Ehlers-Danlos Syndrome

The 10 clinical forms of Ehlers-Danlos syndrome have the common features of hyperextensible skin, joint laxity, and soft tissue fragility. In addition, bleeding episodes and cardiovascular complications are characteristic of some forms of the disorder. The skin of patients with Ehlers-Danlos syndrome is hyperextensible when stretched but snaps back with normal resiliency, in contrast to the skin in patients with **cutis laxa,** which hangs in redundant folds. In some forms the skin also is excessively fragile, and stellate, atrophic scars are found over the knees and elbows. Associated findings may include short stature, scoliosis, soft tissue contractures, multiple dislocations, periodontosis, eye defects, megacolon, and aortic aneurysms. All forms of the disease are inherited; some are autosomal dominant traits, others are autosomal recessive, and two forms are X-linked. Biochemical studies have confirmed specific enzyme defects for types IV, VI, VIIA, VIIB, VIIC, and IX.

Cutis Laxa (Generalized Elastolysis)

Cutis laxa may be congenital or acquired and is a heterogeneous group of disorders. Cutis laxa may be an isolated finding or a feature of several malformation syndromes. There are three major forms of congenital cutis laxa: one is an autosomal dominant, and two are autosomal recessive. In all forms of the disease, affected children have diminished resilience of the skin, which hangs in folds, resulting in a "bloodhound" appearance. The joints are not hypermobile, and there is no tendency to increased bruising as in Ehlers-Danlos syndrome. Elastic tissue may be greatly diminished in the dermis and is of poor quality. In the autosomal dominant form there are few complications, and the life span is usually normal. In the generalized recessive type of cutis laxa,

elastic fibers elsewhere in the body are defective, resulting in inguinal, diaphragmatic, and ventral hernias, rectal prolapse, diverticula of the gastrointestinal and genitourinary tracts, pulmonary emphysema, and aortic aneurysms. Cardiorespiratory complications may cause death in early childhood. The recessive form, cutis laxa with retarded growth and skeletal dysplasia, is typified by intrauterine growth retardation, congenital dislocation of the hips, and a peculiar facies with frontal bossing, antimongoloid slanting of the palpebral fissures, and widening of the fontanels. Unlike other loose-skin syndromes, cutis laxa shows almost normal wound healing. Therefore, affected children are good candidates for cosmetic plastic surgery and its attendant psychologic benefits.

REFERENCES

Behrman RE, Kliegman RM, Jenson HB, editors: *Nelson textbook of pediatrics,* ed 16, Philadelphia, 2000, WB Saunders, Chapters 663, 665.

Freyer DR, Kennedy R, Bostrom BC, et al: Juvenile xanthogranulomas: forms of systemic disease and their clinical implications, *J Pediatr* 129(2):227–237, 1996.

Hernandez-Martin A, Baselga E, Drolet BA: Juvenile xanthogranuloma, *J Am Acad Dermatol* 36(3 Pt 1):355–367, 1997.

DISORDERS OF THE SUBCUTANEOUS FAT

Subcutaneous Fat Necrosis

The lesions of subcutaneous fat necrosis appear 1–4 weeks after birth as solid nodules or plaques and are found on the cheeks, buttocks, back, arms, and thighs. The affected fat is firm, and the overlying skin may appear reddish or violaceous in color, with the texture of an orange peel. Usually the lesions resolve in several weeks or months without complications. Subcutaneous fat necrosis has been associated with hypercalcemia. Infants with this disorder often have a history of birth trauma or neonatal hypoxia. Additional possible precipitating causes of fat necrosis are cold exposure, asphyxia, cardiac surgery, and peripheral circulatory collapse.

Panniculitis

Panniculitis is a descriptive term applied to a broad group of disorders in which the primary pathology is inflammation of the subcutaneous fat. It may occur as an isolated and well-localized disease or may be the manifestation of an underlying systemic disorder.

Because the site of pathology of panniculitis is the subcutaneous fat, the overlying epidermis and dermis obscure the clinical view. This compromises the clinician's ability to accurately diagnose a specific type of panniculitis by physical examination. The lesions appear as red or violaceous nodules or plaques. Occasionally they may have a blue hue or be hyperpigmented; ulceration is common. They tend to be discrete and well circumscribed. They occur most frequently on the legs and abdomen. Although some diagnostic considerations may be made based on the distribution, history of onset, and other known underlying disorders, a definitive diagnosis relies on biopsy and histologic examination.

Cold Panniculitis

Cold panniculitis is seen at all ages but is most common in newborns and children less than 1 year old. The subcutaneous tissue of neonates and infants is relatively high in saturated fats compared with older children and adults. It is believed that crystallization of fat may occur with subsequent fat necrosis when exposed to low ambient temperatures. It has been described in a variety of settings, including ambient cold exposure and application of ice to induce hypothermia before cardiac surgery and to abort supraventricular tachycardia. The term "popsicle panniculitis" refers to a subset of infants in whom buccal panniculitis was triggered after the infants sucked on flavored ice.

Symmetric, tender, indurated, red to violaceous plaques and nodules typically occur on the cheeks 1–3 days after exposure to cold. The diagnosis is made with a suggestive history and examination. Results of such laboratory studies as cold agglutinins, cryoglobulins, basic chemistries, and a complete blood count are usually normal.

The skin lesions are self-limited and usually resolve over 2–4 weeks without scarring. No treatment is necessary, but early recognition of cold panniculitis is important in reassuring parents and avoiding undue anxiety or laboratory studies.

Erythema Nodosum

Erythema nodosum (EN) is a cutaneous, delayed cell-mediated hypersensitivity reaction. The clinical eruption usually presents as symmetric, tender, red, 1–5-cm discrete nodules and plaques on the anterior shins. Occasionally, lesions may occur on the thighs, ankles, knees, arms, face, and neck. Ulceration and draining are not typical of erythema nodosum. Fever, chills, and generalized malaise are usually present, with associated leukocytosis during the initial onset of new lesions. The erythema usually evolves into a brownish red or bluish bruise-like color 1–2 weeks after initial onset; the lesions usually resolve in 3–6 weeks without scarring.

Erythema nodosum is associated with a wide range of systemic diseases and is the most common form of skin hypersensitivity to tuberculosis. After the diagnosis of EN has been made, an investigation for a possible underlying cause is essential. Although the associations are numerous in children (tuberculosis, β-hemolytic streptococcal infections, other respiratory infections, inflammatory bowel disease, invasive fungal diseases, and drugs [oral contraceptives]), in many no etiology is identified.

EN can occur at any age, but has the highest incidence between the ages of 20–30 years. Adult females are three times more often affected than males; in children, girls are only slightly more affected.

Diagnosis of EN may generally be based on the characteristic physical examination. Definitive diagnosis requires a deep skin biopsy, including the subcutaneous fat. The erythrocyte sedimentation rate is elevated. A chest radiographic examination and complete blood counts should be performed, as well as an ASO titer, throat culture, PPD, and possibly fungal antigen skin tests.

Treatment is based on the identification and management of the underlying disorder. Bed rest with leg elevation and wet dressings help reduce the pain. In severe cases NSAIDs are helpful. Systemic corticosteroids are also quite effective but are potentially dangerous if an underlying infection is present. Intralesional corticosteroids are useful for individual lesions.

REFERENCES

Behrman RE, Kliegman RM, Jenson HB, editors: *Nelson textbook of pediatrics,* ed 16, Philadelphia, 2000, WB Saunders, Chapter 666.

Cribier B, Caille A, Heid E, et al: Erythema nodosum and associated diseases, *Int J Dermatol* 37:667–672, 1998.

Ter Poorten JC, Hebert AA, Ilkiw R: Cold panniculitis in a neonate, *J Am Acad Dermatol* 33:383–385, 1995.

White JW Jr, Winkelmann RK: Weber-Christian panniculitis: a review of 30 cases with this diagnosis, *J Am Acad Dermatol* 39:56–62, 1998.

DISORDERS OF HAIR

Hair loss is a dramatic cutaneous condition. Hair loss is divided into scarring and nonscarring alopecia. The evaluation should include a complete history with special attention to nutrition, infectious contacts, family history of hair loss or autoimmune disorders, and recent illness (within 3 months). Physical examination should include evaluation of the scalp and the hair shaft. Are the hair shafts falling out, or are there broken, frayed tips of the hair shaft, which would suggest trauma? Is there significant scaling, erythema, or scarring of the scalp, which would suggest hair loss secondary to a primary skin disease of the scalp? Regional lymph-

TABLE 20–9
Differential Diagnosis of Hair Loss

Disease	Age of onset	Clinical Features	Associated Findings	Prognosis
Alopecia areata	Variable	Discrete 2–5-cm round, coin-shaped patches of hair loss; may progress to total alopecia	May see loss of eyebrows, eyelashes Nail pits	Variable
Monilethrix	Infancy	Dull, dry brittle hair that breaks easily	Follicular keratosis	May improve slightly as child ages
Tinea capitis	2–7 yr of age	Ill-defined round patches of hair loss with scaling and crusting of the scalp	May have tinea infection of face or neck Posterior cervical lymphadenopathy	Complete recovery after antifungal treatment
Telogen effluvium	Variable, more prominent in toddlers	Diffuse thinning of the hair, without discrete patches of alopecia Scalp normal	Follows severe illness or high fever by 3–6 mo	Resolves spontaneously over several months
Loose anagen syndrome	6 mo–6 yr	Seen in fair, blonde children Presenting complaint is that the hair is easily and painlessly pulled from the scalp in clumps Scalp normal	None	Improves with age
Trichotillomania	10–16 yr	Circumscribed, irregular areas of hair loss with broken or frayed hair shafts Excoriations in scalp	Obsessive-compulsive disorder in older children	Improves with behavior modification
Traction alopecia	2–8 yr	Patchy, thinning of hair with broken hair shafts Scalp is normal	Trauma (e.g., tight braiding of the hair)	Improves slightly with age

adenopathy suggests an occult infection. Examination of the nails is helpful because most disease processes will affect both the hair and the nails (Table 20–9).

CUTANEOUS BACTERIAL INFECTIONS

See Chapter 10.

FUNGAL INFECTIONS OF THE SKIN

See Chapter 10.

CUTANEOUS VIRAL INFECTIONS
Warts

Warts are a common cutaneous infection caused by the human papilloma virus. Warts can occur at any age. The most typical lesion is a small (2–5-mm) papule with a papillated or verrucous surface. Warts are classically distributed on the fingers, toes, elbows, and knees. Warts may also be found on the nose, ears, and lips. Filiform warts are 2-mm verrucous, exophytic, papules that have a narrow or pedunculated base. Flat warts are multiple 2–4 mm, flat-topped papules clustered on the dorsal surface of the hands or on the face. Warts are typically self-limited and resolve spontaneously over a period of years. The only treatment options that are currently available are destructive modalities such as liquid nitrogen; these are painful and are not 100% effective. The human papilloma virus infects the keratinocytes of the skin and mucous membranes and cannot cause systemic disease.

Molluscum Contagiosum

The lesions of molluscum contagiosum are small, 2–4-mm, pearly white papules. These papules are dome shaped with a central umbilication and occur in moist, intertriginous regions such as the axillae, groin, and neck. Rarely they may occur on the face in the periocular region. The infection typically affects toddlers and young children. The lesions are caused by infection with a pox virus and are self-limited, resolving over a period of months. Infection with molluscum contagiosum may be complicated by a surrounding dermatitis; systemic disease does not occur. Severely immunocompromised patients or those with extensive atopic dermatitis often have numerous, widespread lesions. Treatment options are limited to destructive modalities such as liquid nitrogen, cantharidin, or curettage.

Herpes Simplex

See Chapter 10.

CUTANEOUS INFESTATIONS

Arthropods are common in the environment. Although many can bite or sting humans, very few infest humans. Arachnids (mites) are the most common, and they parasitize humans and animals by burrowing into the skin and depositing eggs within the skin.

Scabies

Scabies is the most common infestation. The clinical presentation varies, depending on the age of the patient, duration of infestation, and immune status of the patient. Severe and paroxysmal itching is the hallmark. The patient's complaints of itching are frequently worse than the eruption would suggest. Most children exhibit an eczematous eruption composed of red, excoriated papules and nodules. The classic linear papule or burrow is often difficult to find. Distribution is the most diagnostic finding; the papules are found in the axillae, umbilicus, groin, penis, instep of the foot, and web spaces of the fingers and toes. Infants infested with scabies have diffuse erythema, scaling, and pinpoint papules. Pustules and vesicles are much more common in infants and are found in the axilla, groin, palms, and soles. Although the face and scalp are spared in adults and older children, infants usually are affected in these regions. The diagnosis of scabies should be considered in any child with severe itching, and a thorough search for an infested contact should be undertaken. Diagnosis can be confirmed by microscopic visualization of the mite, eggs, or feces of the mite with a scabies preparation. The disease is caused by *Sarcoptes scabiei*. The female mite burrows into the skin and deposits her eggs, which mature in 10–14 days. The disease is highly contagious, because infested humans do not manifest the typical signs or symptoms for 3–4 weeks, facilitating the transmission. Curative treatment is achieved by a 12-hour application of permethrin 5% lotion. Gamma-benzene hexachloride should be avoided in young children because there is a small risk of central nervous system toxicity. The parents and all caregivers should be treated simultaneously. All clothing and bedding should be washed and dried (heat is the most effective scabicide); items that cannot be washed should be placed in a plastic bag for 24 hours. The family should be provided with accurate education material that clearly details mode of transmission and the treatment regimen. They should also be aware of the fact that the itching persists for 7–14 days after the mites have been killed.

Pediculoses

Head lice are most frequently seen in young, school-age children. Caucasians and females are at the greatest risk. Pediculosis differs from scabies infestation in that the louse resides in the hair or clothing and intermittently feeds upon the host by piercing the skin. The "bite" causes small urticarial papules or erosions and itching. Diagnosis can be confirmed by visualizing the live louse. The head louse is a six-legged insect that measures 1–3 mm in size. Nits represent the outer casing of the louse ova; brown nits located on the proximal hair shaft suggest active infestation. White nits located on the hair shaft 4 cm or greater from the scalp indicate previous infestation. Treatment of head lice is controversial, because resistance to many established options has been demonstrated. Permethrin (1%) and pyrethrin-based products are the first choices of therapy. Malathion (0.5%) may be indicated for resistant cases. Removal of viable ova is of utmost importance and is best achieved by wetting the hair and combing the hair with a fine-tooth, metal comb. Topical insecticides are then applied to kill the live louse. Infestation with the head louse may be asymptomatic and has very little morbidity. Families, school nurses, and other health care professionals need to be educated about the mode of transmission and precise diagnosis before treatment of contacts is instituted.

REFERENCES

Behrman RE, Kliegman RM, Jenson HB, editors: *Nelson textbook of pediatrics,* ed 16, Philadelphia, 2000, WB Saunders, Chapter 674.

Crissey JT: Common dermatophyte infections: a simple diagnostic test and current management, *Postgrad Med* 103:191, 197, 205, 1998.

Solomon AR, Rasmussen JE, Varani J, et al: The Tzanck smear in the diagnosis of cutaneous herpes simplex, *JAMA* 251:633–635, 1984.

Tanphaichitr A, Brodell RT: How to spot scabies in infants, *Postgrad Med* 105:191–192, 1999.

SELECTED GENETIC DISORDERS
Hypohidrotic Ectodermal Dysplasia

Diminution or absence of sweating, hypotrichosis, and defective dentition are the most striking features of hypohidrotic ectodermal dysplasia, which usually is an X-linked recessive. The facies is distinctive because of frontal bossing and depression of the bridge of the nose. Eyebrows and lashes are absent or sparse. The skin around the eyes is wrinkled and frequently hyperpigmented. The skin elsewhere is thin, dry, and hypopigmented, and the cutaneous vasculature is more visible. The scalp and body hair is sparse, and the ears and chin are prominent. The lips are thick and everted and may show pseudorhagades. Dental anomalies range from total anodontia to hypodontia with peg-shaped teeth.

The most striking physiologic abnormality is the diminution or absence of sweating. Sweat pore counts usually will demonstrate decreased to absent sweat pores on the fingertips. Absence or hypoplasia of eccrine glands can be confirmed by skin biopsy. Other glandular structures also may be absent or hypoplastic. Less constant findings are conductive hearing loss, gonadal abnormalities, stenotic lacrimal puncta, corneal dysplasia, and cataracts. Mental development is normal. Marked heat intolerance is caused by an inability to regulate the body temperature adequately by sweating. Fever occurs with increases in ambient temperature and exercise, and responds quickly to environmental cooling and rest; however, some febrile reactions may be caused by recurrent upper respiratory tract infections. Because the respiratory mucosa also may be deficient in mucus-secreting glands, viral respiratory tract infections in affected patients tend to linger and become complicated by secondary bacterial infections. To avoid severe hyperthermia, the condition must be diagnosed in infancy.

Every effort should be made to moderate extreme environmental temperatures by using air conditioning. Deficient lacrimation can be palliated by the regular use of artificial tears. The nasal mucosa also must be protected by intermittent saline solution irrigations and application of petrolatum. Affected children must have a thorough dental evaluation during the first years of life, and dental prostheses should be provided even for toddlers so that adequate nutrition is maintained. Reconstructive procedures can be performed later in life to improve the facial configuration. A wig may be required for patients with scant scalp hair.

The incidence of atopic diseases, asthma, allergic rhinitis, and atopic dermatitis is increased in patients with anhidrotic ectodermal dysplasia. Atopic manifestations should be managed as they would be in otherwise healthy infants and children. Accurate carrier detection and early neonatal and prenatal diagnosis are now feasible for many families at risk for this condition.

Numerous other types of ectodermal dysplasia have been defined, including hidrotic ectodermal dysplasia, the ectrodactyly ectodermal dysplasia cleft palate (EEC) syndrome, the ankyloblepharon ectodermal dysplasia cleft palate (AEC) syndrome, the ectodermal dysplasia cleft palate midfacial hypoplasia (Rapp-Hodgkin) syndrome, and chondroectodermal dysplasia (the Ellis–van Creveld syndrome). Some of these may present with scalp erosions or pyodermas in the neonate. Isolated lack of sweat glands occurs in congenital familial anhidrosis.

Xeroderma Pigmentosum

Xeroderma pigmentosum is a rare, hereditary, autosomal recessive genetic disorder. The disease results in marked hypersensitivity to ultraviolet light. After birth, the infant develops erythema, speckled hyperpigmentation, atrophy, actinic keratoses, and cutaneous malignancies. Squamous cell carcinomas, basal cell carcinomas, melanomas, and other rare skin malignancies have all been described in children with xeroderma pigmentosa. The outcome is often fatal by the second decade of life as a result of metastatic disease. The underlying abnormality is a deficiency in an endonuclease that is responsible for the repair of DNA damaged by ultraviolet light. Genetic heterogeneity has been demonstrated, and nine complementation groups have been identified, each with a characteristic range of DNA repair rates. Patients in each of these groups differ with regard to clinical features and epidemiologic patterns. Protection from ultraviolet light exposure is mandatory because this will prevent much of the skin damage and the development of tumors.

Incontinentia Pigmenti

Incontinentia pigmenti is a rare, X-linked dominant disorder that affects the skin, bones, eyes, and central nervous system. Almost all patients are female, but rare affected males have been reported and are thought to represent genetic mosaicism or Klinefelter syndrome.

The cutaneous lesions are usually present at birth and have three distinct morphologic stages. Initially there are 2–4-mm, clear to yellow vesicles that are clustered in a linear configuration. These vesicular lesions appear in crops during the first few weeks of life and most commonly occur on the trunk and limbs. At times they appear distinctly pustular or crusted. Gray to brown, warty, linear and swirled plaques develop next. These are most prominent on the distal limbs. The third stage consists of patterned, macular brown hyperpigmentation in streaks and whorls on the trunk and extremities. Occasionally pigmentation may accompany some of the early lesions, and all three morphologies may be present at the same time. A fourth stage consisting of atrophic, hypopigmented streaks has been described during adulthood in some individuals. Nail hypoplasia, areas of alopecia, and ocular and skeletal abnormalities also may be detected. Delayed dentition, partial anodontia, and abnormalities of the CNS can occur but may not be apparent during the neonatal period. Peripheral eosinophilia is often present during the vesicular phase of the disease. The diagnosis should be considered when inflammatory vesicles arranged in lines are seen in a newborn female infant. Biopsy of a small blister demonstrates a subcorneal vesicle filled with eosinophils. No specific therapy is required for the skin lesions; if inflammation becomes excessive during the vesicular phase, treatment with compresses and topical steroids may be helpful. An ophthalmologic examination is indicated for all infants with this disorder.

CUTANEOUS SIGNS OF SYSTEMIC DISEASES

The skin is the most accessible organ system and frequently provides a window into the child with systemic disease. Skin findings play a major diagnostic role in many neurologic diseases (neurocutaneous syndromes), such as tuberous sclerosis and neurofibromatosis. Likewise, many rheumatologic and infectious disorders will present with cutaneous findings (Table 20–10) (see Chapter 10). The skin also may provide clues to nutritional and immunodeficiency disorders (Table 20–11).

Langerhans Cell Histiocytosis

Langerhans cell histiocytosis is a rare proliferative disorder most often seen in young infants. The disease is caused by infiltration of the skin, bone, and viscera with histiocytes. It is variable in presentation, and the clinical course varies from self-limited skin nodules to progressive multisystem disease. In the newborn, 2–4-mm hemorrhagic vesicles with a central umbilication are the most common. They may occur at any site but have a predilection for the groin, palms, and soles. Rarely, larger ulcerated nodules or tumors may be present. Older infants exhibit an eczematous eruption in the groin and scalp. The scalp or diaper dermatitis often mimics poorly healing and chronic seborrheic dermatitis. Oral lesions result in gingival hyperplasia, ulceration, and natal teeth. Extracutaneous findings include lytic bone le-

sions, exophthalmos, diabetes insipidus, lymphadenopathy, hepatosplenomegaly, and infiltration of the lungs and gastrointestinal tract. Diagnosis is made by skin biopsy, which typically reveals dermal infiltrate of histiocytes that are S-100 and Cd1a positive. Evaluation of an infant with documented cutaneous Langerhans cell histiocytosis includes a complete blood count, measurement of serum electrolyte levels, assessment of liver function, a skeletal survey, and chest radiographic examination. Systemic chemotherapy is used for treatment but is dependent on the extent of internal disease.

REFERENCES
Schmitz L, Favara BE: Nosology and pathology of Langerhans, cell histiocytosis, *Hematol Oncol Clin North Am* 12:221–246, 1998.

Cutaneous Reactions to Drugs

Cutaneous eruptions are relatively common, potentially life-threatening reactions to medications. There are five major subtypes: morbilliform; urticarial; serum-sickness-like; Stevens-Johnson syndrome and toxic epidermal necrolysis; and drug-induced hypersensitivity reaction with systemic involvement. One of the most useful elements in the diagnosis of drug eruptions is recent history of starting an oral medication. On initial exposure to a medication, the eruption will begin 5–10 days after starting the medication. If the child has taken the drug before, the reaction is observed 1–5 days after initiation. Certain drugs are much more likely to cause cutaneous reactions; antibiotics, anticonvulsants, and nonsteroidal antiinflammatory agents appear to be the most common such agents in children.

Urticarial drug eruptions are the most frequent reaction pattern in the pediatric population. They manifest as multiple, 1–4-cm, red, edematous papules that often coalesce into bizarrely shaped annular and serpiginous plaques. The chest and proximal extremities have the highest concentration of lesions. Swelling of the periocular region, lips, and extremities may also be present. The lesions of urticaria are transient; thus individual lesions do not last longer then 24 hours. Viral or bacterial (e.g., *Streptococcus* or *Mycoplasma*) infections may cause an identical urticarial eruption, and it is often difficult to determine the exact etiology of the urticaria. Oral antihistamines will produce a temporary but dramatic improvement in both the symptoms and appearance of the eruption (see Chapter 8).

Morbilliform drug eruptions are characterized by the acute onset of pruritic, 2–4-mm, red, blanching macules. The lesions are distributed symmetrically and diffusely but concentrated on the chest and

TABLE 20–10
Rheumatologic Diseases with Cutaneous Findings

Disease	Age	Cutaneous Findings	Distribution	Associated Findings
Juvenile rheumatoid arthritis	2–16 yr	Red, faint, polycyclic, evanescent eruption with minimal scaling	Upper arms, torso, and face	Transient rash associated with fever
Rheumatic fever	5–16 yr	Erythema marginatum; rapidly enlarging, red polycyclic plaques	Face, torso, and proximal extremities	Fever, carditis, arthritis, rheumatic nodules, chorea ASO elevated Positive culture for group A streptococcus
Systemic lupus	10–12 yr	Photosensitivity that results in diffuse erythema "Butterfly rash" on the face Diffuse hair loss and periungual telangiectasia Rarely urticaria	Malar erythema of the face, anterior chest, and dorsal arms	Arthritis, fever, fatigue, weight loss, uveitis, positive ANA, proteinuria, serositis
Dermatomyositis	8–12 yr	*"Heliotrope rash"* (purplish discoloration and swelling of the eyelids) *"Gottron papules"* (red, scaling papules over the metacarpophalangeal and proximal interphalangeal joints, elbows, and knees) Photosensitivity		Myositis resulting in symmetric proximal weakness, elevated muscle enzymes, malaise
Henoch-Schönlein purpura	4–10 yr	*"Palpable purpura"* (red, nonblanching papules) Edema of the scalp, periorbital region, scrotum, and lips	Lower legs, buttocks, ears, and lower abdomen	Periarticular swellings, cramping abdominal pain, and glomerulonephritis
Wegener's granulomatosis	8–16 yr	*"Palpable purpura"* (leukocytoclastic vasculitis resulting in red, nonblanching papules 0.5–4 cm in size) Rarely, larger necrotic ulcerations	Lower extremities	Upper respiratory granulomas; renal, pulmonary, and gastrointestinal involvement
Neonatal lupus	0–4 mo	Annular, red, scaling plaques Telangiectasia and photosensitivity	Classically in the periocular region, "raccoon eyes," also on chest and back	Congenital heart block, thrombocytopenia, positive maternal anti-SSA and anti-Sb antibodies
Kawasaki disease	<4 yr	Variable cutaneous findings, diffuse scarlatiniform or urticaria eruption, perineal desquamation, edema and desquamation of the palms and soles, conjunctival injection, and swollen bright red lips	Characteristic desquamation of the perineal region (early)	Fever, irritability, strawberry tongue, lymphadenopathy, thrombocytosis (late), coronary aneurysms (late)

TABLE 20–11
Selected Immunodeficiencies with Cutaneous Findings

Disease	Cutaneous Findings	Associated Features
Ataxia-telangiectasia	Conjunctival telangiectasia, telangiectasia on face, neck, and upper chest, 4–8-cm red, granulomatous plaques with ulceration Photosensitivity and severe radiation sensitivity	Cerebellar ataxia, low IgA, IgE, recurrent sinopulmonary pyogenic infections Decreased DNA repair, which results in increased risk of cancer
Wiskott-Aldrich syndrome	Severe and recalcitrant eczema that often is hemorrhagic	Hypogammaglobinemia, thrombocytopenia, X-linked recessive
Chronic granulomatous disease	Eczema, frequent cutaneous bacterial abscesses	Osteomyelitis, sinusitis, abnormal nitroblue tetrazolium test
Chédiak-Higashi syndrome	Pigmentary dilution resulting in fair skin and silvery gray hair	Neutropenia, recurrent bacterial infection, neuropathy, and malignancy
Job syndrome	Severe, early-onset eczema; recurrent non-inflammatory infectious nodules; *"cold abscesses"* of the skin	
Cystic fibrosis	Perioral and perineal erosive dermatitis, generalized dermatitis	Pulmonary, gastrointestinal, and nutritional complications
Complement deficiency C2, C4	Palpable purpura, photosensitivity, malar or butterfly rash	Systemic lupus-like picture
Complement deficiency C1	Urticaria and angioedema	
Complement deficiency C5–9	Purple, angular, depressed plaques on the extremities caused by acute or chronic meningococcal or gonococcal infections	Recurrent meningococcal and gonococcal infections
Severe-combined immunodeficiency	Diffuse eczematous eruption often perioral and perineal in distribution; 4–8-cm red, granulomatous plaques with central ulceration Cutaneous graft-versus-host reaction in the neonate period or after transfusion	Severe immunodeficiency

proximal extremities. The palms and soles are usually involved. Scaling and hyperpigmentation may be observed late in the disease. Oral antihistamines decrease the itching but do not change the cutaneous eruption. Fever, malaise, and lymphadenopathy may be associated with this reaction.

Serum sickness–like reaction has been observed with many medications, most of which are antibiotics. Serum sickness–like reaction parallels urticarial reactions in many ways but is often the result of complement activation by immune complexes, not of preformed IgE (urticaria). It is more frequently observed in younger children and presents with systemic complaints of fever, malaise, and arthralgias 3–14 days after offending medication is initiated. Dramatic, usually large, 4–10-cm, red, edematous plaques with a central blue-red discoloration are present. This central color change is often mistaken for erythema multiforme. The lesions tend to last longer than typical urticaria. A bizarre blue-gray or bruise-like pigmentation is left behind as the cutaneous lesions fade. Extremity and periarticular swelling and hematuria are common. Oral antihistamines are helpful in alleviating symptoms.

A severe multisystem reaction known as **drug-induced hypersensitivity syndrome** has been described in association with aromatic anticonvulsants (phenytoin, phenobarbital, and carbamazepine). This syndrome has also been induced by sulfonamides, minocycline, and allopurinol. The patients present with fever, rash, lymphadenopathy, and signs of internal organ involvement. Unlike other reactions, this syndrome presents 2–12 weeks after starting the medication. The cutaneous eruption is usually morbilliform, but may progress to confluent erythema or toxic epidermal necrolysis. There are dramatic facial edema, pharyngitis, and erythema of the lips. Severe hepatitis and pulmonary, renal, and hematologic abnormalities account for the major morbidity and mortality. Symptoms typically persist for weeks to months after discontinuation of the medication. Oral or intravenous steroids may be beneficial when there is severe internal organ involvement.

ACNE

Acne is the most common adolescent skin disorder and occurs in up to 40% of teenagers. It is a disorder of pilosebaceous units and affects areas with the greatest concentration of sebaceous glands, such as the face, chest, and back. The pathogenesis of acne is multifactorial, with sex, age, genetic factors, and environment all major contributing factors. The primary event is the obstruction of the sebaceous follicle. Androgens are a potent stimulus of the sebaceous gland. Overgrowth of the normal bacterial skin flora may account for the inflammatory component and pustule formation.

Superficial plugging of the pilosebaceous unit results in small (2–3 mm) open (blackhead) and closed (whitehead) comedones. Comedones are the earliest lesion of acne and are typically found over the nose, chin, and central forehead. Inflammatory papules and pustules occur in the same distribution. Larger (1–3 cm), skin-colored or red cysts and nodules represent deeper plugging and are usually found over the cheeks, perinasal region, and back. Cystic acne has the highest incidence of scarring because rupture of a deep cyst may cause inflammation into the dermis and subcutaneous tissues. In a susceptible individual, scarring may follow pustular or even comedonal acne. Certain areas, such as the glabellar region of the forehead and lateral cheeks, appear to scar more frequently.

Acne is a disease of adolescence but may start as young as 8 years of age. Classically, acne lasts 3–5 years; some individuals may have disease for as long as 15–20 years. Neonatal acne occurs in infants 2–4 weeks of age and is thought to be a response to maternal androgens. The primary lesion is a pinpoint, red, inflammatory lesion found on the lateral cheeks and occasionally on the chest or back. These lesions usually resolve spontaneously over a period of months. Infantile acne is an eruption that is observed in older, usually male infants. These children have more typical lesions of acne such as comedones, papules, and cysts. The cyst formation may be dramatic, with severe facial scarring. Topical treatments or oral antibiotics may be indicated.

The mainstay of treatment of acne is topical keratolytic agents and topical antibiotics. The keratolytic agents produce superficial desquamation and subsequently relieve the follicular obstruction. Keratolytic agents are available in several different formulations, with varying degrees of efficacy. The more potent the keratolytic cream or gel, the more irritating the product. Likewise, a variety of topical antibiotics are used and are available in many different vehicles. Oral antibiotics should be instituted for deeper cystic lesions. Antibiotics from the tetracycline family appear to be the most effective because they also have significant antiinflammatory activity. For recalcitrant, severe acne, oral isotretinoin may be instituted. This medication is given at a dose of 1 mg/kg/day for a 20-week period. Isotretinoin has an approximately 80% efficacy rate, but unfortunately has a high side effect profile. Isotretinoin should be used only by physicians familiar with all the potential side effects. Patients using this medication need to be evaluated on a monthly basis, and laboratory monitoring should be performed before treatment is instituted and monthly thereafter. Isotretinoin is teratogenic and must not be used immediately before and during pregnancy.

REFERENCES

Behrman RE, Kliegman RM, Jenson HB, editors: *Nelson textbook of pediatrics*, ed 16, Philadelphia, 2000, WB Saunders, Chapter 675.

Drug Doses*

Drugs Listed Alphabetically by Generic Name

KEY: KEY:

NB	Newborn (birth to end of first mo)	PR	Per rectum
IN	Infant (1–12 mo)	SC	Subcutaneous
CH	Child (1–12 yr)	SL	Sublingual
AD	Adult	sol	Solution
caps	Capsules	susp	Suspension
div	Divided	tabl	Tablets
DW	Dextrose in water	g	Gram
IM	Intramuscular	mg	Milligram = 10^{-3} g
inj	Injection	μg	Microgram = 10^{-6} g (sometimes abbreviated "mcg")
IV	Intravenous	ng	Nanogram = 10^{-9} g
LO	Linguo-occlusal	kg	Kilogram = 10^{3} g
ointm	Ointment	mL	Milliliter = 10^{-3} liter $\simeq$ cm^3 = cc (cubic centimeter)
PO	Per os, oral	Rx	Prescription

Modified from Behrman RE, Kliegman RM, Arvin AM, editors: *Nelson textbook of pediatrics*, ed 15, Philadelphia, 1996, WB Saunders.

*No attempt has been made to reproduce a comprehensive list of adverse side effects or of formulations available for the drugs listed. For these, the reader again is referred to standard textbooks of pharmacology, to the package inserts accompanying the commercial preparations of each drug, and to *Physician's Desk Reference*, distributed annually in the United States by Physician's Desk Reference, Box 210, Westwood, NJ 07675.

Dosages listed in the table are not specifically intended for premature and newborn infants unless so indicated.

All doses are average doses and are approximate. Variability of individual response may require alteration of dosage upward or downward. Doses based on different criteria (e.g., body weight, surface area) frequently do not correspond. Surface area may be calculated from Figure AP-1, p. 909.

Doses generally are expressed as grams or milligrams per kilogram of body weight per 24 hours (g or mg/kg/24 hr), even for drugs ordinarily administered on a p.r.n. (as needed or indicated) basis.

For teratogenic effects of drugs, see Chapter 6, package inserts, and *Physican's Desk Reference*.

Because of the multiplicity of proprietary names and formulations of the drugs listed, only a few representative examples have been given of the many proprietary preparations available in most instances. We have intended no bias in selecting the proprietary names used, and we make due apology to any manufacturers and distributors whose products may appear to have been slighted.

See KEY to abbreviations, above; for further information about drugs, see package inserts.

I. ANTIBIOTICS

Acyclovir; antiviral agent against herpes simplex and varicella-zoster virus by selective inhibition of viral DNA synthesis

℞ in clinical herpes simplex infection in neonates: NB = IV (over 60 min): 10–15 mg/kg/dose every 8 hr, for 14–21 days

Dosing interval should be increased to 24 hr if renal function is less than 25% of normal

℞ in immunocompromised individuals with herpes simplex or varicella-zoster virus infection: CH = IV (over 60 min): 7.5–10 mg/kg per dose every 8 hr for 7 days. PO: 7.5–20 mg/kg per dose administered 4–5 times per day. AD = IV (over 60 min); PO: 800 mg 5 times/day for 7–10 days

℞ mucocutaneous herpes simplex virus (HSV) infection: CH = IV (over 60 min) 5 mg/kg per dose every 8 hr for 7 days; HSV encephalitis: 10 mg/kg per dose every 8 hr for 10–14 days; varicella-zoster infection: 5 mg/kg per dose every 8 hr for 7 days

℞ IV prophylaxis in bone marrow transplant recipients: HSV seropositive 4.5–5 mg/kg every 8–12 hr

℞ in severe first episode of herpes genitalis: CH, AD = LO: 5% ointm

Caution: Acyclovir dosing should be adjusted for patients with renal insufficiency (i.e., glomerular filtration rates <50 mL/min in patients >6 mo of age).

Amikacin sulfate; antimicrobial aminoglycoside effective primarily against gram-negative microorganisms

NB <7 days: <28 wk = IM, IV (over 30–60 min): 7.5 mg/kg once daily; 28–34 wk, 7.5 mg/kg every 18 hr; >34 wk, 10 mg/kg every 12 hr

NB >7 days: <28 wk, 7.5 mg/kg every 12 hr; 28–34 wk, 7.5 mg/kg every 12 hr; >34 wk, 10 mg/kg every 8 hr

IN, CH = IM, IV 15–25 mg/kg/24 hr. AD = IM, IV 15 mg/kg/24 hr every 8–12 hr.

Serum concentrations should be monitored; therapeutic peak concentration 25–40 mg/L, trough concentration <10 mg/L

Amoxicillin; acid-resistant ampicillin congener

IN, CH = PO: 20–50 mg/kg/24 hr, div, every 8–12 hr; high dose 80–90 mg/kg/24 hr for otitis media; AD = 250–500 PO q8–12 hr

Amoxicillin + clavulanic acid; combination of a β-lactam antibiotic with a β-lactamase (penicillinase) inhibitor.

℞ for otitis media, sinusitis, lower respiratory tract, skin, soft tissue, and urinary tract infections: CH = PO: amoxicillin 20–45 mg/kg/24 hr + clavulanic acid 5–10 mg/kg/24 hr, div, every 8–12 hr; higher dose for otitis media 80–90 mg/kg/24 hr

Note: May cause diarrhea, abdominal pain, urticaria and other rashes, possibly because of clavulanic acid alone.

Amoxicillin is available as single component.

AUGMENTIN: tabl of 2 strengths: 250 mg amoxicillin + 125 mg clavulanic acid, and 500 mg amoxicillin + 125 mg clavulanic acid; oral susp with amoxicillin 125 mg + clavulanic acid 31.25 mg/5 mL, or amoxicillin 250 mg + clavulanic acid 62.5 mg/5 mL

Ampicillin; acid-resistant penicillin congener

NB (≤7 days old) = IV (over 15–30 min), IM: 50 mg/kg/24 hr, div, every 12 hr

℞ for meningitis: IV: 100–200 mg/kg/24 hr, div, every 4 hr

NB (>7 days old) = IV (over 15–30 min), IM: 100 mg/kg/24 hr, div, every 8 hr

℞ for meningitis: IV: 200–400 mg/kg/24 hr, div, every 4 hr

℞ for septicemia: IV (over 15–30 min), IM: 100–200 mg/kg/24 hr, div, every 4 hr (IV) or every 6 hr (IM)

℞ for meningitis: IV (over 15–30 min): 300–400 mg/kg/24 hr, div, every 4 hr

Azithromycin; macrolide antibiotic indicated for the treatment of mild to moderate upper and lower respiratory tract infections and infections of the skin caused by susceptible bacteria. *Chlamydia trachomatis, Haemophilus influenzae, Moraxella catarrhalis, Mycoplasma pneumoniae, Staphylococcus aureus, Streptococcus pneumoniae.* Less gastrointestinal distress than associated with erythromycin

CH = PO, 10 mg/kg day 1 followed by 5 mg/kg/day administered once daily for 5 days. Suspected streptococcal infection: 12 mg/kg/24 hr for 5 days.

AD = 500 mg/day 1 followed by 250 mg once daily for 5 days

Caution: Coadministration with aluminum- or magnesium-containing antacids may decrease azithromycin peak serum concentrations by 25%.

Carbenicillin disodium; semisynthetic penicillin susceptible to destruction by penicillinase

℞ for systemic use: NB = IV (over 15–30 min), IM: initial dose 100 mg/kg, followed by maintenance therapy according to the following criteria:

≤2000 g + ≤7 days old: 225 mg/kg/24 hr, div, every 8 hr

≤2000 g + >7 days old: 400 mg/kg/24 hr, div, every6 hr

>2000 g + ≤7 days old: 300 mg/kg/24 hr, div, every 6 hr

>2000 g + >7 days old: 400 mg/kg/24 hr, div, every 6 hr

IN, CH = IV (over 15–30 min), IM: 400–600 mg/kg/24 hr, div, every 4 hr (IV) or every 6 hr (IM)

1 g carbenicillin disodium contains 6.5 mEq Na$^+$

℞ for treatment of urinary tract infection only: CH = PO: 10–30 mg/kg/24 hr, div, every 6 hr carbenicillin indanyl sodium

Cephalosporins; semisynthetic derivatives of 7-amino-cephalosporanic acid, structurally related to penicillins

a. First-generation cephalosporins: active against most gram-positive cocci (excluding enterococci and methicillin-resistant *S. aureus*), some strains of *Escherichia coli, Klebsiella pneumoniae,* and *Proteus mirabilis*

Note: First-generation drugs do not cross the blood-brain barrier and therefore are ineffective for treatment of infections within the central nervous system.

Cefadroxil: relatively resistant against β-lactamases; absorption appears unaffected by food intake; minimal inhibitory concentrations for *E. coli, P. mirabilis, Klebsiella* species may be maintained in urine for about 20 hr after single dose

℞ CH = PO: 30 mg/kg/24 hr, div, every 12 hr

Cefazolin sodium: NB = IV (over 15–30 min), IM: 40 mg/kg/24 hr, div, every 12 hr; IN, CH = IV (over 15–30 min), IM: 50–100 mg/kg/24 hr, div, every 6 hr

Cephalothin: NB = IV (over 15–30 min), IM: <7 days old: 40 mg/kg/24 hr, div, every 12 hr; >7 days old: 60 mg/kg/24 hr, div, every 8 hr; IN, CH = IV: 80–160 mg/kg/24 hr, div, every 4 hr

b. Second-generation cephalosporins: more active against gram-negative bacteria such as *H. influenzae* type b, *Neisseria gonorrhoeae,* and enteric gram-negative bacilli

Cefaclor: effective against some β-lactamase–producing, ampicillin-resistant strains of *H. influenzae;* absorption not affected by food intake

℞ for treatment of otitis media and infections of the upper and lower respiratory tracts, urinary tract, skin, and soft tissues with susceptible organisms: IN, CH = PO: 20–40 mg/kg/24 hr, div, every 8 hr

Cefoxitin: IN (>3 mo old), CH = IV, IM: 80–160 mg/kg/24 hr, div, every 4–6 hr

Note: May cause renal impairment and cross-reaction with penicillin.

c. Third-generation cephalosporins: less active against gram-positive cocci than older cephalosporins but more active against most strains of enteric gram-negative bacilli, moderately active against *Pseudomonas aeruginosa,* highly active against *H. influenzae* and *N. gonorrhoeae*

Ceftriaxone sodium: biliary and renal excretion

℞ misc. infection 50–75 mg/kg/24 hr (not to exceed 2 g), div, every 12 hr; meningitis 100 mg/kg/24 hr (not to exceed 4 g) divided every 12 hr

Cefotaxime: IN, CH = IV, IM: 100–150 mg/kg/24 hr, div, every 4–6 hr

℞ in meningitis: NB = IV 200 mg/kg/24 hr, div, every 6 hr

Note: May cause hypersensitivity reactions in penicillin-sensitive patients. Adjust dose with renal failure. Nephrotoxicity may develop with combined use of a cephalosporin and an aminoglycoside.

Ceftazidime: possesses antipseudomonal activity

NB = IV, IM: <7 days <2000 g, 100 mg/kg/24 hr, div, every 12 hr; >2000 g, 100 mg/kg/24 hr, div, every 8 hr; >7 days, 100–150 mg/kg/24 hr, div, every 8 hr

IN, CH = IV, IM: 100–150 mg/kg/24 hr, div, every 8 hr (meningitis, 150 mg/kg/24 hr, div, every 8 hr)

Chloramphenicol; derivative of dichloracetic acid combined to a structure containing a nitrobenzene ring

NB = IV over 15–30 min loading dose 20 mg/kg then in 12 hr:

Postnatal age ≤7 days, 25 mg/kg/day IV q24h; >7 days ≤2000 g, 25 mg/kg/day IV, q24h

Children: 50–75 mg/kg/day IV, PO divided q 6–8h (meningitis 75–100 mg/kg/day IV divided q6h).

Adults: 50 mg/kg/day IV, PO divided q6h (max dose 4 g/day)

Caution: Newborn infants susceptible to development of high blood levels and gray-baby syndrome on usual doses; therefore, careful monitoring of blood levels, if available, mandatory. Dose-duration–related suppression of erythrocyte production universal; weekly hematocrit or hemoglobin and reticulocyte count mandatory. Idiosyncratic aplastic anemia occasionally occurs without warning and may be lethal. **Use only when specifically indicated.** Target serum levels peak 20–30 mg/L, trough 5–10 mg/L

Chloroquine; a 4-aminoquinoline antimalarial agent; drug of choice for the treatment of attacks of malaria caused by *Plasmodium vivax, Plasmodium ovale, Plasmodium malariae,* and susceptible strains of *Plasmodium falciparum.* Not advised for use in treatment of juvenile rheumatoid arthritis.

℞ oral treatment of uncomplicated attacks (excluding those caused by chloroquine-resistant *P. falciparum*):

Chloroquine diphosphate: CH = PO:

Malaria prophylaxis:

Child: 5 mg/kg/wk PO (max dose 300 mg/dose)

Adult: 300 mg/wk PO

Acute malarial treatment:

Child: 10 mg/kg PO initial dose (max dose 600 mg): 5 mg/kg 6 hr later then 5 mg/kg PO once daily for 2 days; IM 5 mg/kg initial dose, 5 mg/kg 6 hr later (max IM dose 10 mg/kg/24 hr)

Adult: 600 mg initially, 300 mg 6 hr later then 300 mg PO once daily for 2 days

Extraintestinal amebiasis:

Child: 10 mg/kg PO daily for 2–3 wk (max daily dose 300 mg)

Adult: 600 mg PO once daily for 2 days then 300 mg once daily for 2–3 wk

Caution: Irreversible retinal damage may occur with prolonged use; frequent ophthalmologic examination necessary to detect early changes.
Note: Chloroquine does not cause hemolysis in individuals with G-6-PD deficiency.

Chlortetracycline: see Tetracyclines

Clarithromycin; macrolide antibiotic indicated for the treatment of mild to moderate upper and lower respiratory tract infections and infections of the skin structure caused by susceptible bacteria, *C. trachomatis, H. influenzae, M. catarrhalis, M. pneumoniae, S. aureus, S. pneumoniae, Legionella* spp. Less gastrointestinal distress than associated with erythromycin. CH = PO 15 mg/kg/24 hr, div, every 12 hr. AD = PO 250–500 mg/24 hr, div, every 12 hr
   Note: Dose adjustment is necessary with renal disease, creatinine clearance <30 mL/min. May interfere with the hepatic metabolism of certain drugs (e.g., carbamazepine, theophylline).

Clindamycin: semisynthetic derivative of lincomycin
   NB <7 days <2000 g, 10 mg/kg/24 hr, div, every 12 hr
   NB >7 days <2000 g, 15 mg/kg/24 hr, div, every 8 hr
   NB <7 days >2000 g, 15 mg/kg/24 hr, div, every 8 hr
   NB >7 days >2000 g, 20 mg/kg/24 hr, div, every 6 hr
   IN, CH: 20–45 mg/kg/24 hr, div, every 6–8 hr
   Note: Therapy may be associated with the development of pseudomembranous colitis.

Cloxacillin sodium monohydrate; penicillinase-resistant penicillin
   IN, CH = PO: 50–100 mg/kg/24 hr, div, every 6 hr (expressed in terms of the base)

Demeclocycline: see Tetracyclines

Dicloxacillin sodium monohydrate; penicillinase-resistant penicillin
   IN, CH = PO: 12.5–100 mg/kg/24 hr, div, every 6 hr

Doxycycline; see Tetracyclines

Erythromycin; macrolide antimicrobial agent
   IN, CH = PO: 30–50 mg/kg/24 hr, div, every 6 hr; IV: 20–50 mg/kg/24 hr, div, every 6 hr

Ethambutol hydrochloride; antituberculous agent used concomitantly with isoniazid
   ℞ in the treatment of tuberculosis as part of multiple drug regimen. Conditions for safe use in children not firmly established. In adults: 15 mg/kg/24 hr, as single daily dose, for course of treatment or retreatment. *Because of rare side effects of optic neuritis and decreased visual acuity,* eye examinations are indicated before inception of treatment and at monthly intervals thereafter.

Fluconazole; synthetic broad spectrum *bis*-triazole antifungal drug. Selective inhibitor of fungal cytochrome P_{450} sterol C-14 α-demethylation; limited data in pediatrics available.
   Neonate: thrush 6 mg/kg, IV, PO qd first day then 3 mg/kg/day qd for 14–21 days
   Systemic infections: postnatal age <14 days 6–12 mg/kg/day PO, IV q72h; >14 days once daily
   Children: 6–12 mg/kg/day IV, PO qd; cryptococcal meningitis 12 mg/kg/day first day then 6–12 mg/kg/day IV, PO q day

Fluoroquinolones; antimicrobial agents that inhibit the action of microbial DNA gyrase (topoisomerase 2). Drugs in this class include ciprofloxacin, enoxacin, norfloxacin, ofloxacin, and so on. Many of these drugs possess potent activity against a wide range of pathogens, including *P. aeruginosa,* and are available for oral administration. The use of these drugs in pediatrics, primarily for the treatment of children with cystic fibrosis, has been limited because of concern about possible fluoroquinolone-induced joint damage. Toxicity studies in animals have shown destructive lesions of growing cartilage following administration of these agents. Reports of arthropathy in teenage patients with cystic fibrosis have appeared in the literature, suggesting caution in the use of this class of compounds in patients whose skeletal growth is incomplete.
   Ciprofloxacin: CH = PO 20–30 mg/kg/24 hr, div, every 8–12 hr. Usual maximum dose 1.5 g/24 hr. IV (over 60 min) 4–15 mg/kg/24 hr, div, every 8–12 hr. Dose should be adjusted in patients with creatinine clearance <20 mL/min.

Gentamicin sulfate; antimicrobial aminoglycoside
   Neonates: IM, IV (over 30–60 min): *Postnatal age ≤7 days 1200–2000 g:* 2.5 mg/kg q12–18h; *>2000 g:* 2.5 mg/kg q12h; *postnatal age >7 days 1200–2000 g:* 2.5 mg/kg q8–12h; *>2000 g:* 2.5 mg/kg q8h
   Children: 2.5 mg/kg/day divided q8–12h
   Alternatively may administer 5–7.5 mg/kg/day IV once daily. *Intrathecal:* Preservative-free preparation for intraventricular or intrathecal use: neonate 1 mg/day; child 1–2 mg/day; adult 4–8 mg/day
   Adults: 3–6 mg/kg/day divided q8h
   Serum concentrations should be monitored, therapeutic peak concentration 5–10 mg/L, trough <2 mg/L. Dosage and interval may require modification for treatment of patients with cystic fibrosis.
   Caution: Ototoxic, nephrotoxic

Griseofulvin; antifungal agent
   ℞ against deep-seated mycotic infections (skin, hair, nails) with organisms of the species *Microsporon, Trichophyton, Epidermophyton:*

Children: microsize 10–20 mg/kg/day PO divided
q12–14h; ultramicrosize 5–10 mg/kg/day
PO divided q12h

Adult: microsize 500–1000 mg/day PO divided
q12–24 h; ultramicrosize 330–375 mg/day PO
divided q12h

Isoniazid (INH), isonicotinic acid hydrazide; tuberculostatic agent

Ŗ in the treatment of active tuberculosis, in combination with other antituberculous drugs:
IN, CH = PO, IM: 10–20 mg/kg/24 hr, div, every 12–24 hr; maximum daily dose: 300 mg/24 hr. AD = PO, IM: 5 mg/kg/24 hr, div, every 24 hr; maximum daily dose: 300 mg/24 hr

Ŗ for prophylaxis of complications in recent conversion to positive tuberculin reaction (primary tuberculosis), or after suspected exposure: IN, CH = PO: 5–10 mg/kg/24 hr, as single dose, or div, every 12 hr; maximum daily dose: 300 mg/24 hr

Note: "Slow" acetylators (homozygous) need only about 0.20–0.50 of this dose to reach therapeutically effective plasma concentrations achieved by "rapid" acetylators (homozygous and heterozygous). Higher than necessary plasma concentrations of unmetabolized isoniazid seem not to be associated with risk of isoniazid hepatotoxicity.

Caution: Formation of toxic metabolite in some patients may lead to hepatic necrosis with usual doses (rare under 20 yr of age).

Kanamycin sulfate; antimicrobial aminoglycoside

NB = IM, IV (over 20–30 min):
≤2000 g and ≤7 days old: 15 mg/kg/24 hr, div, every 12 hr
≤2000 g and >7 days old: 20 mg/kg/24 hr, div, every 12 hr
>2000 g and ≤7 days old: 20 mg/kg/24 hr, div, every 12 hr
>2000 g and >7 days old: 30 mg/kg/24 hr, div, every 8 hr
IN, CH = IM, IV (over 20–30 min): 15 mg/kg/24 hr, div, every 8–12 hr. Usual duration therapy: 7–10 days; not indicated in long-term therapy because of ototoxic hazard.

Caution: Ototoxic, nephrotoxic

Ketoconazole; imidazole antifungal agent used for prophylaxis and treatment of a variety of mild to moderate fungal infections. Is not effective against infections arising within the central nervous system as the drug does not penetrate the blood-brain barrier.

CH = PO 5–10 mg/kg/24 hr, div, every 12–24 hr. Usual max 800 mg/24 hr.
AD = PO 200–400 mg/24 hr administered once daily.

Note: Gastric acidity is necessary for best oral absorption; thus avoid drug administration with antacids or H_2 receptor antagonists. Numerous potential drug interactions, including ketoconazole-induced increases in serum drug concentrations of astemizole, cyclosporine, phenytoin, terfenadine, theophylline, warfarin. Use may be associated with hepatotoxicity.

Mebendazole; antihelmintic agent that blocks glucose uptake by the susceptible parasites and interferes with their survival

Ŗ against pinworms (*Enterobius vermicularis;* cure rate 90–100%): CH = PO: 100 mg/dose, as single dose; against whipworms (*Trichuris trichiura;* cure rate 61–75%), roundworms (*Ascaris lumbricoides;* cure rate 91–100%), and hookworms (*Ancylostoma duodenale, Necator americanus;* cure rate 96%); alternative method = PO: 100 mg/24 hr, div, every 12 hr, for 3 consecutive days. If patient is not free of parasites 3 wk after treatment, a second course is indicated.

Note: Not extensively studied in children under 2 yr of age.

Methicillin sodium; semisynthetic penicillinase-resistant penicillin

Neonates: Postnatal age IM, IV ≤7 days 1200–2000 g: 50 mg/kg/day q12h (meningitis 100 mg/kg/day divided q12h); *>2000 g:* 75 mg/kg/day divided q8h (meningitis 150 mg/kg/day IV divided q8h); *postnatal age >7 days 1200–2000 g:* 75 mg/kg q8h (meningitis 150 mg/kg/day divided q8h); *>2000 g:* 100 mg/kg IV divided q6–8h (meningitis 200 mg/kg/day IV divided q6h).

Children: 150–200 mg/kg/day divided q4–6h (meningitis 200–400 mg/kg/day IV divided q4–6h).

Adults: 4–12 g/day divided q4–6h (max dose 12 g/day).

Metronidazole hydrochloride; synthetic antibacterial agent highly active against most obligate anaerobes, including *Bacteroides* species such as *B. fragilis*, and *Clostridium* and *Peptostreptococcus* species. The drug also is effective in the treatment of amebiasis, *Giardia*, and *Trichomonas.*

Neonate: 0–4 wk <1200 g: 7.5 mg/kg PO, IV q48h; *postnatal age ≤7 days 1200–2000 g:* 7.5 mg/kg/day PO, IV q24h; *2000 g:* 15 mg/kg/day PO, IV divided q12h. *Postnatal age >7 days 1200–2000 g:* 15 mg/kg/day PO, IV divided q12h; *>2000 g:* 30 mg/kg/day PO, IV divided q12h

Children: 30 mg/kg/day PO, IV divided q6–8h

Adults: 30 mg/kg/day PO, IV divided q6h. Max dose 4 g/day.

Caution: Patient should not ingest alcohol for 24 hr after receiving a dose of this drug (disulfiram-type reaction). Drug interactions possible; may prolong anticoagulant effect of warfarin-type anticoagulants.

Minocycline; see Tetracyclines

Nafcillin sodium; semisynthetic penicillinase-resistant penicillin

NB = IM, IV (over 15–30 min); ≤7 days old: 40 mg/kg/24 hr, div, every 12 hr; >7 days old: 60 mg/kg/24 hr, div, every 8 hr

IN, CH = PO: 50–100 mg/kg/24 hr, div, every 6 hr; IM, IV (over 15–30 min): 100–200 mg/kg/24 hr, div, every 6 hr (IM) or every 4 hr (IV)

Nystatin; antifungal agent; 1 mg = 2000 units; seems to be active by altering permeability of cell membrane of yeasts

℞ for topical treatment of candidosis of the buccal cavity (thrush) and the gastrointestinal tract. Very poorly absorbed. In oral candidosis, spread nystatin suspension into recesses of mouth:

NB (<2000 g) = PO: 200,000–400,000 units/24 hr, div, every 4–6 hr

NB (>2000 g), IN = PO: 400,000–800,000 units/24 hr, div, every 4–6 hr

CH = PO: 800,000–2,000,000 units/24 hr, div, every 4–6 hr

Oxacillin sodium; semisynthetic penicillinase-resistant penicillin

Neonates: postnatal age IM, IV ≤7 days 1200–2000 g: 50 mg/kg/day q12h; *>2000 g:* 75 mg/kg/day divided q8h; *postnatal age >7 days ≤1200 g:* 50 mg/kg/day IV divided q12h; *1200–2000 g:* 75 mg/kg/day q8h; *>2000 g:* 100 mg/kg/day IV divided q6h

Infants: 100–200 mg/kg/day divided q4–6h

Children: PO 50–100 mg/kg/day divided q4–6h

Adults: 2–12 g/day divided q4–6h (max dose 12 g/day)

Penicillin G, benzylpenicillin; potassium penicillin G (1 mg = 1595 units); sodium penicillin G (1 mg = 1667 units). One million units of these salts of penicillin contain either 1.68 mEq K^+ or Na^+; in other terms, 1 g contains either 2.7 mEq K^+ or 2.8 mEq Na^+.

NB = IV (over 15–30 min), IM:

<2000 g: 50,000 units/kg/24 hr, div, every 12 hr

℞ for meningitis: 100,000–200,000 units/kg/24 hr, div, every 12 hr

>2000 g: 75,000 units/kg/24 hr, div, every 8 hr

℞ for meningitis: 200,000–300,000 units/kg/24 hr, div, every 8 hr

IN, CH = PO, IM, IV (15–30 min): 100,000–250,000 units/kg/24 hr, div, every 4–6 hr

℞ for meningitis: 200,000–300,000 units/kg/24 hr, div, every 4 hr

(The higher doses should be chosen for meningitis caused by group B streptococci.)

IN, CH = PO, IM, IV (over 15–30 min) (minor infections): 25,000–50,000 units/kg/24 hr, equivalent to 15.5–31 mg/kg/24 hr, div, every 4–6 hr; if given PO,

administer penicillin G 0.5 hr before or 2 hr after the meal

℞ for prophylaxis of rheumatic fever; PO: 200,000 units/dose, equivalent to 125 mg/dose, twice daily, spaced from meals

Penicillin G benzathine, for injection; combination of 1 mole of dibenzylethylenediamine with 2 moles of penicillin G; 1 mg = 1211 units

℞ for prophylaxis of rheumatic fever: CH = IM: 600,000–1,200,000 units, equivalent to 500–1000 mg penicillin G, once a month

Penicillin G procaine, for injection; combination of penicillin G with procaine, mole for mole (1 mg = 1009 units)

NB = IM: 50,000 units/kg/24 hr, equivalent to 50 mg/kg/24 hr, in single daily dose

IN, CH = IM: 25,000–50,000 units/kg/24 hr, equivalent to 25–50 mg/kg/24 hr, in single daily dose

Penicillin V, phenoxymethyl penicillin; acid-resistant penicillin; 1 mg = 1695 units

IN, CH = PO: 25,000–50,000 units/kg/24 hr, equivalent to 15–30 mg/kg/24 hr, div, every 6–8 hr

Note: 400,000 units = 250 mg (approx.)

Primaquine; 8-aminoquinoline antimalarial agent, used for prophylaxis against *P. vivax, P. ovale,* and *P. malariae* and for "radical" cure for *P. vivax* and *P. ovale.*

IN, CH = PO: 0.55 mg/kg/24 hr (equivalent to 0.3 mg/kg/24 hr of base), as single daily dose, for 14 days

Note: Degree of intravascular hemolysis in individuals with G-6-PD deficiency is related to dosage and particular variant of the deficiency.

Pyrantel pamoate; antihelmintic agent effective by means of neuromuscular paralysis of the parasite

℞ against pinworms (*E. vermicularis*), roundworms (*A. lumbricoides*), and hookworms (*N. americanus, A. duodenale*): pyrantel pamoate has not been extensively studied in infants and children below 2 yr of age, hence particular attention should be given to children of this age group during treatment of parasitic infestation with pyrantel. CH = PO: 11 mg/kg/dose, as single dose and without regard to food intake or time of day; purging not necessary before, during, or after therapy

Note: In pinworm infestation, in which possibility of reinfection with eggs from the host exists, a second treatment 2–3 wk after the first might be indicated.

Pyrimethamine; inhibitor of dihydrofolate reductase, antimalarial agent; for use in treatment of toxoplasmosis

℞ for clinical prophylaxis of malaria, especially effective against *P. falciparum:* IN, CH = PO: 0.5–0.75

mg/kg/dose, once every 7 days. Begin prophylaxis 2 wk before entering malarious area and continue for 8 wk after leaving. To eradicate *P. vivax* and *P. ovale* infections, treatment for 14 days with primaquine should be considered immediately on leaving malarious area while pyrimethamine prophylaxis is still in effect.

Note: Hematologic abnormalities (anemia, thrombocytopenia, leukopenia) secondary to folic and folinic acid depletion can be prevented or reversed by IM administration of folinic acid (leucovorin) without affecting the efficacy of pyrimethamine.

Quinacrine hydrochloride, mepacrine hydrochloride; acridine derivative formerly used as antimalarial agent and against infestation with tapeworms, presently regarded as drug of choice against giardiasis
 ℞ against *Giardia lamblia*: CH = PO: 6 mg/kg/24 hr, div, every 8 hr, for 5 consecutive days; maximum daily dose: 300 mg/24 hr

Rifampin; macrocytic antimicrobial and antimycobacterial agent, interfering with RNA-polymerase of infecting organisms
 ℞ in treatment of tuberculosis, in conjunction with at least 1 other antituberculous agent (isoniazid) and
 ℞ in carriers of *Neisseria meningitidis* resistant to sulfonamide; treatment course of 4 consecutive days (possibility of rapid emergence of resistance); IN, CH = PO: 10–20 mg/kg/24 hr, in single daily dose (1 hr before or 2 hr after meal): maximum daily dose: 600 mg (= adult dose)

Sulfonamides; analogs of *para*-aminobenzoic acid, interfering with the synthesis of tetrahydrofolic acid in sensitive bacteria
 Sulfamethoxazole: IN, CH = PO: 50–60 mg/kg/24 hr, div, every 12 hr
 Trimethoprim/sulfamethoxazole (combination of TMP + SMX): IN (>2 mo old), CH = PO: 6–12 mg TMP + 30–60 mg SMX/kg/24 hr, div, every 12 hr
 ℞ in severe urinary tract or *Shigella* infection: CH = PO, IV: 8–10 mg TMP + 40–60 mg SMX/kg/24 hr, div, every 6–8 hr
 ℞ against *Pneumocystis carinii*: CH = PO, IV: 15–20 mg TMP + 75–100 mg SMX/kg/24 hr, div, every 6–8 hr
 Caution: Do not use in infants less than 2 mo old. Reduce dose in severe renal insufficiency. May cause bone marrow depression.

Tetracyclines; a group of derivatives of polycyclic naphthacenecarboxamide
 Chlortetracycline hydrochloride: CH = PO: 25–50 mg/kg/24 hr, div, every 6 hr
 Doxycycline monohydrate and *doxycycline hyclate:* CH = PO: 2–5 mg/kg/24 hr (max dose 200 mg/24 hr), div, every 12–24 hr

Minocycline hydrochloride: CH = PO, IV: initial dose 4 mg/kg, followed by 4 mg/kg/24 hr, div, every 12 hr
 Oxytetracycline, oxytetracycline hydrochloride, oxytetracycline calcium: same dosage as tetracycline hydrochloride: tabl, inj (IM)
 Tetracycline hydrochloride: CH = PO: 25–50 mg/kg/24 hr, div, every 8 hr; IM (often very painful): 15–25 mg/kg/24 hr, div, every 8–12 hr; IV: 10–20 mg/kg/24 hr, div, every 12 hr
 Note: Tetracyclines have limited indications in infancy and childhood because of their accumulation in bone and teeth and their potential to interfere with growth. Their use should be avoided insofar as possible until formation of dental enamel is complete in most permanent teeth (at about 8 yr), to avoid unsightly discolored, pitted teeth. Tetracyclines may cause increased intracranial pressure in infants (pseudotumor cerebri).

Ticarcillin disodium; semisynthetic penicillin susceptible to penicillinase; each gram of drug contains 5.2 mEq of sodium.
 NB = IV (over 20–30 min), IM:
 <7 days <2000 g; 150 mg/kg/24 hr, div, every 12 hr;
 <7 days >2000 g; 225 mg/kg/24 hr, div, every 8 hr;
 >7 days <2000 g; 225 mg/kg/24 hr, div, every 8 hr;
 >7 days >2000 g; 300 mg/kg/24 hr, div, every 8 hr
 IN, CH = IV (over 20–30 min), IM: 200–300 mg/kg/24 hr, div, every 4–6 hr. IM injection is painful.

Ticarcillin + clavulanic acid; combination of a β-lactam antibiotic (ticarcillin) with a β-lactamase (penicillinase) inhibitor (clavulanic acid). The addition of clavulanic acid extends the activity of ticarcillin to include β-lactamase–producing strains of *H. influenzae* and other drug-resistant pathogens. Doses administered as either IM or IV are the same as those for ticarcillin noted above.

Tobramycin sulfate; antimicrobial aminoglycoside
 Neonates: IM, IV (over 30–60 min): *postnatal age ≤7 days, 1200–2000 g:* 2.5 mg/kg q12–18h; *>2000 g:* 2.5 mg/kg q12h; *postnatal age >7 days, 1200–2000 g:* 2.5 mg/kg q8–12h; *>2000 g:* 2.5 mg/kg q8h.
 Children: 2.5 mg/kg/day divided q8–12h. Alternatively may administer 5–7.5 mg/kg/day IV qd. Preservative-free preparation for intraventricular or intrathecal use: neonate 1 mg/day; child 1–2 mg/day; adults 4–8 mg/day
 Adults: 3–6 mg/kg/day divided q8h
 Caution: Ototoxic, nephrotoxic

Vancomycin; complex glycopeptide that inhibits synthesis of cell wall in gram-positive bacteria and is effective against methicillin-resistant staphylococci; in oral application effective in pseudomembranous colitis caused by toxin-producing bacteria such as *C. difficile* and *S. aureus;* excreted mainly by kidneys

NB = IV (slow over 1 + hr) <7 days, <1200 g, 15 mg/kg/24 hr administered once daily; <7 days, >1200 g, 30 mg/kg/24 hr, div, every 12 hr; >7 days, <1200 g, 15 mg/kg/24 hr administered once daily; >7 days, >1200 g, 30–45 mg/kg/24 hr, div, every 8–12 hr

IN, CH (<12 yr of age) 45–60 mg/kg/24 hr, div, every 6–8 hr

AD = IV 0.5 g every 6 hr to 1 g every 12 hr

℞ for *C. difficile*–associated pseudomembranous colitis in CH = PO: 40–50 mg/kg/24 hr, div, every 6–8 hr.

Caution: Combined administration with an aminoglycoside enhances nephrotoxic potential of both drugs. **Note:** Reduced dosage in renal insufficiency. Therapy may be associated with ototoxicity and renal impairment, skin rashes ("red man" syndrome), and hematologic side effects. Serum concentration should be monitored, therapeutic peak concentration 30–40 mg/L, trough 5–10 mg/L.

Vidarabine; antiviral agent used for treatment of neonatal herpes simplex infections

IN = IV: 15–30 mg/kg infused over 12 hr every 24 hr for 14–21 days

Note: May rarely cause hepatic and hematologic toxicity.

II. DRUGS OTHER THAN ANTIBIOTICS

Acetaminophen, paracetamol

℞ antipyretic, analgesic: IN, CH = PO: 60 mg/kg/24 hr, div, every 4–6 hr, prn

Caution: Massive overdose may cause hepatic necrosis through formation of a toxic metabolite. Lesser overdoses frequently cause reversible jaundice.

Acetylcysteine; mucolytic agent; detoxifying agent in acetaminophen overdose

℞ in acetaminophen overdose: CH, AD = PO: 140 mg/kg first dose, followed by 70 mg/kg/dose every 4 hr for a total of 17 doses

MUCOMYST: vials 10% (100 mg/mL) or 20% (20 mg/mL)

Acetylsalicylic acid (ASA)

℞ antipyretic, analgesic, anti-inflammatory: IN, CH = PO: 30–65 mg/kg/24 hr, div, every 4–6 hr, prn. This dosage corresponds to 27–58 mg salicylate sodium/kg/24 hr, or 20–50 mg salicylic acid/kg/24 hr

℞ antirheumatic: CH = PO: 65–130 mg/kg/24 hr, div, every 4–6 hr

Caution: Acute or chronic overdose may cause life-threatening poisoning syndrome. Use in children <16 yr with varicella or a flu-like illness is associated with Reye syndrome.

Activated charcoal; adsorbent for treatment of oral drug overdose PO: 10 times (by weight) estimated quantity of drug ingested or 1 g/kg orally; may repeat every 4 hr when necessary

Adenosine; endogenous nucleoside; treatment of choice to terminate supraventricular tachycardia; causes acute transient AV nodal conduction block

NB, IN, CH = IV; 0.05 mg/kg/dose rapid injection (1–2 sec), increase by 0.05 q2min to 0.25 mg/kg/dose if prior dose is ineffective

Albuterol; catecholamine analog; β-adrenergic receptor agonist with preferential effect on β_2-adrenergic receptors

℞ bronchodilator: CH = PO: 0.1–0.2 mg/kg, div, every 8 hr; 6–12 yr, 2 mg 3–4 times/24 hr

Nebulization:

Neonates: 0.1–0.5 mg/kg/dose prn or q2–6h

Children: 1.25–2.5 mg prn or q4–6h

Adults: 1.25–5 mg prn or q4–6h

Atropine sulfate, anticholinergic agent used mainly in premedication for anesthesia, as antiarrhythmic agent, and as antispasmodic.

Neonates and children:

<5 kg: 0.2 mg/kg 30 min preop then every 4–6 hr

>5 kg: 0.1–0.2 mg/kg/dose (max 0.4 mg/dose)

Adults: 0.4–0.6 mg IV or SC 30 min preoperatively

℞ treatment of sinus bradycardia:

Neonates and children: 0.02 mg/kg (min dose 0.1 mg); IV or intratracheal (max 0.5 mg); may repeat 5 min later, one time

Adults: 0.5–1 mg every 5 min (max total dose 2 mg)

℞ antidote to organophosphate poisoning: 0.02–0.05 mg/kg every 10–20 min until atropine effect (tachycardia, mydriasis, fever), then every 1–4 hr for at least 24 hr

Betamethasone; long-acting antiinflammatory corticosteroid with little to no sodium retention potential. CH = IM: 0.0175–0.2 mg base/kg/24 hr, div, every 6–12 hr; PO: 0.0175–0.25 mg/kg/24 hr div every 6–8 hr. AD = IM: 0.6–9 mg/24 hr, div, every 12–24 hr; PO: 2–5 mg/24 hr, div, every 12–24 hr

Note: For more information on steroid medications, see Corticosteroids.

Captopril, competitive inhibitor of angiotensin I–converting enzyme, antihypertensive agent, congestive heart failure

℞ for cardiovascular response:

NB = PO: 0.05–0.1 mg/kg/dose administered every 6–24 hr

IN = PO: 0.5–0.6 mg/kg/24 hr, div, every 6–12 hr

CH = PO: 0.15 mg/kg every 4–8 hr; dose may be slowly increased to desired effect: max pediatric dose 6 mg/kg/24 hr

AD = PO: 6.25–12.5 mg/dose every 8–12 hr; usual AD max 450 mg/24 hr.

Note: May cause renal impairment, neutropenia, immunodeficiency, rashes, disturbances of taste. Adjust dose with renal failure.

Carbamazepine, anticonvulsant agent; structurally related to tricyclic antidepressants

IN, CH = PO: initially 5–10 mg/kg/24 hr, div, every 8–12 hr; to be increased progressively, if needed, to 20 mg/kg/24 hr, div, every 12 hr or as a single daily dose, if tolerated. Usual maintenance dose range 20–30 mg/kg/24 hr CH (>12 yr), AD = PO: initially 200 mg every 24 hr, titrated as needed, max 800–1200 mg/24 hr

Note: Carbamazepine is a potent inducer of hepatic microsomal metabolizing enzymes that may stimulate the metabolism of numerous other drugs metabolized via the liver.

Chloral hydrate; trichloro derivative of acetaldehyde; tolerance to its hypnotic effect may develop

℞ for sedation: IN, CH = PO: 25 mg/kg/24 hr, div, every 6–8 hr

℞ for sleep: IN, CH = PO, (PR): 25–100 mg/kg/dose, to be repeated prn after 12–24 hr

Chlorothiazide; saluretic, inhibiting sodium reabsorption and interfering with dilution of urine

IN, CH = PO: 20–40 mg/kg/24 hr, div, every 12 hr

Chlorpromazine; phenothiazine with aliphatic side chain

℞ for sedation: CH = PO: 2 mg/kg/24 hr, div, every 4–6 hr, prn; IM: 2 mg/kg/24 hr, div, every 6–8 hr, prn

Caution: Overdose may produce parkinsonian syndrome. Diphenhydramine may be antidotal.

Cimetidine, H_2-receptor antagonist competitively inhibits secretion of gastric acid

℞ for treatment of duodenal and gastric ulcers and for relief of symptoms caused by gastroesophageal reflux: compatible with concomitant treatment with oral antacids (which should be administered at frequent intervals and in adequate doses) or other therapeutic modalities

NB = PO, IM, IV: (15–20 min) 5–10 mg/kg/24 hr, every 8–12 hr;

IN, CH = IV, PO: 20–40 mg/kg/24 hr, div, every 4–6 hr

Note: Cimetidine may compete with hepatic metabolism of other hepatically metabolized drugs. Many possible drug interactions. May cause gynecomastia, rash, and neutropenia. Reduce dose in renal insufficiency.

Relative Potencies of Corticosteroids

Drug	Antiinflammatory Effect (mg)	Sodium-Retaining Effect (mg)
Hydrocortisone (cortisol)	100	100
Cortisone	80	80
Prednisolone	20	100
Prednisone	20	100
Methylprednisolone	16	0
Triamcinolone	16	0
Dexamethasone	2	0
Desoxycorticosterone	0	2

Clonazepam; benzodiazepine with selective anticonvulsant effect

CH = PO: start with 0.01–0.05 mg/kg/24 hr, div, every 8 hr, and progressively increase up to 0.3 mg/kg/24 hr, div, every 8 hr, if needed.

Caution: Concomitant use of clonazepam and valproate sodium may lead to petit mal status.

Codeine phosphate or sulfate; narcotic analgesic

℞ as antitussive: CH = 1–1.5 mg/kg/24 hr, div, every 4 hr prn

℞ against moderately severe pain: CH = PO: 4 mg/kg/24 hr, div, every 4–6 hr, prn; SC: 3 mg/kg/24 hr, div, every 4–6 hr, prn

Corticosteroids

℞ physiologic replacement

Cortisone: PO 1 mg/kg/24 hr, div, every 8 hr; IM: 0.5 mg/kg/24 hr, every 24 hr

Note: "Increased demand" under stressful situation (e.g., in children with congenital adrenogenital syndrome, receiving replacement therapy, for stressful situation in which 2 mg/kg/24 hr of cortisol may be safer)

℞ use in pharmacologic doses (leukemia, lymphoma, nephrosis, rheumatic carditis, certain types of tuberculosis, immunologic reactions, and other types of autoimmune disease): adjust dosage to the specific situation

Cortisone: PO: 10 mg/kg/24 hr, div, every 6–8 hr; IM: 3–6 mg/kg/24 hr, div, every 12 hr

Prednisone: PO: 2 mg/kg/24 hr, div, every 6–8 hr (or analog in equally effective dosage; see Table)

(For continued treatment after initial response, adjust dosage, frequency of administration, and duration of treatment according to type of disease and side effects to be avoided.)

℞ in status asthmaticus refractory to other types of treatment: methylprednisolone IV: 2–4 mg/kg/dose every 4–6 hr

Caution: May inhibit clinical signs of infection.

Cromolyn sodium

℞ topical prophylaxis of bronchial asthma, allergic rhinitis: not useful in the treatment of acute asthmatic attack because it is not a bronchodilator.

Children and adults:

Asthma: 1–2 puffs (MDI) or 2 ml (nebulizer solution) 3–4 daily

Rhinitis: 1 spray each nostril 3–4 times daily

Conjunctivitis: 1–2 drops 4–6 times daily

Mastocytosis, food allergy:

Children: 100 mg/dose 4 times daily (max 40 mg/ kg/day)

Adults: 200 mg/dose 4 times daily (max 400 mg/dose 4 times daily)

Cyproheptadine hydrochloride; piperidine; serotonin and histamine antagonist with mild anticholinergic and mild sedative effect

℞ antiallergic effect:

Children 2–6 yr: 2 mg/dose every 8–12 hr

>7 yr and adults: 4 mg/dose every 8–12 hr (max 0.5 mg/kg/day)

Deferoxamine; chelating agent for treatment of iron intoxication; may cause hypotension; contraindicated in renal failure or acute anuria unless concomitant hemodialysis is used.

IV: 15 mg/kg/hr infusion

Desmopressin acetate; synthetic analog of vasopressin indicated as replacement therapy in the management of central diabetes insipidus. Toxicities include headache, abdominal cramping, excessive water retention. Nasal insufflation: 0.03–0.05 mL, div, bid or tid dose determined by patient response.

DDAVP: 0.1 mg/mL for nasal insufflation

Dexamethasone: see Corticosteroids

Diazepam; benzodiazepine with anxiolytic and muscle-relaxant effects

Infants and children:

Status epilepticus:

IV: 0.05–0.3 mg/kg/dose given over 2–3 min may repeat every 30 min to max total dose of 5–10 mg

Rectal: 0.5 mg/kg, then 0.25 mg/kg in 10 min if needed

Sedation: Oral: 0.2–0.3 mg/kg (max 10 mg); IM/IV: 0.04–0.3 mg/kg (max 0.6 mg/kg/8 hr)

Adults:

Status epilepticus: IV: 5–10 mg every 30 min (max 30 mg/8 hr)

Anxiety, sedation, muscle relaxant: Oral/IM/IV: 2–10 mg 2–4 times daily

Caution: Confusion and prolonged extreme drowsiness may follow overdose or concurrent ingestion of alcohol in any form.

Digoxin; cardiac glycoside with rapid onset of action and half-life of approximately 48 hr

Neonate: 10–30 µg/kg IV load, then 5–10 µg/kg/day maintenance dose

1 mo–2 yr: 30 µg/kg load, then 10–15 µg/kg/day maintenance dose

2–10 yr: 30 µg/kg load, then 5–10 µg/kg/day maintenance dose

Child >10 yr: 10 µg/kg load, then 2–5 µg/kg/day maintenance dose

Adult: 10–15 µg/kg load, then 0.1–0.5 mg/day maintenance dose

Adjust doses for reduced renal function: CrCl 10–50 mL/min: reduce dose to 25–75%; CrCl <10 mL/min: reduce dose to 10–25% of normal

Note: Digitalizing and maintenance doses must be adjusted to the condition of the patient.

Caution: Fatal arrhythmia may follow overdose.

Diphenhydramine hydrochloride; ethanolamine; antihistamine with mild anticholinergic, sedative, antiemetic, and antitussive effects

℞ antiallergic effect; sometimes used as sedative. IN, CH = PO, IM, IV: 5 mg/kg/24 hr, div, every 6–8 hr

Edetate calcium disodium (EDTA), a heavy metal–chelating agent with greatest affinity for lead. Used in the diagnosis and treatment of lead poisoning. EDTA-lead chelate excreted from the body via the kidney. Drug has affinity for calcium, which is the reason for administering the drug as the calcium (disodium) salt.

℞ for lead poisoning. Many regimens have been suggested; CH = IM, IV (over 1 hr to continuous 24-hr infusion): 50–75 mg/kg/24 hr, div, every 4–6 hr or by continuous IV infusion

℞ as a diagnostic test for lead body burden. CH = IM, IV: 500 mg/m² and collect all urine excreted over the next 8–24 hr to determine EDTA:lead ratio.

Note: Painful on IM injection. For comfort, may add 1 mL of 1% lidocaine with each 1 mL of EDTA injection. Dose must be adjusted for patients with renal disease.

Epinephrine racemic; inhalation treatment of acute spasmodic croup

Inhalation: 0.25–0.5 mL of 2.25% solution diluted in 3 mL of saline given via nebulizer

Furosemide; saluretic with a duration of action of about 2 hr when given IV; inhibits chloride and sodium reabsorption and interferes with concentration of urine

IN, CH = PO: start with 1–2 mg/kg/dose; if needed, increase progressively to 3–6 mg/kg/dose, at intervals of 6–8 hr; IV: start with 1 mg/kg/dose; if needed, increase progressively to 6 mg/kg/dose, with an interval of at least 2 hr between doses

Hydralazine hydrochloride; phthalazine derivative; causes relaxation of vascular smooth muscles, especially of arterioles

℞ as antihypertensive in long-term treatment: CH = PO: initially 0.75 mg/kg/24 hr, div, every 6 hr; increase progressively until desired response or daily maximum dose of 7.5 mg/kg/24 hr is reached

℞ for emergency reduction of hypertension: IV (immediate onset of action), IM (onset of action after 15–20 min): 0.15 mg/kg/dose; repeat prn every 30–90 min up to daily dose of 1.7–3.6 mg/kg/24 hr; switch to oral administration if conditions permit

Note: Hydralazine may produce sodium retention and usually increases plasma renin activity.

Caution: May induce lupus erythematosus–like syndrome: frequency related to dosage.

Hydrochlorothiazide; saluretic, inhibiting sodium reabsorption and interfering with dilution of urine

IN, CH = PO: 2–4 mg/kg/24 hr, div, every 12 hr

Hydroxyzine hydrochloride; neuroleptic agent of the piperazine type, with sedative and antihistamine effects

℞ for sedation and/or antihistamine effect: CH = PO: 2 mg/kg/24 hr, div, every 6–8 hr, prn

Ibuprofen; nonsteroidal antiinflammatory agent of the propionic acid class that possesses analgesic and antipyretic activities. The drug's mechanism of action remains to be described but may involve prostaglandin synthetase inhibition. Pharmacologic effect appears to be equivalent to that of equipotent doses of acetaminophen or aspirin.

℞ as antipyretic or for mild analgesia: CH = PO: 10–15 mg/kg/dose at intervals of 4–6 hr

℞ for juvenile rheumatoid arthritis: CH = PO: 30–70 mg/kg/24 hr, div, every 4–6 hr

Note: Complete scope of associated adverse reactions in infants and children remains to be described. Adverse effects appear to be similar to those associated with aspirin administration, including gastritis, platelet dysfunction, and possible compromise in renal function. Drug should be used cautiously in patients with renal insufficiency.

Ipecac; emetic agent used in the adjunctive management of poisoning or intoxication. Active ingredient emetidine produces local gastric irritation and central effect, resulting in emesis, which usually occurs within 15–35 min of drug administration

℞ to induce vomiting:

IN >8 mo of age, CH = PO: 15–30 mL/dose; if no effect occurs same dose may be repeated in 30 min

N <8 mo of age = PO: 1 mL/kg single dose

Note: Children usually vomit 3–5 times within 1 hr of receiving Ipecac. Ipecac should be available in all households with young infants and children but should not be administered except on the advice of a physician or a poison control center.

Iron preparations

℞ daily maintenance iron requirement, as elemental iron: PO: 0.5–1 mg/kg/24 hr, in single dose or divided

℞ in iron deficiency anemia, as elemental iron: PO: 6 mg/kg/24 hr, div, with meals

Note: Iron supply at this dosage level ought to be continued for 2–3 mo to compensate for the deficits in erythrocytes and iron stores. Only iron in the ferrous form (Fe^{2+}) is absorbed from the gastrointestinal tract. The content of elemental iron in different preparations varies. The percentage of dry weight as elemental iron of ferrous choline citrate is 20; ferrous fumarate, 33; ferrous gluconate, 12; ferrous lactate, 19; ferrous sulfate, 20; and iron-dextran complex (ferric hydroxide), 2.

℞ dose calculation for parenteral iron administration: elemental Fe deficit = 2.5 mg/kg × deficit of hemoglobin concentration (in g/dL) in blood. (The deficit of the hemoglobin concentration is obtained as the difference between the measured and the desirable value, expressed in g/dL.) When iron must be supplied by the parenteral route, deep IM injection is preferable to IV administration. In either case, a test dose of approximately 25 mg elemental Fe in the form of the dextran complex should precede the administration of the total dose. If the total dose is large, it should be divided in separate daily doses of which none should exceed 5 mg/kg/24 hr of elemental iron.

Note: An additional 20–30% of the calculated deficit is needed to restore the tissue iron reserves.

Caution: Acute overdose may lead to shock, CNS depression, death.

Ketorolac tromethamine; nonsteroidal antiinflammatory drug (NSAID) available for oral or parenteral administration; possesses analgesic and antipyretic activities; mechanism of action most likely inhibition of prostaglandin synthesis via antagonism of cyclooxygenase activity

CH = PO, IM: 2 mg/kg/24 hr, div, every 6 hr; many centers have administered the IM formulation via the IV route over 15–20 min

Note: As with all NSAIDs, the use of these drugs may be associated with gastritis, reversible antiplatelet activity, and possible compromised renal function; should be used cautiously in NB and other patients with decreased renal function.

Lidocaine hydrochloride; anesthetic agent used systemically for its antiarrhythmic effects: delayed slow diastolic depolarization, diminished automaticity. Does not affect normal conduction but seemingly improves conduction velocity in damaged areas of myocardium. In therapeutic doses does not depress myocardial contractility or atrioventricular conduction.

℞ against ventricular tachyarrhythmia: IN, CH = IV (slowly, as 20 mg/mL sol): 1 mg/kg/dose, to be repeated prn after 20 min, or continuous IV infusion as 1 mg/mL sol: 0.020–0.050 mg/kg/min, to a maximum total dose of 5 mg/kg/24 hr

Caution: Excessive depression of cardiac conductivity may occur; ECG monitoring indicated during treatment.

Mannitol; osmotic diuretic

℞ test dose for oliguria: CH = IV: 0.2 g/kg/dose, injected within 3–5 min

℞ in cerebral edema: CH = IV: 0.5–1 g/kg/dose, injected as 15–25% sol over 30–60 min

Meperidine hydrochloride; synthetic narcotic analgesic agent; addictive

℞ against severe pain: CH = PO, SC, IM: 6 mg/kg/24 hr, div, prn every 4–6 hr (maximum single dose: 100 mg)

Caution: May produce respiratory depression, seizures, coma in some sensitive patients. Test dose advisable. Naloxone is antidote.

Metaproterenol sulfate; catecholamine analog; β-adrenergic receptor agonist with relatively selective effect on β_2-adrenergic receptors

℞ bronchodilator: IN, CH (<6 yr of age) = PO: 1.3–2.6 mg/kg/24 hr, div, every 6–8 hr; >6 yr of age: 10–20 mg/dose administered 3–4 times daily

Methylphenidate hydrochloride; piperidine derivative structurally related to amphetamine; CNS stimulant with more prominent effects on mental than on motor activities

℞ in minimal brain dysfunction (MBD): drug treatment of MBD not recommended below the age of 3 yr or in nonstructured therapeutic situation. CH (over 3 yr) = PO: initiate treatment with 5 mg dose given at the onset of daytime activities and again 4–6 hr later; if needed, increase the dose at weekly intervals by increments of 5 mg/dose and adjust the size of the respective doses (early morning and midday) according to the response in the patient; daily dose usually should not exceed 2 mg/kg/24 hr. To avoid insommia, do not administer closer than 6 hr before bedtime.

Caution: Reduction of growth rate and weight gain might accompany prolonged use. Chronic abuse can lead to tolerance.

℞ in narcolepsy: PO: proceed for dosage adjustment as in MBD, with correction of the abnormal symptomatology as the end point.

Metoclopramide hydrochloride; gastrointestinal prokinetic agent that increases lower esophageal sphincter pressure and rate of gastric emptying, and augments gastrointestinal peristaltic activity. Use of this drug for the treatment of symptomatic gastroesophageal reflux in infants and children remains controversial. Drug is also used for the treatment of diabetic gastroparesis and as an adjunctive measure facilitating small bowel intubation when the tube does not pass the pylorus with conventional maneuvers. High-dose metoclopramide therapy has been shown to be an effective aid in the adjunctive management of nausea and vomiting associated with cancer chemotherapy.

℞ for gastroesophageal reflux or gastrointestinal dismotility: CH = PO: 0.1 mg/kg/dose administered 4 times a day

℞ for prevention of chemotherapy-induced emesis: 2–3 mg/kg/dose administered before and after chemotherapeutic drug; timing of dose and actual regimen are dependent on the specific chemotherapeutic agent administered.

Caution: Metoclopramide possesses dopamine receptor antagonist activity; thus acute dystonic reactions may occur and are relatively frequent with high-dose therapy. Diphenhydramine may be used to treat metoclopramide (or phenothiazine)-induced acute dystonic reaction. It may be appropriate to coadminister diphenhydramine with high-dose metoclopramide to prevent dystonic reactions in patients receiving this therapy for nausea and vomiting associated with cancer chemotherapy.

Mineral oil; indigestible liquid hydrocarbon with limited absorbability; lubricant

℞ mild laxative: PO: 0.5 mL/kg/dose

Morphine sulfate; narcotic analgesic agent; addictive

℞ against severe pain: CH = SC: 0.6–1.2 mg/kg/24 hr, div, prn every 4 hr, equivalent to 0.1–0.2 mg/kg/dose, to be repeated prn every 4 hr

Caution: Overdose produces severe respiratory depression, hypothermia, coma. Naloxone antidotal.

Naloxone hydrochloride; opioid antagonist; nonaddictive

℞ in respiratory depression because of opioids: NB, IN, CH = IV, IM, SC: 0.1 mg/kg/dose, to be repeated prn after 2–3 min, up to 3 times. After satisfactory response, the dose must be repeated every 1–2 hr as long as opioid depression persists.

Phenobarbital, central nervous system depressant of barbiturate class with long duration of action; initially, hypnotic effect of 8–12 hr; tolerance to hypnotic effect may develop on continued use

R for sedation: IN, CH = PO, IM: 2–3 mg/kg/24 hr, div, every 8–12 hr

R for sleep: IN, CH = PO, IM: 2–3 mg/kg/dose, repeat prn after 12–24 hr

R as anticonvulsant. Status: IV (rate <1 mg/kg/min or 50 mg/min for patients weighing >60 kg). Loading dose: NB = 15–20 mg/kg in single or div dose; IN, CH, AD = 15–18 mg/kg in single or div dose. Maintenance dosing NB = PO, IV: 3–4 mg/kg/24 hr, div, every 12–24 hr; IN, CH: 5–8 mg/kg/24 hr, div, every 12–24 hr. CH (>12 yr of age), AD = PO, IV: 1–3 mg/kg/24 hr

R hyperbilirubinemia: CH (<8 yr of age) = PO 3–8 mg/kg/24 hr, div, every 8–12 hr

Note: Dosing may be guided by serum concentration monitoring, therapeutic values 15–40 mg/L.

Caution: All barbiturates, including phenobarbital, are respiratory depressants. Serum concentrations should be monitored.

Phenytoin, diphenylhydantoin; anticonvulsant agent; effective also in certain types of cardiac arrhythmias; antiarrhythmic effects similar to those of lidocaine; delayed slow diastolic depolarization, diminished automaticity; may facilitate conduction in damaged myocardial areas; does not depress myocardial activity

R as anticonvulsant. Status: IV (rate <1–3 mg/kg/min or 50 mg/min); NB = 15–20 mg/kg in single or div dose; IN, CH, AD = 15–18 mg/kg in single or div dose. Maintenance dosing IV, PO = NB: 5 mg/kg/24 hr, div, every 8–12 hr; IN, CH: 5–10 mg/kg/24 hr, div, every 8–12 hr; CH (>12 yr of age): 5 mg/kg/24 hr, div, every 12 hr

R for arrhythmias. CH, AD = IV: 1.25 mg/kg IV (over 1–3 min) every 5 min prn, up to total loading dose of 15 mg/kg

Note: Anticonvulsant effects may be guided by monitoring serum phenytoin concentrations, therapeutic 10–20 mg/L.

Note: Phenytoin disposition is most often characterized by nonlinear (Michaelis-Menten) pharmacokinetics. Phenytoin is highly protein-bound (>90%) and may be associated with protein-binding displacement interaction; therapy is associated with unpredictable effects on the activity of hepatic drug-metabolizing enzymes. Caution should be used in generic substitution because all generic preparations may not be bioequivalent.

Caution: Imbalance in phenytoin protein binding reflected by abnormally low but therapeutic free serum phenytoin concentrations in patients with renal dysfunction and critically ill with acute head trauma.

Procainamide hydrochloride; antiarrhythmic agent with general cardiodepressant effects; diminished myocardial excitability (decreased threshold potential, pro-longed refractory period), reduced conduction velocity, diminished automaticity; decreases myocardial contractility; effects similar to those of quinidine

R for ventricular tachyarrhythmia: IN, CH = IM: 20–30 mg/kg/24 hr, div, every 4–6 hr; IV loading dose 10–15 mg over 30 min followed by continuous IV maintenance infusion of 20–80 µg/kg/min; PO: 15–50 mg/kg/24 hr, div, every 3–6 hr. Serum concentration should be monitored for both procainamide and its active metabolite N-acetyl procainamide (NAPA).

Propranolol hydrochloride; β-adrenergic blocking agent (β_1 and β_2); racemic mixture of D- and L-propranolol, of which only L form has adrenergic blocking activity

R against selected forms of supraventricular and ventricular tachycardia: IN, CH = IV: 0.01–0.10 mg/kg/dose given slowly; repeat every 6–8 hr prn PO: 0.5–4 mg/kg/24 hr, div, every 6–8 hr

R as antihypertensive in long-term therapy. CH = PO: initially 1 mg/kg/24 hr, div, every 6 hr, and progressive increase of dosage, if needed up to 5 mg/kg/24 hr, div, every 6 hr.

Combination with diuretic and/or hydralazine indicated, because propranolol blocks physiologic compensatory mechanisms such as adrenergic inotropic and chronotropic responses, as well as renin activity.

R for prevention of migraine attack in severe cases and to combat the manifestations of thyrotoxicosis: Propranolol requirements vary widely from patient to patient because of individual differences in severity of underlying disease, endogenous sympathetic neuronal activity, sensitivity of β-adrenergic receptors to blockade, degree of protein binding, and hepatic blood flow. For comparable effect, oral dose 6–10 times higher than intravenous dose in spite of good absorption from the gut because of inactivation of important fraction of propranolol in liver after entrance through portal vein.

Measures in case of exaggerated response: against bradycardia, atropine, if no response, isoproterenol, *cautiously;* against cardiac failure, digitalization, and diuretics; against hypotension, epinephrine; against bronchospasm, isoproterenol, theophylline (aminophylline)

Spironolactone; aldosterone antagonist and potassium-sparing diuretic, which interferes with sodium reabsorption

R as diuretic in selected cases (with normal renal function), most effective in combination with a potassium-wasting diuretic: CH = PO: 1.5–3 mg/kg/24 hr, div, every 4–8 hr

Note: Monitoring of serum concentration of potassium, of potassium intake, and of renal function is indicated during treatment with spironolactone.

Terbutaline sulfate, catecholamine; β-adrenergic receptor agonist with preferential effect of β₂-adrenergic receptors

> ℞ bronchodilator: Dosage in pediatric age group not firmly established. PO: 0.10–0.15 mg/kg/24 hr, div, every 8 hr. β_2-Selectivity is reduced with increasing dosage or on parenteral administration. SC: 0.005–0.01 mg/kg/dose (max 0.4 mg), to be repeated prn after 20 min, once only

Theophylline; methylxanthine commonly used in acute and chronic management of reversible airways disease (asthma), and neonatal apnea, bronchopulmonary dysplasia, among others. Cellular mechanism of action originally believed to be a result of phosphodiesterase inhibition; however, pharmacologic effect is most likely a result of adenosine receptor antagonism.

> *Neonates:*
> Apnea, bronchodilation: loading dose 6–10 mg/kg, maintenance dose 2–4 mg/kg/dose every 12 hr
> *Infants and Children:*
> *6 wk–6 mo:* 10 mg/kg/day
> *6 mo–1 yr:* 12–18 mg/kg/day
> *1–9 yr:* 20–24 mg/kg/day
> *9–12 yr:* 16 mg/kg/day
> *12–16 yr:* 13 mg/kg/day
> *Adults:* 10 mg/kg/day
> (Dosing may be increased for smokers and enzyme-inducing drugs; decrease dose if enzyme inhibitors, liver disease, heart failure, or hypothyroid).
> **Note:** The content of theophylline in the following formulations: theophylline (anhydrous), 100%; aminophylline, 85%; theophylline monoethanolamine, 75%; dihydroxypropyltheophylline, 70%; oxtriphylline, choline salt, 64%; theophylline sodium glycinate, 50%; theophylline calcium salicylate, 48%. Serum concentration should be monitored; therapeutic range for neonatal apnea, 7–13 mg/L; in the management of bronchospasm, 10–20 mg/L.
> **Caution:** Circulatory collapse, seizures, coma may result from acute or chronic overdose.

Valproate sodium, dipropylacetate sodium; anticonvulsant agent with singular mode of action (effective probably by increasing γ-aminobutyric acid in brain tissues)

> ℞ in the treatment of simple petit mal and of complex absence seizures, either alone or in combination with other drugs (see reservation below) according to the results: CH = PO: start with 15 mg/kg/24 hr, div, every 8–12 hr; if needed, dosage increased by weekly increments of 5–10 mg/kg/24 hr up to a maximum recommended dose of 30 mg/kg/24 hr, div, every 8 hr
> **Caution:** Concomitant use of valproate sodium and clonazepam might result in petit mal status. Blood concentrations of phenobarbital and phenytoin may be affected by addition of valproate sodium to the regimen.

Verapamil; calcium channel blocker; toxic effects include allergic reactions, urticaria, bronchospasm, hypotension, decreased cardiac output, and asystole. Cardiac monitoring should be used during administration.

> Doses in infants and young children not well established:
> *Infants:* 0.1–0.2 mg/kg and children 0.1–0.3 mg/kg per dose IV repeated to desired effect
> *Children:* 4–8 mg/kg/day PO q6–8h; usual dose 5 mg/kg/day
> *Adults:* 240–480 mg/day PO divided q6–8h; q12h with extended-release products
> May sprinkle contents of capsule onto soft food without affecting absorption.

Drug Interactions of Potential Importance in Pediatric Practice
Partial Listing*

Interacting Agent	Adverse Effect
Acetaminophen	
Alcohol	Hepatotoxicity
Oral anticoagulants	↑ Anticoagulation
Probenecid	↑ Acetaminophen toxicity
Zidovudine	Granulocytopenia
Acyclovir	
Narcotics	↑ Narcotic toxicity?
Zidovudine	Lethargy
Alcohol	
Antidepressants (tricyclic)	↑ Toxicity
Barbiturates	↑ CNS depression (acute)
Benzodiazepines	↑ CNS depression
Cephalosporins (not all)	Disulfiram effect
Chloral hydrate	↑ CNS depression
Doxycycline	↓ Antibiotic effect
Isoniazid	↑ Hepatotoxicity
Metronidazole	Disulfiram effect
Phenothiazines	Impaired coordination
Phenytoin	↑ Phenytoin toxicity
Allopurinol	
Aluminum hydroxide	↓ Allopurinol absorption
Ampicillin	Rash
Anticoagulants (oral)	↑ Anticoagulant effect
Azathioprine	↑ Azathioprine toxicity
Captopril	↑ Cutaneous hypersensitivity
Cyclophosphamide	↑ Cyclophosphamide toxicity
Theophylline	↑ Theophylline toxicity
Thiazide diuretics	↑ Allopurinol toxicity

Modified from Rizack M, Hillman C: *The Medical Letter handbook of adverse drug interactions,* New Rochelle, NY, 1989, The Medical Letter.
A-V, Atrioventricular; *CNS,* central nervous system; *INH,* isoniazid; *?,* possible effect.
*When possible, an alternate drug combination should be given. If not possible, drug levels *and* signs of toxicity must be monitored.

Continued

Interacting Agent	Adverse Effect
Aminoglycoside Antibiotics	
Amphotericin B	↑ Nephrotoxicity
Bumetanide	↑ Ototoxicity
Cisplatin	↑ Nephrotoxicity
Cyclosporine	↑ Nephrotoxicity
Furosemide	↑ Nephrotoxicity and ototoxicity
Magnesium	↑ Neuromuscular blockade
Neuromuscular blocking agents	↑ Blockade
Vancomycin	↑ Nephrotoxicity?
Antacids	
Beta-adrenergic blockers	↓ Absorption
Captopril	↓ Absorption
Cimetidine	↓ Absorption
Corticosteroids	↓ Absorption
Digoxin	↓ Absorption
Iron	↓ Absorption
Isoniazid	↓ Absorption
Ketoconazole	↓ Absorption
Nonsteroidal antiinflammatory agents	↓ Absorption
Phenytoin	↓ Absorption
Salicylates	↓ Absorption
Tetracycline	↓ Absorption
Theophylline	↑ Toxicity
Aspirin	
Anticoagulants (oral)	↑ Bleeding
Captopril	↓ Antihypertensive effect
Barbiturates	
Anticoagulants (oral)	↓ Anticoagulation
Beta-adrenergic blockers	↓ Beta-blockade
Carbamazepine	↑ Production of carbamazepine epoxide
Chloramphenicol	↑ Barbiturate toxicity
Contraceptives (oral)	↓ Contraception
Corticosteroids	↓ Steroid effect
Influenza vaccine (viral)	↑ Barbiturate toxicity
Rifampin	↓ Barbiturate effect
Theophylline	↓ Theophylline effect
Valproate	↑ Barbiturate toxicity
Bleomycin	
Oxygen	↑ Pulmonary toxicity
Captopril	
Allopurinol	↑ Cutaneous hypersensitivity
Aspirin	↓ Antihypertensive effect
Cimetidine	Neuropathy

Modified from Rizack M, Hillman C: *The Medical Letter handbook of adverse drug interactions*, New Rochelle, NY, 1989, The Medical Letter.
A-V, Atrioventricular; *CNS,* central nervous system; *INH,* isoniazid; *?,* possible effect.

Interacting Agent	Adverse Effect
Captopril—cont'd	
Nonsteroidal antiinflammatory agents	↓ Antihypertensive effect
Potassium	Hyperkalemia
Spironolactone	Hyperkalemia
Carbamazepine	
Anticoagulants (oral)	↓ Anticoagulation
Antidepressants (tricyclic)	↑ Both toxicities
Cimetidine	↑ Carbamazepine toxicity
Contraceptives (oral)	↓ Contraception
Corticosteroids	↓ Steroid effect
Cyclosporine	↓ Cyclosporine effect
Erythromycins	↑ Carbamazepine toxicity
Influenza vaccine (viral)	↑ Carbamazepine toxicity
Isoniazid	↑ Both toxicities
Phenytoin	↓ Carbamazepine effect
Theophylline	↓ Theophylline effect
Valproate	↓ Valproate effect
Cimetidine	
Alcohol	↑ Alcohol effect
Antacids	↓ Cimetidine effect
Anticoagulants (oral)	↑ Anticoagulation
Antidepressants (tricyclic)	↑ Antidepressant toxicity
Benzodiazepines	↑ Benzodiazepine toxicity
Beta-adrenergic blocking agents	↑ Beta-blockade toxicity
Captopril	Neuropathy
Carbamazepine	↑ Carbamazepine toxicity
Digoxin	↑ Digoxin toxicity
Ketoconazole	↓ Ketoconazole absorption
Metoclopramide	↓ Cimetidine effect
Phenytoin	↑ Phenytoin toxicity
Theophylline	↑ Theophylline toxicity
Contraceptives (Oral)	
Anticoagulants (oral)	↓ Anticoagulation
Antidepressants (tricyclic)	↑ Antidepressant toxicity
Barbiturates	↓ Contraception
Carbamazepine	↓ Contraception
Griseofulvin	↓ Contraception
Penicillins (ampicillin, oxacillin)	↓ Contraception?
Phenytoin	↓ Contraception
Rifampin	↓ Contraception
Theophylline	↑ Theophylline toxicity
Cyclosporine	
Alkylating agents	↑ Nephrotoxicity
Aminoglycosides	↑ Nephrotoxicity
Amphotericin B	↑ Nephrotoxicity
Carbamazepine	↓ Cyclosporine effect
Erythromycins	↑ Cyclosporine toxicity

A-V, Atrioventricular; *CNS,* central nervous system; *INH,* isoniazid; *?,* possible effect.

Continued

Interacting Agent	Adverse Effect
Cyclosporine–cont'd	
Furosemide	Gout
Ketoconazole	↑ Nephrotoxicity
Metoclopramide	↑ Cyclosporine toxicity
Nafcillin	↓ Cyclosporine effect
Phenytoin	↓ Cyclosporine effect
Rifampin	↓ Cyclosporine effect
Digoxin	
Antacids	↓ Absorption
Anticholinergics	↑ Digoxin toxicity
Cholestyramine	↓ Absorption
Cimetidine	↑ Digoxin toxicity
Diuretics (hypokalemia)	↑ Digoxin toxicity
Phenytoin	↓ Digoxin effect
Quinidine	↑ Digoxin toxicity
Verapamil	↑ Digoxin toxicity
Erythromycins	
Anticoagulants (oral)	↑ Anticoagulation
Astemizole (Hismanal)	↑ Astemizole toxicity: arrhythmias
Carbamazepine	↑ Carbamazepine toxicity
Cyclosporine	↑ Cyclosporine toxicity
Phenytoin	↓ Phenytoin effect
Terfenadine (Seldane)	↑ Terfenadine toxicity: arrhythmias
Theophylline	↑ Theophylline toxicity
Fluoroquinolones	
Antacids	↓ Antibiotic effect
Theophylline	↑ Theophylline toxicity
Griseofulvin	
Anticoagulants (oral)	↓ Anticoagulants
Contraceptive (oral)	↓ Contraceptive
Isoniazid	
Alcohol	Hepatitis
Antacids	↓ INH absorption
Carbamazepine	↑ Toxicity (both)
Ketoconazole	↓ Ketoconazole effect
Phenytoin	↑ Phenytoin toxicity
Rifampin	↑ Hepatotoxicity
Valproate	↑ Hepatic and CNS toxicity
Ketoconazole	
Antacids	↓ Absorption
Anticoagulants (oral)	↑ Anticoagulation
Cimetidine	↓ Ketoconazole effect
Cyclosporine	↑ Nephrotoxicity
Isoniazid	↓ Ketoconazole effect
Phenytoin	Altered metabolism of both drugs
Rifampin	↑ Effects of both drugs

Modified from Rizack M, Hillman C: *The Medical Letter handbook of adverse drug interactions,* New Rochelle, NY, 1989, The Medical Letter.
A-V, Atrioventricular; *CNS,* central nervous system; *INH,* isoniazid; *?,* possible effect.

Interacting Agent	Adverse Effect
Methotrexate	
Blood transfusion	↑ Toxicity
Cisplatin	↑ Methotrexate toxicity
Etretinate	↑ Hepatotoxicity
Nonsteroidal anti-inflammatory agents	↑ Methotrexate toxicity
Trimethoprim/sulfamethoxazole	Megaloblastic anemia
Metoclopramide	
Carbamazepine	Neurotoxicity
Cimetidine	↓ Cimetidine effect
Cyclosporine	↑ Cyclosporine toxicity
Digoxin	↓ Absorption
Narcotics	↑ Sedation
Nifedipine	
Beta-adrenergic blockers	Heart failure, A-V block
Cyclosporine	↑ Gingival hyperplasia
Phenytoin	↑ Phenytoin toxicity
Prazosin	Hypotension
Quinidine	↓ Quinidine effect
Phenytoin	
Alcohol	↑ Toxicity (acute)
Antacids	↓ Phenytoin effect
Anticoagulants (oral)	↓ Phenytoin toxicity, ↑↓ Anticoagulation
Antidepressants (tricyclic)	↑ Phenytoin toxicity
Carbamazepine	↓ Carbamazepine effect
Chloramphenicol	↑ Toxicity (both)
Cimetidine	↑ Phenytoin toxicity
Contraceptives (oral and implant)	↓ Contraception
Corticosteroids	↓ Corticosteroid effect
Cyclosporine	↓ Cyclosporine effect
Digoxin	↓ Digoxin effect
Dopamine	Hypotension
Folic acid	↓ Phenytoin effect
Isoniazid	↑ Phenytoin toxicity
Miconazole	↓ Phenytoin effect
Neuromuscular blocking agents	↓ Blockade
Nifedipine	↑ Phenytoin toxicity
Quinidine	↓ Quinidine effect
Rifampin	↓ Phenytoin effect
Theophylline	↓ Effects (both)
Valproate	↑ Phenytoin toxicity
Quinidine	
Amiodarone	↑ Quinidine toxicity
Anticoagulants (oral)	↑ Anticoagulation
Barbiturates	↓ Quinidine effect
Cimetidine	↑ Quinidine toxicity
Digoxin	↑ Digoxin toxicity
Metoclopramide	↓ Quinidine effect
Phenytoin	↓ Quinidine effect

A-V, Atrioventricular; *CNS,* central nervous system; *INH,* isoniazid; *?,* possible effect.

Continued

Interacting Agent	Adverse Effect
Quinidine—cont'd	
Procainamide	↑ Procainamide toxicity
Rifampin	↓ Quinidine effect
Verapamil	Hypotension
Rifampin	
Anticoagulants (oral)	↓ Anticoagulation
Barbiturates	↓ Barbiturate effect
Beta-adrenergic blockers	↓ Beta-blockade
Chloramphenicol	↓ Chloramphenicol effect
Contraception (oral)	↓ Contraception
Corticosteroids	↓ Corticosteroid effect
Cyclosporine	↓ Cyclosporine effect
Isoniazid	↑ Hepatotoxicity
Ketoconazole	↓ Effects (both)
Phenytoin	↓ Phenytoin effect
Quinidine	↓ Quinidine effect
Theophylline	↓ Theophylline effect
Verapamil	↓ Verapamil effect
Theophylline	
Barbiturates	↓ Theophylline effect
Beta-adrenergic blockers	↑ Theophylline toxicity
Carbamazepine	↓ Theophylline effect
Cimetidine	↑ Theophylline toxicity
Erythromycins	↑ Theophylline toxicity
Fluoroquinolones	↑ Theophylline toxicity
Influenza vaccine (viral)	↑ Theophylline toxicity
Interferon	↑ Toxicity?
Marijuana smoking	↓ Theophylline effect
Phenytoin	↓ Effect (both)
Rifampin	↓ Theophylline effect
Tobacco smoking	↓ Theophylline effect
Troleandomycin	↑ Theophylline toxicity
Trimethoprim/Sulfamethoxazole	
Anticoagulants (oral)	↑ Anticoagulation
Antidepressants (tricyclic)	Depression
Mercaptopurine	↓ Antileukemia effect
Methotrexate	Megaloblastic anemia
Valproate	
Barbiturates	↑ Phenobarbital toxicity
Benzodiazepines	↑ Diazepam toxicity
Carbamazepines	↓ Valproate effect
Cimetidine	↑ Valproate toxicity?
Ethosuximide	↑ Ethosuximide toxicity?
Phenytoin	↑ Phenytoin toxicity

Modified from Rizack M, Hillman C: *The Medical Letter handbook of adverse drug interactions*, New Rochelle, NY, 1989, The Medical Letter.
A-V, Atrioventricular; *CNS*, central nervous system; *INH*, isoniazid; *?*, possible effect.

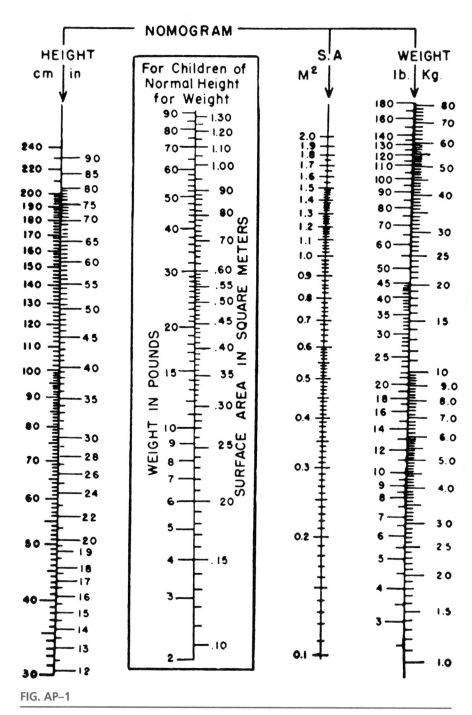

FIG. AP–1

Nomogram for estimation of surface area. The surface area is indicated where a straight line that connects the height and weight levels intersects the surface area column; or the patient is roughly of average size, from the weight alone *(enclosed area)*. (Modified from data of E Boyd by CD West.)

Index

Note: Page numbers followed by f indicate figures; t indicate tables.